Canine Neurology

DIAGNOSIS AND TREATMENT

B. F. HOERLEIN, D.V.M., Ph.D.
Charter Diplomate, American College of
Veterinary Surgery and the American College of
Veterinary Internal Medicine, Neurology Specialty;
Professor and Head of Small Animal Surgery and
Medicine, School of Veterinary Medicine,
Auburn University, Auburn, Alabama

Third Edition

1978
W. B. SAUNDERS COMPANY
PHILADELPHIA • LONDON • TORONTO

W. B. Saunders Company: West Washington Square
Philadelphia, Pa. 19105

1 St. Anne's Road
Eastbourne, East Sussex BN21 3UN, England

1 Goldthorne Avenue
Toronto, Ontario M8Z 5T9, Canada

Library of Congress Cataloging in Publication Data

Hoerlein, B F

Canine neurology.

Includes bibliographies

1. Dogs—Diseases. 2. Veterinary neurology. [DNLM: 1. Dog diseases—Diagnosis. 2. Dog diseases—Therapy. 3. Nervous system diseases—Veterinary. SF991 H694c]

SF992.N3H63 1978 636.7'08'968 77-72825

ISBN 0-7216-4712-X

Canine Neurology: Diagnosis and Treatment ISBN 0-7216-4712-X

Last digit is the print number: 9 8 7 6 5 4 3 2 1

IN MEMORIAM

It is with regret that we announce the death of Mr. K. A. Scott on August 1, 1977. Mr. Scott supported both initial and continued efforts in neurological research at Auburn University and the original development of this textbook.

Also with regret we announce the death of Dean Emeritus James E. Greene on September 20, 1977. In the 40 years of his inspiring service and leadership the development of instruction and research at Auburn University has flourished. Dean Greene was a personal inspiration to the author and supported the development of this textbook.

The contributions of both of these men will long be remembered.

PREFACE TO THE THIRD EDITION

As the interest in the specialty of veterinary neurology has developed, the total body of knowledge in the field has increased tremendously. In this edition special efforts have been made not only to update the information on veterinary neurology in the dog but also to note the unique differences in neurological disorders between the dog and cat, since this book is being developed as a general small pet animal neurology textbook.

A major reorganization of material has resulted in chapters on primary disorders of the central nervous system, which discusses infectious, degenerative, hereditary, vascular, and neoplastic diseases; and a chapter on acute trauma of the central nervous system, which combines material formerly presented in chapters on the brain and spinal trauma. New chapters or sections include localization of CNS lesions, disorders of micturition, neuro-ophthalmology, and behavior. The chapter on behavior includes a section on the new development of electroconvulsive shock therapy for undesirable behavior. This third edition has a total of 21 chapters, a sizable increase in pages, and a 25 per cent increase in total illustrations. The inclusion of data retrieval diagnostic data makes possible a greater appreciation of the incidence of neurological diseases in the dog.

The author is grateful for the expanding interest and competence in veterinary neurology and neurosurgery and the profession's continued support and acceptance of this textbook. It is hoped that the reorganization, updating, and new material in this edition will more completely fulfill the needs of students and practicing veterinarians in small pet animal neurology.

Auburn, Alabama B. F. HOERLEIN

CONTRIBUTORS

J. E. Bartels, B.S., D.V.M., M.S.

Professor, Radiology Section, School of Veterinary Medicine, Auburn University, Auburn, Alabama; Diplomate, American College of Veterinary Radiology

Stephen I. Bistner, B.S., D.V.M.

Associate Professor, Comparative Ophthalmology, School of Veterinary Medicine, University of Minnesota, St. Paul, Minnesota; Diplomate, American College of Veterinary Ophthalmology

J. G. Boring, B.S., D.V.M., M.S.

Assistant Professor, Radiology Section, School of Veterinary Medicine, Auburn University, Auburn, Alabama; Diplomate, American College of Veterinary Radiology

J. M. Bowen, D.V.M., Ph.D.

Professor, Department of Physiology and Pharmacology, College of Veterinary Medicine, University of Georgia, Athens, Georgia

K. G. Braund, B.V.Sc., Ph.D.

Assistant Professor, Department of Small Animal Surgery and Medicine, School of Veterinary Medicine, Auburn University, Auburn, Alabama

E. D. Gage, D.V.M., M.S.

Professor, Department of Urban Veterinary Practice, School of Veterinary Medicine, University of Tennessee, Knoxville, Tennessee; Diplomate, American College of Veterinary Surgeons

Benjamin J. Hart, D.V.M., Ph.D.

Associate Professor, Department of Anatomy, School of Veterinary Medicine, University of California, Davis, California

J. E. Oliver, Jr., D.V.M., M.S., Ph.D.

Professor, Department of Small Animal Medicine, College of Veterinary Medicine, University of Georgia, Athens, Georgia; Diplomate, American College of Veterinary Internal Medicine (Neurology)

R. W. Redding, D.V.M., M.S., Ph.D.

Professor, Department of Physiology and Pharmacology, School of Veterinary Medicine, Auburn University, Auburn, Alabama; Diplomate, American College of Veterinary Internal Medicine (Neurology)

J. S. Spano, D.V.M., Ph.D.

Assistant Professor, Department of Pathology and Parasitology, School of Veterinary Medicine, Auburn University, Auburn, Alabama; Diplomate, American College of Veterinary Pathologists (Clinical Pathology)

S. F. Swaim, B.S., D.V.M., M.S.

Assistant Professor, Department of Small Animal Surgery and Medicine, School of Veterinary Medicine, Auburn University, Auburn, Alabama

Victoria Lea Voith, D.V.M.

Assistant Professor, Department of Anatomy, School of Veterinary Medicine, University of California, Davis, California

T. L. Walker, D.V.M., M.S.

Assistant Professor, Department of Urban Veterinary Practice, School of Veterinary Medicine, University of Tennessee, Knoxville, Tennessee

PREFACE TO THE FIRST EDITION

Much has been written concerning the cause, incidence, epidemiology, immunization, and treatment of the *infectious* neurological diseases of the dog, such as distemper and rabies. Considerable work has been done in classifying and in analyzing neoplasms of the canine brain. However, very little has been done to help the veterinary clinician in the diagnosis and treatment of the *non-infectious* disorders of the nervous system. This lack has stimulated the author's interest and research in these problems for the past 15 years.

Since the animal patient cannot talk and describe his subjective symptoms, objective symptoms must be elicited and evaluated. These clinical signs will most frequently be associated with locomotive dysfunctions. In this text, the physical and radiographic procedures that are helpful in arriving at a differential diagnosis of motor malfunction are emphasized, and the medical and surgical treatment is described.

The reader will find that special attention has been accorded the diagnosis and treatment of cranial and spinal injuries. Lesions involving intervertebral disks are covered in detail, and the treatment methods are discussed and evaluated. A critical evaluation is included of the terminal results in cases of intervertebral disk disease seen by the author over the last 13 years. The chapter on disk disease in the cat stresses the difference in clinical manifestations from those seen in the dog. Methods of diagnosis and surgical treatment of brain tumors and ventricular dropsy are proposed as having an optimistic future application.

The author hopes that the veterinary student and the clinician will find the text most useful in their everyday work. Many chapters, especially those on the spine, contain extensive lists of references that should be of special value to the research worker.

Auburn, Alabama B. F. HOERLEIN

ACKNOWLEDGMENTS

I continue to be indebted to the encouragement of the late Mr. K. A. Scott and the late Dean Emeritus J. E. Greene, who supported and encouraged neurology at this university for so many years. This project has also been enhanced by the ongoing consideration and support of the central administration of Auburn University.

In addition to the marvelous collaborative work of the contributors, I especially appreciate the interest and support of Drs. J. E. Oliver, E. D. Gage, S. F. Swaim, R. W. Redding, and J. E. Bartels. The cooperation of other departmental colleagues too numerous to mention really makes this book a team effort. I would like to acknowledge the expert typing of Mrs. Anne Lynn and Mrs. June Ralston; the administrative help of Mrs. Virginia Klein; the illustrative support of Mrs. Nadine Harper; and the photography of Mr. David Roberts. I am also grateful to Drs. Robert Worthman (neuroanatomy), R. A. Albert (ophthalmology), and Marc Vandevelde (neuropathology) for support in their specialty areas.

I continue to have the highest respect for the W. B. Saunders Company's quality performance and cooperation. The veterinary editor, Mr. Carroll Cann, and the entire staff have been a pleasure to work with. Finally, the patience and encouragement shown by my wife and family during the long hours of preparation of this revision are greatly appreciated.

Auburn, Alabama B. F. Hoerlein

CONTENTS

Part Four

THE CENTRAL NERVOUS SYSTEM IN GENERAL

Part Five

THE SPINE

PART ONE

NEUROLOGICAL EXAMINATION

CHAPTER 1

INTRODUCTION

The nervous system has for centuries been one of the most perplexing systems of the body to understand, and nervous disorders have always been regarded as mysterious and difficult to diagnose. However, in historical times scientists have observed various portions of the nervous system, and these milestones form an appropriate introduction to the various clinical subjects presented in this text.

EARLY HISTORY

The first neurological record was made by the ancient Egyptians about 3000 years BC when they used the term "brain." Hippocrates, Plato, Aristotle, and others in the fifth and fourth centuries BC wrote accounts of neurological disorders such as epilepsy, spinal injuries, and head injuries, as well as descriptions of the brain, its cerebral and cerebellar hemispheres, and its ventricles and membranes.[3]

Despite these observations, the physiological function of the nervous system was not recognized. The brain was believed to be only a gland which secreted "phlegm" into the pituitary gland and nose. The *heart* was the central organ, and the blood vessels, not the nerves, were the channels by which motion and sensation were transmitted. This belief was even shared to some degree by William Harvey some 2000 years later.[3]

The true role of the nervous system was first suspected by Galen of Rome (130–210 AD). He sectioned the spinal cord of newborn pigs and noted the loss of movement and feeling in the limbs. The brain was believed to be the seat of intelligence and imagination, the principal organ for sensory perception. It was also the source of one of the vital spirits that flowed down the nerves' invisible channels, transmitting motion and sensation.[3]

Although the anatomists of the Renaissance—Vesalius, Falloppio, Willis, Sylvius, and Morgagni—laid the foundations for our knowledge of the structure of the nervous system, it was not until the nineteenth century that the mode of transmission of nervous impulses was discovered.[3]

Through the experimental stimulation of exposed tissue of animals and man by mechanical, thermal, and chemical means, the concepts of sensitivity, irritability, and contractility emerged. Nevertheless, the wasting of tissues distal to nerve disruption could still be explained by the loss of nourishing nerve juices which were thought to flow from the brain, although microscopic studies (1674) failed to reveal nerve channels through which they were said to pass.[3]

Physical explanations of anatomy were more persuasive than concepts of the body's humors, and the body was conceived as a machine. Nerve threads connecting the brain to the periphery of the body were supposed to be the bases of movement and sensation. However, the discovery of electricity proved to be a new solution to the mystery of nerve conduction. Galvani (1737–1798) applied this discovery to neurophysiology by using the humble nerve-muscle preparation of the frog to demonstrate that nerve conduction was electrical in nature. Just a century ago it was shown that the nerve impulse results from a self-propagating depolarization of nerve membrane.[3]

The synapse was unknown until Sherrington's work in 1897. The peculiar histology of motor end-plates and the delays in conduction that occurred there raised the possibility of some form of nonelectrical transmission. The roles of adrenalin and acetylcholine in the sympathetic and parasympathetic synapses were discovered by the physiologists Elliott, Loewi, and Dale. The ancient neurohumoral theory thus eventually proved to contain some small truth.[3]

The sequential knowledge of the physiological functions of the spinal cord was made possible by such investigators as Flechsig and Gowers, Schwann and Purkinje, Marchi, Golgi, Cajal, Waller, Brown-Séquard, Magendie, and Bell. Magendie and Bell showed that the spinal roots possessed different functions—the anterior root was a motor nerve, and the posterior root was sensory. The neurohistologists Golgi, Marchi, Weigert, and Cajal, using silver and gold impregnations, aniline dyes, and osmic acid techniques, portrayed the extraordinary complexity of nervous tissue. The development throughout the last century of knowledge of spinal tracts, sensory and motor conduction, and reflex activity of the spinal cord by scientists such as Babinski and Sherrington laid the groundwork for modern neurophysiology and neurological diagnosis.[3]

Although cranial trephination was performed by the ancients, the birth of modern neurosurgery began with Sir William Macewen in 1879. This surgery was based on anatomical, physiological, and clinical observations since the techniques of radiology and the lumbar spinal fluid puncture were unknown before 1891 and 1895 respectively. The ancients studied and named many of the now well known parts of the brain, such as the vein of Galen and the dura and pia mater (the "hard" and "devoted" protecting "mother" membranes). Later, the ventricles were thought to be concerned in the processes of neurological respiration and excretion, which were essential to the Galenical doctrine of the three spirits. The casts and drawings of the ventricles by Leonardo da Vinci (about 1500) were centuries ahead of practical usefulness to medicine. Sylvius, Monro, Magendie, Luschka, and Willis are remembered in the names of the ventricles.[3]

As development of the concepts of the 12 cranial nerves progressed, William Harvey in the seventeenth century was asking whether the substance of the brain or the ventricle had the chief role in mental functions. By 1840, the cells in various parts of the nervous system had been recognized and described. Myelinated and unmyelinated fibers had been demonstrated. By the end of the nineteenth century, Virchow, Waldeyer, Forel, and Cajal had prepared splendid atlases of the gross and microscopic anatomy of the brain, showing that the nervous system was not a simple network of tissue but a highly complex system.[3]

As knowledge of the gross and microscopic anatomy of the brain progressed, functional concepts followed. Through both clinical and experimental studies of ablation and stimulation, visual, auditory, and motor functions were localized in the cortex. The complex functions of facilitation and inhibition and the intricacies of traumatic injuries became understood. Although the electrical currents in the brains of animals were discovered nearly 100 years ago, electroencephalographic signs in man were first recorded only in 1929.[3]

The chemistry of the nervous system is a recent field of neurological study. The chemical constituents of nerve tissue, the activity of electrolytes, enzymes, and lipids, the role of neuroglia, and the blood-brain barrier are assuming increasing importance. Neurochemistry is exerting a profound influence on the whole field of medical research, including genetic and hereditary diseases, pharmacology, and therapy. Thus, although great strides have been made since ancient times in understanding the structure and function of the nervous system, it appears that the future discoveries will be just as astounding as those of the past.[3]

HISTORY OF VETERINARY NEUROLOGY

The history of clinical veterinary neurology has been somewhat slower in development than that of human medicine. Highlights in the history of the various facets of clinical neurology in small pet animals have been mentioned in the various chapters of this book and will not be emphasized here. Since the late 1940's and early 1950's, there has been a tremendous expansion in the field of clinical veterinary neurology. Veterinary colleges have clinical neurologists and neurosurgeons on their faculties; practicing veterinarians are becoming experienced diagnosticians and in some cases neurosurgeons; and in urban areas there is a growing number of specialists in neurology who are devoting the majority of their time to clinical practice. There is a flourishing national association of veterinary neurologists, and recently a specialty board in neurology has been created within the college of veterinary internal medicine. Again, although much has been learned, the surface has just been scratched, and the bright young scientists now emerging in the profession face the challenge of providing more and better clinical service.[3]

INCIDENCE OF NEUROLOGICAL DISEASE

In previous editions of this text, the introductory chapter included discussions of some of the basic concepts of the blood-brain barrier, regeneration of nervous tissue, and differential diagnosis of motor disorders. However, since these topics are discussed in more depth in other areas of the text, a brief discussion of the clinical incidence of neurological disorders[2] may be more appropriate for this chapter and may be enlightening to both student and practitioner.

Statistics from the Auburn University small animal teaching hospital cited in previous editions of this text placed the incidence of neurological diseases at 4.5 per cent in 1961–1962 and 4.8 per cent in 1968–1969. However, in the 1975–1976 annual report of nonsurgical diagnoses, 14.7 per cent of the disorders were neurological in nature. When both surgical and nonsurgical diagnoses are included, a total of 14.8 per cent were neurological. In these statistics, neurological diagnoses comprised 11.9 per cent of genetic disease classification, 9.4 per cent of infectious diseases, 13 per cent of traumatic disorders, and 15.1 per cent of surgical disorders. It is acknowledged that these figures are unusually high because this institution specializes in neurology. However, other statistics also emphasize the importance of clinical neurology in the practice of small animal medicine and surgery.

From the National Cancer Institute Veterinary Medical Data Program (VMDP), which has stored information collected for over 10 years from 12 colleges of veterinary medicine in North America, 8117 cases of intervertebral disk disease were reported in 356,954 dogs.[2] These data show a crude hospital/clinic rate of 23 cases per 1000 dogs per year. In estimated relative risk (R) techniques and chi-square tests of significance, in which an R value of greater than 1 indicates increased relative risk, dachshunds experience an R value of 9.9, Pekingese 3.5, Welsh corgis 2.3, beagles 2.0, small poodles 0.8, and cocker spaniels 0.7. In another study, Goggins[1] found that the dachshund suffered a risk of disk disease that was 12.6 times greater than the risk for all other breeds combined. From other VMDP untreated statistics, 23.8 per cent of the dachshunds, 4.7 per cent of the beagles, and 1.1 per cent of the mixed breed dogs entering these institutional clinics suffered from clinical disk disease.*

As more accurate statistical data are accumulated in veterinary medicine, it is probable that the importance of neurological diseases in veterinary practice will increase as sophistication in diagnosis is developed.

EXPANDING AREAS OF CLINICAL VETERINARY NEUROLOGY

A short discussion of the expanding areas of knowledge in clinical veterinary neurology is appropriate for this introduction to the balance of the text. The neurological examination in recent years has been aided substantially by newer techniques and special diagnostic aids. The ocular fundic changes in infectious, metabolic, and toxic diseases are better documented.

*Data printouts have been furnished by the courtesy of Dr. William A. Priester, Bethesda, Maryland, Veterinary Medical Data Program.

Electromyographic and microchemical techniques and nerve conduction testing have added new dimensions to the diagnosis of neuromuscular disorders. Newer methods of examining cerebrospinal fluid and exfoliative cytology will, by enhancing knowledge of disease processes, bring about improvements in diagnosis and therapy. The continued efforts toward development of a safe, water-soluble contrast medium for myelography and ventriculography will make these procedures more meaningful and practical in diagnosing space-occupying lesions. It is possible that radioisotope scanning of central nervous tissue will eventually become a practical procedure in veterinary neurology.

The study of hereditary and congenital diseases in animals have in some cases become models for the study of the corresponding human disorders. Diseases such as globoid cell leukodystrophy, Down's syndrome (mongolism), neuronal glycoproteinosis (Lafora's disease), and neuronal GM gangliosidosis (Tay-Sachs disease) are examples of animal disorders that are identical to those in man. Likewise, it is increasingly evident that animals may also aid in the study of so-called slow virus diseases in humans. It is possible that there is a relationship between chronic distemper and subacute sclerosing panencephalitis (SSPE) in man. This is only one example of many zoonotic diseases that are becoming more clearly understood in clinical neurology.

The subject of animal behavior has gained prominence in the past few years, and in this edition it is given a separate chapter. The most expedient control of undesirable behavior in pets in the Auburn Clinic is Redding's electroconvulsive shock therapy. This method is proving to be the most practical and effective method of control of undesirable behavioral problems, especially aggressiveness toward persons or other animals.

Much emphasis has been placed recently on traumatic CNS disorders. It has been established that trauma in the CNS excites the release of excessive levels of certain catecholamines and enzymes, which contribute to the hemorrhagic necrosis seen in profound spinal cord injury. Considerable advances are being made in controlling the deleterious effects of edema, swelling, and neurochemical changes by use of anticatecholamines, steroids, and dimethyl sulfoxide. Surgical hypothermia, durotomies, myelotomies, and complete laminectomies have been proposed for severe spinal trauma. Advances in decompression of the cord (ventral cervical) and skeletal immobilization are continuing to provide more effective results in the animal patient. Future research in CNS trauma will lead to a greater basic understanding of the pathogenesis and effective treatment of such problems.

In summary, this chapter has endeavored to present the highlights of the history of neurology, the statistical significance of the incidence of neurological diseases, and several exciting advances in the understanding and treatment of nervous disorders. These advances are given appropriate emphasis in the balance of the text.

REFERENCES

1. Goggins, J. E., Li, A. S., and Franti, C. E.: Canine intervertebral disk disease, characterization by age, sex, breed, and anatomical site of involvement. Am. J. Vet. Res. *9*, 1687, 1970.
2. Priester, W. A., and Mantel, N.: Occurrence of tumors in domestic animals. Data from 12 United States and Canadian colleges of veterinary medicine. J. Natl. Cancer Inst. *47*, 1333, 1971.
3. Spillane, J. D.: *An Atlas of Clinical Neurology*, 2d ed. Oxford University Press, New York, 1975.

CHAPTER 2

ANATOMY AND PHYSIOLOGY

R. W. Redding, D.V.M., Ph.D.

INTRODUCTION

In this chapter we will briefly discuss the anatomy and physiology of the nervous system (structure-function relationship) to provide the reader with a basis for evaluation of the signs shown by an animal with a neurological disease. It is beyond the scope of this chapter either to delve deeply into the intimate anatomical details and the complex physiological functions or to teach neurophysiology, but we will indicate those important features that are necessary for an understanding of the nature of dysfunction in disease.

The nervous system controls such rapid activities of the body as muscular contractions, some rapid visceral reactions, and the rate of secretion of endocrine glands. Since these functions are frequently visible to the observer, they may be used to determine the state of activity of the nervous system. Although it is not possible to observe nerve tissue activity, one may observe the result of that activity as manifested by behavioral attitudes and muscular and glandular reactions. Diseases of the nervous system manifest themselves as abnormalities of behavior, locomotion, sensory responses, and autonomic activity.

THE NERVE

THE NEURON

The neuron, or nerve cell, the functional and structural unit of the nervous system (Fig. 2–1), conducts nerve impulses or communication signals from one part of the body to another. It is so specialized that it sacrifices many other biological functions: It cannot reproduce itself, and its metabolic activity is so simple that it cannot live for more than a few minutes without oxygen or fuel. Therefore, the neuron is the most delicate cell in the whole body and requires an environment more constant than other cells of the body. It is not surprising, therefore, that changes in blood glucose levels, pH, oxygen tension, pCO_2, and other chemical constituents cause a marked alteration of nervous system function.

Neuroanatomists classify neurons according to their location, structure, and function. Basically, there are three types of neurons: (1) the sensory neuron, whose cell body lies outside the central nervous system and whose function is to conduct impulses (information) from the periphery into the central nervous system (CNS); (2) the interneuron, which is located entirely within the central nervous system and whose function is to conduct impulses within the CNS to the motor neurons from sensory neurons and other interneurons, forming highly complex neuron networks (the basis of nervous integration), and (3) the motor neuron, whose cell body is located within the central nervous system and whose function is directly concerned with transmitting signals to the muscles and glands by axons extending outside the central nervous system. Figure 2–2 is a schematic representation of each of these neurons.

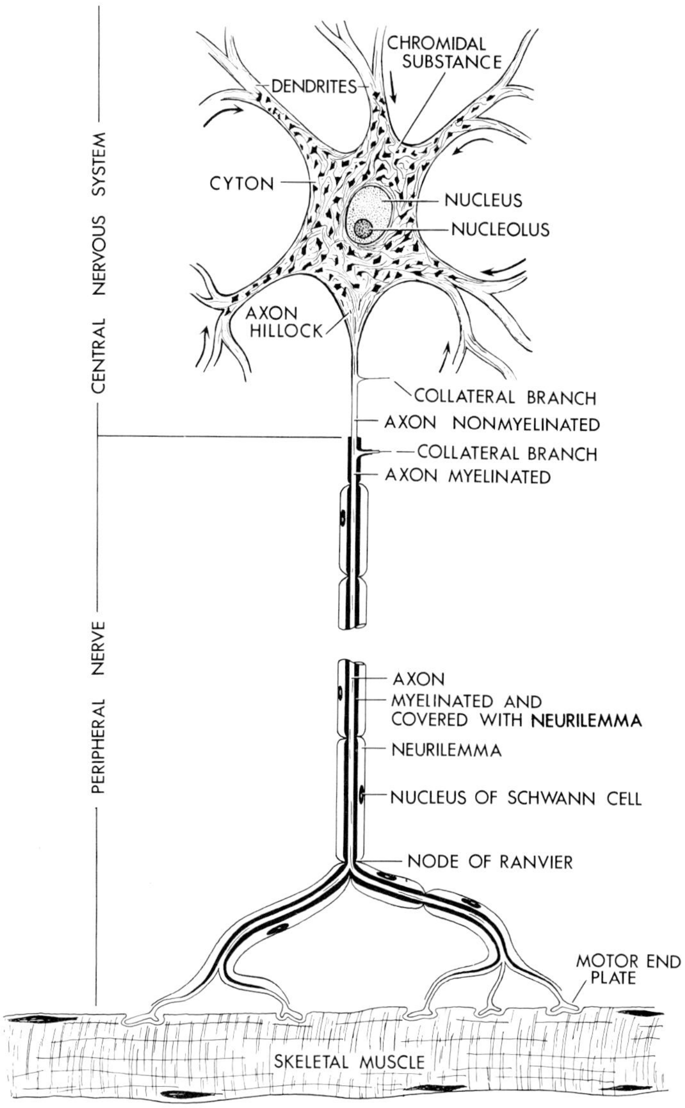

FIGURE 2–1 Schematic drawing of a lower motor neuron. (From Miller, M. E., Christensen, G. C., and Evans, H. E.: *Anatomy of the Dog.* W. B. Saunders Co., Philadelphia, 1964.)

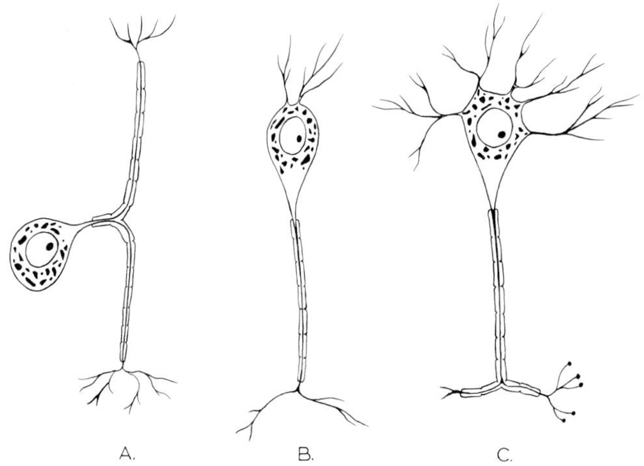

FIGURE 2–2 Schematic drawing of vertebrate neurons. *A*, Sensory neuron. *B*, Interneuron. *C*, Motor neuron.

It is quite obvious that disease processes that affect the neurons can cause different signs, depending upon which type of neuron is involved; e.g., irritative processes will cause hypersensitivity if the sensory neurons are involved, integrative dysfunction if the interneurons are involved, and hyperactivity of muscles and glands if the motor neurons are involved. Conversely, if destructive processes occur, there will be loss of sensory input into the CNS when sensory neurons are involved, loss of integrative control when the interneurons are involved, and loss of function of muscles and glands when the motor neurons are involved. This summary is, of course, an oversimplification, but it serves to point out the causes of various clinical signs.

Neurologists frequently classify motor neurons in two subdivisions: (1) upper motor neurons (UMN), of which the cell bodies and axons lie totally within the central nervous system, the axons forming the descending fasciculi (long tracts). The cell bodies are located in the cerebral cortex or brain stem; and (2) lower motor neurons (LMN), of which the cell bodies are located on the brain stem and spinal cord, and the axons form the motor fibers outside the central nervous system to innervate the muscular structures. Clinical signs associated with diseases of the upper motor neurons are different from those associated with diseases of the lower motor neurons; therefore, clinical neurologists classify clinical signs as "upper motor neuron signs" and "lower motor neuron signs." See Chapter 4 for definition of signs.

If a nerve cell body is destroyed e.g., by anoxia, by toxins, or by virus infection, (such as distemper), the whole neuron dies. If the axon is severed, the neuron may die unless its continuity is re-established. In the case of peripheral axons, new axon filaments will grow along the neurilemmal sheath from the central end and a repair may be effected. However, within the CNS, where there is a differently formed neurilemmal (glial network) sheath, repair is so exceptional that for practical purposes it may be discounted altogether.

NERVE FIBERS

Every axon (and some dendrites) and its branches, as far as the terminal filaments (Fig. 2–1), are covered with a layer of white fatty substance known as *myelin*. The larger the axon, the thicker its myelin sheath. Nerve fibers (axons or dendrites) vary in size from 0.5 μ to 20 μ. The smallest axons have only a very thin film of myelin, which could not be seen with the fat stains formerly used for observation of myelin with the light microscope. To this day small fibers are called "unmyelinated" fibers. In larger axons, both inside and outside the central nervous system, the myelin is arranged in segments separated by the *nodes of Ranvier*. So-called "unmyelinated" fibers have only a continuous thin covering of myelin.

If myelin is not present around the axon, it will not conduct impulses. In young animals, some fibers are not myelinated until several weeks after birth. This explains in part why a newborn or very young animal is not capable of receiving information, analyzing that information, and performing meaningful actions in response to stimuli. Moreover, myelin may be destroyed by such diseases as distemper and allergic reactions, thus preventing the conduction of nerve impulses and producing abnormal clinical signs. Axons (nerve fibers) outside the central nervous system have a further covering outside the myelin, the *endoneurium*.

Nerve Damage and Regeneration

When a nerve fiber is divided, the portion separated from the cell body undergoes degenerative changes. Degeneration does not start at the point of damage only; all parts of the nerve fiber, including the terminals, are involved simultaneously. All parts of the nerve fiber degenerate, with the exception of the neurilemma, until all that remains is the empty neurilemmal tube. Alterations also occur on the proximal side of the damaged nerve fiber (retrograde degeneration). The nerve fiber up to the first node of Ranvier degenerates similarly to the distal portion. In the cell body, the nucleus and cytoplasm undergo swelling. The Nissl substance undergoes chromatolysis. If the cell does not make functional connections with receptors or other neurons, atrophy of the cell body may ultimately result.

Regeneration of peripheral nerve fibers occurs when conditions are suitable; however, in nerve fibers of the central nervous system, glial scarring inhibits the process. Regeneration is accomplished by a downgrowth of neurofibrils from the proximal portion of the severed nerve. These neurofibrils enter the empty neurilemmal sheath in the distal segment and, over a period of time, traverse its entire length. The rate of growth of the new neurofibrils varies from 0.5 mm to 2 mm per day in the dog (see Chapter 10). Restoration of function requires weeks or months, depending upon the distance of the severed nerve from its distal termination.

THE NERVE IMPULSE

The transmission of information from inside and outside of the animal's body (via receptors) to and within the CNS, and out of the CNS to effectors, is accomplished by a self-propagated physiological process called the "nerve impulse." The nerve impulse generation is the mechanism by which all rapid reaction of the animal's body that is necessary for its survival is accomplished. There is a great amount of information available relative to the conduction velocity of various size nerve fibers (thicker ones conduct more rapidly than those of smaller diameter); this information may contribute to the diagnosis and prognosis of disease states of the nervous system of the dog (see Chapter 9).

THE SYNAPSE

Information is transmitted to the CNS through a continuous succession of neurons. The point at which one neuron joins another or joins an effector is called a "synapse" (Fig. 2–3). It is not generally appreciated that these junctions not only may transmit the signal but also may (a) block its transmission from one neuron to another; (b) change it from a single impulse into many repetitive impulses; (c) reduce the number of signals; or (d) integrate the signal with impulses from other neurons. These actions produce highly intricate patterns of impulses in successive neurons, and eventually produce meaningful motor responses. The mechanism by which the presynaptic neuron terminals (Fig. 2–3) excite the postsynaptic neuron is believed to be the release of an excitatory substance called the excitatory transmitter. It is probable that more than one type of excitatory transmitter is released at different synapses in the CNS. A certain quantity of excitatory transmitter must be released per unit time to cause excitation of the postsynaptic neuron and the conduction of a nerve impulse. If the sufficient "quantum" is not released, the postsynaptic neuron does not fire. However, this does not mean that no change has taken place in the postsynaptic cell. It is more easily activated (facilitated) by additional presynaptic discharges than would normally be true. Facilitation in the

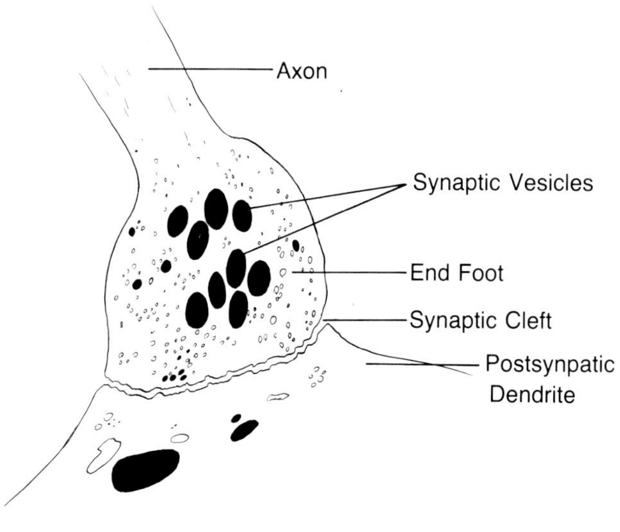

FIGURE 2–3 Schematic diagram of the synapse. (After Ham: *Textbook of Histology*, 6th ed. J. B. Lippincott Co., Philadelphia, 1969.)

CNS is displayed in animals by external signs such as hyperesthesia, hyperalgesia, and excessive motor responses to minimal auditory, visual, and tactile stimuli.

Inhibition can and does occur in the CNS. In fact, if it were not for continual inhibitory activity, the nervous system could not function at all. For instance, all parts of the central nervous system receive a continual barrage of large numbers of incoming signals from peripheral nerves. If it were not for adequate inhibition of most of these input signals, the brain would remain in so great a state of continual excitation that it would be almost useless. Therefore, inhibition plays a role in *selecting* those signals that are important, while blocking those that are unimportant for that particular set of circumstances at that time. An example of the effect of loss of inhibition is the profound abnormal activity (tetanic spasms and muscular rigidity) seen in tetanus and strychnine poisoning. Both tetanus toxin and strychnine depress inhibitory neurons. The responses observed demonstrate clearly that inhibition is a very important part of CNS activity. The inhibitory presynaptic terminals derive from special types of neurons called inhibitory neurons. The terminal fibers from these neurons secrete only *inhibitory transmitter* substance. The exact nature of this substance is controversial.

TABLE 2–1 CLASSIFICATION OF RECEPTORS

Type of Receptor	Special Sense	Receptor End[a]
Mechanoreceptors	Touch	Free nerve endings Meissner's corpuscle
	Pressure	Pacinian corpuscle Hair end organs, Golgi-Massoni corpuscle
	Kinesthetic	Pacinian corpuscles Golgi tendon receptor
	Sound	Cochlea hair cells
	Equilibrium	Macula and ampulla hair cells
	Muscle stretch	Muscle spindles
	Lung stretch	?
	Heart muscle stretch	?
Thermoreceptors	Heat	Special free nerve endings (Ruffini's end organ?)
	Cold	Special free nerve endings (Krause's end organ?)
Chemoreceptors	Pain	Free nerve endings
	Taste	Taste buds
	Smell	Olfactory cells
	Oxygen in blood	Carotid and aortic body chemoreceptors
Electromagnetic radiation receptors	Sight	Rods and cones of eye

[a]Although certain receptors in the past have been associated with special senses it is now believed that some receptor endings serve multiple functions.

SENSORY RECEPTORS

Receptors are bascially transducers; that is, they turn specific forms of energy into nerve impulses. Most receptors are specific—they transmute only a particular form of energy under normal body conditions. Under unusual conditions, other forms of energy at high intensity may initiate nerve impulses from receptors. In general, the receptors are located at the peripheral end of the dendrite of the sensory neuron.

Physiologists classify sensory receptors in several ways: by the location of the receptor, by the site of action of the receptor, by the size of the fiber involved, and by the kind of stimulus necessary to excite the receptors. The last is the most easily understood and will be used in the following discussion.

Table 2–1 depicts the classification. Basically, there are four different types of receptors: (1) mechanoreceptors; (2) thermoreceptors; (3) chemoreceptors; and (4) electromagnetic radiation receptors. It is important to realize that these receptors are purposefully activated during the course of the neurological examination and an understanding of their function is necessary for proper interpretation of the results of this activation. Means of activation during examination may include (1) the use of volatile oils or foods to activate the olfactory receptors (chemoreceptors); (2) the projection of light into the eye to activate the rods and cones (electromagnetic receptors) for evaluation of the direct and consensual light reflex; (3) a pin-prick test of the face to activate the touch and pain receptors for evaluation of the integrity of the trigeminal and facial nerves; (4) activation of the touch and pressure receptors (mechanoreceptors) in placing and hopping reactions to evaluate the functional integrity of the spinal cord and higher centers; (5) activation of the muscle spindles (mechanoreceptors) in the knee jerk reflex to evaluate the functional status of the lumbar cord; and (6) holding a blindfolded animal in the air by the pelvis to evaluate the functional status of the vestibular receptors. These are a few examples of receptor activation utilized by the neurologist in the diagnosis of disease. Disorders of receptors per se are relatively rare, except for some special senses such as rods and cones of the eye and olfactory cells.

EFFECTORS

Parts of the body that can be controlled by the nervous system are called effectors. Certain structures, such as skeletal muscle, cardiac muscle, smooth muscle, and endocrine and exocrine glands, stand out as effectors. Their responses to nerve impulses are visible to the observer and thus serve as visual clues to normality or abnormality.

Skeletal muscle activity is the end result of both reflex activity and highly integrated nervous system functions. The observation of the results of these contractions, as manifested by body movements and reflexes, is used as a clue to the functional activity of the nervous system and of its effectors. It should be pointed out here that such conditions as atrophy and hypertrophy are frequently indications of the status of nervous connections to the skeletal musculature. Atrophy of the temporalis and masseter muscles is suggestive of trigeminal (motor portion) nerve nuclei or peripheral nerve damage, and loss of facial expression and drooping of the upper eyelid and face are suggestive of facial nucleus or peripheral nerve damage.

REFLEXES

An important part of the neurological examination is evaluation of reflexes. The object of reflex evaluation is to determine the presence of a lesion, its location, and the extent of its involvement in the CNS. Reflexes are of two types: pure spinal cord or brain stem reflexes, and reflexes involving the spinal cord or brain stem and the higher centers, i.e., the basal nuclei, cerebrum, and cerebellum.

The components of a reflex system (called a reflex arc) are a receptor, an afferent neuron, one or more synapses within the CNS, and efferent neuron, and an effector. Figure 2–4 is a schematic diagram of a simple reflex system. Reflex systems are seldom as simple as that seen in Figure 2–4, in which the pathways are shown only as abstractions. Functionally, they rarely, if ever, operate in such simple form. The observed response of an animal to stimulation of a receptor is called a reflex act. It should be realized that the relatively fixed pattern of response or behavior for any given stimulus is an inborn (inherited) phenomenon, and as such, is—fortunately for the clinician—a reliable test of normality. Any deviation from the stereotyped pattern is suggestive of a dis-

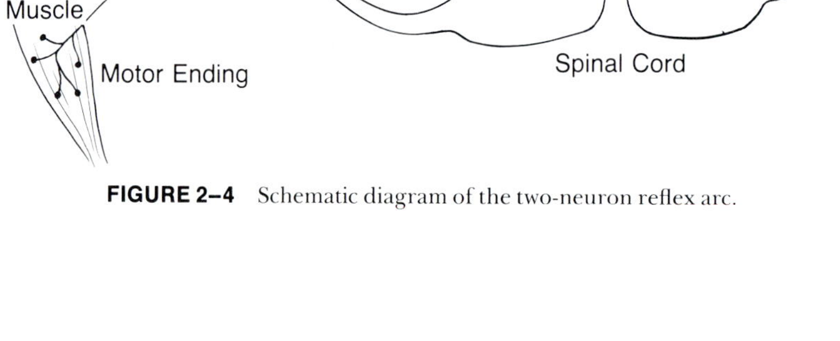

FIGURE 2–4 Schematic diagram of the two-neuron reflex arc.

eased state of the tissues involved. An understanding of the normal response to a specific stimulus (standardized reflex test) is mandatory for diagnosticians in the evaluation of a patient.

TYPES OF REFLEX NEURONAL NETWORKS

A two-neuron system, as shown in Figure 2–4, shows the simplest reflex arc that has clinical significance. This reflex arc is known as the *myotatic* or *stretch reflex.* The most common application of this reflex is seen in the knee jerk test, in which a tap on the tendon of the quadriceps femoris muscle below the patella elicits a quick reflex muscular contraction (called a jerk), causing the stifle joint to go into extension. As shown in Figure 2–4, the receptor is the neuromuscular spindle located in the belly of the muscle. When this spindle stretches, it sends a nerve impulse to the spinal cord via the sensory neurons that synapse with the large motor neurons in the ventral gray horns. The axons of these cells transmit impulses to the lengthened muscle, which now contracts to return to its original length, causing the "jerk." The foregoing is a description of a method of eliciting, in an exaggerated form, an otherwise nonrecognizable normal activity of the body. The stretch reflex is constantly functioning when an animal is standing, sitting, or in motion. Muscles are stretched when their antagonists contract, and when joints are flexed, as a result of gravity acting upon the body and limbs. It is believed that the muscle spindles in antigravity muscles are very sensitive and are responsible for what is known as *muscle tone.*

A system involving three or more neurons (Fig. 2–5) is best exemplified by the withdrawal reflex (toepinch reflex), a response to a painful stimulus. The impulses originating in the pain receptors travel centrally and are widely distributed in the spinal cord. After passage through many interneurons (only one is shown in the simplified schematic diagram), they activate many motor neurons, thus causing reflex flexion at several joints and withdrawal of the limb. This sequence appears to be a simple and relatively isolated mechanism; however, involvement of the opposing muscles makes the whole reaction more complex, as described in the next paragraph.

COORDINATION OF REFLEXES

Reflex responses involve not only contractions but also relaxations of opposing muscles. The production of this relaxation is an *inhibitory* function of the synapses and interneurons in the spinal cord. Figure 2–6 is a schematic representation of inhibition mechanisms within the gray matter of the spinal cord. Figure 2–7 demonstrates multisegmental and contralateral responses.

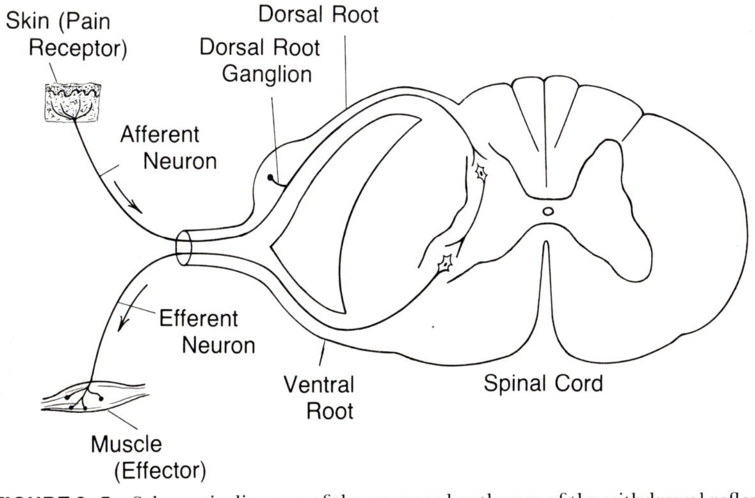

FIGURE 2–5 Schematic diagram of the neuronal pathways of the withdrawal reflex.

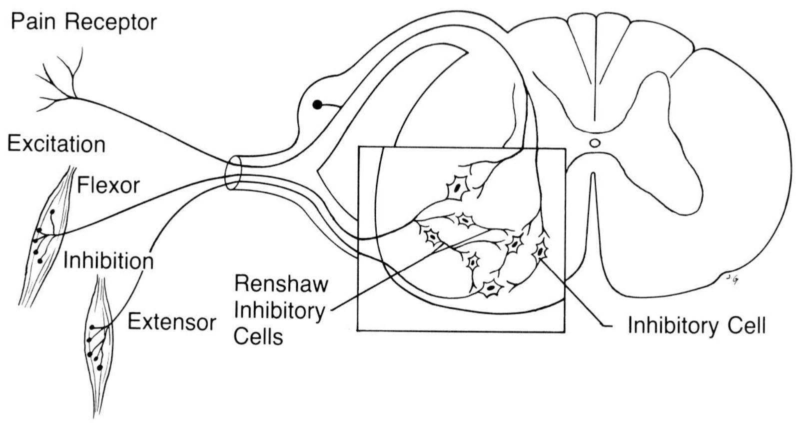

FIGURE 2–6 Schematic diagram of the inhibition mechanisms in the gray matter of the spinal cord. (Modified from Gardner, E. D.: *Fundamentals of Neurology*. W. B. Saunders Co., Philadelphia, 1968.)

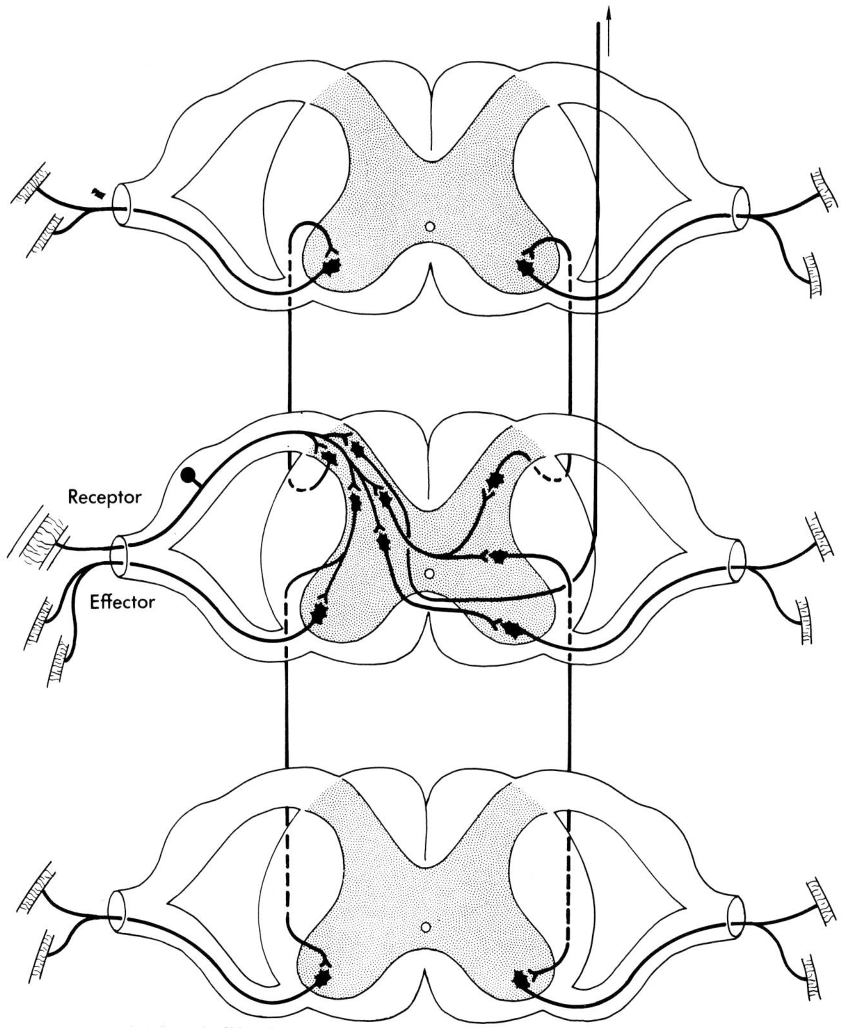

FIGURE 2–7 Diagram of the connections by which impulses from a receptor reach motor neurons at various levels of both sides of the spinal cord. This accounts for multisegmental, ipsilateral and contralateral responses. (From Gardner, E. D.: *Fundamentals of Neurology*, 6th ed. W. B. Saunders Co., Philadelphia, 1975.)

The preceding discussion of reflex systems serves to point out the components of spinal cord reflexes, which are a basis of more highly integrated reflexes involving the higher center. In Chapter 3, the pathways involved in each useful diagnostic reflex, both those involving only the spinal cord and those involving higher centers, will be discussed or diagrammed.

NEUROGLIA

Lying among the nerve cells of the CNS and providing a supporting framework (in addition to other functions) are the cells known collectively as the *neuroglia* or *glial cells.* Glial cells vary in size and shape, and classification of them is based upon structure (Fig. 2–8). All of the cells have processes that weave around nerve cells and nerve fibers and that frequently attach themselves to the walls of blood vessels. In the gray matter, the processes of these cells so completely surround the blood vessels and neurons that there is practically no extracellular space.

There are three distinctive, recognizable types of neuroglia. (1) *Astrocytes,* so named because of their shape, are presumed to serve the function of mechanical support and to provide nutrition for the nerve cells, and they may be involved in the so-called blood-brain barrier. Astrocytes also proliferate in response to many types of injury to the central nervous system. (2) *Oligodendroglia* are believed to play an important role in the formation of myelin material of nerve fibers in the central nervous system, and as such may play an important role in diseases involving myelin formation and destruction. (3) *Microglia* are considered to be reticuloendothelial cells. They are migratory and phagocytic, wandering into the nervous tissue from the vascular components of the CNS. In inflammatory processes, these cells increase in number and are capable of removing degenerating nervous tissue after destruction or injury.

In contrast to neurons, all glial cells can divide mitotically. They are particularly important clinically because approximately 50 per cent of brain tumors are of neuroglial origin, i.e., astrocytomas, oligodendrogliomas, and glioblastomas.

MENINGES

The brain and spinal cord are surrounded by three membranes called meninges. The *dura mater* is the tough, dense, fibrous outermost membrane. It is practically impossible for fluids to penetrate it. The cranial dura mater is composed of periosteal and meningeal layers, within which lie the dural sinuses. Spinal dura mater is often regarded as a single meningeal layer directly surrounding the spinal cord. (2) The *arachnoid* is a thin membrane just inside the dura mater. The potential space between the arachnoid and the dura mater is termed the *subdural* space. Around the brain, a delicate network of connective tissue trabeculae connects the arachnoid to the innermost membrane, the *pia mater.* (3) The *pia mater* is a very delicate membrane that is closely applied to the brain and spinal cord, covering all the folds and sinking into the various fissures along its surface.

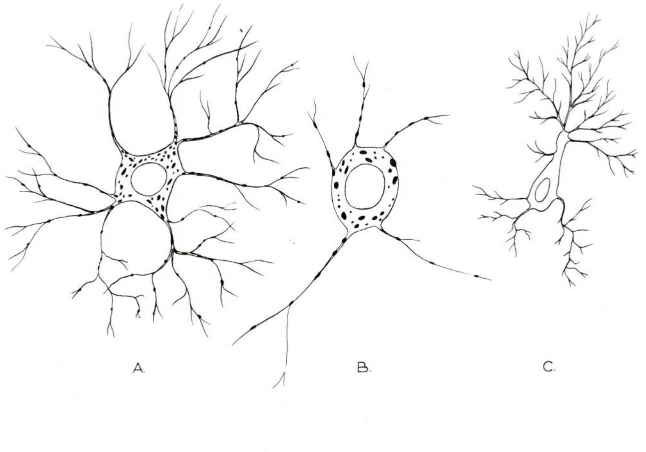

FIGURE 2–8 Neuroglial cells of the central nervous system. *A,* Astrocyte. *B,* Oligodendroglia. *C,* Microglia cell. (After Ham: *Textbook of Histology,* 6th ed. J. B. Lippincott Co., Philadelphia, 1969.)

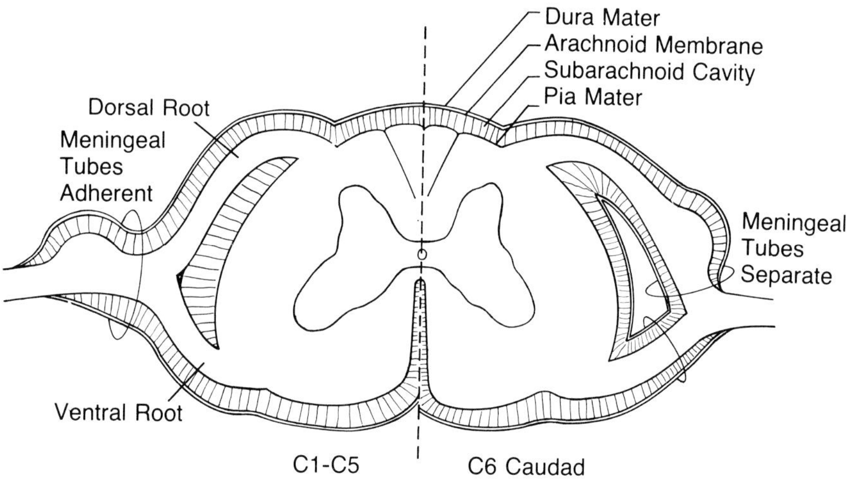

FIGURE 2–9 Schematic drawing of the meninges of the spinal cord.

This arrangement of arachnoid and pia mater permits the existence of a space called the *subarachnoid space,* which contains extraventricular cerebrospinal fluid. (For a more complete discussion of the meninges, see Chapter 17).

Figures 2–9 and 2–11 show the arrangement of the meninges around the brain and spinal cord. It is obvious from the anatomical structure that the meninges protect the delicate nervous tissue by supporting it in a fluid medium that acts as a shock-absorber against the everyday bumps and jolts of an animal in motion. In addition to their protective function, the meninges, with the accompanying blood vessels, serve as a lymph drainage system, since the brain and spinal cord do not have lymph vessels.

INTERNAL CAVITIES OF THE BRAIN

Within the cerebrum and brain stem there is a communicating system of four cavities filled with cerebrospinal fluid (CSF). These cavities are designated as the two lateral ventricles and the third and fourth ventricles (Fig. 2–10). Both lateral ventricles communicate through the interventricular foramen (foramen of Monro) with the anterior aspect of the third ventricle. The third ventricle is a narrow, vertical, cleft-like structure between the two lateral ventricles.

Three openings communicate with the third ventricle. Two communicate with the lateral ventricles, and one is a posterior opening into a narrow aqueduct (aqueduct

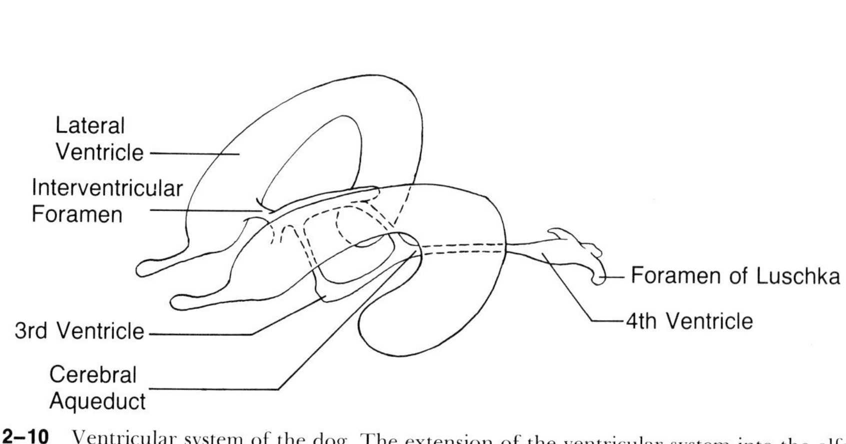

FIGURE 2–10 Ventricular system of the dog. The extension of the ventricular system into the olfactory bulbs is not commonly seen in ventriculograms.

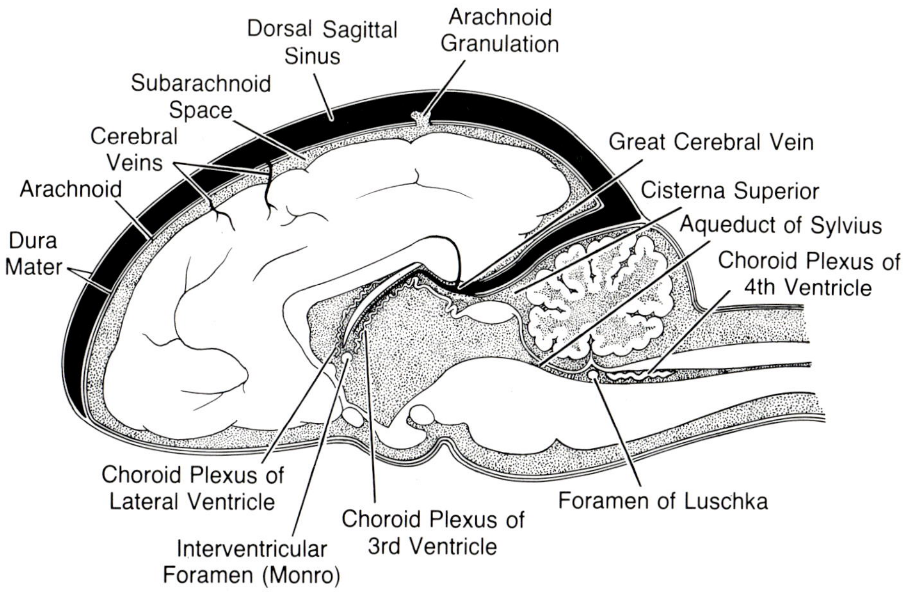

FIGURE 2–11 Meninges and choroid plexuses of the dog. The existence of the arachnoid granulations of this species is controversial.

of Sylvius or cerebral aqueduct) that connects the third and fourth ventricles. The fourth ventricle lies under the cerebellum and is bounded ventrally by the pons and medulla. It is continuous with the cerebral aqueduct anteriorly and with the central canal of the spinal cord posteriorly. In addition to the two connections mentioned, the fourth ventricle has two other communicating openings. Each lateral portion of the fourth ventricle communicates with the subarachnoid space near the cerebellum through the lateral apertures (foramina of Luschka). The medial aperture (foramen of Magendie), an opening in the posterior portion of the roof of the fourth ventricle in primates, is not present in the dog.[41] (For additional information on the ventricular system, see Chapters 5 and 21.)

Each of the four cavities of the ventricular system has highly vascular, fringe-like processes of pia mater projecting into it, which are covered by an epithelial layer of ependymal cells. These processes are called the choroid plexuses of the lateral, third, and fourth ventricles (Fig. 2–11).

CEREBROSPINAL FLUID

Cerebrospinal fluid (CSF) is present in the ventricular system, the central canal of the spinal cord, and the external system: the subarachnoid spaces, including the dilated portions known as the cisterns. (See Chapter 5 for cisterna magna puncture.) Communication between the internal and external systems occurs through the lateral apertures of the fourth ventricle (foramina of Luschka).

CSF is believed to originate primarily in the choroid plexuses through an active secretory process of the cells of the plexuses. There is some evidence that CSF may also come from the brain tissue. In addition, fluid may be derived from the pial and ependymal vessels.

It is postulated that an active circulation of CSF occurs. Fluid forms in the lateral ventricles, circulates through the interventricular foramina into the third ventricle, and moves by way of the cerebral aqueduct into the fourth ventricle. The fluid escapes from the fourth ventricle via the lateral apertures (foramen of Luschka) into the subarachnoid spaces, where it diffuses over the brain and spinal cord. The CSF is believed to be absorbed primarily by the veins in the arachnoid or subarachnoid villi (the existence of which is questionable in the dog), which project into the dural venous sinuses. A small portion of the fluid may be absorbed by the epidural tissue of the cranial and spinal nerves.

The cerebrospinal fluid system is believed to act as the lymphatic system of the central nervous tissue, since no lymphatic structures are present. Probably an equally important, if not more important, function of the ventricular and cerebrospinal fluid system is that of protecting the delicate nervous tissue. It acts as a hydraulic cushion around and within the brain and spinal cord, which "float" in this fluid medium, preventing or diminishing the transmission of shocking or jarring forces. Its role in metabolic transfer is not completely understood. Conceivably, it may convey nutrients to the CNS and carry away products of metabolism.

An understanding of the ventricular system and the formation and flow of CSF is essential in comprehending the problems associated with diseases of the CNS. An appreciation of the small size of such ducts as the cerebral aqueduct in the miniature breeds (Chihuahua and Pomeranian) makes one aware of the possibility of occlusion, with resultant development of hydrocephalus, following even a slight injury to the cerebrum. Acquired hydrocephalus is a common problem in small breeds (see Chapters 7 and 21).

BLOOD-BRAIN, BLOOD-CEREBROSPINAL FLUID, AND CEREBROSPINAL FLUID-BRAIN BARRIERS

It is known that many materials and drugs that are readily delivered to most tissues of the body through the blood stream do not easily enter the central nervous system tissue. Based upon this knowledge, the concept of the *blood-brain barrier* has been developed. Materials and drugs may also enter the nervous tissue via the cerebrospinal fluid system. However, there is a barrier to the transfer of such substances at the choroid plexus; this has been called the *blood-cerebrospinal fluid barrier*. A third barrier to the transfer of substances from the cerebrospinal fluid to the substance of the brain and spinal tissue called the *cerebrospinal fluid-brain barrier* also exists.

The *blood-brain barrier* consists structurally of pedicular processes of astrocytes which cover the capillaries of the central nervous system. This interposition of glial processes provides selectivity for the entrance of materials into the CNS tissue. The *blood-cerebrospinal fluid barrier* is based upon the organization of the choroid epithelium and its associated capillaries to allow selective permeability for the passage of materials from the blood into the cerebrospinal fluid. The *cerebrospinal fluid-brain barrier* is due in part to the selectivity of the ependymal cells lining the ventricles and the cerebral aqueduct and the astrocytes adjacent to the ependyma.

In certain regions of the nervous system these barrier systems are markedly reduced for purposes of physiological regulation. These areas include the pineal body, the wall of the optic recess of the third ventricle, the saccular eminence of the hypophyseal stalk, the area postrema of the fourth ventricle, and, most importantly, the posterior lobe of the hypophysis.

Because of these barriers certain therapeutic agents that are usually effective against microorganisms that may involve the CNS are ineffective.

BRAIN CIRCULATION

ARTERIAL CIRCULATION

Arterial blood transports oxygen, electrolytes, nutrients, and other substances necessary for the function of the brain. The needs of the brain are critical compared to those of other tissues, and a constant flow of blood must be maintained at all times.

The principal arteries to the cerebrum are the anterior, middle, and posterior cerebral arteries. The cerebellum obtains its major blood supply from the anterior and posterior cerebellar arteries (Fig. 2–12). All of the above cerebral arteries are derived from the arterial circle of the brain (circle of Willis) formed by the right and left internal carotids and the basilar artery. The cerebellar arteries are derived from the basilar artery and the arterial circle of the brain (Fig. 2–13). It is important for the clinician who utilizes cerebral angiograms for diagnostic purposes to recognize the normal vascular pattern (see Chapter 5). Figure 2–14 shows the areas of the cerebrum supplied by the cerebral arteries. It is interesting to speculate on whether cere-

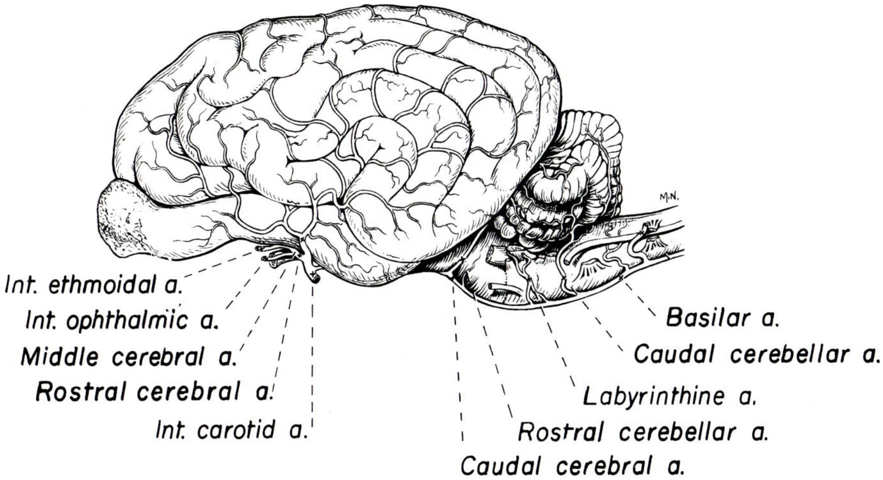

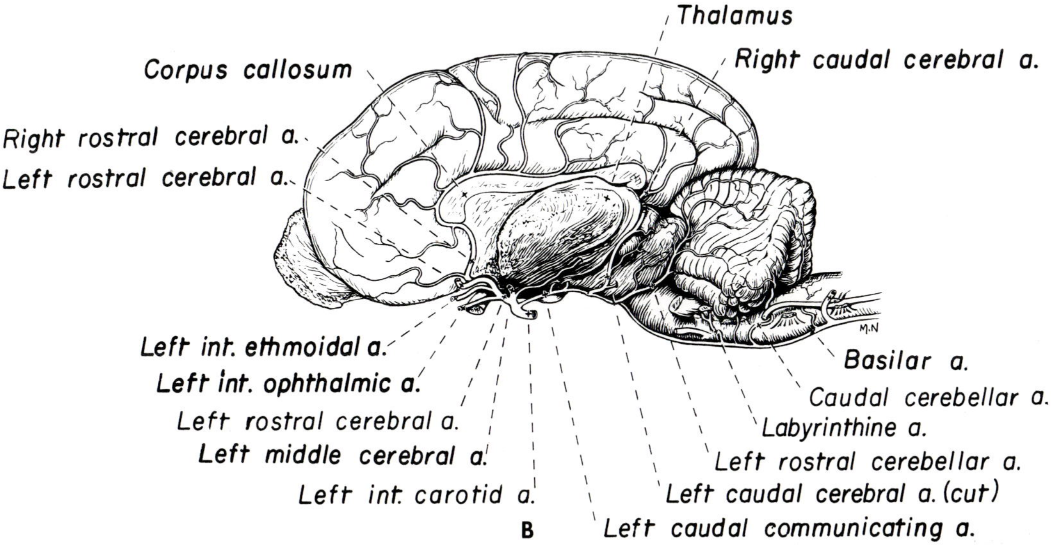

FIGURE 2–12 *A,* Distribution of the middle cerebral artery, lateral aspect. *B,* Arteries of the cerebellum and medial surface of cerebrum. (Adapted from Miller, M. E., Christensen, G. C., and Evans, H. E.: *Anatomy of the Dog.* W. B. Saunders Co., Philadelphia, 1964.)

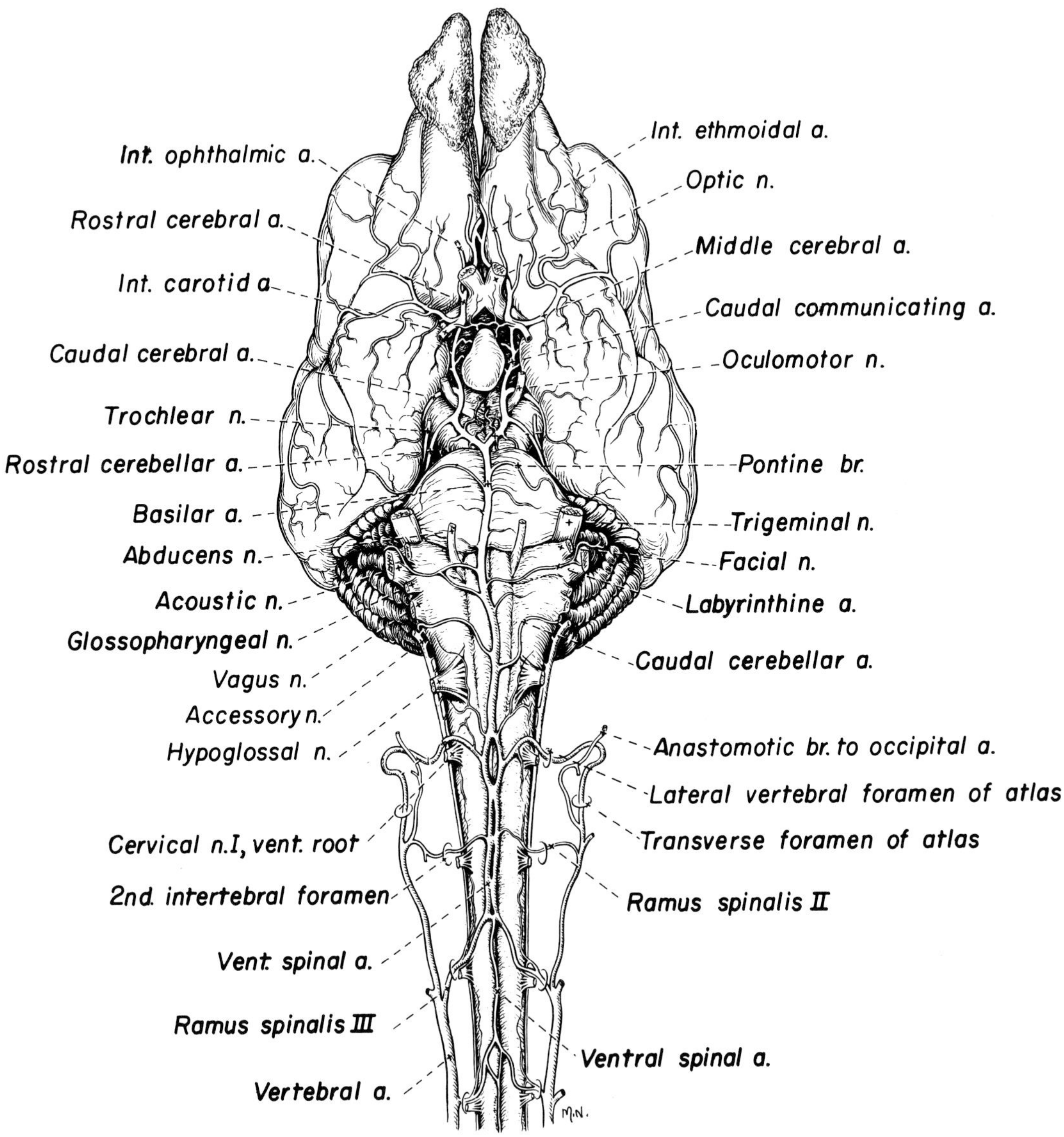

FIGURE 2–13 Arteries of the brain and cervical spinal cord, ventral aspect. (Adapted from Miller, M. E., Christensen, G. C., and Evans, H. E.: *Anatomy of the Dog*. W. B. Saunders Co., Philadelphia, 1964.)

brovascular accidents (CVA) similar to those described in man occur in dogs. Unlike man, the dog is not primarily a cortical animal, as far as gross motor activity goes, but a diencephalic-mesencephalic motor animal, and this reduces the likelihood that a dog will show the dramatic clinical signs seen in man. However, clinical cases presented with a flaccid hemiparesis of sudden onset strongly suggest an acute vascular accident. More work to determine the nature of these cases is needed. The presence of clinical syndromes suggests that the possibility of occlusion or hemorrhage of blood vessels to the basal nuclei, interbrain, and midbrain structures exists.

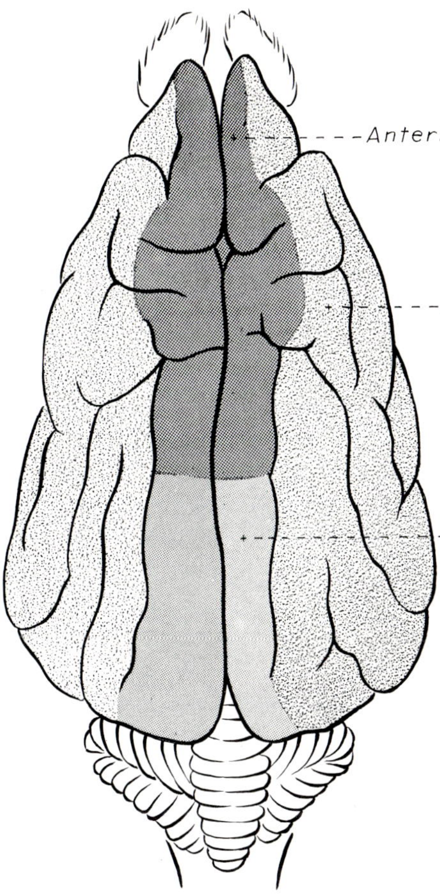

FIGURE 2–14 Areas supplied by the cerebral arteries, dorsal aspect. (From Miller, M. E., Christensen, G. C., and Evans, H. E.: *Anatomy of the Dog*. W. B. Saunders Co., Philadelphia, 1964.)

VENOUS CIRCULATION

The venous drainage from the brain is primarily in the vascular channels within the structure of the dura mater known as the dural sinuses. Figures 2–15 and 2–16 are diagrams of the major sinuses of the brain. During cerebral angiography (see Chapter 5), abnormalities may be seen on the venous side of the injection flow, or the so-called venogram.

PHYSIOLOGY OF CEREBRAL CIRCULATION

The vital requirements of brain tissue for oxygen becomes evident upon examination of experimental findings of many workers who have found severe permanent lesions in the cortex of the cat after circulation has been stopped for 3 to 6 minutes. In the dog, however, occlusion of some of the major vessels has not produced profound changes or severe damage.[45] Brain metabolism comprises approximately 14 per cent of the total oxygen consumption of the body. A large part of this oxygen utilization is for oxidation of glucose. In the brain, carbohydrate is the chief source of energy. It has been estimated that at any one time the brain contains only enough oxygen to last, at normal rates of metabolism, for about 10 seconds.[15] It is not surprising that the survival time of cerebral cortical tissue in the face of an oxygen deficit is quite short.

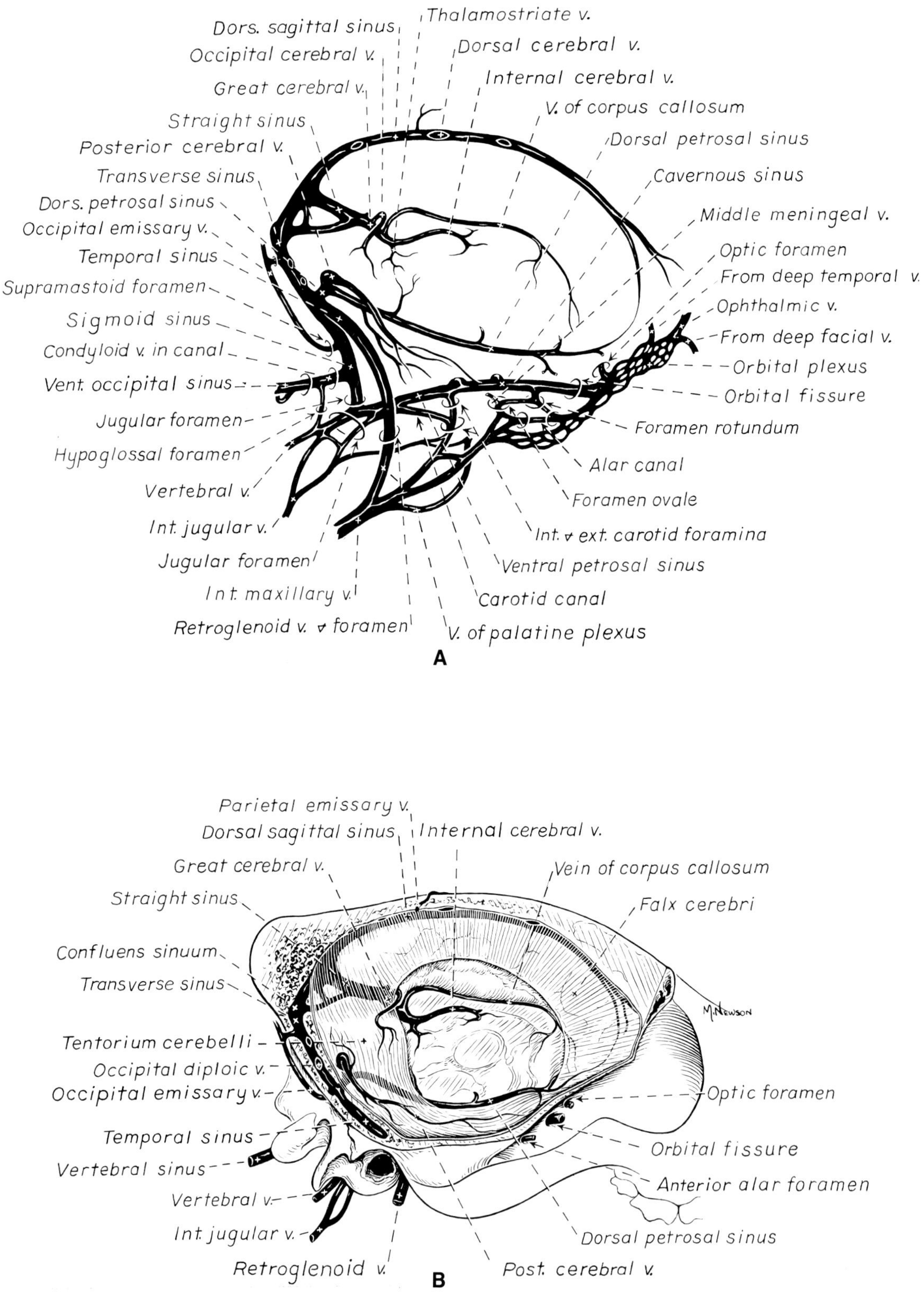

FIGURE 2–15 *A*, Diagram of the cranial venous sinuses, lateral aspect. *B*, Cranial venous sinuses, lateral aspect. (Right cerebral hemisphere removed.) (From Reinhard, K. R., Miller, M. E., and Evans, H. E.: The craniovertebral veins and sinuses of the dog. Amer. J. Anat. *111*, 67, 1962.)

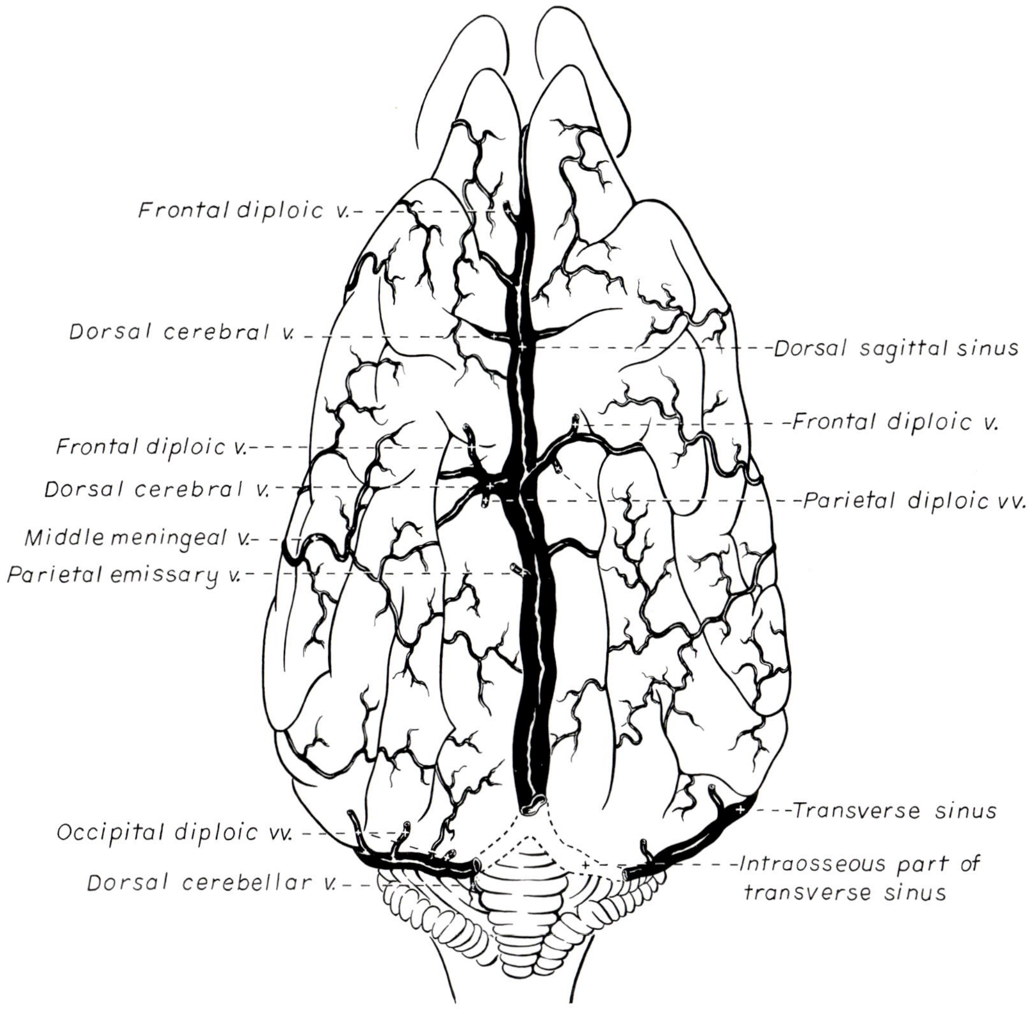

FIGURE 2–16 Veins of the brain, dorsal aspect. (From Miller, M. E., Christensen, G. C., and Evans, H. E.: *Anatomy of the Dog.* W. B. Saunders Co., Philadelphia, 1964.)

AUTOREGULATION OF CEREBRAL BLOOD FLOW

It is believed that the brain circulation is somewhat controlled by the sympathetic and parasympathetic autonomic systems. Actually, autoregulation occurs in the brain. Both the oxygen and the carbon dioxide concentrations are believed to operate, but the concentration of carbon dioxide is dominant. When the brain pCO_2 increases, the blood vessels dilate, allowing rapid blood flow to remove the excess carbon dioxide and, at the same time, other tissue metabolites, which tends to bring the pCO_2 back to normal value. Conversely, a decrease in pCO_2 causes vasoconstriction, which allows carbon dioxide levels to increase toward the normal value. This is an important type of regulation for the brain, since carbon dioxide influences the degree of activity of all neurons drastically.

One of the problems associated with surgery of the brain is brain edema. To combat brain edema, it is common to hyperventilate the animal with approximately 96 per cent oxygen (the remaining 4 per cent is the inhalation anesthetic and nitrogen). Hyperventilation increases the concentration of oxygen at the tissue site, causing vasoconstriction, which in turn reduces the blood flow to the tissue, resulting in some decrease in the size of the brain. Hyperventilation also "washes out" the carbon dioxide, reducing the pCO_2, which *also* causes vasoconstriction and further reduces brain size. This effect aids the surgeon in tissue manipulation and hemostasis, but it can produce other CNS problems if it is excessive.

THE CEREBRAL HEMISPHERES

The two cerebral hemispheres that make up the largest portion of the brain are separated by a deep longitudinal fissure. An extension of the dura mater called the *falx cerebri* projects into this longitudinal fissure. An interconnecting bridge of nerve fibers (white matter) called the *corpus callosum* connects the two hemispheres at the midline (Fig. 2–17). The surface of each hemisphere features a number of convolutions called *gyri*, which are separated from each other by valleys called *sulci*.

The surface of each hemisphere is divided into four lobes: the frontal, parietal, temporal, and occipital (Fig. 2–18). The boundaries of these lobes are not anatomically distinct. There is considerable variation in the sulcal and gyral patterns of individuals in the canine species, making it difficult to describe distinct borders for the

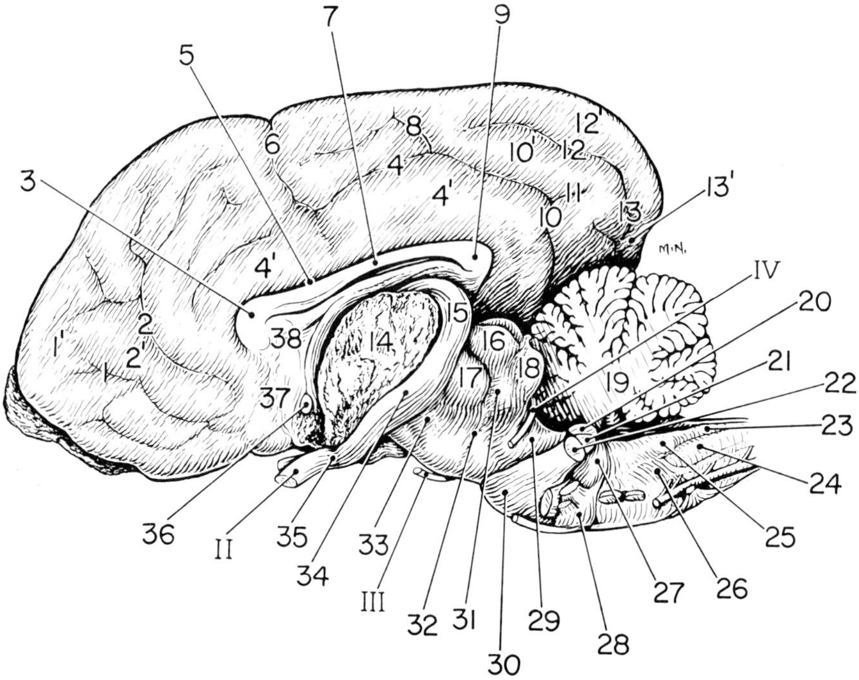

FIGURE 2–17 Medial surface of the right cerebral hemisphere and lateral surface of the brain stem. (From Miller, M. E., Christensen, G. C., and Evans, H. E.: *Anatomy of the Dog*. W. B. Saunders Co., Philadelphia, 1964.)

1. Ectogenual sulcus
1′. Ectogenual gyrus
2. Genual sulcus
2′. Genual gyrus
3. Genu of corpus callosum
4. Cingulate sulcus
4′. Cingulate gyrus
5. Callosal sulcus
6. Cruciate sulcus
7. Body of corpus callosum
8. Lesser cruciate sulcus
9. Splenium of corpus callosum
10. Splenial sulcus
10′. Splenial gyrus
11. Posterior horizontal ramus of splenial sulcus
12. Suprasplenial sulcus
12′. Suprasplenial sulcus
13. Postsplenial sulcus
13′. Postsplenial gyrus
14. Cut surface between cerebrum and brain stem
15. Lateral geniculate body
16. Superior colliculus
17. Medial geniculate body
18. Inferior colliculus
19. Arbor vitae cerebelli
20. Superior cerebellar peduncle
21. Inferior cerebellar peduncle
22. Middle cerebellar peduncle
23. Fasciculus cuneatus
24. Spinal tract of trigeminal nerve
25. Accessory cuneate nucleus
26. External arcuate fibers
27. Cochlear nuclei
28. Trapezoid body
29. Lateral lemniscus
30. Transverse fibers of pons
31. Brachium of inferior colliculus
32. Transverse peduncular tract
33. Crus cerebri
34. Left optic tract
35. Optic chiasm
36. Anterior commissure
37. Paraterminal gyrus
38. Septum pellucidum
II. Optic nerve
III. Oculomotor nerve
IV. Trochlear nerve

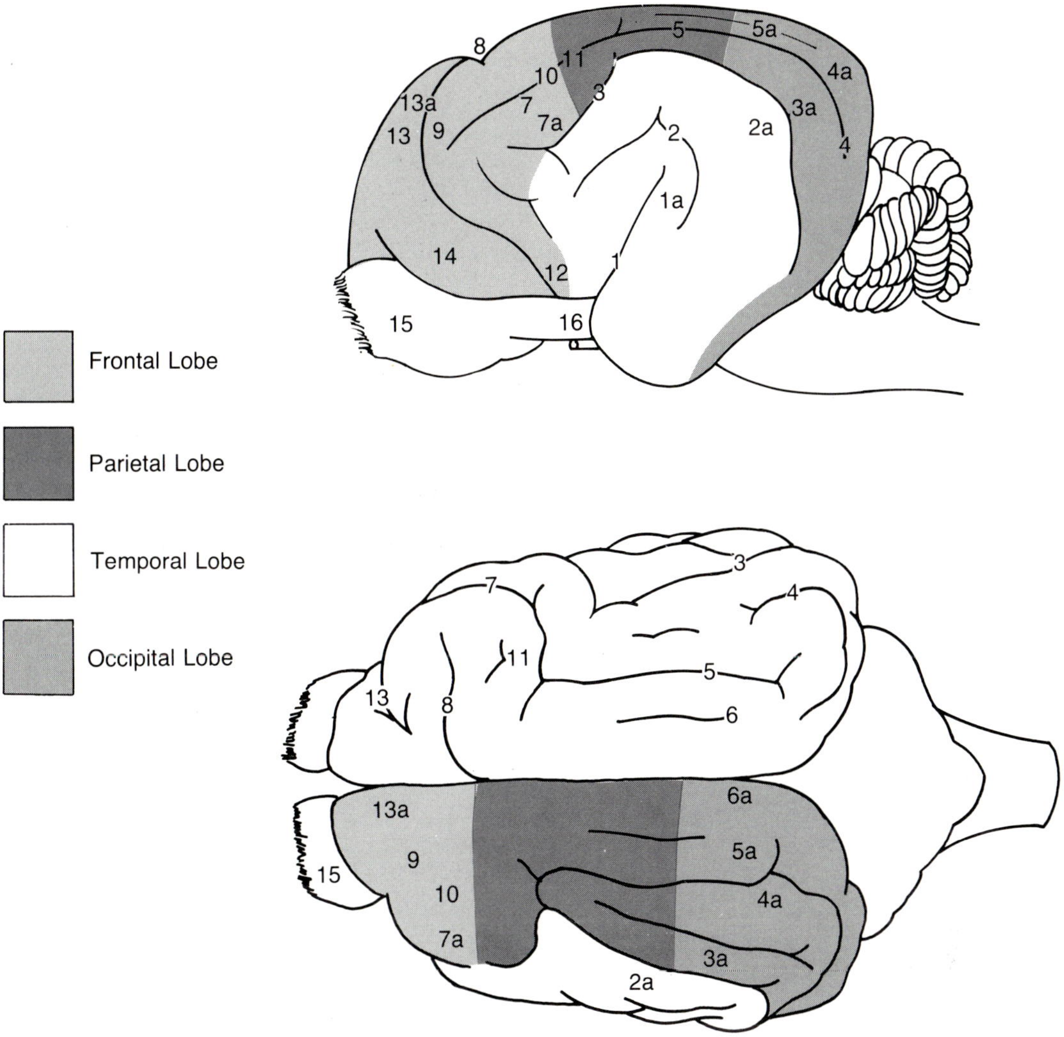

FIGURE 2–18 The lobes of the dog's brain. (1) Sylvian sulcus; (1a) sylvian gyrus; (2) ectosylvian sulcus; (2a) ectosylvian gyrus; (3) suprasylvian sulcus; (3a) suprasylvian gyrus; (4) ectolateral sulcus; (4a) ectolateral gyrus; (5) lateral sulcus; (5a) lateral gyrus; (6) entolateral sulcus; (6a) entolateral gyrus (marginal gyrus—Kreiner); (7) coronal sulcus; (7a) coronal gyrus; (8) cruciate sulcus; (9) anterior sigmoid gyrus; (10) posterior sigmoid gyrus; (11) postcruciate sulcus (central sulcus—Kreiner); (12) presylvian sulcus; (13) prorean sulcus; (13a) prorean gyrus; (14) prorean gyrus (orbital gyrus—Kreiner).[36] (15) olfactory bulb; (16) piriform area.

lobes. However, there are a few particularly distinct sulci which form a basic pattern. These sulci serve as a reference point for surgical and physiological procedures and research. The major reference sulci are shown in Figure 2–18.

The outer layers of the cerebrum comprise what is known as the cerebral cortex. The cerebral cortex is not as important in the dog as it is in higher animals, such as the primates. Experimental removal of the cortex in the dog does not prevent the animal from carrying out many complex motor functions. For example, the animal is able to run, walk, maintain equilibrium, and right itself.[40] It cannot seek out and eat food, although it will eat food placed in its mouth. The intellectual functions are lost. The animal cannot recognize its owner, develop conditioned reflexes, or perform skilled movements.

The functional areas of the cerebral cortex have been determined by experimental means. Electrical stimulation of specific areas to observe the responses and surgical removal of specific areas to observe the resultant deficits are the methods used. Certain areas have been found to be responsible for motor control of skeletal muscle and other areas to control sensory perception. The cortex anterior, around the base, and some areas ventroposterior to the cruciate sulcus house the motor cortex (Fig. 2–19). Removal of this cortical area results in the loss of specific responses, such as placing and hopping reactions. It should be noted that there is no flaccid or spastic paralysis, such as that seen in primates. Paresis is present in the dog following surgical removal of this area for a period of time varying from 3 days to 3 weeks, after which complete recovery from the paresis occurs.[61]

Posterior to the cruciate sulcus (parietal lobe) is the sensory cortex (somesthetic area), which is responsible for the perception of general somatic sensibilities. Unfortunately, we are not able to communicate with animals who have lesions of the parietal lobe to determine if there is truly a situation comparable to that in man, i.e., paresthesia, numbness, formication, and electric shock-like and "pins-and-needles" sensations on the side of the body opposite to that of the lesion.

The temporal lobes are presumed to serve memory and auditory function. Experimental removal of the cortex from these areas does not produce complete deafness.

The occipital lobe houses the visual reception and visual interpretation areas. Re-

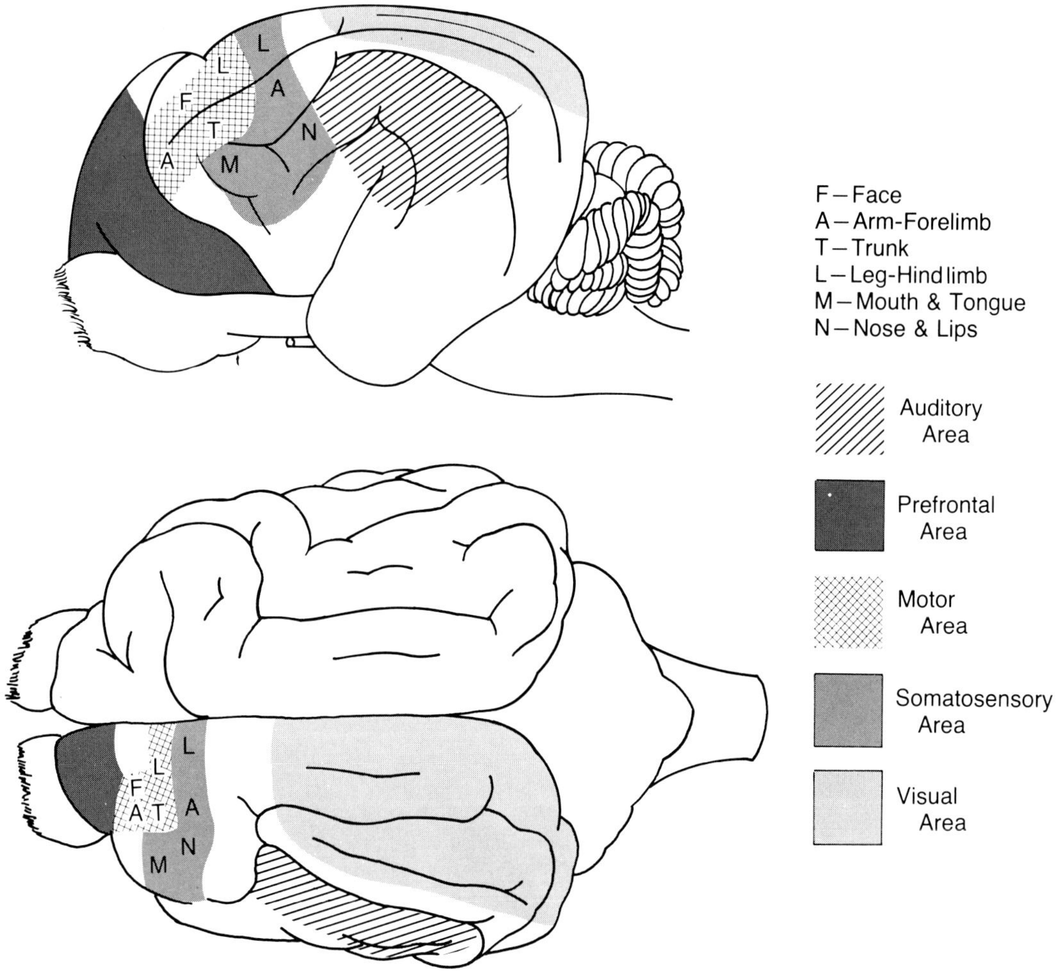

FIGURE 2–19 Motor and sensory areas of the cerebral cortex of the dog.

moval of all of the occipital cortex results in total blindness.

The frontal area serves as the psychic level of the dog and is therefore a very important area. Destructive lesions of this area cause marked changes in personality. The animal may fail to recognize its owner, is unable to perform previously learned tasks (conditioned reflexes), loses some of its ability for contact and pressure appraisal, and frequently becomes impulsive and ill-tempered.

THE SUBCORTICAL STRUCTURES

Deep to the cerebral cortex are a number of nuclei that, in conjunction with other parts of the brain, mediate complex motor activity and play an important role in integrating and coordinating movements. These nuclei perform a great number of the sensory and motor functions in the dog. Most, if not all, of the unconscious movements of the animal are initiated in these nuclei. Experimental destruction of these structures and naturally occurring lesions caused by vascular accidents and tumor growth produce a profound loss of motor control. In the experiments by Few,[22] only very large lesions caused motor loss.

THE BASAL NUCLEI

The basal nuclei are subcortical masses of neurons (Fig. 2–20) that serve as motor nuclei. They make nervous connections with the motor cortex and in themselves serve as major motor nuclei for what is known as the extrapyramidal system. It is believed that in lower animals, such as birds, which have a very thin cerebral cor-

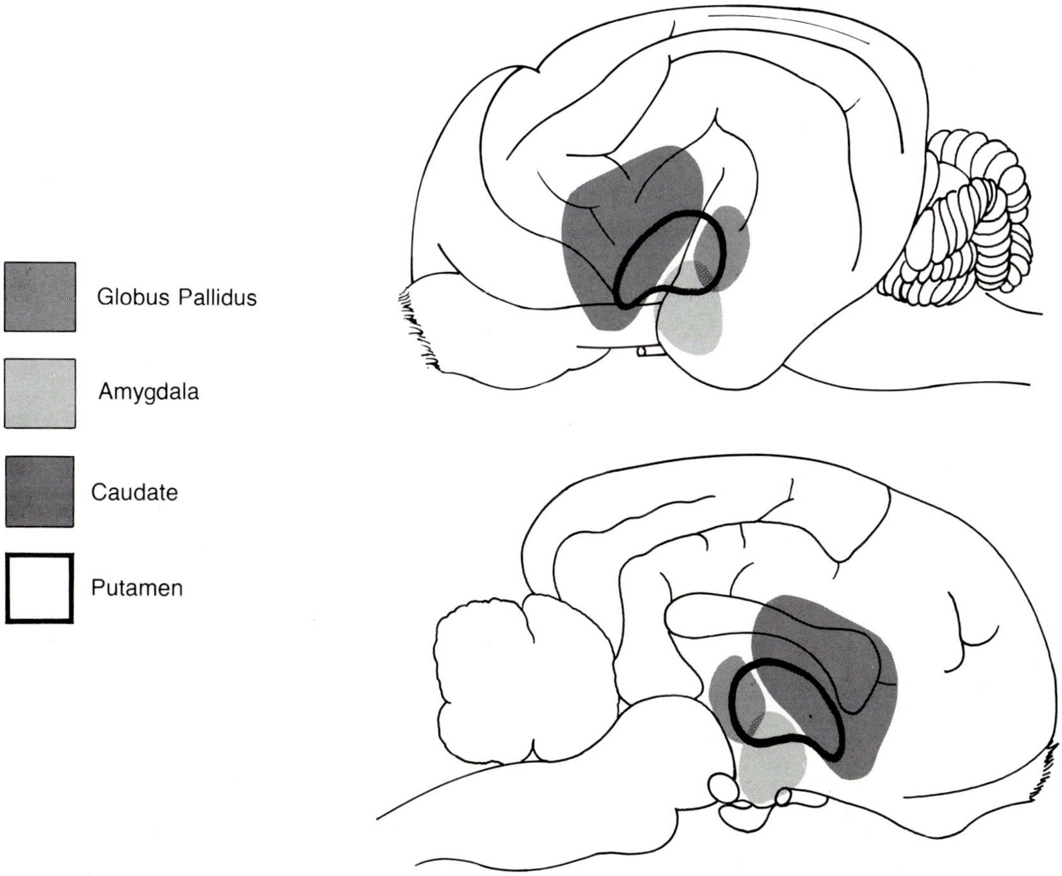

FIGURE 2–20 The basal nuclei of the dog. (After Kreiner, J.: Homologues of the fissural and gyral pattern of the hemispheres of the dog and monkey. Acta Anat., *70*, 137, 1968.)

tex, well-coordinated behavior and movements are initiated by these structures. The functional organization of the basal nuclei is poorly understood in the dog. The basal nuclei are difficult to reach without destroying other parts of the nervous system. Electrical stimulation has not revealed concise information about their functions. It is the opinion of the author that the basal nuclei serve as major motor nuclei for the dog in the initiation of general muscular activity and some specific movements. This opinion is based upon the fact that removal of the motor cortex of the dog does not produce a loss of the gross musculature activity. Wright[61] removed the motor cortex of the dog after first establishing conditioned reflexes for fine graded movements of the fore limbs. A loss of the fine graded movements resulted, but gross movement of the fore limbs was not affected. In fact, the animals appeared normal in every respect except for the trained movements.

Motor disorders associated with diseases in the basal nuclei of man, such as Parkinsonism, athetosis, true chorea (not the rhythmic muscular spasms seen in the dog that are erroneously called chorea), and hemiballismus are not recognized as clinical syndromes in the dog. Apparently the functional activity of these structures is not comparable to that in man. Lesions of the basal nuclei induced experimentally by Few[22] produced paresis, abnormal turning movements, and loss of motor control to the limbs and trunk, suggesting that the

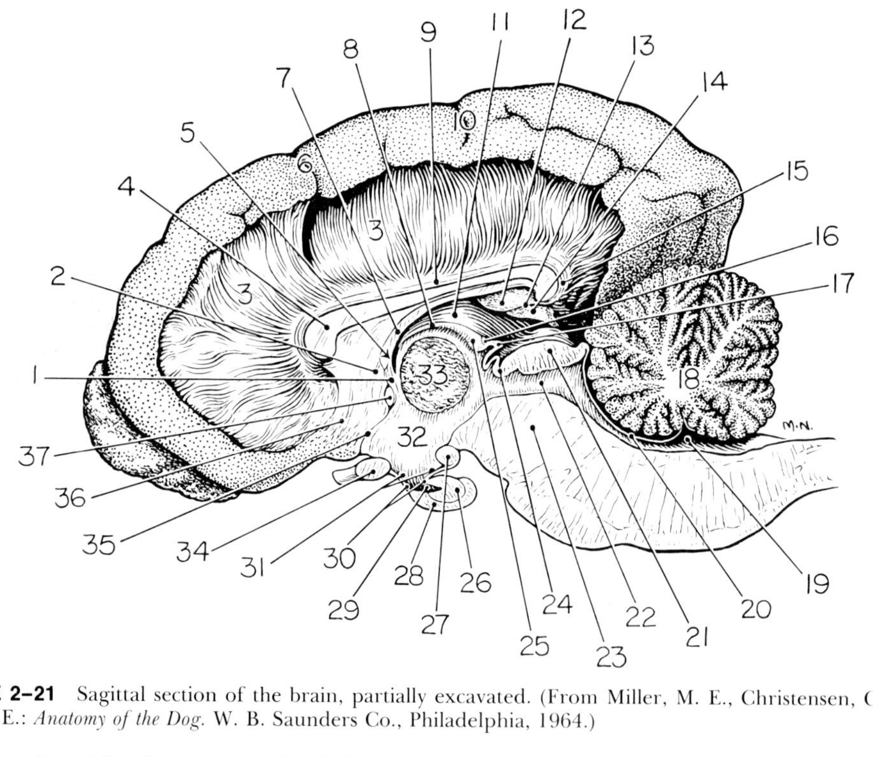

FIGURE 2–21 Sagittal section of the brain, partially excavated. (From Miller, M. E., Christensen, G. C., and Evans, H. E.: *Anatomy of the Dog*. W. B. Saunders Co., Philadelphia, 1964.)

1. Postcommissural fornix
2. Precommissural fornix
3. Fibers of corpus callosum
4. Genu of corpus callosum
5. Interventricular foramen
6. Cruciate sulcus
7. Fornix
8. Stria medullaris thalami
9. Indusium griseum
10. Lesser cruciate sulcus
11. Dorsal aspect of thalamus
12. Tubercle of dentate gyrus
13. Subsplenial flexure of dentate gyrus
14. Callosal gyrus
15. Gyrus fasciolaris
16. Habenular commissure
17. Pineal body or epiphysis
18. Cerebellum
19. Fourth ventricle
20. Anterior medullary velum
21. Tectum of mesencephalon
22. Cerebral aqueduct
23. Cerebral peduncle
24. Posterior commissure
25. Habenular nucleus
26. Neurohypophysis
27. Mammillary body
28. Pars glandularis
29. Infundibular recess of third ventricle
30. Infundibular stalk of hypophysis
31. Tuber cinereum
32. Third ventricle
33. Interthalamic adhesion (intermediate mass)
34. Optic chiasm
35. Lamina terminalis
36. Paraterminal gyrus
37. Anterior commissure

basal nuclei are primary motor centers for skeletal muscular activity.

It is suspected by the author that the "stroke-like" syndrome seen in dogs, which is similar to that seen in man, may very well be the result of a vascular accident involving the blood supply to the basal nuclei or the internal capsule. However, morphological proof for this assumption is lacking.

THE THALAMUS

Each cerebral hemisphere surrounds a relatively large ovoid mass of nuclei, called the thalamus, that is located on either side of the third ventricle. The two thalami are connected together at the midline by the interthalamic adhesion (massa intermedia) (Fig. 2–21).

The thalamus serves both as a relay center for all sensory input to the cerebral cortex and as a recognition center for some specific sensations. In both man and dog, when there is a loss of the sensory cortex, the tactile, thermal, and pain sensibilities remain. It is believed that pain impulses entering only the thalamus will cause conscious perception of pain, and that only the cortical areas are involved in localizing the pain. Damage to the thalamus may be associated with a peculiar overreaction to minimal stimulation of pain receptors known in man as the *thalamic syndrome.* The author has observed two dogs with a similar syndrome. The dogs were extremely sensitive to touching and patting and would howl and cringe as if being touched were a painful stimulus. Unfortunately, proof of a thalamic lesion was not obtainable by necropsy. In man, this condition is usually due to a blockage of the thalamogeniculate branch of the posterior cerebral artery, with subsequent damage to the posterior thalamic nuclei. In man, minor peripheral stimuli lead to prolonged, severe, and very unpleasant pain.[15, 25]

THE HYPOTHALAMUS

The hypothalamus is a collection of nuclei located ventral to the thalamus and forming the floor and part of the lateral

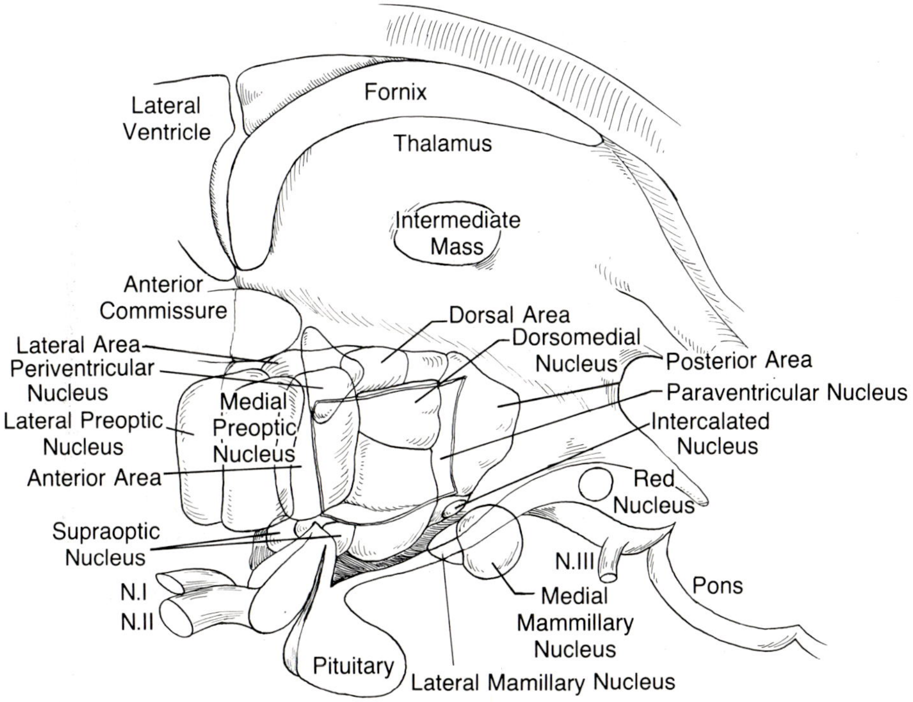

FIGURE 2–22 The hypothalamus. (Modified from an original by Netter in Ciba Clinical Symposia, copyright 1956, Ciba Pharmaceutical Co.)

walls of the third ventricle. It includes the *supraoptic nuclei mammillary bodies, tuber cinereum,* and the *infundibulum,* which is a hollow process extending to the posterior lobe of the hypophysis (Fig. 2–22). Afferent connections are made with most of the subcortical structures, and cortical impulses arrive indirectly at the hypothalamus. Efferent tracts send impulses to the pituitary, thalamus, tegmentum, lower brain levels, and the limbic system.

The functions of the hypothalamus are many and diversified. A summary of the hypothalamic-regulating mechanisms is seen in Table 2–2. Lesions of the hypothalamus may produce a variety of signs, including diabetes insipidus, changes in sexual behavior, loss of temperature control, changes in the sleep and wakefulness patterns, polyuria, polydipsia, and hyperphagia and obesity (or the opposite—anorexia and loss of weight). Personality changes with fear and rage have been produced by experimental destruction of the pathways from the cerebral cortex.

THE MIDBRAIN

The midbrain is the short portion of the brain between the pons and the diencephalon. The dorsal portion (the tectum) contains the four corpora quadrigemina (the anterior and posterior colliculi). The anterior colliculi are associated with the optic system and the posterior colliculi are associated with the auditory system. The ventral portions of the midbrain contain the two cerebral peduncles that connect the ce-

TABLE 2–2 SUMMARY OF HYPOTHALAMIC REGULATORY MECHANISMS*

Function	Afferents From	Integrating Centers
Temperature regulation	Cutaneous cold receptors; temperature-sensitive cells in hypothalamus	Anterior hypothalamus, response to heat; posterior hypothalamus, response to cold
Neuroendocrine control of:		
Catecholamines	Emotional stimuli, probably via limbic system	Dorsomedial and posterior hypothalamus
Vasopressin	Osmoreceptors, "volume receptors," others	Supraoptic nuclei
Oxytocin	Touch receptors in breast, uterus, others (?)	Paraventricular nuclei
Thyroid-stimulating hormone (TSH)	Temperature receptors, perhaps others (?)	Anterior median eminence and anterior hypothalamus
Adrenocorticotropic hormone (ACTH)	Limbic system (emotional stimuli); ascending reticular system ("systemic" stimuli); hypothalamic or anterior pituitary cells sensitive to circulating blood corticoid level; others (?)	Middle portion of median eminence
Follicle-stimulating hormone (FSH) and luteinizing hormone (LH)	Hypothalamic cells sensitive to estrogens; eyes, touch receptors in skin and genitalia of reflex ovulating species	Posterior median eminence, other areas
Luteotropic hormone (LTH)	Unknown receptors	Posterior median eminence (hypothalamus inhibits secretion)
Growth hormone	Unknown receptors	Anterior median eminence
"Appetitive" behavior:		
Thirst	Osmoreceptors	Lateral superior hypothalamus
Hunger	"Glucostat" cells sensitive to rate of glucose utilization	Ventromedial satiety center, lateral hunger center, also limbic components
Sexual behavior	Cells sensitive to circulating estrogen and androgen, others	Anterior ventral hypothalamus, plus, in the male, pyriform cortex
Defensive reactions:		
Fear, rage	Sense organs and neocortex, paths unknown	Diffuse, in limbic system and hypothalamus

*From Ganong, W. F.: *Review of Medical Physiology,* 2nd ed. Lange Medical Publications, Los Altos, 1965, p. 168.

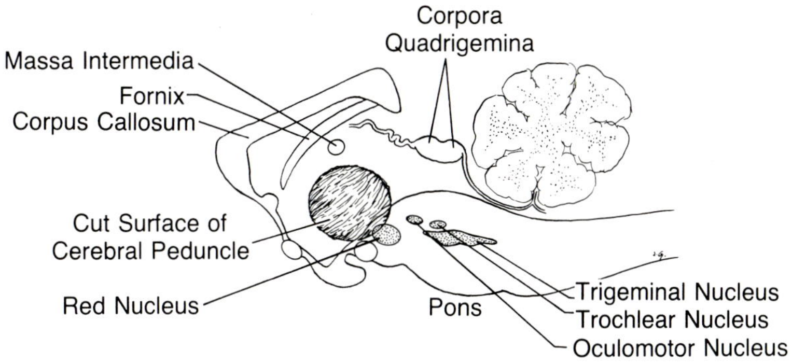

FIGURE 2–23 Midbrain structures.

rebral hemisphere with the brain stem. The tegmentum, the dorsal part of the cerebral peduncles, contains the fiber tracts for sensory information bound for the thalamus and motor tracts bound for the spinal cord. The tegmentum also contains the *red nucleus* from which arise the rubrospinal tract and some reticulospinal fibers, the proposed major motor tracts for the dog.[16] In addition, the nuclei of the *trochlear, oculomotor,* and *mesencephalic* root of the *trigeminal nerves* are located in the midbrain (Fig. 2–23).

The clinical findings associated with lesions of the midbrain have not been described in detail in the dog. Since the structures contained in the midbrain apparently have the same functions in both man and dog, it is not unreasonable to expect signs similar to those in man in the dog. Experimental lesions in the cat produce signs similar to those elicited by naturally-occurring disease of the same areas in man. Destruction of the third and fourth cranial nerves gives rise to the classical signs of paralysis of these nerves. For a more complete discussion, see Chapter 4.

THE PONS

Just below the midbrain lies the pons (Fig. 2–24), composed of fiber tracts and a number of nuclei. Fibers run transversely across the pons and through the middle cerebellar peduncle into the cerebellum; as the external fibers cross over, they have the bridge-like appearance that give the pons its name. Nuclei of the fifth, sixth, seventh, and eighth cranial nerves are located in the upper part of the pons. In addition, an important nucleus called the *pneumotaxic center,* which functions in the control of respiration, is present in the pons. (See Chapters 3 and 4 for discussion of the functions of the cranial nerves.)

Lesions in the area of the pons do occur in dogs. They produce signs associated with

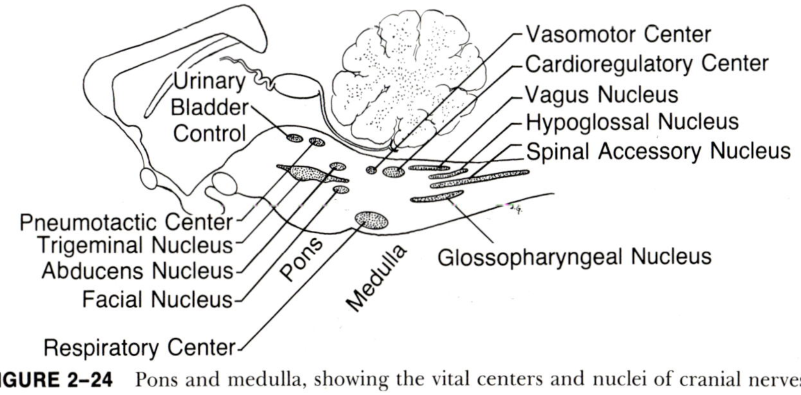

FIGURE 2–24 Pons and medulla, showing the vital centers and nuclei of cranial nerves.

dysfunction of the cranial nerves whose nuclei are located in the pons. The author has seen a syndrome in dogs similar to that reported in man involving the sensory portion of the trigeminal nerve. The syndrome is called *trigeminal neuralgia* or *tic douloureux* In two cases the animal was exquisitely sensitive to touch on one side of the face. The application of a cold spoon to that side resulted in what appeared to be a sudden attack of excruciating pain of short duration.

THE MEDULLA OBLONGATA

The medulla oblongata or bulb is the most posterior part of the brain that attaches to and is continuous with the spinal cord. It is separated from the pons anteriorly by a transverse groove (Fig. 2–24). The bulb is composed of projection tracts and the nuclei of the eighth, ninth,* tenth, eleventh,† and twelfth cranial nerves (see Chapters 3 and 4). In addition, the medulla contains the nuclei for many autonomic reflex centers. Some of these perform functions so necessary for life that they are called *vital centers.* They are the cardiac, vasomotor, and respiratory centers (inspiratory, expiratory, and apneustic). Because the medulla contains these centers, it is the most vital part of the entire brain—so vital that injury or disease of the bulb often proves fatal. In addition, the bulb functions in many reflexes such as vomiting, coughing, sneezing, hiccoughing, and swallowing.

On each side of the dorsal posterior part of the medulla are two prominent nuclei, the *nucleus gracilis* and the *nucleus cuneatus,* concerned with the synaptic transmission of touch, pressure, and kinesthetic sensations bound for the thalamus, cerebellum, and cerebral cortex. All projection tracts between the spinal cord and the brain necessarily pass through the bulb. Therefore, it is involved in a great many sensory and motor mechanisms.

*The glossopharyngeal nerve does not have a definitive central nucleus, except the inferior salivatory, but it has instead a string of cells in the reticular formation of the bulb near the olivary and ambiguus nuclei.[21]

†The spinal accessory nerve nucleus is primarily located in the ventral horn of the upper cervical spinal cord.[21]

THE CEREBELLUM

The cerebellum, the second largest part of the brain, is located posterior to the cerebrum. A transverse fissure separates the cerebellum from the cerebrum (see Figs. 2–17 and 2–21). Like the cerebrum, the cerebellar surface is grooved with numerous sulci, but its convolutions are more slender and less prominent than those of the cerebrum.

Projection tracts connect the cerebellum with other parts of the brain and spinal cord. These enter or leave the cerebellum by way of its three pairs of peduncles as follows: (1) *Posterior cerebellar peduncles* (restiform bodies)—composed of tracts into the cerebellum from the medulla and cord (spinocerebellar, vestibulocerebellar and reticulocerebellar, and olivocerebellar). Out-

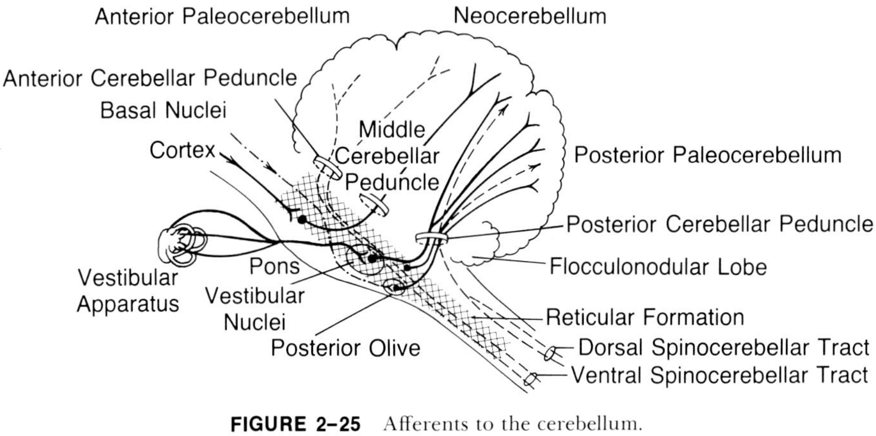

FIGURE 2–25 Afferents to the cerebellum.

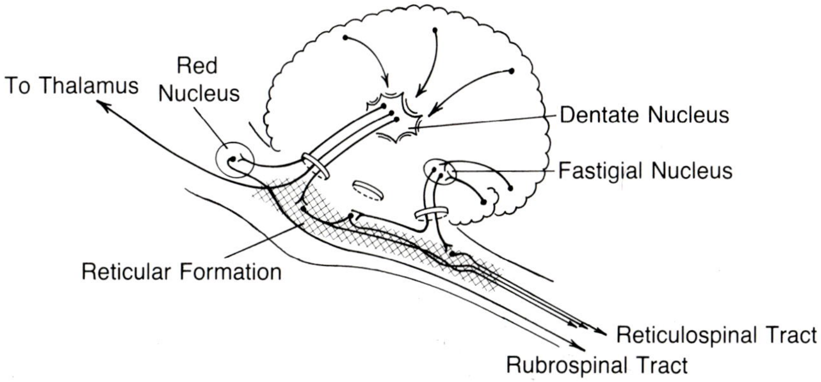

FIGURE 2–26 Efferents from the cerebellum.

flow tracts send fibers to the reticular formation and the vestibular nuclei. (2) *Middle cerebellar peduncles* (brachia pontis)—composed of the tracts into the cerebellum from the pons (pontocerebellar tracts). (3) *Anterior cerebellar peduncles* (brachium conjunctivum)—composed of tracts from the cerebellar dentate nuclei to the red nucleus, cerebral cortex, and thalamus. By means of these tracts, the cerebellar impulses influence the basal nuclei and the motor cortex of the cerebrum. Impulses travel also in the reverse direction from the spinocerebellar tracts.

Figures 2–25 and 2–26 show the input and output of the cerebellum.

FUNCTIONS OF THE CEREBELLUM

The cerebellum performs three general functions, all of which are related to the control of skeletal muscle activity: (1) it acts with the cerebral cortex and the basal nuclei to produce accurately controlled coordinated movements of groups of muscles; (2) it controls skeletal muscle to provide assistance in maintaining equilibrium, with the assistance of impulses from the vestibular apparatus; and (3) it functions to control posture.

All of the activities of the cerebellum are carried on below the level of consciousness, making body and limb movements smooth instead of jerky, steady instead of trembling, and efficient and coordinated instead of ineffective, awkward, and uncoordinated. If there is one key word to describe the function of the cerebellum, it is *coordination.* The cerebellum accomplishes this by comparing the *intent* (of muscle activity) originating in the cerebral cortex and basal nuclei with the *performance* and automatically making the proper adjustments by facilitation or inhibition.

Lesions of the cerebellum produce signs of dysmetria and ataxia. Hypermetria, a form of dysmetria, is predominant. It is characterized by such overreaction as lifting the limbs too high and putting them down with excessive force when walking. Another example would be moving the head too far when trying to eat or drink, so that the animal's head hits the edge of the dish or is jammed into the food or water.

THE VESTIBULAR SYSTEM

Vestibular sensations are used primarily for the control of muscles involved in maintaining equilibrium, positioning the head, and regulating eye muscle movement. Such impulses, however, reach the sensory cortex and inform the animal of its relationship to gravity and the position of its body during motion.

The vestibular system (Fig. 2–27) consists of a bilateral complex of receptors, nuclei, and neuronal pathways. There are two kinds of receptors in the vestibular labyrinth: *cristae* in the semicircular canals and *maculae* in the utriculi and sacculi. Each crista contains hair cells embedded in a gelatinous substance (cupula). The flow of fluid in the semicircular canals (endolymph) past the crista when the head is moved (because the fluid has inertia) stimu-

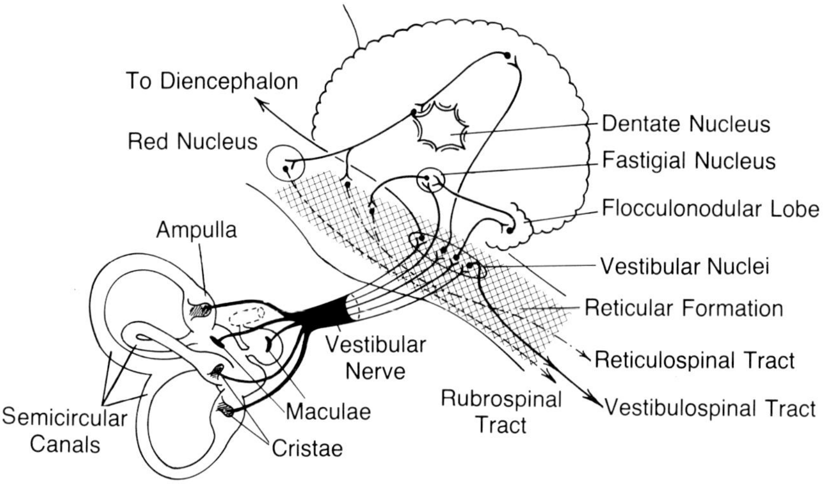

FIGURE 2–27 Neuronal connections of the vestibular system in the central nervous system.

lates the hair cells, which send impulses by way of the vestibular nuclei. The maculae in utriculi and sacculi are so arranged that they are roughly at right angles to each other. Each macula contains hair cells embedded in a thin layer of gelatinous material that has *otoconia,* small grains of calcium carbonate sometimes called "ear dust," over its free surface. Gravitational pull on the otoconia causes them to press continually on the macular hair cells in the utriculus, and this constantly apprises the central nervous system of the position of the head with respect to gravity (static equilibrium). The function of the sacculus is controversial. When the body of an animal is suddenly accelerated or decelerated forward or backward, the otoconia, which have greater inertia than the surrounding fluids, press on the hair cells and inform the central nervous system of the linear motion. Thus the otoconia operate to maintain equilibrium.

A very important function of the semicircular canals is the detection of the *onset* of so-called angular acceleration. When the head *begins* to rotate in any direction, the hair cells in the ampulla transmit signals to the vestibular nuclei. In addition, signals are sent when rotation of the head stops. Furthermore, the semicircular canals respond to rotation of the head in any plane—coronal, horizontal, or vertical—because fluid movement occurs in at least one of the semicircular canals. One can explain the function of the semicircular canals during motion by the following: If a hound dog is running forward and then suddenly begins to turn to one side, he will become off-balance and will fall in a second or so unless appropriate corrections are made *ahead of time.* (The utricle *cannot* detect that he is off-balance until *after* it has occurred.) The semicircular canals, however, will have already detected the beginning of the turn because the head turns before the body. Nerve impulses will inform the central nervous system of the fact that the dog *will* be off-balance unless corrective action is taken. In other words, the semicircular canal mechanisms *predict* imminent loss of balance before it occurs, and thereby cause equilibrium centers to make appropriate adjustments in time to prevent the loss of balance.

The vestibular nerve, which carries the messages from the previously mentioned receptors, enters the brain stem (see Fig. 2–27) to terminate either in one of the four vestibular nuclei (anterior, posterior, lateral, or medial) or in the cerebellum.

The cells of the vestibular nuclei send impulses to the cerebellum, the reticular formation, and the lower motor neurons via the vestibulospinal tract. In addition, they convey messages to the nuclei of the eye muscles via the medial longitudinal bundle. The vestibulospinal tract conveys messages to the muscles of the trunk and exerts a powerful influence upon the muscles of the limbs to maintain balance.

Nystagmus always occurs automatically

when the semicircular canals are stimulated (normal physiological nystagmus). When the head rotates, the eyes must rotate in the opposite direction if they are to remain "fixed" on any object to maintain a clear image. After they have rotated far to one side, they jump suddenly in the direction of rotation of the head to "fix" on a new object and then rotate slowly backward. This sudden jumping and slow backward motion is known as nystagmus. The jumping motion is called the *fast component* and the slow movement the *slow component*. In diseases of the vestibular system, including the vestibular nuclei, it is common to see nystagmus independent of head movements, as if the control mechanism had become unlocked, allowing the eye movements to become free-running and out of control.

It should be realized that the cerebellum works in close relationship with the vestibular apparatus in regulating skeletal muscle activity to maintain balance, equilibrium, and coordination. If there is one word that describes the general function of the vestibular system, it is *equilibrium*.

When performing a neurological examination, one purposely activates the vestibular system to determine if it is functioning normally. An understanding of the mechanisms previously described aids greatly in interpretation of one's findings.

RIGHTING MECHANISM OF THE DOG

There are five mechanisms by which a dog maintains its body in the normal position with respect to gravity. These reactions are complex and are dependent upon each other in some instances. The five reflex mechanisms are: (1) vestibular (labyrinthine) righting reflexes acting upon the neck muscles; (2) neck righting reflexes that act upon the body; (3) body righting reflexes that act upon the head; (4) body righting reflexes that act upon the body itself; and (5) optical (visual) righting reflexes. The vestibular mechanisms have already been discussed and are responsible for the position of the head with respect to gravity and linear or angular motion. Head position and the labyrinthine reflexes act upon the neck muscles to turn the head toward its natural position in the dimensions of space. Following this, the proprioceptive reflexes of the neck muscles bring the body into its normal relationship to the head.

In addition to the previously discussed mechanisms, there are touch and pressure receptors (contact pressure appraisal), which inform the animal of its position relative to some form of rigid support. The animal can be standing or in any recumbent position and be apprised of its relationship to support so that it may right itself. Optical (visual) righting reflexes are initiated by visual clues. Such visual impressions play an important role in the orientation of the head of the dog.

The veterinary neurologist utilizes three basic mechanisms in the differential diagnosis of vestibular, cerebellar, and cerebral disease. By eliminating either visual or contact pressure appraisal (or both), allowing one of the mechanisms to become dominant in maintaining equilibrium, a differential diagnosis may be made. For example, if a normal animal is held by the pelvis with its head down, it will automati-

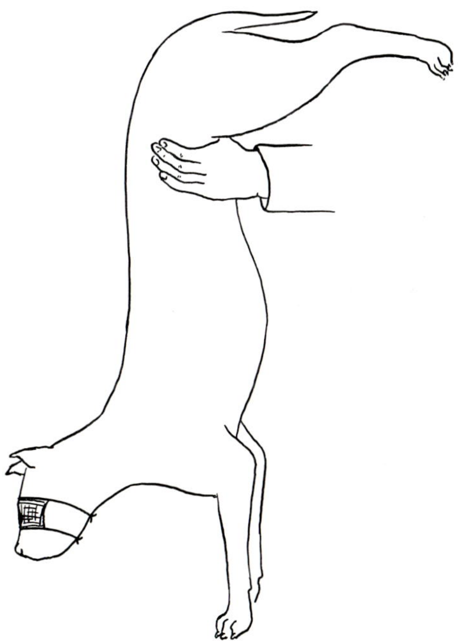

FIGURE 2–28 Position sense of a dog using the vestibular mechanisms only. The visual and contact appraisal receptors are non-functional since the animal is blindfolded and suspended in the air. A dog with normally functioning vestibular mechanisms will assume the position shown in the diagram. If the vestibular mechanism is diseased, the animal will turn to one side or writhe about.

cally tend to assume a 45-degree angle toward the horizontal (Fig. 2–28) without turning to either side. This is accomplished through both vestibular and visual mechanisms (the contact pressure appraisal has been eliminated). If the animal is blindfolded and the visual clues eliminated, however, the animal still assumes the same position using the vestibular mechanisms only. If there is disease of the vestibular mechanism, the animal will immediately be "lost" in space, since the other two mechanisms are not functioning. The presence of these signs suggests a diagnosis of vestibular disease. Other methods of testing these systems are: (1) The dog is dropped in an upside-down position from a height sufficient to allow vestibular righting reactions to occur, allowing the animal to land on its feet. (The author does not consider this test reliable or esthetically proper.) (2) The animal is placed forcibly upon its sides to see if it will right itself. Unless the animal is blindfolded, this test is of little value, since visual righting mechanisms play a very important role in the dog. (3) Ice water is syringed into the ear canal (the caloric test). A normal reaction is nystagmus within 3 to 4 minutes.

THE RETICULAR FORMATION

The reticular formation is a system of interlacing fibers and nerve cells that form the central core of the brain stem, extending between and functionally connecting the thalamus and the spinal cord (Fig. 2–29).

The reticular formation and its multiple connections with nuclei in the brain stem, spinothalamic, auditory and visual tracts, thalamus, and hypothalamus jointly constitute what is known as the *reticular activating system* (RAS). This system provides the background of neuronal activity essential to consciousness, integrated movements, and some visceral activity. Consciousness and the state of wakefulness are maintained by a continual flow of impulses from the thalamic portion of the reticular formation to the cerebral cortex. Feedback from the cerebral cortex via the thalamus maintains the reticular activating system in an excited state. Other feedback loops from the spinal cord contribute to the input of the RAS. The reticular activating system may be considered essential for arousal from sleep, for wakefulness, for alerting or focusing of attention, and for perceptual association; its impaired function may be associated with comatose states and anesthesia. When this system is excited, a sleeping animal arouses, and electrocortical tracings (EEG—see Chapter 7) change from a sleeping to waking pattern.

Hypnotic, anesthetic, and tranquilizer drugs selectively block transmission of impulses in the reticular activating system; awakening from the effects of these drugs is associated with normal nervous activity of this system. Destruction of the area containing the reticular activating system in animals results in permanent coma similar

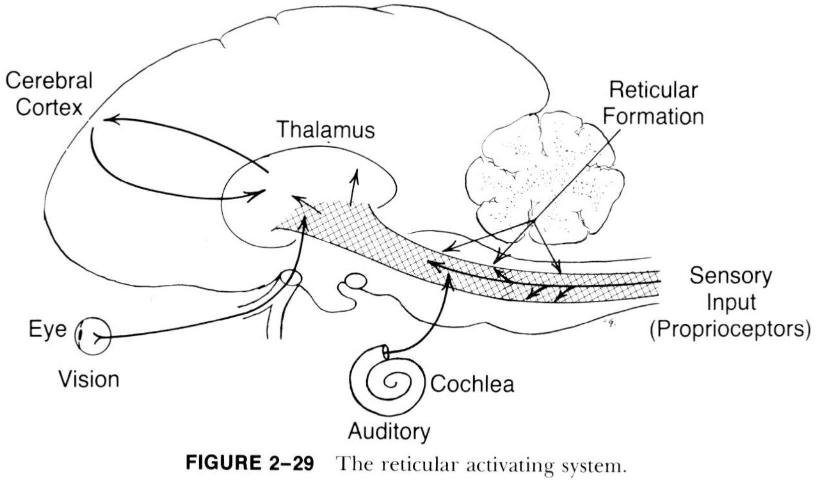

FIGURE 2–29 The reticular activating system.

to that seen in man when injury or disease (sleeping sickness) destroys the functional capacity of this system.

THE SPINAL CORD

The spinal cord is a cylindrical continuation of the bulb that is contained within the vertebral canal. In the dog it extends posteriorly to the level of the fifth or sixth lumbar vertebra.[41] Fibers in the dorsal roots receive sensory (afferent) impulses that travel through motor or reflex centers in the spinal cord or pons and on to higher cranial centers. Through the ventral roots, nerve fibers carry motor (efferent) impulses to the muscles and glands of the body (Fig. 2–30).

The spinal cord is anatomically functionally connected with the brain by many ascending and descending tracts that connect with those functional centers in the cerebrum and cerebellum that are necessary for the animal's functional existence. Ascending and descending tracts also connect various segments of the spinal cord with each other. The spinal cord has been divided anatomically into segments. Each segment is that portion of the spinal cord where nerve fibers in the rootlets of a pair of spinal nerves enter and leave the cord. The dog usually has 36 spinal cord segments: 8 cervical, 13 thoracic, 7 lumbar, 3 sacral, and 5 coccygeal.[41] Like the brain, the spinal cord is surrounded and supported by the meninges (Fig. 2–30).

A transverse section of the spinal cord reveals a butterfly-shaped central core of gray matter (mostly the cell bodies of neurons) (Fig. 2–31). The wings of the gray matter are referred to as dorsal and ventral horns. Surrounding the gray matter is the white matter (consisting primarily of nerve fiber tracts), arranged into so-called columns or funiculi. The dorsal gray horns approach the surface of the cord, and the white matter between the horns of the two sides forms the dorsal columns. The ventral horns project toward the ventral surface of the spinal cord, forming imperfect boundaries between the lateral and ventral columns. There is a sulcus in the white matter ventrally that does not reach so far centrally as the gray matter, enabling nerve fibers to cross from one side of the spinal cord to the other in this bridge, which is called the ventral white commissure. There is a dorsal septum that reaches as far centrally as the gray matter; there is therefore no dorsal white commissure.

Since a large number of white fibers in the cord either ascend from the spinal cord to higher centers in the brain or descend from the brain to lower centers in the cord, it is obvious that the amount of white mat-

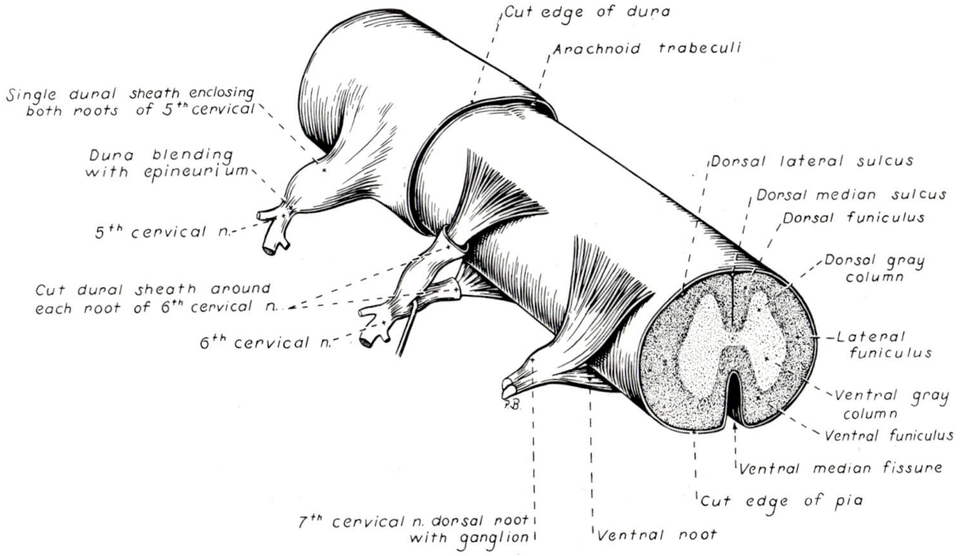

FIGURE 2–30 Cross section of spinal cord and meninges. (From Miller, M. E.: *Guide to the Dissection of the Dog.* Edwards Bros., Ann Arbor, Mich. 1952 © Dr. Malcolm E. Miller.)

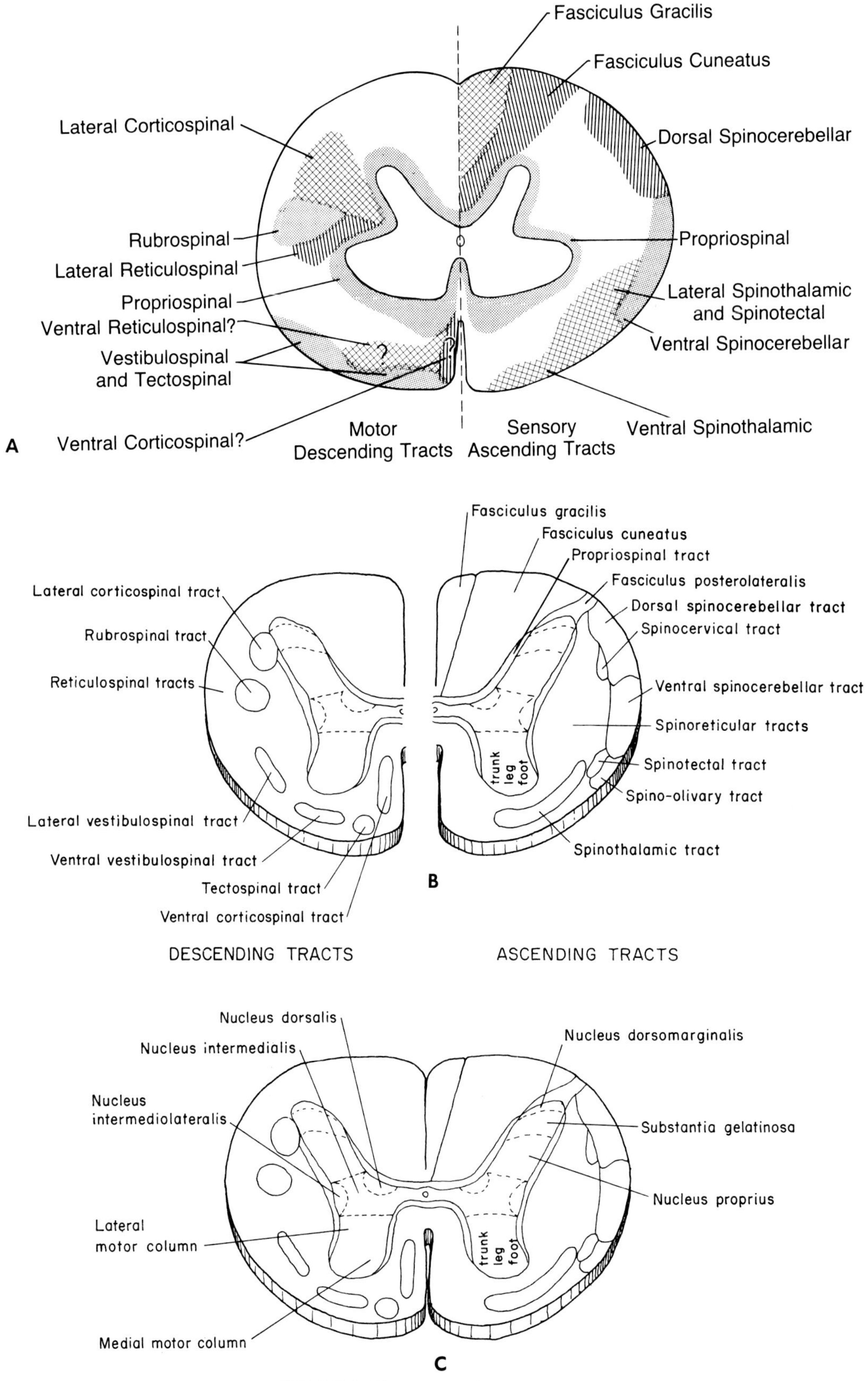

FIGURE 2–31 *See legend on opposite page.*

ter is greatest at the cervical levels and least at the lumbar levels. The gray matter, however, is a continuous core of cells that varies in amount at different levels. It is greatest in amount where the largest nerve roots enter or leave the spinal cord. These enlargements are called the cervical and lumbar enlargements.

A physiological functional separation of the cell bodies in the gray matter can be made. Most of the cells in the ventral gray horn are motor in function (motoneurons); their axons terminate at the motor end plates in striated muscle. There are two types of motor neurons: large *alpha*-motoneurons, whose fibers innervate voluntary striated muscle, and small *gamma*-motoneurons, whose fibers innervate the intrafusal muscle fibers of muscle spindles. These are involved in the maintenance of muscle tone, especially that of antigravity muscles.

Most of the cells in the dorsal gray horns are relay neurons, receiving impulses from peripheral afferent processes and connecting to other spinal neurons or to higher centers in the brain stem, cerebellum, or cerebrum. These comprise approximately one half of the total number of nerve cells in the spinal gray matter. The remaining cells are internuncial in function, connecting with relay neurons and motor neurons in the spinal cord itself. The neurons around the central canal are homologous and continuous with the reticular formation in the brain stem. Between the first thoracic and the fourth or fifth lumbar segments of the spinal cord and in the sacral segments are special motor neurons, smaller than those in the ventral gray horn, found in the lateral part of the gray matter (sometimes called the intermediolateral cell column). These neurons give rise to axons that emerge in the ventral root and are distributed as the *white rami communicantes* to the ganglia of the autonomic nervous system.

The bundles of nerve fibers entering and leaving the spinal cord are called spinal nerves. Every spinal nerve has a *dorsal* (sensory) and a *ventral* (motor) root (see Fig. 2–30). The ventral root consists of fibers (axons) from ventral horn cells that emerge as distinct bundles of fibers gathered together at the root. After the ventral root exits from the dura mater, its fibers join those of the dorsal root to form a mixed nerve (motor and sensory).

The fibers of the dorsal roots conduct impulses from the periphery toward the central nervous system. The afferent nerve cell bodies are not located within the central nervous system but instead are found in the dorsal root ganglia (see Fig. 2–30), which are encapsulated collections of nerve cell bodies lying in a pouch of dura mater just proximal to the junction of the dorsal and ventral roots. The dorsal root fibers do not enter the spinal cord in clumps but enter in a continuous row, like an extended fan.

THE FIBER TRACTS OF THE SPINAL CORD

The foregoing description of the ascending and descending "tracts" in the spinal cord creates the impression that they occupy distinct or specific areas in the white matter; however, with the possible exception of the dorsal columns, this is not true. The fibers of all of the tracts are mixed to a certain extent, especially at the areas where they adjoin each other (see Fig. 2–31).

THE ASCENDING TRACTS

Dorsal Columns (Fasciculus Cuneatus and Fasciculus Gracilis)

Fibers carrying impulses associated with discrete touch, pressure, and kinesthetic senses are transmitted in the *fasiculus gracilis* and *fasciculus cuneatus.* The former transmits from the caudal portion of the body and the latter from the cranial. The cells of origin of these tracts are located outside the spinal cord in the spinal ganglia. Processes from these cells enter the spinal cord and ascend on the same side to

FIGURE 2–31 *A,* Transverse section of the spinal cord showing the sensory (ascending) tracts on the right and the motor (descending) tracts on the left. The question marks indicate that the existence of these tracts in the dog is questionable. *B* and *C,* Diagrammatic cross sections of the spinal cord. *B,* Ascending and descending fiber systems. *C,* The location of identifiable nuclei within the gray matter. (From Breazile, J. E.: Textbook of Veterinary Physiology. Philadelphia, Lea & Febiger, 1971.)

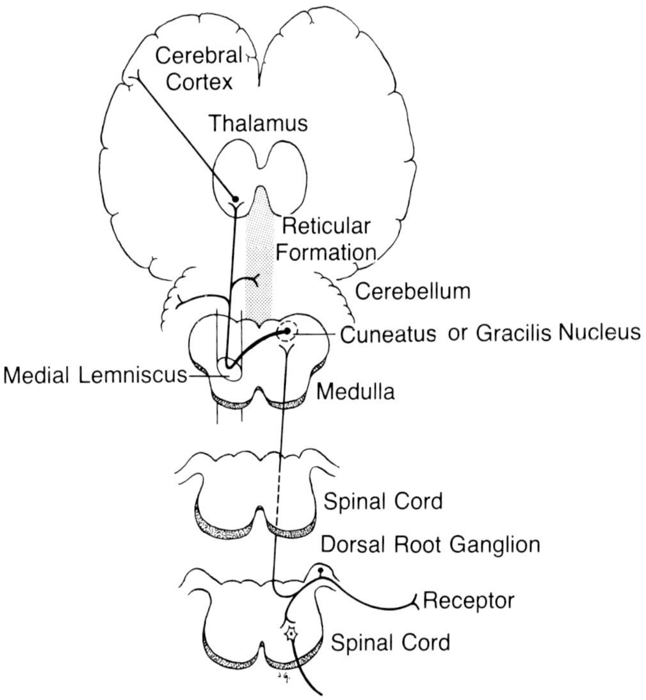

FIGURE 2–32 Transmission of touch, pressure, and kinesthetic sensations in the dorsal column system. Note that the fibers do not cross to the opposite side until after synapsing in the cuneatus or gracilis nuclei.

terminate in the *cuneate* and *gracile nuclei* on the dorsal aspect of the medulla oblongata. Impulses are then transmitted to the thalamus, where a second synapse is made to transmit impulses to the cerebral cortex (Fig. 2–32).

Besides connecting to the cerebral cortex, some fibers make synapses with spinal motor neurons, the reticular formation, and the cerebellum. Lesions of these tracts or of the nuclei in the medulla oblongata result in signs of disturbed movement regulation. Undoubtedly, some loss of cutaneous sensitivity occurs; however, this is difficult to evaluate in the dog because of lack of communication between the examiner and the patient. Since the kinesthetic senses (muscle and joint movement, tension, and position) may be lost, the animal may have difficulty moving.

LATERAL SPINOTHALAMIC TRACT. In man, the sensations of pain, heat, and cold are transmitted in the lateral spinothalamic tracts to the thalamus, and from there to the cerebral cortex (Fig. 2–33*A*). Both the dog and the cat perceive the above sensations; however, the transmission of these sensations may involve other pathways. The cells of origin of these tracts are in the dorsal gray columns (input is from the dorsal-root-ganglion cells).

The axons from these doral gray column neurons may cross over to the opposite side of the spinal cord immediately, or they may ascend a few segments before crossing over via the white commissure. Approximately 50 per cent of the fibers of this tract terminate in the spinal cord for reflex functions, and the remaining fibers terminate in the reticular activating system and in the subthalamic nuclei (Fig. 2–33*A*).

Because of the great clinical importance of this pathway and the transmission of pain to higher centers, several researchers have attempted to evaluate the transmission of pain in the dog and cat. Kennard[33] performed degeneration experiments on the spinal cord of the cat to determine the location of pain pathways. Kennard also found that there is great difference between the cat and man in the transmission of painful stimuli, and that in the cat pain transmission in the spinal cord is much more diffuse. She found that the response to painful stimuli cannot be altered in the cat by hemisection, bilateral ventral section, or unilateral dorsal section of the spinal cord. She concluded that pain is conveyed

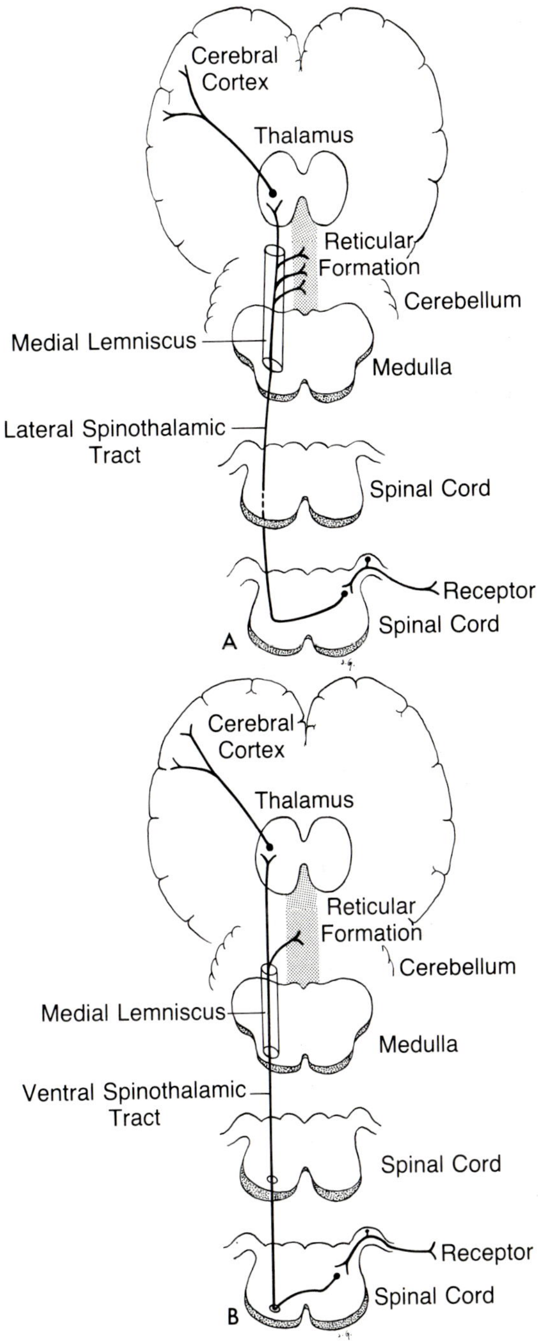

FIGURE 2–33 *A*, Transmission of heat, cold, and pain sensations in the lateral spinothalamic tract. Note that the fibers cross over soon after entering the spinal cord. They may ascend or descend two or three spinal segments before crossing to the opposite side. *B*, The ventral spinothalamic tract (man). Crude pressure, crude touch, and sexual sensations are transmitted by this tract in man. The transmission of these sensations in the dog may be in a similar tract, but it is not yet described *per se*. Many authors do not list this tract in the dog.[16, 35, 40, 47] Miller states that it has not been clearly defined in the dog.[41]

in the cat bilaterally, chiefly by way of the dorsal lateral pathways.

Apparently, domestic animals have diffuse and bilateral representation of somatic pain fibers in the spinal cord, in contrast to man, who has specific pathways which are unilateral in transmission. Lesions involving the lateral portion of the spinal cord may produce hyperesthesia to pain (hyperalgesia) and temperature sensations in the early stages of the disease process. This is frequently seen in the protruding intervertebral disk syndrome, in spinal cord tumors, and following trauma. The loss of pain and temperature sensations on the opposite sides of the body below the level of a unilateral destructive lesion of the spinal thalamic spinal tract has not been reported in animals as it has in man. Since research has indicated that pain is bilaterally represented because of multiple connections, this is not a surprising finding.

VENTRAL SPINOTHALAMIC TRACT. The existence of the ventral spinothalamic tract as a separate tract in the dog is doubtful.[41] Some authors simply do not list this tract, indicating by its omission that crude touch, crude pressure, and sexual sensations are not perceived by the dog (this seems highly unlikely), or that the transmission of these sensations is by some other ascending tract (Fig. 2–33).

Dorsal and Ventral Spinocerebellar Tracts

The spinocerebellar tracts carry impulses arising in the proprioceptors of muscles, tendons, and joints. The information is transmitted to the cerebellum for the subconscious adjustment of skeletal muscle tone and synergizing of muscle actvity during both motionlessness and activity (Fig. 2–34). It is important to note that as these tracts conduct more rapidly (up to 150 meters per second) than other ascending tracts, they are therefore of vital significance to the animal for rapid adjustment, especially during motion. These sensations are transmitted in the spinal cord mainly on the same side of the body as that on which they originate; however, some fibers do cross over and ascend on the opposite side to terminate in the opposite cerebellar cortex.

Since these tracts are vital to the animal in muscular adjustments, damage to them will result in loss of coordination and ataxia. Unilateral section of the dorsal spinocerebellar tract in the dog caused the animal to fall toward the side of the lesion and to have hypotonus of the muscles of the limbs on that side.[47] Proprioception is one of the most important sensory functions in the dog because of its influence in locomotion, and the afferent tracts responsible for it are well developed in this species.

Spinotectal Tracts

Although it is well known that the dog uses auditory and visual clues (which probably utilize both the tectospinal and spinotectal tracts) in avoidance and attentive reactions, there is little information about this pathway. Miller lists this tract as one of the

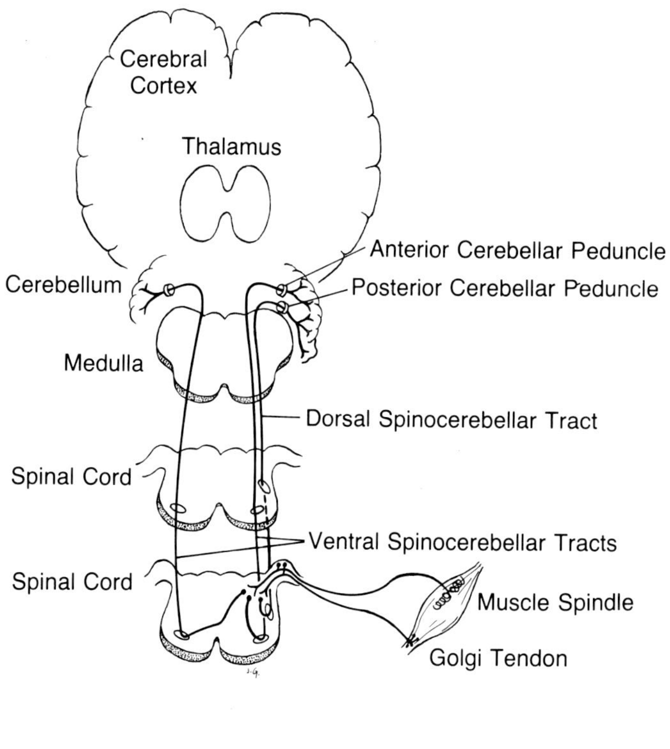

FIGURE 2–34 The dorsal and ventral spinocerebellar tracts. The subconscious transmission of proprioception (muscle, tendon, and joint receptors) for cerebellar integration is via these tracts.

TABLE 2–3 ASCENDING TRACTS OF THE SPINAL CORD

Name	Function	Location	Origin	Terminations	Final Termination
Fasciculus cuneatus and gracilis	Conscious fine touch, pressure and kinesthetic, deep touch and pressure (same side)	Dorsal white columns	Dorsal root ganglia of same side	Medulla oblongata, cuneate, and gracile nucleus	Sensory cortex of cerebrum, cerebellum, spinal motor neurons
Lateral spinothalamic	Pain and thermal sensations (opposite side)	Lateral white columns	Dorsal gray column, opposite side	Thalamus, spinal cord	Thalamus, cerebral cortex(?)
Ventral spinothalamic[a]	Crude touch, pressure, and sexual sensations (opposite side)	Ventral white columns	Dorsal gray column, opposite side	Thalamus, spinal cord, reticular formation	Thalamus, reticular formation, cerebral cortex(?)
Dorsal spino-cerebral and ventral spinocerebellar	Subconscious kinesthetic sensations	Lateral white columns	Dorsal gray column	Cerebellum	Cerebellum
Spinotectal*	Subconscious visual and auditory reflexes	Ventral white columns	Dorsal gray column	Tectum	Tectum
Propriospinal (ground substance) (fasciculi)	Ascending and descending fibers of the spinal cord itself, pain transmission, reflex centers—coordinate body movements	Surrounding gray matter of spinal cord	Dorsal gray column and internuncial cells	Other spinal segments, reticular formation(?)	Motor neurons, thalamus(?)

[a]Not proved with certainty in the dog.[41]

ascending tracts in the dog.[41] Other authors fail to mention its existence or function.

Table 2–3 gives a summary of the ascending tracts.

THE DESCENDING TRACTS

Lateral Corticospinal Tract

The lateral corticospinal tract (Fig. 2–31) originates in the cerebral cortex and terminates in interneurons which synapse with the cell bodies of the lower motor neurons in the ventral horn of the spinal cord gray matter. The general anatomic plan of the corticospinal tract can be seen in Figure 2–35. From the cerebral cortex, the axons converge and descend through the internal capsule, through the basis pedunculi of the midbrain and the basal portions of the pons and then into the medulla, where the corticospinal tracts become visible on the ventral surface of the pyramids.

In the medulla, most of the fibers cross at the pyramidal decussation and descend into the cord at the lateral corticospinal tract in the lateral portion of the spinal cord on the opposite side. The minority of fibers, which do not cross at the medullary level, descend into the ventral portion of the spinal cord as the ventral corticospinal tract, which borders the ventral median fissure. During the descent of the fibers from the cerebral cortex, many collateral fibers terminate in the basal nuclei, reticular formation, and olivary nuclei.

Ventral Corticospinal Tract

There is considerable controversy in the literature about the size, extent, and even the existence of the ventral corticospinal tract in animals. A report by Nyberg-Hanson and Brodal[42] indicates that these authors found descending fibers in both the lateral and ventral portions of the cord, even to the lowest lumbar segments.

Several authors state that they were unable to identify a ventral corticospinal tract in the dog; others simply failed to mention its existence in the discussion of the motor

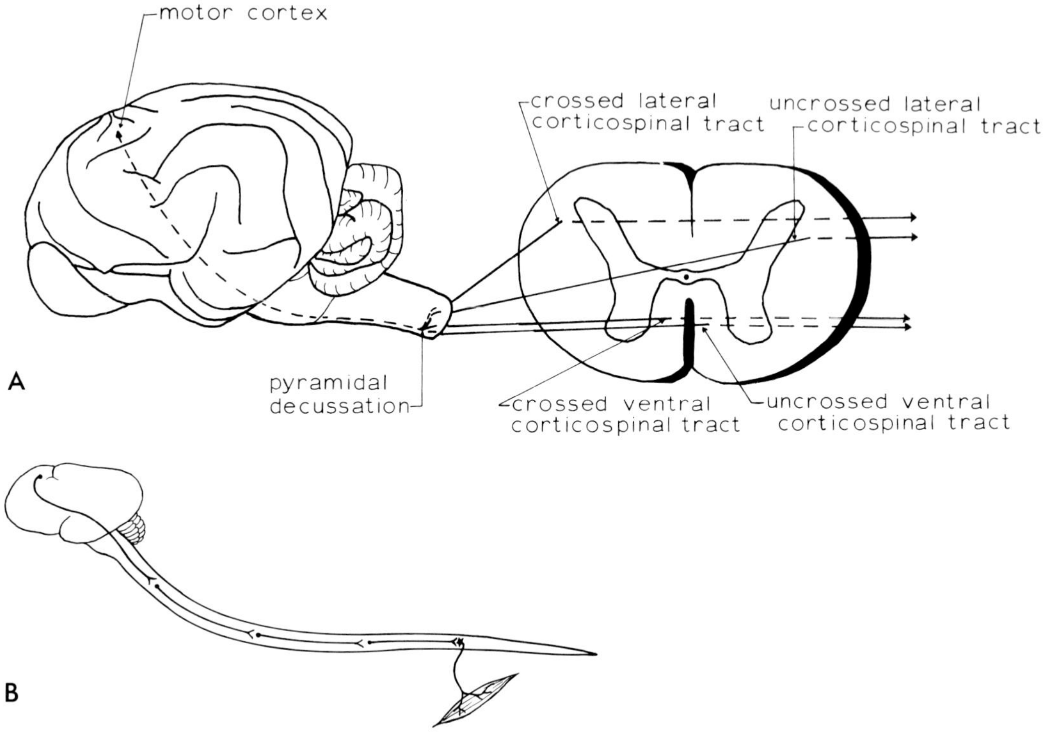

FIGURE 2–35 *A*, Diagrammatic illustration of the corticospinal tracts arising from one cerebral hemisphere in the dog. (From Breazile, J. E.: *Textbook of Veterinary Physiology*. Lea & Febiger, Philadelphia, 1971.) *B*, Proposed multisynaptic corticospinal system of the dog. (Modified from Palmer; *Introduction to Animal Neurology*. F. A. Davis Co., Philadelphia, 1965.)

tracts. The previous discussion of the ventral corticospinal tract in the cat suggests that it may exist; however, positive proof of a continuous tract is still lacking in the dog.

The corticospinal system is phylogenetically a newer acquisition of the nervous system and, therefore, it is not surprising that its greatest physiologic expression is found in the higher primates. As might be expected, clinical deficits that result from lesions of this system are less dramatic in subprimates (i.e., dog and cat) than in the primates. In man, a unilateral brain lesion at the origin of the corticospinal tracts results in a contralateral spastic paralysis with increased deep reflexes, loss of superficial reflexes, and the presence of a positive "babinski" sign (a fanning of the toes and dorsiflexion of the great toe when stimulus is applied to the sole of the foot). This is the typical upper-motor-neuron paralysis as seen in many hemiplegics who have suffered a stroke or cerebrovascular accident.

In contrast to the paralysis and obvious incapacitation described for man as a result of corticospinal lesions, Buxton and Goodman[11] report the following signs as a result of unilateral removal of the motor cortex in the dog. There is no overtly abnormal deportment; that is, the animals appeared to walk, sit, and recline normally. Testing of these dogs revealed, however, that unilateral motor cortex destruction caused hypotonia, hypokinesia, and some dysmetria on the opposite side and greater functional deficits in the hind limb than in the fore limb; however, there was no obvious paralysis in the dogs.

Wright[61] experimentally conditioned adult dogs to perform a lever-pushing maneuver to obtain food. After experimental bilateral destruction of the motor cortex, the animals could not perform the previously learned task even though they obviously tried to perform this task. In addition, voluntary control of the hind limbs apparently was decreased for several days after the abolition experiment. There was no paralysis in either of these experiments or in other reported studies.

Rubrospinal Tract

The rubrospinal tract arises from cells throughout the red nucleus located in the midbrain tegmentum (Figs. 2–31, 2–36). The fibers immediately cross to the opposite side, descend in the lateral brain stem, and continue down the lateral portion of the spinal cord. The rubrospinal fibers are ventrolateral to and partially intermingled with the descending fibers of the lateral corticospinal tract. The fibers descend to the level of lumbar segments. During their descent, they give off fibers at various levels where they terminate on interneurons controlling the lower motor neurons.

Input to the red nucleus originates from the cerebrum, cerebellum, basal nuclei, and reticular formation. This multiplicity of input suggests its vital function in the initiation and coordination of some voluntary and involuntary movements in the dog. Discrete bilateral lesions in the red nucleus of the dog result in hypokinesia; voluntary motor control is apparently not impaired, but the animal shows disinclination to move when stimulated.

It is generally agreed that the cardinal function of the rubrospinal tract is the control of muscle tone in the flexor muscles.

Lateral Reticulospinal Tract (Medullary Reticulospinal Tract)

The fibers that make up this tract originate in cells scattered throughout the medullary reticular formation of the brain stem. It is probable that some of these fibers cross and others remain uncrossed. The reticulospinal fibers descend and terminate primarily on the spinal cord interneurons to both facilitate and inhibit motor neurons in the automatic regulation of muscle tone and coordination in reflex action (Fig. 2–31 *B*).

Ventral Reticulospinal Tract (Pontine Reticulospinal Tract)

Although this tract is described in primates, it has not been clearly defined or described in the dog. Jenkins[32] mentions this tract in his anatomic discussion but does not identify with certainty its existence in the dog or cat.

Vestibulospinal Tracts

There are two vestibulospinal tracts: the medial and the lateral (Fig. 2–31 *A* and *B*). The medial vestibulospinal tract arises from the medial vestibular nucleus and descends on both sides, but mostly on the same side of the spinal cord. The lateral vestibulospinal tract is minor and extends only to the midthoracic region of the spinal

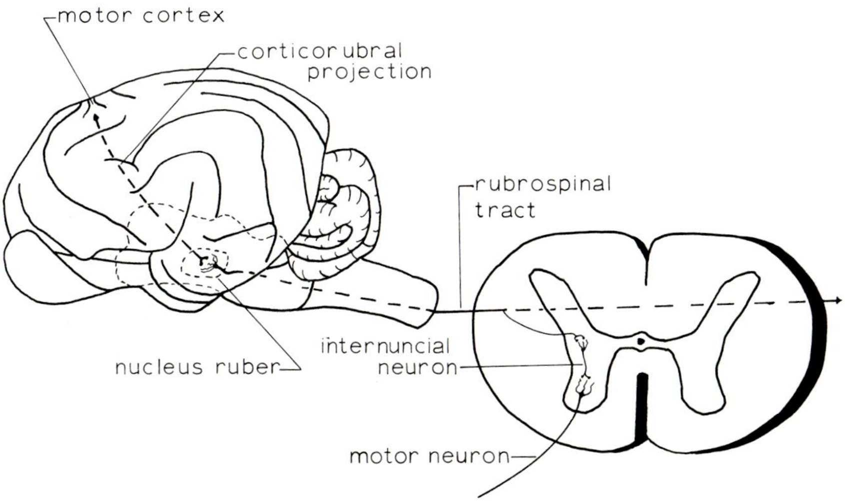

FIGURE 2–36 Illustration of the corticorubrospinal pathway for somatic motor control. (From Breazile, J. E.: *Textbook of Veterinary Physiology*. Lea & Febiger, Philadelphia, 1971.)

cord. The nomenclature of these tracts is inconsistent, and sometimes they are classified as lateral and ventral vestibulospinal tracts.

Phylogenetically, these tracts are very old. They conduct nerve impulses from the vestibular system and indirectly from the cerebellum, and are concerned with the regulation of equilibrium, coordination, and synergy of muscular activity. They act in synergy with the reticulospinal tracts to increase the extensor tonus of muscles on the same side and decrease the flexor and extensor tonus of muscles of the opposite side.

Tectospinal Tract

The tectospinal tract arises from the superior and inferior colliculi of the midbrain tectum (Fig. 2–31 *A* and *B*). The fibers pass to the opposite side and descend in the ventral portion of the spinal cord. The majority of the fibers terminate with internuncial neurons to the lower motor neurons in the upper four cervical segments. The function of the tectospinal tracts is to convey impulses for immediate reflex action for both visual and auditory stimuli. Clinically, the neurologist uses auditory and visual stimuli to determine the functional integrity of these tracts and, conversely, to determine visual and auditory acuity by observation of the motor responses to these stimuli.

Medial Longitudinal Fasciculus

The medial longitudinal fasciculus, phylogenetically, is a very old tract that extends from the level of the midbrain caudally throughout the brain stem and continues in the ventral portion of the spinal cord. In the dog, this tract has been traced caudally as far as the lumbar spinal segments. In the cat, however, the majority of the fibers end at the level of the thoracic segments. The cells of origin of this tract are in multiple locations in the diencephalon and mesencephalon. This tract serves as a connector

TABLE 2–4 DESCENDING TRACTS OF THE SPINAL CORD

Name	Function	Location	Origin	Terminations	Final Terminations
Lateral corticospinal (crossed pyramidal)	Voluntary movement of small groups of muscles (skilled movements)	Lateral white columns	Motor area of cerebral cortex (opposite side)	Motor neurons or interneurons (short relay system?)	Motor neurons
Ventral corticospinal		Not proved to be present in the dog			
Rubrospinal	Voluntary movement, subconscious movement, co-ordination of muscle groups	Lateral white columns	Red nucleus (receives input from cerebrum, basal nuclei, and cerebellum), opposite side	Spinal cord, interneurons	Motor neurons
Lateral reticulospinal	Facilitatory and inhibitory influence on motor neurons and autonomic nervous system	Lateral white columns	Reticular formation	Spinal cord, interneuron	Motor neurons
Ventral reticulospinal		Not proved to be present in the dog			
Vestibulospinal tracts, lateral and ventral	Facilitatory and inhibitory influence on motor neurons (equilibrium)	Ventral and lateral white columns	Vestibular nuclei	Spinal cord, interneurons	Motor neurons
Tectospinal	Visual and auditory reflexes	Ventral white columns	Gray matter of tectum	Spinal cord, interneurons	Motor neurons

between the vestibular and motor nuclei of the cranial nerves and is involved in vestibular reflexes involving eye movements.

Olivospinal Tract

The existence of the olivospinal tract is questionable and has not been substantiated by experimental studies in the dog and cat.

The Dorsal, Lateral, and Ventral Fasciculus Proprius (Propriospinal) Tracts

The propriospinal tracts are also known as intersegmental fasiculi, ground bundles, spinospinal tracts, and the fasciculus proprius. They consist of short, ascending and descending fibers that begin and end in the gray matter and connect the different segments of the spinal cord (Fig. 2-31 *A* and *B*). These tracts are concerned with intersegmental spinal reflexes and perhaps with the transmission of specific modalities, such as pain, to the higher centers.

The Dorsolateral Fasciculus of Lissaeur

This tract is composed of thinly myelinated and nonmyelinated fibers of the lateral division of the dorsal root, which acts principally as a relay interneuron system to convey impulses of pain and temperature sense. Tables 2-3 and 2-4 show the functions of the ascending and descending tracts.

BEHAVIOR AND EMOTION

In the past few years, much has been written about the behavior—normal and, especially, abnormal—of dogs. Most of the papers written are concerned with descriptions of experimentally produced abnormal behavior and the naturally occurring behavioral and emotional reactions of this animal. The term *veterinary ethology* means a scientific study of animal behavior. The reader is referred to the work of Fox[23] and Campbell[13] for a comprehensive review of the abnormal behavior in animals. There is no doubt that behavioral problems exist in some of the patients presented to the practitioner; he is urged therefore to familiarize himself with the diagnosis and possible treatment of such patients.

That emotional activity and resultant behavioral problems exist is beyond doubt, but where do these phenomena reside? Undoubtedly, they are caused by the central nervous system. At the present time, it is believed that they are for the most part associated with the deeper structures of the brain and medial cortical structures known collectively as the "limbic system."

THE LIMBIC SYSTEM

A medial complex of the cerebral cortex, the subcortical nuclei, and the tracts that connect these structures to the hypothal-

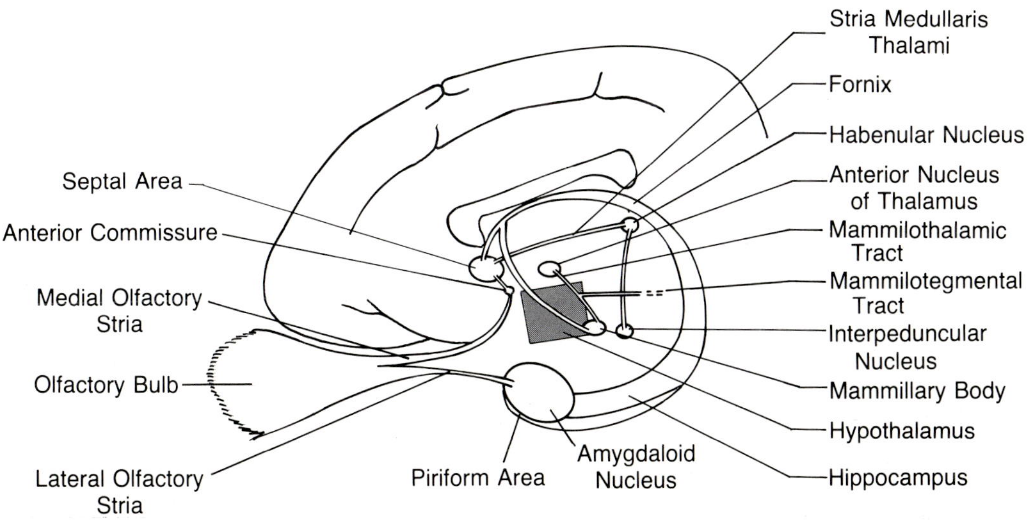

FIGURE 2-37 Deep structures of the limbic system. (After Papez: A proposed mechanism of emotion. Arch. Neurol. Psych. *38*, 725, 1937.)

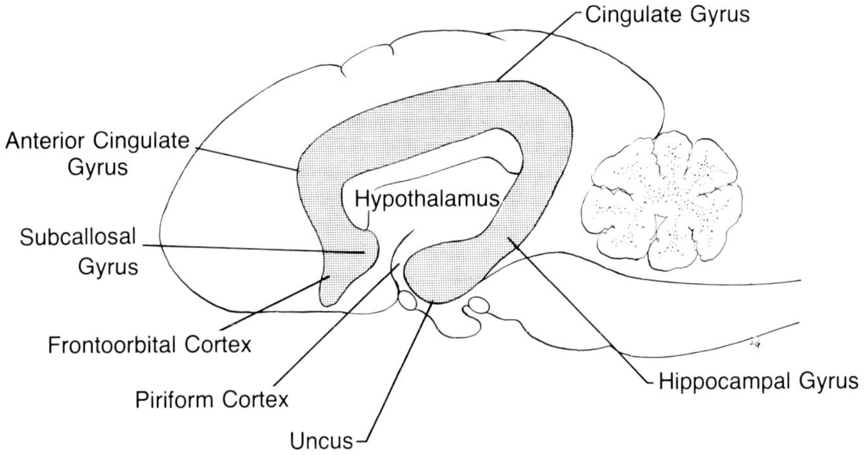

FIGURE 2–38 View of the medial surface of one hemisphere. Shaded area represents the limbic cortex.

amus and the rhinencephalon is known collectively as the *limbic system.* The term *limbus,* meaning "border" or "marginal," refers to the structures surrounding the ventricular cavities and the border of the cerebral cortex around the subcortical structure (Figs. 2–37 and 2–38).

The locus of specific areas of the limbic system for specific emotional responses has been determined by experimental destruction of that area and by electrical stimulation via implanted electrodes. There are many technical difficulties involved in such procedures, and as a result the findings of such studies vary with the different investigators. However, some concepts regarding the general functions of a number of the structures have been formed.

THE HYPOTHALAMUS

Although the hypothalamus is a relatively small structure (Fig. 2–39), it contains the loci for many kinds of emotional behavior and, in addition, behavior for such actions as feeding and drinking. The following generalization as to the probable function of the subdivision of the hypothalamus are based upon ablation and stimulation experiments.

Ventromedial Nuclei

The ventromedial nuclei (see Fig. 2–22) are believed to be responsible for tameness and emotional stability (i.e., they restrain emotional behavior). When this area is destroyed, animals that were previously tame display varying degrees of wildness and savageness.[4, 27, 31, 51] They will attempt to escape, will growl, and may attack savagely if approached. In addition, animals with destructive lesions of these nuclei have a voracious hunger drive that is extremely hard to satisfy. As a result, they eat so much that they become excessively obese.

Posterior Hypothalamus

The posterior hypothalamus (see Fig. 2–22) is involved in alertness, attention, and awareness of environment. Destruction of this region results in general stolidity and inactivity, with a tendency to sleep most of the time.[25] Cataplexy has also been associated with destructive lesions of this area.[15]

Lateral Hypothalamus

The lateral hypothalamic region (see Fig. 2–22) is in some way related to hunger and appetite. Destructive lesions of these areas abolished the urge to eat, resulting in extreme emaciation and eventually death.[15]

THE MIDTHALAMUS

The midthalamus, which surrounds the descending column of the fornix (see Fig. 2–37), including the preoptic and ventral

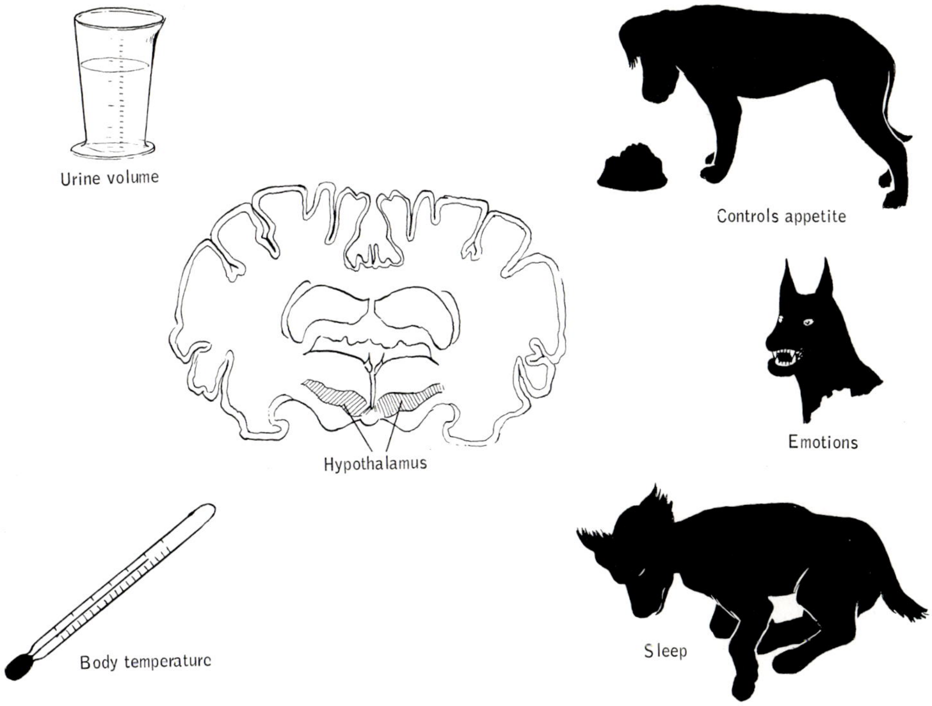

FIGURE 2–39 Functions of hypothalamus. Controls appetite, emotions, sleep, body temperature, and urine volume.

septal areas, is believed to be concerned with fright and flight reactions.[31]

AMYGDALA

The amygdala (see Fig. 2–37) appears to be related to the emotional behavior of fear or wariness. Removal of the amygdala from dogs produced passiveness or unresponsiveness.[34] The dogs approached objects or strange persons, which normally excited wariness or fear, without hesitation and without vocalization or facial expression. Removal of the amygdala nuclei and the overlying cerebral cortex in cats made them exceedingly docile.[50-53]

THE HIPPOCAMPUS

Although at one time it was believed that the hippocampus (see Fig. 2–37) was related to fearlessness and, to some extent, to tameness, it is now believed that this structure does not execute any gross emotional behavior.[50] However, this does not mean that the hippocampus is not involved in CNS activity. It is suggested that this structure plays the role of correlating sensory information and sending it to the hypothalamus and other centers of attention and learning.[29]

THE LIMBIC CORTEX

The most poorly understood portion of the limbic system is the ring of cerebral cortex called the *limbic lobe* (see Fig. 2–38), which surrounds the subcortical structures. The fact that the limbic cortex is connected to the subcortical structures by fiber tracts suggests that the cortex may direct the emotion elicited by the subcortical structures. However, ablation of some cortical structures has produced behavioral changes.

Anterior Cingulate Gyri

Bilateral removal of the anterior portion of the cingulate gyri has eliminated the rage reaction. The animal lacked fear in situations in which fear existed prior to the surgical abolition.[25]

Posterior Fronto-orbital Cortex

Bilateral abolition of the posterior portion of the fronto-orbital cortex caused an increased motor activity. The animal was restless and was frequently unable to sit or lie still. Persistent restlessness and continuous movement are characteristic after such an operation.[9, 25]

Piriform Area

Experimental lesions of the piriform cortex of the cat, rat, and monkey have produced tame, fearless animals that no longer recognize their natural enemies.[25, 52, 54] In addition, in male animals these lesions were associated with hypersexual behavior. It is interesting to note that androgenic hormone, either endogenous or exogenous, was necessary for this reaction to be displayed. Reports of this experimental procedure on the dog are lacking.

Surgical and Naturally Occurring Limbic Damage

Rage attacks in response to trivial stimuli have been observed many times in human patients with brain damage.[25] This change in behavior has been associated with pituitary surgery in which there has been inadvertent damage to the limbic areas of the brain. It may also follow a number of diseases of the nervous system (especially encephalitis and epidemic influenza) that destroy neurons in the limbic system and hypothalamus. It is not unusual to observe behavioral changes in dogs following distemper encephalitis (see Chapter 7 for EEG). The possibility of limbic system damage certainly exists in these cases.

Table 2–5 is a summary of limbic structures and associated emotional activity.

CONCLUSIONS

It is not unreasonable to suspect an abnormality of one or more of the limbic system structures whenever gross abnormal

TABLE 2–5 LIMBIC SYSTEM STRUCTURES AND ASSOCIATED EMOTIONAL ACTIVITY OF THE DOG

Structure	Effect of Destruction	Effect of Stimulation
Ventromedial nucleus of hypothalamus	Rage, savageness, hyperphagia, obesity	— — —
Posterior hypothalamus	Inactivity, somnolence	Wakefulness, alertness, excitement
Anterior hypothalamus	— — —	Somnolence and sleep
Lateral hypothalamus	Inappetence, emaciation, death from starvation	— — —
Midthalamus	— — —	Defense reactions, fight and flight
Amygdala	Passiveness, unresponsiveness, docility	Fear, wariness, rage(?)
Septal region	Excitement, savageness, less fearfulness and anxiety	— — —
Pyriform cortex	Hypersexuality; if subcortical structures removed also, tameness and fearlessness	— — —
Anterior cingulate gyri	Fearlessness	— — —
Posterior fronto-orbital cortex	Increased motor activity, listlessness, unable to stand or sit	

behavioral changes occur in a patient. Unfortunately the veterinary literature is deficient in reports on the naturally occurring lesions of the limbic system that are associated with behavioral changes. Perhaps this deficiency is due to the difficult and time-consuming aspects of neuropathological examination of this system and to the fact that the lesions may be biochemical in nature and therefore not observable under the microscope. There is certainly a need for productive research in this area.

REFERENCES

1. Baker, A. B.: *An Outline of Neurology.* William C. Brown, Dubuque, Iowa, 1958.
2. Best, C. H., and Taylor, N. B.: *The Physiological Basis of Medical Practice,* 7th ed. The Williams & Wilkins Co., Baltimore, 1961.
3. Bowsher, D.: *Introduction to the Anatomy and Physiology of the Nervous System.* Blackwell Scientific Publications, Oxford, 1967.
4. Brady, J. V., and Nauta, W. J. H.: Subcortical mechanisms in emotional behavior. J. Comp. Physiol. Psychol., *46,* 339–346, 1953.
5. Brook, G. B.: *Experimental and Clinical Studies of the Spine of the Dog.* Baillière, Tindall, and Cox, London, 1936.
6. Breazile, J. E.: *Textbook of Veterinary Physiology.* Lea and Febiger, Philadelphia, 1971.
7. Breazile, J. E., Blaugh, B. D., and Nail, N.: Experimental study of canine distemper myoclonus. Am. J. Vet. Res., *27,* 1375, 1966.
8. Breazile, J. E., and Thompson, W. D.: Motor cortex of the dog. Am. J. Vet. Res., *28,* 1483–1486, 1967.
9. Brutkowski, S.: Functions of prefrontal cortex in animals. Physiol. Rev. *45,* 721–746, 1965.
10. Bucy, P. C.: The human neural mechanisms controlling skeletal muscuiar activity. *In* Mosberg, W. H. (ed.): *Clinical Neurosurgery.* The Williams & Wilkins Co., Baltimore, 1962.
11. Buxton, D. F., and Goodman, D. C.: Motor function and the corticospinal tracts in the dog and raccoon. J. Comp. Neurol. *129,* 341–360, 1967.
12. *Canine Medicine.* 1st Catcott Ed. American Veterinary Publications, Inc., Santa Barbara, 1968.
13. Campbell, W. E.: *Behavior Problems in Dogs.* American Veterinary Publications, Inc., Santa Barbara, Cal., 1975.
14. Chang, H.-T.: Choreiform movements in a dog suffering from cortico-striatal disease. J. Neurophys. *8,* 89, 1945.
15. Chusid, J. G., and McDonald, J. J.: *Correlative Neuroanatomy and Function Neurology,* 13th ed. Lange Medical Publications, Los Altos, 1967.
16. Clark, C. H.: In Hoerlein, B. F. (ed.): *Canine Neurology.* W. B. Saunders Co., Philadelphia, 1966.
17. Crosby, E. C., Humphrey, T., and Lauer, E. W.: *Correlative Anatomy of the Nervous System.* Macmillan, New York, 1962.
18. Denny-Brown, D.: *The Basal Ganglia.* University Press, Oxford, 1962.
19. Dow, R. S., and Moruzzi, G.: *The Physiology and Pathology of the Cerebellum.* University of Minnesota Press, Minneapolis, 1958.
20. Eccles, J. C., et al.: *The Cerebellum as a Neuronal Machine.* Springer-Verlag, New York, 1967.
21. Elliott, H. C.: *Textbook of Neuroanatomy.* J. B. Lippincott Co., Philadelphia, 1963.
22. Few, A. B.: A study of the clinical signs and necropsy findings resulting from experimentally produced lesions in the canine brain. Thesis, Auburn University, 1964.
23. Fox, M. W.: *Abnormal Behavior in Animals.* W. B. Saunders Co., Philadelphia, 1968.
24. Fox, M. W.: Postnatal development of the EEG in the dog. I, II, III. J. Small Anim. Pract. *8,* 71–112, 1967.
25. Ganong, W. F.: *Review of Medical Physiology,* 2nd ed. Lange Medical Publications, Los Altos, 1965.
26. Gardner, E.: *Fundaments of Neurology,* 6th ed. W. B. Saunders Co., Philadelphia, 1975.
27. Grinker, R. R., and Sahs, A. L.: *Neurology.* Charles C Thomas, Springfield, Ill., 1966.
28. Guyton, A. C.: *Function of the Human Body,* 4th ed. W. B. Saunders Co., Philadelphia, 1974.
29. Guyton, A. C.: *Textbook of Medical Physiology,* 5th ed. W. B. Saunders Co., Philadelphia, 1976.
30. Hamuy, T. Pinto, Bromiley, R. B., and Woolsey, C. N.: Somatic afferent areas I and II of dog's cerebral cortex. J. Neurophysiol. *19,* 485, 1956.
31. Hunsperger, R. W.: Affektreaktionen auf electrische Reizung in Hirnstamm der Katz. Helv. Physiol. Acta *14,* 70–92, 1956.
32. Jenkins, T. W.: *Functional Mammalian Neuroanatomy.* Lea & Febiger, Philadelphia, 1972.
33. Kennard, M. A.: The course of ascending fibers in the spinal cord of the cat essential to the recognition of painful stimuli. J. Comp. Neurol. *100,* 511, 1954.
34. Kluver, H., and Buncy, P. C.: Preliminary analysis of functions of temporal lobes of monkeys. Arch. Neurol. Psychiat. *42,* 979–1000, 1939.
35. Knecht, C. D., and Small, E.: *Clinical neurology.* In *Canine Medicine.* 1st Catcott Ed. American Veterinary Publications, Santa Barbara, 1968.
36. Kreiner, J.: Homologies of the fissural and gyral pattern of the hemispheres of the dog and monkey. Acta Anat. *70,* 137–167, 1968.
37. Lassek, A. B., Dowd, L. W., and Weil, A.: The quantitative distribution of the pyramidal tract in the dog. J. Comp. Neurol. *51,* 153, 1930.
38. Laughton, N. B.: Studies on the occurrence of extensor rigidity in mammals as a result of cortical injury. Amer. J. Physiol. *85,* 78, 1928.
39. Mettler, F. A., and Goss, L. J.: Canine chorea due to striocerebellar degeneration of unknown etiology. J.A.V.M.A. *108,* 377–384, 1946.
40. McGrath, J. T.: *Neurologic Examination of the Dog.* Lea & Febiger, Philadelphia, 1956.
41. Miller, M. E., Christensen, G. C., and Evans, H. E.: *Anatomy of the Dog.* W. B. Saunders Co., Philadelphia, 1964.
42. Nyberg-Hansen, R., and Brodal, A.: Sites of termination of corticospinal fibers in the cat. An experimental study with silver impregnation methods. J. Comp. Neurol. *122,* 369, 1964.
43. Ochs, Sidney: *Elements of Neurophysiology.* John Wiley and Sons Inc., New York, 1965.

44. Oliver, J. E., Jr.: Canine cranial surgery. Thesis, Auburn University, 1966.
45. Oliver, J. E., Jr.: Brain tumor in a dog. Vet. Med. Small Anim. Clin. *61*, 29–34, 1966.
46. Prynn, R. B.: The effect of intra-carotid injections of ceramic microspheres on the electroencephalogram of the dog. Ph.D. Dissertation, Ohio State University, 1969.
47. Palmer, A. C.: *Introduction to Animal Neurology.* F. A. Davis Co., Philadelphia, 1965.
48. Palmer, A. C.: *Introduction to Animal Neurology,* 2d ed. Blackwell Scientific Publications, London, 1976.
49. Renfrew, S.: *An Introduction to Diagnostic Neurology.* Vol 1. Livingstone, Edinburgh, 1967.
50. Ruch, T. C., and Patton, H. D.: *Physiology and Biophysics,* 20th ed. W. B. Saunders Co., Philadelphia, 1976.
51. Schreiner, L., and Kling, A.: Rhinencephalon and behavior. Amer. J. Physiol. *184,* 486–499, 1956.
52. Schreiner, L., and Kling, A.: Effects of castration on hypersexual behavior induced by rhinencephalic injury in the cat. Arch. Neurol. Psychiat. *72,* 180–186, 1954.
53. Schreiner, L., and Kling, A.: Behavioral changes following thalamic injury in the cat. J. Neurophysiol. *16,* 643–659, 1953.
54. Sherrington, G. S.: On secondary tertiary degenerations in the spinal cord of the dog. J. Physiol. *6,* 177, 1885.
55. Sodeman, W. A., and Sodeman, W. H., Jr.: *Pathologic Physiology,* 5th ed. W. B. Saunders Co., Philadelphia, 1974.
56. Stone, A. B.: Variant lesions in the central nervous system of dogs and cats. J. Small Anim. Pract. *10,* 287–294, 1969.
57. Turbes, C.: Studies on involuntary movements at rest in the dog. Anat. Rec. *118,* 362, 1954.
58. Verhaart, W. J. C.: The pyramidal tract, its structure and functions in man and animals. World Neurology, *3,* 43, 1962.
59. Verhaart, W. J. C.: Se faisceau rubro-spinal, son origine, sa localisation, sa structure fibrellaire et ses contingents se terminant dans le bulbe. Le système mésencéphalo-bulbocérèbelleux. C. R. Ass. Anat., 45th meeting, 768, 1958.
60. Woolsey, C. N.: Postural regulations of the frontal and motor cortex of the dog. Brain *56,* 353–370, 1933.
61. Wright, J. S.: Ablative and stimulative studies of certain areas on the motor cortex of trained dogs. Ph.D. Dissertation, Auburn University, 1970.

CHAPTER 3

NEUROLOGICAL EXAMINATION

R. W. REDDING, D.V.M., PH.D.
K. G. BRAUND, B.V.SC., PH.D.

INTRODUCTION

The objectives of the neurological examination are threefold: (1) to determine the presence or absence of a nervous system malfunction; (2) to establish the location and extent of involvement of the nervous system if a lesion is present; and (3) to arrive at a tentative differential diagnosis and a prognosis. The neurological examination forms an integral part of the overall diagnostic process and provides a foundation for further ancillary investigation. Not only is it of value in understanding the nature of the disease process, but it also provides information concerning the state of the disease (progressive or static) and the efficacy of medical or surgical management. An outline summary of the complete neurological examination is shown in Table 3–1.

DIAGNOSTIC EQUIPMENT

A minimum of special equipment is required for the clinical examination. Basic needs are: (1) reflex hammer; (2) 18-gauge hypodermic needle; (3) pen light or other source of focal beam of light; (4) nonirritating volatile oil or food; (5) blindfold; and (6) hemostatic forceps. At the conclusion of the examination, it may be apparent that specialized tests are required to substantiate a clinical diagnosis; e.g., electroencephalography (EEG), electromyography (EMG), electroretinography (ERG), nerve conduction velocity studies (NCV), spinal fluid analysis, radiography, pneumoencephalography, cerebral angiography, and myelography.

ANAMNESIS

An important adjunct to the neurological examination is a complete and chronological anamnesis which in itself may suggest a tentative diagnosis. One should not, however, ignore other possible causes of the signs described by the owner or observed by the clinician. Certain disorders are often related to (1) breed—e.g., intervertebral disk disease in the dachshund, epilepsy in the poodle, hydrocephalus in the Chihuahua, and spinal dysraphism in the Weimaraner; (2) age—e.g., hereditary and inflammatory diseases in young animals, and degenerative and neoplastic disorders in older animals; (3) functional use of the animal—e.g., hypoglycemia-related CNS disturbances in pointers.

The rapidity of onset of an abnormality may be important in the differential diagnosis; for example, acute onset may suggest (1) toxicosis, (2) trauma, (3) vascular accident, or (4) a fulminating inflammatory eti-

TABLE 3–1 SUMMARY OF NEUROLOGICAL EXAMINATION

A. History: *Date* ______

B. Mental Status: *Case No.* ______

C. Locomotion:

D. Postural Reactions:
1. Wheelbarrowing
2. Hemistanding
   L R
3. Hemiwalking
   L R
4. Hopping
   LF RF LH RH
5. Proprioception
   LF RF LH RH
6. Extensor postural thrust
   LF RF LH RH
7. Righting
8. Placing
   tactile LF RF LH RH
   visual LF RF LH RH
9. Tonic neck
10. Tonic eye

E. Cranial Nerves:
- I. Olfactory
- II. Optic
  - Menace
  - Following
  - Obstacle
- III. Oculomotor
  - Pupillary
    - direct
    - consensual
    - sympathetic
  - Strabismus
- IV. Trochlear
- V. Trigeminal
  - Motor
  - Sensory
    - maxillary ophthalmic
    - corneal
    - palpebral
- VI. Abducent
  - Strabismus
- VII. Facial
- VIII. Vestibulocochlear
  - Cochlear
  - Vestibular
    - nystagmus
      - physiological
      - spontaneous
      - positional
- IX. Glossopharyngeal
- X. Vagus
- XI. Spinal accessory
- XII. Hypoglossal

F. Muscle Tonus

G. Spinal Cord Reflexes:
1. Tendon
   patellar: L R
   gastrocnemius: L R
   bicipital: L R
   tricipital: L R
2. Flexor
   hindlimb: L R
   forelimb: L R
3. Crossed extensor
4. Panniculus
5. Anal

H. Pain Perception:
1. Head: L R
2. Fore limb: L R
3. Hind limb: L R
4. Trunk: C T L/S
5. Perineal
6. Tail

ology. On the other hand, a more chronic course will suggest a degenerative, neoplastic, or low grade inflammatory process. It is important to ascertain whether the condition has progressed, as in German shepherd myelopathy; remained static, as in a post-traumatic condition; or demonstrated periodic relapses, as in intervertebral disk disease.

Information related to the first abnormal signs and any subsequent signs noted in a patient may differentiate between a focal and a multifocal disease process. In an animal in which the first signs are posterior paresis or paralysis with subsequent forelimb involvement, a multifocal progressive process is suggested—e.g., ascending viral myelitis.

Some diseases, such as idiopathic epilepsy in poodles and German shepherds, have a familial relationship. Accordingly, detailed information about lineage may aid in establishing a basis for a suspected hereditary disorder.

Behavioral and personality changes or abnormalities should be ascertained when taking the history as an aid in differential diagnosis; for instance, sudden onset of periods of fear or aggression may suggest a psychomotor-like epilepsy or a space-occupying mass of the telencephalon.

METHOD OF EXAMINATION

The examination should be undertaken in a systematic manner. A routine should be established and adhered to so that no part of the examination is omitted. One method is to evaluate the nervous system from the higher to the lower centers of integration.

The examination should include assessment of (1) mental status, (2) gait, (3) postural reactions, (4) craniospinal reflexes, and (5) muscle tonus (see Tables 3–1, 3–2, and 3–3). The order of the examination may depend upon the clinical condition and cooperative attitude of the patient—tests which may cause undue excitation (such as nociceptive assessment of the limbs) should not be performed on anxious patients early in the examinations.

TABLE 3-2 SUMMARY OF CRANIAL NERVE EVALUATION

Nerve	Clinical Signs of Dysfunction	Clinical Tests	Normal Response	Abnormal Response
I. Olfactory	Hyposmia or anosmia	Smell of food or non-irritating volatile substance	Food: interest or attempt to eat. Volatile substance: sniffing, recoil, and nose lick	No reaction
II. Optic	Visual impairment, hesitancy in walking	1. Obstacle test 2. Visual placing test 3. Menace reaction 4. Following movement (ophthalmoscopic examination)	1. Avoidance of obstacle 2. Visual placing of limbs 3. Eye blink 4. Follows motion of object (normal retina)	1. Bumping objects 2–4. No reaction (retinal lesions)
	Anisocoria Mydriasis	Point source of light in each eye	Direct and consensual pupillary reflexes	On affected side, direct and consensual pupillary reflexes absent; on unaffected side, direct and consensual pupillary reflexes present
III. Oculomotor	Anisocoria Mydriasis Ptosis Strabismus (ventrolateral)	1. Point source of light in each eye 2. Observation of eye when following a moving object in horizontal/vertical planes	1. Direct and consensual pupillary reflexes 2. Normal medial, dorsoventral ocular movement	1. On affected side, direct pupillary reflex absent, consensual reflex present; on unaffected side, direct pupillary reflex present, consensual reflex absent 2. Impaired ocular movement in vertical plane and impaired ocular adduction in horizontal plane (unable to follow upward, downward, or medially)
IV. Trochlear	Strabismus (dorsomedial)	–	–	–
V. Trigeminal (motor)	Masseteric and temporalis muscle atrophy; inability to open and close jaws	1. Jaw tonus 2. Palpation of masseter and temporalis muscles	1. Resistance to opening jaws 2. Normal contour/muscle resilience	1. Lack of resistance or supranormal resistance 2. Hypotonia, atrophy
(sensory)		3. Maxillary-ophthalmic reflex 4. Palpebral reflex 5. Corneal reflex	3–5. Eye blink	3–5. No reaction; intense discomfort, recoil, vocalization
VI. Abducens	Strabismus (medial)	Observation of eye when following moving object in horizontal plane	Normal lateral ocular movement	Impaired ocular abduction (unable to follow laterally)
VII. Facial	Asymmetry of facial expression, inability to close eyelids, lip commissure paralysis, auricular paralysis	1. Maxillary-ophthalmic reflex 2. Palpebral reflex 3. Corneal reflex 4. Menace reflex 5. Handclap	1–4. Eye blink 5. Auricular contraction	No reaction
VIII. Vestibulocochlear				
(Cochlear)	Deafness	1. Handclap 2. EEG alerting	1. Startle reaction, eye blink, auricular contraction 2. EEG alert recordings	1–2. No reaction
(Vestibular)	Circling, head tilt, nystagmus, loss of balance	1. Rapid head movement in horizontal/vertical planes 2. Caloric test 3. Rotatory test 4. Righting reactions	1–2. Physiologically induced nystagmus 3. Postrotatory nystagmus 4. Normal righting	1–4. No reaction; spontaneous/positional nystagmus; strabismus (ventrolateral) upon dorsal head extension
IX. Glossopharyngeal	Dysphagia	Gag reflex	Swallow	No reaction
X. Vagus	Dysphagia	1. Gag reflex 2. Laryngeal reflex 3. Oculocardiac reflex	1. Swallow 2. Cough 3. Bradycardia	1–3. No reaction
XI. Spinal accessory	Dorsolateral neck muscle atrophy; torticollis	Palpation of cervical musculature	Resilience of normal contour muscle	Hypotonia, muscle atropy
XII. Hypoglossal	Deviation of tongue (contralateral deviation occurs early in diseases; ipsilateral deviation atrophy, and epithelial corrugation occur in chronic disease)	Tongue stretch	Retraction	No retraction

TABLE 3–3 SPINAL CORD REFLEXES

Reflex	Peripheral Nerve	Cord Segment
Patella	Femoral	L4-6
Gastrocnemius	Tibial	L5-7, S1
Bicipital	Musculocutaneous	C6-8
Tricipital	Radial	C7-8, T1-2
Flexor reflex (fore limb)	Axillary	C6-8
	Musculocutaneous	C6-8
	Median/ulnar	C8, T1-2
Flexor reflex (hind limb)	Sciatic	L5-7, S1
Panniculus	Spinal	C8, T1
Anal	Pudendal	S1-3
Micturition	Pelvic	S1-2

MENTAL STATUS (LEVEL OF CONSCIOUSNESS)

The level of consciousness is influenced by the functional relationship between the active brain stem and the higher cortical centers. Normal mental status is present in animals which are bright and alert and react to visual, auditory, and tactile stimuli. Abnormal or altered mental status (hysteria, depression, confusion, delirium, or coma) may be present in animals with acute encephalitis, toxicoses, cerebral trauma or neoplasms. The mental status in individual cases will depend upon the duration and severity of the disease, and may be altered by previous medical treatment.

LOCOMOTION

While in motion, the animal utilizes the motor cortex to initiate some motor movements, the subcortical nuclei to regulate and initiate gross movements, the cerebellum to coordinate these movements, the vestibular system to maintain balance, and the spinal cord to conduct nerve impulses from the higher centers to the lower motor neurons and skeletal muscle and to conduct proprioceptive signals back to the cerebellum and cerebrum for proper integration. It is obvious that many areas of the nervous system are functioning simultaneously during locomotion and that it requires additional testing to locate the specific focus of the disease if it exists.

The owner or an assistant should induce the animal to walk, run, and, if possible, ascend and descend steps. In addition, the animal can be led or directed toward objects it must avoid by visual means. This portion of the examination allows the clinician to evaluate the function of four systems: (1) visual, (2) motor, (3) vestibular and cerebellar, and (4) proprioceptive.

Some of the signs that indicate diseases of these systems follow.

1. Bumping into objects or reluctance to ambulate suggests a disease of the visual system.
2. Hypermetria, hypometria, or lack of coordination indicates disease of the cerebellum or its pathways.
3. Loss of balance, circling, or falling to one side suggests a disease of the vestibular system or subcortical nuclei.
4. Paresis or paralysis of one or more limbs suggests spinal cord or peripheral nerve disease.

These observations serve to focus attention on the specific systems that must be evaluated carefully as the examination is continued.

POSTURAL REACTIONS

Postural reactions such as wheelbarrowing, hemistanding, hemiwalking, hopping, righting, and placing assess reflex pathways (including touch/pressure, stretch receptors in joints, muscles, and tendons) as well as ascending and descending fiber tracts in the spinal cord and higher centers. The main value of postural reaction testing is to detect subtle asymmetrical deficiencies that may go unnoticed in the gross examination of locomotion. Individual reactions do not specifically localize a lesion; however, when combined with other reactions and signs they are of diagnostic value.

Wheelbarrowing

Normal walking reactions under the control of the spinal cord may be tested by supporting the patient under the abdomen so that the pelvic limbs do not touch the ground and forcing the patient to walk on its pectoral limbs (Fig. 3–1). Normal animals will walk with a symmetrical, alternate, forelimb movement with the head extended in a normal position. Patients with lesions of the peripheral nerves, cervical spinal cord, brain stem, or higher centers may show asymmetrical movements, stumbling, or knuckling. More severe lesions involving the cervical spinal cord produce a tendency to carry the head flexed with the nose close to and occasionally touching the ground for support. This test is useful in differentiating diseases of the brachial plexus and cervical spinal cord from those associated with the thoracolumbar cord. In the latter, the wheelbarrowing reaction should be symmetrical.

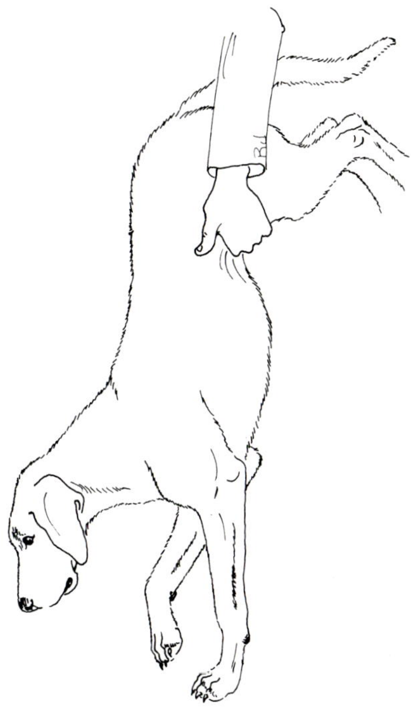

FIGURE 3–1 Wheelbarrowing. The animal is supported under the abdomen so that it is forced to walk on its pectoral limbs. Normal animals walk with a symmetrical, alternate fore limb movement.

Hemistanding and Hemiwalking

Hemistanding and hemiwalking reactions test the patient's ability to stand or walk with the pelvic and pectoral limbs on one side only. These can be evaluated by holding the hind and front limbs of the same side off the ground and forcing the patient to move either forward or sideways (Fig. 3–2). This particular test determines the functional integrity of the motor cortex and the spinal cord. The animal's normal response is to position the limbs vertical to the axial plane of the body and to move them in a symmetrical fashion when forced to move. A patient with a unilateral disease of the motor cortex or internal capsule may have a normal gait when all four limbs are used but during hemiwalking will frequently show a deficit—e.g., scuffing of the limb, knuckling, or a delayed limb position-

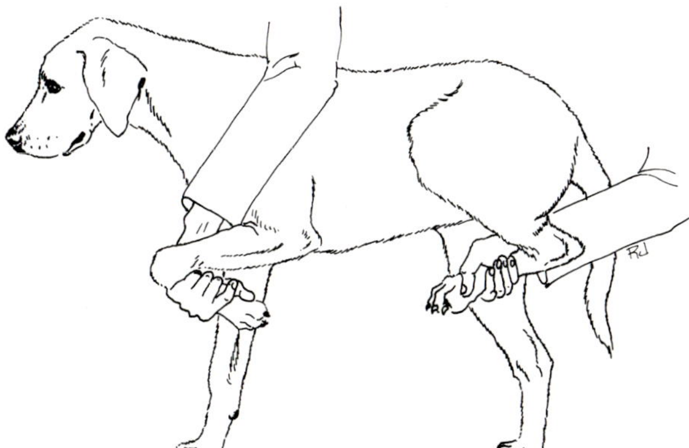

FIGURE 3–2 Hemistanding and hemiwalking. The animal is forced to stand and walk on the front and hind limbs of the same side. This test determines the functional integrity of the motor cortex and spinal cord.

ing reaction. With severe cervical and thoracic cord lesions, the limbs on the same (ipsilateral) side may be unable to support the animal when it is in a hemistanding position. An exaggerated or hypermetric response may be observed in animals with disorders of the cerebellum or the cerebellar pathways.

Hopping Reactions

These reactions depend upon a great number of CNS structures and are some of the most complex of the reactions tested. They involve the cerebrum, cerebellum, brain stem, spinal cord, and touch-pressure/pressure-stretch receptors in the joints, muscles and tendons.

These reactions are tested by holding the animal in a horizontal position. Three of the limbs should be elevated so that they do not touch the examination table or floor, and the animal is supporting its weight on one limb. Move the animal forward, backward, and to each side (Fig. 3–3). The animal should hop on the supporting leg in the direction of the displacement, keeping the foot directly under its body to support its weight. This reaction should be attempted on each of the four limbs. A variety of abnormal responses similar to those in the hemiwalking test may be observed.

Proprioception

Proprioceptive-positioning tests evaluate the afferent system that determines the patient's ability to recognize the position of the limb when it has been flexed or extended, and the efferent response that returns the limb to a normal position. The animal's paw is placed in a flexed position, and the response is observed. A normal animal should return the paw to its usual position so that it will support itself against gravity. The reaction time is considered normal when the response occurs within 1 to 3 seconds. Patients with peripheral nerve pathology or unilateral lesions of the spinal cord or higher ascending and descending pathways may fail to show the proprioceptive-positioning reaction.

Extensor Postural Thrust Reaction

This reaction involves touch, pressure, and stretch receptors. The cerebrum, vestibulocerebellar system, and spinal cord must be intact for this reaction to occur. The animal is held by the axillae and lowered until its hind limbs touch the floor or a solid supporting surface (Fig. 3–4). The limbs should stiffen in extension and support weight. If the lesion is in the spinal cord but is incomplete and unilateral, only

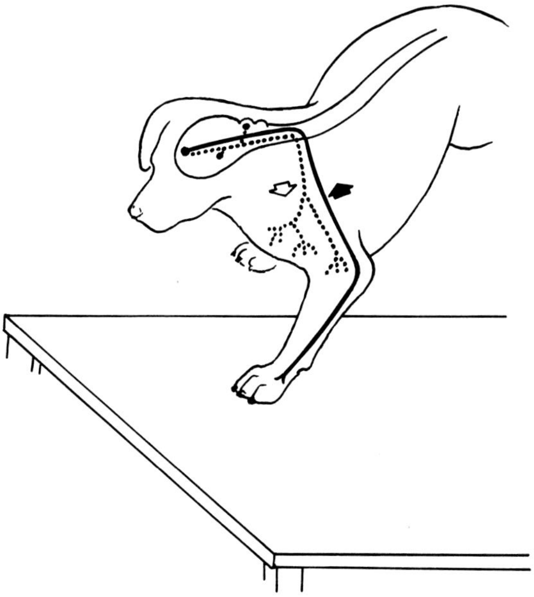

FIGURE 3–3 The hopping reaction. Pressure and stretch receptors are activated by the movement of the animal's body while it is supporting its weight on one limb. Afferent pathways (solid line) terminate in the cerebrum, reticular formation, and cerebellum. Efferent impulses (dotted line) originate in the cerebrum, basal nuclei, and reticular formation. These impulses cause appropriate muscular activity to bring the limb into proper position for the efficient support of weight.

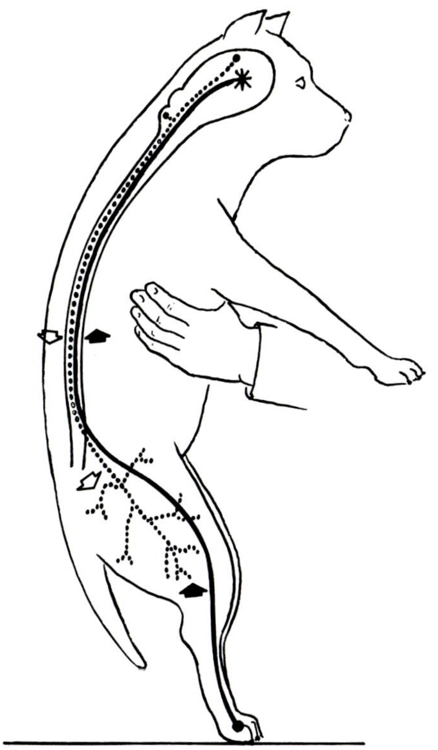

FIGURE 3–4 The extensor postural thrust reaction. When touch and pressure receptors are activated, afferent impulses (solid line) arrive at the cerebral cortex via the spinal cord tracts. Efferent impulses (dotted line), both cortical and subcortical in origin, are transmitted to the extensor muscles to support weight.

one limb will react. If the lesion is complete, there will be no extension on either side. If there is a cerebral lesion, the contralateral side may be abnormal, and if the dog has a vestibulocerebellar lesion, the ipsilateral side may be abnormal. This reaction is assessed in the fore limbs by supporting the animal by the pelvis (Fig. 3–5).

Righting Reactions

The ability of an animal to maintain its normal position in relation to gravity and during motion involves three physiological mechanisms: the visual system, the vestibular system, and the contact-pressure proprioceptive system. When evaluating righting reactions, it is necessary to eliminate one or two of the three in order to properly evaluate the remaining system or systems.

Test

1. The animal is suspended by the pelvis and the position of the head observed. The head should assume a position in space at approximately a 45-degree angle to the horizontal and in a line with its body, not rotating to one side or the other, and the limbs should be held in an extended position. To test vestibular function alone the animal should be blindfolded (Fig. 3–6).

2. The animal is placed in a lateral recumbent position on each side, and the animal's ability to right itself is noted. The contact-pressure–appraisal receptors on the side of the body will be stimulated, and the animal should right itself normally by extension and flexion of uppermost and lowermost limbs, respectively. If unilateral vestibular pathology is present, this righting reaction will be abnormal on the ipsilateral side.

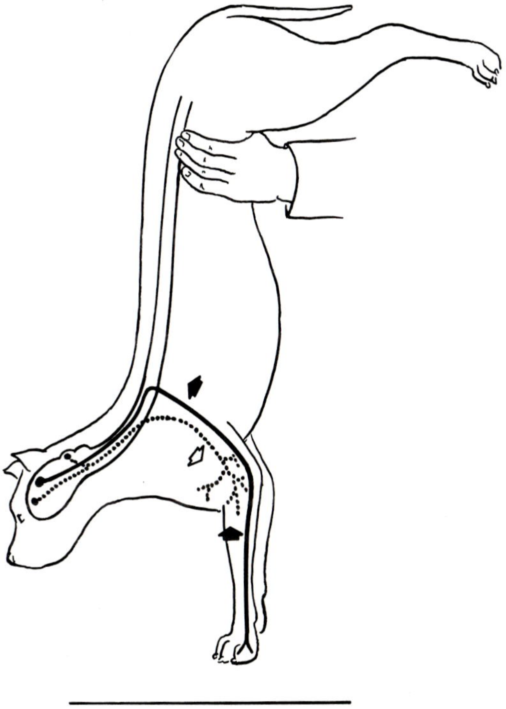

FIGURE 3–5 Testing the righting mechanism and the contact-placing reaction. The righting mechanism utilizes the vestibular and visual systems and the contact-placing reaction utilizes touch receptors. Afferent pathways (solid line) to the cerebrum transmit the recognition of touch. Efferent pathways (dotted line) pass from the cerebrum to the extensor muscles. Blindfolding the animal will eliminate the visual mechanisms and allow evaluation of the vestibular mechanisms alone.

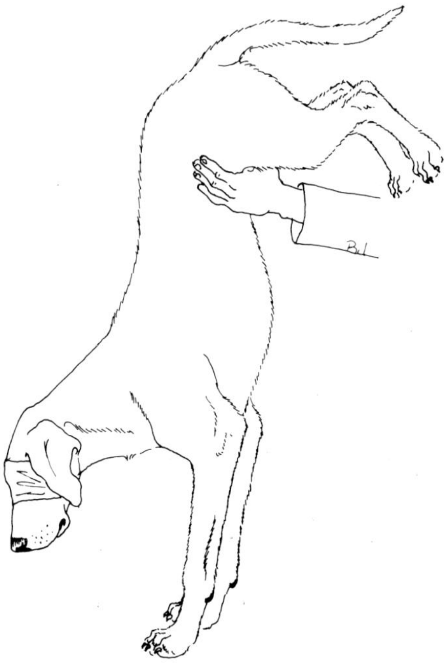

FIGURE 3–6 Vestibular righting reaction. The animal is blindfolded and suspended by the pelvis, and the position of the head is noted. A normal animal assumes a head position at approximately 45 degrees to the horizontal and in line with its body.

Placing Reactions

Placing reactions involve both tactile and visual pathways. In the former, the reactions are initiated by touch and pressure stimulation, and in the latter the initiating stimulus originates in the visual centers.

Tactile Placing Reactions (Animal Blindfolded)

The blindfolded animal is grasped under the thorax and held in a horizontal position in the air with the fore limbs hanging. It is then moved toward the edge of a solid object such as a table edge in order to initiate contact with the anterior surface of the fore limbs. The slightest contact should result in accurate and immediate placing of the paws in a supporting position on the table surface (Fig. 3-7*A*). The fore limb response is tested in both limbs at the same time and then in each limb separately. The hind limb responses are tested in a similar manner. These reactions may be difficult to elicit upon repeated testing.

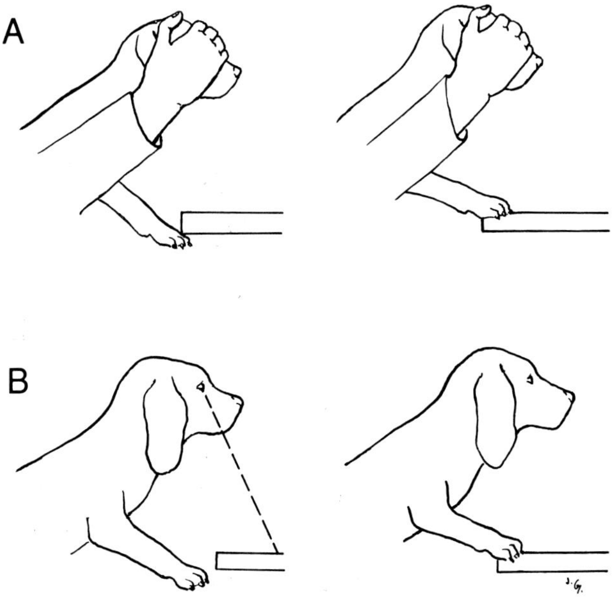

FIGURE 3–7 *A*, Tactile placing reaction. This reaction tests voluntary motor ability. The blindfolded animal feels the table (left), then voluntarily places its leg on the table. *B*, Visual placing reaction. This reaction tests the ability of an animal to move its legs voluntarily. The animal sees the table and voluntarily places its foot on it.

Visual Placing Reaction

The animal is supported in the same way as for the tactile placing reaction test. As the table is approached the animal's normal response is to place both paws on the surace (Fig. 3–7*B*). Each limb should be tested individually.

Tonic Neck Reactions

The dog is placed in a standing position and the head is raised. The normal dog will exhibit extensor tonus of the fore limbs and partial flexion of the hind limbs. When the head is flexed downward, semiflexion of the fore limbs and extension of the hind limbs are normal responses. When the head is rotated to the right and to the left, extensor tonus on the side to which the head is rotated is a normal response. These complex responses are a result of the coordination of the vestibular centers with neck muscle and joint receptors.

Abnormalities

Frontal lobe lesions may cause contralateral abnormalities, and vestibular lesions may cause ipsilateral abnormalities. A patient with disease of the general proprioceptive system in the cervical spinal nerves, cord, or medulla may fail to extend the fore limbs, and these joints may passively flex so that the weight is borne on the dorsal surface of the paw.

Tonic Eye Reactions

Tonic eye reactions involve joint and muscle proprioceptors in the cervical areas which make connections with the vestibular system and the nuclei of cranial nerves III, IV, and VI for conjugate ocular movement postural control.

The test consists of flexion, extension, and rotation of the head and neck. The normal response is for the eyes to fix on an object throughout deviation of motion. If the head is elevated, the eye actually remains fixed but appears to move downward. Similarly, if the head is lowered, the eyes appear to move upward. If the head is rotated laterally, the eyes appear to move in the opposite direction.

After the animal has been observed in motion and the postural reactions have been evaluated, it should be placed on an examination table to facilitate examination of the sensory-motor pathways of the craniospinal systems.

EXAMINATION OF THE CRANIAL NERVES

The cranial nerves, which are conventionally numbered I through XII, comprise those that are attached to the brain stem. The olfactory nerve (I) fibers enter the olfactory bulb of the hemispheres, and the spinal accessory nerve (XI) attaches to the cervical spinal cord but enters the skull and re-emerges from it. The optic nerve (II) is not a true peripheral nerve developmentally, structurally, or in its pathological manifestations.

It should be realized that clinical deficiency phenoma (lower motor neuron signs—for instance, hypotonia, flaccid paralysis, and hyporeflexia) are commonly observed in disorders of the cranial nerves. Release phenomena such as hypertonia, hyperreflexia, and spastic paralysis (characteristic of upper motor neuron disease, as seen in spinal pathology) are infrequently detected in the cranial-neuromuscular system of animals.

The cranial nerves should be examined in sequence from I to XII so that none are omitted.

Olfactory Nerve (Tracts)

The use of a nonirritating volatile substance may be employed to test the functional integrity of the olfactory system. Most animals will recoil and lick their noses after sniffing the substance when it is placed near the external nares. However, some animals will not respond sufficiently for diagnostic purposes. The ability of a hungry animal to detect the smell of food is frequently a more reliable reaction of olfactory acuity. Disorders of the sense of smell (hyposmia/anosmia) are relatively rare in the dog but do occur. They may be caused by conditions that affect the primary olfactory receptors in the nasal mucosa, such as severe bacterial infections. Occasionally, the virus of distemper may destroy these cells.

The neurons of the olfactory bulb and tract may also be affected; however, this is relatively rare. Lesions of the uncus, a part of the olfactory system, may cause hallucinations of smell, and the owner may report that the animal continually appears to be smelling something that is not present.

Optic Nerve and Associated Pathways

For normal sight the retina, optic nerves, optic tracts, lateral geniculate bodies, optic radiations, and occipital lobes must all be functional. Determination of the visual acuity of an animal is sometimes difficult because of tactile or auditory sense compensation. The fundus should be examined by either direct or indirect ophthalmoscopy (see Chapter 18 for a discussion of this portion of the examination). In addition, the following tests may be used to evaluate the visual pathways:

Menace Reaction

A threatening gesture toward the eye will result in a blink response of the eye and some head recoil. The eyes should be tested individually. The menace reaction is mediated by cranial nerves II and VII. This test is conducted using a sheet of transparent material between the examiner and the animal to prevent air currents and the induction of another reflex (from nerves V and VII).

Following Movements

The following movement test evaluates the integrity of cranial nerve II and the corticomesencephalic integrative centers. (1) Move the hand in front of the animal and note whether its eyes follow the hand. (2) Cotton balls may be tossed toward or in front of animal's face. The normal animal will follow the trajectory of the cotton ball once it has entered its visual field.

Obstacle Test

Lead the animal through an obstacle course in both bright and reduced light conditions.

Visual Placing Reactions

(See earlier discussion of placing reactions.)

Abnormalities of the Optic Nerve

(1) Visual impairment. (2) Mydriasis—iris is unresponsive to stimulation by bright light.

Oculomotor Nerve

The somatic portion of the oculomotor nerve innervates all the extrinsic ocular muscles except for the lateral rectus, retractor bulbi, and superior oblique. In addition, this nerve has a parasympathetic component which is concerned with pupillary-motor control and accommodation.

Pupillary Light Reflexes

The pupillary light reflexes depend upon the functional integrity of the oculomotor nerve and the optic nerve together with the midbrain integrative centers (pretectal and Edinger-Westphal nuclei) and sympathetic pathways.

TEST. When light is focused on the retina using a brilliant point-surface of light, the normal iris constricts, causing the pupil to become smaller (direct pupillary reflex). When the light is withdrawn the iris relaxes, and the pupil becomes larger. Because of the neuronal cross-connections in the optic chiasm and tectum, the opposite pupil should also respond to the light in a similar manner, even though the light is directed into only one eye. This response is called the consensual or indirect pupillary reflex (see Fig. 3–8).

ABNORMALITIES OF PARASYMPATHETIC FUNCTION. (1) There is an unresponsive, dilated pupil in the eye tested but a normal consensual response in the contralateral eye. Stimulation of the contralateral eye will result in a normal direct response but an absent consensual in the affected eye. (2) Transient unilateral or bilateral miosis due to irritation and stimulation of the midbrain integrative structures may be seen early in the acute phase of cranial trauma. Later, as midbrain compression

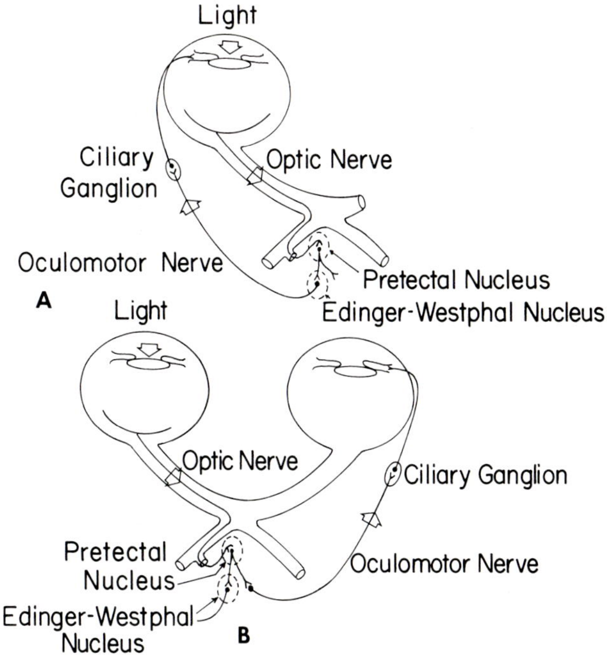

FIGURE 3–8 Pupillary light reflexes. The arrows indicate the direction of impulse transmission. *A*, Direct pupillary light reflex. *B*. Consensual pupillary light reflex.

progresses, the pupils may become dilated and unresponsive to direct light stimulation. In such cases absence (bilateral) of the consensual response will be evident.

Somatic Motor Function

Somatic motor function can be tested by slowly rotating the head in both horizontal and vertical planes and observing ocular movement.

ABNORMALITIES OF SOMATIC MOTOR FUNCTION. (1) Venotrolateral strabismus. (2) Reduced or absent adduction of the eye in the horizontal plane and reduced ocular movement (dorsal and ventral) in the vertical plane of the eye. (3) Paralysis of the upper eyelid of affected side (ptosis), resulting in a narrowed palpebral fissure.

Sympathetic Control

The sympathetic pathways begin in the hypothalamus and pass through the brain stem and cervical cord to synapse with cell bodies located in the intermediolateral gray matter of the spinal cord in T1 and T2 segments. Fibers from these neurons travel via the vagosympathetic trunk to the cranial cervical ganglia where synapse occurs. Postganglionic fibers continue through the middle ear to innervate eventually the dilator pupillae muscle and the smooth muscle of the lids and periorbita.

Lesions at any level of the sympathetic pathways may produce a group of signs known as Horner's syndrome.

ABNORMALITIES OF SYMPATHETIC CONTROL. (1) Pupillary miosis. (2) Ptosis (the ptosis noted in sympathetic dysfunction is less than that which occurs with impaired somatic oculomotor function). (3) Enophthalmus. (4) Prolapse of the third eyelid.

Trochlear Nerve

Disorders of this nerve or its central nuclei rarely produce clinical signs in animals. There may be a slight dorsomedial rotation of the affected eye due to paresis or paralysis of the superior oblique muscle.

Trigeminal Nerve

The trigeminal nerve is both motor and sensory. The motor portion innervates the muscles of mastication (temporalis, masseter, medial and lateral pterygoid, and anterior portion of the digastric; the sensory portion supplies the face, eyelids, cornea, oral cavity structures, and the mucosa of the nasal septum inside the nares.

Sensory Tests

(1) Maxillary/ophthalmic reflex: stimulation of the cutaneous skin receptors with a needle over the maxillary and periorbital area will result in a blink reflex of the tested side. (2) Corneal reflex: stimulation of the cornea with a moistened cotton swab will induce an ipsilateral blink reflex. (3) Palpebral reflex: stimulation of the margins of the palpebral fissure will also produce an ipsilateral blink response.

All of the above tests are mediated via the trigeminal (V) nerve (sensory), and the facial (VII) nerve (motor).

The menace reaction (via cranial nerves II and VII) may be elicited if these tests are performed too aggressively.

Sensory Abnormalities

(1) Absence of the previously mentioned reflexes. (2) Hypoalgesia or analgesia of the affected side. (3) Hyperesthesia (a trigeminal neuralgia-like syndrome) with intense discomfort induced by mild sensory stimulation.

Motor Tests

Open and close the dog's mouth and note the resistance. Normal trigeminal nerve motor control will be evident by resistance to opening the mouth. Palpate the temporalis and masseter muscles for evidence of atrophy or fibrosis.

Motor Abnormalities

(1) Inability to close the jaws, as seen in the early phase of bilateral trigeminal motor paralysis, e.g., rabies. (2) Restricted range of jaw mobility, usually seen in the chronic stages of trigeminal paralysis with associated muscle fibrosis. (3) Trismus (tetanus).

Abducent Nerve

The abducent nerve is the remaining cranial nerve associated with extrinsic ocular muscle innervation. This nerve supplies the lateral rectus muscle and the retractor bulbi muscle.

Abnormalities

(1) Medial strabismus of the affected side. (2) Impaired abduction of the globe of the affected side.

Facial Nerve

This nerve supplies motor innervation to the muscles of facial expression and the posterior portion of the digastric muscle. It also supplies the anterior two-thirds of the tongue for taste sensation and all major exocrine glands of the head (lacrimation, salivation) except the parotid.

Tests

(1) The menace response (nerves II and VII). (2) Maxillary/ophthalmic, corneal, and palpebral reflexes (nerves V and VII).

Abnormalities

(1) Inability to close the eye. (2) Paresis or paralysis of the lip commissure of the affected side. (3) Impaired auricular movement on the affected side. (4) Widening of the palpebral fissure on the affected side.

Clinical signs will depend upon the level of the lesion. If the lesion is external to the stylomastoid foramen the above signs will be seen; however, if it is more centrally located (at or before the level of the geniculate ganglion in the genu of the facial canal), these signs together with reduced or absent lacrimation will lead to dryness of the eye with potential keratitis sicca of the cornea.

Trauma to the facial nerve where it curves around the mandible is the most common cause of facial paralysis. Extension of inflammatory conditions from the external to the middle ear may also involve the facial nerve. Occasionally, space-occupying lesions (tumors) in the pons may be responsible for facial paralysis. When this occurs, however, usually some other cranial nerve abnormality will be seen as well.

Vestibulocochlear Nerve

This nerve has two subdivisions and serves two functions. The cochlear nerve serves in a sensory capacity for hearing, and the vestibular nerve is proprioceptive for equilibrium and posture control.

Cochlear Nerve

TESTS. (1) Clapping the hands behind the head of the animal. Normally, the animal responds by turning the head toward the source of sound, blinking the eyes, and moving the ears. (2) Electroencephalographic audiometry is a test which is more definitive for a partial auditory impairment (see Chapter 6).

ABNORMALITIES. (1) Lack of startle response or turning toward the source of the sound. The clapping test is less objective than the electroencephalographic test.

Vestibular Nerve

The vestibular system of each side consists of the end organs (utricle, saccule, and three semicircular canals), the vestibular nerve, and four brain stem nuclei, all of which govern primarily ocular responses, head and neck, and trunk and limb posture.

TESTS. (1) Rapid movement of the head in the horizontal and vertical planes, normally produces a physiological nystagmus in each plane. (2) Caloric test—the installation of cold or warm water into the ear canal for 3 to 5 minutes—will produce physiological nystagmus. (3) Postrotatory nystagmus test. This test is conducted by spinning the animal on a rotatable object such as a swivel chair for 30 to 60 seconds and then stopping suddenly. Upon cessation of rotation a nystagmus will appear with the fast component toward the direction opposite that of body rotation. (4) Vestibular righting test. To perform this test the animal is supported by the pelvis and held suspended for a period of 20 to 30 seconds. The normal response noted is fore limb extension, the head held at approximately a 45 degree angle with the nose directed vertically (Fig. 3–6).

ABNORMALITIES. (1) Lack of induction of physiologic nystagmus. (2) Spontaneous nystagmus—vertical, horizontal, or oscillating. In the dog the most common type is horizontal. It may have an equal rate of ocular movement in each direction, (pendular nystagmus), or it may be unequal with fast-slow components (jerking nystagmus). In jerking nystagmus the direction of the quick phase is by convention the direction of the nystagmus. In vestibular disorders the direction of the quick phase is opposite the side of involvement. In these disorders the slow component is abnormal, and the fast phase is compensatory. The nystagmus may be present at rest, or it may be induced by manipulation of the head (positional nystagmus). (3) Head tilt toward the side of the vestibular disease (ipsilateral). (4) Falling or rolling or both (ipsilateral). (5) Tight circling toward the side of the lesion. (6) Vestibular strabismus on the same side as the abnormality. This is a ventrolateral strabismus which may be apparent when the head is dorsally extended.

Diseases of the flocculonodular lobe of the cerebellum may simulate the vestibular signs mentioned earlier.

Glossopharyngeal Nerve

The glossopharyngeal nerve innervates the musculature of the pharyngeal and palatine structures, and the parotid gland, and provides sensory innervation to the posterior third of the tongue (taste).

Test

Gag reflex. When pressure is applied externally to the pharyngeal area, swallowing is the normal response. This reflex can also be initiated by direct digital pharyngeal stimulation.

Abnormalities

(1) Absence of gag reflex. (2) Reduced pharyngeal tone. (3) Dysphagia.

Vagus Nerve

The vagus nerve has many functions, both somatic and visceral. The sensory and motor functions are similar to those of the glossopharyngeal nerve with regard to swallowing and the gag reflex. Vocalization and sensory innervation of the skin of the external ear are somatic functions of the vagus. The autonomic function of the vagus is cardioregulation and innervation of the thoracic and abdominal viscera. In tests for glossopharyngeal nerve function, the vagus is also involved.

Tests

(1) Gag reflex. (2) Laryngeal reflex. Moderate external pressure over the laryngeal area normally results in a slight coughing response. (3) Oculocardiac reflex. Direct pressure applied to both eyeballs simultaneously results in reflex bradycardia (this reflex is mediated by cranial nerves V and X).

Abnormalities

(1) Absence of the above reflexes. (2) Dysphagia. (3) Altered vocalization. (4) In bilateral vagal disorders cardiopulmonary and gastrointestinal signs may also be noted.

Spinal Accessory Nerve

This nerve supplies innervation to certain muscles of the neck (trapezius, sternomastoid, cleidomastoid, omotransversarius, and cleidocervicalis).

Tests

Muscle tone assessment of these muscles by palpation and flexion of the head and neck.

Abnormalities

(1) Muscle atrophy. (2) Torticollis in chronic unilateral disorders.

The incidence of pure, bilateral damage to the spinal accessory nerve or nucleus is exceedingly rare.

Hypoglossal Nerve

The hypoglossal nerve is the motor nerve to the musculature of the tongue.

Test

Manual stretching of the tongue induces a voluntary retraction.

Abnormalities

(1) Lack of retraction in response to stretch. (2) Lateral deviation of the tongue; in the early stage of unilateral hypoglossal paralysis, the deviation is on the side opposite the lesion (flaccid paralysis of the muscles of the diseased side enables the contralateral muscles to act unopposed). In chronic paralysis, atrophy and fibrotic contraction result in a corregated appearance of the tongue, and the deviation occurs on the affected side.

MUSCLE TONE

Muscle tonus depends primarily upon the integrity of the muscle spindles and their segmetal connections, and on the influence of higher facilitory centers (reticular formation and vestibular nuclei) and inhibitory centers (red nucleus, cerebral cortex, and reticular formation).

Tests

(1) Passive manipulation of limbs (flexion and extension). (2) Individual muscle palpation (paraspinal, appendicular, etc.). Normal response to manipulation is an increase in resistance. Normal muscles exhibit a degree of resilience and tension when palpated (normotonia).

Abnormalities

(1) Absence of tone (atonia). (2) Reduced tone (hypotonia). (3) Increased tone (hypertonia). (4) Exaggerated tone (spasticity/clasp-knife effect). The first two abnormalities represent "deficiency" phenomena characteristic of lower motor neuron (LMN) disease. Neurogenic segmental muscular atrophy may be associated with these signs. Hypertonia and spasticity are "release" phenomena characteristic of disorders involving upper motor neuron (UMN) pathways.

SPINAL CORD REFLEXES

Spinal reflexes form the basic unit of CNS integration and function. In most cases reflex testing does not test any other portion of the CNS except those cord segments in which the reflexes are involved. It should be realized that all reflexes are influenced by higher centers of control.

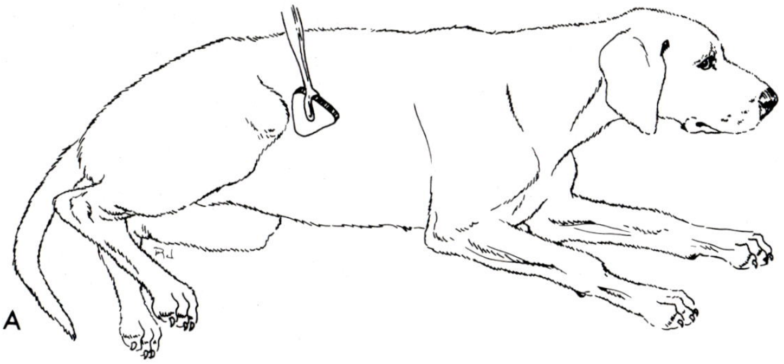
A

FIGURE 3–9 Patellar reflex (knee jerk)—a myotatic reflex. *A*. The straight patellar ligament is lightly tapped, using a percussion hammer. A normal response is a quick extension of the stifle joint. *B*. Mechanism of reflex. Muscle spindle receptors are activated to elicit this reflex. Afferent pathways (solid line) terminate in monosynaptic spinal cord reflex centers. Efferent impulses (dotted line) originate in the motor neurons of the spinal cord, causing extensor muscles that were originally stretched to contract, extending the stifle joint.

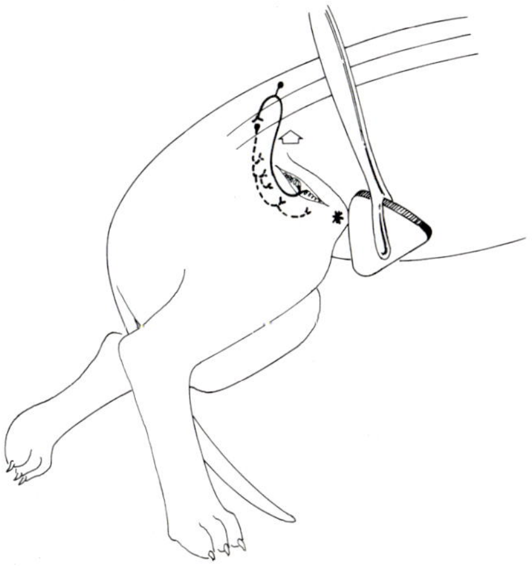
B

These reflexes may be elicited when the animal is either in a lateral recumbent position or supported upright by an assistant. When the animal is supported, it may become excited, and this will interfere with the reactions. The animal must be relaxed if the reflexes are to be elicited in their normal form. It is best to start with the reflexes least likely to disturb the animal and then proceed to those initiated by pain. Spinal reflexes are more easily elicited in the larger breeds.

Tendon Reflexes (Myotatic)

Tendon reflexes are initiated by stimulation of muscle spindle activity through muscle stretch.

PATELLAR REFLEX. The patellar reflex is the most reliable tendon reflex in the dog and is mediated via the cord segments L4 to L6.

Tests. With the hind limb in a relaxed, semiflexed position, the straight patellar ligament is lightly tapped with a percussion hammer (Fig. 3–9 *A* and *B*). The normal response is a quick extension of the stifle joint.

Abnormalities. (1) Absence of response (areflexia). (2) Depressed response (hyporeflexia). (3) Increased response (hyperreflexia). (4) Repetitive response (clonus). As in assessment of muscle tone, the first two abnormal reflexes are seen with LMN disorders, while increased reflexes are usually seen with UMN involvement.

GASTROCNEMIUS REFLEX. This reflex is mediated via tibial branches of the sciatic nerve and cord segments L5 to L7 and S1. Using the reflex hammer, a sharp tap is applied to the examiner's forefinger, which is placed over the gastrocnemius tendon. The normal response is a reflex extension of the hock, followed by flexion.

Abnormalities. Same as those for the patellar reflex.

BICIPITAL AND TRICIPITAL REFLEXES. In the front limb these reflexes can be elicited in dogs that are lying relaxed in a lateral recumbent position.

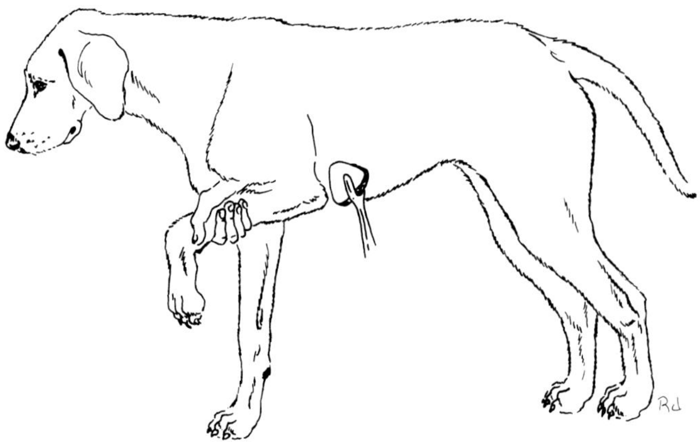

FIGURE 3–10 Tricipital reflex. The tendon of the insertion of the triceps muscle proximal to the olecranon is lightly tapped, using a percussion hammer. The normal response is a slight extension of the elbow.

The bicipital reflex is mediated by the musculocutaneous nerve and cord segments C6 to C8.

Test. Tap the distal end of the bicipital and brachial muscles at the level of the elbow. A slight flexion of the elbow will occur in a normal animal.

The tricipital reflex is mediated by the radial nerve and cord segments C7–8 and T1–2.

Test. Tap the tendon of insertion of the triceps proximal to the olecranon (Fig. 3–10). The normal response is a slight extension of the elbow.

At times it is difficult to see these fore limb reflex reactions; however, if the respective muscles are palpated during the test, the contraction may be felt.

Abnormalities. Same as those for the tendon reflexes.

Flexor Reflexes

The flexor reflexes are initiated by painful stimuli and determine the integrity of the reflex arc and the spinal cord centers, as well as the pathways in the CNS that are concerned with the patient's response to a painful stimulus.

The *hind limb flexor reflex* is mediated by the sciatic nerve and its branches and by cord segments L5–7 and S1.

The *fore limb flexor reflex* is mediated by the axillary, musculocutaneous, and medial/ulnar nerves and by cord segments C6–8 and T1–2.

TEST. Stimulation of pain receptors by compression of foot pads (Fig. 3–11), interdigital tissue, or the nail-skin junction results in reflex flexion of the appropriate limb. Intense stimulation will result in vocalization and turning of the head toward the stimulus (see section on pain perception).

ABNORMALITIES. (1) Areflexia. (2) Hyporeflexia. (3) Hyperreflexia. (4) Clonus. (5) Crossed extensor reflex.

Crossed Extensor Reflex

When a painful stimulus is applied to one limb, the opposite (contralateral) limb will extend. The crossed extensor reflex is

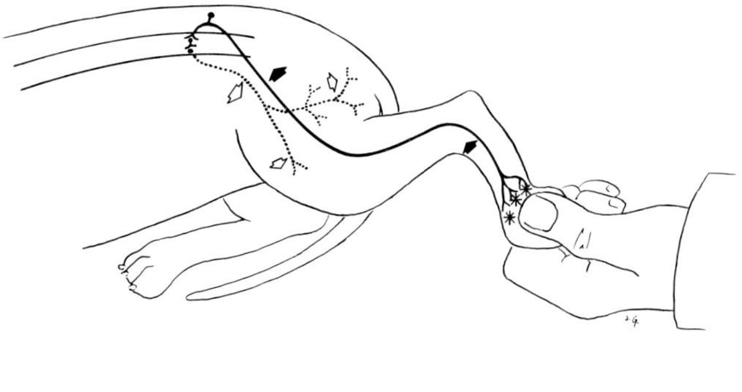

FIGURE 3–11 The flexor reflex (toepinch). Pain receptors are activated to elicit this reflex. Afferent pathways (solid line) terminate in multisynaptic spinal cord reflex centers. Efferent impulses (dotted line) originate in the spinal cord centers to cause contraction of the flexor muscles, resulting in withdrawal of the limb. Pain impulses are also transmitted to the thalamus via the lateral spinothalamic tracts (not shown on diagram). Voluntary withdrawal of the limb may also occur as a result of impulses from the higher centers.

not seen in a normal animal. Its presence is indicative of spinal cord pathology above the spinal cord segments controlling the reflex, and it is associated with an absence of contralateral inhibition.

Panniculus Reflex

The panniculus reflex tests the integrity of the innervation of the musculature of the subcutaneous trunk. The afferent limb of this reflex is mediated via the segmental sensory nerves, and the efferent component is mediated via C8 and T1 motor nerves.

TEST. A tactile stimulus is applied to the dorsal midline of the thoracolumbar region with a sharp, pointed instrument. The normal response is a reflex contraction of the subcutaneous musculature at the point of stimulation.

ABNORMALITIES. (1) Absent/depressed reflex caudal to the level of a spinal lesion. (2) Exaggerated response at the level of or immediately above the area of cord involvement.

Anal Reflex

The anal reflex is mediated via the pudendal nerve and cord segments S1–3.

TEST. (1) Tactile stimulation of the perianal region. (2) Compression of the glans of the penis in males. The normal response is a contraction of the external anal sphincter.

ABNORMALITIES. (1) Areflexia. (2) Hyporeflexia.

SENSORY EVALUATION

Sensory pathways include all the structures leading from a peripheral field of stimulation to the cerebral cortex. With the exception of olfaction, all sensory pathways include the sense organs, peripheral nerves, dorsal root ganglia, ascending tracts in the CNS, synapses in the thalamus, and thalamocortical radiations. Sensory pathways include those of both general and special senses (olfactory, visual, auditory, gustatory, and vestibular). General sensory pathways mediate (1) the primitive (protopathic) sensations—pain, temperature, and crude touch and pressure via the spinothalamic tracts, and (2) discriminative (epicritic) sensations—fine touch-pressure and kinesthetic senses via the dorsal column system. These pathways transmit conscious sensations to the higher centers. In animals objective sensory evaluation is limited to the modalities of pain and perhaps kinesthesia (proprioception). Pathways that do not mediate conscious sensations, e.g., those to the cerebellum (spinocerebellar tracts), are extremely difficult to evaluate in animals. Apart from conscious proprioception (the tests for which have already been given in the section on postural reactions), evaluation of the sensory system in

TABLE 3–4 DERMOTOMAL ASSESSMENT

	Dermotomal Area	Sensory Nerve	Brain Stem/Spinal Cord Segments
Head	Face, nasal/oral cavities	Sensory trigeminal	Pons–medulla, upper cervical cord
Pectoral limb	Dorsal surface of paw	Radial	C7-8, T1-2
	Palmar surface of paw	Median and ulnar	C8, T1-2
	Craniolateral surface of forearm	Radial	C7-8, T1-2
	Caudal surface of forearm	Ulnar	C8, T1-2
	Medial surface of forearm	Musculocutaneous	C6-8
	Lateral surface of brachium	Axillary	C6-8
Pelvic limb	Dorsal/cranial surface of paw, hock, stifle	Peroneal	L5-7, S1
	Plantar surface of paw	Tibial	L5-7, S1
	Medial surface of paw, hock, stifle, thigh	Saphenous	L4-6
	Caudolateral surface of hock, stifle, thigh	Sciatic	L5-7, S1
Trunk	Paraspinal surface	Spinal	C1-S1
Perineal	Perianal	Pudendal	S1-3
Tail	Dorsal, ventral, lateral	Coccygeal	Cy1-(n)

animals is largely dependent upon tests for pain perception.

Test

Stimulation of superficial and deep pain receptors by compression.

Normal Response

Retraction of the limb, head recoil, vocalization, turning of the head toward the site of stimulus.

Abnormalities

(1) Absence of pain (analgesia). (2) Reduced pain sensation (hypalgesia). (3) Increased pain sensation (hyperalgesia). (4) Muscle spasm (e.g., paraspinal) and restricted range of joint mobility (e.g., cervical articulating articulations). In certain circumstances when light touch (tactile stimulation) evokes an exaggerated localized cutaneous response, it seems appropriate to term this response "hyperesthetic." Testing for pain perception over recognized dermatiomal areas will provide useful information about the integrity of the sensory nerves and associated cord segments and brain stem nuclei (see Table 3–4).

REFERENCES

1. Clark, C. H.: Basic concepts in neurologic diagnostics. In Hoerlein, B. F. (ed.): *Canine Neurology.* 1st ed. Philadelphia. W. B. Saunders Company, 1965.
2. de Lahunta, A.: Small animal neurologic examination. Vet. Clin. N. Amer. *1*, 191, 1971.
3. Knecht, C. D., and Small, E.: Clinical neurology. In Catcott, E. J. (ed.), *Canine Medicine.* American Veterinary Publications, Inc., Santa Barbara, California, 1968.
4. McGrath, J. T.: *Neurologic Examination of the Dog.* Philadelphia, Lea & Febiger, 1956.
5. Oliver, J. E.: Neurologic examinations. Vet. Med. Small Anim. Clin. *67*, 433–434, 654, 658, 882–884, 1105–1106, 1327–1328, 1972; *68*, 151–154, 383–385, 763, 1973; *69*, 295–298, 607–610, 1974.
6. Palmer, A. C.: *Introduction to Animal Neurology.* Philadelphia, F. A. Davis Company, 1965.
7. Redding, R. W.: Neurological examination. In Hoerlein, B. F. (ed.): *Canine Neurology,* 2d ed. Philadelphia, W. B. Saunders Company, 1971.
8. Redding, R. W.: Neurological examination. In Ettinger, S. J. (ed.): *Textbook of Veterinary Internal Medicine.* Philadelphia, W. B. Saunders Company, 1975.

CHAPTER 4

LOCALIZATION OF LESIONS IN THE NERVOUS SYSTEM

J. E. OLIVER, JR., D.V.M., M.S., PH.D.

NEUROLOGICAL DIAGNOSIS

The complexity of clinical signs, history, and laboratory data which may be compiled on an individual patient can make the diagnosis of a disease seem to be impossible. Weed[87] has demonstrated the value of listing all of the problems of the patient and analyzing each of them independently. There is a minimum amount of data which is necessary to solve any medical problem. The actual amount of data to be gathered may be modified because of risk, cost, or accessibility as opposed to the severity of the disease. Priorities can be established for collection of data which will rule out the most probable causes of a given clinical sign early while reserving until last tests for rare diseases.

Weed's problem oriented system is eminently suited for neurological diagnosis. The steps necessary for diagnosis of a neurological problem are listed in Table 4-1.

TABLE 4-1 OUTLINE OF NEUROLOGICAL DIAGNOSIS

Collect minimum data base
Identify problems
Identify one or more problems related to nervous system
Localize level of lesion
Estimate extent of lesion within that level
Determine cause or pathology
Determine prognosis with and without therapy

MINIMUM DATA BASE

The initial evaluation of a patient with neurological signs, including the history and physical examination, will usually provide evidence of a neurological problem (Table 4-2). Some problems are difficult to classify—for example, syncope versus convulsions, or weakness versus paresis. The initial physical examination of every patient should include a screening neurological examination designed to detect the presence of neurological abnormality in most cases. This examination should include (1) observation of mental status, gait, and posture; (2) superficial examination of cranial nerves II (vision), III (pupils), V (sensation of face, ability to open and close the mouth), and VII (facial expression, palpebral reflex); (3) proprioception of all four limbs; (4) placing reactions; and (5) hopping reactions (see Chapter 3). Most of these tests are performed in the course of a routine physical examination. Animals that have no abnormalities in this examination rarely have other neurological deficits.

The minimum data base recommended for an animal with a neurological problem is shown in Table 4-3. The chemistry pro-

TABLE 4-2 CLINICAL PROBLEMS IN THE NERVOUS SYSTEM

Problem	*Localization*
Usually CNS origin	
1. Convulsions	1. Cerebrum, diencephalon
2. Altered mental status	2. Cerebrum, limbic system
a. Stupor or coma	a. Brain stem reticular formation
b. Behavior	b. Limbic system
3. Paresis, paralysis	3. See Tables 4–5 and 4–7
4. Proprioceptive deficit	4. Similar to UMN—see Tables 4–5 and 4–7
5. Ataxia	5.
a. Head tilt, nystagmus	a. Vestibular system
b. Intention tremor, dysmetria	b. Cerebellum
c. Proprioceptive deficit, no head involvement	c. Spinal cord
6. Hypesthesia, analgesia	6. See Figure 4–4, cranial nerve V
Possible CNS origin	
1. Syncope	1. Usually cardiovascular or metabolic
2. Weakness	2. See Tables 4–5 and 4–7; metabolic or muscular
3. Lameness	3. Orthopedic—see Table 4–4
4. Pain, hyperesthesia	4.
a. Generalized	a. Thalamus, meningitis
b. Localized	b. See Fig. 4–4, cranial nerve V
5. Blindness	5.
a. Pupils normal	a. Occipital cortex (contralateral)
b. Pupils abnormal	b. See Fig. 4–10
6. Hearing deficit	6.
a. No vestibular signs	a. Cochlea
b. Vestibular signs	b. Cranial nerve VIII, labyrinth
7. Anosmia	7. Nasal passages, cranial nerve I
8. Visceral dysfunction	8. See Chapter 2

file is recommended if automated analysis is available so that cost is not a major factor. Otherwise, these chemical tests should be selected according to the problems present. Additional tests will be recommended for specific problems.

PROBLEM LIST

A problem list is formulated from information in the minimum data base. For each problem a diagnostic plan is developed. A diagnostic plan for a neurological problem includes the following steps. (1) Localize the level of the lesion with a neurological examination. Confirmation of the lesion may require survey or contrast radiography. (2) Estimate the extent of the lesion both longitudinally and transversely. The neurological examination provides most of this information, but ancillary diagnostic procedures may be of assistance. (3) Determine the cause of the pathological process involved. The history is useful in establishing the class of disease (e.g., neoplasia, infectious disease, trauma).[64] Laboratory, radiographic, or electrophysiologic tests may be necessary to substantiate the diagnosis. From this information the clinician can establish a prognosis with and without appropriate therapy based on what is known about the disease (Table 4–1).

TABLE 4-3 MINIMUM DATA BASE: NEUROLOGICAL PROBLEM

History
Physical examination
Neurological examination
Clinical pathology
CBC
Urinalysis
Chemistry profile
BUN
SGPT
Calcium
Alkaline phosphatase
Fasting blood glucose

FUNCTIONAL ORGANIZATION OF THE NERVOUS SYSTEM

A comprehensive knowledge of the anatomy and physiology of the nervous system is very useful in clinical neurology. However, the majority of neurological problems in clinical practice can be diagnosed and managed without knowing the names of neural tracts or nuclei. This section is intended to provide a guide to the localization of lesions with minimal knowledge of neuroanatomy. Refer to Chapter 2 for details.

LOWER MOTOR NEURON AND SEGMENTAL SIGNS

The lower motor neuron (LMN) is an efferent neuron connecting the central nervous system (CNS) to an effector muscle or gland. Any activity of the nervous system must ultimately be expressed through an LMN to be recognized as a movement or secretion. The cell bodies of the LMN are located in all spinal segments in the intermediate and ventral horns of the gray matter, and in the nuclei of the cranial nerves (III, IV, VI, VII, IX, X, and XII) (see Chapters 2 and 9) in the brain stem. The axons extending from these cells form the peripheral and cranial nerves (Fig. 4–1).

Sensory neurons are located in the ganglia of the dorsal roots along the spinal cord and in the ganglia of some of the cranial nerves, with the exception of the special sensory pathways (olfaction, vision, hearing, balance).

The nervous system is arranged in a segmental fashion. A spinal cord segment is demarcated by a pair of spinal nerves, each spinal nerve having a dorsal (sensory) and a ventral (motor) root (Fig. 4–2). The brain has less uniform segmentation, but anatomically and functionally distinct segments can be identified (Fig. 4–3). The muscle or group of muscles innervated by one spinal nerve is called a myotome. Myotomes are arranged segmentally in the paraspinal muscles but are more irregular in the limbs. Comparison of clinically affected groups of muscles with tables of distribution of spinal nerves can be used to localize a lesion of a spinal nerve or ventral root.

The area of skin innervated by one spinal nerve is called a dermatome. Dermatomes are also arranged in a regular, segmental fashion except on the limbs, where there is some variation (Fig. 4–4). Alterations in sensation of a dermatome can be used to localize a lesion of a spinal nerve or dorsal root.

Lesions of the LMN, whether of the cell body or the axon, produce a characteristic group of clinical signs. LMN signs include (1) paralysis of the muscles innervated, (2) areflexia, (3) early and severe muscle atrophy (neurogenic), (4) flaccidity of muscle, loss of tone, and loss of resistance to passive manipulation, (5) electromyographic (EMG) changes after 5 to 7 days (fibrillation potentials and positive sharp waves; see Chapter 9), and (6) contracture and fibrosis of the muscles after several weeks (Table 4–4).

LMN signs are easily recognized on the

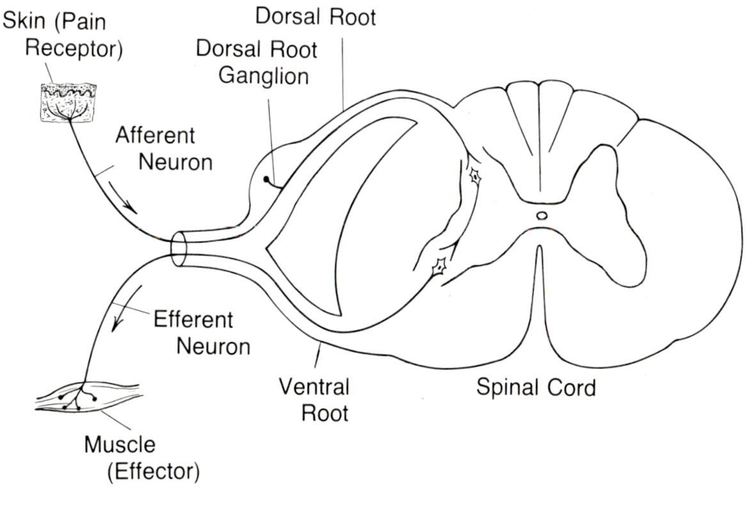

FIGURE 4–1 Schematic diagram of the neuronal pathways of the withdrawal reflex. The efferent neuron is the lower motor neuron (LMN).

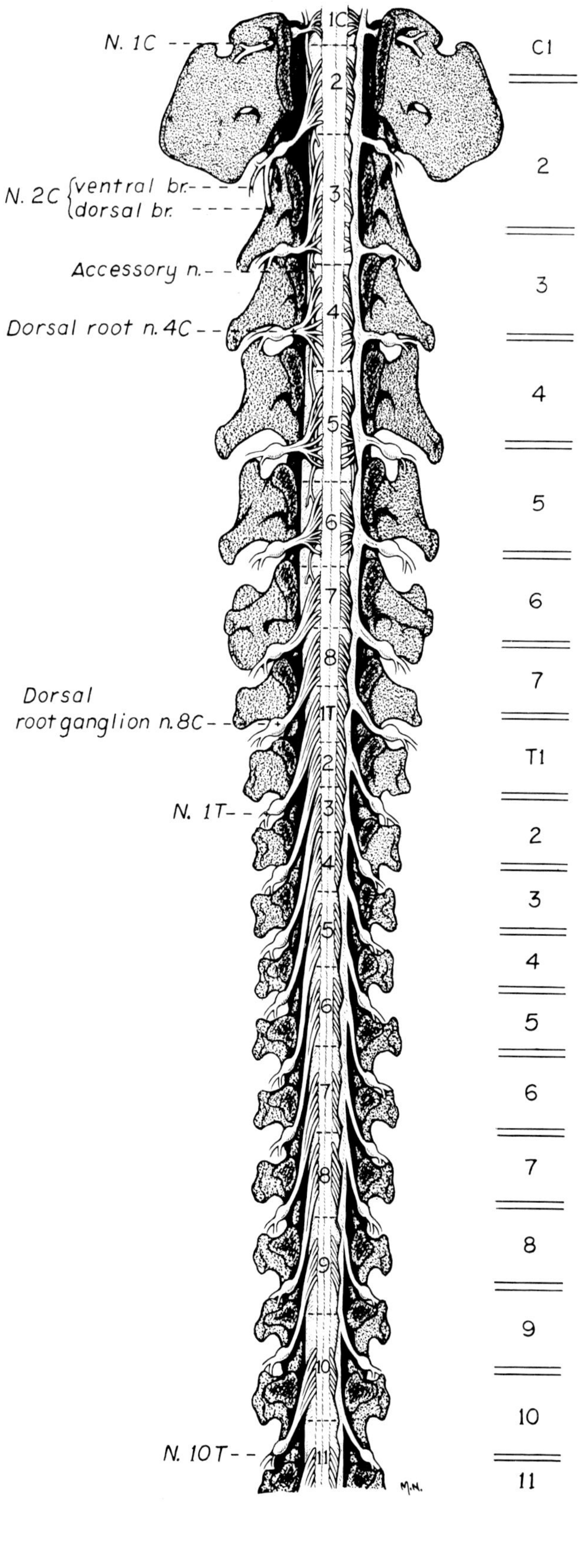

FIGURE 4–2 *A.* Dorsal roots of spinal nerves and spinal cord segments, cervical 1 to thoracic 11. Dorsal aspect. The dura mater has been removed except on the extreme right side. (The figures on the right represent levels of the vertebral bodies.) (From Fletcher, 1964. Thesis, University of Minnesota.)

Figure continued on opposite page

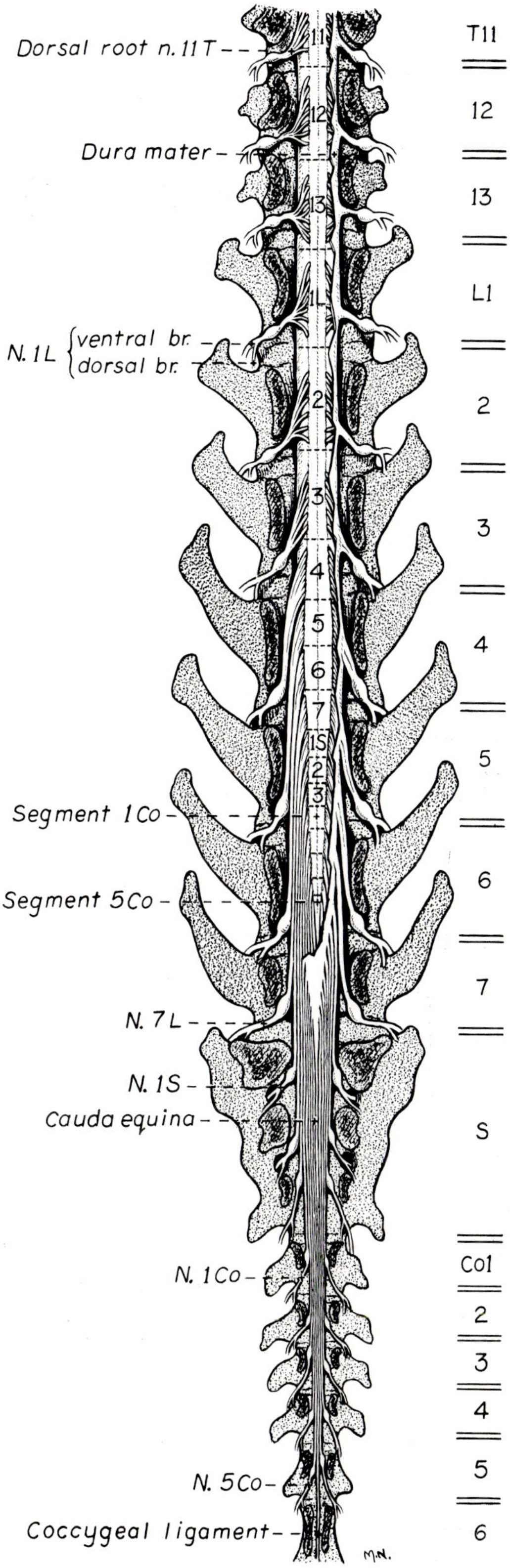

FIGURE 4–2 *B.* Dorsal roots of spinal nerves and spinal cord segments, thoracic 11 to coccygeal 5. Dorsal aspect. The dura mater has been removed except on the extreme right side. (The figures on the right represent levels of the vertebral bodies.) (From Fletcher, 1964. Thesis, University of Minnesota.)

Figure continued on following page

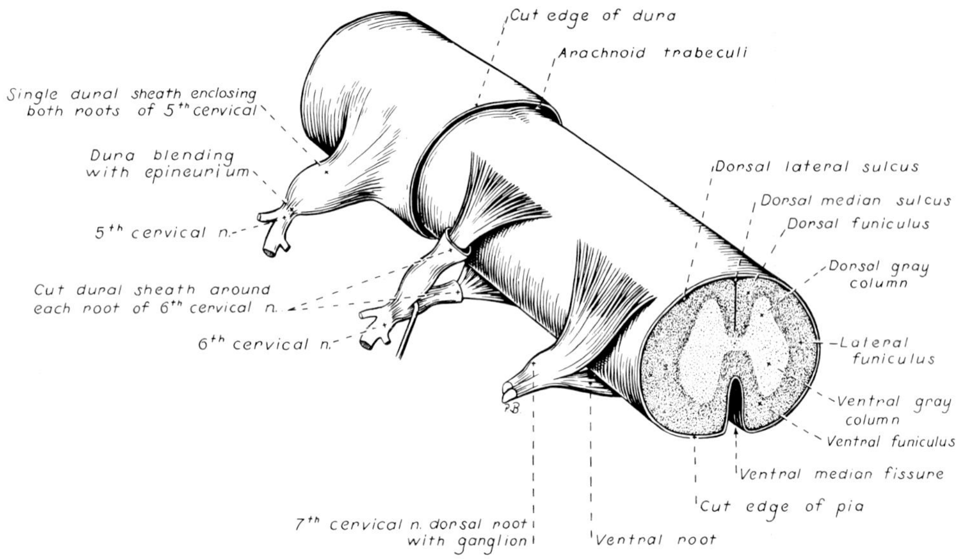

FIGURE 4–2 *C.* Cross section of spinal cord and meninges. (From Miller, M. E.: *Guide to the Dissection of the Dog.* Edwards Bros., Ann Arbor, Mich. 1952 © Dr. Malcom E. Miller.)

neurological examination. Paralysis, loss of tone, and loss of reflexes are present immediately after the neuron is damaged. LMN signs are especially significant in localizing a lesion. The differentiation of a lesion of the cell body or nerve root (spinal cord or brain stem) or of the axon (peripheral or cranial nerve) is made on the basis of distribution of signs.

Lesions of the sensory neurons also produce characteristic clinical signs. Segmental sensory signs include (1) anesthesia (complete lesion), (2) hypesthesia, or decreased sensation (partial lesion), (3) hyperesthesia, or increased sensation or pain (irritative lesion), or (4) loss of reflexes. Increased or decreased sensation of a dermatome can be mapped by pinpricking the skin (Chapter 3). With practice, lesions of sensory roots can be accurately mapped to within three spinal cord segments.[65]

UPPER MOTOR NEURON (UMN) AND LONG TRACT SIGNS

The collective term upper motor neuron (UMN) is applied to the motor systems in the brain which control the lower motor neurons. The UMN systems are responsible for initiation and maintenance of normal movements and for maintenance of tone in extensor muscles used to support the body against gravity. The cell bodies are located in the cerebral cortex, basal nuclei, and brain stem. The pathways include: the corticospinal and corticorubrospinal tracts, which are primarily responsible for voluntary motor activity, and the reticulospinal and vestibulospinal tracts, which are primarily responsible for muscle tone and posture (see Chapter 2 for details).

Sensory pathways of clinical significance

TABLE 4–4 SUMMARY OF LMN vs. UMN SIGNS

	Lower Motor Neuron—Segmental Signs	Upper Motor Neuron—Long Tract Signs
Sensory	Anesthesia of innervated area (dermatome); paresthesia or hyperesthesia of adjacent areas	Decreased proprioception; decreased perception of superficial pain and deep pain
Motor	Paralysis—loss of muscle power, flaccidity; loss of muscle tone	Paresis to paralysis; loss of voluntary movements
Muscle atrophy	Early and severe: neurogenic	Late and mild: disuse
Reflexes	Areflexia	Hyperreflexia, especially myotatic reflexes

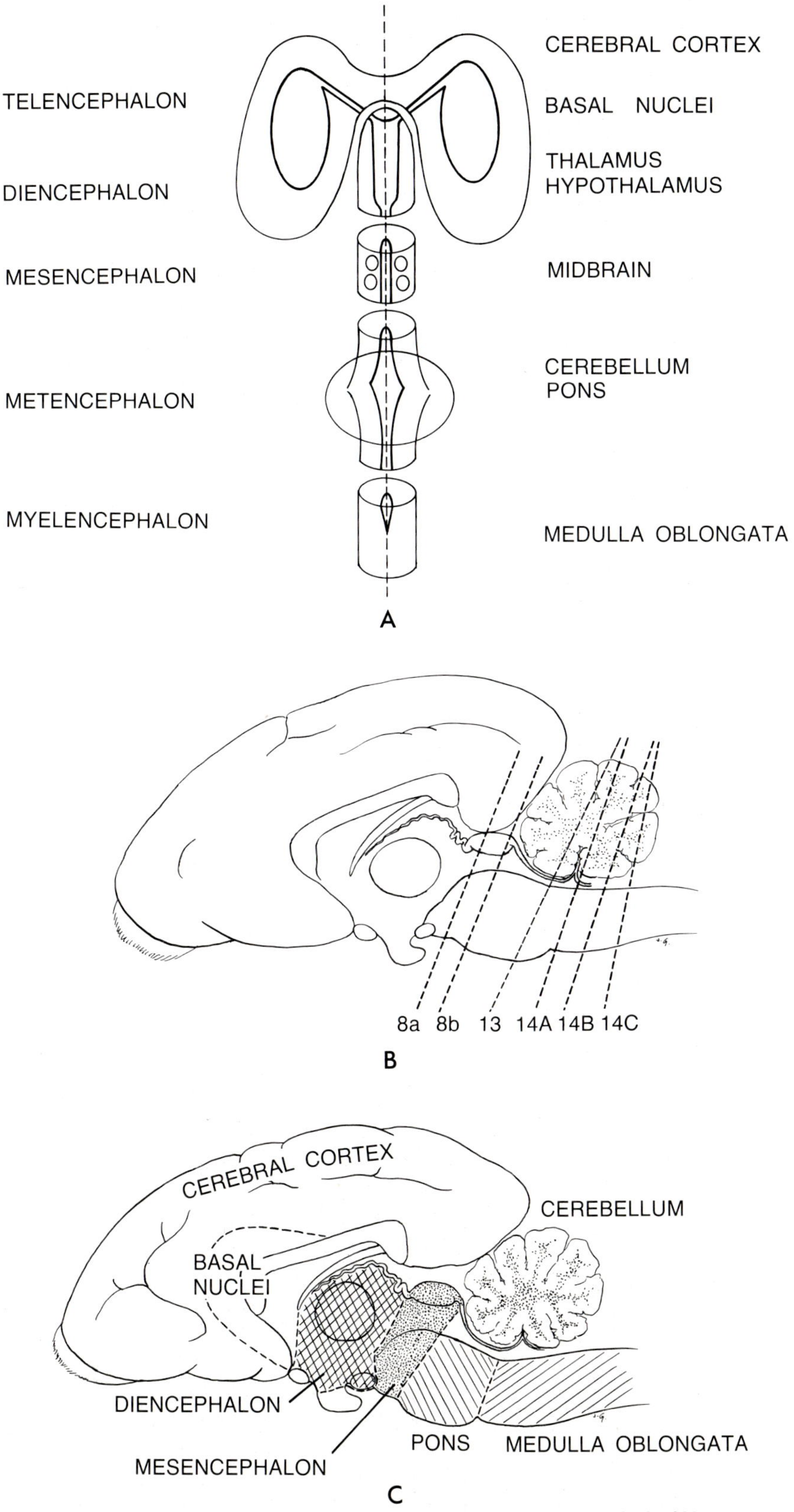

FIGURE 4–3 Subdivisions of the brain. ([*A*] modified from Elliott, H. C.: *Textbook of Neuroanatomy.* J. B. Lippincott Co., Philadelphia, 1963.)

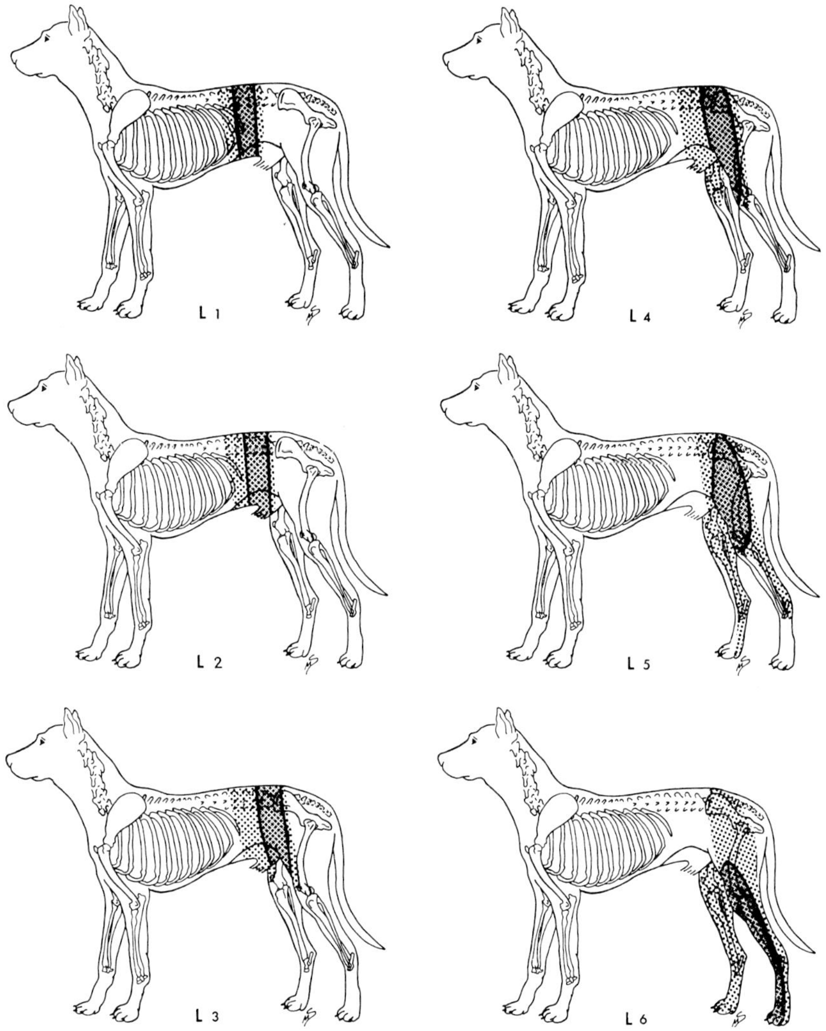

FIGURE 4–4 The tactile dermatomes are illustrated in relation to skeletal landmarks. Superimposed on the most common distribution for each dermatome is the region of maximal innervation (darker area) depicted on the lateral surface only, through it continued symmetrically to the ventral (or medial) surface. The maximal innervation zones were not prominent caudal to S_1. (From Fletcher, T. F., and Kitchell, R.: The lumbar, sacral, and coccygeal dermatomes of the dog. J. Comp. Neurol. *128*, 171, 1966.)

Figure continued on opposite page

include those responsible for proprioception (position sense) and pain. Sensory neurons from the body are located in the dorsal root ganglia and synapse in the spinal cord gray matter (Fig. 4–1). Proprioceptive pathways are found in the dorsal and dorsolateral portions of the spinal cord. Relays are present in the brain stem and thalamus before projecting to the cerebellum and cerebral cortex. Superficial pain pathways (discrete pain, pin prick, skin pain) are primarily located in the ventrolateral portion of the spinal cord with a relay in the thalamus.[34] The pathway ultimately extends to the cerebral cortex for conscious recognition of pain. The deep pain pathway (which includes severe or crushing pain and joint, bone, or visceral pain) is a bilateral, multisynaptic system which projects to the reticular formation, thalamus, and cerebral cortex.[6, 37]

Lesions of the UMN, whether of the origin of the pathway in the brain or of some portion of the tract in the brain or spinal cord, produce a characteristic group of clinical signs. UMN signs include: (1)

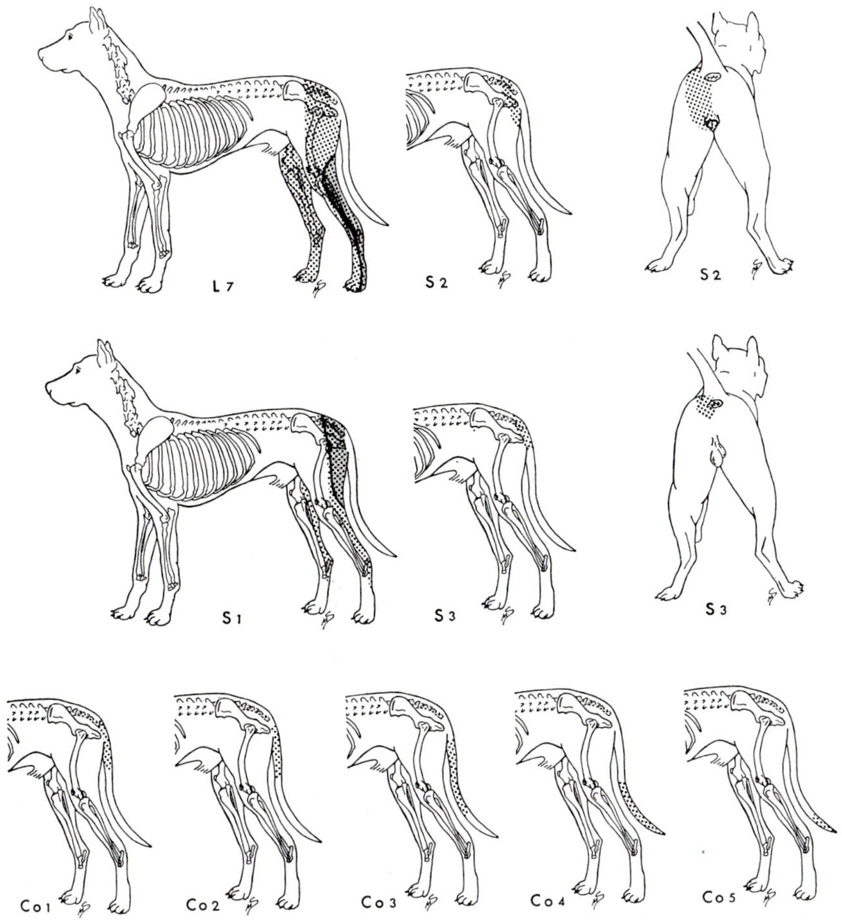

FIGURE 4–4 *Continued.*

paresis or paralysis of voluntary motor function, (2) intact, often hyperactive spinal reflexes, (3) increased tone in extensor muscles (spasticity), and (4) abnormal reflexes, e.g., crossed extensor reflex or extensor toe response (Table 4–4). UMN signs are present caudal to the level of the lesion.

UMN signs are more common than LMN signs in neurologic diseases. They are not as useful in localizing a lesion as LMN signs, but localization to a *region* of the CNS is possible on the basis of UMN signs.

Signs of sensory long tract lesions are valuable for prognosis of CNS disorders, although they are not usually of much help in localization. Proprioceptive deficits are usually the first signs observed with compressive lesions of the spinal cord. Abnormal positioning of the feet and ataxia may be present before there is any significant loss of voluntary motor activity. Superficial pain (conscious perception of pin prick) is often lost at about the same time as voluntary motor activity. Deep pain (strong pinch of bone or joint) is the last clinically useful sign to be lost when the spinal cord is compressed.[81] Sensory long tract signs are present caudal to the level of the lesion.

LOCALIZATION OF LESIONS

MOTOR SIGNS

After the neurological examination is completed, the fore and hind limbs should be classified as normal or characterized by LMN or UMN signs (Table 4–4). Briefly, LMN signs consist of weakness, loss of reflexes, and loss of tone. UMN signs include loss of voluntary motor activity, increased tone, and exaggerated reflexes.

TABLE 4–5 LOCALIZATION OF LESIONS BASED ON MOTOR FUNCTION

- Hind limbs
  - Normal
    - Fore limbs
      - Normal
        - Normal motor function of spinal cord
      - UMN signs
        - (Rare) brain or C1–5
          - (1) *Recheck* Hind limbs, cranial nerves, other brain fn.
          - (2) Orthopedic problems
      - LMN signs
        - Brachial plexus
          - (1) See Table 4–6
          - (2) Sensory exam
  - UMN (Table 4) signs
    - Fore limbs
      - Normal
        - T2–L3
          - (1) See Fig. 4–4
      - UMN signs
        - Brain or C1–5
          - (1) Check cranial nerves exam
          - (2) Sensory
      - LMN signs
        - C6–T2
          - (1) See Table 4–6
          - (2) Sensory exam
  - LMN (Table 4) signs
    - Fore limbs
      - Normal signs
        - L4–S2
          - (1) See Table 4–6
          - (2) See Fig. 4–4
      - UMN signs
        - L4–S2 and brain or C1–5
          - Multifocal or systemic disease
      - LMN
        - L4–S2 and C6–T2
          - Complete spinal cord destruction, respiration(?) or generalized peripheral neuropathy

UMN = Upper motor neuron; LMN = lower motor neuron; C = cervical; T = thoracic; L = lumbar; S = sacral spinal cord segments.

Table 4–6 SPINAL REFLEXES

Reflex	Muscle	Peripheral Nerve	Spinal Cord Segments
Myotatic (stretch)	Biceps brachii	Musculocutaneous	C(6), 7–8, (T1)
	Triceps brachii	Radial	C7–8, T1–(2)
	Extensor carpi radialis	Radial	C7–8, T1–(2)
	Quadriceps	Femoral	L4–6
	Cranial tibial	Peroneal (sciatic)	L6–7, S1
	Gastrocnemius	Tibial	L6–7, S1
Flexion (withdrawal)	Fore limb	Radial, ulnar, median, musculocutaneous	C6–T2
	Hind limb	Sciatic	L6–S1
Perineal	Anal sphincter	Pudendal	S1–2

Localization to a region of the spinal cord or brain can be made using these findings in combination with Table 4–5. For example, the presence of UMN signs in both fore and hind limbs indicates a brain or C1–5 lesion. Table 4–5 lists, under the location of the lesion, suggested procedures to further localize the lesion. In this case, the cranial nerves should be reviewed to rule out brain stem disease, and the sensory examination should be reviewed for possible signs related to C1–5.

Using only the information related to LMN and UMN signs of the limbs it should be possible to localize the lesion to one of the following regions: (1) brain, (2) C1–5, (3) C6–T2—brachial plexus (fore limb), (4) T2–L3, (5) L4–S2-lumbosacral plexus (hind limb), (6) S1–3, (7) Cyl–5.

If LMN signs are present in the limbs, the lesion can be localized further by identifying the muscles affected. Table 4–6 lists the spinal cord segments (roots) and peripheral nerves affected in some of the most commonly tested reflexes. It may be possible to localize the lesion within two to four segments if LMN signs are present.

Spinal cord segments do not correlate directly to vertebral levels. When the spinal cord level is determined, refer to Figure 4–2 for an estimation of the vertebral level.

SENSORY SIGNS

Proprioception

For purposes of localization, abnormalities of proprioception are interpreted exactly the same as UMN signs. For example, loss of proprioception in the hind limbs with normal fore limbs indicates a lesion in the region of T2 to L3 (Table 4–5). Spinal nerve or peripheral nerve lesions may cause a loss of proprioceptive positioning, but the LMN signs should be obvious.

Pain

Hyperesthesia (increased sensitivity) is a very useful localizing sign and may be present when there is little or no motor deficit. The animal's limbs and trunk, especially the vertebral column, should be palpated and manipulated while watching for signs of pain. Obvious reactions may include vocalization or aggressive or fearful behavior. More subtle reactions may include resistance to movement and tensing of the muscles. By placing one hand on the abdomen and squeezing each vertebral segment in turn with the other a tensing of the abdominal muscles can be felt as painful areas are palpated. The skin is pricked with an 18 gauge needle after palpation is completed. The skin should be pricked gently so that there is no significant reaction in normal areas. Areas of hyperesthesia will elicit a skin twitch or a behavioral response. Pin pricking should be performed in a caudal to cranial direction, since areas below a lesion will usually have decreased sensation. Normal or increased sensation can be ascertained by these methods. If a spinal lesion is present, the sensory area affected should have the conformation of a dermatome (Fig. 4–4).[65]

The panniculus (cutaneous muscle) reflex is elicited with the needle in the same manner as that just described. The pathway of cutaneous sensation begins at the spinal cord at each segment (dermatome) and ascends to the brachial plexus (C8–T1) to the *lateral thoracic nerve*, which innervates the cutaneous trunci (panniculus carnosus) muscle. Contraction of the cutaneous muscle causes a skin twitch. A segmental lesion will block the ascending afferent stimulus, abolishing the reflex. Pin pricking the skin in a caudal to cranial direction will identify the first level at which the reflex can be elicited. This segment is normal, and the lesion will be one segment caudal to it. The superficial pain pathways must be blocked to abolish the reflex. Normally the panniculus reflex is most apparent in the thoracolumbar (saddle) area. Minimal response is obtained from a stimulus in the sacral or caudal region, and no response is obtained from a cervical stimulus.

Hypesthesia (decreased sensation) or anesthesia (no sensation) may be useful localizing signs also. Single nerve root lesions will not usually produce a clinically detectable area of decreased sensation because of the overlapping pattern of cutaneous innervation (Fig. 4–4). Multiple nerve roots may be involved in some lesions, especially in the area of the cauda equina. Lesions of the spinal cord may result in decreased perception of pain caudal to the lesion. Determination of the level of decreased sensation has already been discussed, and prognostic implications of loss of sensation will be discussed later.

In the motor examination the lesion should have been localized to one of six regions of the spinal cord or to the brain (Table 4–7). In a carefully performed sensory examination the lesion should be localized to within *three segments of the spinal cord* or to a peripheral nerve (see Chapter 9).

TABLE 4–7 SIGNS OF LESIONS IN NERVOUS SYSTEM

Cyl–5	LMN—tail
S1–3	UMN—tail
Pelvic plexus	LMN—anal sphincter, bladder
L4–S1	UMN—tail, bladder, sphincter
Lumbosacral plexus	LMN—hind limbs
T3–L3	UMN—hind limbs, bladder, sphincter LMN—segmental spinal muscles
C6–T2	UMN—hind limbs, bladder
Brachial plexus	LMN—fore limbs
C1–C6	UMN—all four limbs, bladder
Brain stem	UMN—unilteral or bilateral fore and hind limbs LMN—cranial nerves
Cerebellum	Ataxia, tremor, dysmetria Wide based stance
Vestibular system	Turning or circling Nystagmus, head tilt Ipsilateral weakness
Cerebrum	Behavior, seizures, Vision—normal pupils Placing reaction, contralateral

LOCALIZATION IN BRAIN

If the lesion was localized to the brain, the next step is to determine what part of the brain is involved. Localization to one of four regions of the brain can be made on the basis of clinical signs (Table 4–7).

1. Brain stem lesions will produce UMN signs in all four limbs (tetraparesis) or in the fore and hind limbs on one side (hemiparesis). Cranial nerve signs are produced by brain stem lesions of significant size and provide good localizing signs (LMN or sensory). Refer to Chapters 2, 3, and 8 for evaluation of the cranial nerves. Cranial nerve signs are ipsilateral to the lesion, whereas motor signs may be ipsilateral or contralateral, depending on the level and pathways involved.

2. Vestibular lesions may be central (brain stem) or peripheral (labyrinth). Clinical signs include turning or circling, nystagmus, and head tilt. Lesions of the labyrinth may involve the facial nerve.[3] Peripheral vestibular lesions usually produce horizontal or combined horizontal-rotatory nystagmus which is not altered by changes in head position. Central vestibular lesions may produce nystagmus in vertical, diagonal, or horizontal directions which is altered by changing the position of the head. UMN signs or ipsilateral weakness are frequently present with brain stem lesions.[36]

3. Cerebellar lesions may be unilateral or bilateral, depending on etiology. Characteristic signs include ataxia, wide based stance,

dysmetria, and intention tremor with little weakness. Involvement of the head differentiates cerebellar lesions from spinal tract lesions, which may produce some of these signs in the limbs. For example, dysmetria is usually recognized as "goose-stepping" in the limbs. Dysmetria of the head can be recognized as a severe head drop when the head is elevated and suddenly released, or the animal will thrust his nose too far into the water dish when drinking or may even hit the edge of the dish. Intention tremors are tremors which become much worse when the animal initiates an activity such as eating or drinking.

4. Cerebral lesions usually produce alterations in behavior or mental status, seizures, loss of vision with intact pupils, or mild hemiparesis with deficits in placing and hopping reactions. Only one or two of these signs may be present, since the cerebrum is a relatively large structure with localized functional areas. Signs are generally contralateral to the lesion.

Localization to one of the four regions of the brain is usually adequate for a clinical diagnosis. Cranial nerve signs provide positive evidence for precise localization within the brain stem. Combinations of signs also allow precise localization. Tables 4–8 and 4–9 list specific signs associated with each area, and Table 4–10 lists relatively common combinations of signs.

Clinical signs referable to several parts of the nervous system suggest diffuse or multifocal disease such as infection, metabolic disorder, or malignant neoplasia.

In the following paragraphs some of the more vital areas of the brain and the signs associated with their destruction are briefly discussed. In Table 4–2 the most common signs of CNS disease with the most probable location have already been listed. This section can be used to review other signs likely to be present if a lesion is in the area suggested by the table. The structures and references included are selective, not comprehensive. As far as possible, the material selected is that which is most likely to have some clinical application. It is important to

TABLE 4–8 LEVEL OF LESION IN THE BRAIN[a]

I. Cerebral cortex
   A. Deficiency of placing and hopping reactions (contralateral)
   B. Alteration of mental function (recognition of owner, house training)
   C. Vision impaired
   D. Seizures
   E. Hypertonia or hypotonia in extensors (contralateral)
   F. Deficiency in voluntary movements
II. Basal nuclei
   A. Deficiency of nonvisual placing and hopping reactions
   B. Adversive turning movements
   C. Hyperkinesias (unilateral or bilateral)
   D. Hypertonia in contralateral limb
III. Diencephalon
   A. Pain, generalized or contralateral; may be intermittent
   B. Hypothalamic disorders. Changes in: eating, drinking, sleeping, or sexual behavior; cardiovascular and temperature regulation; endocrine activity
   C. Visual field defects—optic tract or chiasm
IV. Midbrain
   A. Cranial nerve III or IV
   B. Spasticity, deficiency in voluntary movement
   C. Decreased sensation (contralateral)
V. Cerebellum
   A. Ataxia—incoordination of body movements, station and gait
   B. Extensor hypertonus, acute opisthotonos
   C. Chronic muscle weakness
   D. Dysmetria—tremor with movements and other disturbances of phasic movements in chronic disorder
   E. Cerebellar nystagmus
VI. Pons
   A. Cranial nerves V, VI, VII
   B. Decreased sensation (contralateral)
   C. Deficiency of voluntary movements, spasticity (may be hypotonia if caudal pons, vestibular nucleus, or fastigial nucleus is involved)
VII. Medulla oblongata
   A. Cranial nerves VIII, IX, X, XI, XII
   B. Vestibular signs
   C. Decreased sensation
   D. Hemiparesis or tetraplegia, usually decreased tonus
   E. Cardiovascular or respiratory abnormalities, or both

[a]The best evidence of the level of brain stem lesion is cranial nerve involvement. The cranial nerves listed under each level signify their possible involvement in a lesion and not necessarily the anatomical origin of the nerve. One or more of the signs listed may not be present in a particular lesion. Losses may be total or partial.

TABLE 4-9 LOCALIZATION WITHIN A REGION

- I. Cerebral cortex
  - A. Frontal lobe
    - 1. Prefrontal cortex (See Figure 4-6)
      - a. Ablation
        - (1) Medial surface – drive disinhibition
        - (2) Lobectomy – impaired delayed response (learning), hyperactivity, forced pacing, circling, inattention
    - 2. Motor cortex
      - a. Ablation – contralateral extensor hypotonus of limbs and trunk, some weakness and incoordination, poor proprioception, dysmetria, hyperative stretch reflexes, deficient placing and hopping reactions
      - b. Stimulation – movement of appropriate part (see Figs. 4-6 and 4-7). Possible Jacksonian seizure.
  - B. Parietal lobe
    - 1. Somatosensory cortex (see Fig. 4-6)
      - a. Ablation – transitory contralateral loss of tactile conditioned response
  - C. Occipital lobe
    - 1. Visual cortex (see Figs. 4-6 and 4-9)
      - a. Ablation – loss of ability for pattern discrimination, contralateral hemianopia with large lesions
  - D. Temporal lobe
    - 1. Auditory cortex (see Fig. 4-6)
      - a. Ablation – bilateral lesion required for hearing deficit (higher threshold); unilateral lesion alters auditory orientation reactions
    - 2. Deeper structures – temporal lobe seizures
- II. Basal nuclei (see Fig. 4-14)
  - A. Caudate nucleus
    - 1. Anteroventral ablation – hyperkinesia, adversive turning movements
  - B. Lesions involving several nuclei – deficiency of nonvisual placing and hopping, adversive turning movements. Bilateral lesions – choreiform movements.
- III. Thalamus
  - A. Central pain syndrome
- IV. Hypothalamus
  - A. Discrete nuclei – probably not clinically significant
  - B. Ablation – disturbance of: eating, drinking, sleeping or sexual behavior; cardiovascular and temperature regulation; endocrine activity
- V. Midbrain (see Fig. 4-15)
  - A. Cranial nerves III and IV and nucleus of Edinger-Westphal
    - 1. Ablation (see Chapter 8)
  - B. Rostral colliculus
    - 1. Ablation – impairment of visual orientation reactions

- V. Midbrain (Continued)
  - C. Pretectal area
    - 1. Ablation – oculomotor and pupillary changes
  - D. Tegmentum
    - 1. Mass – obstructs cerebral aqueduct, produces hydrocephalus
    - 2. Ablation – large lesions produce coma and decerebrate rigidity. Smaller lesions, destroying medial longitudinal fasciculus, alter vestibular origin eye movements. May produce cerebellar signs due to disruption of cerebro-cerebellar pathways.
  - E. Crus cerebri
    - 1. Ablation – contralateral deficiency of voluntary movements, deficiency of placing and hopping reactions
- VI. Pons
  - A. Cranial nerves IV, V, VI, VII (see Chapter 8)
  - B. Tegmentum
    - 1. Large rostral lesion – coma, loss of micturition reflex, decerebrate rigidity
    - 2. Caudal lesion – may be conscious, spastic, or flaccid, depending on extent of lesion
    - 3. Smaller lesions – cerebellar signs due to disruption of cerebro-cerebellar pathways
- VII. Cerebellum
  - A. Total ablation
    - 1. Acute – opisthotonos, extensor hypertonus of the fore limbs, incoordination of movements, clonic spasms of hind limbs
    - 2. Chronic – ataxia, incoordination, dysmetria, wide based stance
  - B. Unilateral
    - 1. Falls to affected side, ipsilateral signs as above
  - C. Flocculonodular lobes
    - 1. Vestibular signs – head tilt, turning, nystagmus
- VIII. Medulla oblongata
  - A. Cranial nerves VI, VII, IX, X, XI, XII (see Table 4-10 and Chapter 8)
  - B. Vestibular system
    - 1. Nerve – ipsilateral head tilt and weakness of limbs, abnormal righting reflex, abnormal caloric response
    - 2. Nucleus – ipsilateral head tilt, turning, rolling, weakness of limbs, nystagmus. Contralateral extensor hypertonus. Abnormal righting reflexes, abnormal postrotation nystagmus and caloric response.
    - 3. Nucleus or medial longitudinal fasciculus – abnormal eye movements
  - C. Large lesions
    - 1. Flaccid tetraplegia, loss of micturition reflex, abnormal cardiovascular response, abnormal respiration, death

TABLE 4–10 LOCALIZATION BY COMBINATION OF SIGNS

I. Near cribriform plate
   A. *Signs*—anosmia, blindness, no pupillary reflex, mental changes
   B. *Anatomy*—cranial nerves I, II, frontal lobe
II. Pituitary fossa
   A. *Signs*—blindness or visual field defects, no pupillary reflexes. Hypothalamic signs: changes in: eating, drinking, sleeping, or sexual behavior, cardiovascular and temperature regulation; endocrine activity
   B. *Anatomy*—optic chiasm, oculomotor nerve, hypothalamus
III. Ventrolateral posterior fossa
   A. *Signs*—ipsilateral: head tilt, circling, weakness, nystagmus, depressed reflexes in extensor muscles, abnormal tonic neck and eye reflexes, and abnormal righting reflexes
   B. *Anatomy*—flocculonodular lobes of cerebellum, vestibular nerve, and nuclei
IV. Medulla oblongata
   A. *Signs*—poor gag reflex, dysphagia, dysphonia, paresis of tongue, poor righting response
   B. *Anatomy*—cranial nerves VII, IX, X, XII
V. Tentorial herniation
   A. *Signs*—earliest: dilated pupil, ipsilateral. Later: ptosis, lateral strabismus, progressive loss of consciousness. Loss of placing reaction may be ipsilateral or contralateral.
   B. *Anatomy*—cranial nerve III, reticular formation, ipsilateral motor pathways or contralateral cerebral peduncle (see Fig. 4–10)
VI. Cranial nerves VI and VII
   A. *Signs*—contralateral conjugate deviation of eyes, ipsilateral facial paralysis
   B. *Anatomy*—nucleus of VI, including parabducens nucleus, genu of VII
VII. Cranial nerves III, IV, VI
   A. *Signs*—strabismus, altered mobility of eyes depending on degree of damage
   B. *Anatomy*—intracranial course of the nerves on the floor of the cranial fossa and in the cavernous sinus or in orbit
VIII. Horner's syndrome
   A. *Signs*—miosis, ptosis, enophthalmos
   B. *Anatomy*—sympathetic pathway to pupil (see Fig. 4–11), lesion in hypothalamus, lateral medulla, cervical spinal cord, anterior cervical ganglion, or postganglionic fibers. Associated signs required for localization.
IX. Cerebellopontine angle
   A. *Signs*—ipsilateral: facial paralysis, paralysis of muscles of mastication, anesthesia of head cranial to occiput, head tilt, deafness. Occasionally, atrophy and deviation of tongue, motor abnormalities.
   B. *Anatomy*—cranial nerves V, VII, VIII, sometimes XII, late compression of brain stem

recognize that the clinician should be able to localize the lesion to the extent outlined in Tables 4–5 and 4–7 without this much detailed information.

Cerebral Cortex

The cerebral cortex has long been considered the site of such higher mental functions as memory, learning, and voluntary actions. Phylogenetically, the cortex is of major significance only in the mammals; it increases in complexity from the more primitive species through carnivores to primates, and it reaches its greatest development in man. The dog, along with other carnivores, has a convoluted cortex differing from that of primates principally in the lack of the large "association" areas (mainly the frontal and parietal lobes) (Fig. 4–5).

Cortical maps, defining specific activities for specific areas, have been made using histological, stimulation, evoked response, and ablation techniques. Figure 4–6 is a diagram of the cerebral cortex of the dog, representing the various motor and sensory areas as defined by a number of investigators.[7, 25, 31, 72, 89-91] An area may be responsible for a specific action when stimulated and yet not be the only area in the brain that produces that action. Generally there are several areas involved in a function, any one of which may or may not be essential for its performance. For example, when the cortical motor area is stimulated, movement of a limb can be elicited. However, the area can be ablated and the animal will still walk. Only with careful clinical examination can a deficit in motor function be detected in such cases.

The dog functions remarkably well without a cerebral cortex.[28] Walking is still possible, although there is some loss of agility; e.g., the dog cannot step on a horizontal ladder.[85] Vision is severely impaired,[74, 77, 78] although touch is relatively unaffected[28] and the hearing threshold (loudness) is only slightly elevated.[52] However, learning is virtually absent, and behavior is inappropriate and stereotyped.[28] According to Goltz, the dog responded to threats as little as to caresses.[13]

Frontal Lobe

Prefrontal Cortex (see Fig. 4–6). Small lesions in the prefrontal regions are not likely to produce detectable signs in the dog. Drive disinhibition, the release of activity normally inhibited by this area, is a

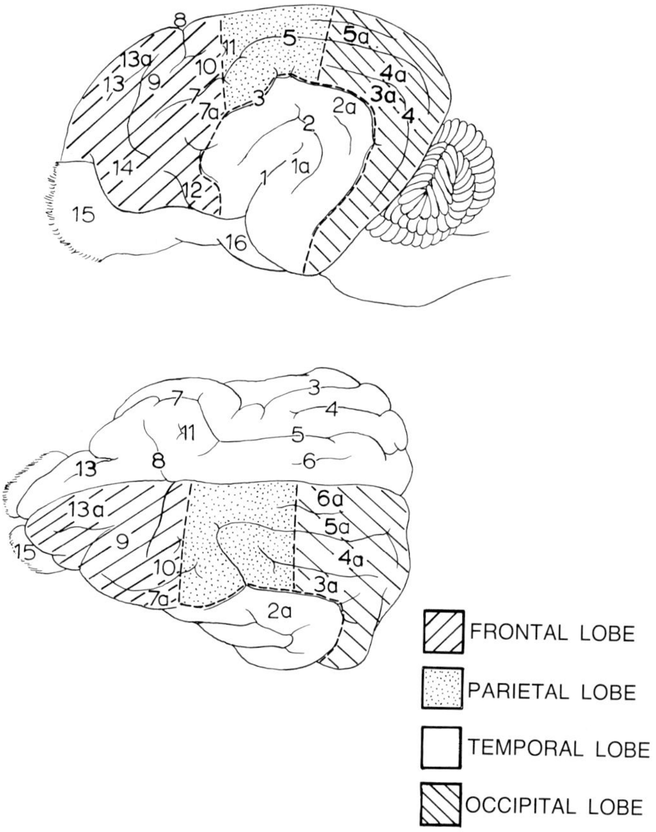

FIGURE 4–5 Cerebral cortex. Lobes are approximate, based primarily on Kreiner.[98, 99, 101–105] (Modified from Miller, M. E., Christensen, G. C., and Evans, H. E.: *Anatomy of the Dog.* W. B. Saunders Co., Philadelphia, 1964.) Legend: (1) sylvian sulcus; (1a) sylvian gyrus; (2) ectosylvian sulcus; (2a) ectosylvian gyrus; (3) suprasylvian sulcus; (3a) suprasylvian gyrus; (4) ectolateral sulcus; (4a) ectolateral gyrus; (5) lateral sulcus; (5a) lateral gyrus; (6) entolateral sulcus; (6a) entolateral gyrus (marginal gyrus—Kreiner); (7) coronal sulcus; (7a) coronal gyrus; (8) cruciate sulcus; (9) anterior sigmoid gyrus; (10) posterior sigmoid gyrus; (11) postcruciate sulcus (central sulcus—Kreiner); (12) presylvian sulcus; (13) prorean sulcus; (13a) prorean gyrus; (14) prorean gyrus (orbital gyrus—Kreiner); (15) olfactory bulb; (16) periform area.

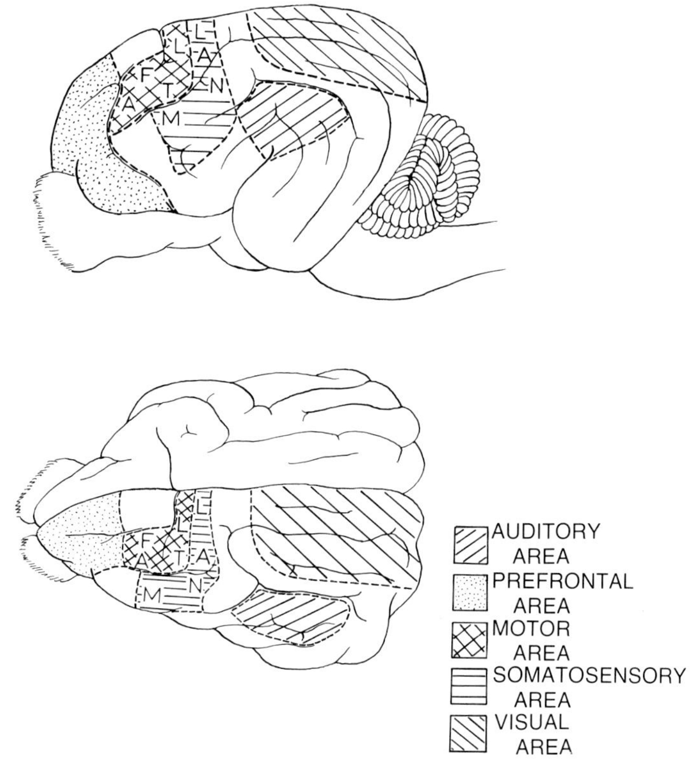

FIGURE 4–6 Functional areas of the cerebral cortex. See text for details F=Face, A=Arm (forelimb), T=Trunk, L=Leg (hindlimb), M=Mouth and tongue, and N=Nose and lips. (Modified from Miller, M. E., Christensen, G. C., and Evans, H. E.: *Anatomy of the Dog.* W. B. Saunders Co., Philadelphia, 1964.)

common finding of many investigators. The impaired delayed response is probably due to lack of inhibition. (Delayed response is the ability to perform a task after a delay; e.g., to find a food reward that has been placed under a cup or two cups after a delay of several seconds.) Hyperactivity, forced pacing, circling (unilateral lesion), and inattention, the clinical signs most often seen with lesions in the prefrontal region, are principally signs of release of inhibition. Augmentation of most emotional states has also been described.[8]

MOTOR CORTEX. The data available on the functions of the motor cortex of the dog are somewhat conflicting.[7, 22, 25, 72, 89, 91] Areas that elicit muscular response when stimulated electrically can be defined (see Fig. 4–7). Movements can also be elicited by stimulation of sensory areas, and this fact probably explains some of the difference of opinion as to the exact extent of the motor area. A precise distinction between these reactions is not possible. The motor area as shown in Figure 4–6 is a composite of results of several investigators; this type of experimentation has numerous variables.

The presence of a motor area in the cortex as defined by electrical stimulation is of clinical interest in relation to Jacksonian seizures. Focal motor seizures that affect only a part of the body or limbs and progress to full grand mal seizures are called Jacksonian seizures (after Hughlings Jackson, who first described them). A true Jacksonian seizure requires a somatopic arrangement of the motor area, so that as the seizure discharge spreads from a focus in one area it will gradually involve other areas and finally the entire body. Jacksonian seizures are seen infrequently in dogs, but they do occur.[51] The portion of the body involved in the early part of the seizure is strongly suggestive of the location of the lesion.

Ablation of the motor area results in abnormal reactions in the contralateral limbs. Many of these signs are virtually undetectable after 2 or 3 weeks owing to compensation. The most significant signs, all contralateral, include: extensor hypertonus when lifted from the floor, abnormal positioning (proprioception), weakness, deficiency in voluntary activity, hyperactive stretch reflexes (e.g., knee jerk), and deficiency of placing and hopping reactions.[89] Hypotonia rather than hypertonia has been described in dogs, cats, and raccoons after motor cortex[9, 10] or pyramidal tract[82] section. On the basis of available evidence, lesions that are limited strictly to the motor cortex will probably produce hypotonia rather than hypertonia. Dysmetria has also been described in these animals. Lesions in the motor cortex cause considerable loss of dexterity in species that are able to manipulate their distal extremities, such as primates and raccoons.[10]

Parietal Lobe

Most of the parietal lobe has sensory or "association" functions, modalities that are especially difficult to evaluate in animals.[14] Only the somatosensory cortex will be discussed here.

SOMATOSENSORY CORTEX (see Fig. 4–6). The postcruciate sulcus,[54] which has been

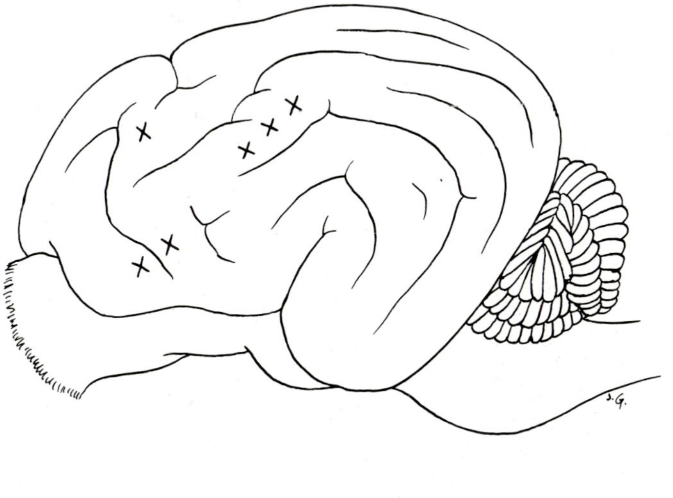

FIGURE 4–7 Location of areas in the cerebral cortex of the dog that produce eye movements when stimulated electrically. (After Miller, M. E., Christensen, G. C., and Evans, H. E.: *Anatomy of the Dog.* W. B. Saunders Co., Philadelphia, 1964.)

called the central sulcus by Kreiner,[43, 44, 47] separates the motor cortex from the somatosensory cortex (see Figs. 4–5 and 4–6). The limbs, body, and head are represented somatotopically with the hind foot on the medial surface and the head situated most laterally. The nose, mouth, and lips have the largest representation, as these areas are the most important in cutaneous sensibility in the dog.[2, 31, 89]

Unilateral ablations of the somatosensory cortex cause transient impairment of contralateral tactile response. Bilateral ablations produce more severe deficits, but even these are transitory.[60]

Isolated lesions of this area probably are not detectable clinically.

Occipital Lobe[46]

VISUAL CORTEX. Vision is the major function of the occipital cortex. Primary and secondary visual areas have been described (see Figs. 4–5 and 4–6). Lesions large enough to produce clinical signs would probably have to involve most of the occipital lobe. Relatively large unilateral lesions involving occipital, parietal, and temporal lobes have produced contralateral hemianopias, which required careful testing to detect.[77, 78] The deficit was more marked when part of the temporal lobe was ablated than when it was not. Other investigators have found a loss of visual pattern discrimination[74] or of brightness discrimination[73] following bilateral visual cortex ablation.

Clinical testing for visual deficits must be performed carefully and patiently. With proper care, visual fields can be plotted with a fair degree of accuracy if the dog is alert enough to respond. Moving objects or pieces of food brought into the field of vision from the lateral side, or from behind a 4-foot square piece of plywood placed in front of the dog will evoke a head and eye movement in most dogs. Several repetitive examinations may be needed to verify results on each eye. Evoked response techniques using computer averaging offer promise for more effective evaluation of the visual system.[33]

Complete hemianopias in the ipsilateral eye would not be expected because the optic nerve fibers from the temporal part of the retina are both crossed and uncrossed. Because all of the nasal part of the retinal fibers is crossed, the hemianopia

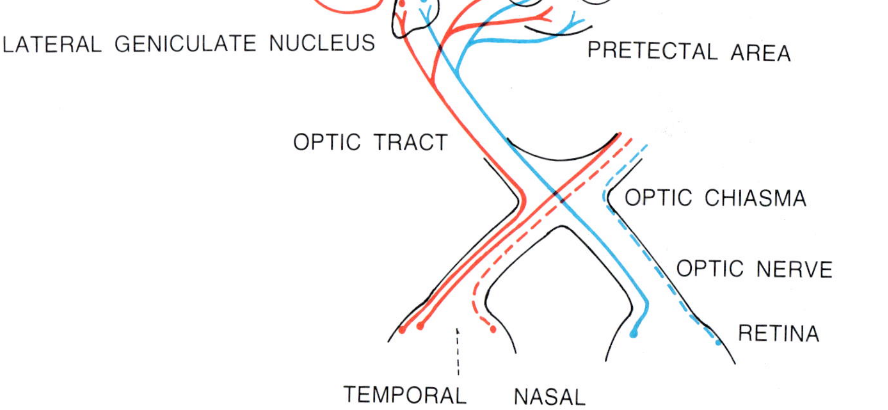

FIGURE 4–8 Visual pathway. Fibers from the nasal half of the retina cross in the optic chiasm and ascend in the contralateral optic tract. Approximately 25 per cent of the fibers from the temporal half of the retina cross and ascend in the contralateral half of the retina; the remainder ascend in the ipsilateral optic tract.[77, 80]

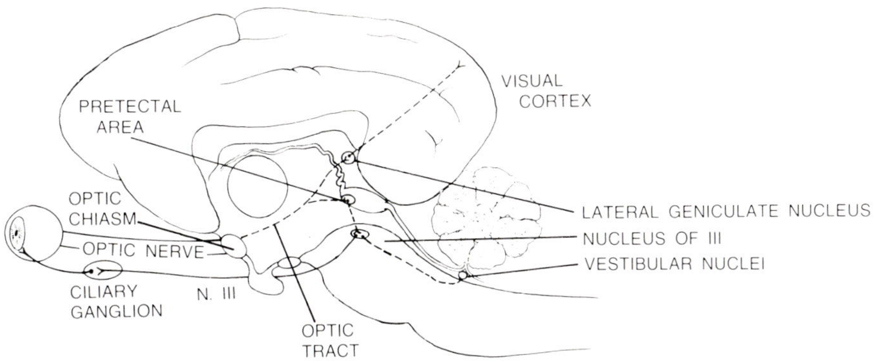

FIGURE 4–9 Diagrammatic representation of the sensory and motor pathways of the visual system. Notice that both the sensory (to cortex) and the motor (from vestibular nuclei) systems traverse the length of the brain and are thus susceptible to damage to lesions in many areas.

should be worse in the contralateral eye (Fig. 4–8).[80]

Cortical lesions usually do not affect pupillary responses (see Section III and Figs. 4–9 to 4–11).

Temporal Lobe[45]

Auditory Cortex. The auditory cortex is located primarily on the ectosylvian gyrus in the dog and cat (see Figs. 4–5 and 4–6).[1, 83, 84, 91] A tonotopic pattern has been found, with high frequencies represented at the anterior end of the auditory area and low frequencies at the posterior end.[83, 84]

The auditory system is a complex series of pathways with multiple synapses and multiple crossings; therefore, complete loss of hearing with unilateral lesions rostral to the cochlear nucleus is virtually impossible.

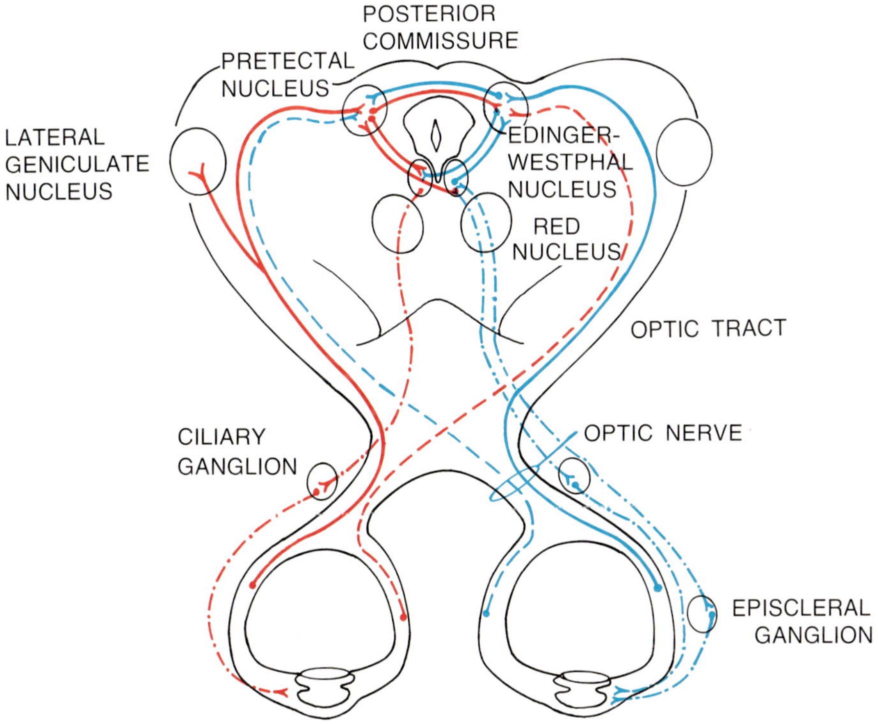

FIGURE 4–10 The oculomotor pathway involved in pupillary constriction. The clinician should be able to predict direct and consensual pupillary responses and visual deficits with lesions in the optic nerve, optic tract, pretectal area, or oculomotor nerve. (After Crosby, E. C., Humphrey, L., and Laver, E. W.: *Anatomy of the Nervous System.* Macmillan Co., New York, 1962.)

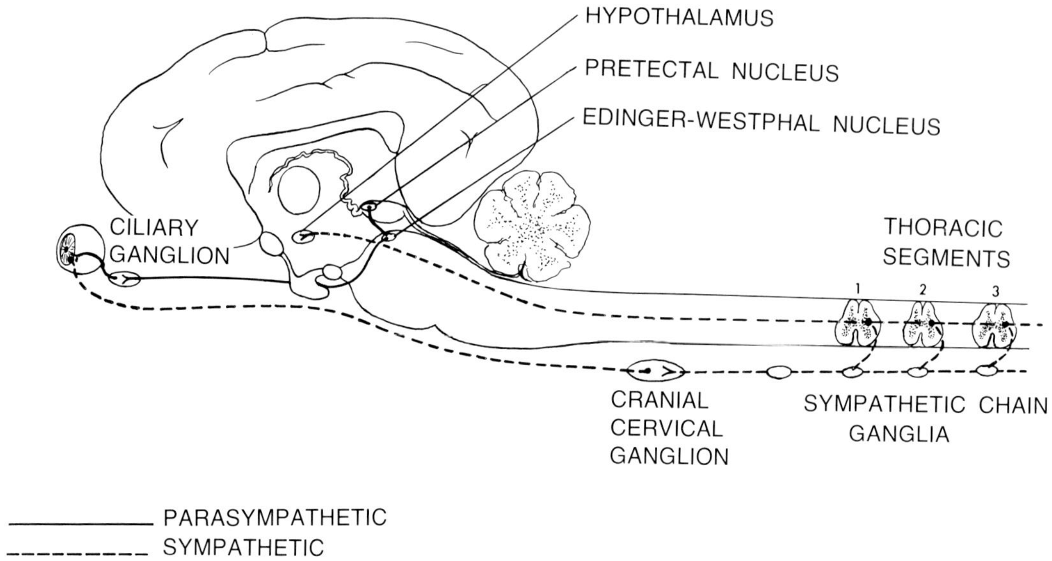

FIGURE 4–11 The motor pathways to the iris: parasympathetic-constrictor and sympathetic-dilator.

The decorticate animal can still hear, although there is a loss of ability to orient toward the sound, even with unilateral lesions,[77, 78] and the hearing threshold is raised.[52]

Inclusion of auditory cortex in ablations of visual cortex increases the severity of visual deficit, resulting in almost complete hemianopia.[77, 78] Clinical detection of hearing deficits caused by cortical damage is unlikely except with newer techniques using computer averaging of the evoked cortical response.

Deeper Structures. The amygdaloid nucleus, hippocampus, and associated cortex are part of the complex limbic system.[41, 66] They are considered here because of their involvement in so-called temporal lobe seizures.

The limbic system is a complex circuit uniting parts of the rhinencephalon with the hypothalamus and other structures listed in Figure 4–12. Experimental ablations of portions of this system have caused severe alterations in behavior. For example, bilateral injury to the amygdaloid nuclei in cats produced increased motor activity, exaggerated oral and vocal behavior, docility, and hypersexuality.[75] Movements of the mouth and alterations in visceral activity

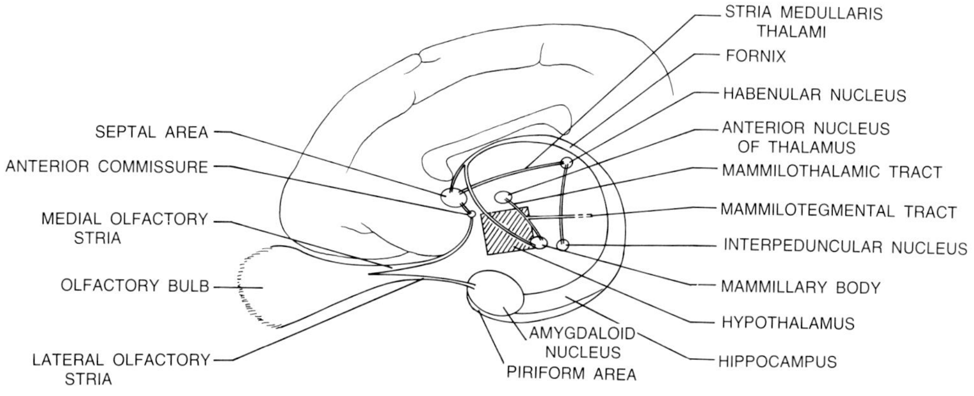

FIGURE 4–12 Schematic diagram of the complex circuits in the limbic system. Alterations in behavior are associated with lesions in this system. (After Papez, J. W.: A proposed mechanism of emotion. Arch. Neurol. Psychol. *38*, 725, 1937.)

have also been produced by electrical stimulation or destruction of some of these structures.[21, 38, 68]

Temporal lobe epilepsy is probably common in dogs.[26, 51] "Chewing-gum" convulsions and "running fits" are apparently forms of temporal lobe seizures. Damage to the brain is thought to occur in the course of trauma (birth injury) or infection (distemper), which produce cerebral edema. The parahippocampal gyri tend to herniate through the tentorial opening, causing necrosis of the cortex (Fig. 4–13).[61] The injured area has the potential for becoming an epileptic focus. The lesion may be bilateral, or if seizures are present for an extended period, a mirror focus may develop.[29, 30] Mirror focus is a seizure discharge in a similar area of contralateral hemisphere.

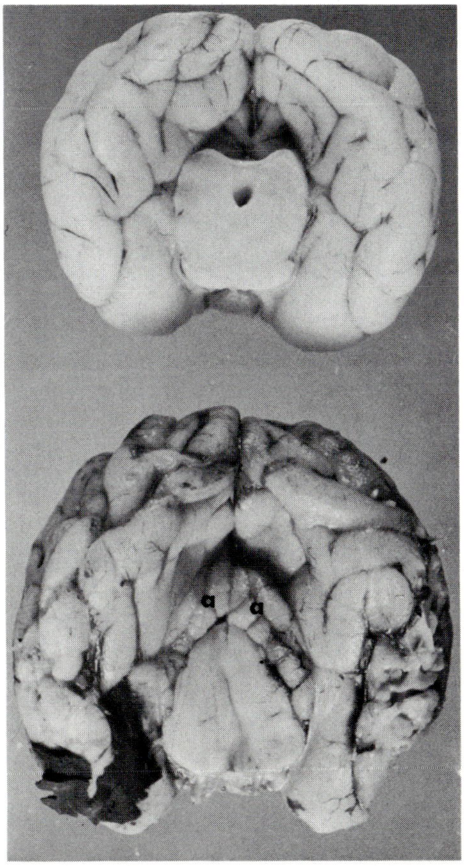

FIGURE 4–13 Caudal view of brain transected at mesencephalon. *Top:* Normal brain. *Bottom:* Severe cerebral edema has caused herniation of the cerebrum (a) under the tentorium cerebelli, compressing and distorting the brain stem. The cerebral aqueduct is closed, resulting in further increases in cranial pressure. (From Oliver, J. E., Jr.: Principles of canine brain surgery. Animal Hosp. *2*, 73, 1966.)

Temporal lobectomy has been used to control this type of seizure in man when medication has failed. Bilateral removal is necessary in some cases of bilateral or mirror focus lesions, a relatively rare problem.[29] Behavioral deficits following surgery are greater when large portions of the hippocampus are excised,[27, 30] especially when the excision is bilateral.[75]

Basal Nuclei

The caudate nucleus, putamen, and globus pallidus are the most important structures in what are generally termed the basal nuclei (Figs. 4–3 and 4–14). Anatomically, the basal nuclei may include the claustrum and amygdala. Physiologically, the subthalamic nucleus, substantia nigra, red nucleus, and parts of the reticular formation and cerebellum are included in the so-called extrapyramidal system.

The function of this system, which is relatively large anatomically, has been surprisingly difficult to analyze experimentally. Much of the literature is confusing and even contradictory. Species differences, such as those between carnivores and primates, are apparently important in the function of the extrapyramidal system.[15] Stimulation of the caudate nucleus generally produced turning of the head and body contralaterally and flexion of the contralateral limbs.[23, 57] Large destructive lesions usually caused the dog to turn ipsilaterally, although occasionally contralateral turning was seen.[55] Liles and Davis[49] could produce contralateral turning, permanent loss or depression of nonvisual placing and hopping reactions, and hypertonia in the contralateral limbs with lesions in the anteroventral caudate nucleus. In addition, some of the animals developed hyperkinesias, either athetoid or choreiform in character. Location of the lesion is apparently very critical. Lesions placed more caudally abolished the hyperkinetic activity. Two areas have been identified in the caudate nucleus: the anteroventral one is "inhibitory" and the caudodorsal one is "facilitatory."[48, 49] These experiments in cats demonstrate a potential in the carnivore for syndromes of extrapyramidal diseases de-

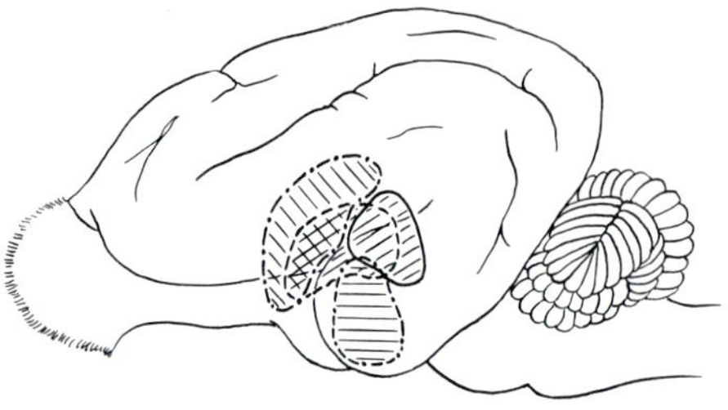

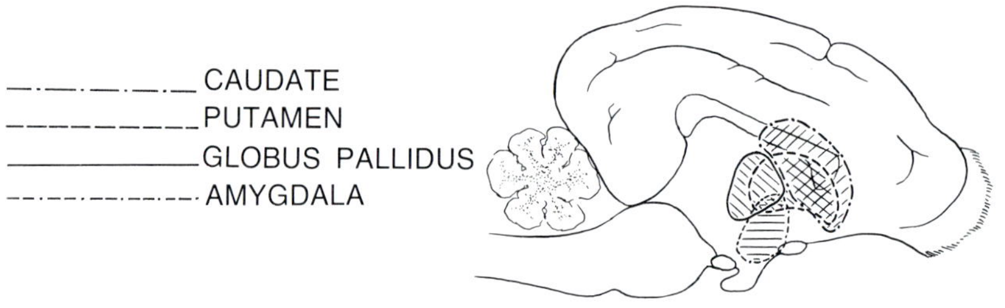

FIGURE 4–14 The basal nuclei are located deep to the cerebral cortex, approximately as shown. (After Kreiner, J., and Maksymowicz, K.: A three-dimensional model of the striated nuclei in the dog's brain. Acta Biol. Exp. *22*, 69, 1962.)

scribed in man (e.g., Parkinson's disease). It is likely that some of the myoclonic activity that remains after canine distemper has its origin in this system.[12, 53] However, research findings indicate that many, if not most, cases of distemper myoclonus in the dog are caused by abnormal activity in the spinal cord and will persist even after complete spinal transection.[5, 88]

Clinically, lesions of the basal nuclei will produce circling (ipsilateral or contralateral), deficiency of nonvisual placing and hopping reactions, hypertonia in the contralateral limbs, and possibly hyperkinesias such as athetosis or chorea.

Diencephalon (Fig. 4–3)

Thalamus

The thalamus is the major relay and integrating center for the cerebral cortex. Large spinal pathways, such as the spinothalamic tracts, have synapses in the thalamus. Thalamic neurons then send fibers to the cerebral cortex. Conversely, the cerebral cortex sends many fibers to the thalamus.

Lesions of the thalamus usually produce signs related to the system affected. For example, lesions of the lateral geniculate nucleus produce visual defects. The various systems are discussed in Chapter 2.

Central pain phenomena (the thalamic syndromes) are well documented in man.[11] Lesions producing pain usually involve the relay nuclei or pathways of the lateral spinothalamic system.[86] However, interpretation of sensory signs in dogs is very difficult. McGrath described a Boston terrier that whined and cried continuously, as if it were in pain. A brain tumor was found in the left thalamus on necropsy.[51]

Hypothalamus

The hypothalamus is a very small but extremely important part of the brain (see Fig. 4–3). Numerous "centers" regulating behavioral and autonomic functions have been defined. Such functions as eating, drinking, sexual behavior, anger, blood pressure, respiration, and pupillary size can be altered by stimulation or destruction of discrete areas in the hypothalamus. The hypothalamus influences almost every activity of the body through the production of hormones that are released in the pituitary gland.

Pathologic lesions affecting hypothalamic function are not usually discrete, so a variety of functional abnormalities may be seen. Behavioral and autonomic disorders related to hypothalamic lesions include changes in eating (polyphagia, dysphagia), drinking (polydipsia), and sleeping habits;

alterations in blood pressure, pulse rate, and temperature regulation; behavioral disturbances, such as rage; and Horner's syndrome (see Chapter 18 and Fig. 4–11).

The hypothalamus may be affected by inflammatory processes, such as encephalitis; circulatory disorders, especially hemorrhage; and neoplasms, especially pituitary tumors.

Mesencephalon (Midbrain)

The midbrain consists of the tectum, tegmentum, and basis pedunculi cerebri (Fig. 4–15). The tectum is characterized by the paired rostral and caudal colliculi, which are concerned with visual and auditory pathways (see Fig. 4–1 and Chapter 2). The tegmentum, comprising the area between the tectum and the crus cerebri, consists of long tracts (see Chapter 2), red nuclei, and reticulary formation. The crus cerebri includes substantia nigra, a part of the extrapyramidal system previously discussed, and the descending cortical pathways to the brainstem, cerebellum, and spinal cord (pyramidal and extrapyramidal systems). Cranial nerves III (oculomotor) and IV (trochlear) originate in the midbrain (see Chapter 16 and Figs. 4–16 and 4–17). The cerebral aqueduct traverses the length of the mesencephalon (Figs. 4–15 and 4–17).

Most of the signs of midbrain damage are referrable to the long tracts, cranial nerves, and reticular formation. Complete transection at this level produces the classical intercollicular decerebration.[76] Such a preparation typically results in marked extensor hypertonus with exaggerated stretch

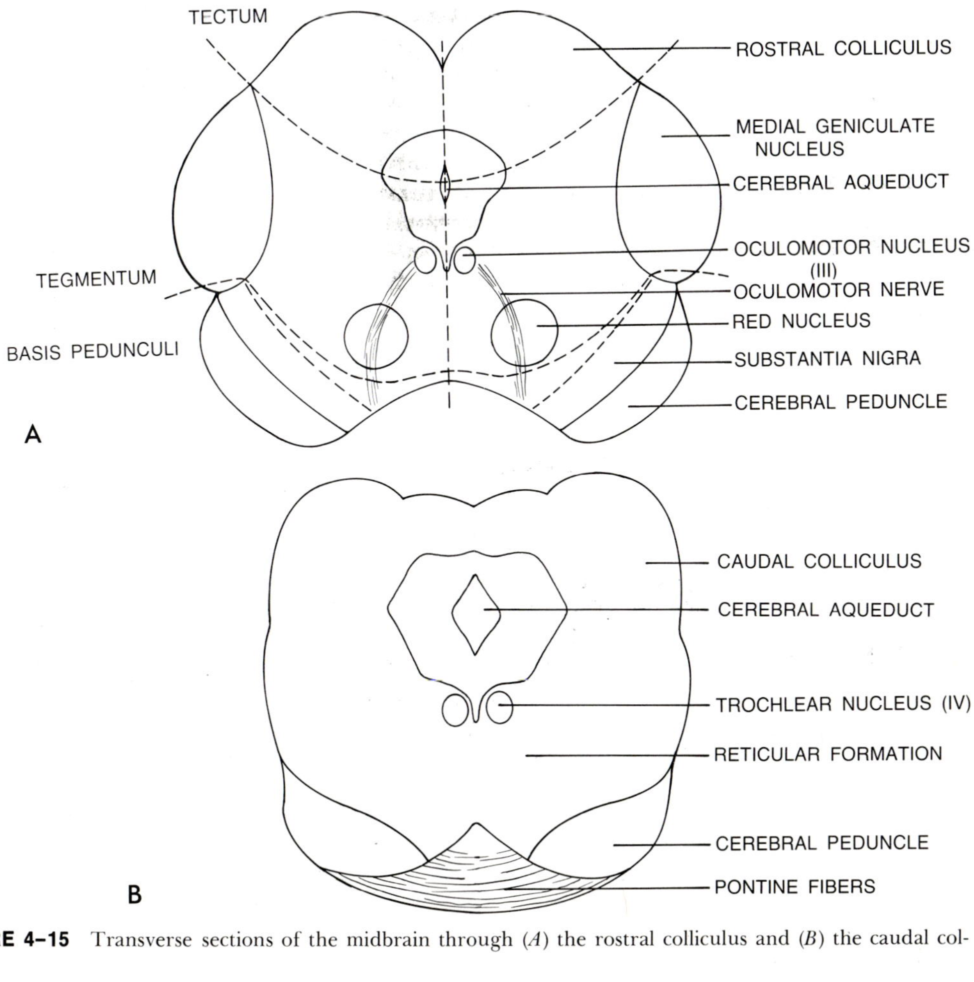

FIGURE 4–15 Transverse sections of the midbrain through (*A*) the rostral colliculus and (*B*) the caudal colliculus.

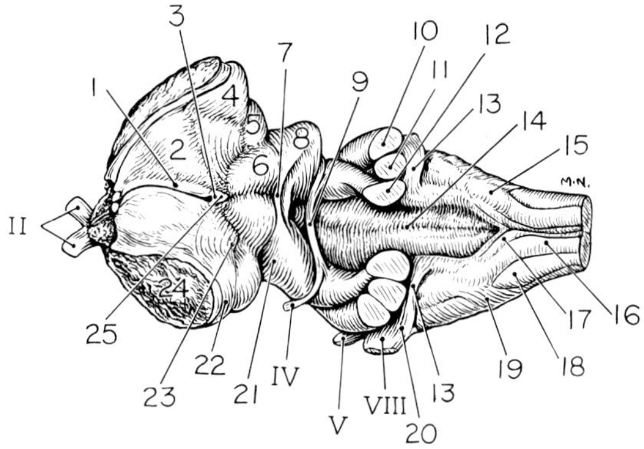

FIGURE 4–16 Dorsolateral view of the brain stem. (From Miller, M. E., Christensen, G. C., and Evans, H. E.: *Anatomy of the Dog.* W. B. Saunders Co., Philadelphia, 1964.)

1. Stria medullaris thalami
2. Dorsal aspect of thalamus
3. Habenular commissure
4. Lateral geniculate body
5. Medial geniculate body
6. Superior colliculus
7. Commissure of inferior colliculi
8. Inferior colliculus
9. Crossing of trochlear nerve fibers in anterior medullary velum
10. Middle cerebellar peduncle
11. Inferior cerebellar peduncle
12. Superior cerebellar peduncle
13. Dorsal cochlear nucleus
14. Dorsal median sulcus in fourth ventricle
15. Accessory cuneate nucleus
16. Fasciculus cuneatus
17. Fasciculus gracilis
18. Spinal tract of trigeminal nerve
19. External arcuate fibers
20. Left ventral cochlear nucleus
21. Brachium of inferior colliculus
22. Optic tract
23. Brachium of superior colliculus
24. Cut surface between cerebrum and brain stem
25. Pineal body or epiphysis

II. Optic nerves
IV. Trochlear nerve
V. Trigeminal nerve
VIII. Vestibulocochlear nerve

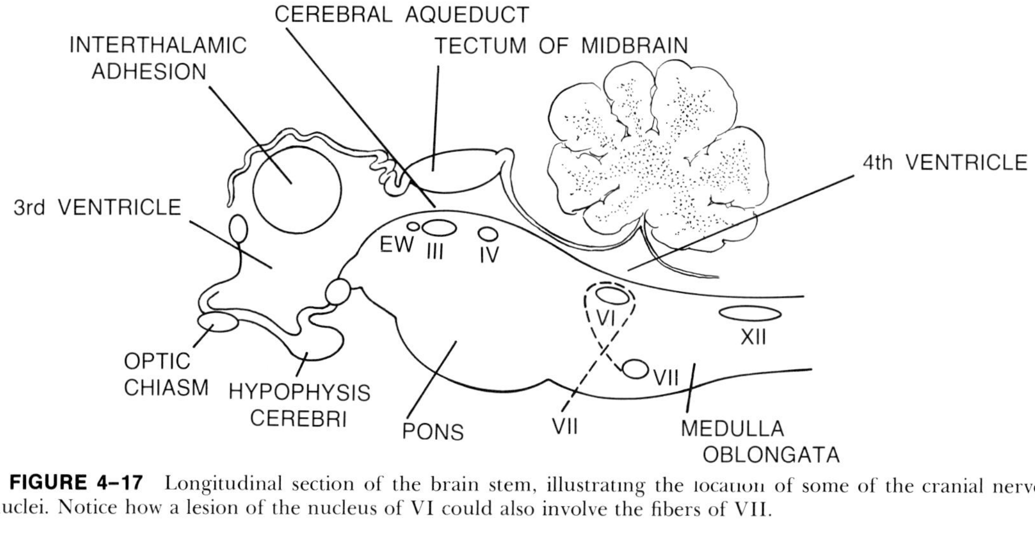

FIGURE 4–17 Longitudinal section of the brain stem, illustrating the location of some of the cranial nerve nuclei. Notice how a lesion of the nucleus of VI could also involve the fibers of VII.

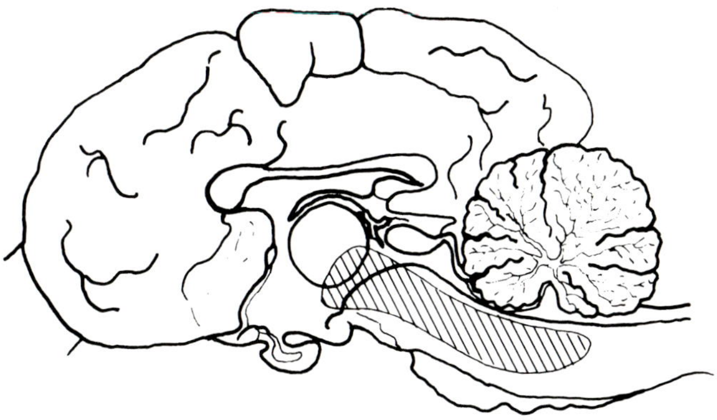

FIGURE 4–18 Longitudinal section of brain, illustrating the approximate extent of the reticular formation. Large lesions in the rostral portion will cause coma. (From Oliver, J. E., Jr.: Surgical management of acute head injury. Proceed. 19th Gaines Vet. Symposium, 1969.)

reflexes. The animal does not move spontaneously and does not right itself if placed on its side.[71, 85] Large lesions involving the tegmentum produce loss of consciousness because of destruction of the rostral reticular formation (Fig. 4–18).

Cerebral edema or large masses in the rostrotentorial compartment (Fig. 4–19) frequently cause herniation of the cerebrum under the tentorium cerebelli. The pressure is transmitted to the midbrain (which lies immediately beneath the tentorium), causing distortion, pressure necrosis, and interference with the blood supply (see Fig. 4–13). The result is usually coma with decerebrate rigidity and signs of oculomotor paralysis. Smaller lesions may produce less severe signs. Dilation of the ipsilateral pupil is usually the earliest sign of impending tentorial herniation.[35]

Lesions that occlude the cerebral aqueduct produce obstructive hydrocephalus with dilation of the lateral and third ventricles.

Small lesions in the tegmentum may produce signs associated with any of the long tracts. Midline lesions may interrupt the medial longitudinal fasciculus, producing abnormal eye movements—especially those of vestibular origin ("doll's eye," abnormal caloric test).[67]

Pons

The pons consists of a tegmentum and a basilar portion (Fig. 4–20). The tegmentum consists of long tracts, the reticular formation, and part of the nuclei of the trigeminal nerve (V). The basilar portion is

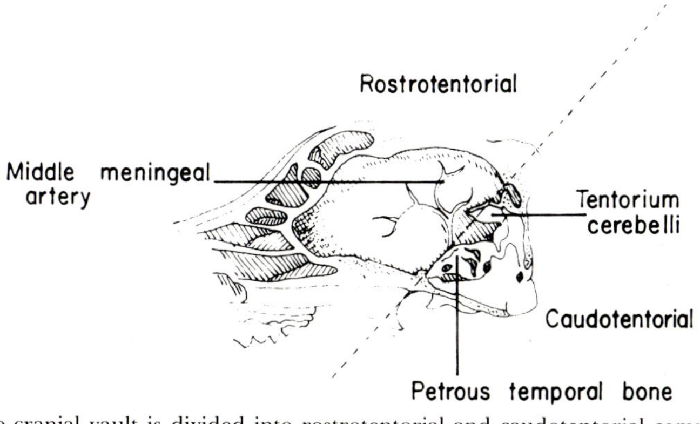

FIGURE 4–19 The cranial vault is divided into rostrotentorial and caudotentorial compartments by the tentorium cerebelli and petrous ridge. (From Oliver, J. E., Jr.: Surgical management of acute head injury. Proceed. 19th Gaines Vet. Symposium, 1969.)

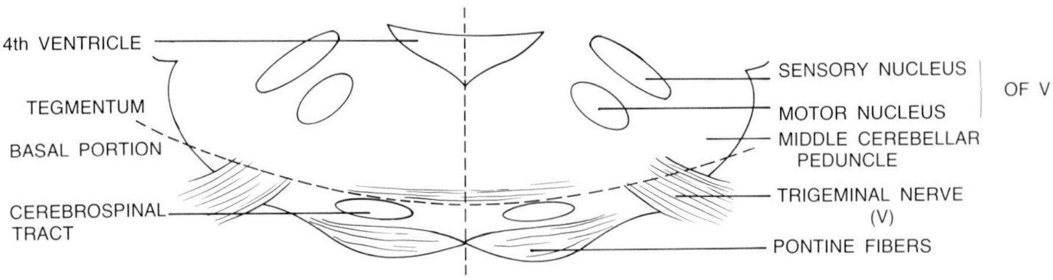

FIGURE 4–20 Transverse section of the pons through the trigeminal nerve.

composed of the continuation of the longitudinal fibers of the crus cerebri, the pontine nuclei and their projection fibers, and the transverse pontine fibers that form the brachium pontis (middle cerebellar peduncle).

Lesions in the pons may interfere with cranial nerves IV, VI, and VII, as well as V. The motor nucleus of V is most likely to be damaged, producing paralysis of the muscles of mastication. Large lesions of the pons may abolish the micturition reflex and produce coma. Smaller lesions may produce cerebellar signs or interfere with the long tracts of the brain stem.

Cerebellum

The cerebellum has received considerable attention from anatomists and physiologists, who have been trying to clarify the intricacies of its function.[18, 24] Yet, for the clinician, the ablation experiments of Luciani,[50] Dusser deBarenne,[17] and Rademaker,[69] which were carried out 35 to 70 years ago, are still relevant. Their descriptions of the signs of decerebellation and hemidecerebellation are classic. Roberts has lucidly summarized the literature and included his personal observations to provide the best description of cerebellar function in carnivores currently available.[71]

Removal of the cerebellum, unlike removal of the cerebral hemispheres, does not alter the animal's sensory processes to any significant degree. Voluntary activity is still possible; however, the normal integration of posture and phasic movement is seriously disturbed. Immediately after decerebellation, the animal is unable to stand, extends the fore limbs, dorsiflexes the neck (opisthotonos), and paddles with the hind legs. In a few days the animal regains some control; it still falls frequently, but it can swim quite well. The major persisting abnormality is dysmetria. Movements are exaggerated; for example, in walking the limbs are lifted too high and put down with too much force. The head is apt to hit the water dish instead of stopping at the proper level for drinking. The animal learns to move cautiously, using the wall for support.[71]

Most of the signs of cerebellectomy are the result of loss of inhibition. The loss is more obvious in unilateral lesion: extensor hypertonus of the ipsilateral limbs is seen when the animal is placed on its back. When the animal is upright, it falls to the ipsilateral side because the limbs on this side are inhibited by a spinal reflex from the normal side.[71]

Several weeks after cerebellectomy the animal has residual characteristic responses that are usually permanent. A broad-based stance is adopted to maintain an upright posture. Most reactions are exaggerated. For example, the hopping reaction (Chapter 3) is slow in onset, the dog takes a higher step than normal, and the limb is not accurately placed in a new supporting position. Coarse tremors are evident as movements are initiated and persist through the maneuver. Dysmetria is usually obvious when the animal walks, as the feet are lifted very high with each step. The gait is erratic; the body shifts grossly from side to side.

Unilateral lesions generally produce similar signs confined to the ipsilateral side. With compensation, the animal often tends to turn to the affected side because of the ipsilateral weakness.

Violent twisting or circling movements usually occur only if the vestibular nuclei are damaged.

As indicated by the description of the

cerebellectomized animal, the function of the cerebellum is to improve the smoothness of reactions, much in the manner of a servo-control system. Small lesions can be expected to produce a variety of signs, depending on the area affected. Various parts of the body are represented in various areas of the cerebellum. The relationship of this somatotopic organization and the clinical signs resulting from cerebellar lesions is not at all clear, however. For most clinical purposes, signs of cerebellar damage can be expected to be ipsilateral to the lesion. The major clinical signs are ipsilateral weakness and dysmetria in all of its manifestations, including tremors on movement ("intention tremors"). Acute cerebellar lesions may produce extensor hypertonus and opisthotonos. According to Roberts, opisthotonos is never present when the anterior lobe of the cerebellum is intact.[71]

The clinician should also be aware that the cerebellum is involved in autonomic function. Evoked responses can be recorded from the cerebellum when visceral nerves are stimulated,[4, 58, 59] and stimulation of the cerebellum can alter autonomic function.[44, 51] For example, stimulation of the fastigial nucleus depresses the micturition reflex by depressing motor activity in the pelvic nerve, whereas ablation of the anterior vermis results in a hyperactive micturition reflex.[4]

Medulla Oblongata

The most caudal portion of the brain stem, the medulla oblongata, is continuous

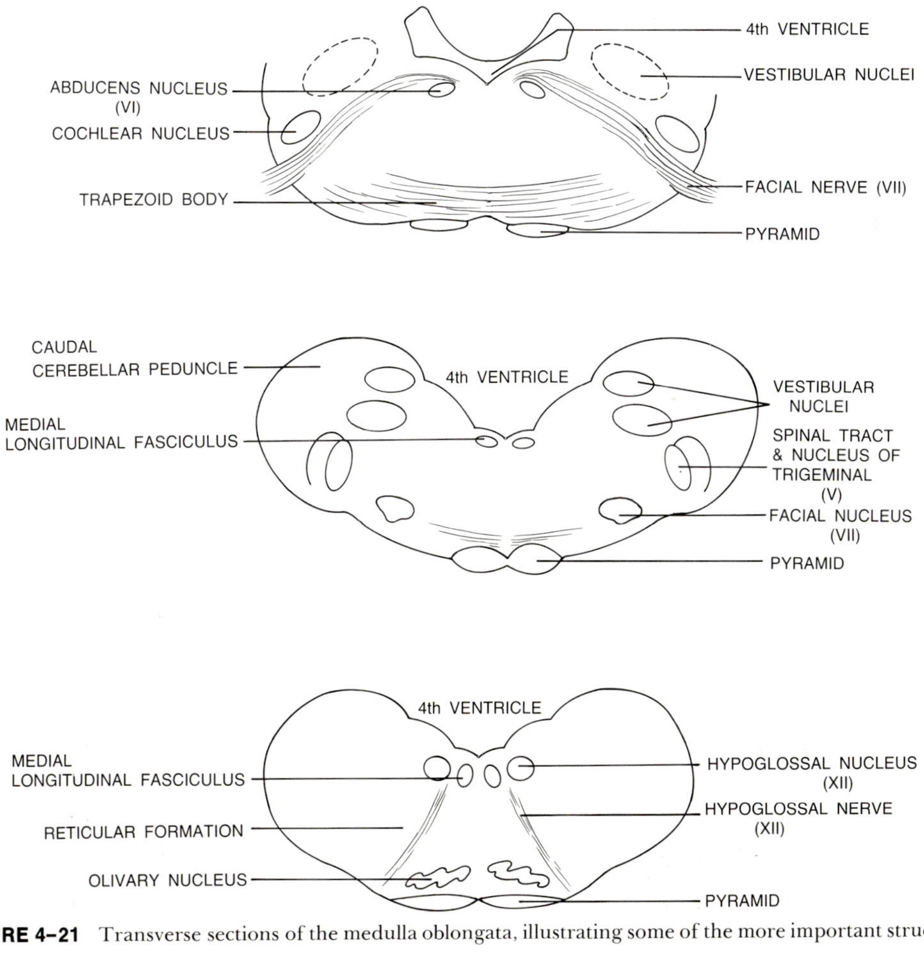

FIGURE 4–21 Transverse sections of the medulla oblongata, illustrating some of the more important structures.

with the spinal cord. Nuclei of cranial nerves V to XII, all ascending and descending pathways between brain and spinal cord, and some important portions of the reticular formation are contained in this area (Figs. 4–17 and 4–21).

A response that is similar to the Babinski response in man (extension of the digits in response to a light touch on the foot pads or the dew claw) has been described in dogs and cats whose brain stem has been transected between the medulla and pons.[32] Presumably this response requires only destruction of pyramidal and extrapyramidal pathways (upper motor neuron lesions).[39]

Important cardiovascular and respiratory centers are located in the medullary reticular formation. Because of the close proximity of so many important structures, lesions will generally produce a variety of signs, Extensive destructive lesions produce respiratory paralysis, the cause of death in so-called "bulbar paralysis."

Vestibular signs predominate in many smaller lesions and are discussed in Chapters 2 and 3. Cranial nerve signs are discussed in Chapter 8.

ETIOLOGY

To make statements about prognosis, the clinician must first localize the lesion and then determine the etiology. Localization of the lesion has been discussed from the standpoint of clinical signs and neurological examination.

The etiology of the disease process is determined by comparing the history, physical examination, neurological examination, and ancillary studies (e.g., cerebrospinal fluid analysis, radiologic studies, and electroencephalographic (EEG) studies). The neurological examination is used to determine the location of the lesion, an important part of the diagnosis. Radiology, CSF, and EEG are discussed in separate chapters; specific changes are listed in the discussion of individual diseases. The physical examination may reveal a fever, indicating possible infection, bruises, indicating trauma, and so forth.

The history may well be the most important factor—and unfortunately, the most neglected. Some CNS diseases, such as epilepsy, may have to be diagnosed and

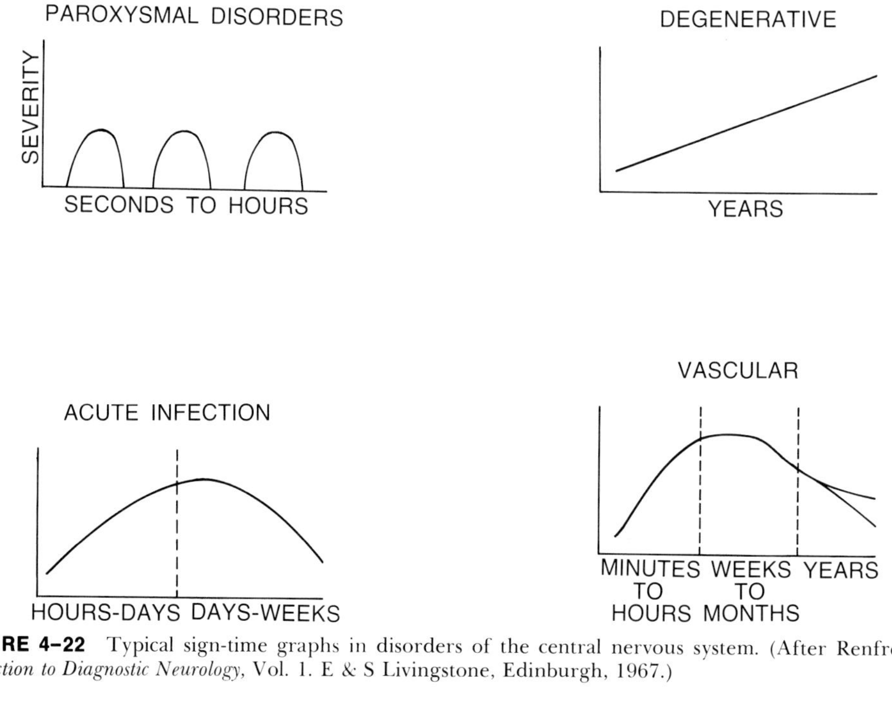

FIGURE 4–22 Typical sign-time graphs in disorders of the central nervous system. (After Renfrew, S.: *An Introduction to Diagnostic Neurology,* Vol. 1. E & S Livingstone, Edinburgh, 1967.)

treated entirely from the history, which is admittedly a risky venture. However, many dogs have seizures infrequently, with no warning; the clinician may never actually observe one. Most diseases are not as difficult to observe as epilepsy, but the history may still hold the clue to diagnosis.[64]

Obtaining a good, complete, reliable history is an art best learned from a skilled clinician. No attempt will be made here to outline a guide for taking the history; rather, some important points and their significance will be mentioned.

The course of the disease is often the most essential item gleaned from the history. Time and rate of onset, frequency of attacks, and progression of signs can be charted in the form of a sign-time graph.[70] The relative severity of signs is plotted on the ordinate and the time on the abscissa. Typical graphs are illustrated in Figure 4–22. All diseases may not conform exactly to these graphs, but the majority will be similar. Obviously, the experienced clinician does not have to draw a graph for each case; the concept is built into his reasoning processes. The graphs do illustrate one of the more important items to be obtained in the history, however.

Because of the prevalence of canine distemper, the history should always include dates of vaccinations, exposure to sick animals, and recent illnesses. Many animals with postviral CNS disease have had distemper vaccine at least once and have not had typical systemic signs of distemper. Other viral encephalitides may be responsible in some cases.[79]

PROGNOSIS

Providing the animal's owner with a reasonably accurate prognosis is an essential part of clinical neurology. Prognosis is influenced by many variables. Some of these include the age, breed, and sex of the animal and the location, extent, and cause of the lesion.

The clinical course of the problem provides insight into the prognosis. A disease that has been slowly progressive for an extended period of time has a much poorer prognosis than one that has passed its peak and shows signs of recovery (Fig. 4–23).

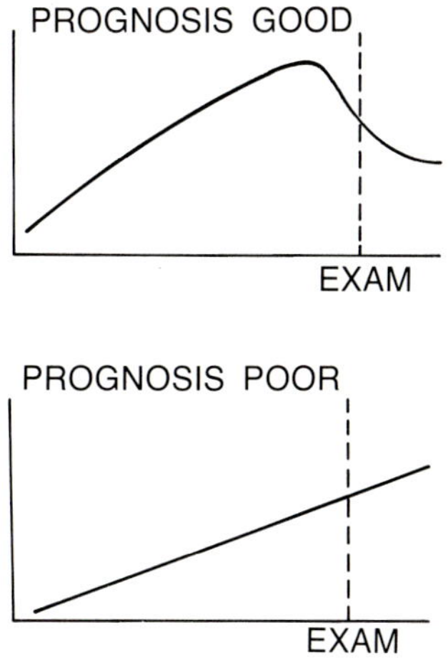

FIGURE 4–23 Estimation of prognosis based on sign-time graph.

Degenerative and neoplastic diseases are examples of progressive diseases.[64]

Clinical signs are also valuable clues to prognosis. Spinal cord compression produces signs which vary with increasing compression, as outlined in Table 4–11. Functional recovery is frequently possible until the response to deep pain is lost. An animal with no response to deep pain has a very low probability of recovery. Those that do recover frequently have relatively severe motor deficits.

The duration of the lesion is also a significant factor in prognosis. Nervous tissue tolerates injury for only a short time before cellular death. Spinal cord compression has been studied more thoroughly than most injuries to the CNS. It has been demonstrated that a compression of the spinal cord severe enough to abolish voluntary motor function but not the response to deep pain has a reasonably good prognosis if decompression is accomplished within 5 to 7 days. However, the longer compression exists, the slower the recovery. If de-

TABLE 4–11 PROGRESSION OF SIGNS IN SPINAL CORD COMPRESSION[a]

Proprioceptive deficit
Loss of voluntary motor function
Loss of superficial pain responses
Loss of deep pain responses

[a] All signs caudal to the level of the lesion.

compression is delayed more than 7 days, the probability of recovery is approximately the same whether decompression is accomplished or not. Compression that causes loss of deep pain has a very poor prognosis after only 2 to 4 hours.

Prognoses of the many disorders affecting the nervous system are discussed throughout the text.

REFERENCES

1. Ades, H. W.: The acoustic projection system, a comparative study. J. Neurophysiol., *8*, 463, 1945.
2. Adrian, E. D.: Afferent discharges to the cerebral cortex from peripheral sense organs. J. Physiol. *100*, 159, 1941.
3. Blauch, B., and Strafuss, A. C.: Histologic relationship of the facial (7th) and vestibulocochlear (8th) cranial nerves within the petrous temporal bone in the dog. Am. J. Vet. Res. *35*,481–486, 1974.
4. Bradley, W. E., and Teague, C. T.: Cerebellar influence on the micturition reflex. Exp. Neurol., *23*, 399–411, 1969.
5. Breazile, J. E., Blaugh, B. D., and Nail, N.: Experimental study of canine distemper myoclonus. Am. J. Vet. Res. *27*, 1375, 1966.
6. Breazile, J. E., and Kitchell, R. L.: A study of fiber systems within the spinal cord of the domestic pig that subserve pain. J. Comp. Neurol. *133*, 373–382, 1968.
7. Breazile, J. E., and Thompson, W. D.: Motor cortex of the dog. Am. J. Vet. Res. *28*, 1483–1486, 1967.
8. Brutkowski, S.: Functions of prefrontal cortex in animals. Physiol. Rev. *45*, 721–746, 1965.
9. Bucy, P. C.: The human neural mechanism controlling skeletal muscular activity. *In* Mosberg, W. H. (ed.): *Clinical Neurosurgery.* The Williams & Wilkins Co., Baltimore, 1962.
10. Buxton, D. F., and Goodman, D. C.: Motor function and the corticospinal tracts in the dog and raccoon. J. Comp. Neurol., *129*, 341–360, 1967.
11. Cassinari, V., and Pagni, V.: *Central Pain, A Neurosurgical Survey.* Harvard University Press, Cambridge, Mass., 1969.
12. Chang, H. T.: Choreiform movements in a dog suffering from cortico-striatal disease. J. Neurophysiol. *8*, 89, 1945.
13. Clarke, E., and O'Malley, C. D.: *The Human Brain and Spinal Cord.* University of California Press, Los Angeles, 1968.
14. Crosby, E. C., Humphrey, T., and Laver, E. W.: *Anatomy of the Nervous System.* Macmillan Co., New York, 1962.
15. Denny-Brown, D.: *The Basal Ganglia.* University Press, Oxford, 1962.
16. Dow, R. S., and Moruzzi, G.: *The Physiology and Pathology of the Cerebellum.* University of Minnesota Press, Minneapolis, 1958.
17. Dusser de Barenne, J. G.: Experimentelle Physiologie des kleinhirns. *In* Bumke, W.: Foersters Handbuch Neurol. *2*, 235–267, 1937.
18. Eccles, J. C., *et al.: The Cerebellum as a Neuronal Machine.* Springer-Verlag, New York, 1967.
19. Elliott, H. C.: *Textbook of Neuroanatomy.* J. B. Lippincott Co., Philadelphia, 1963.
20. Emerson, J. D., Bruhn, J. M., Foley, J. O., and Emerson, G. M.: Autonomic responses to chronic electrode stimulation of cerebellum. Am. J. Physiol., *201*, 697–699, 1961.
21. Fennegan, F. M., and Puiggari, M. J.: Influence on gastric motility in dogs. J. Neurosurg. *24*, 497–504, 1966.
22. Ferrier, D.: *The Functions of the Brain,* 2d ed. Smith, Elder, London, 1886.
23. Forman, D.: Responses to electrical stimulation of caudate nucleus in cats in chronic experiments. J. Neurophysiol. *20*, 230, 1957.
24. Fox, C. A., and Snider, R. S.: *The Cerebellum.* American Elsevier, New York, 1967.
25. Fritsch, G., and Hitzig, E.: Ueber die elektrische Erregbarkeit des Grosshirns. Arch. Anat. Physiol. Wissensch. Med. *37*, 300–332, 1870.
26. Gastaut, H., Bernard-Badier, M., Darraspen, M., and van Bozaert, L.: Anatomic and clinical study of 19 epileptic dogs. *In* Baldwin, M., and Bailey, P. (eds.): *Temporal Lobe Epilepsy.* Charles C Thomas, Springfield, Ill., 1958.
27. Gol, A., and Faibish, G. M.: Effects of human hippocampal ablation. J. Neurosurg. *26*:390–398, 1967.
28. Goltz, F.: Der Hunde ohne Grosshirn. Pfugers Arch. Ges. Physiol. *51*, 570–614, 1892.
29. Green, J. R., and Scheetz, D. G.: Surgery of epileptogenic lesions of the temporal lobe. Arch. Neurol. *10*, 135–148, 1964.
30. Green, J. R.: Temporal lobectomy, with special reference to selection of epileptic patients. J. Neurosurg. *26*, 584–593, 1967.
31. Hamuy, T. P., Bromiley, R. B., and Woolsey, C. N.: Somatic afferent areas I and II of dog's cerebral cortex. J. Neurophysiol., *19*, 485, 1956.
32. Hoff, H. E., and Breckenridge, C. G.: Observations on the mammalian reflex prototype of the sign of Babinski. Brain *79*, 155, 1956.
33. Howe, J. W., Crombie, A. L., and Harcourt, R. B.: Electrophysiological examination of the visual system in paediatric practice. Develop. Med. Child Neurol. *17*, 719–725, 1975.
34. Illingworth, R. D., and Molina-Negro, P.: Spontaneous and electrically-evoked activity in the anterolateral column of the spinal cord in dogs. J. Neurosurg. *40*, 58–64, 1974.
35. Jennet, W. B., and Stern, E. W.: Tentorial herniation, the midbrain and the pupil. J. Neurosurg. *17*, 598, 1960.
36. Jongkees, L. B. W.: Vestibular tests for the clinician. Acta Otolaryngol. *97*, 77–80, 1973.
37. Kennard, M. A.: The course of ascending fibers in the spinal cord of the cat essential to the recognition of painful stimuli. J. Comp. Neurol. *100*, 511–524, 1954.
38. Kluver, H., and Bucy, P. C.: Preliminary analysis of function of the temporal lobes in monkeys. Arch. Neurol. Psychol. *42*, 979–1000, 1939.

39. Kneller, S. K., Oliver, J. E., Jr., and Lewis, R. E.: Differential diagnosis of progressive caudal paresis in an aged German shepherd dog. J. Am. Anim. Hosp. Assoc. *11*, 414–417, 1975.
40. Kreiner, J.: The myeloarchitectonics of the frontal cortex of the dog. J. Comp. Neurol. *116*, 117, 1961.
41. Kreiner, J.: Myeloarchitectonics of the cingular cortex in the dog. J. Comp. Neurol. *119*, 255–267, 1962.
42. Kreiner, J., and Maksymowicz, K.: A three dimensional model of the striatal nuclei in the dog's brain. Acta Biol. Exp. *22*, 69–79, 1962.
43. Kreiner, J.: Myeloarchitectonics of the parietal cortex in dog. Acta Biol. Exp. *24*, 195–212, 1964.
44. Kreiner, J.: Myeloarchitectonics of the sensorimotor cortex in dog. J. Comp. Neurol. *122*, 181–200, 1964.
45. Kreiner, J.: Myeloarchitectonics of the perisylvian cortex in dog. J. Comp. Neurol. *123*, 231–242, 1964.
46. Kreiner, J.: Myeloarchitectonics of the occipital cortex in dog and general remarks on the myeloarchitectonics of the dog. J. Comp. Neurol. *127*, 531–558, 1966.
47. Kreiner, J.: Homologies of the fissural and gyral pattern of the hemispheres of the dog and monkey. Acta Anat. *70*, 137–167, 1968.
48. Liles, S., and Davis, G. D.: Interrelation of caudate nucleus and lateral thalamus in regulation of somatic motor activity in anesthetized and awake cat. Fed. Proc. *27*, 387, 1968.
49. Liles, S. L., and Davis, G. D.: Athetoid and choreiform hyperkinesias produced by caudate lesions in the cat. Science *164*, 195–197, 1969.
50. Luciani, L.: *Human Physiology,* Vol. 1–5. Translated by F. A. Welby. Macmillan, London, 1915.
51. McGrath, J. T.: *Neurologic Examination of the Dog,* 2nd ed. Lea & Febiger, Philadelphia, 1960.
52. Mettler, F. A., Finch, G., Girden, E., and Culler, E.: Acoustic value of the several components of the auditory pathway. Brain *57*, 475–483, 1934.
53. Mettler, F. A., and Goss, L. J.: Canine chorea due to strio-cerebellar degeneration of unknown etiology. J.A.V.M.A. *108*, 377–384, 1946.
54. Miller, M. E., Christensen, G. C., and Evans, H. E.: *Anatomy of the Dog.* W. B. Saunders Co., Philadelphia, 1964.
55. Morgan, L. O.: Corpus striatum. A study of secondary degenerations following lesions in man and of symptoms and acute degenerations following experimental lesions in cats. Arch. Neurol. Psychol. *18*, 495–549, 1927.
56. Moruzzi, G., and Magoun, H. W.: Brain stem reticular formation and activation of the EEG. EEG Clin. Neurophysiol. *1*, 455–473, 1949.
57. Mountcastle, V. B.: Somatic functions of the nervous system. Ann. Rev. Physiol., *20*, 487, 1958.
58. Newman, P. P., and Paul, D. H.: The representation of some visceral afferents in the anterior lobe of the cerebellum. J. Physiol. *182*, 195–208, 1966.
59. Newman, P. P., and Paul, D. H.: The projection of spanchnic afferents on the cerebellum of the cat. J. Physiol. *202*, 223–238, 1969.
60. Norrsell, U.: A conditioned reflex study of sensory defects caused by cortical somatosensory ablations. Physiol. Behav. *2*, 73–81, 1967.
61. Oliver, J. E., Jr.: *Canine Cranial Surgery.* Thesis, Auburn University, Auburn, Alabama, 1966.
62. Oliver, J. E., Jr.: Principles of canine brain surgery. Anim. Hosp. *2*, 78–88, 1966.
63. Oliver, J. E., Jr.: Management of the patient with acute head injury. Proc. 19th Gaines Veterinary Symposium, Lafayette, Indiana, Sept. 26, 1969.
64. Oliver, J. E., Jr.: Neurologic examination, I. Taking the history. Vet. Med. Small Anim. Clin. *67*, 433–434, 1971.
65. Oliver, J. E., Jr.: Neurologic examination, X. Sensation: pain. Vet. Med. Small Anim. Clin. *70*, 607–610, 1974.
66. Papez, J. W.: A proposed mechanism of emotion. Arch. Neurol. Psychol. *38*, 725–744, 1937.
67. Plum, F., and Posner, J. B.: *The Diagnosis of Stupor and Coma.* F. A. Davis Co., Philadelphia, 1966.
68. Pribram, K. H., and Kruger, L.: Functions of the olfactory brain. Ann. N.Y. Acad. Sci. *58*, 109–138, 1954.
69. Rademaker, G. G. J.: *Das Stehen.* Springer-Verlag, Berlin, 1931.
70. Renfrew, S.: *An Introduction to Diagnostic Neurology,* vol. 1. E. & S. Livingstone, Edinburgh, 1967.
71. Roberts, T. D. M.: *Neurophysiology of Postural Mechanisms.* Plenum Press, New York, 1967.
72. Schafer, E. A.: *Textbook of Physiology,* vol. 2. Young J. Pentland, Edinburgh, 1900.
73. Schilder, P.: Loss of a brightness discrimination in the cat following removal of the striate area. J. Neurophysiol. *29*, 888, 1966.
74. Schneider, G. E.: Two visual systems. Science *163*, 895–902, 1969.
75. Schreiner, L., and Kling, A.: Behavioral changes following rhinencephalic injury in cat. J. Neurophysiol. *16*, 643–659, 1953.
76. Sherrington, C. S.: *Selected Writings of Sir Charles Sherrington.* Edited by D. Denny-Brown, Paul B. Hoeber, Inc., New York, 1940.
77. Sprague, J. M.: Interaction of cortex and superior colliculus in mediation of visually guided behavior in the cat. Science *153*, 1544–1547, 1966.
78. Sprague, J. M.: Visual, acoustic, and somesthetic deficits in the cat after cortical and midbrain lesions in the thalamus. *In* Purpura, D. P., and Yahr, M. (eds.): *Thalamus,* Columbia University Press. New York, 1966.
79. Stone, A. B.: Variant lesions in the central nervous system of dogs and cats. J. Small Anim. Pract. *10*, 287–294, 1969.
80. Stone, J.: The naso-temporal division of the cat retina. J. Comp. Neurol. *126*, 585–600, 1966.
81. Tarlov, I. M.: Spinal cord compression, mechanism of paralysis and treatment. Charles C Thomas, Publishers, Springfield, Ill., 1957.
82. Tower, S. S., and Hines, M.: Dissociation of the pyramidal and extrapyramidal functions of the frontal lobe. Science *82*, 376, 1935.
83. Tunturi, A. R.: A study of the pathway from the medial geniculate body to the acoustic cortex in the dog. Amer. J. Physiol. *147*, 311–319, 1948.
84. Tunturi, A. R.: Physiological determination of the arrangement of the afferent connections to the middle ectosylvian area in the dog. Amer. J. Physiol. *162*, 489–502, 1950.

85. Walsh, E. G.: *Physiology of the Nervous System*, 2d ed. Longmans, Green and Co., London, 1964.
86. Waltz, T. A., and Ehni, G.: The thalamic syndrome and its mechanism. J. Neurosurg. *24*, 735, 1966.
87. Weed, L. L.: *Medical Records, Medical Education and Patient Care.* Press of Case Western Reserve University, Cleveland, 1969.
88. Whittier, J. R.: Flexor spasm syndrome in the carnivore I, II, III. Am. J. Vet. Res. *17*, 720, 1956.
89. Woolsey, C. N.: Postural regulations of the frontal and motor cortex of the dog. Brain *56*, 353–370, 1933.
90. Woolsey, C. N.: Second somatic receiving area in the cerebral cortex of cat, dog, and monkey. Fed. Proc. *2*, 55, 1943.
91. Woolsey, C. N.: Some observations on brain fissuration in relation to cortical localization of function. *In* Tower, D. B., and Schade, J. P. (eds.): Structure and Function of the Cerebral Cortex. Elsevier Publishing Co., Amsterdam, 1960.

CHAPTER 5

NEURORADIOGRAPHY

J. E. Bartels, B.S., D.V.M., M.Sc.
B. F. Hoerlein, D.V.M., Ph.D.
J. G. Boring, B.S., D.V.M., M.S.

The fundamental concepts of diagnostic radiography suggested for the general practitioner also apply in the science and art of neuroradiography.[17] Radiographic procedures supplement the physical neurological examination and its interpretation and special tests such as electrodiagnostic and laboratory procedures. Radiographic examination will not be helpful if the basic procedures discussed in Chapters 1 through 4 are not carefully performed. To this end, radiography must be used only to confirm a tentative physical or clinical diagnosis.

The equipment necessary for neuroradiography should be superior to that generally available in general practice. The x-ray machine itself should be of 300 ma and 100 kvp minimum capacity, with a table that can be tilted and is equipped with a Potter-Bucky diaphragm. The latter could be readily replaced by a high-quality, high-ratio parallel or focused grid or grid cassette. Each grid or grid system has its own particular advantages and disadvantages; its basic purpose is to reduce secondary scattered radiation, thereby preventing "film fogging" and loss of detail. A minimal Bucky exposure of 1/10 of a second is desirable but not necessary. Generally speaking, unless a photo-timer is employed, 1/10 of a second will be the best Bucky exposure available. Again, the use of some type of grid is emphasized. Grid cassettes can be acquired readily in lieu of previously described types; however, the initial cost is considerably more. The tube head should be easy to position and should be supplied with a satisfactory cone, diaphragm, or, preferably, a well-designed collimator to delineate the x-ray field and to reduce secondary scattered radiation. Most diaphragms and collimators are equipped with a centering light to determine the exact position of the central ray. The latter provides for precise positioning of the area of the animal to be portrayed on the film.

The accessory devices or equipment are of equal importance in the production of superior quality diagnostic radiographs in neuroradiology. All cassettes and intensifying screens should be clean and of good quality. The types of screen should be properly adjusted to the capacity of the equipment and speed of the film. Basically, film detail is determined by screen crystal size. As the speed of screens increases, the ultimate film detail is decreased. Three screen speeds are generally available for routine radiography. These are: detail or high-definition screens, which are slow speed; general purpose or par speed screens; and high-speed screens, which lack a proportionate amount of detail. It can be inferred that the best quality radiographs can most easily be obtained by the proper combination of film speed, speed of screens, and output of equipment. This combination should be determined by an experienced technician or veterinary radiologist. As outlined by Schebitz and Wilkens, the use of high-definition screens and detail film will produce superior quality diagnostic films.[86] The use of nonscreen film for neuroradiology will be considered later in this chapter.

Other devices should include: radiolucent foam cushions to assure and maintain proper positioning, accurate calipers to measure part thickness, film markers and identification, lead aprons, gloves, and film badges to enforce radiation protection. Lastly, an up-to-date, clean, adequately equipped darkroom is a must for the production of quality diagnostic radiographs.

SPINAL CORD AND VERTEBRAL RADIOGRAPHY

Most spinal lesions are minute in size and are of extremely low radiographic density; therefore, superior quality diagnostic films, as well as multiple views, are required to

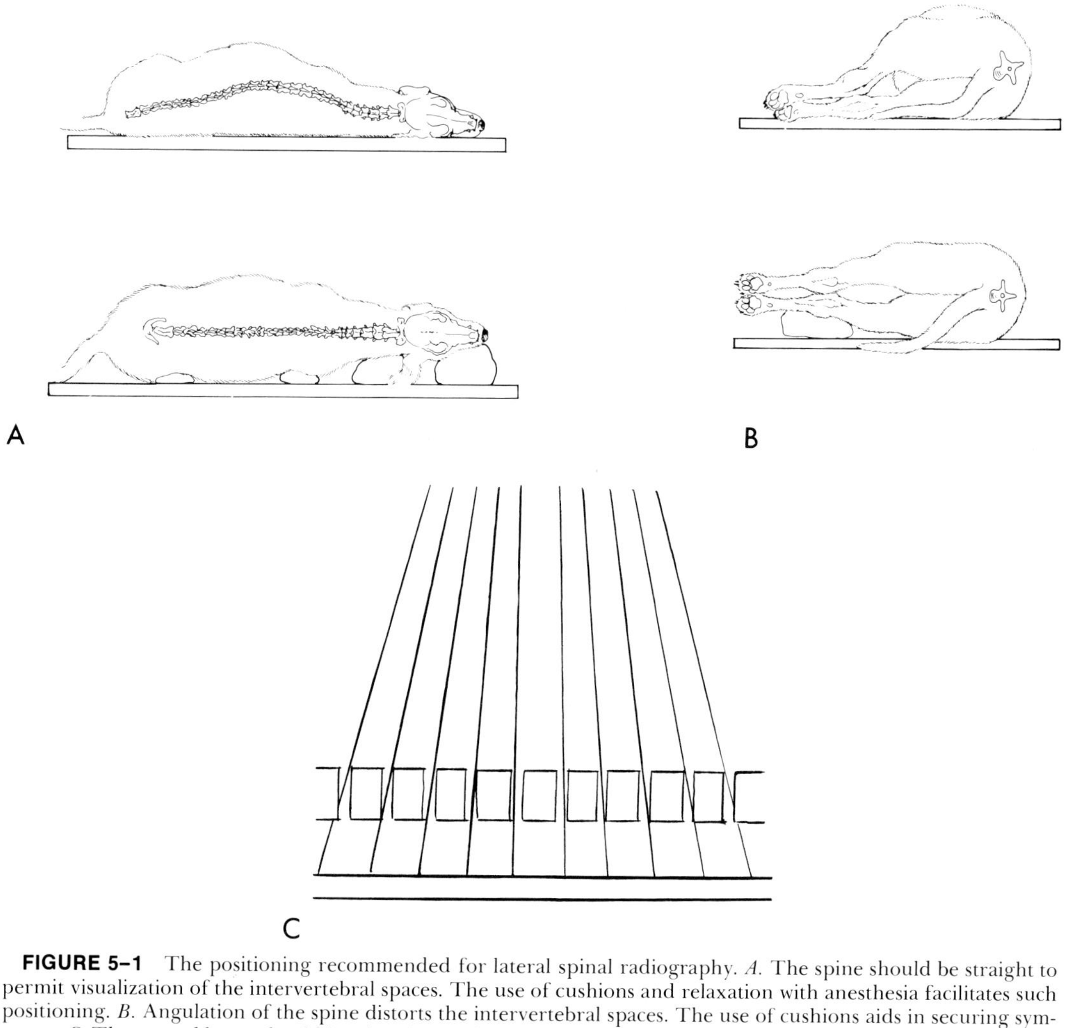

FIGURE 5–1 The positioning recommended for lateral spinal radiography. *A.* The spine should be straight to permit visualization of the intervertebral spaces. The use of cushions and relaxation with anesthesia facilitates such positioning. *B.* Angulation of the spine distorts the intervertebral spaces. The use of cushions aids in securing symmetry. *C.* The central beam should be placed over the suspected disk lesion so that vertebrae are not pictured overlying each other, as this would partially obliterate the intervertebral space. (Based on Douglas, S. W., and Williams, H. D.: *Principles of Veterinary Radiology*. The Williams & Wilkins Co., Baltimore, 1963.)

demonstrate these lesions. When not medically contraindicated, a tranquilizer, sedative such as oxymorphone hydrochloride (Numorphan) (except in metrizamide [Amipaque] myelography), or short-acting anesthetic such as thiopental sodium (Pentothal) is mandatory; these agents limit or stop motion and therefore contribute to greater film detail. Involuntary muscle contractures must be eliminated, and exact positioning must be attained.

CONVENTIONAL FILMS

Positioning

The basic positions of the animal are the lateral (Lat) recumbent, and ventrodorsal (VD) views. Placing a cushion under areas of uneven flesh distribution, such as the neck, will allow the spine to be parallel to the film and will facilitate a direct lateral view, so that distortion is avoided and perfect superimposition of bilaterally symmetrical parts occurs—e.g., both intervertebral foramina will appear as one foramen (Figs. 5-1 to 5-3). This facilitates the interpretation of the relative width of disk spaces and the presence of protrusions into the spinal canal. Normally, lateral views of the spine should be taken in a normal position, that is, not flexed or hyperextended. However, occasionally moderate flexion and extension is helpful to demonstrate vertebral instability that may be associated with a disk disorder. The VD view places the spine closest to the film, so that maximal detail will be seen with minimal distortion. The VD view should be taken with the dog in a bilaterally symmetrical position. Scoliosis and rotation of the trunk can be avoided

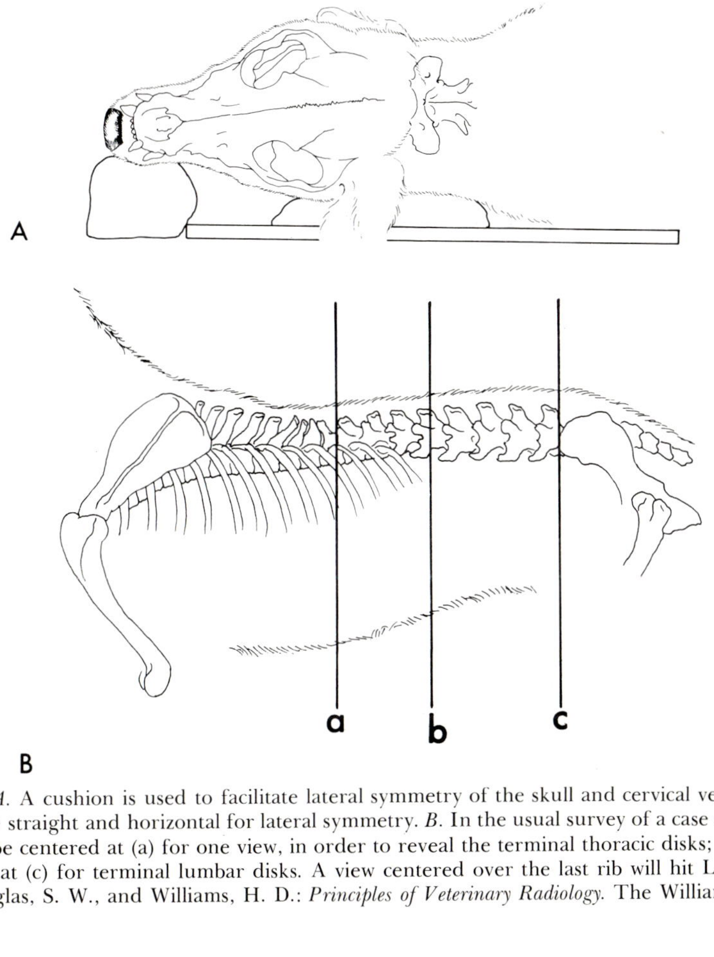

FIGURE 5-2 *A*. A cushion is used to facilitate lateral symmetry of the skull and cervical vertebrae. The skull and spine must be straight and horizontal for lateral symmetry. *B*. In the usual survey of a case of disk paraplegia, the beam should be centered at (a) for one view, in order to reveal the terminal thoracic disks; at (b) for anterior lumbar disk, and at (c) for terminal lumbar disks. A view centered over the last rib will hit L1-2 or L2-3 disk. (*A*. based on Douglas, S. W., and Williams, H. D.: *Principles of Veterinary Radiology*. The Williams & Wilkins Co., Baltimore, 1963.)

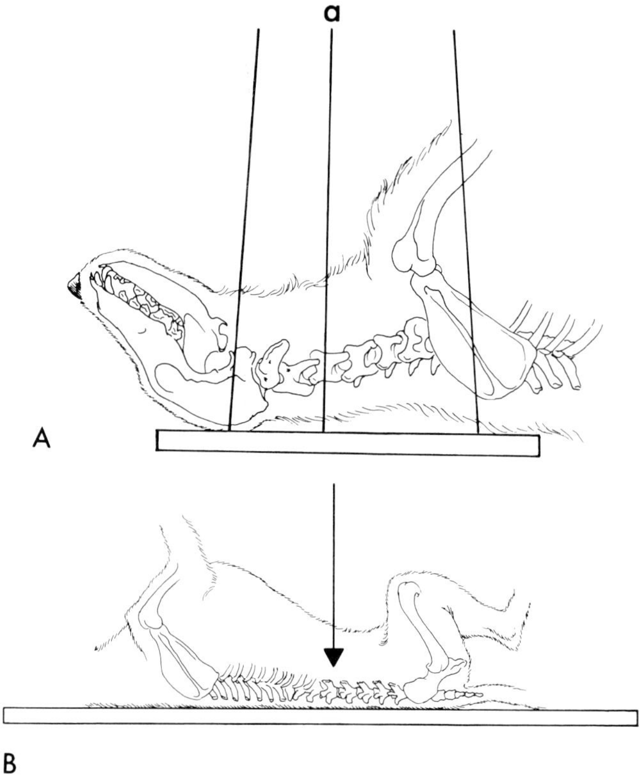

FIGURE 5–3 *A*. The VD view of the cervical disk spaces can at times be viewed most effectively by a 5 to 10 degree angulation of the central beam of the x-ray (a). *B*. Diagram demonstrating the position in a VD spinogram. (Based on Douglas, S. W., and Williams, H. D.: *Principles of Veterinary Radiology*. The Williams & Wilkins Co., Baltimore, 1963.)

completely with the use of anesthetic and positioning cushions (Figs. 5–1 and 5–2). Oblique views, either by patient positioning or by angling the tube head, can be used to supplement the two standard views. Geary has effectively used this technique to isolate spinal lesions.[45, 46]

Technique

The complete spinal survey provides patient information on possible future spinal problems. It also allows valid comparison of the width of no more than three or four disk spaces on one view, and is nearly devoid of distortion and superimposition of vertebral bodies. The divergent characteristic of x-ray demands that the latter technical aspect of film quality be considered closely.[29, 45, 51, 52]

For general spinal radiography, cassettes with par speed intensifying screens are adequate. Detail and high detail screens, as previously mentioned, will yield excellent quality or detail films. Survey radiography can be accomplished on any size cassette, but 10 by 12 inches is a convenient size and yields spinal segmentation without gross distortion of the osseous anatomy. The latter depends, of course, upon the size of the dog. Screen cassettes can be easily divided with a leaded sheet, thus allowing two views per cassette.

Any soft tissue part thickness measuring more than 9 cm requires the use of a grid or grid system. This is particularly true of the spine and any neuroradiographic procedure. The use of a Bucky or a parallel or focused grid to limit scattered radiation is mandatory. The grid ratio should range from 8:1 to 12:1, with 60 to 80 lines per inch, and preferably, a variable latitude focus-film distance. Because of the absorption of the primary ray, the use of a grid requires the addition of 10 to 13 kvp to attain comparable quality films.

Two views at 90 degrees to each other—i.e., Lat and VD—are necessary to appreciate spatial relationships and geometry. Generally, the VD film of the spine requires a proportionately greater exposure per centimeter of thickness than the lateral view. This exposure is usually attained by an increase in kvp.

The development of the nonscreen Bucky technique for spinal radiography has served its usefulness in diagnostic neuroradiology. Screen film radiography with newer composition screens provides nearly equal detail. Characteristically, nonscreen film yields extreme latitude of exposure densities and therefore finite detail.

Both Geary[45] and the authors of this chapter have found that if a high-capacity 300 ma unit is available, the variable screen technique can easily be performed.

Modern processing equipment and precise techniques must be used to demonstrate the minimal lesions that are frequently seen in cord and vertebral disorders. Effective solutions, proper processing intervals, and thorough washing should be applied to all films. Films should be entirely dry before interpretation is attempted.[17]

MYELOGRAPHY

Contrast Media

Ideally, four criteria are employed for the selection of the most suitable or practical contrast medium for this special procedure. The radiopaque media should be (1) relatively nontoxic, and (2) readily absorbed; (3) it should provide superior contrast or opacity, and (4), it should have satisfactory viscous properties to allow free, even flow and distribution throughout the subarachnoid space.[33]

Theoretically, three types of media are miscible with spinal fluid: water-soluble agents, aqueous suspensions of finely divided opaque particles, and emulsions of an opaque oil in water. In general, agents prepared in a water base give the best radiographic detail and possess even flow characteristics and good radiopacity, but they tend to be toxic. Convulsions, muscle spasms, paresthesia, and death have been reported to result from water-soluble media.[5, 25, 39, 64] These contrast agents are hypertonic and are usually irritating to the meninges, and they are rapidly absorbed from the cerebrospinal fluid. A pronounced vasospasm has also been associated with their use.

According to Lasser, the degree of toxicity depends on three factors that comprise the total response: (1) hypersensitivity; (2) true chemotoxicity, which has a direct relationship to peripheral vasodilation as well as the blood brain barrier, manifested by an increased permeability of cerebral capillaries; and (3) the hyperosmolarity-pH relationship, in which the hypertonicity of the medium results in tissue dehydration and meningeal irritation.[31]

From 1949 to 1952, Hoerlein evaluated the use of a recently developed iodized oil contrast medium, ethyl iodophenylhundecylate (Pantopaque), in several hundred experimental and clinical cases in dogs requiring cisternal myelography. At the same time, some evaluation was made of an aqueous suspension of 25 per cent thorium dioxide (Thorotrast). Thorotrast had much superior flow characteristics but was toxic clinically and histopathologically,[50] After this study, several other available radiopaque contrast media were tested experimentally for myelographic suitability in dogs.[53] Briefly, the trade names of these products tested and reported in 1953 were (some are still available): (1) iodized oils—Iodochloral, and Lipiodol, and (2) aqueous iodine preparations—Neo-Ipax (75 per cent), Skiodan (20 per cent), and Diodrast (35 per cent). The oil preparations showed inferior flow characteristics compared to Pantopaque; they caused little immediate clinical toxicity but produced some chronic fibrotic leptomeningitis. The aqueous preparations, when introduced in the cisterna, were very toxic clinically and in some cases proved fatal. Skiodan (Kontrast U), reevaluated more than 10 years later by Funkquist was at that time shown to be less fatal than other media but produced severe reactions. Based on these results, Pantopaque has been used by the authors steadily since the 1950's until a few years ago, when lumbar administration of Skiodan became more feasible.[53]

As mentioned, Pantopaque has proved to be the standard myelographic agent in humans since its development in 1944. In the dog, the medium has the disadvantage of slow and inaccurate flow characteristics, and tends to break up in droplets instead of remaining a bolus. Pantopaque will demonstrate gross compressive lesions and produces an excellent radiopaque image. It is slowly absorbed, and causes a chronic fibrotic nonpurulent leptomeningitis, which peaks in 5 days and then regresses[99] and is rarely important clinically[53, 55] (Fig. 5–4).

Thorium dioxide (Thorotrast) is no longer used since it is radioactive, and toxemia has occurred 2 to 6 years after administration[78] (Fig. 5–5).

The use of Skiodan (Kontrast U) in lumbar administrations has been common in the past few years based on work by Funkquist.[34–41] The various mixtures of agents used with Skiodan and other means of controlling clinical reactions will be discussed in the next section of myelographic techniques.

Continued efforts to utilize water-soluble media for myelography have been documented.[14, 42, 72, 73, 80, 81] Investigators have modified techniques in cisternal and lumbar taps and have varied the dose, rate of administration, per cent concentration, pre-medication anesthesia, post-medication, and positioning. These modifications were made in an attempt to reduce or suppress untoward sequelae from toxicity, which were manifested as seizures, general muscular fasciculation, cord malacia, irritibility, and death.[7, 8]

These efforts have resulted in a new product called metrizamide (Amipaque), which is a non-ionic, biologically inert preparation. It is of the lowest possible osmolarity and is reported to be nonirritating to the meninges; it also has less immediate clinical toxicity and no apparent long-term effects. Clinical trials have been performed in several veterinary centers, and the drug has been approved for clinical trials in humans in the United States, Canada, and Europe.[1, 2, 7, 11, 15, 64, 65] Bartels finds an approximate seizure incidence of 20 per cent in dogs, but others suggest an incidence of 0 to 10 per cent in dogs and cats. It is hoped that metrizamide or a similar preparation will be clinically available for canine myelography in the relatively near future.

Air has been reported as a satisfactory contrast medium in cervical myelography in man.[75] In pneumoventriculograms of the dog, air has been observed occasionally in the cerebral, cerebellar, and cervical subarachnoid spaces. However, more investigation is needed to determine whether air can be used effectively to demonstrate cervical compression in the dog.

Fig. 5–4

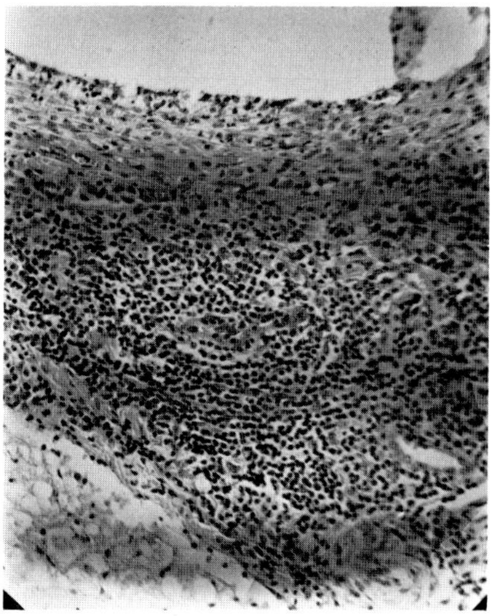

Fig. 5–5

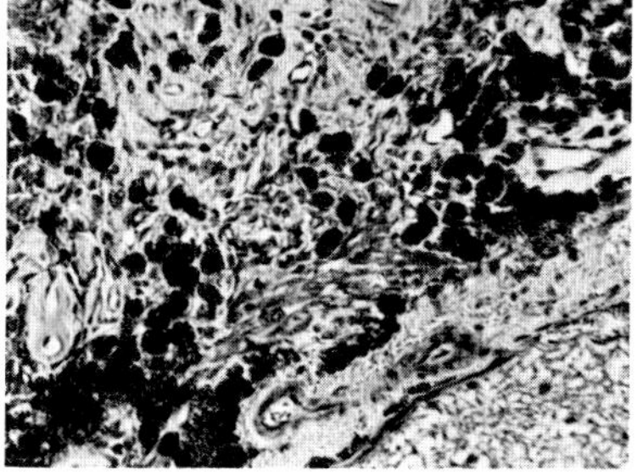

FIGURE 5–4 An advanced case of fibrotic arachnoiditis caused by the myelographic administration of Pantopaque.

FIGURE 5–5 Arachnoiditis caused by the myelographic use of Thorotrast.

Myelographic Techniques

In a case of spinal compression resulting from a disk protrusion, a malformation of the cervical spinal canal (wobbler), or a meningeal tumor, conventional films may not diagnose adequately the site or extent of the lesion. Subarachnoid myelography may be desirable only if the lesion is clinically determined to be a reversible one and one which requires decompressive surgery for recovery. In such instances, a myelographic examination (using subarachnoid administration of a contrast medium) is helpful.

Cisternal Technique

Cisternal administration of contrast medium has been described adequately by Brooks.[13] In this method, an anesthetized dog is placed in a sternal recumbent position with his head held firmly at an angle of approximately 90 degrees to the cervical spine. The hair is clipped, and the skin is aseptically prepared for introduction of the needle. A 3-inch, 22-gauge spinal needle with stylet is inserted in the dorsal midline, midway between the occipital protuberance and the most palpable part of the wings of the atlas. The needle is directed perpendicularly to the spinal column, through the dorsal skin and musculature and into the atlanto-occipital interspace. At this point, the needle pierces the rather tough ligamentum flavum. The dura mater lies just below this firm structure when the head is held in the position just mentioned. As the needle pierces the dura mater, a cutaneous "flinch" is frequently seen. The stylet of the needle is then withdrawn, and one watches for bubbling of spinal fluid out of the needle hub. If the needle is not in the correct position, synovial fluid may be retrieved from the atlanto-occipital joint. A syringe is attached and the fluid is slowly withdrawn. With the bevel of the needle directed posteriorly, the oil contrast medium is slowly injected (0.5 ml/min) into the subarachnoid space. It has been our experience that if the medium is rapidly injected, it will be forced into the fourth ventricle and over the cerebellar hemisphere. An aqueous medium such as metrizamide may be injected at 2 ml per minute with no sequelae. The amount of spinal fluid with-

Fig. 5–6

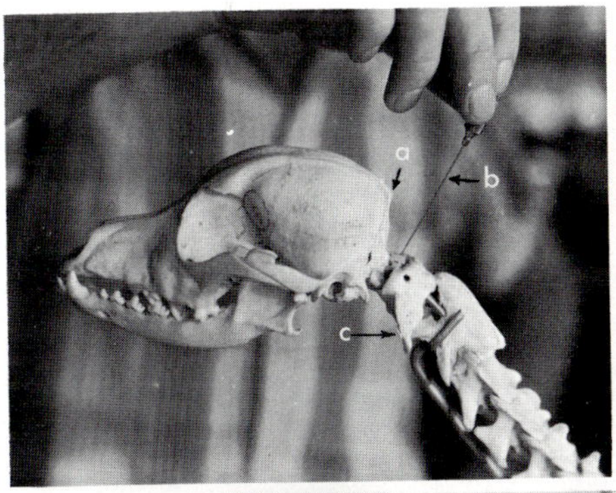

Fig. 5–7

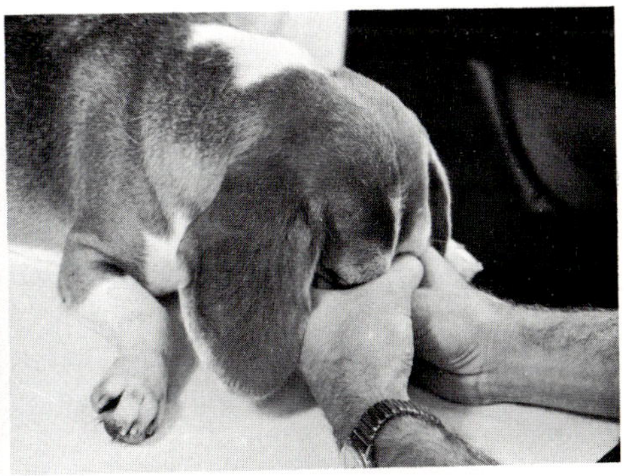

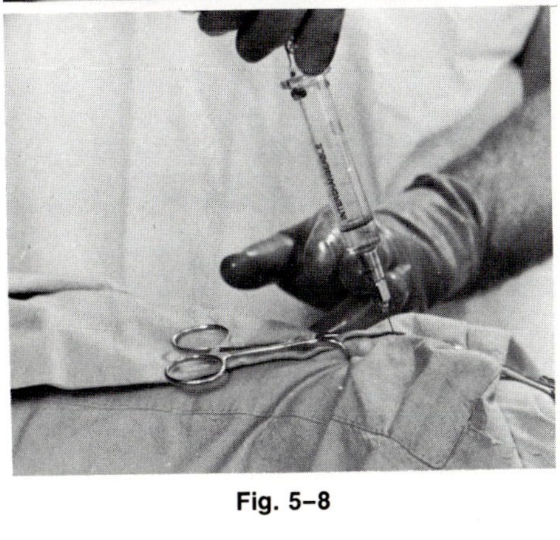

Fig. 5–8

FIGURE 5–6 The landmarks for a cisternal tap: (a) occipital protuberance; (c) most prominent area of the wings of the atlas; (b) midway between (a) and (c) on the dorsal midline with the needle (2-inch 22-gauge Quincke) directed at right angles to the cervical spine.

FIGURE 5–7 The head is firmly positioned at right angles to the cervical spine. The dog is placed in the sternal recumbent position for a cisternal tap.

FIGURE 5–8 Slow withdrawal of spinal fluid from the cisterna magna in a cisternal tap. In myelography, the quantity of contrast medium injected should equal the amount of spinal fluid withdrawn.

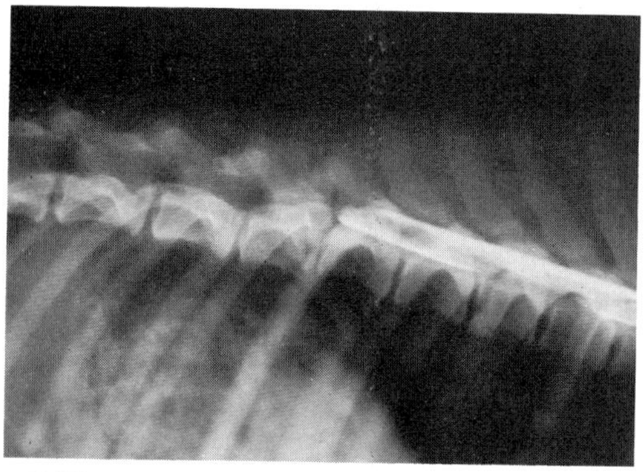

FIGURE 5–9 Lateral view of subarachnoid (cisternal) administration of Pantopaque, showing a complete blockage at T10–11 interspace. This lesion is a fracture of T11 vertebra.

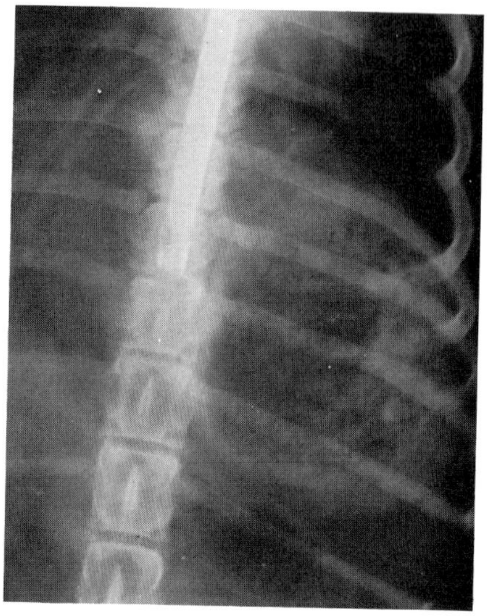

FIGURE 5–10 Ventrodorsal view of Figure 5–9.

drawn should approximate the amount of medium administered, usually 1 to 3 ml of an oil medium or 0.3–0.5 ml/kg body weight of a water-contrast medium[13, 21, 52, 55] (see Figs. 5–6 to 5–8).

When the spinal needle has been withdrawn, the head of the dog should be elevated as the neck is rotated and moved about gently to promote caudal migration of the oily medium. The table is tilted to a 60-degree angle, keeping the dog's head uppermost. Periodic films are taken with the dog in a dorsoventral (DV) position until posterior migration of the contrast medium has stopped. At this point, a lateral exposure is made in order to obtain additional information about the flow pattern. If the veterinarian prefers, the lateral film may precede the DV exposure. The total time consumed by a myelographic examination with an iodized oil medium is expected to be 30 to 45 minutes,[52, 55] or approximately 7 to 20 minutes with an aqueous medium. Since aqueous media flow so quickly, the head should be elevated slightly, but films must be made immediately after injection for cervical lesions (Figs. 5–9 to 5–11).

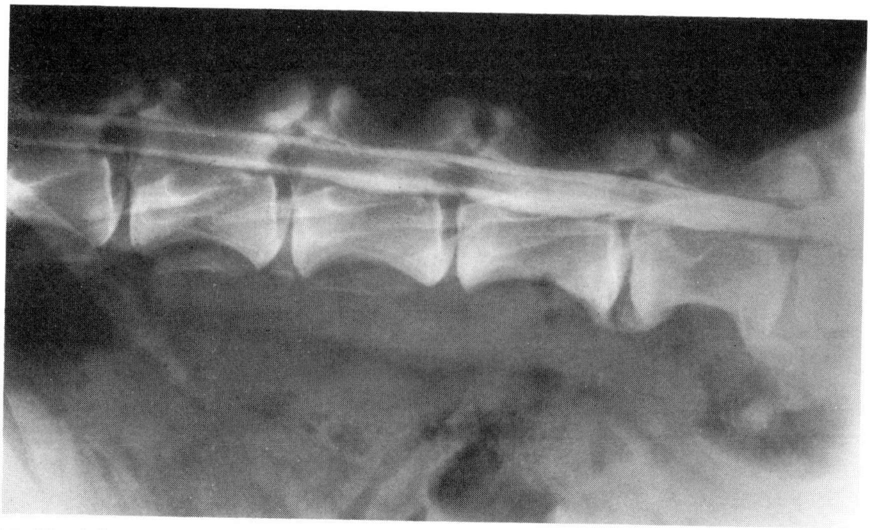

FIGURE 5–11 A lateral view of a metrizamide myelogram given by cisternal injection. Notice that there is no marked abnormality of flow in the spondylytic areas.

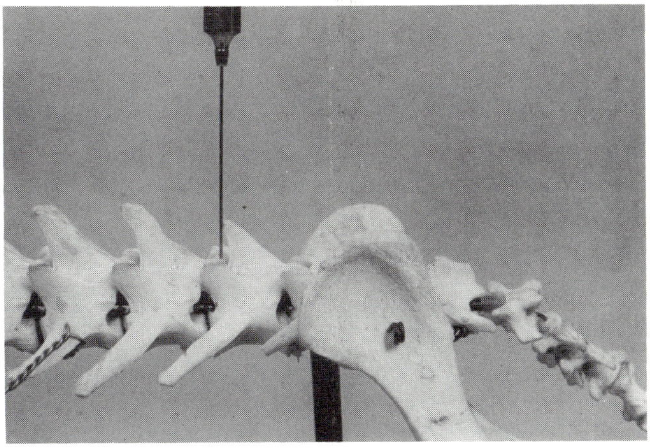

FIGURE 5–12 The lumbar puncture is generally made at L4–5 or L5–6. This picture shows the spinal needle at L5–6.

Lumbar Technique

In some cases, the lumbar route may be selected for subarachnoid administration of the contrast medium. This procedure has the disadvantage of being more difficult, and the quantity of spinal fluid available is considerably smaller than by the cisternal route. The possible advantages of this site are the possibility of a quicker examination and the use of less contrast medium.

In a dorsal subarachnoid lumbar tap, the anesthetized dog is placed in either a lateral or a flexed sternal recumbent position. The table may be tilted, keep the dog's head uppermost, to a 45 to 60 degree angle in order to promote an accumulation of spinal fluid in the lumbar area. If the dog is in a sternal recumbent position, a sling placed around its perineum helps to maintain the dorsal arch in the spine and tends to minimize the tension of the supporting cords on the forelegs. If in a lateral recumbent position, the hind legs should be brought forward between the front limbs in order to flex the spine. The lumbar subarachnoid space can be punctured as far posteriorly as the L4–5 or L5–6 interspace. Ordinarily, a site posterior to the lesion is most desirable for a myelographic examination (Figs. 5–12 and 5–13).

The spinal needle should be inserted in the dorsal midline just anterior to the spine of the vertebra and pushed downward until bone is reached. Ticer suggests passing a needle lateral to the dorsal spine of L6 and directing it medioventral to enter the spinal canal. The small interarcual space between the vertebrae is palpated with the needle, and at this point the needle is forcibly inserted into the dorsal subarachnoid space. Spinal fluid is withdrawn in the manner described for the cisternal tap. The medium is injected with the bevel of the

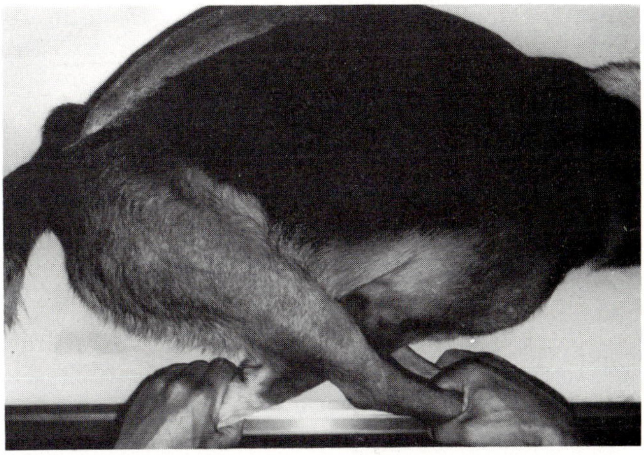

FIGURE 5–13 The lumbar tap can be made in the flexed spinal position in either the lateral or sternal recumbent position. This illustration shows a means of flexing the spine in order to open the interarcual spaces to allow passage of the needle.

needle point directed toward the suspected lesion. The table can be flattened in most cases or tilted in the head-downward position at a 10- to 20-degree angle to promote anterior flow of the medium. Flow of medium into the cranium should be avoided.[52, 54, 55]

Funkquist[34] inserts a metal bar, grooved on both sides, through the incised skin and fascia along the anterior surface of the spine until the vertebral arches are reached; the bar acts as a guide so that the needle can be inserted more easily into the ventral subarachnoid space. The spine is straightened and the medium is injected while the dog's forequarters are slightly elevated.

As mentioned previously, Funkquist developed a method of using an aqueous contrast medium, Kontrast U, which had been previously investigated by Hoerlein as Skiodan (sodium iodomethanesulfonate). Funkquist considered Kontrast U to be satisfactory when introduced into the subarachnoid spaces in the posterior lumbar area in the following manner.[34] (1) A light plane intravenous barbiturate anesthesia is employed; (2) A lumbar tap at L4–5 is made, as previously described; (3) A single, fast injection of 20 per cent Kontrast U with the addition of 1 mg Xylocaine* per ml of contrast medium is made. A dosage rate of 0.3 ml/kg body weight should be used; (4) The injection time is 10 seconds, and films are taken immediately thereafter.

Injections of Kontrast U were made in a total of 151 dogs, including 136 dachshunds, with clinical signs of cord compression of varying degrees. Myelographic changes corresponded closely to those seen at either necropsy or surgery. The characteristic toxic effects caused by Kontrast U were severe muscle spasms, which Xylocaine tended to alleviate. However, Xylocaine was shown to cause a marked fall in blood pressure, especially in extensive cases of myelomalacia.[37] Noradrenaline injections should be administered for such reactions. Muscle contractions can be avoided if succinylcholine chloride is administered before the contrast-Xylocaine mixture. Neurological deterioration was seen when the medium was present in the central canal. Histopathologically, the contrast medium caused various degrees of edematous foci in the white substance, the larger foci having necrotic centers. The number and degree of these lesions were greatest in dogs that had suffered the greatest fall of blood pressure.[41]

Funkquist[40] also used the same technique for demonstrating cervical cord lesions. The cervical subarachnoid space was filled with the contrast-Xylocaine mixture by making a lumbar injection. However, after the injection and the cisternal withdrawal of spinal fluid, the hindquarters of the dog were elevated. The films were taken in the lateral recumbent position. Muscle relaxation was promoted by use of succinylcholine. Toxic effects were no greater than those seen in thoracolumbar procedures.

Several variations of the technique described by Funkquist have been tried. A spinal "cocktail" may be prepared by mixing equal parts of 40 per cent Skiodan and cerebrospinal fluid from the animal to be examined and adding 1 mg of 5 per cent Xylocaine in a 75 per cent dextrose solution to the Skiodan mixture just before injection. For thoracolumbar myelography 0.3 ml/kg of the mixture is used, and for cervical examination 0.45 ml/kg is used.[22] Others have used glucocorticosteroids prior to injection, keeping diazepam (Valium) ready for immediate intravenous administration to control convulsive activity.[7, 9, 74, 95] If the animal is scheduled for immediate surgery, the danger of convulsive seizures is less with prolonged surgical anesthesia.

Recent work[9] indicates that 40 per cent sodium methiodal can be administered via the cisternal route with no more sequelae than those with the previously described mixtures. Myelography using this technique has been performed on 115 clinical and experimental cases. Unaltered 40 per cent sodium methiodal was administered by the cisternal route in a dose of 0.12 ml per pound of body weight, with volatile gaseous anesthesia and no premedication with corticosteroids. Immediately after injection the table was tilted to 40 degrees, and the medium flowed to the cauda equina in 5 to 7 minutes. Minor bulbar fasciculation and muscle contractures were noted with rare

*Xylocaine hydrochloride is the hydrochloride of diethylaminoaceto-2, 6-xylidide, Astra Pharmaceutical Products, Inc., Worcester, Massachusetts.

grand mal seizures. Valium was utilized in the latter instances.[9]

Transmedullary Lumbar Myelography

The technique for performing transmedullary lumbar myelography by inserting a spinal needle through the spinal cord and injecting the contrast medium into the ventral subarachnoid space has been described by others.[6, 81, 95, 96] In some diagnostic laboratories this technique has been proposed for routine practice in veterinary neuroradiology instead of the traditional method of inserting the needle into the dorsal subarachnoid space (not penetrating the spinal cord).

Histopathologic studies were performed on spinal cords on which ventral subarachnoid spinal taps had been performed at L4–5.[12] Some dogs were given contrast media and others were not. Myelomalacia causing considerable destruction of the dorsal and ventral columns was seen in the cord along the needle tract. The cord myelomalacia was more extensive than the expected size of the needle tract. When no contrast medium was injected, the lesion could not be attributed to a chemical toxic reaction.[12] When contrast medium was injected the reaction was more severe, supporting Parker's observation that any leakage of contrast medium into the cord tissue causes massive destruction of tissue.[81] Cystic necrosis, myelomalacia, demyelination, and axonal necrosis in the periphery of the lesion as well as macrophagic infiltration, vascular reaction, and gliosis were the usual manifestations of transmedullary needle puncture.[12] It is therefore concluded that the trauma associated with a transmedullary spinal tap makes the practice especially dangerous if pathological myelopathy is already present[12] (Figs. 5–14 and 5–15).

Interpretation of Myelograms

Oil contrast myelograms are usually useful only in cases of extradural compression which cause a marked deviation of flow or a complete subarachnoid blockage. However, aqueous contrast media can provide helpful information regarding (1) extradural masses (hematoma, protruded disk, or tumor); (2) intradural–extramedullary

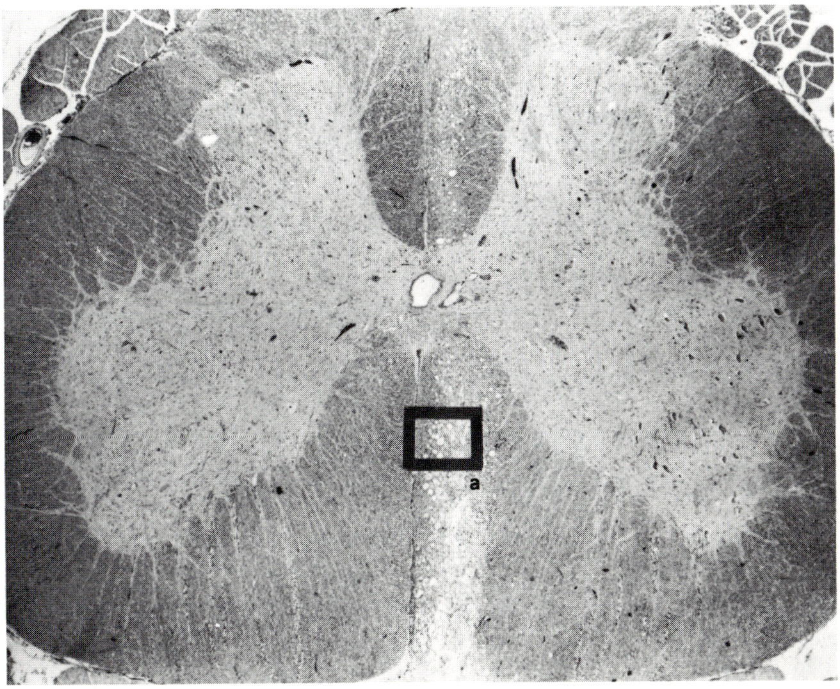

FIGURE 5–14 Myelomalacia caused by introducing a 22-gauge spinal needle into the ventral subarachnoid space at L4–5 interspace.

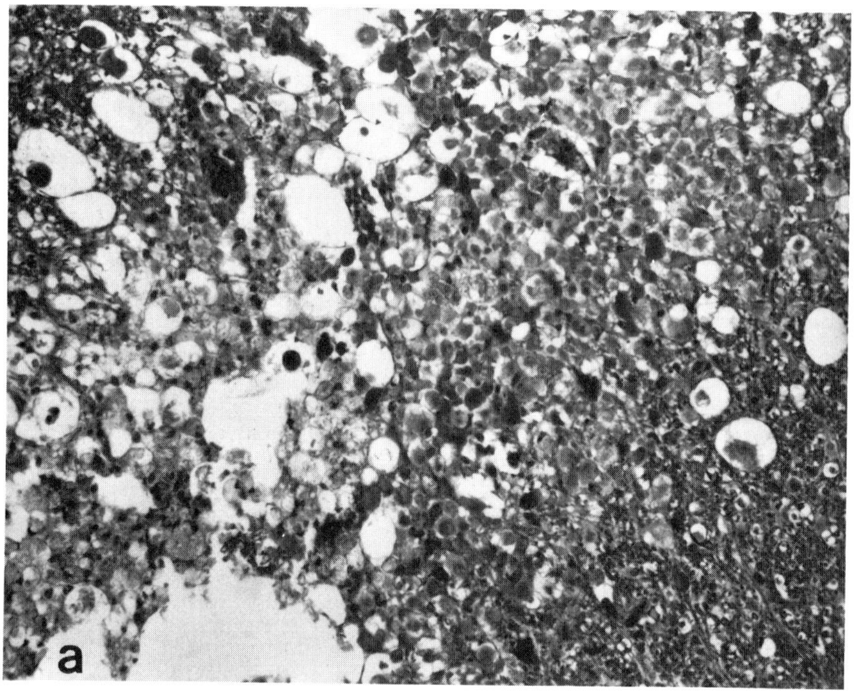

FIGURE 5–15 A high-power examination of area marked (a) in Figure 5–14. Note that cystic necrosis, demyelination, axonal necrosis, and macrophagic infiltration are more extensive than the expected size on the needle tract.

masses (tumor); and (3) intramedullary masses (tumor). These lesions all cause transverse (localized) myelopathies, whereas disseminated myelopathies or meningopathies do not require myelography. The clinician must know the normal enlargements of the spinal cord (cervical and lumbar), the normal slight indentations of the ventral contrast column of the intervertebral disks on lateral views, and other normal peculiarities of aqueous media myelograms. Extradural compressive masses will cause a narrowing and deviation of the subarachnoid space on at least one view. Tumors and wobbler lesions may encircle the cord and cause an hourglass-like constriction. Spinal cord edema causes diffuse enlargement of the diameter of the contrast columns over several vertebral lengths. If the swelling is so great that the entire subarachnoid space is obliterated, only faint contrast or no contrast will be noted in the area. In cases of hematomyelia, necrosis, and degeneration of the spinal cord and meninges, the contrast medium may exhibit a patchy diffuse distribution where it has escaped in spinal cord tissue or pooled between hemorrhagic areas. In intradural–extramedullary masses, the filling defect may have an air-bubble-like appearance. Some of these intradural–extramedullary lesions may resemble an intramedullary mass which causes a widening of the cord image in both views. Most intramedullary lesions cause an increase in cord size (for several vertebral lengths) similar to that seen in cord edema. The history of trauma in a case of cord edema will aid in clinical differentiation of this entity from an intramedullary cord tumor. More specific information of interpretative myelography will be given under the discussions of specific cord lesions[6, 91] (Figs. 5–16 to 5–18).

EPIDURALOGRAMS

This technique originated in humans,[87] and air was initially used as a contrast medium. Lipiodol and Pantopaque were used later, but it was difficult to direct either of these media once it had entered the epidural space.[87] For these reasons, epiduralo-

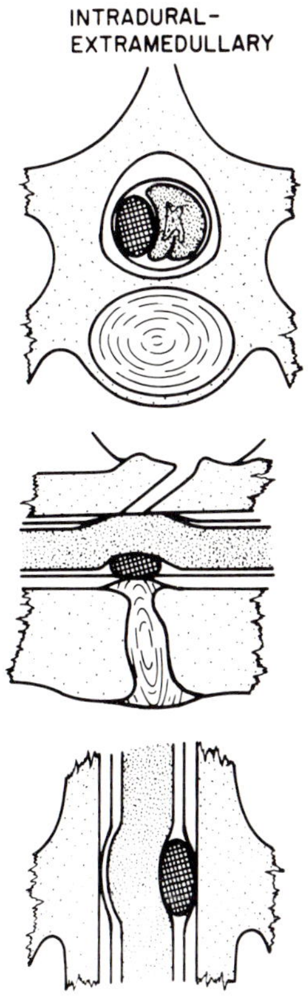

FIGURE 5–16 Line drawing depicting an intradural-extramedullary mass. These masses may compress and deviate the spinal cord and may produce a filling defect in the subarachnoid space. (From Stowalter, J. L., Menhusen, M. J., and Gendreau, C. L.: Canine myelography with Skiodan. Part I. Indications and interpretation. Vet. Med. Small Anim. Clin. *71,* 1207, 1976.)

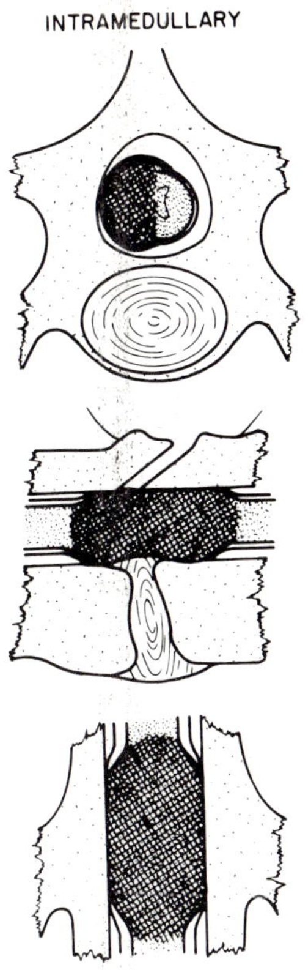

FIGURE 5–17 Line drawing depicting an intramedullary mass. The spinal cord enlarges in all directions, narrowing and often obliterating the surrounding subarachnoid space. (From Stowalter, J. L., Menhusen, M. J., and Gendreau, C. L.: Canine myelography with Skiodan. Part I. Indications and interpretation. Vet. Med. Small Anim. Clin. *71,* 1207, 1976.)

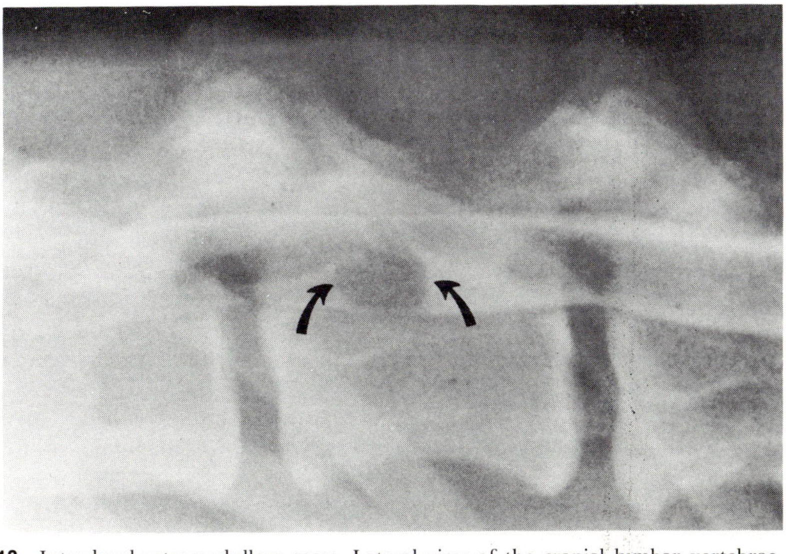

FIGURE 5–18 Intradural-extramedullary mass. Lateral view of the cranial lumbar vertebrae. Water-soluble myelography shows a filling defect in the subarachnoid space at L1, typical of intradural-extramedullary masses (arrows). This 9 year old German shorthair pointer had an acute transverse myelopathy with upper motor neuron signs in the hindlegs. Histologically, the mass was identified as a meningioma. (From Bailey, C. S., and Holliday, T. A.: Diseases of the spinal cord. *In* Ettinger, S. J.: *Textbook of Veterinary Internal Medicine, Diseases of the Dog and Cat.* W. B. Saunders Co., Philadelphia, 1975.)

graphy failed to find a place in the routine examination of the spinal canal.

The procedure has been adapted to the dog and to the technique previously described.[48, 53] Recently, investigators have modified and improved the technique, and suggested that the canine epiduralogram is safe and useful in the diagnosis of space-occupying lesions of the spinal cord.[60] Briefly, 1 ml of 20 to 40 per cent sodium methiodal per 4 to 10 pounds of body weight is injected at the lumbosacral intervertebral space into the epidural space.

These authors preferred the epidural space to the subarachnoid space because technical complications were frequently incurred when the latter was used. Of nine dogs examined fluoroscopically or radiographically by epiduralograms, five had radiographic evidence of a spinal lesion. In none of these was there clinical evidence of the sequelae frequently seen in subarachnoid administration of an aqueous medium[60] when 20 per cent concentrations were used. In two of three dogs, the 40 per cent concentration of the aqueous medium was toxic, causing adverse neurological signs of low lumbar pain.

DISKOGRAPHY

The radiographic procedure used in man to demonstrate disk disease is called diskography. Lindblom first reported on this procedure in 1950.[64] The method was to insert a 19-gauge needle posteriorly between the vertebrae as in a routine spinal tap. As the spinal cord was approached, a 22-to 24-gauge needle was inserted inside the 19-gauge needle and directed through the cord substance into the nucleus of the intervertebral disk. If the disk was ruptured, 2 to 5 ml of 35 per cent Diodrast or another water-soluble medium was injected into the disk, and the abnormality was then demonstrable by subsequent radiography. In a normal disk, only 0.5 to 1 ml could be injected, and a radiograph showed it as a small circumscribed radiopaque object confined to the nucleus.[19, 20]

Diskography has not been employed clinically in the dog. Since the disk is much smaller in the dog than in man, proper insertion of the needle into the nucleus without surgical exposure of the disk is difficult. It appears that the normal canine disk will not accommodate more than 0.1 to 0.5 ml of an aqueous medium, and even this quantity can be inserted only with difficulty. A lateral or dorsolateral insertion of the needle into the disk seems to be preferable to a dorsal piercing of the spinal canal and cord, since most disk lesions in the dog occur anterior to the termination of the spinal cord.[30] No trauma to the cord would be produced by the dorsal lateral insertion.

Reports on diskography in dogs have been published. An incision 2.5 cm long was made in a craniocaudal direction, 3 to 5 cm lateral to the dorsal midline. A 20-gauge spinal needle measuring 7.75 cm in length (with a stylet) was introduced 3 to 5 cm lateral to the cranial aspect of the spinous process of the caudal vertebra, adjacent to the disk to be injected. The needle was introduced at a 45-degree angle from the horizontal and was gently worked into the disk. The stylet was removed and replaced with a 26-gauge needle that was also supplied with a stylet. The second needle was inserted into the nucleus of the disk and 1 ml of methylglucamine diatrizoate was injected. Diskograms were successfully performed in 54 intervertebral disks in 31 dogs.[43]

VENOGRAPHY

Worthman demonstrated that the venous sinuses of the longitudinal vertebrae in the dog could be filled in a retrograde manner if the caudal vena cava was ligated.[100] Following this, Lindblad and associates employed the same method in clinical cases of compression myelitis.[63] The caudal vena cava was compressed by compressing the abdomen with a blunt, rounded, wooden instrument. Eight to 20 ml of 60 per cent urografin was injected into the saphenous vein in an amount proportionate to the size of the dog.

It was concluded that such a method could demonstrate even slighter compressions than could be seen with myelography, but that it was not useful in localization of protrusions. However, venography is a simple method of excluding spinal cord compression, at least below the level of the eleventh or twelfth thoracic vertebra.[63]

More recently, vertebral venography has

been proposed by Blevins to locate compressions of the spinal cord, swelling of the cord, and neoplasia of the cord or vertebrae. For thoracolumbar lesions, a Lundy-Irving needle is used to drill into the body of the L7 vertebra. The needle is introduced ventrolateral beneath the wing of the ilium. In the lateral recumbent position, the head is lowered and 10 ml of an aqueous contrast medium are injected. Normally, the veins will be opacified to the level of the seventh or eighth thoracic vertebrae. For cervical studies, the angularis oculi vein or the nasal or facial veins are used for injection, with concomitant compression of the jugular vein. Visualization is possible to the first or second thoracic vertebra.[4, 22]

RADIOGRAPHY OF THE BRAIN AND SKULL

CONVENTIONAL FILMS

Positioning

The basic positions for skull and brain exposures are the lateral (Lat) and ventrodorsal (VD) or dorsoventral (DV) views. The same precautions mentioned for radiography of the spine apply to the head; that is, lateral symmetry and precise superimposition should be achieved in positioning the animal. Usually the DV position in an anesthetized or deeply tranquilized animal promotes bilateral symmetry. This position accentuates some distortion in the image, since the brain is further from the film than it would be in the VD position (Fig. 5-19). The brachiocephalic breeds that characteristically have a flat calvarium can be easily placed in a symmetrical VD position. A cushion placed under the nose of the animal in a lateral exposure will aid in maintaining superimposition of parts (Fig. 5-20).

Another important position of the head is the anteroposterior or frontal view.[17, 29, 45] The animal is placed in the dorsal recumbent position, the nose is held at a perpendicular angle to the cassette, and the x-ray beam is either centered on the perpendicular plane formed by the hard palate or is 5, 10, or 20 degrees from it.[44] The frontal sinuses and the lateral ventricles may be seen clearly in this view (Figs. 5-21 to 5-23). A frontal open mouth view is frequently used to portray the foramen magnum, the odontoid process, and the bulla ossea. The central x-ray beam should be directed as shown in Figure 5-21.

Oblique views may complement the examination and add to the definite localiza-

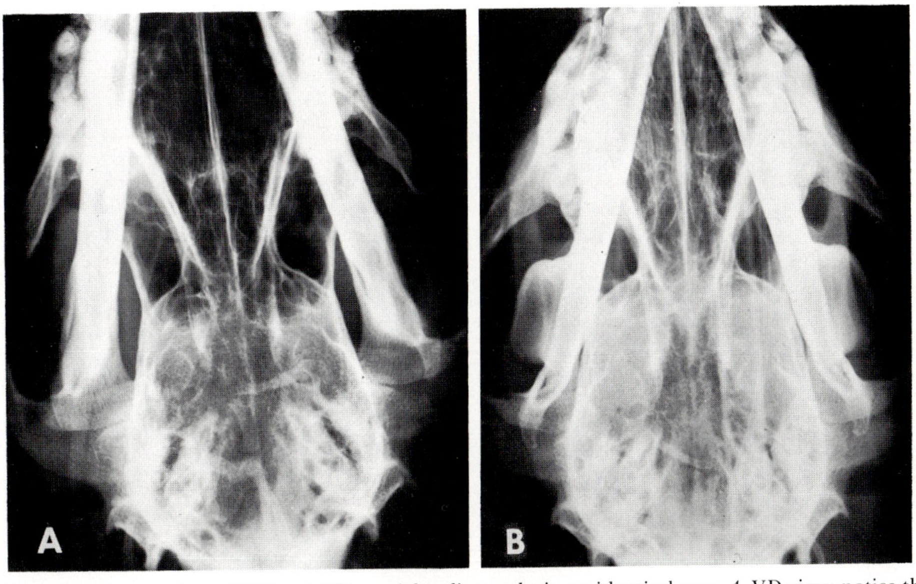

FIGURE 5-19 Comparison of VD and DV cranial radiographs in an identical case. *A.* VD view; notice the lesser distortion and more spacious view of the sinus. *B.* DV view demonstrating greater distortion.

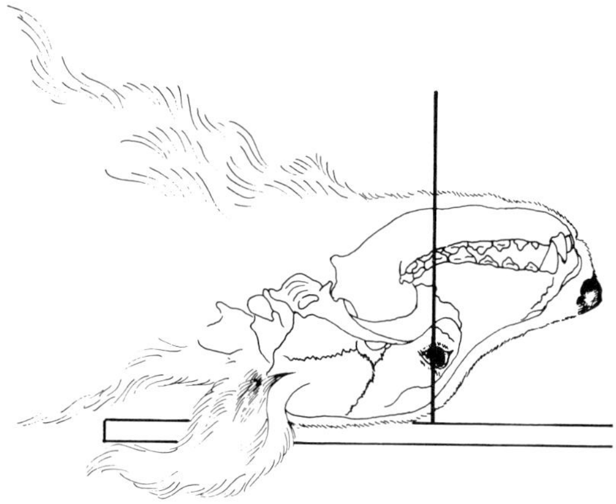

FIGURE 5–20 The proper position for VD or sinuses and frontal and prefrontal brain areas.

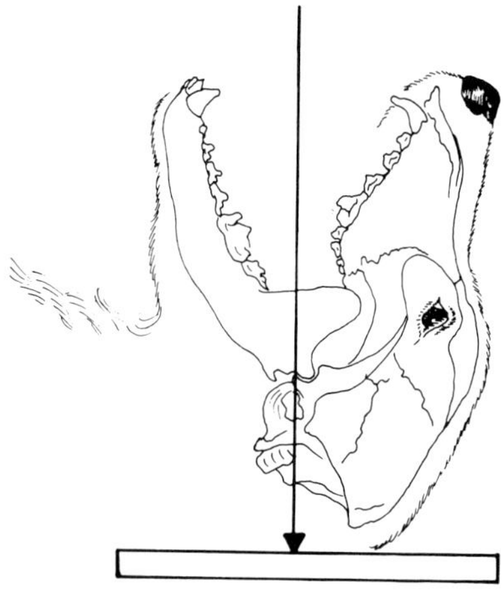

FIGURE 5–21 Open-mouth position shows the odontoid process and the foramen magnum. Direct beam of the x-ray is aimed down the throat.

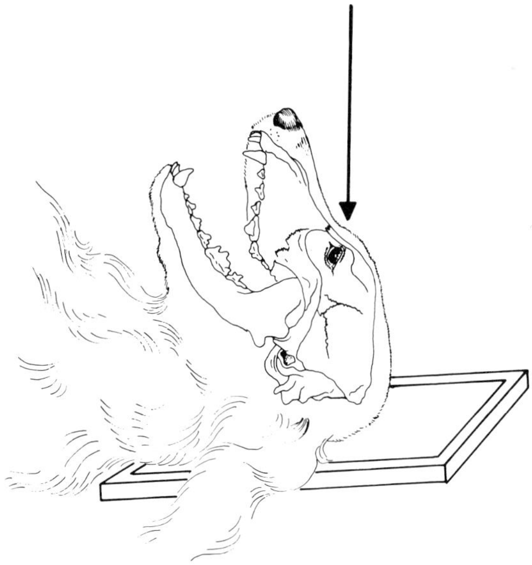

FIGURE 5–22 Standard frontal or AP position. When the head is positioned at right angles or vertically, the central beam of the x-ray is aimed at a 10-degree angle. This position will demonstrate frontal sinuses and contrast-filled lateral ventricles of the brain. (Based on Douglas, S. W., and Williams, H. D.: *Principles of Veterinary Radiology*. The Williams & Wilkins Co., Baltimore, 1963.)

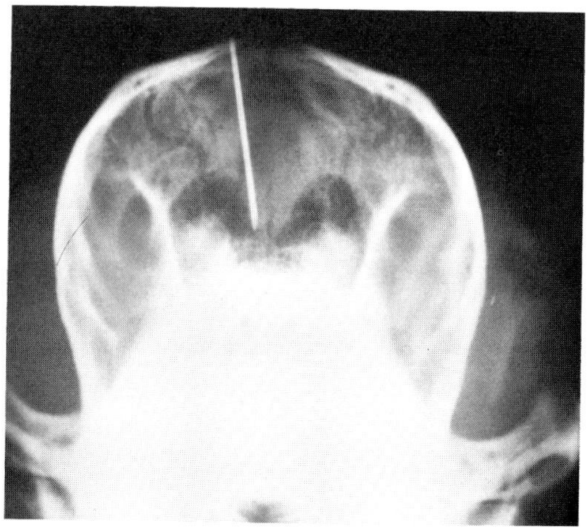

FIGURE 5–23 Frontal view of a pneumoventriculogram using the position shown in Figure 5–22. Notice the bilateral symmetry of the lateral ventricles.

tion of a lesion. This is particularly true of skull fractures and ill-defined neoplastic processes; however, the ancillary views cannot replace the two standard views.

The necessity for precise positioning in radiography has been previously described. The cranial vault, immediate soft tissue, and osseous anatomical structures are extremely compact in the dog. That fact, plus an extreme variability in the size and shape of the skull, brain, and musculature, makes radiography and interpretation a difficult and sometimes discouraging task. The gross anatomy of the skull, brain, and meninges has been well described.[49, 86] The calvarium in the brachycephalic breeds is thinner and more uniform than that in the dolichocephalic breeds. Figures 5–24 and 5–25 show salient features of "landmarks" necessary for interpretive orientation.

In the newborn, sutures between different bones have not ossified, and they show up as radiolucent, serrated-appearing spaces between the respective ossification centers, i.e., frontal, parietal, occipital, temporal, and other bones. These usually close within 3 weeks; the fontanel closes as the animal approaches maturity. Ossification of the intramembranous bones of the calvarium continues until maturity.

Brain tissue, essentially lipid in content, presents a density between fluid and gas.

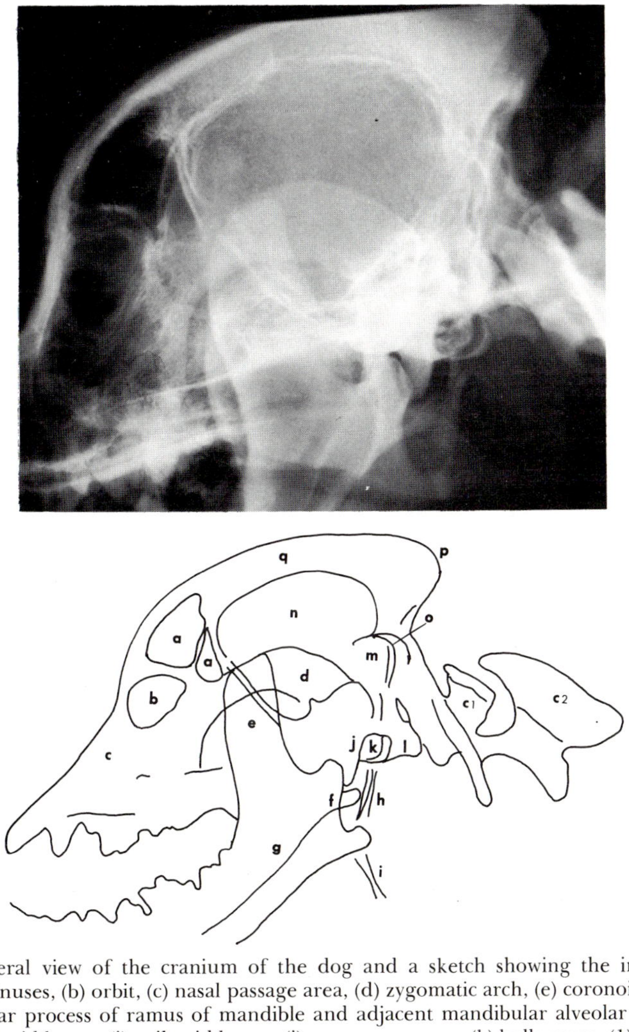

FIGURE 5–24 Lateral view of the cranium of the dog and a sketch showing the important radiographic anatomy. (a) Frontal sinuses, (b) orbit, (c) nasal passage area, (d) zygomatic arch, (e) coronoid process of the ramus of mandible, (f) angular process of ramus of mandible and adjacent mandibular alveolar articulation, (g) ramus of mandible, (h) stylohyoid bones, (i) epihyoid bones, (j) osseous ear area, (k) bulla ossea, (l) occipital condyles, (m) cerebellum, (n) cerebrum, (o) tentorium cerebelli (osseum), (p) occipital protuberance, (q) calvarium, (r) vomer or nasal septum, (s) dorsal sella, (t) palatine bones, perpendicular parts, (u) oval and caudal alar foramina, (v) external carotid foramina.

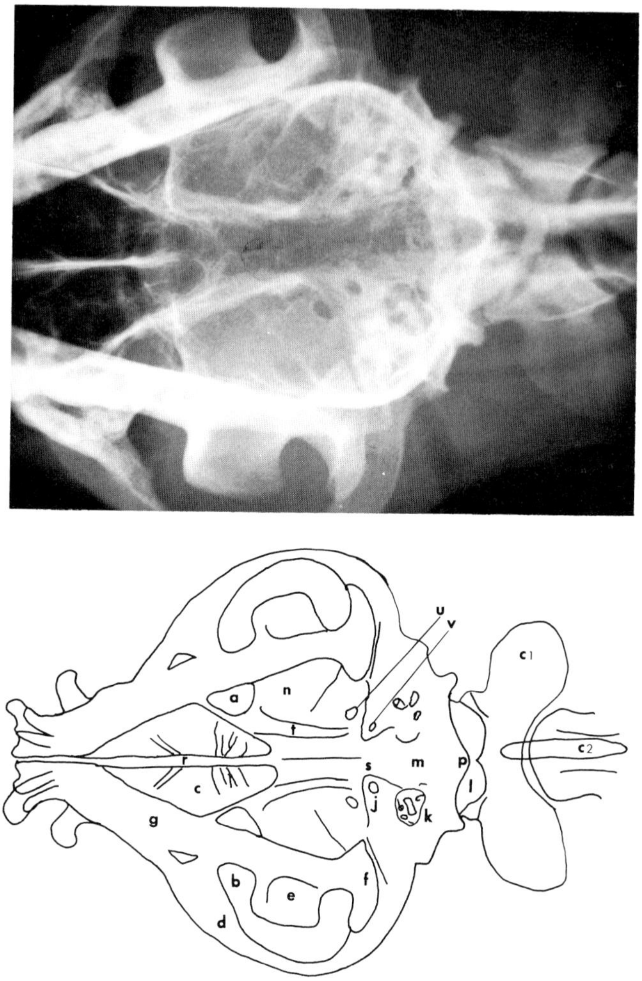

FIGURE 5–25 Ventrodorsal view. (a) Frontal sinuses, (b) orbit, (c) nasal passage area, (d) zygomatic arch, (e) coronoid process of the ramus of mandible, (f) angular process of ramus of mandible and adjacent mandibular alveolar articulation, (g) ramus of mandible, (h) stylohyoid bones, (i) epihyoid bones, (j) osseous ear area, (k) bulla ossea, (l) occipital condyles, (m) cerebellum, (n) cerebrum, (o) tentorium cerebelli (osseum), (p) occipital protuberance, (q) calvarium, (r) vomer or nasal septum, (s) dorsal sella, (t) palatine bones, perpendicular parts, (u) oval and caudal alar foramina, (v) external carotid foramina.

The reflection of endosteum forms the external layer of the cranial dura and is usually visible radiographically. With improved techniques and contrast studies, as described in this chapter, most of the structures can be visualized.

Interpretation

The interpretation of brain and skull radiographs depends on a complete knowledge of radiographic anatomy.[49, 86] Without this knowledge, the study of films will be most confusing, and many diagnostic mistakes will be made. It has already been emphasized that correct positioning is an essential factor in establishing a roentgenographic diagnosis, particularly in the brain. Fortunately, most lesions are unilateral, and when bilateral symmetry has been achieved in positioning, proper exposure and processing techniques make the lesion more easily observed. Critical observation of differences in radiographic density should be noted when comparing symmetry. A diagnostic interpretation can be made only after the history and physical examination are considered.

CONTRAST PROCEDURES

Since these procedures have been in use, they have proved to be of definite practical application, and with familiarization they can be readily achieved. Since the radiographic density of the various parts of the brain is rather uniform, many neurological lesions are difficult to see. In the dog, differences in skeletal density of the skull make this problem even more acute. Dolichocephalic breeds of dogs are characterized by their long, thick cranial bones and by a relatively small cranial cavity. In these breeds, the osseous bullae are situated well toward the midline, and they obscure much of the brain in VD exposures.

However, contrast techniques are being developed to help remedy this situation. Although many of these procedures have been used only a short time, the authors believe that they have a practical application, and they are discussed in that light.

Cerebral Angiography

Technique

Although cerebral angiography has been widely used in medicine for several years, De la Torre,[26] James and Hoerlein,[57] and Clarkson[18] were among the first to apply the technique in the dog.[90] Whiteleather and DeSaussure tested many intravenous contrast agents in dogs and found that diatrizoate sodium (Hypaque*) gave satisfactory results in the cerebrum.[98] James[57,58] used Hypaque and Hypaque M† in 56 injections on 22 experimental animals and developed a practical procedure. He also described in detail the anatomy of cerebral circulation.

The contrast materials used by James caused varying degrees of muscle contractions during their circulation through the brain. These contractions frequently made it difficult to maintain the head in the proper position during radiography. After the injection, apnea frequently occurred for 10 to 15 seconds, followed by hyperpnea for 2 to 3 minutes.[57]

Some animals recovered slowly from anesthesia, and some motor disturbance persisted (Fig. 5–27 and 5–28).

Berstein has proposed the administration of low molecular weight dextran as a deterrent to toxic effects.[10] Ten milliliters per kilogram of body weight of 15 per cent dextran in 5 per cent dextrose in water was

*Hypaque is 50 per cent aqueous solution of diatrizoate sodium. Winthrop Laboratories, New York.

†Hypaque M is 90 per cent aqueous solution containing 30 per cent (W/V) diatrizoate sodium and 60 per cent (W/V) of the N-methylglucamine salt of diatrizoic acid. Winthrop Laboratories, New York.

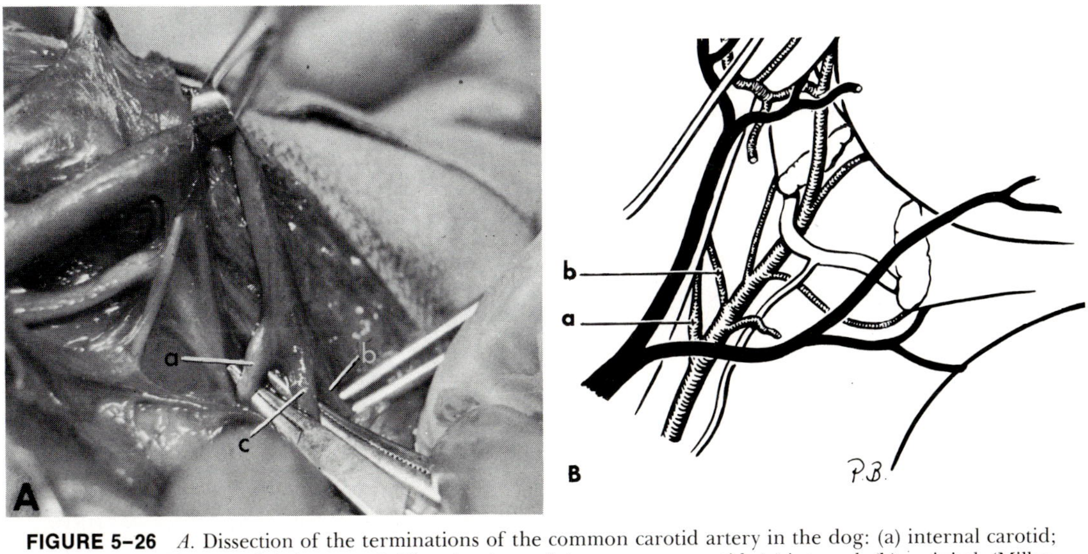

FIGURE 5–26 *A.* Dissection of the terminations of the common carotid artery in the dog: (a) internal carotid; (b) external carotid; (c) occipital artery. *B.* Terminations of the common carotid: (a) internal; (b) occipital. (Miller, M. E.: *Guide to the Dissection of the Dog.* 3rd ed. Edwards Bros., Ann Arbor, Mich. 1952 © Dr. Malcolm E. Miller.)

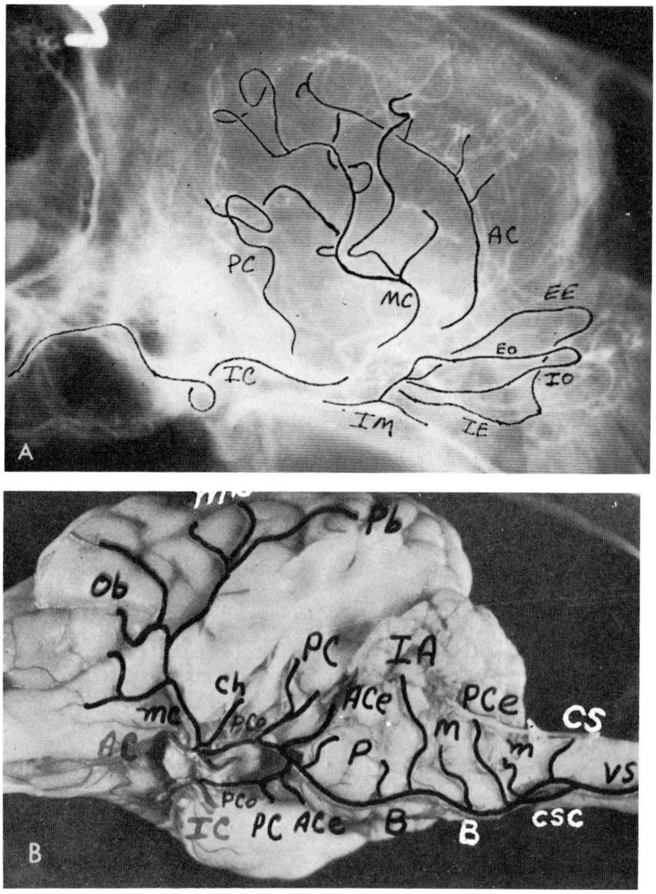

FIGURE 5–27 Arterial supply to brain. *A*. Angiogram. *B*. Specimen injected with latex. (James, C. W.: Radiographic anatomy of the cerebral arterial system of the dog. Thesis, Auburn University, Auburn, Alabama, 1963.)

AC, anterior cerebral artery; ACe, anterior cerebellar artery; ACo, anterior communicating artery; B, basilar artery; CC, common carotid artery; Ch, choroid artery; CS, cerebrospinal artery; CSC, cerebrospinal circle; EE, external ethmoidal artery; EO, external ophthalmic artery; IA, internal auditory artery; IC, internal carotid artery; IE, internal ethmoidal artery; IO, internal ophthalmic artery; M, medullary artery; MB, middle branch of middle cerebral artery; OL, olfactory artery; P, pontine artery; PB, posterior branch of middle cerebral artery; PC, posterior cerebral artery; PCe, posterior cerebellar artery; PCo, posterior communicating artery; V, vertebral artery; VS, ventral spinal artery.

administered intravenously over a 2-minute period, 10 minutes prior to the injeciton of the contrast medium. However, administration of dextran has been seen to lower the radiographic contrast of the medium.

The toxic effect of cerebral angiography has also been of concern in human medicine. Field and co-workers reported complications in 2.1 per cent of 2000 consecutive angiographic examinations, with a fatality rate of 0.34 per cent.[32] A motor deficiency was also a prevalent finding. Shealy found that in his patients, methylglucamine diatrizoate (Renografin) produced less pain in postinjection periods than did Hypaque.[88]

More recently, the use of another methylglucamine diatrizoate preparation (Cardiografin) has been found to produce less immediate reaction upon injection. Since muscle rigidity and movement have not been as severe as with the use of Hypaque, maintaining the position of the head during rapid exposures has not been of major concern. Cardiografin produces satisfactory vascular contrast in radiographs. In clinical cases, an inhalation anesthetic agent, such as halothane, administered in a close system with oxygen, would be less toxic than phenobarbital sodium.

Based on the work of James and earlier investigators,[57,58] Dorn[27,28] modified the technique to perform cerebral angiography successfully in patients with a critically damaged central nervous system. The technique in Dorn's work can be recommended as a basis for canine cerebral angiography, since it was found clinically to be both safe and practical. A basic standard technique also facilitates accurate interpretation.

The modified technique of Dorn consists of the following essential points:

1. The exclusive use of inhalation anesthesia – i.e., methoxyflurane (Metofane) with induction of pentothal sodium (Thiopental).

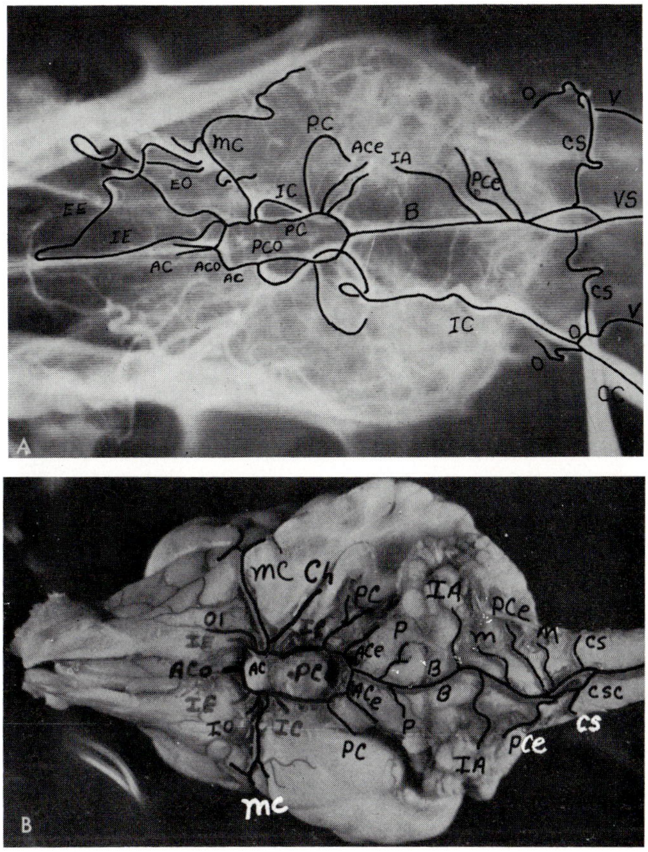

FIGURE 5–28 Arterial supply to brain. *A*. Angiogram. *B*. Specimen injected with latex. (James, C. W.: Radiographic anatomy of the cerebral arterial system of the dog. Thesis, Auburn University, Auburn, Alabama, 1963.)

AC, anterior cerebral artery; ACe, anterior cerebellar artery; ACo, anterior communicating artery; B, basilar artery; CC, common carotid artery; Ch, choroid artery; CS, cerebrospinal artery; CSC, cerebrospinal circle; EE, external ethmoidal artery; EO, external ophthalmic artery; IA, internal auditory artery; IC, internal carotid artery; IE, internal ethmoidal artery; IO, internal ophthalmic artery; M, medullary artery; MB, middle branch of middle cerebral artery; OL, olfactory artery; P, pontine artery; PB, posterior branch of middle cerebral artery; PC, posterior cerebral artery; PCe, posterior cerebellar artery; PCo, posterior communicating artery; V, vertebral artery; VS, ventral spinal artery.

2. Preoperative medication consisting of atropine sulfate (Atropine), antibiotics, and corticosteroids.

3. The use of a ventral midline rather than a lateral surgical approach to the previously described carotid bifurcation.

4. The exclusive use of meglumine iothalamate (Conray-60) at a dosage rate of 1 ml/2.75 kg (6 lb) of body weight. This medium did not produce the severe muscle contractions characteristic of Hypaque; therefore, restraint and positioning of the head were not a problem, as they were in James' work.

5. Ligation of the external carotid artery cranially and the common carotid artery caudally to the proposed catheterization (Fig. 5–26).

6. A French 5 catheter is inserted into the common carotid artery (a French 8 catheter if the dog is large). The catheter is threaded up to the region of the internal carotid and occipital arteries. The artery is ligated around the catheter.

7. Flushing with heparinized saline. One ml of meglumine iothalamate is injected for each 3 kg body weight. One ml is added for the catheter.

8. Two series of six films each for Lat and VD positions are taken at 1-second intervals.

9. Suture or ligation of the common carotid artery; routine closure of other tissues.

The technique of Rising and Lewis[84] has proved to be one satisfactory method of cerebral angiography. Generally, arterial catheterization under image-intensified fluoroscopy (IIF) is more advantageous than cut-down methods. The vertebral, internal carotid, and left vertebral artery can be entered via IIF. Utilizing radiographic magnification and subtraction techniques, the microvasculature can be visualized with clarity in this technique. Complications ensue from repeated injections via the vertebral artery at the C3–4 level. Because the blood-brain barrier is passed, apparently with high concentrations of the aqueous iodine media, hypothermia and seizures result.[84]

Technically, filling of the circle of Willis is not consistent, and therefore bilateral symmetry, vascular blushes, neovascularization, and vascular displacements are difficult to assess.[84]

A technique suggested by Suter[92] probably has more technical merit relative to the hemodynamics of CNS circulation. Utilizing a carotid puncture after cut-down, a small catheter is directed into the internal carotid artery, unilaterally or bilaterally. No extravascular clamping is done, and free-flow injections are made in both VD and lateral projections. The procedure is readily performed and yields excellent quality cerebral angiograms.[92]

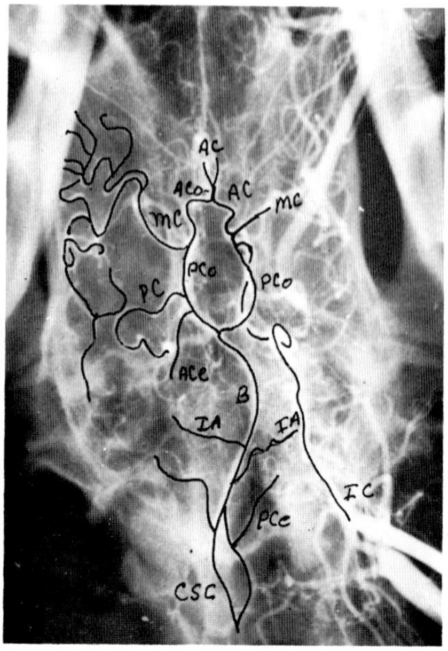

FIGURE 5–29 VD view of a cerebral arteriogram with a deviated basilar artery (B).

Interpretation

The interpretation of cerebral angiograms may present some difficulties. Both James and Dorn have described some rather consistent variations in certain vessels. In James' work, some variation could be attributed to problems of head restraint during injection.[27, 28, 57, 58] Any deviation from a bilaterally symmetrical position of the head will make interpretation difficult (Figs. 5–27 and 5–28).

Common abnormalities that should be observed in the arterial side of the vascular system or in a so-called arteriogram are aneurysms, thromboses, ruptured arteries, and space-occupying lesions that cause displacement of vessels.[18] Dorn further observed cerebrovascular injury, arteriovenous fistula, and neoplasms.[27, 28] Both highly vascular and nonvascular lesions should be discernible in this examination (Figs. 5–29 to 5–33).

The venous phase, venogram, or venous side of the injection flow is and should be an important consideration, as it occurs within 3 to 4 seconds after the initial injection. Highly vascular lesions, such as meningioma, are characterized by retention of the contrast medium for a considerable time after the rest of the brain has been cleared of it (Fig. 5–32).

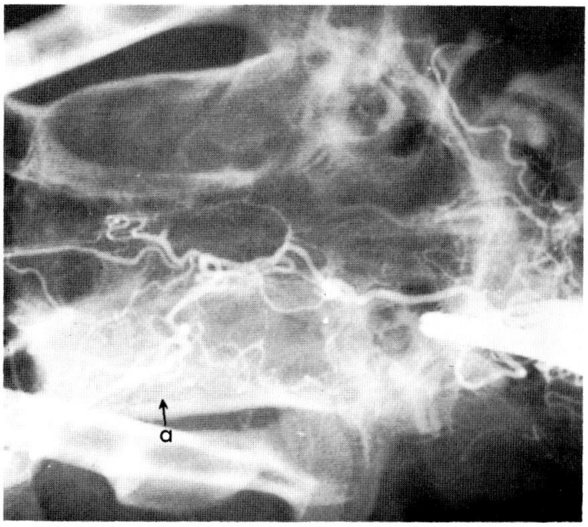

FIGURE 5–30 VD exposure taken 2 seconds after injection of 50 per cent Hypaque in a cerebral arteriogram. The lesion is a meningioma (a).

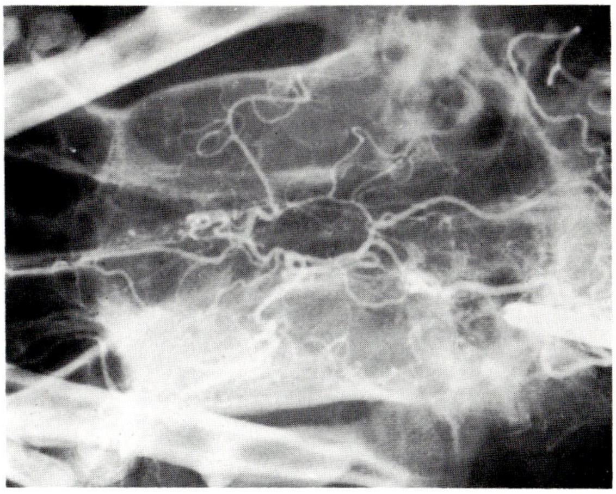

FIGURE 5–31 Exposure taken 4 seconds after injection in the same case as shown in Figure 5–30. Notice that the circle of Willis is well outlined and that more contrast has accumulated in the meningioma.

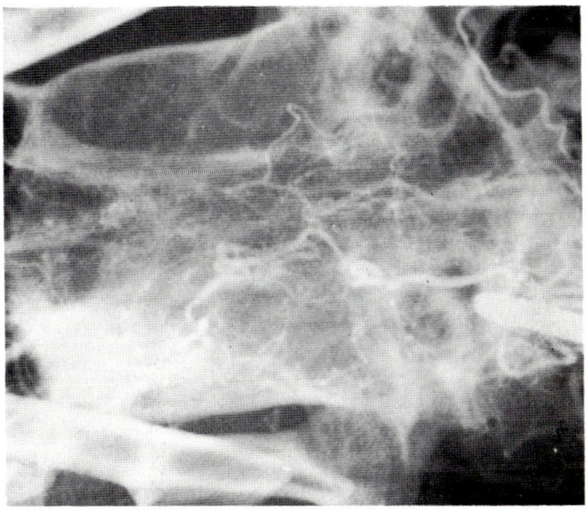

FIGURE 5–32 An exposure taken 10 seconds after injection of a cerebral venogram, same case as shown in Figures 5–30 and 5–31. Notice medium in the lesion.

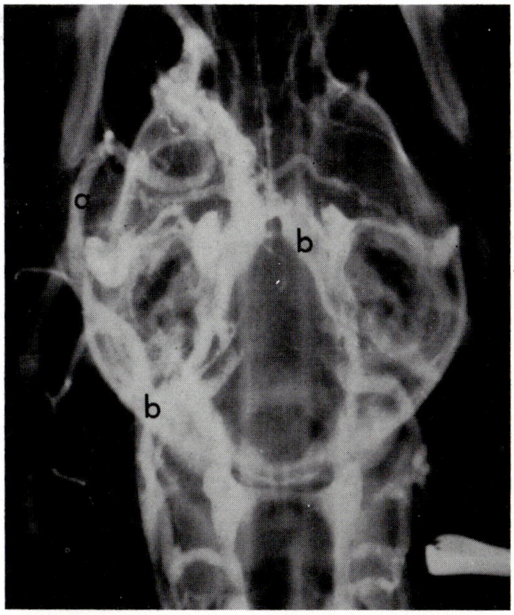

FIGURE 5–33 VD view of an angiogram of a dog with an arteriovenous fistula shows concurrent arterial and venous filling. The external carotid artery (a) is filled, along with the sigmoid and ventral petrosal sinuses (b). (Courtesy of Dr. A. S. Dorn, Auburn University, Auburn, Alabama.)

Cerebral angiography is becoming a practical aid in radiographic diagnoses. Great care in the administration of contrast medium, the proper choice of anesthetic procedure, and the employment of an efficient radiographic technique can make cerebral angiography effective and relatively safe.

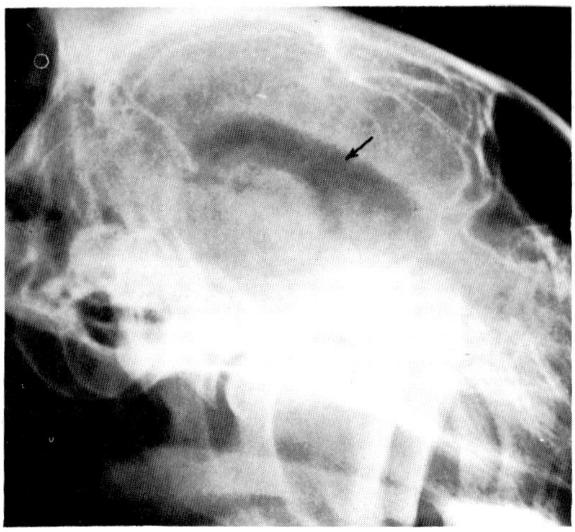

FIGURE 5–34 Lateral pneumoencephalogram taken after 40 ml of air was injected in the L1–2 subarachnoid space. Notice the air in the lateral ventricles.

Pneumoencephalography

Davis credits Dandy with the use of encephalography and ventriculography as early as 1918.[24] Using air as the contrast material, he made a lumbar subarachnoid injection and visualized the cranial subarachnoid spaces and ventricles with the subject in various positions. This procedure was called encephalography. When air, oxygen, or other gases are used, it is correctly called pneumoencephalography.

Air is usually preferred to oxygen as a medium, as it is absorbed much more slowly and radiographic studies can therefore be performed over a longer period. If larger quantities of contrast medium are needed for study, oxygen has the advantage of causing less prolonged postinjection discomfort. Robertson has demonstrated that different head positions are more apt to demonstrate ventricular filling correctly at the various stages of injection.[85] When the head and neck are fully flexed, the cisterna magna, the fourth ventricle, and the cerebral aqueduct are more fully visualized. At a 45-degree angle, more air enters the fourth and third ventricles. At a 25-degree angle, more air enters the third ventricle, and at a 10- to 20-degree angle, most of the air enters the third and lateral ventricles. However, encephalography is currently being performed less frequently than ventriculography in human practice because of its inconsistent filling effects on the ventricular system and because it seems to be more dangerous than other procedures.[25]

The lumbar technique has been described by Hoerlein and Petty,[54] and the cisternal techniques are also described by Cobb.[21] Since these techniques are rarely used in veterinary practice, they will not be discussed in more detail here (Figs. 5–34 to 5–36).

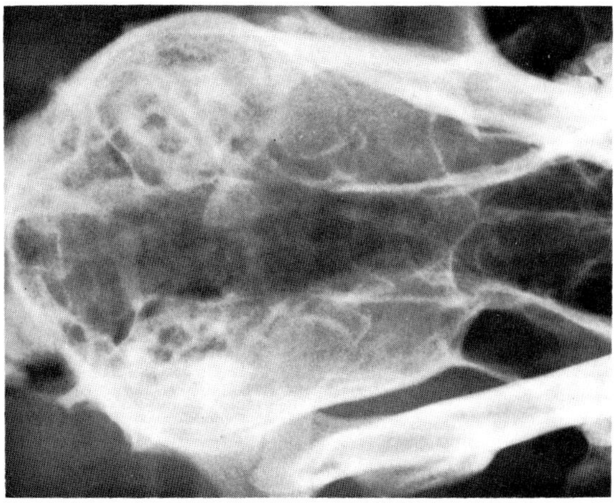

FIGURE 5–35 VD pneumoencephalogram, same case as shown in Figure 5–31. Notice poor definition of ventricles.

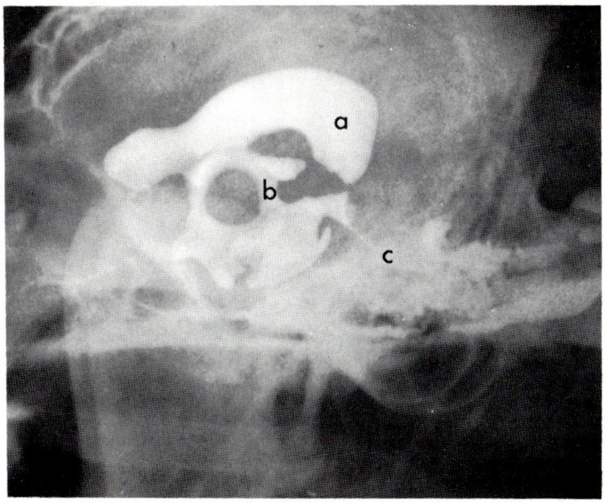

FIGURE 5–36 Lateral ventriculogram taken after injection of 3 ml of Pantopaque. Same case as shown in Figures 5–31 and 5–32: (a) lateral ventricle; (b) third ventricle; (c) fourth ventricle.

Ventriculography

Ventriculography is a radiographic method of demonstrating the ventricles of the brain after the ventricular fluid has been replaced by air or by an opaque medium.[24] As a rule, it is a surgical procedure, since the medium is injected via tubes inserted through trephine holes in the skull. In man, ventriculography requires the use of general anesthesia, whereas encephalography does not. Ventriculography is considered quite safe and is consistently effective in the dog.[54]

Some work has been done with agents other than air. Pantopaque has been used via the lumbar route in a procedure called rhomboencephalography by Mones.[70] Horwitz has used Pantopaque instead of air in ventriculography and found it to be quite satisfactory.[56] Other media, notably Conray-60, have proven to be satisfactory in the dog by Albert.[3]

Technique

The patient is started on glucocorticosteroids 24 hours before ventriculography unless the drug is contraindicated. The dog is given gaseous anesthesia and is placed in a sternal recumbent position. The skin of the calvarium is prepared for surgery in the usual manner. A convenient landmark for entry into the lateral ventricle is situated approximately midway between the lateral canthus of the eye and the external occipital protuberance.[44] A small midline incision 1 to 2 cm in length is made, and the temporal muscles are dissected from the skull cap for a length of about 1 to 2 cm from the midline. Oliver[76] prefers the use of a head holder for pneumoventriculography to facilitate various positioning views of the air bubbles. A small skin incision over the site of puncture is made, and the muscle is penetrated without dissection. In cases of hydrocephalus with open lateral fontanels, no incision is necessary; a needle tap can be made directly through the skin (Fig. 5–37). This applies to young animals or those with extremely thin cortical bone of the calvarium.

In order to penetrate the bone, a small hole is made by means of a sharp intramedullary pin and handchuck, usually about 0.5 to 1 cm from the midline at the previously described landmark. When the hole has barely penetrated the skull, a 22-gauge spinal needle is forced through it. The needle should fit snugly so that its position will be maintained during the procedure. The needle is then slowly forced directly downward, parallel to the midline, for a distance of 1 to 2 cm. The stylet is frequently withdrawn to ascertain presence in the lateral ventricle. Fluid will slowly rise in the needle when the ventricle has been punctured. Negative pressure of the syringe should be used sparingly during the act of locating the ventricle, since this will tend to suck brain material into the needle and plug it. In pneumoventriculography, Oliver[77] prefers tapping each lateral ventricle, compressing each jugular momentarily to increase the CSF pressure while adjusting each needle for ventricular location and withdrawal of fluid; 3 ml of air

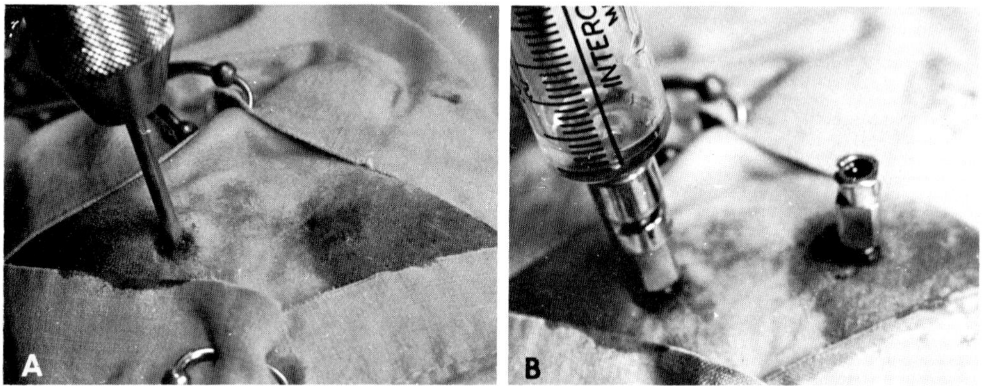

FIGURE 5–37 *A*, Drilling a hole in the skull to allow passage of the spinal needle for a ventriculogram. B, Placing the second needle. Some practitioners use only one drill hole and spinal needle.

are slowly introduced in each needle while the patient's pulse is carefully monitored. Both needles are left in place to equalize ventricular pressure until the injections are complete. The needles are withdrawn and radiographs are taken in various positions of the skull (Figs. 5–37 to 5–39).

A recently modified technique for ventriculography has definite practical use.[3] Meglumine iothalamate 60 per cent (Conray-60) is less toxic than other water-soluble materials, is miscible with CSF, has a high degree of opacity, is free from precipitation, and has a low viscosity. Being water soluble, it is rapidly absorbed from the subarachnoid space. Its relative clinical toxicity has been investigated, as previously described.[3, 16]

In all cases, meglumine iothalamate has produced fair to excellent ventriculograms.[3] Its flow and manipulation characteristics, dose, and capability of use in unilateral ventricular puncture are obvious advantages over other media. Occasionally, patients exhibit postsurgical or anesthetic hypersensitivity to external stimuli, but proceed to recover uneventfully.[3] Histological examination of brain tissue shows no evidence of meningitis (Fig. 5–40).

Interpretation

In the interpretation of ventriculograms, one must understand the anatomy of the ventricular system. It should be noted that the extent of the lateral ventricles in the

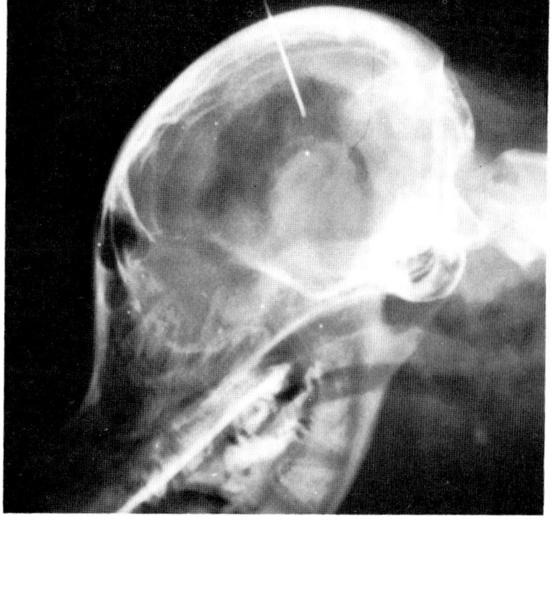

FIGURE 5–38 Lateral view of a pneumoventriculogram.

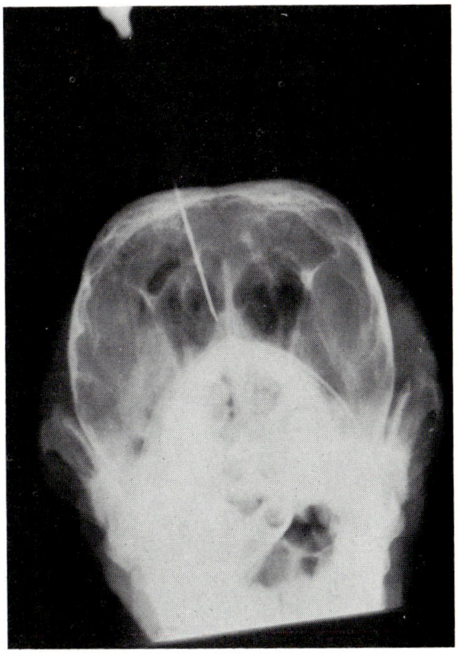

FIGURE 5–39 Frontal view of lateral ventricles distended with air in a pneumoventriculogram.

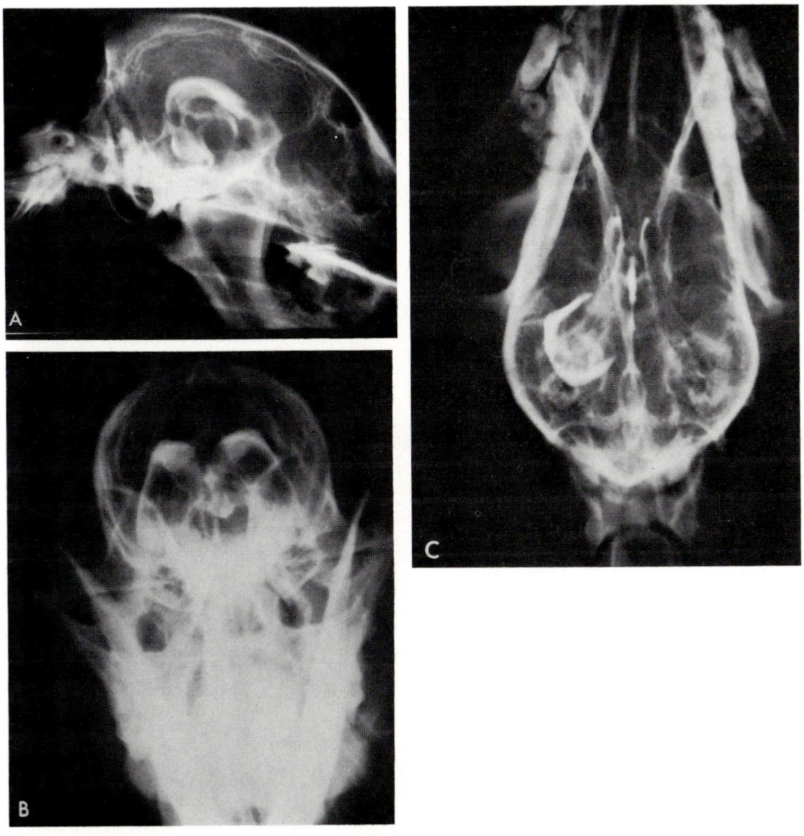

FIGURE 5–40 Normal flow pattern exhibited in the ventricular system with the use of meglumine iothalamate (60 per cent). *A.* Lateral view with superimposition of ventricles. *B.* Frontal view showing the lateral ventricles and the third ventricle or foramen of Monroe. *C.* VD with flow cranially into the olfactory recesses and caudally into the fourth ventricle. (Courtesy of Dr. R. A. Albert, Auburn University, Auburn, Alabama.)

normal animal is substantial. Ventriculography in clinical practice is of value in demonstrating either unilateral or bilateral ventricular dropsy as well as space-occupying lesions (tumors, hemorrhages, abscesses) that either obliterate the normal contour of the ventricles or cause it to deviate. At present, the procedures discussed appear to be both useful and practicable.

Cranial Sinus Venography

Oliver reviewed the existing literature and described two techniques for sinus venography in the dog.[76] The object of the investigation was to determine the advantages of sinus venography over conventional procedures for visualization and delineation of structures of the cranial vault.

Dorsal Sagittal Sinus

The exposure is accomplished by a dorsal midline incision made near the caudal aspect of the frontal sinus (Fig. 5–41). Contrast medium (5 to 10 ml of 60 per cent meglumine iothalamate [Conray-60]) is injected via a catheter placed in the rostral end of the superior sagittal sinus. Figure 5–42 demonstrates the results of the serial radiographs. The dorsal sagittal and transverse sinuses were visualized. Oliver concluded that dorsal sagittal sinus venography is a difficult technique with potentially serious complications.[76]

Cavernous Sinus

The cavernous sinus is outlined by a simple injection of contrast media into the angularis oculi vein (Figs. 5–43 and 5–44). During injection, the external jugular veins were compressed. Cavernous sinus venography was described as a simple, safe technique for visualization of the orbit, ventral cranial sinuses and veins and as far caudal as the cranial third of the thoracic vertebral sinuses. The technique requires no special equipment such as a rapid film changer, power injector, or fluoroscope.[76]

Lee and Griffiths[62] compared the diagnostic value of verebral arteriography and cavernous sinus venography in similar cases of brain lesions. Of the seven cases studied by arteriography, only one showed a radiographic lesion which was substantiated by necropsy. Of nine cases studied by venography, six had positive radiographic findings, five of which were substantiated by necropsy. Because of its ease and safety of performance, it was concluded that cavernous sinus venography might be a practical clinical procedure as an aid in clinical localization of brain lesions.[62]

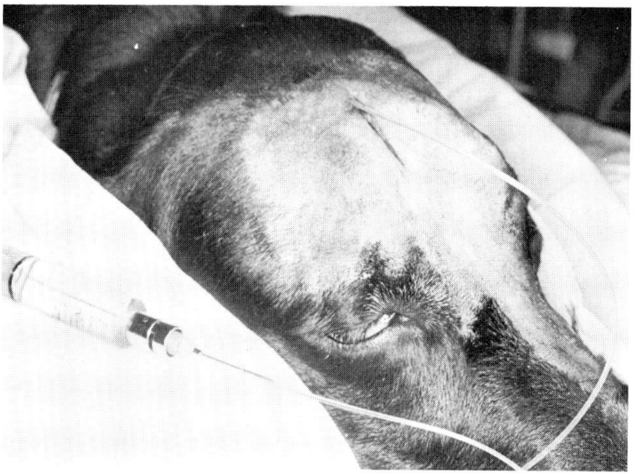

FIGURE 5–41 Polyethylene catheter inserted into the dorsal sagittal sinus. Sterile drapes have been removed to show position of injection site. (Courtesy of Dr. J. E. Oliver, Jr.: J. Am. Vet. Rad. Soc., *10*, 66, 1969.)

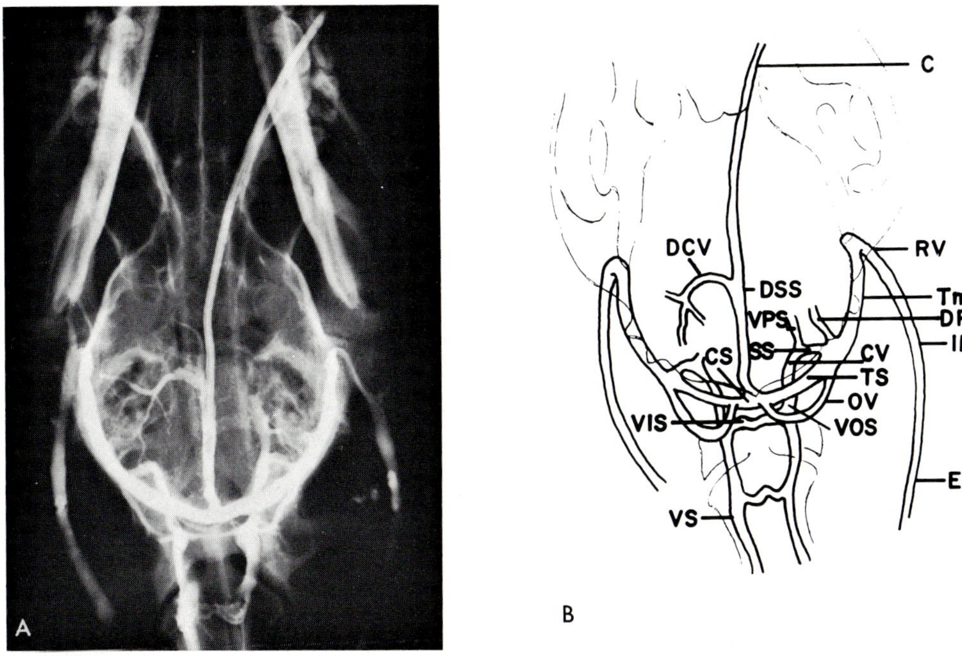

FIGURE 5–42 *A*. DV view, dorsal sagittal sinus venogram. (Courtesy of Dr. J. E. Oliver, Jr.: J. Am. Vet. Rad. Soc., *10*, 66, 1969.) *B*. Tracing of *A*, illustrating sinuses and veins outlined in contrast media.

ABBREVIATIONS FOR FIGS. 5–42 *B*. and 5–44 *B*.

AA, anastomotic artery from external ophthalmic artery; **AICS,** anterior intercavernous sinus; **AOpV,** anastomosis of ophthalmic veins; **AOV,** angularis oculi vein; **BO,** bulla ossea; **C,** catheter; **CS,** confluens sinuum; **CV,** condyloid vein; **CvS,** cavernous sinus; **DCV,** dorsal cerebral vein; **DFV,** deep facial vein; **DPS,** dorsal petrosal sinus; **DS,** dorsum sellae; **DSS,** dorsal sagittal sinus; **EJV,** external jugular vein; **EMV,** external maxillary vein; **FV,** facial vein; **HF,** hypophyseal fossa; **ICA,** internal carotid artery; **IJV,** internal jugular vein; **IMV,** internal maxillary vein; **OP,** orbital plexus; **OpV,** ophthalmic vein; **OV,** occipital vein; **PP,** palatine plexus; **RV,** retroglenoid vein; **SS,** sigmoid sinus; **STV,** superficial temporal vein; **TmS,** temporal sinus; **TS,** transverse sinus; **VIS,** ventral interoccipital sinus; **VOS,** ventral occipital sinus; **VPS,** ventral petrosal sinus; **VS,** vertebral sinus; **VV,** vertebral vein.

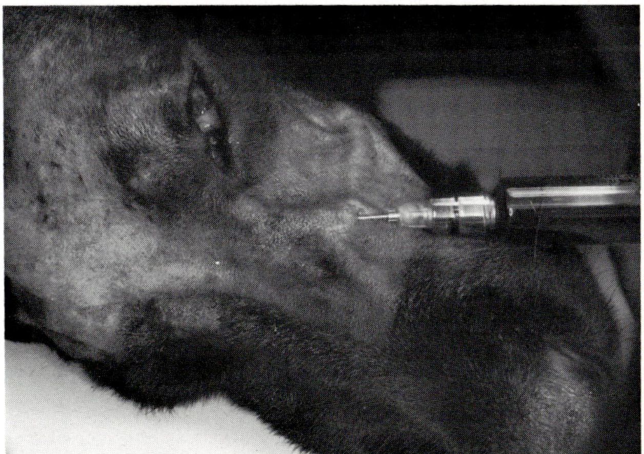

FIGURE 5–43 Injection into the angularis oculi vein for orbital and cavernous sinus venography. (Courtesy of Dr. J. E. Oliver, Jr.: J. Am. Vet. Rad. Soc., *10*, 66, 1969.)

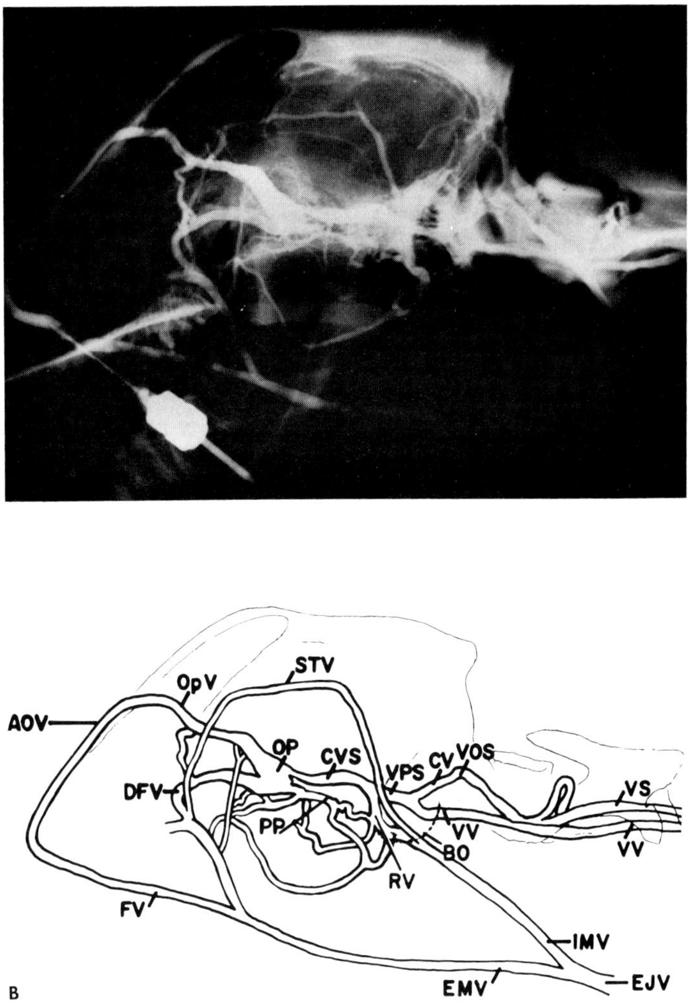

B

FIGURE 5–44 *A*, Lateral view of venogram following injection of contrast media into angularis oculi vein. *B*, Tracing of *A*, illustrating sinuses and veins outlined by contrast media. (Courtesy of Dr. J. E. Oliver, Jr.: J. Am. Vet. Rad. Soc., *10*, 66, 1969.)

Future Neuroradiography

Practical neuroradiology currently being instituted is centered around an all-purpose unit. With cinefluorography, image intensification, and spot filming, precise catheterization of individual vessels is routine. Such catheterization will obviate surgical procedures for catheter placement in cerebral angiography.

Cinefluorography and image intensification will permit serial physiological sequence observation of arterial and venous phase arteriography. Ancillary equipment includes seriographs and automatic injection syringes for the accurate delivery of metered contrast media at a constant pressure. Tomography will continue to gain importance as a diagnostic procedure. The term tomography is applied to a special type of radiography in which the object is "sectioned" by controlled motion during the actual radiographic exposure. This procedure selectively blurs the images of all structures that are not in a predetermined plane. The technique allows demonstration of structures within the living patient, and the image resembles thin-cut sections of the actual anatomical part in question.[38] The new, relatively nontoxic, water-soluble contrast materials will make CNS and spinal contrast procedures routine and will increase their diagnostic value.

The advent of nuclear medicine with its potential of organ-imaging, either static or dynamic, offers yet a new parameter to neurodiagnostics. The normal canine brain scan can then be established and correlated with anatomic and pathologic changes. Initial studies by Kaufeltz, Brawner, Burt, and O'Brien indicate that the canine brain scan utilizing technetium-99m will be of value diagnostically in correlating clinical signs, cerebral angiography, and pathoanatomic functional changes. The rectilinear scan or gamma camera can also provide valuable ancillary information about CNS and neurologic disk problems.

Although not routinely utilized at present, ultrasonography and computerized atial tomography may eventually become available for use in veterinary diagnoses.

REFERENCES

1. Ackerman, M., and Corwin, L. A., Jr.: Myelography with MP20 32-MNG meglumine iocarmate. J. Am. Vet. Rad. Soc. *14*(5), 174, 1975.
2. Metrizamide—a non-ionic water-soluble contrast medium. Experimental and preliminary clinical investigations. Acta Radiol. (Suppl.) *335*, 1973.
3. Albert, R. A.: *Canine Ventriculography and Encephalography.* Thesis (M.S.), Auburn University, Auburn, Alabama, 1967.
4. Amsler, F. R., Jr., and Wilbert, M. C.: Venographic diagnosis of intervertebral disc disease. J. Bone Joint Surg. *49A* (4), 703, 1967.
5. Amundsen, P., Helsinger, P., and Kristiansen, K.: Evaluation of lumbar radiculography (myelography) with water-soluble contrast media. Acta Radiol. *1,* 659, 1963.
6. Bailey, C. S., and Holliday, T. A.: Diseases of the spinal cord. *In* Ettinger, S. J. (ed.): *Veterinary Internal Medicine: Diseases of the Dog and Cat.* W. B. Saunders Co., Philadelphia, 1975.
7. Bartels, J. E., Braund, K. G., and Redding, R. W.: An experimental and clinical evaluation of a nonionic agent Amipaque (metrizamide) as a neuroradiologic medium in the dog. J. Am. Vet. Rad. Soc. In press. 1978.
8. Bartels, J. E., Braund, K. G., and Redding, R. W.: An experimental evaluation of a non-ionic agent Amipaque (metrizamide) as a neuroradiologic medium in the dog. J. Am. Vet. Rad. Soc. In press. 1977.
9. Bartels, J. E., and Boring, J. G.: Experimental data (unpublished). Auburn University School of Veterinary Medicine, Auburn, Alabama, 1974.
10. Berstein, E. F., and Evans, R. L.: Low-molecular-weight dextran. J.A.M.A. *174,* 1417, 1960.
11. Biery, D. N.: Personal communication, 1976.
12. Boring, J. G., Swaim, S. F., and Vandevelde, M.: Transmedullary myelography. J.A.V.M.A. (in press).
13. Brooks, G. B.: *Experimental and Clinical Studies of the Spine of the Dog.* William Wood and Co., Baltimore, 1936.
14. Bullock, L. P., and Zook, B. C.: Myelography in dogs, using water-soluble contrast mediums. J.A.V.M.A. *151*(3), 321, 1969.
15. Burt, J.: Personal communication, 1976.
16. Campbell, R. I., Campbell, J. A., Heinburger, R. F., Kalsbeck, J. E., and Mealey, J., Jr.: Ventriculography and myelography with absorbable radio-opaque medium. Radiology *82,* 286, 1964.
17. Carlson, W. D.: *Veterinary Radiology,* 2d ed. Lea & Febiger, Philadelphia. 1967.
18. Clarkson, T. B., Netsky, M. G., and De la Torre, E.: Chromophobe adenoma in a dog: angiographic and anatomic study. J. Neuropathol. Exp. Neurol. *18,* 559, 1959.
19. Cloward, R. B., and Buzoid, L. I.: Diskography: technique, indications and evaluation of the normal and abnormal intervertebral disc. Am. J. Roentgenol. *68,* 552, 1952.
20. Cloward, R. B.: Cervical diskography: a contribution to the etiology and mechanism of neck, shoulder and arm pain. Ann. Surg. *150*:1052, 1959.
21. Cobb, L. M.: Pneumoencephalography in the dog. Canad. Vet. J. *1,* 444, 1960.
22. Conrad, C. R.: Radiographic examination of the central nervous system. *In* Ettinger, S. J. (ed.): *Textbook of Veterinary Internal Medicine: Diseases of the Dog and Cat.* W. B. Saunders Co., Philadelphia, 1975.
23. Conrad, C. R., and Oliver, J. E., Jr.: Cerebral arteriography. *In* Ticer, J. W. (ed.): *Radiographic Technique in Small Animal Practice.* W. B. Saunders Co., Philadelphia, 1975.
24. Davis, F. M., Llewellyn, R. C., and Kirgis, H. D.: Water-soluble contrast myelography using meglumine iothalamate (Conray) with methylprednisolone acetate (DeproMedrol). Radiology *90*:(4), 705, 1968.
25. Davis, L.: Principles of neurological surgery, 4th ed. Lea & Febiger, Philadelphia, 1953.
26. De la Torre, E., Netsky, M. G., and Meschan, I.: Intracranial and extracranial circulation in the dog: anatomic and angiographic studies. Am. J. Anat. *105*:343, 1959.
27. Dorn, A. S.: A standard technique for canine cerebral angiography. J.A.V.M.A. *161,* 12, 1972.
28. Dorn, A. S.: Cerebral angiography in the dog: tion. Thesis (M.S.), Auburn University, Auburn, Alabama, 1968.
29. Douglas, S. W., and Williamson, H. D.: *Principles of Veterinary Radiography.* The Williams & Wilkins Co., Baltimore, 1963.
30. Erlacher, P. R.: Nucleography. J. Bone Joint Surg. *34B,* 204, 1952.
31. Felson, B.: *Roentgen Techniques in Laboratory Animals.* W. B. Saunders Co., Philadelphia, 1968.
32. Field, J. R., Robertson, J. T., and DeSaussure, R. L.: Complication of cerebral angiography in 2000 consecutive cases. J. Neurosurg. *19,* 775, 1962.
33. Fisher, R. L.: An experimental evaluation of Pantopaque and other recently developed myelographic contrast media. Radiology *85*(3), 537, 1965.
34. Funkquist, B.: Lumbar subarachnoid puncture and injection in the dog. Nord. Vet. Med. *12*:805, 1960.

35. Funkquist, B.: Myelographic localization of spinal cord compression in dogs. A comparison between cisternal and lumbar injection of metrizamide "Amipaque" in diagnosing and locating spinal cord compression. Acta Vet. Scand. *16*, 1–4, 1973.
36. Funkquist, B.: Simplified myelography technique. Svenska Veterinidartining *18*, 587–589, 1974.
37. Funkquist, B.: Tonic muscle spasms and blood pressure changes following the subarachnoid injection of contrast media. Excerptum Acta Radiol. *53*, 337, 1960
38. Funkquist, B.: Thoraco-lumbar myelography with water-soluble contrast medium in dogs. I. Technique of myelography: side effects and complications. J. Small Animal Pract. *3*, 53, 1962.
39. Funkquist, B.: Thoraco-lumbar myelography with water-soluble contrast medium in dogs. II. Appearance of the myelograms in disk protrusion and its relation to functional disturbance and patho-anatomic changes in the epidural space. J. Small Animal Pract. *3*, 67, 1962.
40. Funkquist, B.: Cervical myelography with a water-soluble contrast medium. Excerptum Acta Radiol. *56*, 257, 1961.
41. Funkquist, B., and Obel, N.: Effect on the spinal cord of subarachnoid injection of water-soluble contrast medium. Excerptum Acta Radiol. *56*, 449, 1961.
42. Gage, E. D., and Bartels, J. E.: Water-soluble contrast medium. Excerptum Acta Radiol. *56*, 257, 1961.
43. Garrick, J. G., and Sullivan, C. R.: A technic of performing diskography in dogs. Proc. Mayo Clin. *39*, 270, 1961.
44. Gay, W.: Personal communication.
45. Geary, J. C.: Personal communication.
46. Geary, J. C.: Veterinary tomography. J. Am. Vet. Rad. Soc. *8*, 32, 1967.
47. Goldie, I.: Changes observed in the intervertebral disc after discography. Acta Pathol. Microbiol. Scand. *42*, 192, 1968.
48. Greene, J. E.: Surgical intervention for paraplegia due to herniation of the nucleus pulposus. N. Am. Vet. *32*, 411, 1952.
49. Hare, U. C. D.: Radiographic anatomy of the canine skull. J.A.V.M.A. *133*, 149, 1958.
50. Hoerlein, B. F.: *Intervertebral Disc Protrusions in the Dog: A Clinical and Pathological Study.* Thesis (Ph.D.), New York State Veterinary College, Cornell University, Ithaca, New York, 1952.
51. Hoerlein, B. F.: Clinical spinal radiography in the dog. J.A.V.M.A. *134*, 343, 1959.
52. Hoerlein, B. F.: Intervertebral disc protrusion in the dog. III. Radiological diagnosis. Am. J. Vet. Res. *51*:275, 1953.
53. Hoerlein, B. F.: Various contrast media in canine myelography. J.A.V.M.A. *123*, 311, 1953.
54. Hoerlein, B. F., and Petty, M. F.: Contrast encephalography and ventriculography in the dog—preliminary studies. Am. J. Vet. Res. *22*, 1041, 1961.
55. Hoerlein, B. F.: *Canine Neurology, Diagnosis and Treatment,* 2d ed. W. B. Saunders Co., Philadelphia, 1971.
56. Horwitz, N. J.: Positive contrast ventriculography—critical evaluation. J. Neurosurg. *13*, 388, 1956.
57. James, C. W., and Hoerlein, B. F.: Cerebral angiography in the dog. Vet. Med. *55*, 45, 1960.
58. James, C. W.: *Radiographic Anatomy of the Cerebral Arterial System of the Dog.* Thesis, Auburn University, Auburn, Alabama, 1963.
59. James, C. W.: Personal communication.
60. Klide, A. M., Steinberg, S. A., and Pond, M. J.: Epiduralograms in the dog: the uses and advantages of the diagnostic procedure. J. Amer. Vet. Rad. Soc. *8*, 39, 1967.
61. Kubie, L. S., and Retan, G. M.: Forced drainage of the cerebrospinal fluid. J.A.M.A. *101*, 354, 1933.
62. Lee, R., and Griffiths, I. R.: A comparison of cerebral arteriography and cavernous sinus venography in the dog. J. Small Animal Pract. *13*, 225, 1972.
63. Lindblad, G., Ljunggren, G., and Olsson, S. E.: On spinal cord compression in the dog: an angiographic study. Adv. Small Animal Pract. *3*, 121, 1962.
64. Lindblom, K.: Technic and results in myelography and disc puncture. Acta Radiol. *34*, 321, 1950.
65. Lord, P. F., and Olsson, S. E.: Myelography with metrizamide in the dog: a clinical study on its use for the demonstration of spinal cord lesions other than those caused by intervertebral disc protrusion. J. Am. Vet. Rad. Soc. *18*(2) 42–50, 1976.
66. Lord, P. K.: Personal communication, 1976.
67. Lord, L. H., and Robinson, G. A.: Progressive myelopathy in a dog, caused by thorium dioxide. Can. J. Comp. Med. Vet. Sci. *29*:306, 1965.
68. Manhauser, M. J., and Parker, A. J.: Clinical observations of cardiovascular and respiratory changes during contrast myelography with water-soluble media. J. Am. Animal Hosp. Assoc. *11*, 401–403, 1975.
69. Maupin, R. A., Baker, H. L., and Kerr, F. W. L.: Emulsified Pantopaque. Radiology *86*(3), 509, 1966.
70. Mones, R., and Werman, R.: Pantopaque fourth ventriculography via lumbar route. J. Mt. Sinai Hosp. (N.Y.) *25*, 201, 1958.
71. Morgan, J. P.: *Radiology in Veterinary Orthopedics.* Lea & Febiger, Philadelphia, 1972.
72. Morgan, J. P.: Spinal dural ossification in the dog: incidence and distribution based on a radiographic study. J. Am. Vet. Rad. Soc. *10*, 43, 1969.
73. Morgan, J. P.: Congenital anomalies of the vertebral column of the dog: a study of the incidence and significance based on a radiographic and morphologic study. J. Am. Vet. Rad. Soc., *9*, 21, 1968.
74. Morgan, J. P., Suter, P. F., and Holliday, T. A.: Myelography with water-soluble contrast medium. Acta Radiol. (Suppl.) *319*, 217–230, 1972.
75. Murtagh, F., Chamberlain, W. F., Scott, M., and Wyeiss, H. T.: Cervical air myelography: review of 130 cases. Amer. J. Roentgenol. *74*, 1, 1955.
76. Oliver, J. E., Jr.: Cranial sinus venography in the dog. J. Am. Vet. Rad. Soc., *10*, 66, 1969.

77. Oliver, J. E., and Conrad, C. R.: Cerebral ventriculography. *In* Ticer, J. W. (ed.): *Radiographic Technique in Small Animal Practice.* W. B. Saunders Co., Philadelphia, 1975.
78. Olsson, S. E.: On disc protrusion in the dog (enchondiosis intervertebralis). Acta Orthoped. Scand. Suppl. *8*, 1951.
79. Olsson, S. E.: Disbrack hos hund. Medlemsbl. Sv. Vet. Forbund. *12*, 149, 1960.
80. Olsson, S. E.: The radiologic examination. *In* Pettit, G. D. (ed.): *Intervertebral Disc Protrusion in the Dog.* Appleton-Century-Crofts, New York, 1966.
81. Parker, A. J.: Myelomalacia attributable to intramedullary leakage of sodium methiodal and lidocaine. J. Am. Animal Hosp. Assoc. *11*, 404–406, 1975.
82. Parker, A. J., Park, R. D., and Henry, J. D., Jr.: Cervical vertebral instability associated with cervical disc disease in two dogs. J.A.V.M.A. *163*, 1369–1371, 1973.
83. Patterson, D. E., and Botts, R. P.: A simple cassette changer. Small Animal Clin. *1*, 1, 1961.
84. Rising, J. C., and Lewis, R. E.: Femorovertebral cerebral angiography in the dog. Am. J. Vet. Res. *33*, 665, 1970.
85. Robertson, E. C.: *Pneumoencephalography.* Charles C Thomas, Publishers, Springfield, Ill., 1957.
86. Schebitz, H., and Wilkens, H.: *Atlas of Radiographic Anatomy of Dog and Horse.* Paul Parey, Berlin and Hamburg, 1968.
87. Shapiro, R.: *Myelography.* Year Book Medical Publishers, Inc., Chicago, 1962.
88. Shelay, C. H.: A comparison of Renografin and Hypaque for carotid arteriography. J. Neurosurg. *20*, 137, 1936.
89. Sicard, J. A., and Forestier, J.: Method général d'exploration radiologique par l'hinle iodée (Lipiodol). Bull. Mem. Soc. Med. Hôp. (Paris) *16*, 463, 1922.
90. Spooner, R. L.: Cerebral angiography in the dog. J. Small Animal Pract. *2*, 243, 1961.
91. Stowater, J. L., Menhusen, M. J., and Gendreau, C. L.: Canine myelography with Skiodan. Part I. Indications and interpretations. Vet. Med. Small Anim. Clin. *71*, 1207, 1976.
92. Suter, P. F., Morgan, J. P., Holliday, T. A., and O'Brien, T. R.: Myelograph in the dog: diagnosis of the spinal cord and vertebrae. J. Amer. Vet. Rad. Soc. *12*, 29, 1971.
93. Teplick, J. G., Haskin, M. E., and Skelley, J. F.: Total myelography with radiopaque emulsions. Radiology *90*(4), 698, 1968.
94. Thrall, D. E., Lewis, R. E., Walker, M. A., Kneller, S. K., and Losonsky, J. M.: The basis for dosing water-soluble myelographic medium for lumbar administration: body weight or crown rump length. J. Am. Vet. Rad. Soc. *16*(4), 130, 1975.
95. Ticer, J. W., and Brown, S. G.: Water-soluble myelography in canine intervertebral disk protrusion. J. Am. Vet. Rad. Soc. *14*(1), 3, 1974.
96. Ticer, J. W. (ed.): *Radiographic Technique in Small Animal Practice.* W. B. Saunders Co., Philadelphia, 1975.
97. Vaughan, L. C.: Studies on intervertebral disc protrusion in the dog. II. Diagnosis of disease. Brit. Vet. J. *114*:203, 1958.
98. Whiteleather, J. E., and DeSaussure, R. L.: New contrast medium (Hypaque) for cerebral angriography. Radiology *67*, 537, 1956.
99. Wilson, J. W., Bahr, R. J., Leipold, H. W., and Guffy, M. M.: Acute leptomeningeal reaction to the subarachnoid injection of ethyl iodophenylundecylate in dogs. J.A.V.M.A. *169*, 415, 1976.
100. Worthman, R. P.: The longitudinal vertebral venous sinuses of the dog. II. Functional aspects. Amer. J. Vet. *17*, 349, 1956.

CHAPTER 6

LABORATORY EXAMINATIONS

J. S. Spano, D.V.M., Ph.D.
B. F. Hoerlein, D.V.M., Ph.D.

As the physical and radiographic examination of the neurological patient progresses, certain general laboratory examinations of blood, urine, feces, and spinal fluid specimens are performed. One must emphasize that a wealth of neurological manifestations appear in disorders that are not traditionally considered neurological diseases. Therefore, in order to establish the primary diagnosis and the most effective treatment, the results of the laboratory tests must be correlated with the physical and radiographic findings.

HEMATOLOGY

Confirmatory evidence is often necessary in correlating hematologic results with the findings of the neurological examination. In suspected cases of bacterial meningitis, encephalitis, or abscesses of the central nervous system, leukocytosis could certainly be expected on evaluation of the hemogram. Depending on the degree of involvement, the neutrophil count may be slightly or markedly elevated, and a variable number of immature neutrophils may be present. As with other stress reactions lymphopenia and eosinopenia may also be present. The typical stress picture of leukocytosis, lymphopenia, and eosinopenia also occurs in patients with trauma to the central nervous system without infection and in cases of intervertebral disk protrusion; steroid therapy also produces these signs. Mycotic infections, including cryptococcosis and blastomycosis, may be accompanied by a normal hemogram or one that shows some degree of leukocytosis. Parasitic infections including toxoplasmosis may cause a reaction that ranges from leukopenia to leukocytosis.

Leukopenia may accompany some viral diseases such as canine distemper or infectious canine hepatitis. Overwhelming bacterial infections may also cause a marked decrease in leukocyte numbers.

BIOCHEMISTRY

Abnormal serum calcium levels may cause clinical signs that must be differentiated from those of a primary central nervous disorder. Hypocalcemic tetany is sometimes observed in the lactating bitch and in the stressed hunting dog.

Hypoglycemia may also cause central nervous signs. It may result from hyperinsulinism due to insulin overdose or from an insulin-secreting tumor of the pancreas.

Sudden release of insulin and a transient hypoglycemia may be the cause of the seizures sometimes seen in dogs with acute pancreatitis. However, acute abdominal pain may also be related to this seizure-like activity. Hepatic insufficiency, Gierke-like syndrome in toy breeds, and hypoglycemia in stressed hunting dogs are other possible causes of hypoglycemic convulsions.[14, 21]

The convulsions that are sometimes related to diabetes mellitus and hyperadrenocorticism in the dog are associated with elevated serum glucose levels. Convulsions due to a primary central nervous disorder are often associated with a higher than normal blood glucose level. Blood urea nitrogen, serum creatine, and serum phosphorus are important biochemical determinations used to evaluate the presence of kidney disease. Generalized convulsive seizures and uremic neuropathy are sometimes associated with terminal kidney disease. Nephritis may occur secondary to a spinal lesion that is causing urinary retention, cystitis, and a subsequent retrograde kidney dysfunction.

Serum levels of cholesterol, total bilirubin, glutamic pyruvic transaminase (SGPT), albumin, total protein, and alkaline phosphatase (SAP) are important biochemical determinations to be considered in evaluating liver disease that may be the cause of central nervous depression, disorientation, or convulsions. The early stages of cirrhosis and the hepatoencephalopathy seen with portal caval anomalies may show normal SGPT and SAP, low serum total protein, cholesterol and albumin, and occasionally abnormally low blood urea nitrogen levels. Convulsions, mental confusion, or depression may be seen in conjunction with these findings.[7, 10, 29]

In advanced cirrhosis serum total bilirubin, cholesterol, SGPT, and SAP are usually elevated, while serum total protein and albumin remain depressed. Acute hepatic necrosis characterized by elevated SGPT, SAP, and abnormal serum total protein and albumin may occasionally be accompanied by a hepatocerebral syndrome.

Serum sodium and potassium are other important biochemical tests. Hyperkalemia and convulsions may be associated with acidosis, renal failure, diabetes mellitus, severe dehydration, hypoxia, and sudden withdrawal from steroid therapy. Hyponatremia associated with hypoadrenocorticism or diuretic therapy may cause extreme muscle weakness.

URINALYSIS

A urine specimen of very low specific gravity (<1.008) with clinical polyuria may accompany a pituitary tumor that decreases production of antidiuretic hormone. Glycosuria and ketonuria in a dog with neurologic signs may point to a diabetic ketoacidosis.

SEQUALAE IN STEROID THERAPY

Laboratory findings may be important in evaluating the possible complications that may occur following steroid therapy for decompressive disk surgery. Complications such as gastric, duodenal, and colonic ulcerations have been described. Clinical signs of abdominal pain, vomiting, and diarrhea may be accompanied by an elevated temperature and laboratory signs of hemoconcentration and leukocytosis with a shift to the left. Long-term steroid therapy may also induce pancreatitis accompanied by leukocytosis, as well as elevated SAP, SGPT, and lipase levels.

Excessive hemorrhage and a possible microangiopathic hemolytic anemia have been seen after trauma to the musculature following surgery for decompressive disk surgery. A regenerative anemia was observed in these cases, sometimes accompanied by the presence of fragmented erythrocytes on the peripheral blood smear.[15]

FECES

Fecal examinations are necessary routine procedures for any successful clinician. There have been reports of extreme internal parasitism causing neurological signs such as seizures. However, when such signs occur, it is felt that they are generally associated with secondary critical metabolic disturbances. Parasitic invasion or ascaridal larval migrations in the CNS cause direct neuropathy and clinical signs. Reports of parasitic and protozoan infections in the CNS are becoming more frequent. In light of these factors, a fecal determination is basic to any physical examination and diagnosis.

CEREBROSPINAL FLUID

Hippocrates recognized the presence of a peculiar fluid in the central nervous system in pathologic conditions; Galen is said to have described and studied this fluid under normal circumstances. This unique material has been the subject of study, controversy, and confusion in the intervening centuries.[3]

The cerebrospinal fluid (CSF) is normally a clear watery fluid that bathes the CNS tissue both internally and externally. It has unique properties and physiological functions, which change in the course of the disease. A detailed discussion of CSF appears in Chapter 21; however, those aspects of CSF pertinent to physical examination and laboratory tests will be discussed here.[5]

PRESSURE

Technique of Collecting Fluid and Recording Pressure

The cisternal and lumbar sites for collection of CSF were described in detail in Chapter 5 under myelography. However, since an important phase of the neurological examination is recording the CSF pressure, the subarachnoid tap should be made with the dog in the lateral recumbent rather than the sternal recumbent position called for in myelography. Because CSF pressure varies with differences of technique all details of the procedure should be kept as routinely standard as possible. Also, since the lumbar subarachnoid space is small and the anatomical features in this area make the tap difficult, recording of pressure and securing the CSF sample are better performed in the cisterna magna. The procedure should be carried out in strict asepsis.

Bailey describes CSF manometry in L4–5 or L6–7 ventral subarachnoid taps, using jugular compression to test patency of the spinal subarachnoid space. To the authors' knowledge, this is the only reference to lumbar CSF manometry in veterinary literature.[2]

Clinically, CSF pressure can be most effectively measured by using the Ayer glass or plastic disposable spinal fluid manometer,* which will give a direct CSF pressure reading. Chronological steps in the cisternal procedure are as follows:

1. Give general ultra-short barbiturate anesthesia (gaseous or local anesthesia if patient is in critical condition).
2. Intubate the trachea.
3. Perform aseptic cisternal tap with the dog in the lateral recumbent position, using a 22-gauge spinal needle.
4. Keep the dog in a standard unrestricted position. Exert no pressure on any part of the body; jugular veins must be free of compression that might result from pronounced cervical flexion.
5. Attach the manometer to the needle and a three-way stopcock before any fluid escapes. If infection is suspected, a drop of heparin should be used in the apparatus to prevent any coagulation of fluid. The fluid is allowed to rise to its maximum height and the average reading is recorded.
6. Remove 1 to 2 ml of fluid by means of the three-way stopcock and a syringe; withdraw slowly, not over 1 ml/30 seconds.[25] This fluid can be used for culture and laboratory examination.
7. Record a second pressure immediately thereafter, and observe the subsequent recovery of pressure normalcy.
8. Additional quantities of CSF can be subsequently withdrawn if fluid is readily available and if it is required for laboratory examination. Generally 2 ml is sufficient (Figs. 6–1 to 6–3).

Pressure Readings

As previously emphasized, the variations of technique in performing a spinal tap and CSF pressure recording will contribute to the published variations of normal readings. Pressure recordings obtained by using the authors'

*Becton, Dickinson and Company, Rutherford, New Jersey.

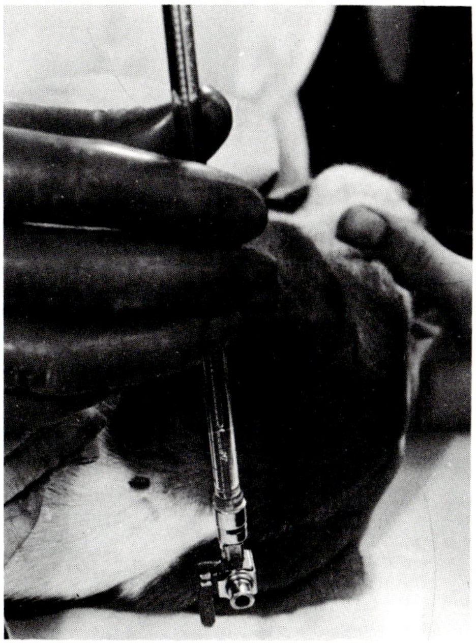

FIGURE 6–1 A clinical method of measuring cerebrospinal fluid pressure using a Becton, Dickinson manometer.

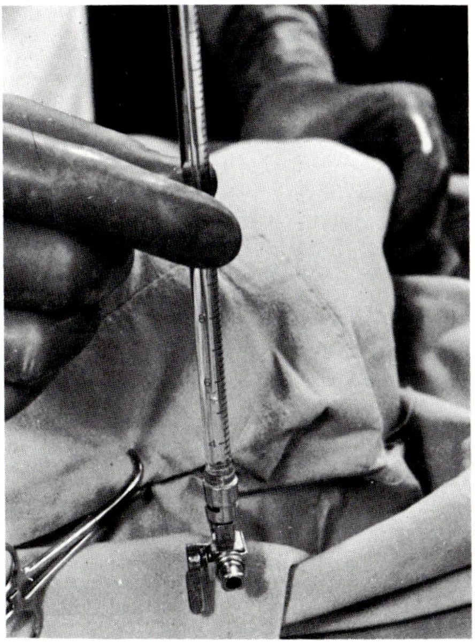

FIGURE 6–2 Use of the apparatus shown in Figure 6–1 on a clinical patient. This procedure must be carried out aseptically.

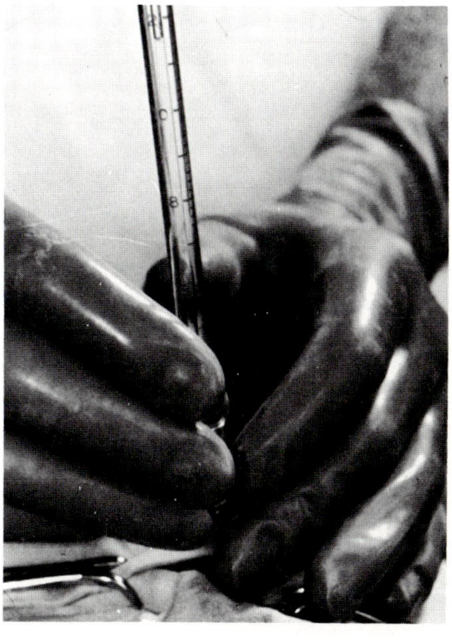

FIGURE 6–3 The cerebrospinal fluid has risen to the 118 mm level. This is a normal reading for an anesthetized dog.

technique, as previously described, will vary from 50 to 140 mm of CSF, with the average around 80 mm. Frauchiger and Fankhauser[11] reported an average of 86.5 mm of saline, while Verwer[32] recorded a range of 24 to 172 mm water, with an average of 86.5 mm. In previous determinations, the authors found the average pressure to be 97 mm of Ringer's solution.[13]

The aforementioned normal CSF pressures were largely single, isolated recordings that were taken while the dog was sedated or anesthetized. An interesting paper by Verdura and co-workers recorded chronic or continuous pressures in a variety of physiological states by means of permanent cannulation of the cisterna through the ventral aspect of the base of the skull.[31] The cannula was attached to a venous-pressure transducer and a multichannel electronic recorder. The average CSF pressure in the awake, unrestrained, ambulatory dog was 135 to 150 mm water. During barking or straining, the values rose by as much as 60 to 80 mm water to values of 195 to 230 mm. Under sodium pentobarbital anesthesia, the readings were 109 to 122 mm water. With temporary hypoxia produced by clamping the endotracheal tube for 1 minute, a sustained increase in pressure to 400 to 475 mm water was recorded.[31]

Neurosurgeons have found that hyperventilation, hypothermia, and intravenously administered hypertonic solutions such as mannitol and urea can lower the CSF pressure appreciably. It has been shown that in anesthetized, hyperventilated, normothermic dogs the CSF pressure could be lowered from 121 mm to 36 mm of water with a fully effective dose of urea. In anesthetized, hyperventilated, hypothermic dogs, the CSF pressure could be lowered from 121 to 77 mm of water. If a full dose of urea was given to these same dogs, their pressure dropped to 18 mm water.[22] Leonard and Redding[20] report a consistent reduction in intraventricular pressure after intravenous injection of mannitol and urea solutions (1.5 gm/kg body weight) within a 15-minute interval. Most pressures were reduced to zero for about an hour and then gradually rose to normal levels. Other methods of combatting clinical brain edema, such as the administration of adrenocortical steroids, will also lower CSF pressure.

As emphasized repeatedly in later chapters, the clinician should not routinely perform a cisternal tap and record CSF pressure or analyze sizable quantities of CSF in patients with acute cerebral trauma. One must establish that intracranial hemorrhage is not occurring before a tap is made. If extradural or subdural hemorrhage is occurring, removal of CSF will promote tentorial herniation and compression of the vital centers in the medulla oblongata. Death usually results. In addition, when the CSF pressure is reduced via a cisternal tap, the brain mass recedes proportionately and hemorrhage is facilitated.

Interpretation of Pressure Recordings

The interpretation of CSF pressure must be attempted with full knowledge of clinical history, physical signs, and the technique of recording. High recordings (up to 550 mm water) may be seen in communicating hydrocephalus, intracranial tumors, abscesses, hemorrhage, meningitis, and cerebral edema. Lower recordings in pressure may occur in noncommunicating, obstructive hydrocephalus, in either congenital or acquired forms. If the initial reading is above normal and the second is abnormally low (after a 2 ml sample of CSF has been taken), there is a small reservoir of fluid, and a space-occupying mass, such as a tumor or abscess, probably is present in the cranial cavity.[25] Severe general dehydration could result in a low recording.[9, 25]

Hoerlein observed little change in CSF pressures in cases of thoracolumbar compression resulting from disk protrusion.[13] A lumbar tap and the jugular pressure test as used in man might aid in establishing a diagnosis of spinal compression in the dog.[2]

LABORATORY EXAMINATION OF CSF

Much fine work on the composition of canine spinal fluid has been done by Frauchiger and Fankhauser,[11] Verwer,[32] and others. Bentinck-Smith[4] summarizes these and original findings in the following chart.

Cerebrospinal Fluid
(mg/100 ml except where indicated)

Quantity	0.9–16.0 ml
Aspect	clear, colorless
Pressure	24–172 mm H_2O
Specific gravity	1.003–1.012
Freezing point depression	–0.61° C to 0.63° C
Alkali reserve	48.5–68.6 vol. per cent
Cells/cu mm	1–8 lymphocytes, occasional endothelial cell
Chloride	761–883 as NaCl mg/100 ml
Sugar	61–116
Phosphorus	2.8–3.5
Magnesium	2.6–3.8
Nonprotein N	below 40
Total protein	11–55
Albumin	16.5–37.5
Globulin	5.5–16.5
Pandy test	negative[2]

In addition, Yeary establishes sodium as 142.0 to 170.6 mEq/l, potassium as 2.8 to 3.4 mEq/l, and calcium as 3.8 to 8.6 mg/100 ml.[35]

Color

Normal CSF is clear and colorless, and it doesn't coagulate. If a bright red color is seen upon withdrawing the sample, probably one of the cervical venous sinuses or anastomosing veins has been punctured by the needle. In this case, the clinician should reposition the needle and make an effort to obtain clear fluid. Blood contamination from needle trauma makes laboratory examination of CSF most difficult.

If the CSF contains blood from trauma of tapping, centrifugation of the sample produces a clear supernatant fluid that can be used for some other tests. A yellowish tinge to the fluid or supernatant portion is called xanthochromia, and it indicates old hemorrhage in the CNS (bilirubin from disintegration of red cells) or a generalized icterus. A dull red to brown color indicates intracranial hemorrhage from brain trauma or hemorrhagic lesion.[6]

Turbidity of CSF generally is due to the presence of cells in excess of 500/cu mm. Bacteria and mycotic organisms can contribute to the turbidity of CSF. Cases of bacterial meningitis may cause only slightly turbid to almost pure pus in CSF, which may cause the CSF to clot. Viral encephalitis, trauma, tumors, or abscesses may produce turbidity in CSF due to large amounts of protein, fibrin, or cells.

Total Cell Count

Cell counting procedures should be performed on the CSF within 20 minutes after collection, since white cells disintegrate upon standing. The preferred method of determining a total cell count and differential estimation in the Neubauer or Zeiss counting chamber is as follows:

1. Draw diluting fluid up to 1 mark on white cell pipette. This diluting fluid consists of 0.1 gm crystal violet, 10 ml glacial acetic acid, and 90 ml distilled water.
2. Draw CSF up to 11 mark on pipette.
3. Mix thoroughly and discard two or three drops. Fill each side of standard hemocytometer and wait 2 minutes for cells to settle. Count all the cells within the ruled areas on both sides of the counting chamber (18 1-mm squares) and multiply by 0.6 to obtain the number of cells per cu mm.[3]
4. Estimate the type of cells by counting the polymorphonuclear cells present under high power of the microscope.
5. If the CSF specimen is contaminated with whole blood, a total red and white cell count should be performed. Since the approximate ratio of RBC to WBC is 500:1 in normal blood, an increase in WBC in CSF can be roughly estimated. An actual RBC:WBC ratio may be calculated from counts made on a concomitant specimen of peripheral blood.[6]

An alternative method of performing a cell count on CSF is to load a standard hemocytometer chamber with well-mixed CSF, using a capillary tube. All the cells are counted in the ruled area of one side of the chamber. This number multiplied by 1.1 gives the number of cells per cu mm. Another capillary tube rinsed in glacial acetic acid is filled with CSF and counted in a similar manner. This will give the number of white blood cells in the sample. The difference between the first and second count is the number of red blood cells.[1]

High counts (pleocytosis) are generally seen in inflammatory or irritative lesions of the meninges, brain, or spinal cord. High counts can be seen in tumors, in chronic, focal, or degenerative lesions, in brain or cord abscesses, and in encephalitis, such as distemper. Extremely high counts are seen in pyogenic meningitis.[6, 23]

Differential Cell Count

A differential cell count should be made in cases of pleocytosis. In counts of less than 500/cu mm, the sample is centrifuged, the supernatant is poured off, and two or three drops of serum are added to the sediment and the cells are resuspended in it. A smear should be made and stained with any polychrome stain used in blood smears. In counts of over 500 cells/cu mm, a direct smear of CSF may be made. A wet coverslip method of Cornelius causes less cellular distortion and disintegration. Three drops of new methylene blue is added to 1 ml of CSF or sediment, a drop of this mixture is placed on a slide, a coverslip is applied, and the slide is examined 5 minutes later.[6, 17]

Normal CSF has only small lymphocytes present. If the increase in cells is predominantly lymphocytic or mononuclear, a viral infection such as distemper, a chronic infection, postvaccinal inflammation, uremic disorder, or a toxic or fungal condition may be present. If the increase is predominantly neutrophilic, a bacterial infection is generally present. Verwer studied 600 CSF samples from healthy and diseased dogs, of which necropsies were performed on 107. The highest percentage of abnormal fluid samples were collected from dogs with meningoencephalitis, brain tumors, distemper, and encephalomyelitis.[6, 9, 23, 32]

Protein

In normal CSF, protein levels are very low and consist almost entirely of albumin. Globulin levels are increased in pathologic conditions. The simplest determination of the globulin level is the Pandy test. Pandy's reagent is prepared by adding 10 gm of carbolic acid crystals to 100 ml of distilled water. A few drops of CSF are added to 1 ml of Pandy reagent in a tube, and the mixture is shaken. Normal CSF may show a very slight hazy turbidity, while pathologic fluid shows a definite white turbidity proportionate to its globulin content. A similar test is the Nonne-Apelt or Ross-Jones test.[6]

More accurate quantitative methods are available for the determination of protein in CSF. These generally require the use of a spectrophotometer. The methodology is described in standard biochemical texts.[12, 24]

Increased levels of globulin are seen in inflammatory disorders such as encephalitis, distemper, brain or cord abscesses, toxoplasmosis, and meningitis. Certain noninflammatory disorders that increase capillary permeability and alter the blood-CSF barrier, such as pneumonia, convulsive states, and uremia, may increase the globulin CSF level. Hemorrhage and edema in CNS may raise globulin levels.[6, 9]

Sophisticated techniques including electrophoresis and immunoelectrophoresis of CSF proteins are currently being used in humans to assess more accurately the globulin fractions. These techniques are beginning to be used in veterinary medicine and may prove useful in the diagnoses of distemper encephalitis and other important CNS lesions.[1, 8]

Chlorides

The procedures for cerebrospinal fluid chloride determination are similar to those for blood. Chloride levels are normally higher in CSF than in blood. The chloride level is usually found to have an inverse relation to total protein levels. Its chief use would be in diagnosing meningitis (low chloride level); however, protein determinations are performed more simply.[6]

Sugar (Glucose)

The concentration of glucose in CSF is dependent upon the blood glucose level, the selective permeability of the CSF barrier, and the presence of glycolytic microorganisms. The last circumstance, which causes a low glucose CSF level, is seen primarily in glycolytic activity of bacteria causing acute pyogenic infections. Therefore, for proper interpretation, glucose determinations should be made on concomitantly drawn specimens of blood and spinal fluid. Slight elevations of glucose have been seen in encephalitis, spinal cord compressions, brain tumors and abscesses.[6] Recent reports have shown that some types of meningeal or intracranial neoplasms have produced sterile CSF, pleocytosis, and a low sugar content, probably due to an impedance of glucose transport across the meningeal membranes infiltrated with neoplasia.[19] Dogs with nervous distemper have a low CSF glucose level.[23]

Other Chemical Tests

The CSF electrolytes—eg., phosphorus, sodium, calcium, potassium, and magnesium—are currently of questionable diagnostic significance in various pathologic disorders. Nonprotein nitrogen levels parallel those found in the blood. Normal cholesterol levels (from none to a trace) have been increased in hemorrhages of the CNS, in tumors, meningitis, and brain abscesses. The CSF transaminases (SGOT and SGPT) have been found to be elevated significantly in cases of distemper,[4–6] purulent meningitis, and experimentally produced cerebral infarctions. Cerebrospinal fluid lactate dehydrogenase and isocitric dehydrogenase have been found to be elevated in man in cases of metastatic carcinoma, subarachnoid hemorrhage, and cerebral infarctoin.[17]

CULTURAL AND CYTOMORPHOLOGICAL EXAMINATIONS OF CSF

Cultural examination for various microorganisms, including fungi and yeasts, should be performed by an experienced microbiologist. The specimen must be obtained aseptically, so it is preferable to do it prior to pressure recordings, unless great care in maintaining asepsis of the manometer has been exercised. Since the techniques of these examinations are beyond the scope of the average clinician, appropriate texts should be consulted for details.

Cytomorphological examinations of CSF are usually infrequently performed because of a lack of interest and qualified personnel. However, in qualified hands, such examinations have been extremely helpful in diagnosing CNS neoplasia, subarachnoid hemorrhage, and inflammatory and demyelinating diseases. The organisms of cryptococcosis, toxoplasmosis, and blastomycosis are occasionally observed in CSF. These are often accompanied by a pleocytosis consisting of mononuclear cells, neutrophils, and often eosinophils. It has been reported that meningiomas and intra-axial gliomas cannot usually be diagnosed by cytomorphological examination.[18] It has been of special value in suspected metastatic or disseminated tumors that are in contact with the ventricles or the subarachnoid space. In one study, tumor cells were found in 24 per cent of specimens from human patients with benign neoplasms, 32 per cent from patients with malignant gliomas, and 29 per cent from patients with metastatic neoplasms.[33]

Special techniques for concentrating cells in CSF are now more widely used in veterinary practice. The most popular techniques include membrane filtration, cytocentrifugation, and sedimentation.[26–28] Each of these procedures has the advantage of collecting cells for careful morphologic studies in cell-poor fluids. Disadvantages for the veterinary clinician include time needed for testing, cost of equipment, and technical staining procedures. Generally these methods are used only by special laboratories, since some degree of expertise is required to perform them and interpret the significance of the cell types observed. These procedures are becoming popular in the clinical pathology laboratories of veterinary schools. The Millipore technique is currently being evaluated in our laboratory.

Vandevelde and Spano[30] report a study of 90 dogs in which the cytomorphology of CSF was examined by membrane filtration. The CSF cells were separated into lymphocytes, monocytes, macrophages, neutrophils, eosinophils, plasma cells and specific cell elements (such as tumor cells). Subsequently, histopathological examination was performed in each case. The results of the CSF findings were grouped into five categories according to the histopathological findings.[30]

The first category was composed of 40 cases of inflammatory disease, including distemper, other viral, granulomatous, and bacterial diseases, cryptococcosis, blastomycosis, and toxoplasmosis. In all inflamma-

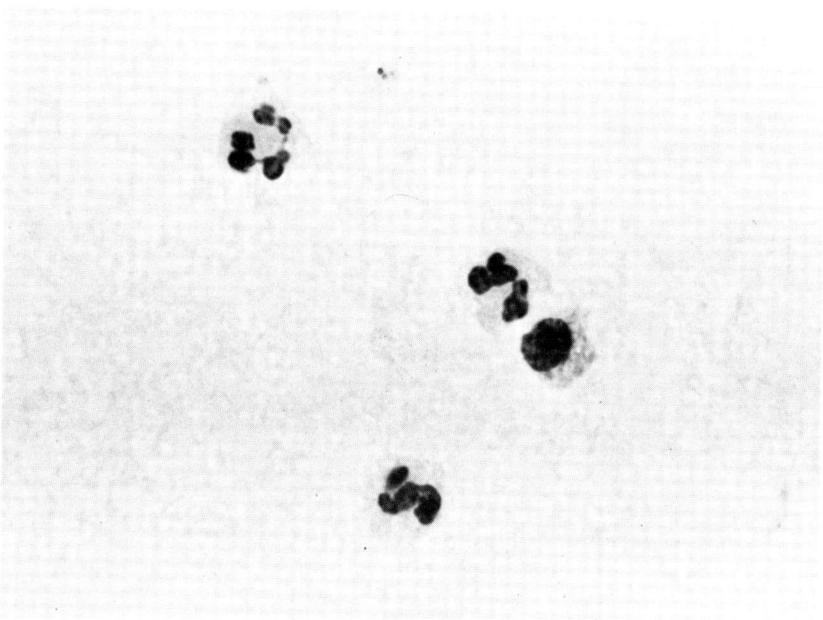

FIGURE 6–4 A case of suppurative meningitis. Note the presence of neutrophils, characteristic of bacteria infections. (In Figures 6–4 to 6–9 the membrane filtration technique of examining CSF has been used; oil immersion Pollaks trichrome stain.)

tory conditions there was an increase in CSF protein and a marked pleocytosis. The cell increase in viral infections was predominantly mononuclear. In bacterial or mycotic infections the polymorphonuclear elements showed a strong increase. In canine distemper-encephalitis the pleocytosis was usually rather moderate and largely due to an increase of lymphocytes. Mycotic organisms were demonstrated in the CSF in one case of blastomycosis and in one case of cryptococcosis. The CSF of the latter

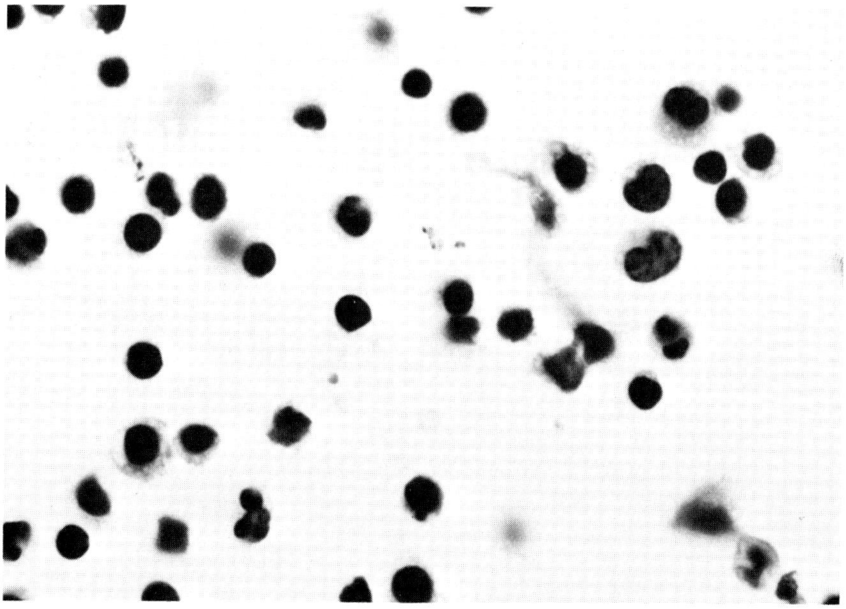

FIGURE 6–5 A confirmed case of rabies. Note the mononuclear cells (both lymphocytes and monocytes) that are characteristic of a viral encephalitis.

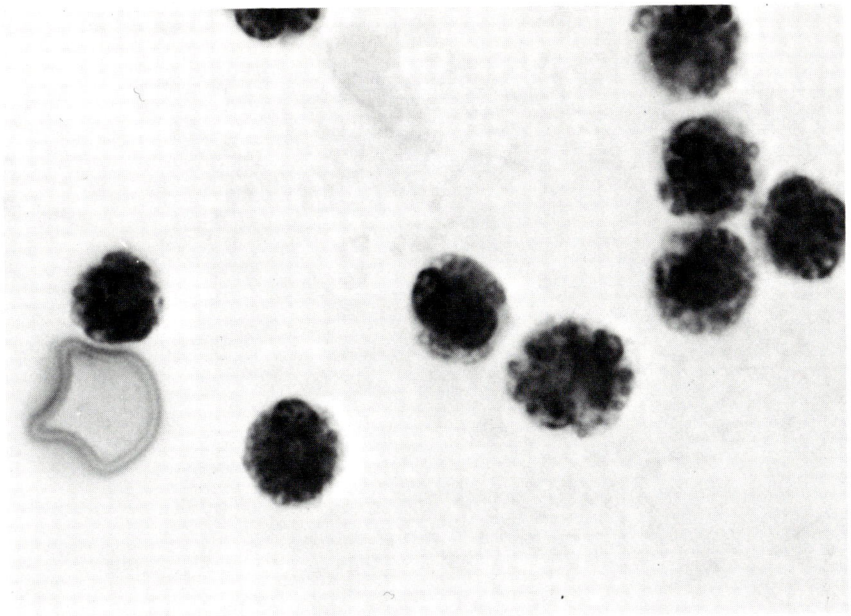

FIGURE 6–6 A case of mycotic meningitis. Note the numerous eosinophils and the large *Cryptococcus neoformans* microorganism in the 7 o'clock position.

case was also strongly eosinophilic[30] (Figs. 6–4 to 6–7).

The second group was composed of 23 cases of CNS trauma, including intervertebral disk protrusion, spinal fractures, tumors of the spine and epidural tissues, spinal cord and cerebral trauma, and vertebral instability. Most of the CSF samples examined in this group were from cases with spinal cord compression of miscellaneous causes. There was usually a slight pleocytosis with a significant increase of neutrophils. In chronic spinal cord compression there was a moderate increase in

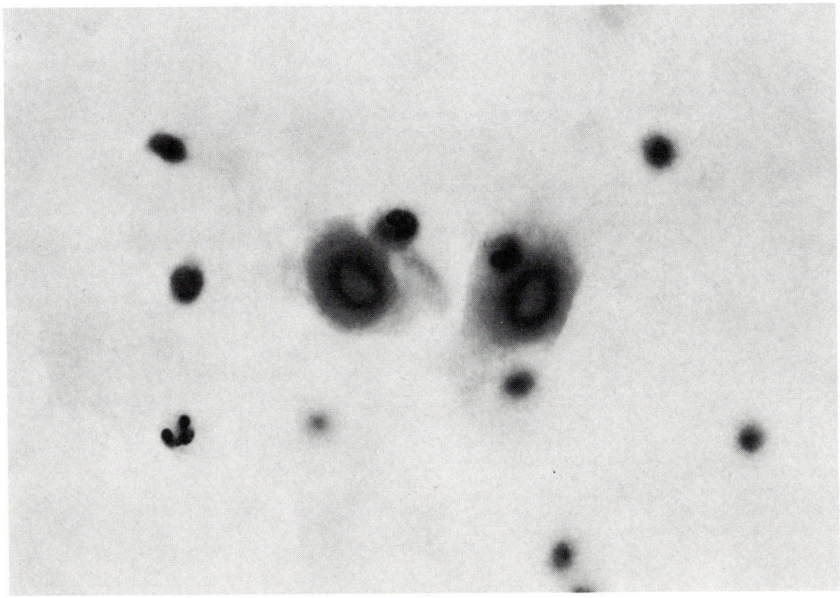

FIGURE 6–7 A case of mycotic meningoencephalitis. Note the two *Blastomyces dermatitides* microorganisms in the center of the photo.

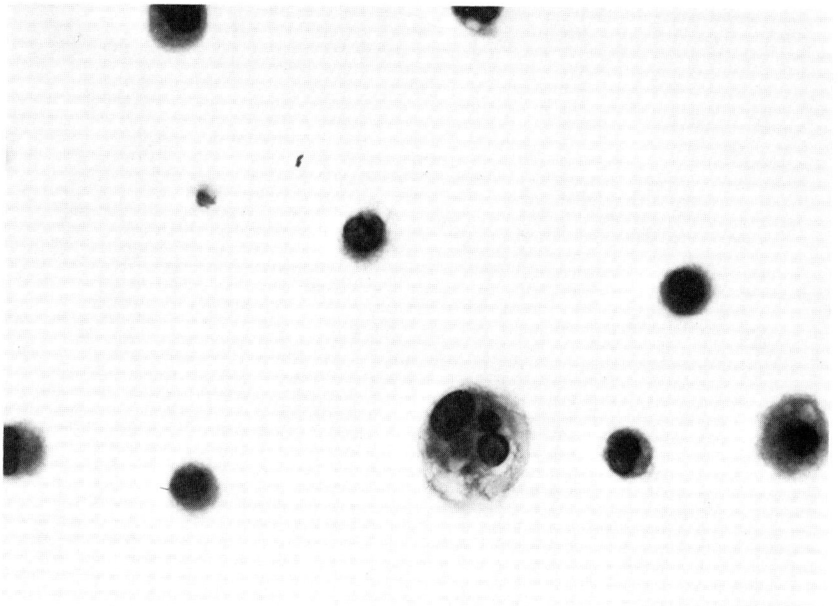

FIGURE 6–8 A case of cerebral hemorrhage examined several days after the trauma. Note the erthrophagocyte in the lower center of the illustration with several other mononuclear cells in other areas.

protein content. It was not possible to relate the CSF changes to the extent of the spinal cord damage. It was felt, however, that CSF examination could help in supporting a diagnosis of physical spinal cord damage to differentiate this entity from muscular neurogenic or other conditions clinically presented as spinal ataxia.[30]

The third group was composed of 12 cases of congenital and degenerative diseases, including congenital malformations, hypomyelinogenesis, cerebrocortical necrosis, Ammon's horn sclerosis, German shepherd myelopathy, polyradiculoneuropathy, and hepatic encephalopathy. This was a heterogeneous group of samples. It

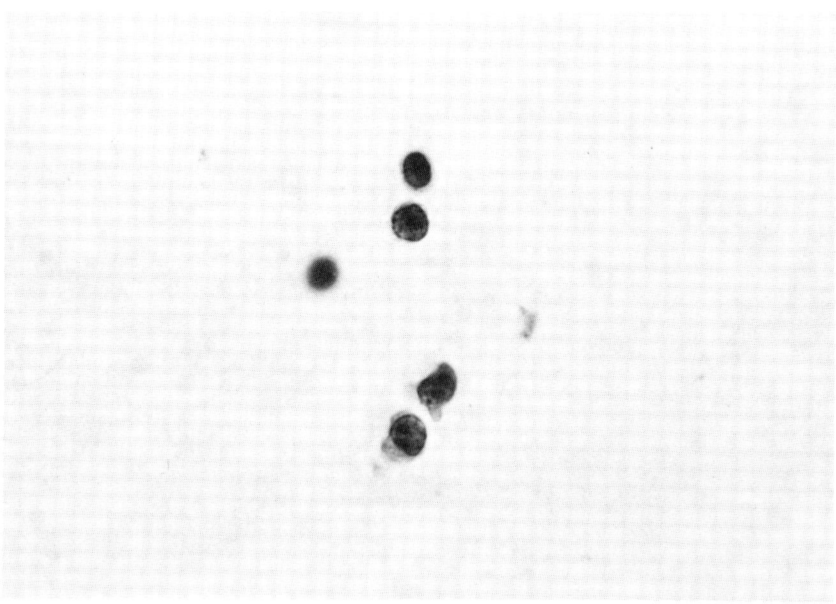

FIGURE 6–9 A case of lymphosarcoma. Note the large numbers of lymphoblastic cells.

was felt that CSF examination could be helpful in differentiating congenital malformations from congenital degenerative diseases. Pleocytosis with neutrophils was found in two cases of cerebrocortical necrosis, and a strong lymphocytic increase was observed in one case of polyradiculoneuropathy.[30]

The fourth group consisted of seven cases of cerebrovascular diseases, including vasculitis, cerebral infarcts, cerebral hemorrhage, and hematomyelia. A strong increase in protein was found in two cases of cerebral vasculitis. Neutrophilic pleocytosis was observed in cerebral infarcts, and erythrophagocytes appeared in cases with cerebral hemorrhage (Fig. 6–8).[30]

The fifth group was composed of 10 cases of tumors, including astrocytoma, oligodendroglioma, neurofibroma, reticulosis, metastatic squamous carcinoma, metastatic renal carcinoma, and lymphosarcoma. A marked increase in CSF protein content was seen in two brain tumor cases. Suspected malignant cells were found in the CSF of one neuroectodermal tumor. In

TABLE 6–1 CEREBROSPINAL FLUID CHANGES IN DISEASE[1, 3, 6, 23, 32]

Disorder	Pressure	Appearance	Cell Count	Cell Type	Protein	Sugar	Other
Encephalitis:							
Bacterial	Elevated	Turbid	Increased	Neutrophil	Increased	Normal to sl. increased	Culture
Viral (distemper)	Sl. elevated	Clear to sl. turbid	Increased	Lymphocytes and mononuclear cells	Increased	Normal to decreased	SGOT, SGPT increased
Meningitis:							
Bacterial	Elevated	Turbid	Increased	Neutrophils	Markedly increased	Sl. to markedly decreased	Culture
Viral	Sl. elevated	Milky-yellow	Increased	Lymphocytes and mononuclear cells	Increased	Normal to decreased	—
CNS abscess	Elevated	Clear to sl. turbid or sl. yellow	Increased	Neutrophils–monocytes	Increased	Normal to sl. increased	Culture
Toxoplasmosis	Sl. elevated	Sl. yellow	Increased	Lymphocytes	Increased	—	Culture
CNS tumor:							
Primary	Elevated	Clear to sl. turbid or sl. yellow	Normal	Tumor cells	Normal to increased	Questionable	—
Metastatic	Elevated	Same	Normal to sl. increased	Lymphocytes, tumor cells	Same	Questionable	—
CNS trauma:							
Hemorrhage	Elevated	Degrees of red-brown or yellow	Increased	Erythrophagocytes, RBC, neutrophils	Increased	—	—
Edema	Elevated	Clear to sl. turbid	Normal to sl. increased	Normal to few RBC, WBC	Sl. increased	—	—
CNS degeneration:							
Encephalomalacia	Normal	Clear	Normal to sl. increased	—	Increased	—	—
Spinal cord compression	Normal to sl. elevated	Clear	Normal to sl. increased	Lymphocytes	Normal to sl. increased	Normal to sl. increased	—
Hydrocephalus:							
Communicating	Elevated	Clear to sl. turbid	Normal to sl. increased	—	Normal to sl. increased	—	—
Obstructive	Lower	Clear to sl. turbid	Normal to sl. increased	—	Normal	—	—

both cases of metastatic carcinoma of the brain large numbers of hemosiderinophages were observed in the CSF. Large numbers of tumor cells were demonstrated in the CSF of two cases with lymphosarcoma[30] (Fig. 6–9).

It was concluded from this study that the examination of CSF, including cytomorphology, is a significant aid in the diagnosis of neurological disease in animals.[30]

The examination of cerebrospinal fluid and the recording of CSF pressure in the dog may be of diagnostic importance. Certainly, the appearance, cell count, and protein determinations of CSF are highly important and are valuable aids in establishing a diagnosis when considered with the balance of the neurological examination.

An attempt to summarize the predominant changes of CSF in disease is presented in Table 6–1.

SPECIAL STUDIES

Conjunctival swabs and transtracheal washings may be valuable in fluorescent antibody (FA) studies for the diagnosis of canine distemper virus infection in these tissues. It has been felt, however, that recent vaccinations (modified live virus type) will cause positive reactions. Rarely, neutrophils or erythrocytes in stained peripheral blood smears or in hematocrit buffy coat smears may show the presence of cytoplasmic inclusions characteristic of distemper. The value of these techniques diminishes as the disease progresses, and viral antigen and virus inclusions are no longer present in peripheral tissues in many cases by the third or fourth week following initial signs of the disease.[34] Fluorescent antibody studies on brain material obtained at necropsy are very useful for retrospective diagnoses.

Confirmation of a diagnosis of toxoplasmosis and blastomycosis may be obtained by demonstration of high or rising titers of antibodies in sera or by cultural techniques.[16]

REFERENCES

1. Averill, D. R., Jr.: Examination of the cerebrospinal fluid. *In* Kirk, R. W. (ed.): *Current Veterinary Therapy V.* W. B. Saunders Co., Philadelphia, 1974.
2. Bailey, C. S.: Lumbar puncture for collection of cerebrospinal fluid. Proc. Am. Anim. Hosp. Assoc. *289*, 1973.
3. Benjamin, M. M.: *Outline of Veterinary Clinical Pathology,* 2d ed. Iowa State Press, Ames, Iowa, 1961.
4. Bentinck-Smith, J.: A roster of normal values. *In* Kirk, R. W. (ed.): *Current Veterinary Therapy III.* W. B. Saunders Co., Philadelphia, 1968, p. 699.
5. Bowsher, D.: *Cerebrospinal Fluid Dynamics in Health and Disease.* Charles C Thomas, Publishers, Springfield, Ill., 1960.
6. Coles, E. H.: *Veterinary Clinical Pathology,* 2d ed. W. B. Saunders Co., Philadelphia, 1974.
7. Cornelius, L. M., Thrall, D. E., Holliwell, W. H., Frank, G. M., Kern, A. J., and Woods, C. B.: Anomalous portosystemic anastomoses associated with chronic hepatic insufficiency in six young dogs. J.A.V.M.A. *167,* 220, 1975.
8. Cutler, R. W. P., and Averill, D. R., Jr.: Cerebrospinal fluid gamma globulins in canine distemper encephalitis. Neurology *19,* 1111, 1969.
9. de Lahunta, A.: Examination of spinal fluid. *In* Kirk, R. W. (ed.): *Current Veterinary Therapy III.* W. B. Saunders Co., Philadelphia, 1968, p. 470.
10. Ewing, G. O., Suter, P. F., and Bailey, C. S.: Hepatic insufficiency associated with congenital anomalies of the portal vein in dogs. J. Am. Anim. Hosp. Assoc. *10,* 463, 1974.
11. Frauchiger, E., and Fankhauser, R.: *Die Nervenkrankleiten Unserer Hunde.* Schmid und Cie., Bern, 1949.
12. Henry, R. J.: *Clinical Chemistry, Principles and Technics,* 2d ed. Harper and Row, New York, 1974.
13. Hoerlein, B. F.: Intervertebral disc protrusions in the dog. A clinical and pathological study. Thesis, Cornell University, Ithaca, New York, 1952.
14. Hoerlein, B. F.: *Canine Neurology, Diagnosis and Treatment,* 2d ed. W. B. Saunders Co., Philadelphia, 1971.
15. Hoerlein, B. F., and Spano, J. S.: Nonneurological complications following decompressive spinal cord surgery. Arch. Am. Coll. Vet. Surg. *4,* 11, 1975.
16. Jungerman, P. F., and Schwartzman, R. M.: *Veterinary Medical Mycology.* Lea & Febiger, Philadelphia, 1972.
17. Kaneko, J. J., and Cornelius, C. E.: *Clinical Biochemistry of Domestic Animals,* 2d ed. Academic Press, New York, 1970.
18. Kolar, O., and Zeman, W.: Spinal fluid cytomorphology. Arch. Neurol. *18,* 44, 1968.
19. Laszlo, M. H., and LeVine, M. A.: Low cerebrospinal-fluid sugar content in meningeal and intracranial neoplasia. J.A.M.A. *193,* 834, 1965.
20. Leonard, J. L., and Redding, R. W.: Effects of hypertonic solutions on cerebrospinal fluid pressure in the lateral ventricle of the dog. Am. J. Vet. Res. *34,* 213, 1973.
21. Lord, P., Olsson, S. E., and Audell, L.: Acute pulmonary edema and seizures in hunting dogs. Nord. Vet. Med. *27,* 112, 1975.
22. Lund, L. O., Beckwitt, H. J., Grover, R. F., and Virtue, R. W.: Effects of hyperventilation, hypothermia, and urea on circulation and cerebrospinal fluid pressure in the dog. Anesthesiology *26,* 45, 1965.
23. Markiewicz, K.: Examination of the blood and cerebrospinal fluid of dogs with the nervous

form of distemper. Medcyna. Wet. *21,* 528, 1965.
24. Pesce, M. A., and Strande, C. S.: A new micromethod for determination of protein in cerebrospinal fluid and urine. Clin. Chem. *19,* 1265, 1973.
25. Roberts, R. M.: Personal communication.
26. Roszel, J. F.: Membrane filtration of canine and feline cerebrospinal fluid for cytologic evaluation. J.A.V.M.A. *160,* 720, 1972.
27. Roszel, J. F., Steinberg, S. A., and McGrath, J. T.: Periodic acid-Schiff-positive cells in cerebrospinal fluid of dogs with globoid cell leukodystrophy. Neurology, *22,* 738, 1972.
28. Steinberg, S. A., and Vandevelde, M.: A comparative study of two methods of cytological evaluation of spinal fluid in domestic animals. Folia Vet. Latina *4,* (2), 1974.
29. Strombeck, D. R., Weiser, M. G., and Kaneko, J. J.: Hyperammonemia and hepatic encephalopathy in the dog. J.A.V.M.A. *166,* 1105, 1975.
30. Vendevelde, M., and Spano, J. S.: Cerebrospinal fluid cytology in canine neurological diseases. In press.
31. Verdura, J., White, R. J., and Albin, M.: Chronic measurements of cerebrospinal-fluid pressure in the dog; a new method and results. J. Neurosurg. *21,* 1047, 1964.
32. Verwer, M. A. J.: Weitere ergebnisse; liquoruntersuchungen bei gesunden und kranken hunden. Kleint-Praxis *10,* 33, 1965.
33. Wilkins, R. H., and Odom, G. L.: Cytological changes in cerebrospinal fluid associated with resections of intracranial neoplasms. J. Neurosurg. *25,* 24, 1966.
34. Wright, M. G., Cornwell, H. J. C., Thompson, H., and Lauder, I. M.: Canine distemper: current concepts in laboratory and clinical diagnosis. Vet. Rec. *94,* 86, 1974.
35. Yeary, R. A., Shannon, C. L., and Pregmone, J. R.: Cerebrospinal fluid electrolytes in the dog. Am. J. Vet. Res. *31,* 306, 1960.

CHAPTER 7

CANINE ELECTROENCEPHALOGRAPHY

R. W. REDDING, D.V.M., PH.D.

THE PRODUCTION OF THE ELECTROENCEPHALOGRAM

If electrodes are placed on the scalp of the dog over an area in which the cerebral hemispheres are near the surface, one can record, with appropriate amplifiers and writing instruments, oscillations of electrical potential which arise from the cerebral cortex. This activity consists of alternations in electrical potential from 3 microvolts to 300 microvolts recurring at frequencies of ½ to 40 hertz (Hz). A recording of such activity is called the electroencephalogram (EEG).

At the present time there are at least three tenable theories concerning the production of the EEG.[6, 18, 23, 25, 29, 36, 45] One theory visualizes each EEG wave as the algebraic sum of many individual spike discharges originating from cell bodies of cortical neurons and their processes, resulting in a vector which has magnitude, direction, and polarity. The recording instrument graphs this vector in the form of a wave, tracing time on the abscissa and voltage on the ordinate.

Another theory is based upon the results of research using microelectrodes in proximity to the body of a neuron or apical dendrite within the cerebral cortex. It has been found that a variable "standing" potential develops in the vicinity of the nerve cells. According to this theory, the EEG is the instantaneous summed effect of these potential changes on surface electrodes as they are recorded according to a standard procedure, and does not necessarily depend on spike elicitation or propagation.

A third theory proposes that the EEG is a summated composite of all the excitatory postsynaptic potentials (EPSP's) and inhibitory postsynaptic potentials (IPSP's) within the range of the recording electrodes.

These theories may serve to establish the relative site of origin of electrical components of the EEG. However, they do not explain the phasic activity seen or the rhythmicity observed. Two theories of regulation have been proposed. One theory is that the neurons of the cerebral cortex have an intrinsic basic rhythm that "fires off" spontaneously as a result of the individual cell or cells reaching threshold value. Preparations of cortical tissue in which the tissue has been isolated from all neuronal attachments but has retained its blood supply show rhythmical electrical activity.

The other theory visualizes the control of cortical cells by discharges from deeply located structures such as the thalamus. This is the pacemaker theory, for which there is considerable support. The following phenomena give support to the pacemaker theory. Implanted electrodes in the thalamus can be used to stimulate the surrounding thalamic tissue to discharge at a rate of approximately 6 hertz (Hz). If recordings are made from the surface of the cerebral cortex they are found to fall in phase with the thalamic tissue, and 6 Hz are recorded from the cortex. Stimulation of the reticular activating system in the sleeping animal causes an arousal pattern to replace the sleep pattern. On the other hand, destructive lesions of the brain stem result in EEG patterns of slow wave form suggestive of sleep. Rhythmicity then is believed to be the result of influences originating in both the subcortical structures such as the thalamus and the reticulator formation of the brain stem.

It would appear that the production of the EEG is based upon the sum of changing potential differences arising from the cortical cells, their synapses, and their processes, and that these structures are under the control of subcortical nuclei and reticular substance in the medulla which probably act as pacemakers according to the physiological state of the animal.

INSTRUMENTS AND RECORDING TECHNIQUE

THE ELECTROENCEPHALOGRAPH

The electroencephalograph is an electronic device that amplifies and graphically records potential alternations from the cerebral cortex. Many types of amplifier-recording systems are commercially available. It is beyond the scope of this text to discuss the various instruments in detail. All the devices consist of a lead system, preamplifiers, amplifiers, and a penwriting galvanometer, as shown in Figure 7–1. The amplifiers are so designed as to give an amplification of approximately one million times. This is necessary since the magnitude of the voltages from the surface of the scalp ranges from 3 to 300 microvolts. All the EEG machines available have incorporated a reference signal which can be used to standardize each channel of the machine simultaneously. The usual standardization signal is 50 to 100 microvolts. The amplifiers are adjusted so that the standardization signal causes a deflection on the vertical scale of the galvanometer of 5 to 10 mm. With this standardization, the range of voltage available from the surface of the scalp will be accurately recorded without distortion due to the limits of the galvanometer. Some animals with thick skulls and heavy musculature may require an EEG amplifier with increased sensitivity to reflect the actual cortical potentials.

ELECTRODES

An electroencephalogram obtained without harm to the patient is necessary for evaluation of the physiological status of the cerebral hemispheres in an animal suspected of having a cerebral disorder. Several types of electrodes that are available for use in man have been used on animals with varying degrees of success. None of them has been found to be completely satisfactory. Such electrodes are Reymond tripods, silver disk electrodes, and needle

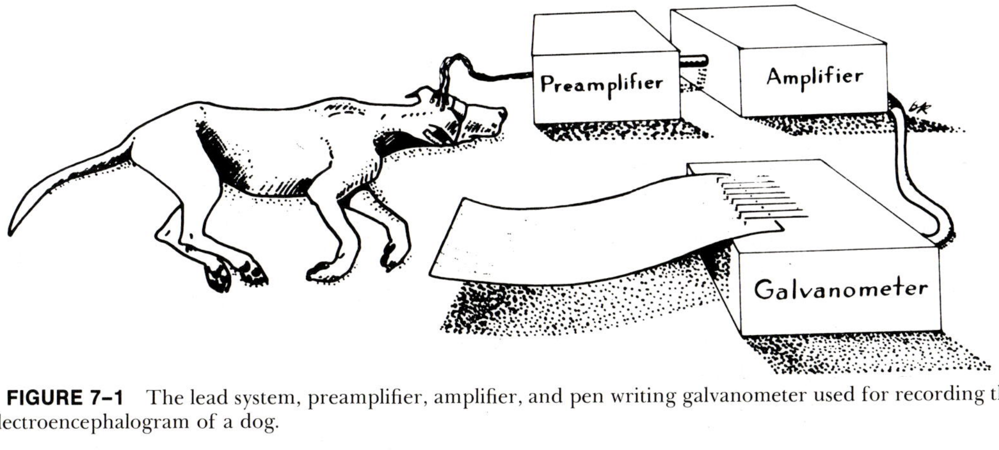

FIGURE 7–1 The lead system, preamplifier, amplifier, and pen writing galvanometer used for recording the electroencephalogram of a dog.

electrodes. The electrode must be attached easily, must be secure to the skin over the cranium, and must have a low stable resistance. None of the aforementioned types meets all these critieria when used on the dog. The electrode found to be most suitable is a small copper or cadmium-plated battery or alligator clamp that grasps a portion of the skin firmly and securely. It makes good electrical contact with the skin when used with electrode gel to assure the best conduction of the electrical impulses generated by the cerebral cortex.[52] Needle electrodes are more suitable in very small animals because of the close proximity of the electrodes on the scalp. The electrode resistance is usually high, 35,000–50,000 ohms. This high resistance may cause undesirable baseline fluctuations.

TECHNIQUE OF APPLYING ELECTRODES

It is not necessary to clip the hair from the head of the animal. To assure good electrical contact with clamp electrodes, the scalp is first defatted by being rubbed vigorously with acetone or alcohol. To prevent pain when the electrode clamps are applied to the skin over the scalp, it is necessary to infiltrate the skin and subcutaneous tissue at the point of application of the electrode with a long-acting local anesthetic solution such as 0.5 per cent lidocaine (this diluted concentration is sufficient for local anesthesia but will not produce toxic side reactions when absorbed). When infiltrating the subcutaneous tissue with the local anesthetic solution, it is convenient to infiltrate also the skeletal musculature of the head immediately under the point of application of the electrode, to eliminate the muscle potential artifact that might otherwise be recorded during electroencephalography.

After the skin and skeletal muscle have been anesthetized, the electrode gel is applied and rubbed into the area in which the electrodes are to be attached. It is necessary to make certain that the adjacent areas treated with electrode gel do not come in contact with each other, as this will cause a shorting of the circuit. The gel is applied, and the skin is grasped with the electrode and squeezed tightly. The resistance should be checked between the adjacent electrodes to assure good electrical contact. A resistance of 10,000 ohms or less is desirable for recording the EEG with clamp electrodes.

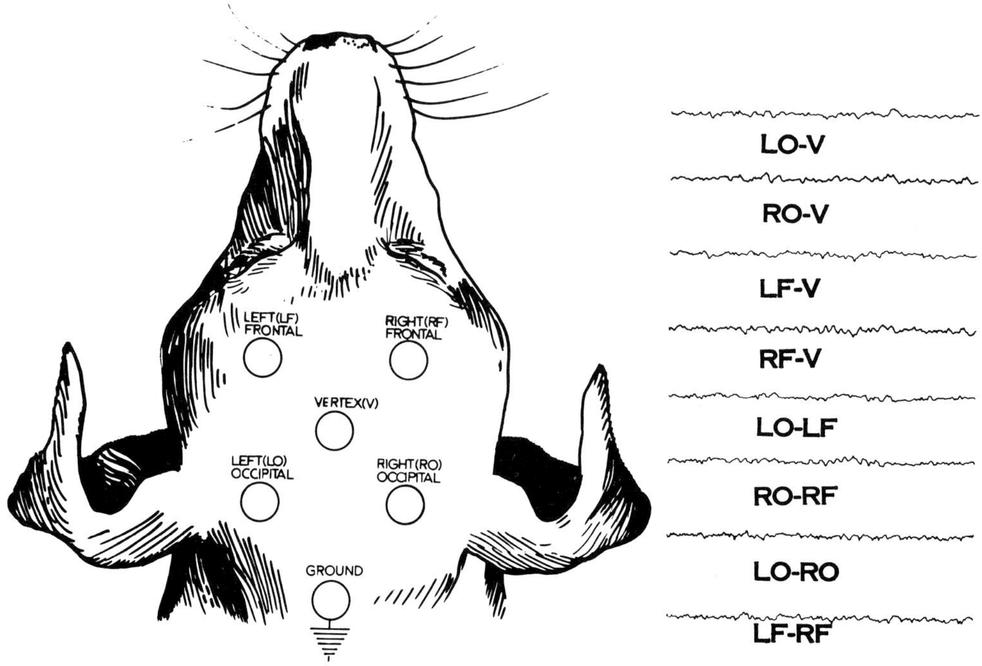

FIGURE 7–2 Points of electrode attachment for recording the electroencephalogram. Recordings obtained from a combination of the lead points are shown on the right.

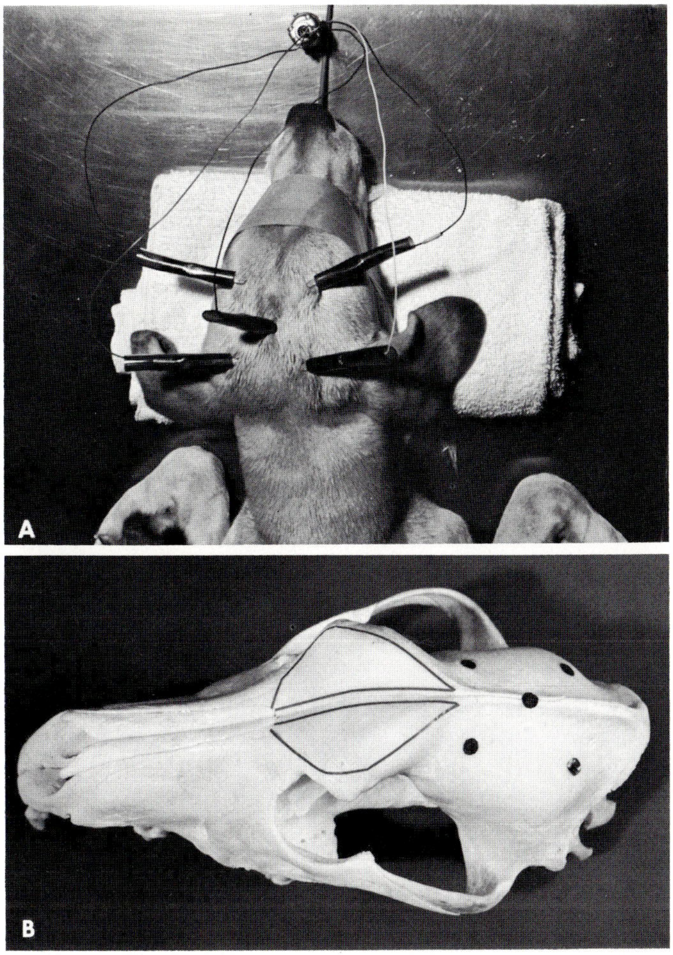

FIGURE 7–3 *A*. Clip electrodes attached to the scalp of the dog. The ground lead is not shown. *B*. The skull of a dog showing the points from which the recordings are made. The frontal sinus is outlined. Electrodes must be placed posterior to the sinuses to obtain a recording of the cortical potentials.

ELECTRODE PLACEMENT

There are various methods called "montages" for electrode placement on the scalp. Each montage has its own merits, and each individual electroencephalographer has his or her own frame of reference for detecting abnormalities. No one method is perfect, and the best aspects of each should be utilized in electroencephalography.

A suitable electrode arrangement for recording the EEG of the dog consists of two electrodes on the frontoparietal areas, two over the occipital areas, and one over the vertex. A ground electrode is also necessary. This may be attached to the skin over the external occipital protuberance (Figs. 7–2 and 7–3). With these five electrode recording points it is possible to record the following: the four areas of the cerebral hemispheres against the vertex lead as a common reference; transoccipital leads; transfrontal leads; left hemispheric leads, occipital to frontal; and right hemispheric leads, occipital to frontal. When an eight-channel EEG recording system is used, one can record simultaneously all these leads. Simultaneously recorded leads are of great clinical significance. To evaluate a cerebral abnormality properly, one must compare both hemispheres simultaneously. The localization of focal lesions is accomplished much more easily with the use of simultaneous recordings—in fact, it is considered essential.

RESTRAINT OF THE PATIENT

It is desirable to restrain the patient without the use of any chemical agent, since any such agent causes alteration of cortical activity. One type of restraint is a mechanical one. The pectoral limbs are bound together with tape, as are the pelvic limbs. The eyes are covered to prevent visual stimuli from affecting the cortical potentials (Fig. 7–4*A*). It is also desirable to decrease auditory perception by placing a large pledget of cotton in each external auditory canal, and it is essential to obtain the recording in an environment free of noise and at a temperature at which the animal neither shivers nor pants. With the aforementioned restraint, an assistant holds the animal in a lateral recumbent position or the animal may be secured to a table with a "seat belt" type strap. Most patients when so restrained struggle for only a short time, then relax so that a recording may be made. Some patients actually doze or sleep for a short period if the room is quiet and dark. This is very useful for the interpretation of the record, since abnormalities frequently are displayed when the animal is relaxed. Another form of physical restraint that may be used on small uncooperative animals is the restraint bag—a flexible plastic bag filled with tiny polyurethane balls. The restraint bag is molded around the animal, leaving the head exposed, and the air is exhausted using a vacuum, causing the bag to solidify and securely restrain the patient (Fig. 7–4*B*). A run of approximately 20 minutes usually is sufficient for most clinical cases. Figure 7–5 *A-C* shows a typical recording obtained from a normal adult dog when alert, relaxed, and in light sleep.

Other methods of restraint have been

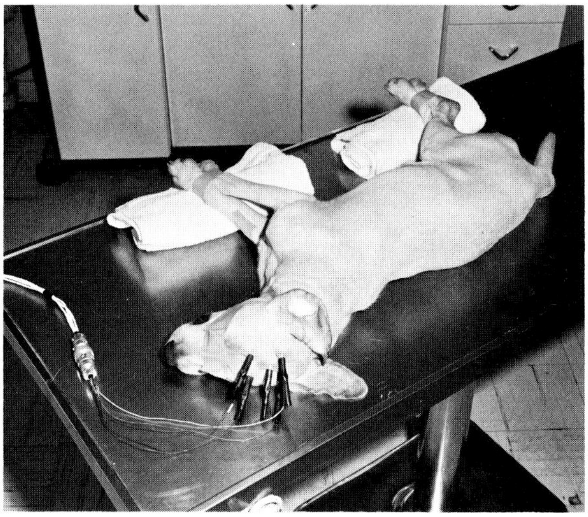

A

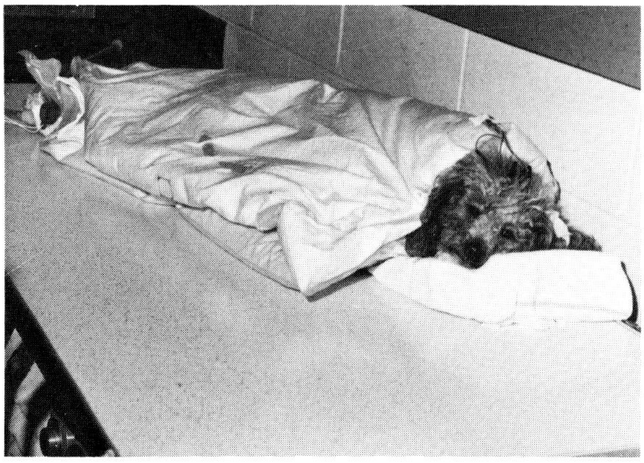

B

FIGURE 7–4 *A*. Restraint of dog for recording the electroencephalogram. *B*. Physical restraint using a restraint bag.

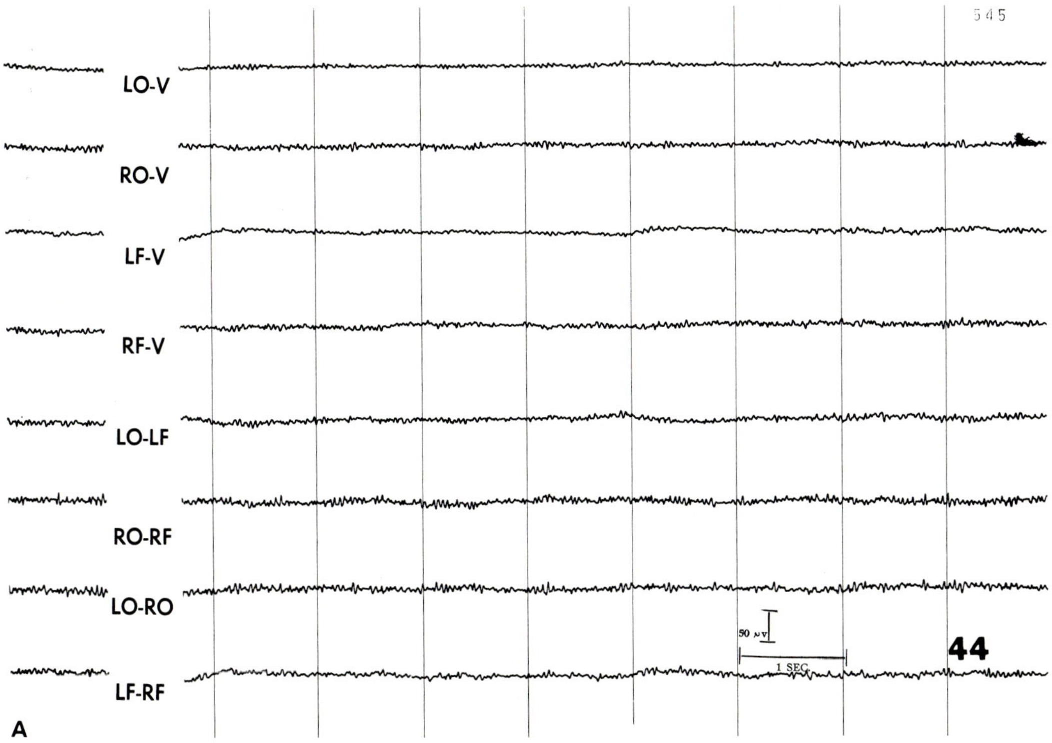

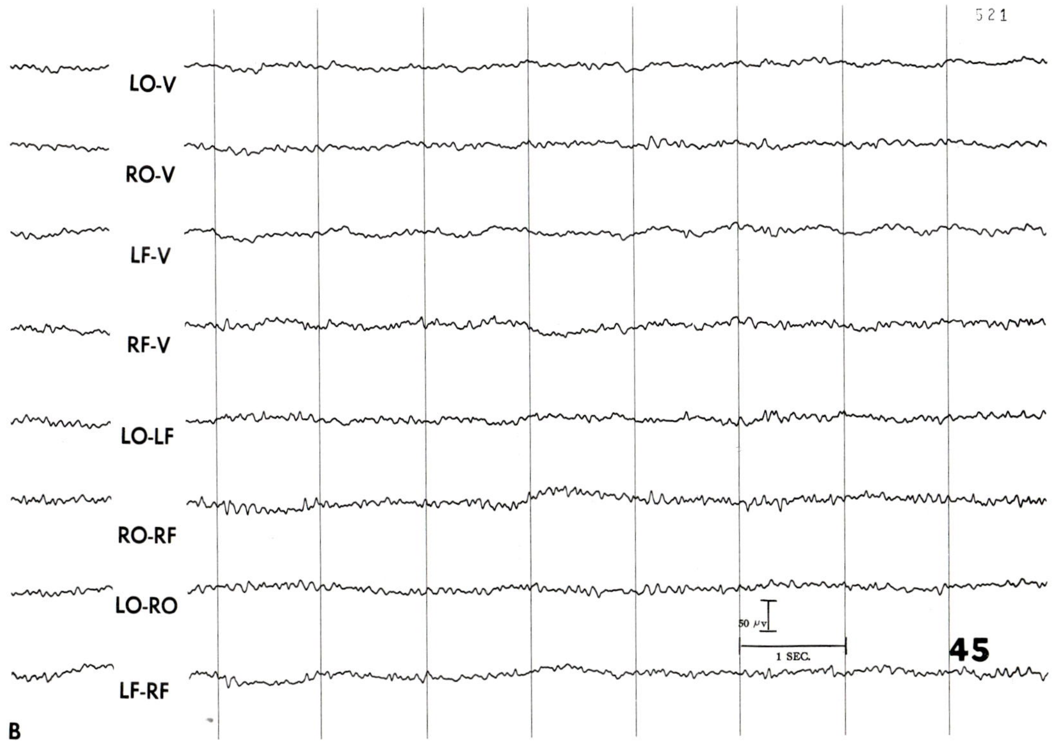

FIGURE 7–5 Normal adult animal. *A.* An alert animal, showing activity of 15–30 Hz, 3–10 microvolts. *B.* A relaxed animal, showing activity of 5–15 Hz, 10–25 microvolts.

Figure 7–5 continued on following page

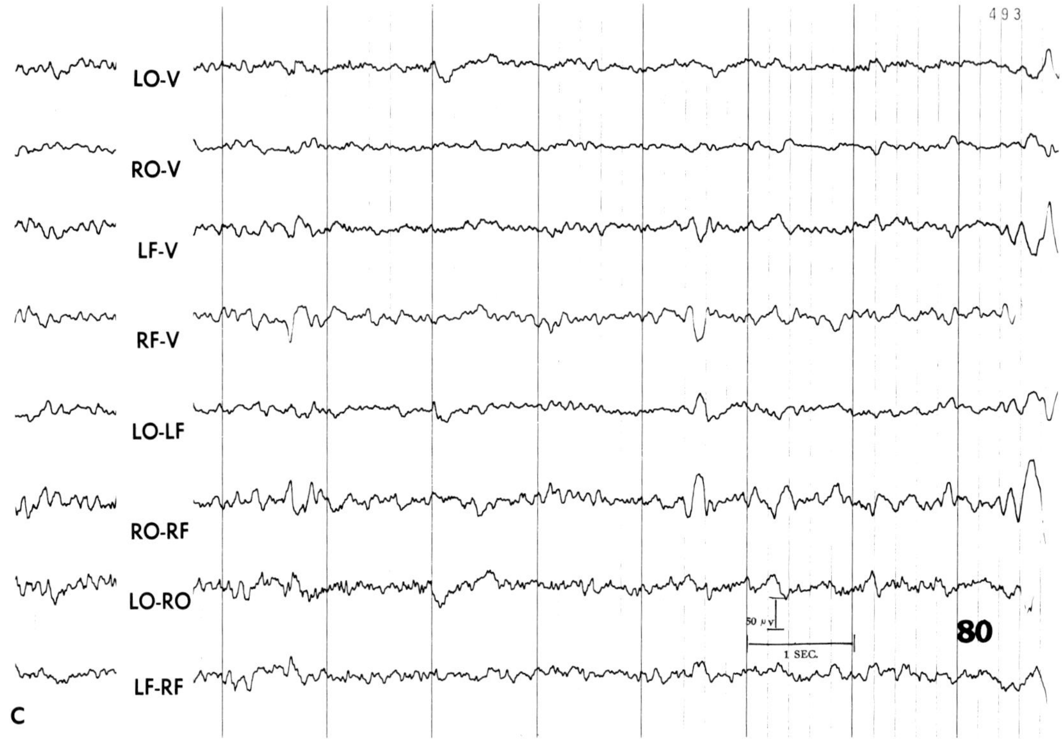

FIGURE 7–5 *Continued* *C*. An animal in light sleep, showing activity of 3–15 Hz, 10–80 microvolts.

proposed. Klemm[35, 36, 43] prefers to use barbiturate anesthesia. Herin et al.[28] utilizes gallamine triethiodide, a skeletal muscle paralyzing agent, and artificial respiration during the recording of the EEG.

Approximately 10 per cent of the animals resist mechanical restraint to the degree that a clinically useful EEG is not obtainable. The author has found that giving the dog ethchlorvynal (Placidyl) by mouth in a dose of 10 to 20 mg/lb (20–40 mg/kilo) body weight 45 minutes prior to attempting a recording will result in sufficient relaxation to obtain a diagnostic EEG. The animal tends to drift into a light sleep. However, arousal can be accomplished easily by an auditory or tactile stimulus, so that one can obtain both awake and light sleep recordings for interpretation.

THE BREED DIFFERENCE IN RECORDING

Some breeds of dogs, such as the boxer and hound, have heavy musculature over the portion of the scalp from which the EEG is to be recorded. In these animals, it is very difficult to obtain good recordings, especially of the occipital areas. Occasionally it is necessary to use insulated needle electrodes inserted through the temporalis muscle to the calvarium to obtain good recordings. Increasing the gain of the amplification system when using scalp electrodes may aid in obtaining a diagnostic EEG tracing. Some species of dogs have a rather large and extensive frontal sinus, which may extend over a portion of the frontal cortex and interfere with the recordings being made over the frontoparietal area. Care must be taken to assure proper placement of the electrode so that it does not overlie a frontal sinus. Figure 7–3*B* depicts the extent of the frontal sinus in some animals.

PHYSIOLOGICAL STATES AFFECTING THE ELECTROENCEPHALOGRAM

It should be appreciated that cortical electrical activity is influenced by physiological variables. The age of the patient must be known, along with the state of consciousness at the time the recording is made.[8, 21, 48]

AGE OF THE INDIVIDUAL

The stage of maturation of the cerebral cortex and other subcortical structures of the central nervous system influences the EEG pattern.[6, 8, 21, 24, 25, 36, 48, 59, 60, 66] In the very young animal, from birth to approximately 7 days, very little cortical activity is seen. Random bursts of 5 to 10 Hz activity with voltages of approximately 25 microvolts may be seen. There is no correlation between the two hemispheres in this burst of activity. When the animal is approximately 3 weeks of age, the pattern has developed to a medium voltage potential of low frequency. The medium voltage, low frequency pattern gradually matures during puppyhood and adolescence, progressing to an adult alert pattern of approximately 10 to 30 Hz with a voltage of approximately 5 to 15 microvolts. This pattern is acquired by about 22 to 30 weeks of age, depending upon sex and breed. The basis for this change to an adult pattern is not well understood, but it is probably due to increased arborization of a dendritic network and myelinization of the tracts within the central nervous system. The light sleep pattern of a mature animal is shown in Figure 7–5*C*. Figure 7–6 *A–C* shows the typical pattern at various age levels in both the alert and sleep states.

During the maturation process, the wave forms change considerably, and some of the normal frequencies and amplitudes seen are very similar to, if not indistinguishable from, those symptomatic of disease. It becomes very obvious that the age of the animal must be known in evaluating a tracing, so that a normal recording at a specific age will not be misinterpreted as a disease process.

THE LEVEL OF CONSCIOUSNESS

The EEG is markedly influenced by the level of consciousness.[21, 48, 52] Awareness produces a high frequency, low voltage pattern. A relaxed but not somnolent state

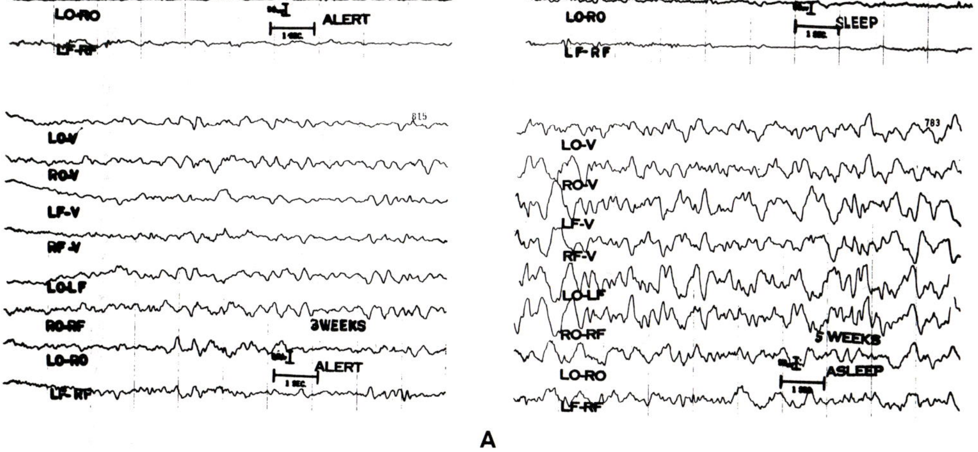

A

FIGURE 7–6 *A* and *B*. The maturation of the electroencephalogram of a puppy from the age of 1 week to 52 weeks. (*A*, 1 to 5 weeks; *B*, 13 to 17 weeks; and *C*, 22 to 52 weeks.) The "alert" electroencephalogram is shown on the left side of the illustration and the "somnolent" on the right.

Figure 7–6 continued on following page

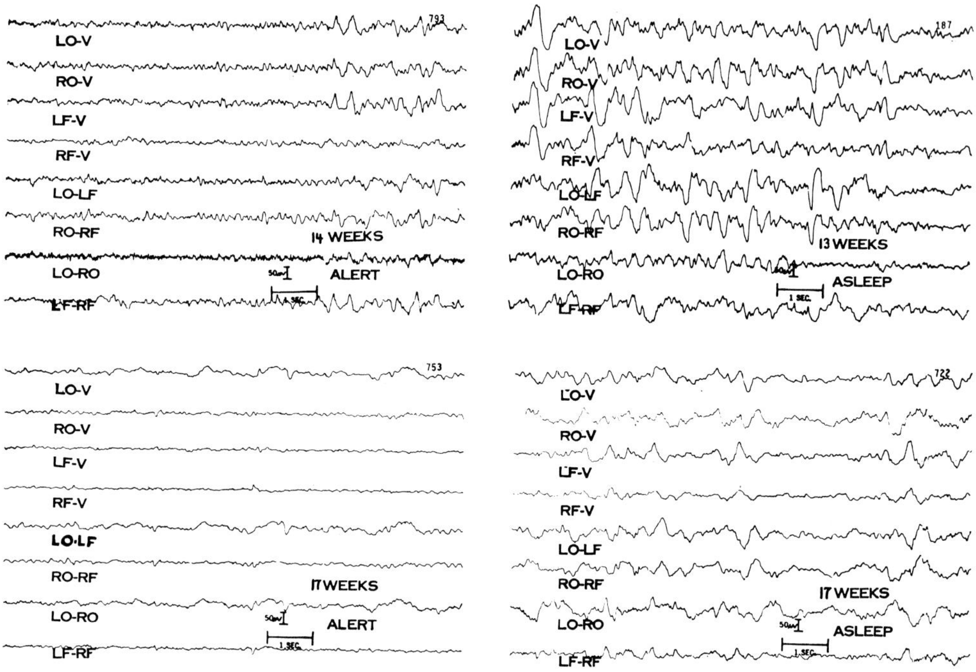

B

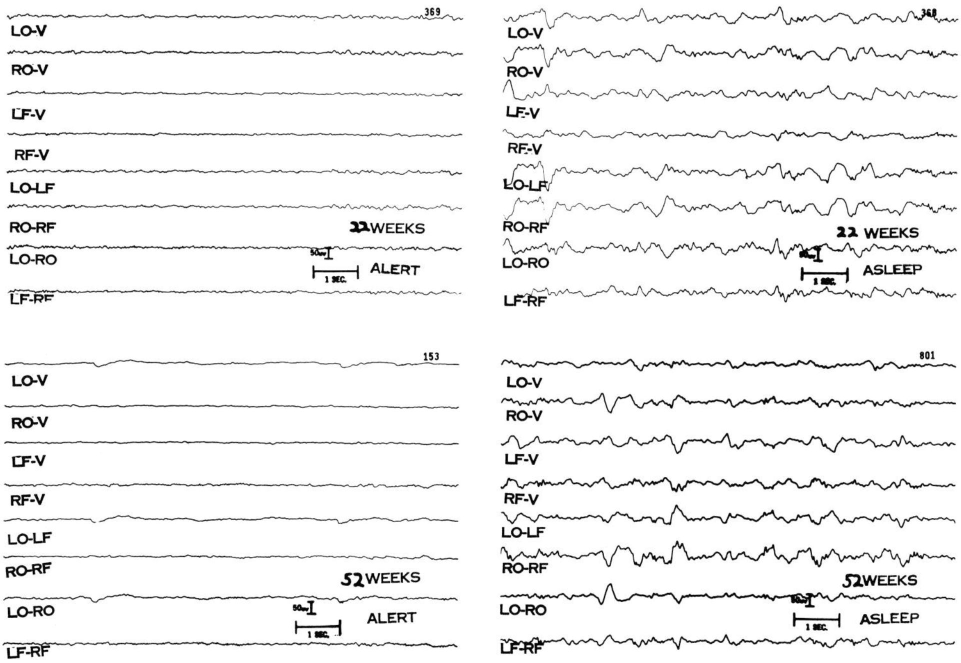

C

FIGURE 7–6 *Continued*

produces a higher voltage, lower frequency pattern. Drowsiness is characterized by an even slower frequency and higher voltage; light sleep—a continuation of drowsiness—by frequencies of 4 to 6 Hz and voltages of 75 to 100 microvolts. Deep sleep is characterized by very high voltage, 150 to 200 microvolts, and slow frequency discharge, 1 to 3 Hz. Deep sleep patterns are seldom recorded under clinical examination conditions.

ARTIFACTS

Electroencephalographic tracings of the patient may contain artifacts[34] that may, if improperly interpreted, lead to an erroneous diagnosis of a disease that the animal does not have. *Muscle potentials,* especially over the occipital areas, are frequently encountered (Fig. 7–7). These muscle potentials may be mistaken for high-voltage spikes thought to originate in the occipital cortex. Occasionally, electrodes placed over the frontal sinuses show no activity or very little activity (Fig. 7–7). This should not be mistaken for a disease state in which very low voltages are encountered.

Ear movements cause a shift in the baseline of the recording made adjacent to that ear (Fig. 7–7). Eye blinks and the eyeball movements are frequently seen in the frontal recordings. They may be unilateral or bilateral (Fig. 7–7).

Licking, chewing, and swallowing movements cause a characteristic overall baseline shift (Fig. 7–7).

Many dogs of the toy breeds shiver periodically and produce characteristic oscillations of the base (Fig. 7–7).

Electrodes have poor contact with the skin or those having poor electrical contacts in the wiring show rapid shifts in the baseline or spike-like discharges. These should not be mistaken for spiking activity originating in the cerebral cortex (Fig. 7–7). Canine choreiform movements may cause the entire body or a portion of the body to shift slightly during each spasm. This spasm will cause a baseline shift in the recording.

A very common artifact that may simulate slow wave activity is that produced by *panting,* which is readily recognized by si-

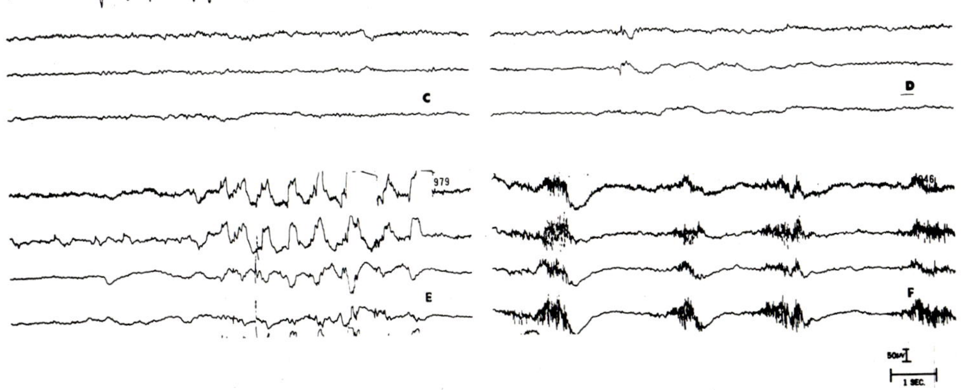

FIGURE 7–7 Artifacts seen in electroencephalogram of the dog. *A.* Skeletal muscle potentials. *B.* Electrode indicated by arrow placed at edge of frontal sinus. Note reduced voltage compared to lower tracing of opposite side. *C.* Upper tracing indicates movement of the left ear. *D.* Eyelid blinks followed by eyeball movement. *E.* Licking, chewing, and swallowing movements. *F.* Shivering with muscle potentials in bursts.

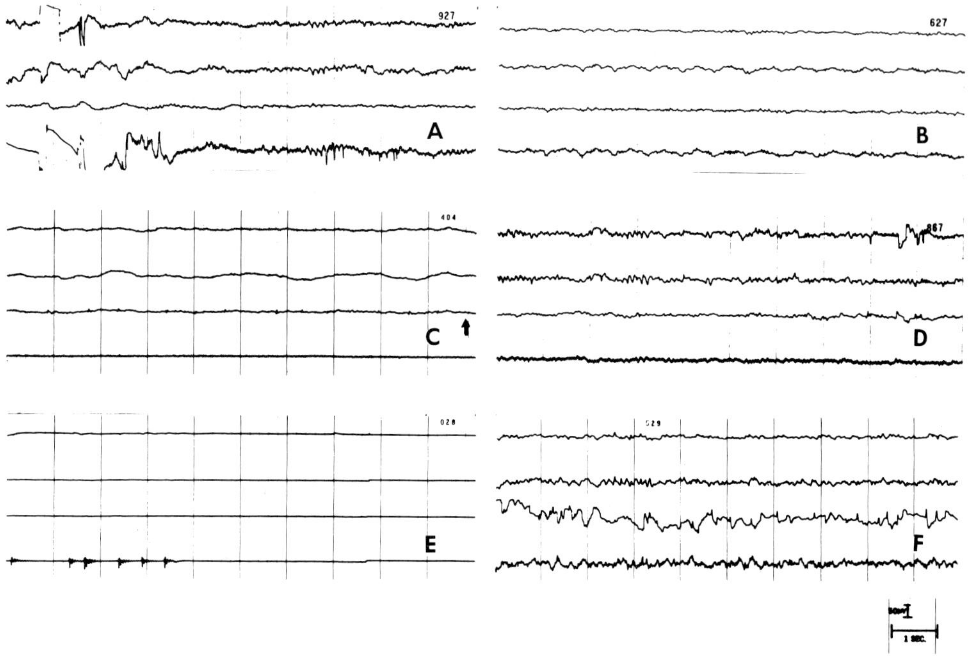

FIGURE 7–8 Artifacts seen in EEG recording of the dog. *A*. Loose electrode wire causing spike-like activity. *B*. Panting: note the rhythmic one cycle per second waves in the second and fourth tracings. *C*. Electrocardiogram in tracing indicated by arrow. *D*. Alternating current interference can be seen in the lower tracing. *E*. Microphonic tube in amplifier. *F*. Noise in one amplifier due to defective connection. Third tracing.

multaneous observation of the animal and the recording (Fig. 7–8).

The electrocardiogram (ECG) may be seen as a rhythmic spike-like activity in the tracing and should not be mistaken for spikes that originate in the cerebral cortex. The appearance of this artifact may be due to the reference electrode being applied to the ear, or the animal may have a *wet haircoat.* The identification of this artifact can be confirmed by simultaneously recording the ECG on one channel of the EEG machine.

Interference due to alternating current is occasionally encountered, and the use of a shielded room or a cage may be necessary to eliminate it completely. Modern EEG machines adequately reject 60 Hz interference. The typical pattern of alternating current interference is shown in Figure 7–8.

Noise originating within the channels or wiring of the EEG may in itself present difficulties. Such noise may be that of a microphonic tube in the amplifier or a poor wiring connection within the circuit itself (Fig. 7–8).

THE NORMAL ELECTROENCEPHALOGRAM

The definition of normality is difficult to state, since it depends upon the method of restraint used to make the recording (chemical or physical restraint). Each method of restraint influences the type of recording obtained. In addition, the frequency and amplitude vary from one animal to another and from one breed to another. For example, thin-skulled animals (such as the Chihuahua) show relatively higher voltages and slower frequencies than do heavy-skulled, heavy-muscled animals (such as the boxer).

The interpreter of the EEG must have a clear mental picture of what is considered normal before he can interpret the tracing with any degree of accuracy. The tracings included in this section are to be compared with Figure 7–5 *A–C*, which shows normal EEGs obtained without chemical restraint. Electroencephalograms are reported in frequency amplitude, with the frequency on the abscissa and the amplitude on the ordinate of the graph. An adult alert pattern is approximately 8 to 38 Hz, with voltages from 3 to 15 microvolts.

Once the patterns seen in an electroencephalographic tracing have been learned, visual analysis of the electroencephalogram becomes a relatively simple task of recognition—very much like learning to read a new language with an unfamiliar alphabet and a different kind of script. To gain proficiency in interpreting electroencephalograms, practice is necessary. The sample tracings in this chapter will provide the reader with some concept of normality and abnormalities.

THE ELECTROENCEPHALOGRAM IN DISEASE

The EEG may be used in clinical medicine as one more diagnostic aid in evaluating the patient's neurological status.[9-12, 16, 20, 22, 34, 36, 51, 53, 54, 57, 62] In diseases of the cerebral hemispheres and in generalized metabolic disturbances, the EEG pattern is altered. The interpreter of an EEG must have a clear mental picture of the normal pattern variations that will serve as a reference for comparison with EEGs from animals with suspected brain disease. The patient's age and state of awareness must be taken into consideration when one evaluates such records. In general the abnormal record shows excessively slow or excessively fast activity for the physiologic state under which the recording was made. The records may demonstrate focal abnormalities of various types such as spiked discharges, paroxysmal bursts of either slow or fast activity, or generalized slowing with the greatest slowing over specific areas.

Some general conclusions concerning abnormalities can be stated. The most fundamental conclusion is that disease causes changes in either amplitude or frequency and occasionally in both. Of the two changes, amplitude changes are the most dramatic indicator of disease. Frequency changes, on the other hand, are relatively more reliable. The following is a list of conclusions formulated by Klemm and Hall[42] as they relate to animal electroencephalography:

1. Low voltage–fast activity (LVFA) and spikes indicate an ongoing irritative process due to a variety of causes.
2. High voltage–slow waves (HVSA); if persistent, indicate death of many neurons due to a variety of causes.
3. LVFA and HVSA are not pathognomonic of any given disease but are suggestive of several diseases.
4. Local EEG abnormalities indicate a cortical rather than a subcortical lesion.
5. Common causes of local cortical lesions are vascular (infarct), hemorrhage, an early tumor, or focal necrosis.
6. Generalized EEG abnormalities can indicate that a lesion is either (1) generalized in the cortex or (2) focal subcortically.
7. Common causes of generalized lesions are (1) infections, (2) trauma, (3) space-occupying lesions (tumor, hydrocephalus), or (4) idiopathic epilepsy.
8. Cerebral recordings during illness can indicate the effectiveness of therapy in the progress of the disease process.

Low voltage–fast activity and high voltage–slow activity are not necessarily characteristic of specific diseases. However, abnormal brainwave activity is useful in indicating what kind of disease process is involved and whether the process is acute or chronic, improving or regressing. Acute inflammatory diseases such as canine distemper encephalitis cause low voltage–fast activity and spikes in the initial stages. As the disease progresses, the pattern converts from low voltage–fast to high voltage–slow, upon which there may be superimposed fast activity. On the other hand, high voltage–slow wave activity is produced by various degenerative diseases such as trauma, vascular disorders, and hydrocephalus. Tumors generally show abnormally slow waves with occasional spikes in the area upon which the tumor is encroaching. If the tumor is deeply located, it will cause generalized slow wave activity and occasionally some superimposed spikes.

The electroencephalographic abnormalities just described can occur throughout any area of the cerebral cortex, or they may be localized at a few points and detectable by proper electrode placement. If the abnormality is localized, the lesion is also localized and most probably in the cerebral cortex. Most EEG recordings are obtained from the cortical tissue, and lesions in one area of the cortex will cause local EEG abnormalities. If the abnormality is below the cortex, the EEG abnormality will most likely appear in several areas of the cortex because the subcortical brain tissue sends projecting fiber tracts to scattered areas on the cerebral cortex.

Knowledge of the focal or diffused nature of EEG abnormalities suggests certain conclusions about potential causes of neuropathies. Focal brain damage can be caused by vascular disorders, such as small infarcts or hemorrhages, an early tumor, or a focal necrosis of hematogenous origin. In dogs and cats, focal brain damage appears to be relatively rare except in cases of trauma. Diffuse brain damage, however, is often seen in the dog and cat and is usually caused by viral, protozoan, fungal, or bacterial infections and by space-occupying lesions located deep within the diencephalon. To follow the course of any encephalopathy, it is important to make serial recordings of the EEG, since such recordings can indicate whether the disease is progressing, resolving, or remaining unchanged. In addition, the effectiveness of therapy is easily evaluated by serial recordings.

THE ENCEPHALOPATHIES

Distemper Encephalitis

Perhaps one of the most useful tools in the diagnosis of encephalitis[9, 10, 20, 22, 43, 53, 54, 57, 62] is the electroencephalogram. What appears to be encephalitis on clinical observation may be proved beyond doubt when the EEG is obtained from the animal. Early encephalitis is characterized by a 3 to 5 cycle pattern upon which is superimposed a 20 to 30 cycle spike discharge (Fig. 7–9 *A-C*). An acute case of encephalitis is characterized by very slow 2 to 3 Hz activity with voltages of approximately 100 to 200 microvolts (Fig. 7–9 *D-G*). Late encephalitis is characterized by 4 to 7 Hz with voltages of 10 to 15 microvolts (Fig. 7–9 *H, I*). The pattern is relatively consistent, and can be altered for only a few seconds[57] by either auditory or visual stimulation, after which it returns to the characteristic pattern for that stage of the disease. Since the slowing takes on a character somewhat similar to that of sleep, one must be certain of the state of awareness when interpreting the record.

Text continued on page 171

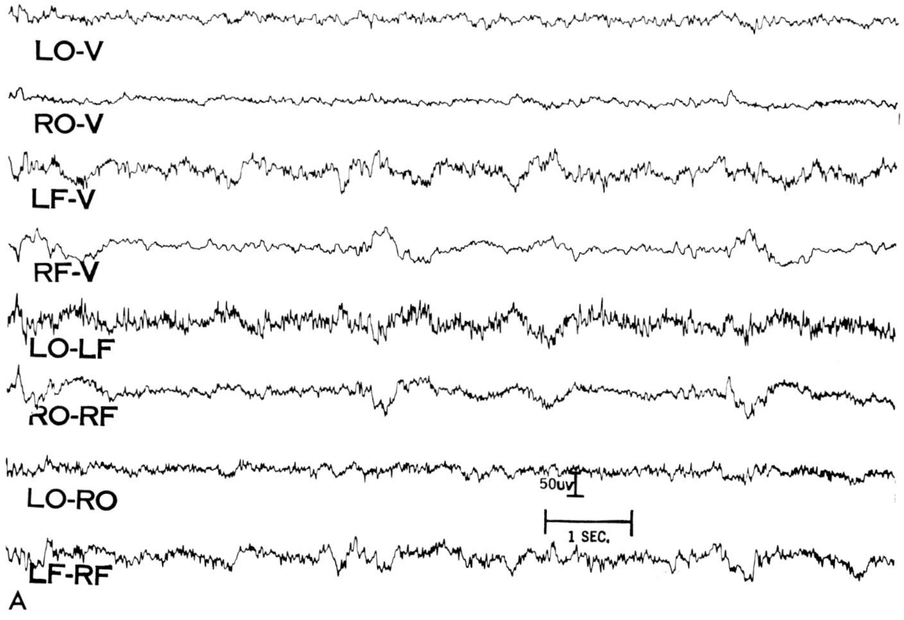

FIGURE 7–9 *A*, *B*, and *C*. Characteristic pattern seen in early encephalitis. *A* and *B* show the 20–30 Hz spike discharge pattern. *C* is in the transition stage toward the acute phase of disease.

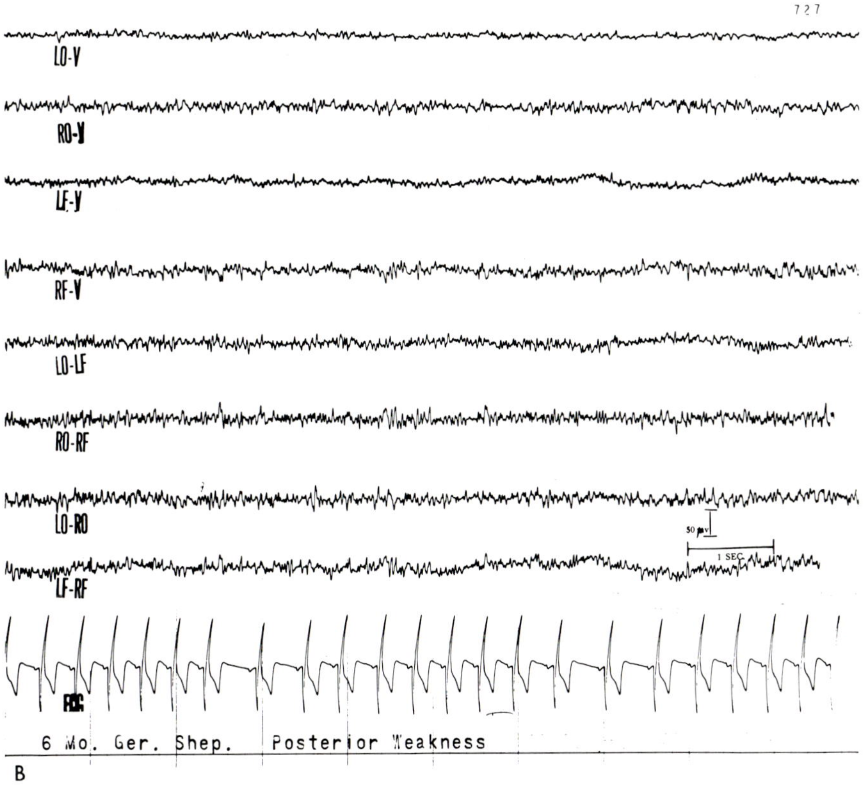

B

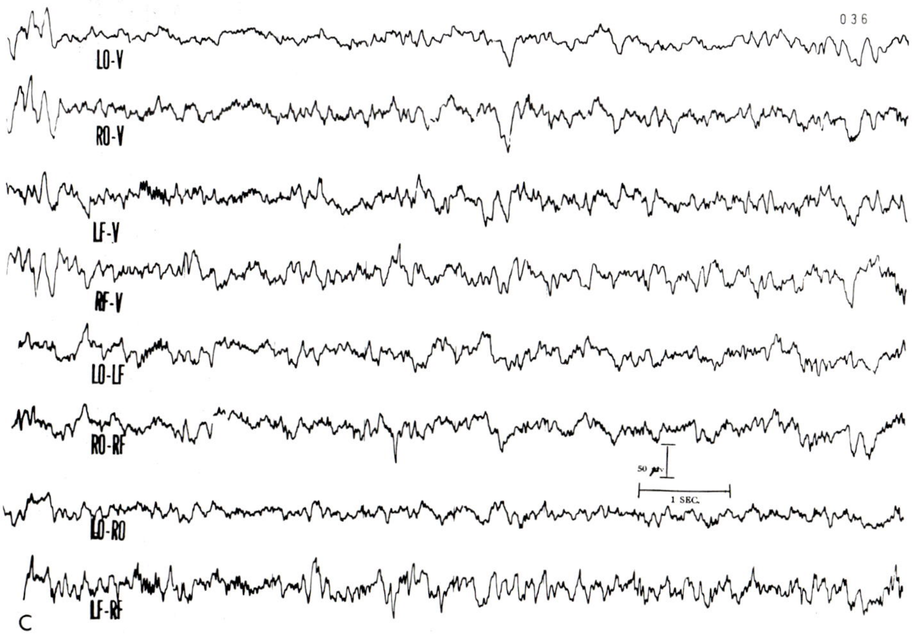

C

FIGURE 7–9 *Continued See legend on opposite page*

Figure 7–9 continued on following page

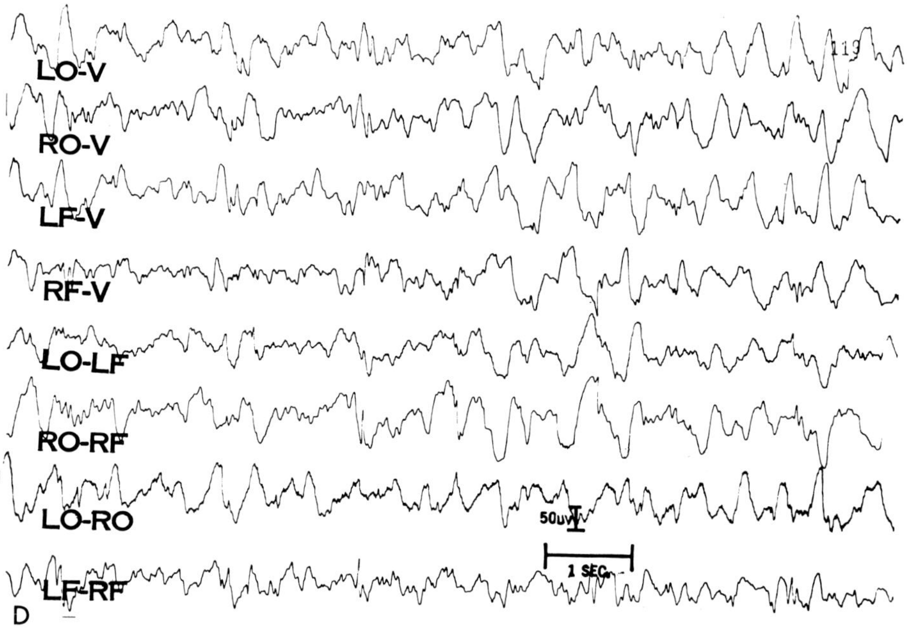

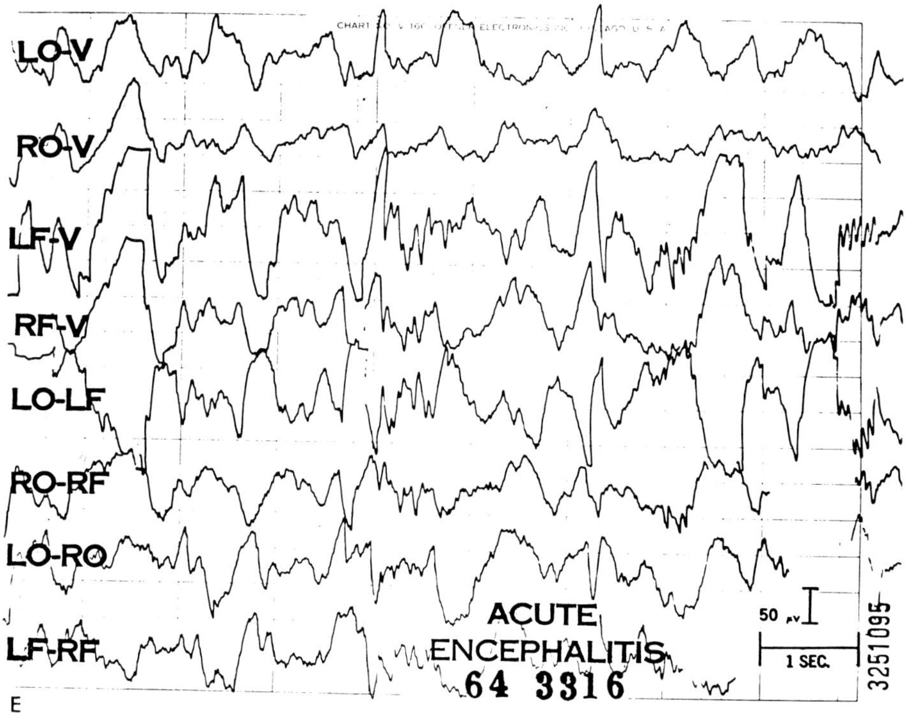

FIGURE 7–9 *Continued D–G.* Characteristic pattern seen in the acute stage of encephalitis. Clinical signs of cerebral involvement are evident at this time. Note the extremely high voltage synchronous slow wave activity in *D, E,* and *F. G* is a recording of a "larval" seizure. No motor manifestation was observed at the time of the recording.

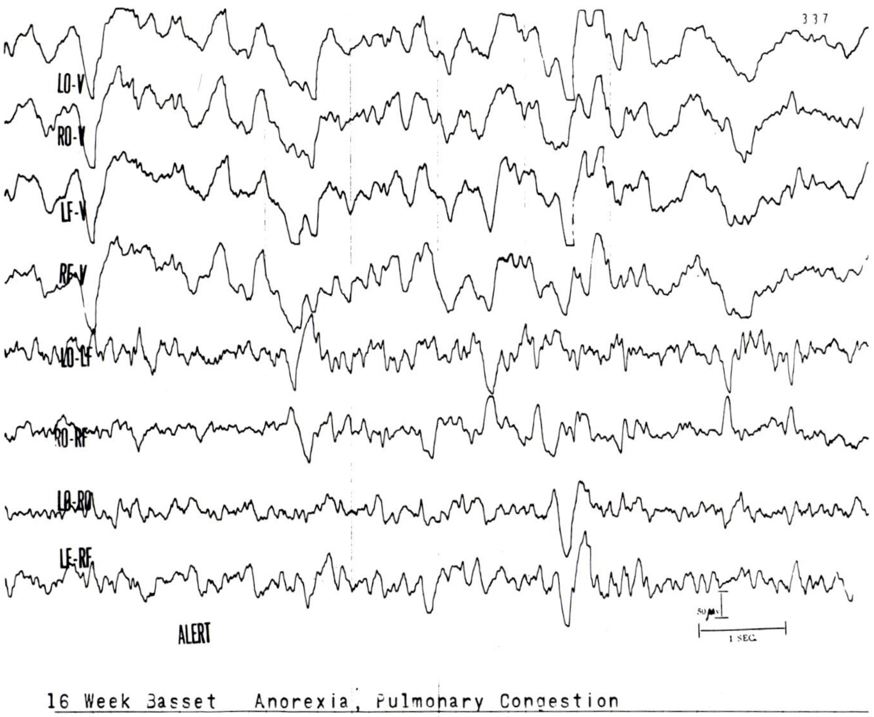

F

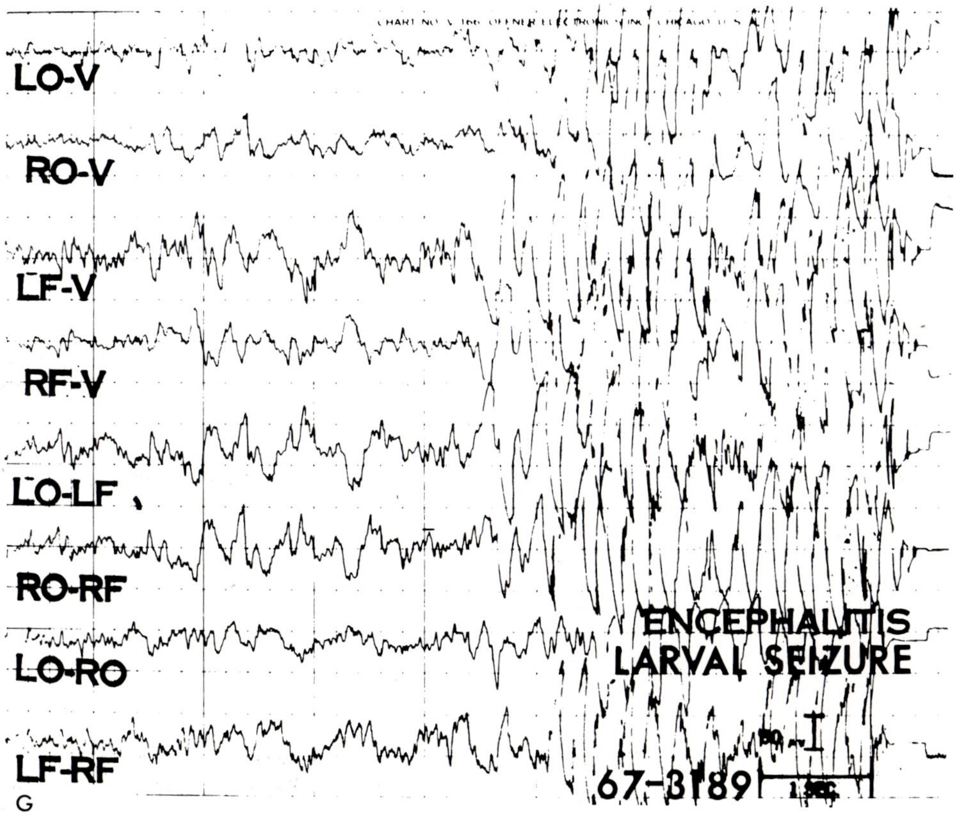

G

FIGURE 7–9 *Continued*

Figure 7–9 continued on following page

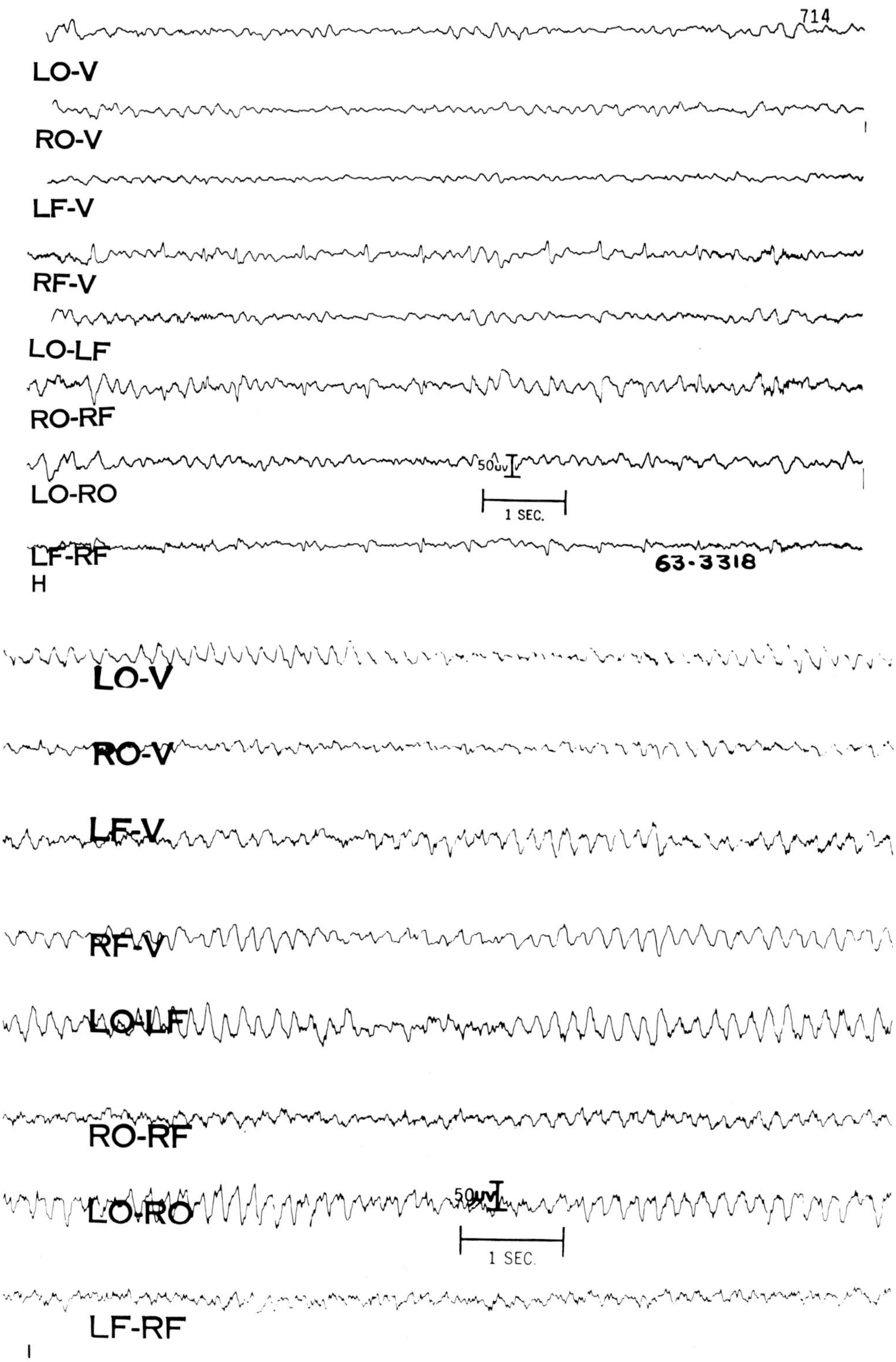

FIGURE 7–9 *Continued* *H* and *I*. Characteristic pattern seen during the recovery stage of encephalitis (late encephalitis). Persistent activity of 4–6 Hz 50–100 microvolts is dominant during this stage of the disease.

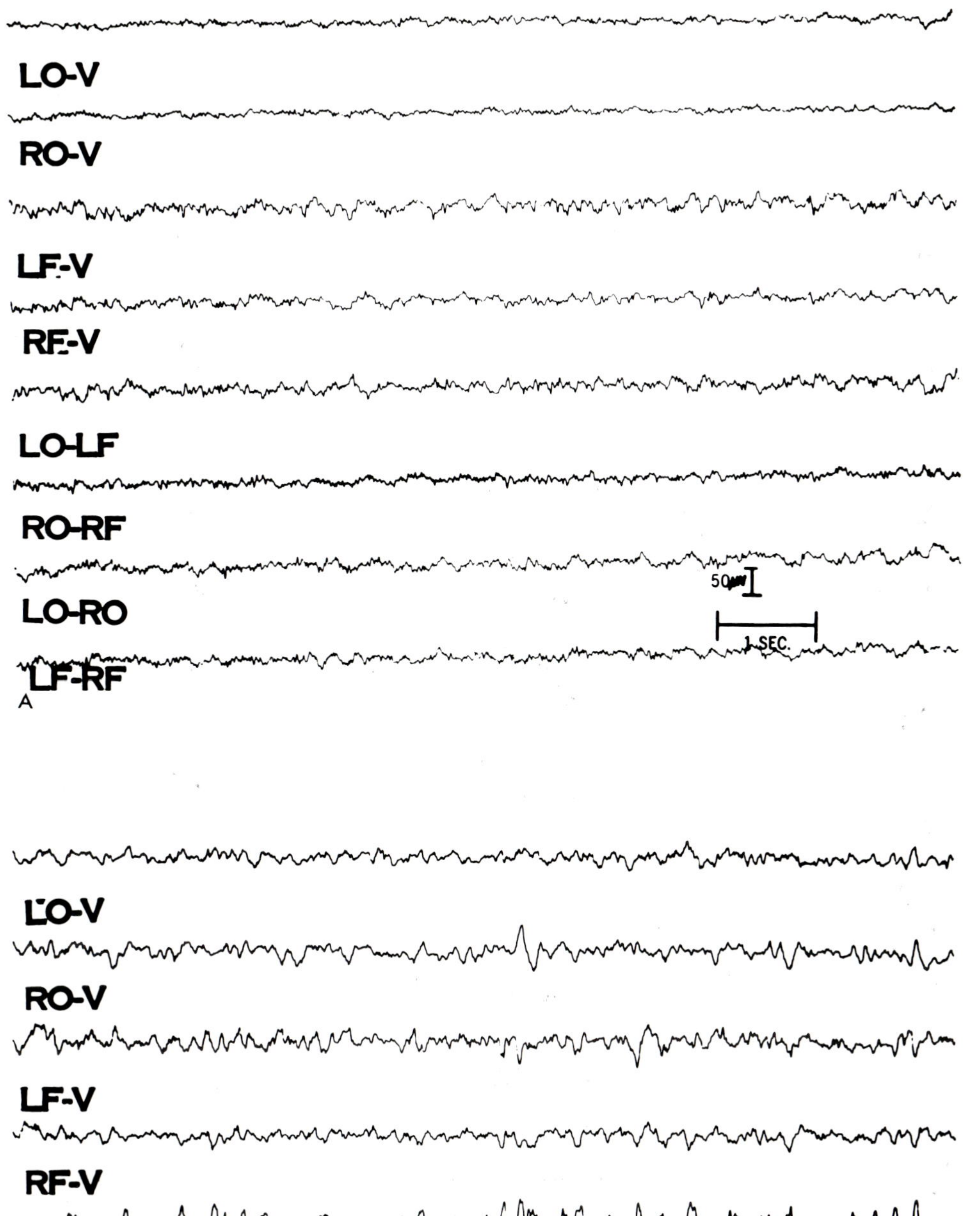

FIGURE 7–10 *A–H.* A series of recordings obtained from a patient during the course of distemper encephalitis. *A.* Animal presented for examination because of anorexia and depression; early encephalitis. *B.* Five days after first EEG recording—transition from early to acute stage.

Figure 7–10 continued on following page

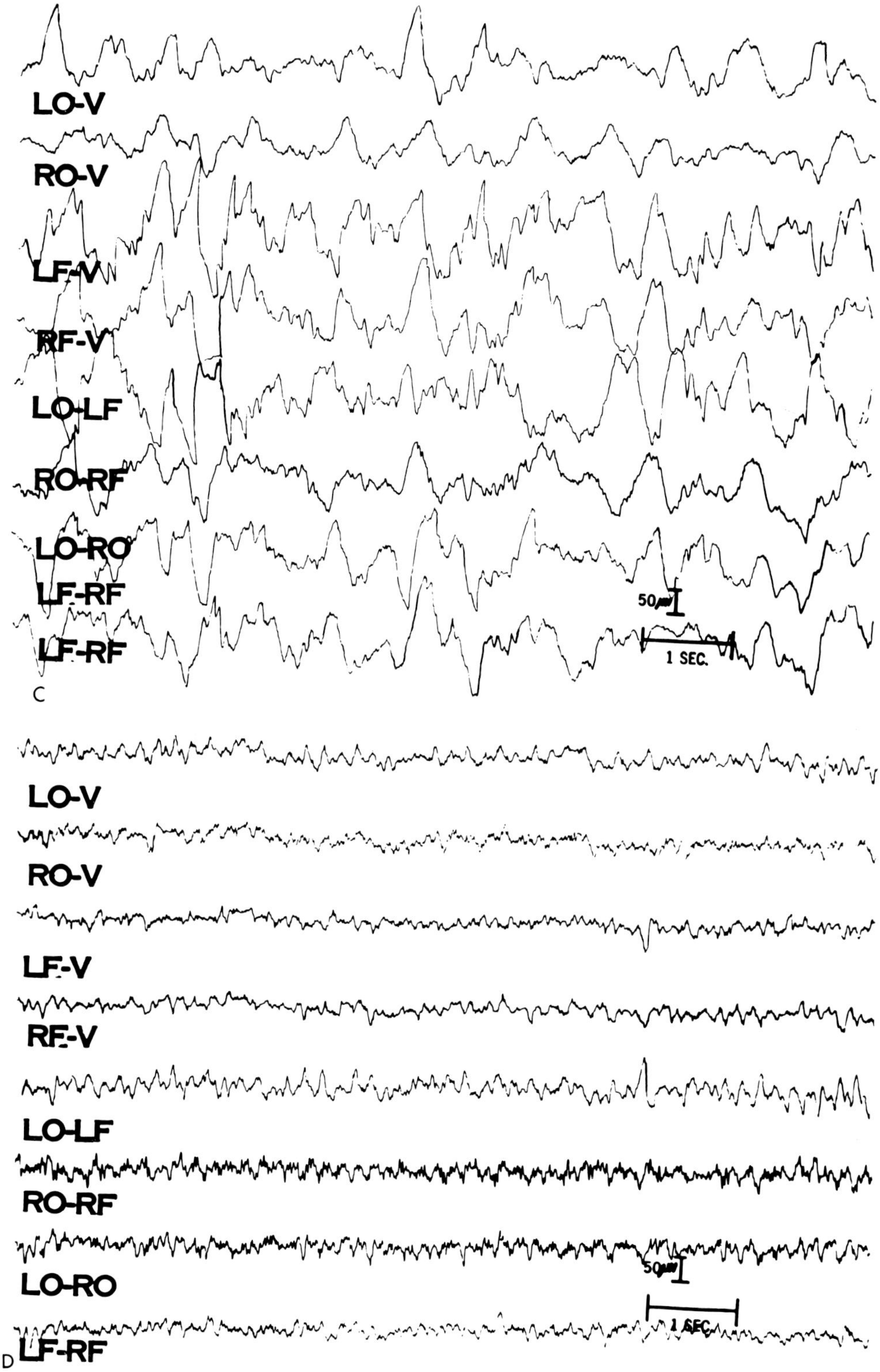

FIGURE 7–10 *Continued* *C*. Seven days after first EEG examination—acute stage of encephalitis. Two weeks after *C*, clinical recovery was complete. *D*. Two weeks after clinical recovery—beginning of late encephalitis pattern.

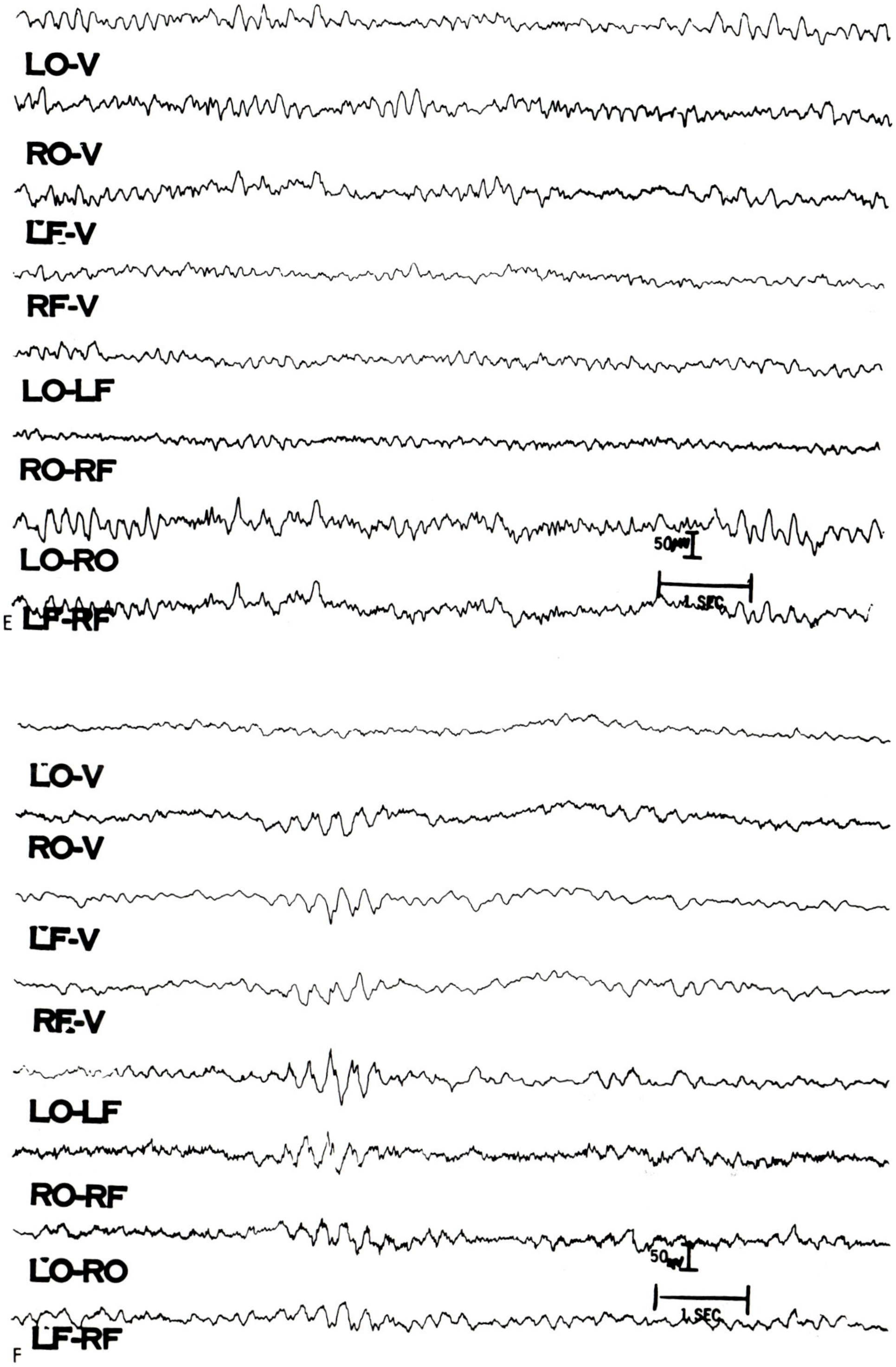

FIGURE 7–10 *Continued* *E.* Two months after clinical recovery. *F.* Four months after clinical recovery—genesis of the burst of 4 Hz activity unknown.

Figure 7–10 continued on following page.

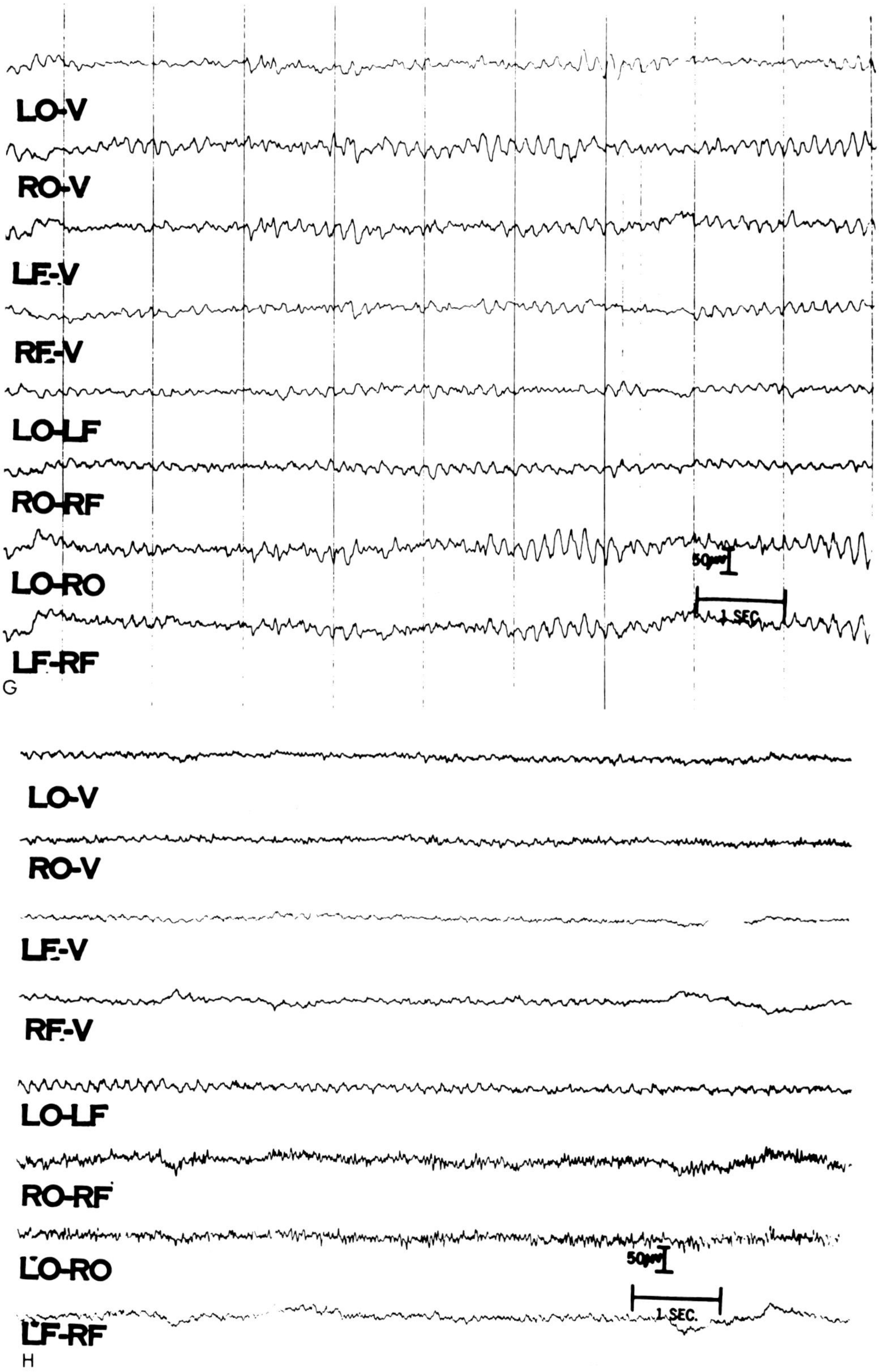

FIGURE 7–10 *Continued* *G.* Five months after clinical recovery. *H.* Six months after clinical recovery with some residual 6 Hz low voltage activity present. Some muscle artifact seen in occipital areas.

However, with experience there is little difficulty in differentiating the two.

Residual slow wave activity of the EEG is present in postencephalitic patients for as long as one year after clinical recovery. The clinical signs of recovery can be correlated with lessening of slow wave activity and the return to normal frequencies. Persistent abnormal slow wave activity is frequently associated with seizures; therefore its presence can be helpful in the differential diagnosis of seizures. Figure 7–10 *A-H* shows sequential recordings from a case of distemper encephalitis, from the early stages of the disease to complete clinical recovery. Residual slow wave activity was still present 6 months after recovery. Occasional seizures were seen in this case and were controlled with anticonvulsant drugs.

Chronic Encephalitis

Occasionally a confirmed case of encephalitis fails to show the progression of changes just described under distemper encephalitis. This is more commonly seen in older dogs and has been termed "old dog encephalitis." Repeated sequential EEG tracings show an almost consistent medium voltage–slow wave activity (Fig. 7–11). The pattern does not change over months of time. The dog frequently has seizures which are difficult to control with medication. In addition, the animal may show generalized depression. Distemper inclusion bodies may be found in these cases.

Other Encephalopathies

There are many histopathological classifications of other confirmed cases of encephalopathies. They include: panencephalitis (Fig. 7–12 *A*), meningoencephalitis (Fig. 7–12 *B*), poliomeningoencephalomyelitis (Fig. 7-12 *C*), encephalomalacia (Fig. 7–12 *D*), meningoencephalomyelitis (Fig. 7–12 *E*), polioencephalitis (Fig. 7–12 *F*), and encephalomyelitis (Fig. 7–12 *G*). There are no specific patterns for any one of these. They all show abnormal slow wave activity with

Text continued on page 175

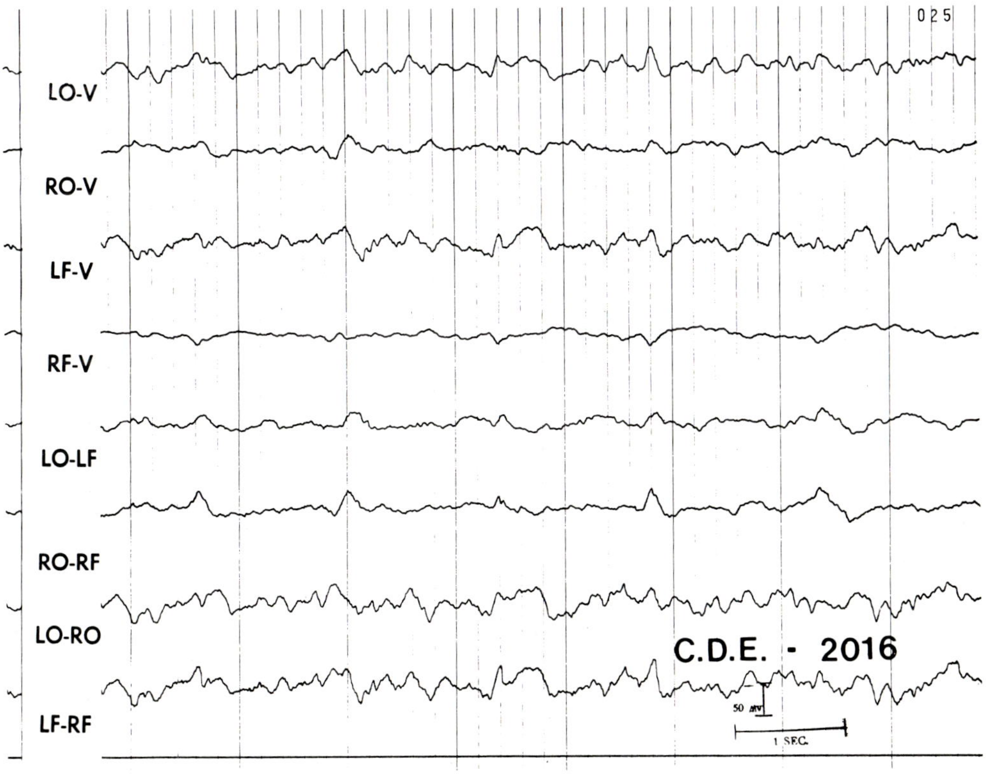

FIGURE 7–11 Tracing obtained from an 8½-year-old male poodle that suffered from depression and frequent seizures.

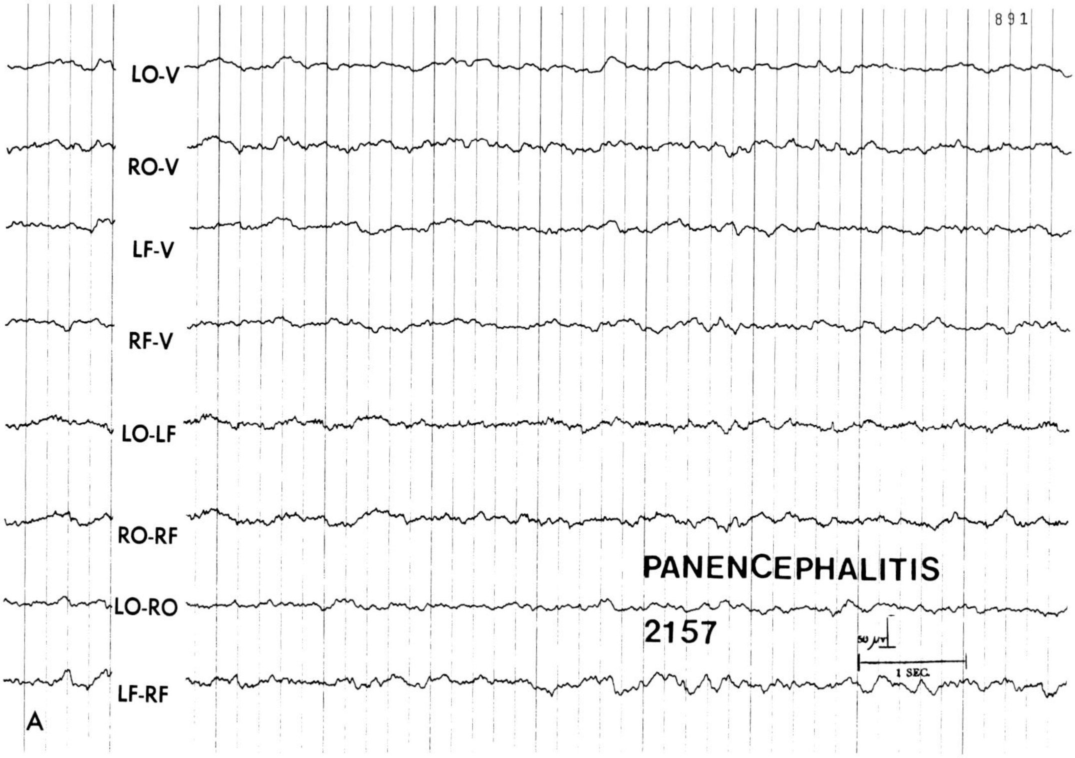

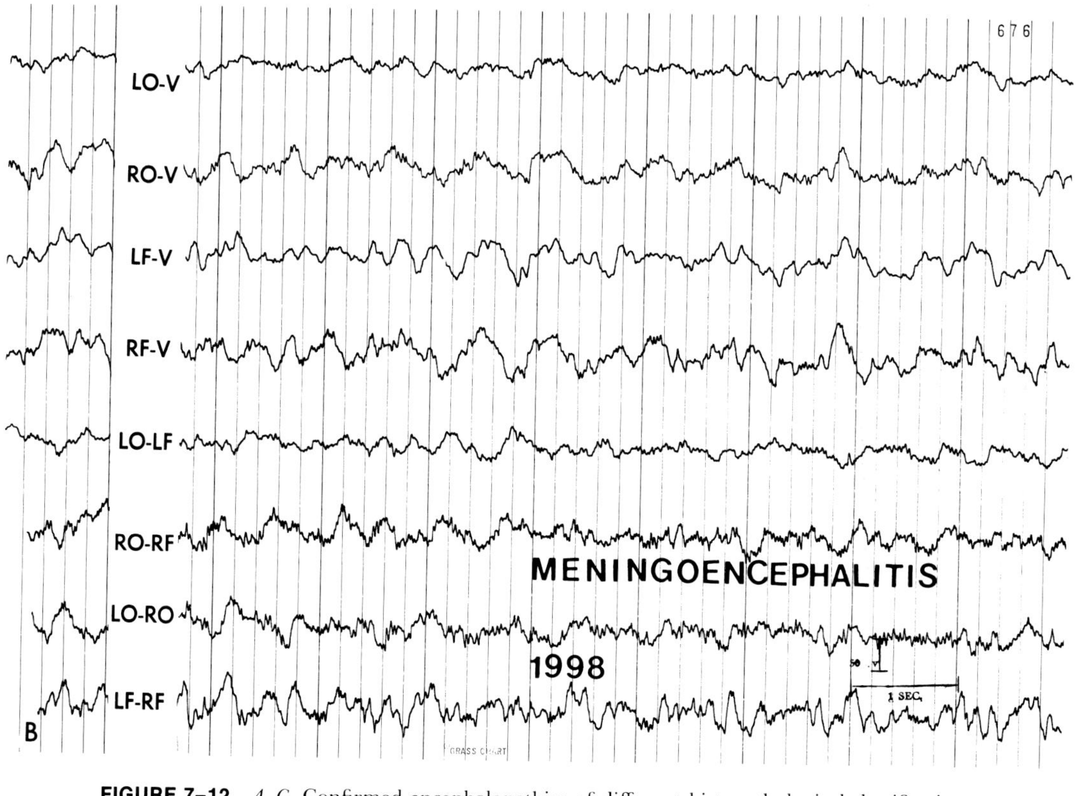

FIGURE 7–12 *A–G.* Confirmed encephalopathies of different histopathological classifications.

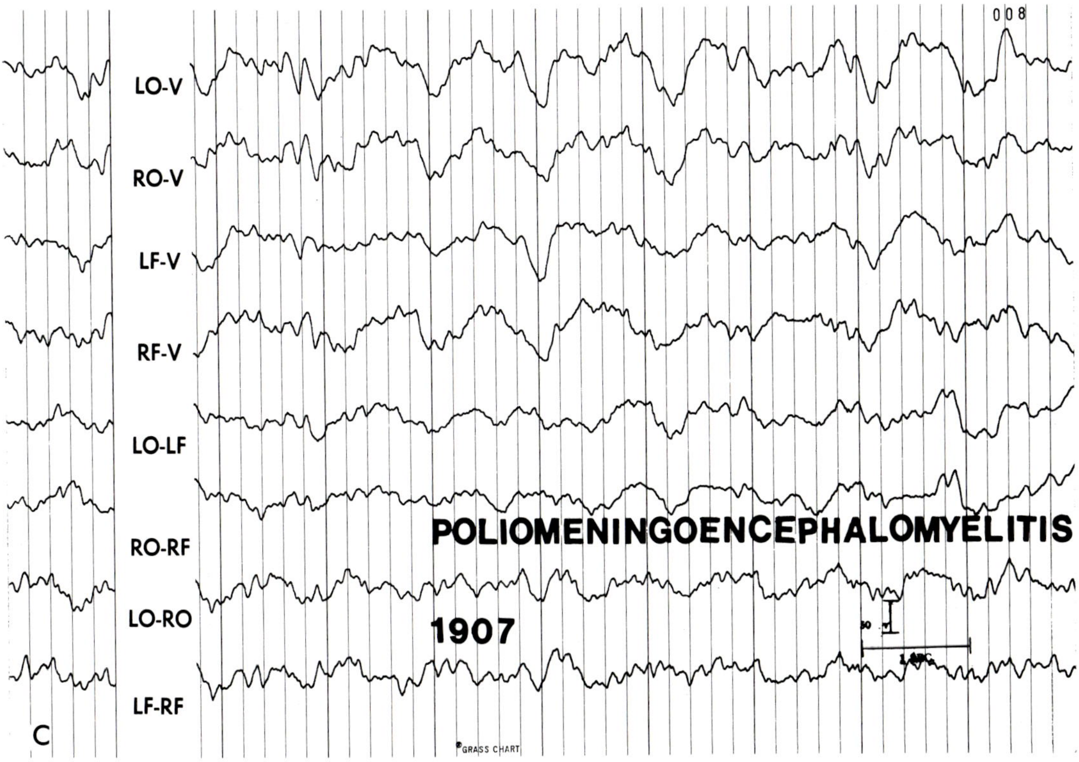

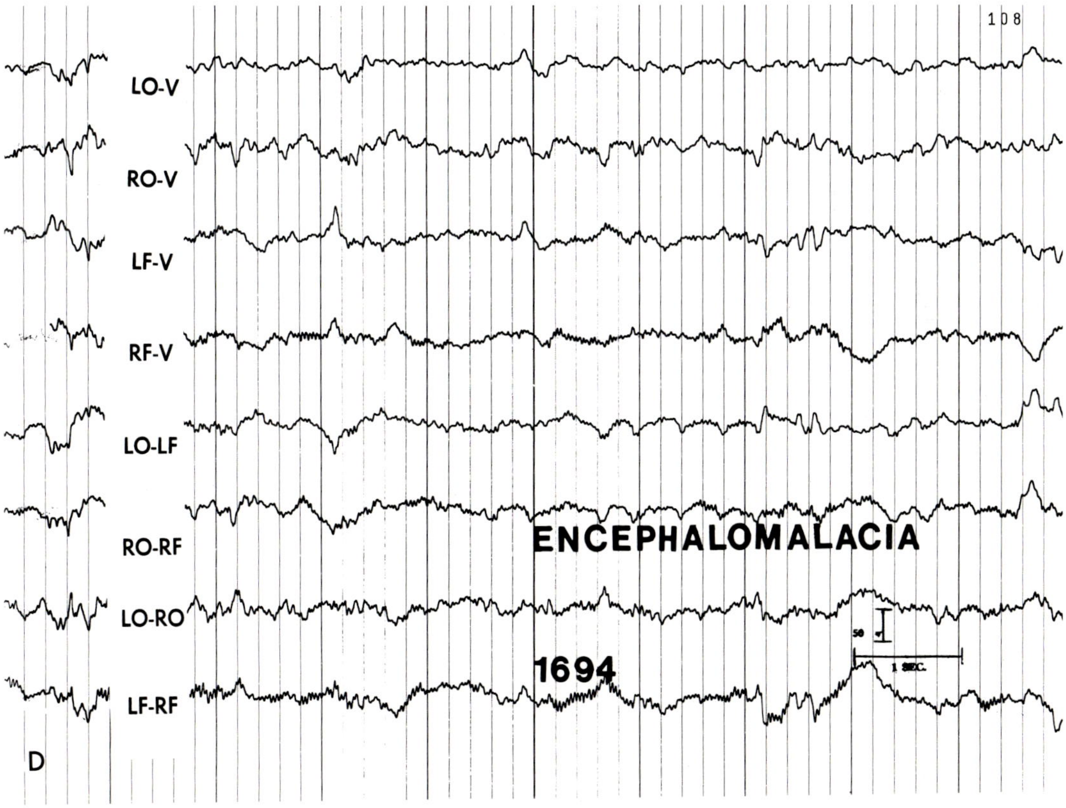

FIGURE 7–12 *Continued*

Figure 7–12 continued on following page

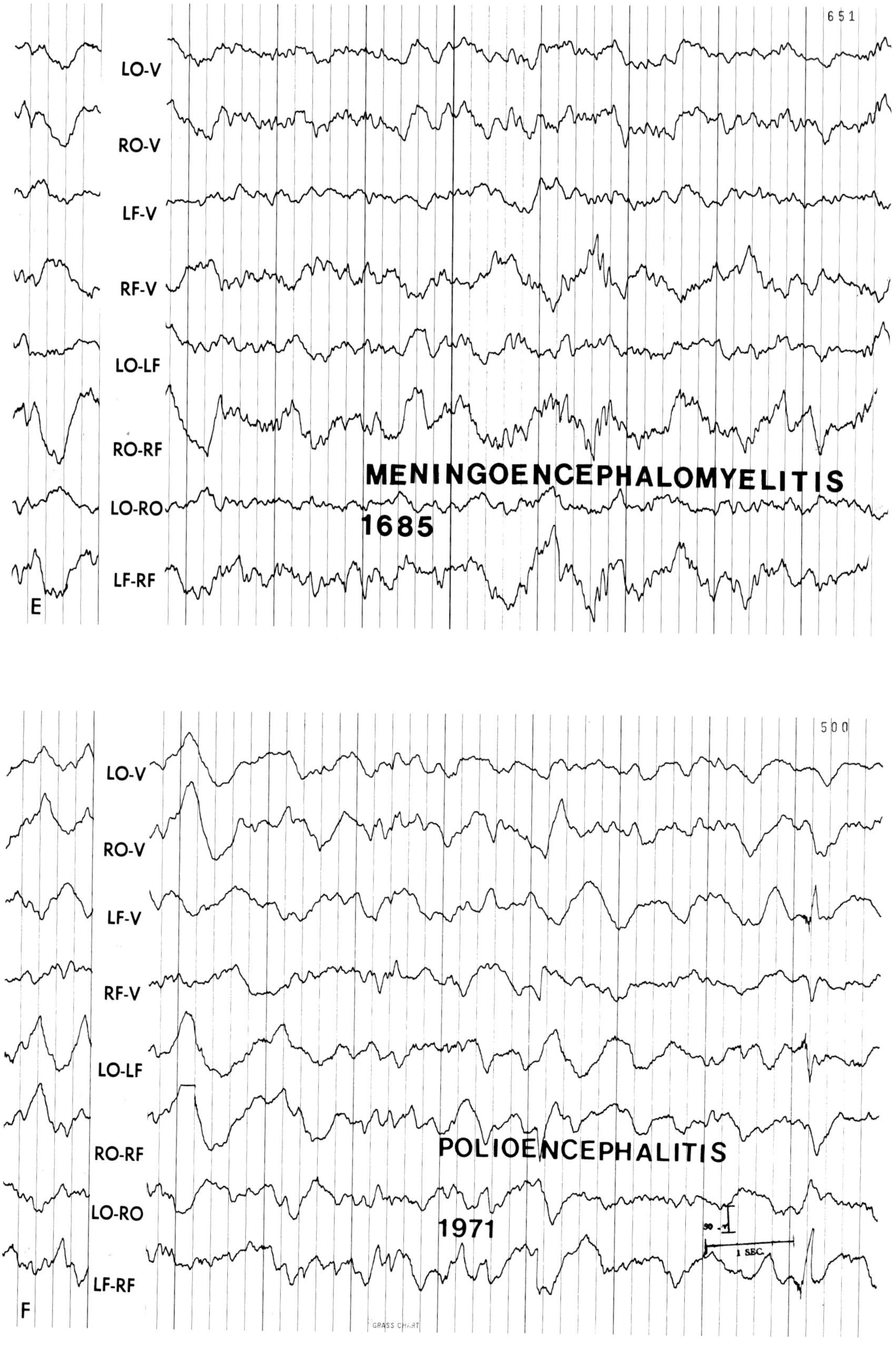

FIGURE 7–12 *Continued*

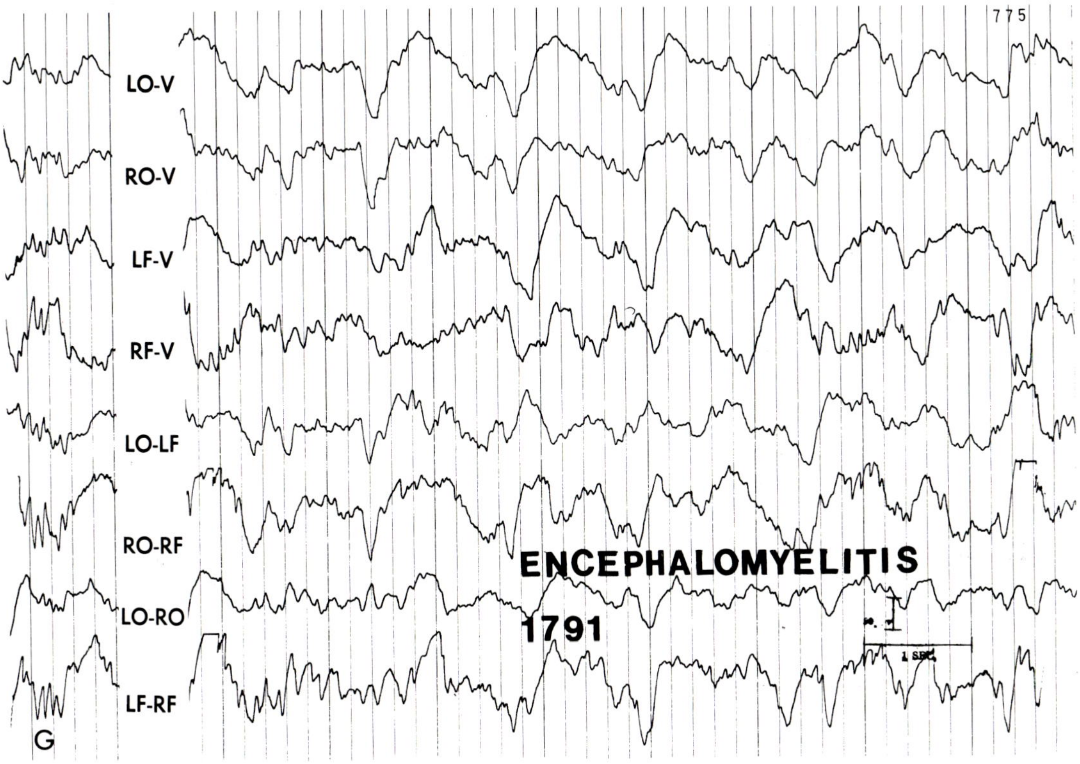

FIGURE 7–12 *Continued*

superimposed fast waves or paroxysmal discharges. The voltages vary from medium to high, 25 to 150 microvolts.

Hepatoencephalopathy

Hepatoencephalopathy is characterized electroencephalographically by medium to fast frequencies of 5 to 20 Hz and medium voltages of 15 to 50 microvolts. Figure 7–13 is a tracing obtained from an animal in the latter stages of the disease.

Lissencephaly

Lissencephaly, an abnormality of cerebral cortical development frequently seen in the Lhasa apso breed, is characterized by irregular random slow waves with a marked lack of symmetry between comparable cortical areas (Fig. 7–14).

LEUKODYSTROPHY

Electroencephalographic studies from three dogs afflicted with globoid-cell leukodystrophy have been reported by Fletcher.[19] Electroencephalographic abnormalities seen in this disease consist of generalized cerebral hemispheric asymmetry, asymmetrical spindling and spikes, excessive high-voltage, low-frequency activity, and a decrease in EEG arousal to auditory stimuli (Fig. 7–15). Apparently the EEG is a useful diagnostic tool in the early stages of globoid-cell leukodystrophy because it can reveal diffuse cerebral hemisphere disorders before they are identified clinically.

SEIZURE DISORDERS

One of the most common reasons for electroencephalographic examination is to determine the cause of seizures.[54] Among the many causes of seizural activity are encephalitis, hydrocephalus, post-traumatic lesions, brain tumors, vascular disorders, metabolic diseases, toxins, and bacterial infections. The wave forms seen with these disturbances have been or will be discussed. The following are additional seizure disorders yielding abnormal EEG findings.

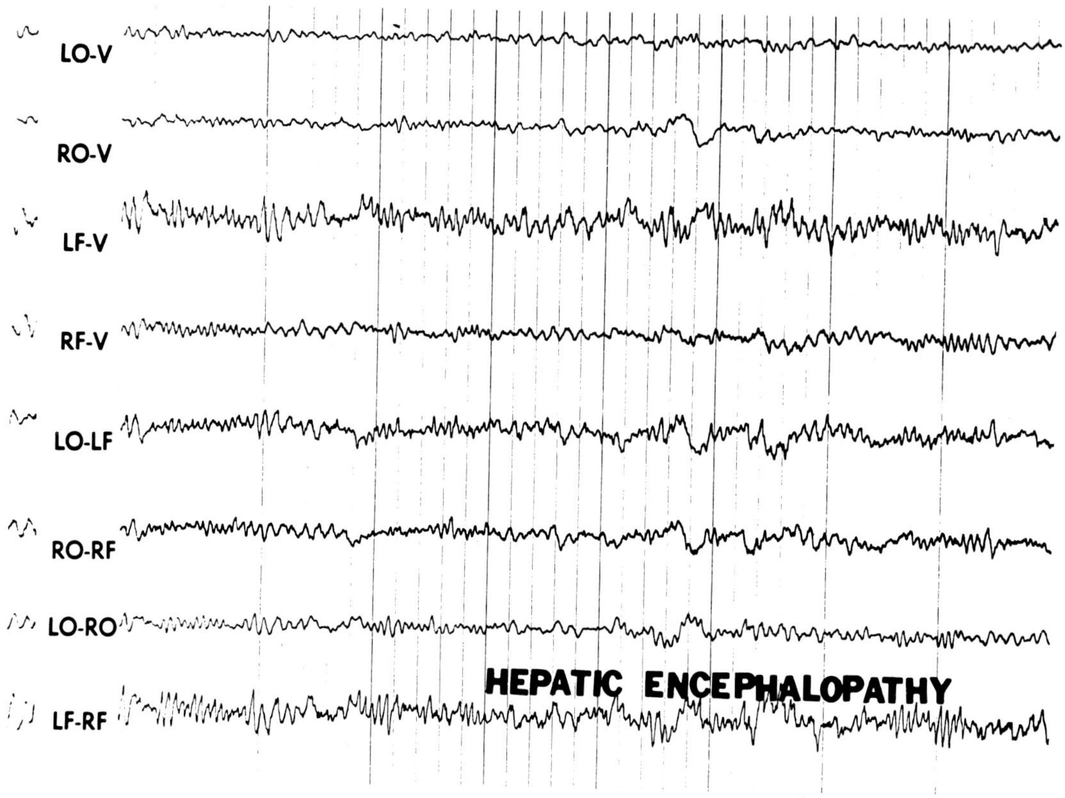

FIGURE 7–13 Tracing obtained from an animal with hepatic encephalopathy in the latter stages of the disease.

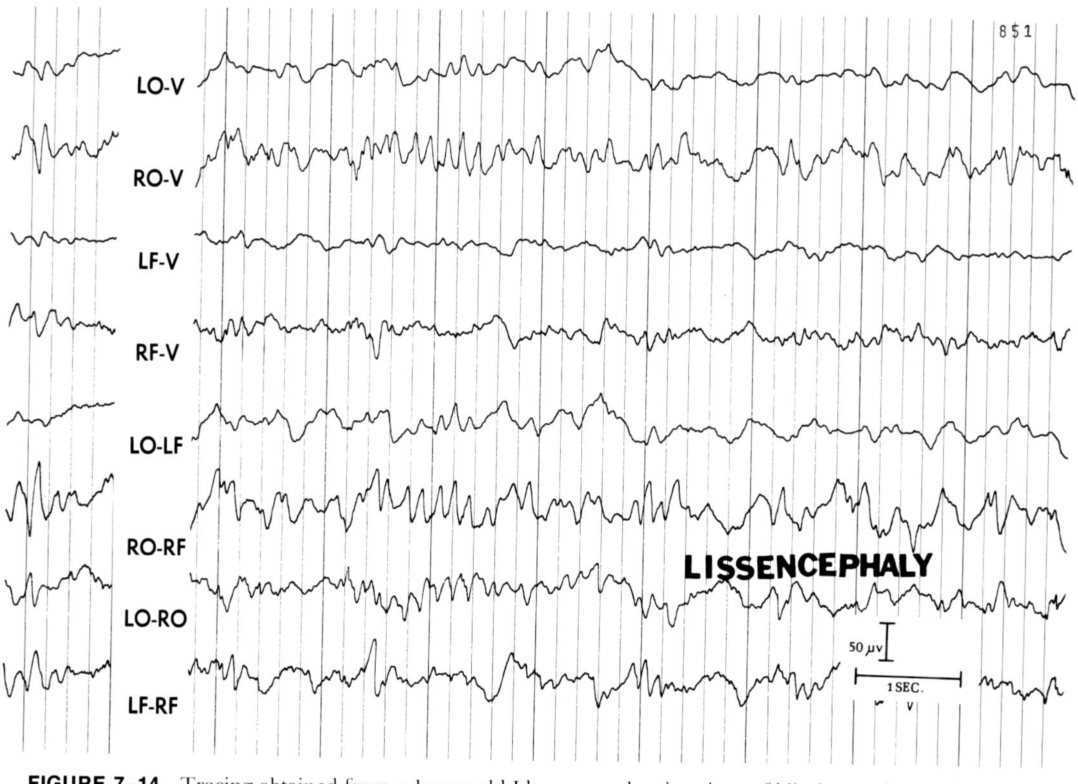

FIGURE 7–14 Tracing obtained from a 1-year-old Lhasa apso showing signs of blindness, abnormal aggressive behavior, syncope, and seizures. The gross and histopathological diagnosis was lissencephaly.

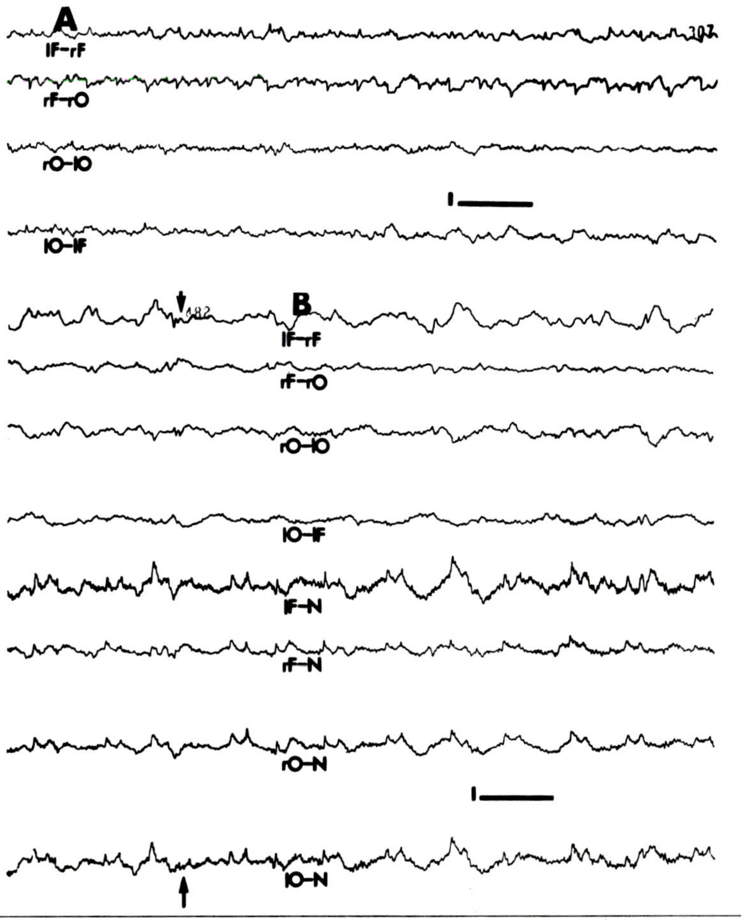

FIGURE 7–15 Recordings obtained from a dog with globoid-cell leukodystrophy. *A*. During the sixth week of the disease; dog alert. Excessive, high-voltage–low-frequency pointed waves are evident, particularly from the right frontal region. *B*. During the ninth week of the disease; dog drowsy. The introduction of a sudden noise (arrows) produced EEG arousal that lasted only about half a second. Calibrations: 50 μV, 1 second. (From Fletcher, T. F.: Electroencephalographic features of leukodystrophic disease in the dog. J.A.V.M.A., *157*, 194, 1970.)

Psychomotor-like Epilepsy

Psychomotor-like epilepsy EEG tracings reveal bursts of medium slow wave activity and are frequently associated with behavior changes of a paroxysmal nature (Fig. 7–16).

Petit-Mal Epilepsy

In man, typical spike and wave patterns are characteristic of petit-mal epilepsy. Less frequently, a comparable electroencephalographic pattern is seen in dogs (Fig. 7–17). This pattern is usually associated with the petit-mal type of seizural activity in which the animal has a transient loss of contact with reality and may show minor motor signs.

Grand-Mal Epilepsy

Tracings recorded from physically restrained animals are very disappointing because the pattern typically seen in human grand-mal epilepsy is seldom, if ever, obtained. The pattern seen in man consists of high voltage–high frequency activity with frequent spikes. Klemm[43] has reported high frequency–high voltage spikes in animals with grand-mal epilepsy when using barbiturate anesthesia to activate abnormal foci. Apparently, chemical restraints may

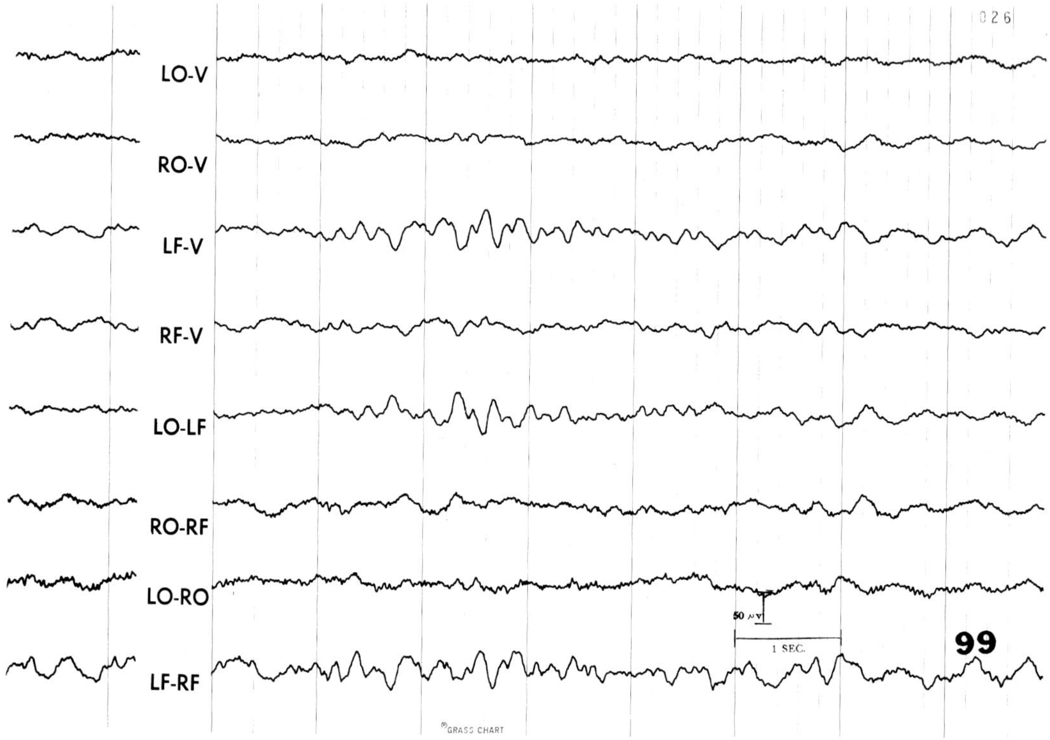

FIGURE 7–16 Tracing obtained from a dog with a periodic behavior change signaled by signs of fear followed by aggression. Note the paroxysm of slow waves in the left frontal lead.

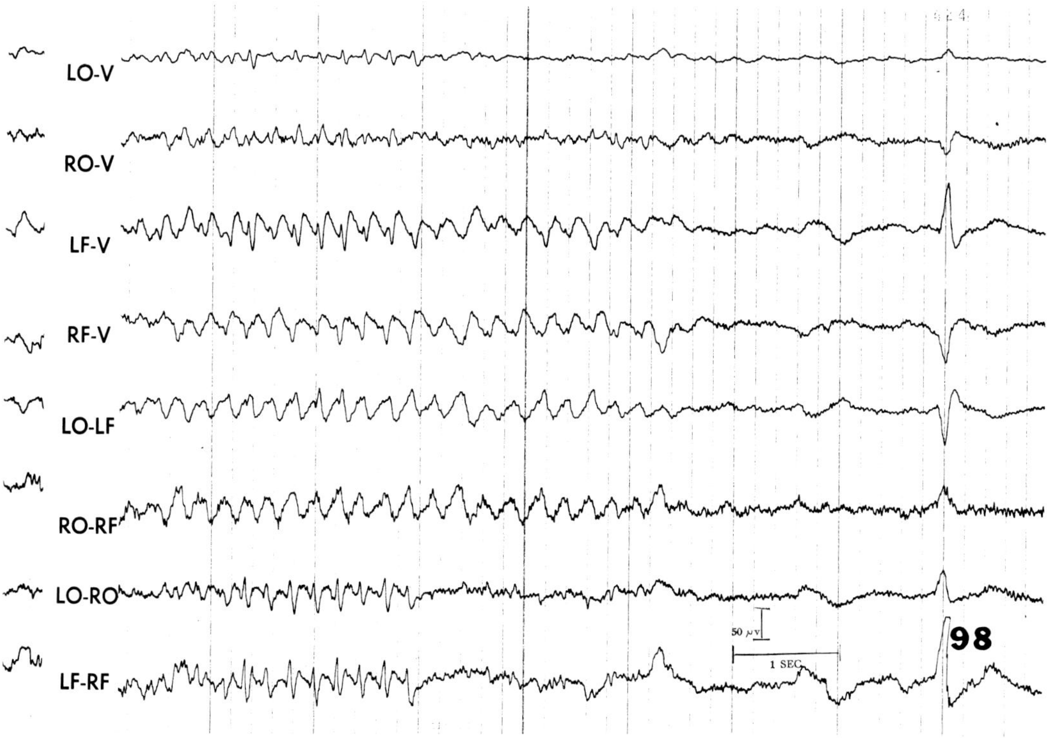

FIGURE 7–17 Tracing obtained from a 3-year-old poodle with frequent signs of a transient loss of contact with reality signaled by staring. Note the spike and wave forms that last for approximately 3 to 4 seconds. The animal did not show abnormal clinical signs at the time of the tracing.

be necessary to activate abnormal, grand-mal epileptic seizural activity that may be recorded on the EEG.

Idiopathic Epilepsy

Idiopathic epilepsy frequently occurs in the dog and has familial tendencies. The interictal EEG pattern is usually nondiagnostic. Occasionally, however, paroxysmal spindles will be recorded. Figure 7–18 is a tracing from a dog with idiopathic epilepsy showing the spindle-type wave forms. This particular pattern is also recorded when the animal shivers. Careful observation of the patient is necessary during the recording period to be sure that the spindle wave form is not an artifact.

Emotional Disorders

Turbes and Jobe[65] have studied the EEG changes in emotional disorders of the dog and cat. Of 83 dogs studied, 51 showed some dysrhythmia, with the major abnormality being recorded in the temporal-occipital regions and usually consisting of abnormal slow-wave activity. However, no specific pattern was related to any one individual behavior problem. Electroencephalographic tracings obtained by the author from animals with abnormal behavior have been disappointing in that very few abnormalities were seen.

CEREBRAL TRAUMA

Cerebral trauma results from head injuries, and the abnormality varies depending upon the degree of injury to the brain tissue (Fig. 7–19 *A–E*). Damage to the cerebral hemispheres, especially to the more superficial portions, is more accessible to EEG examination. Recordings made immediately following cerebral trauma (mild concussion) show characteristic low voltage–slow waves at first, but these are rapidly

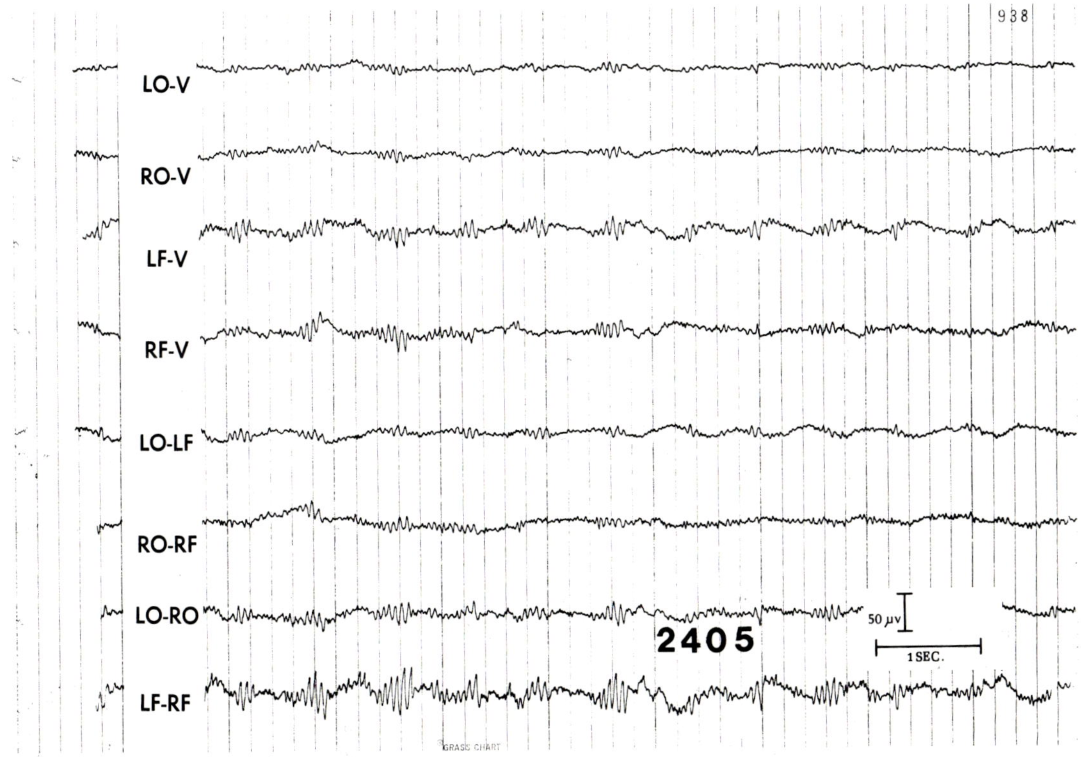

FIGURE 7–18 Tracing obtained from a 1½-year-old poodle with a history of idiopathic epilepsy. The spindle formation is marked. Many idiopathic epileptics have the same wave form but less frequently.

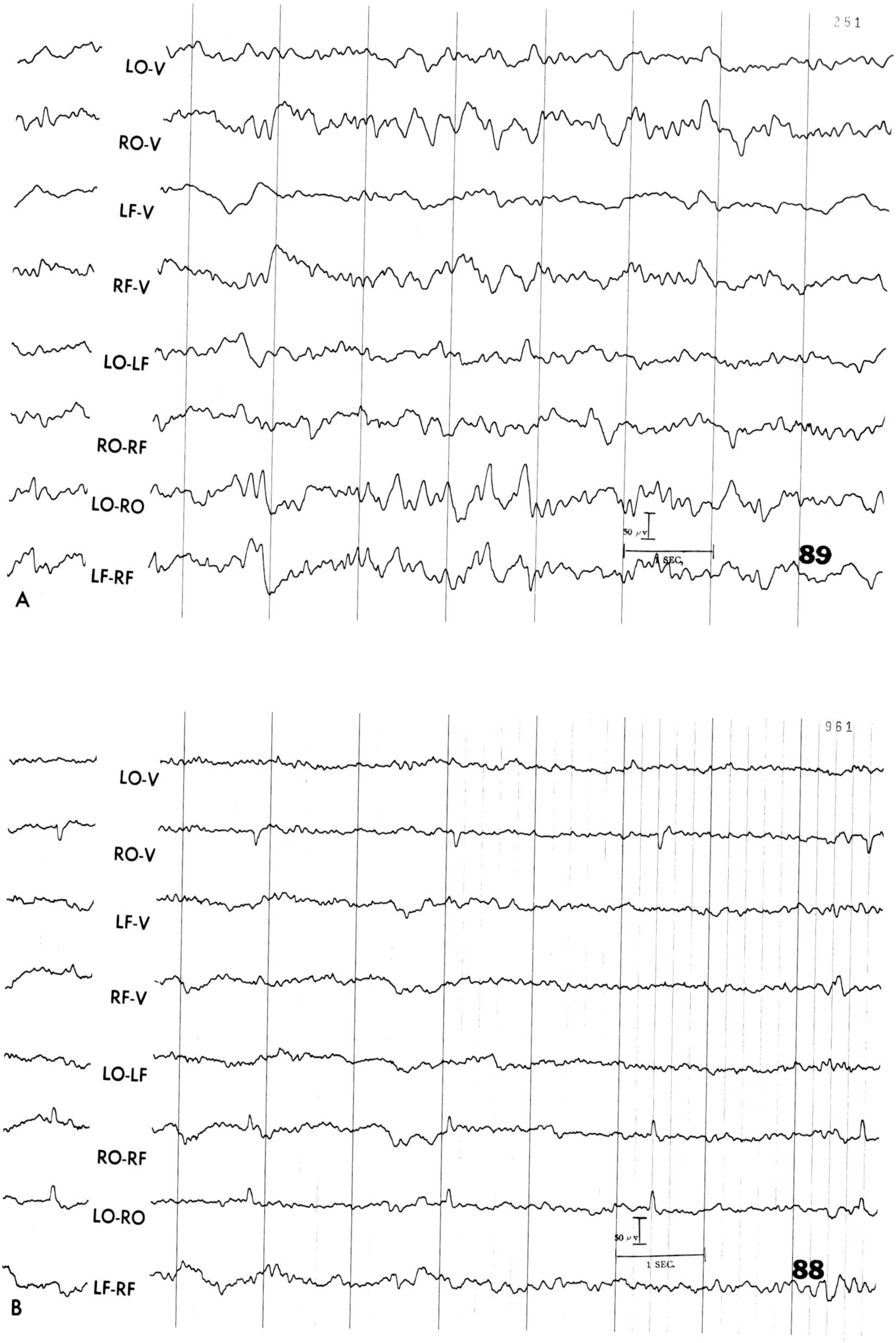

FIGURE 7–19 Electroencephalograms obtained from patients suffering from various head injuries and resultant cerebral trauma. *A*. Animal had been dropped on its head 4 days prior to presentation. *B*. Animal was hit by a basketball 5 days before tracing was made.

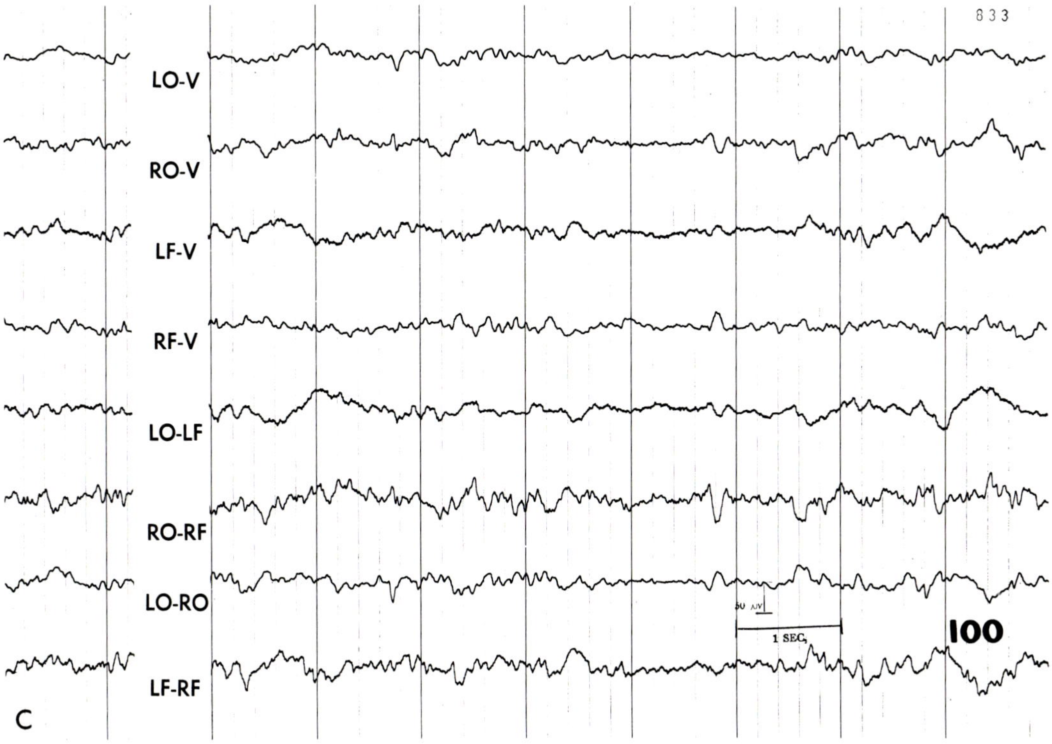

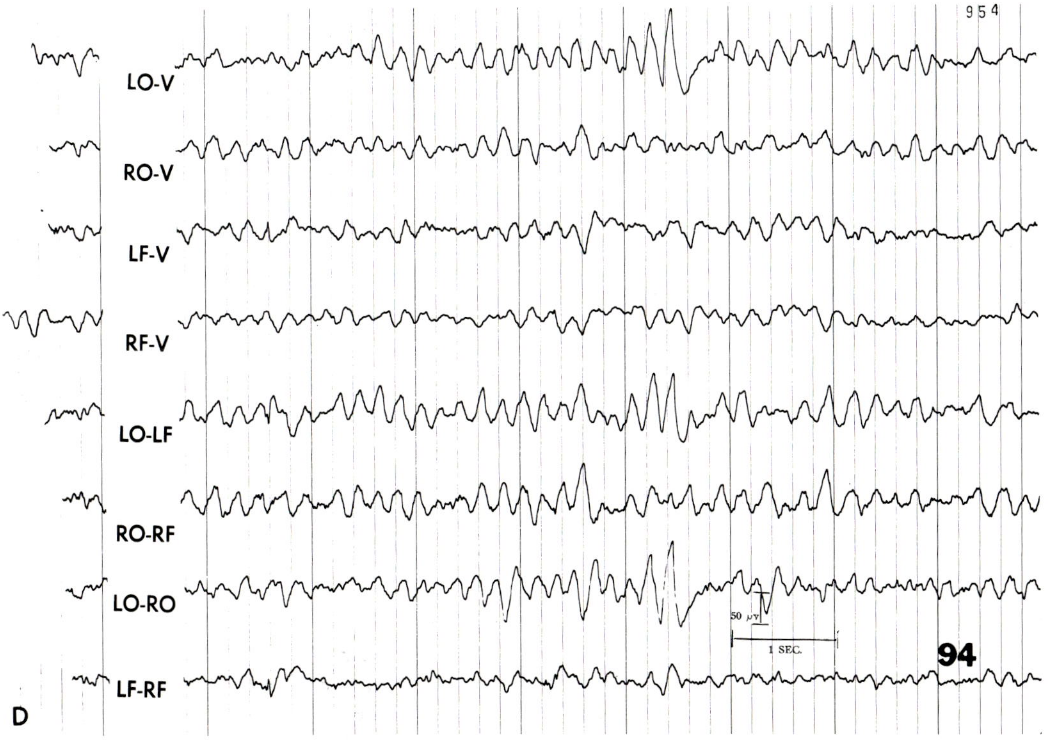

FIGURE 7–19 *Continued* C. Animal was hit by a car 4 to 6 weeks prior to tracing. *D.* Animal was hit by a car and suffered fractured skull.

Figure 7–19 continued on following page

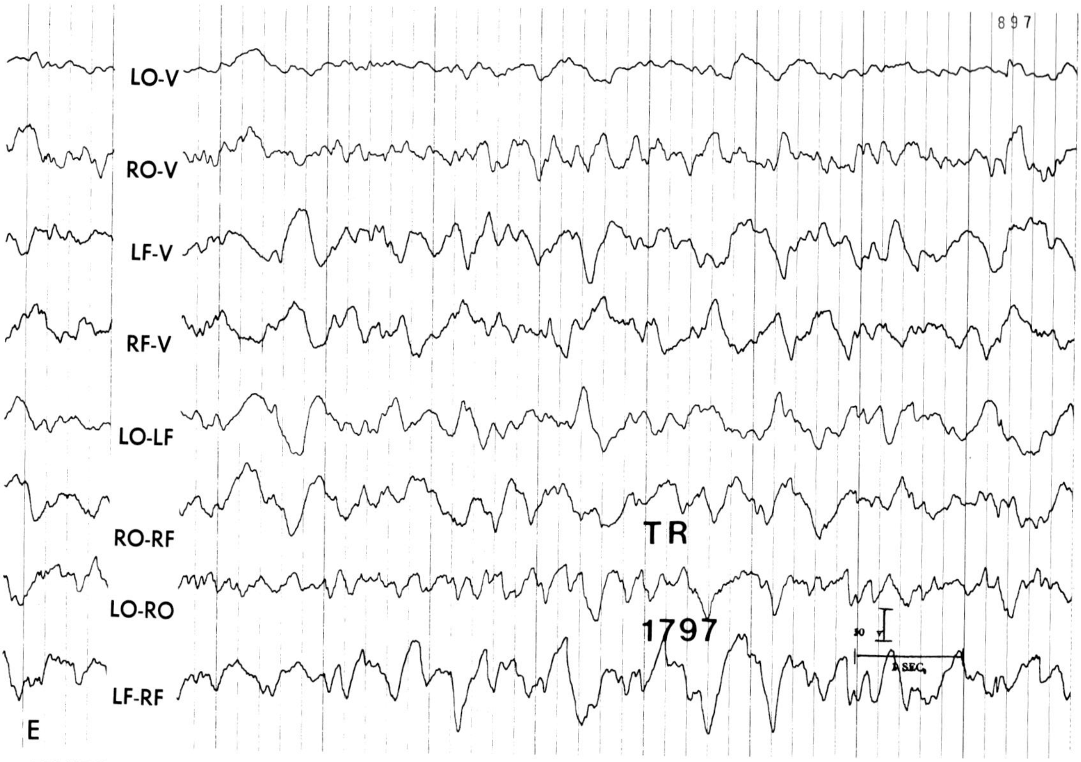

FIGURE 7–19 *Continued* *E.* Animal had been struck by a car 3 days prior to presentation. The animal showed clinical blindness and depression. Note the asymmetry between the occipital leads and the lower voltages.

replaced by high voltage–slow waves. If a lesion is localized, focal high-amplitude activity is produced by the damaged tissue. Occasionally the high voltage–slow wave activity is accompanied by a high frequency component riding on the slow wave activity in the area of damage. Structures in the posterior fossa may also be damaged by head injuries. EEG recordings of animals with posterior fossa damage may not show any gross abnormality; some slowing, however, may be noted and is probably associated with damage to the reticular activating system in the anterior portion of the brain stem that influences the thalamic or diencephalic structures.

In localized brain damage, the focal electric high voltage activity may not be seen at first. Instead, there is generalized slowing, indicative of the general brain edema, which gradually disappears and allows the focal damaged area to persist and to be demonstrated electroencephalographically. The focal abnormality may persist for weeks or even months. The damaged area may act as a focal point for epileptic seizures that occur 3 to 5 months following the injury.

Head injuries may also cause vascular lesions, such as cerebral hemorrhage or subdural hematoma. One might suspect that cerebral hemorrhage would result in a localized abnormality, but it has been the author's experience that it is difficult to establish a localized abnormality using an electroencephalogram in cerebral hemorrhage following trauma. In subdural hematomas, the pattern may show generalized high voltage–slow wave activity as shown in Figure 7–20 *B*. Occasionally random spiking is seen in subdural hematomas (Fig. 7–20 *A*).

HYDROCEPHALUS

Hydrocephalus, like distemper encephalitis, is very easily diagnosed through the use of the electroencephalogram and can be confirmed by radiographic studies.[34, 51] However, it is not often necessary to use radiographic studies to establish a diagnosis

Text continued on page 186

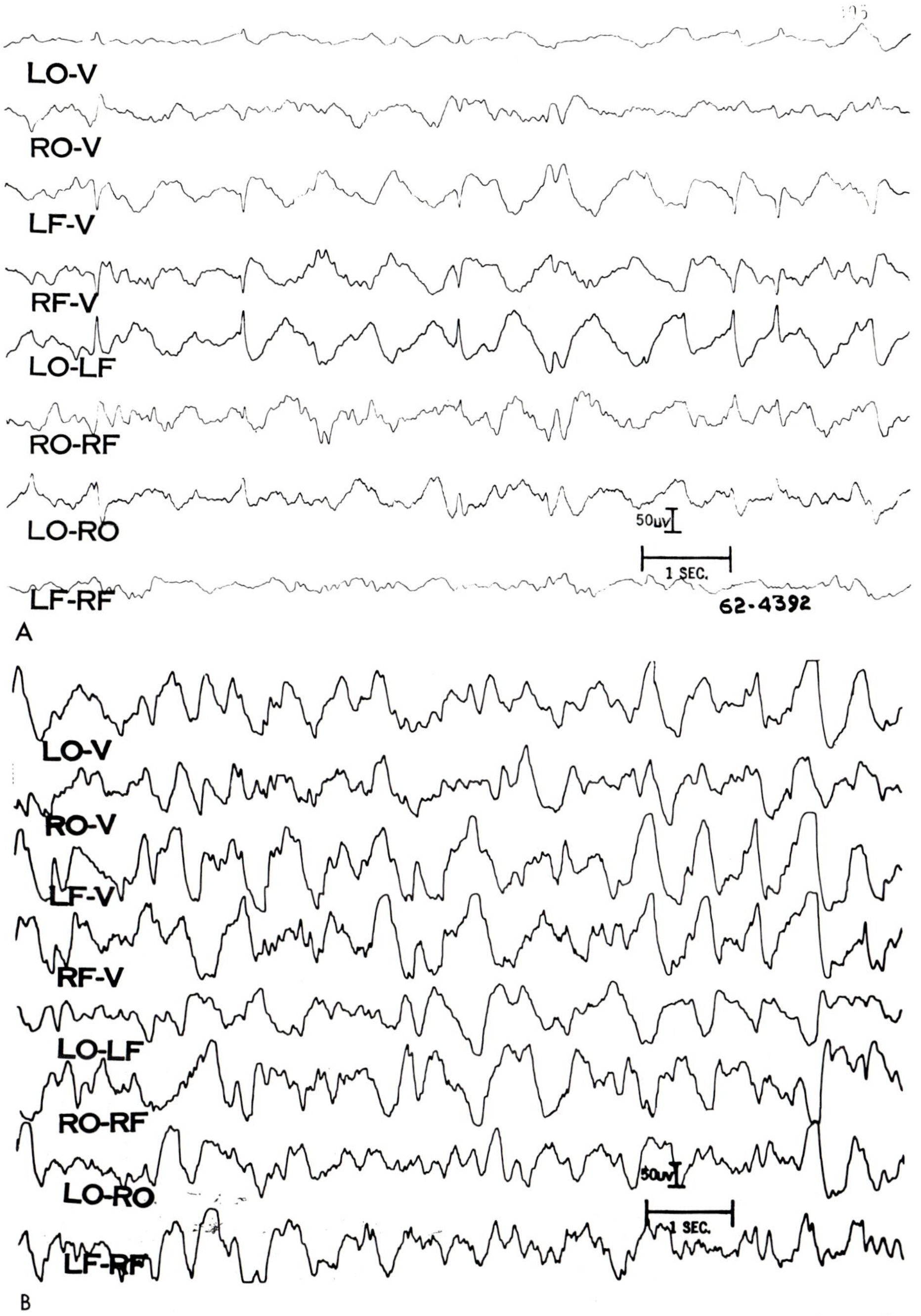

FIGURE 7–20 *A*. Subdural hematoma. The animal from which this recording was made had a massive subdural hematoma over the frontoparietal region. *B*. Recording obtained from an animal with a massive diffuse subdural hematoma (confirmed at necropsy).

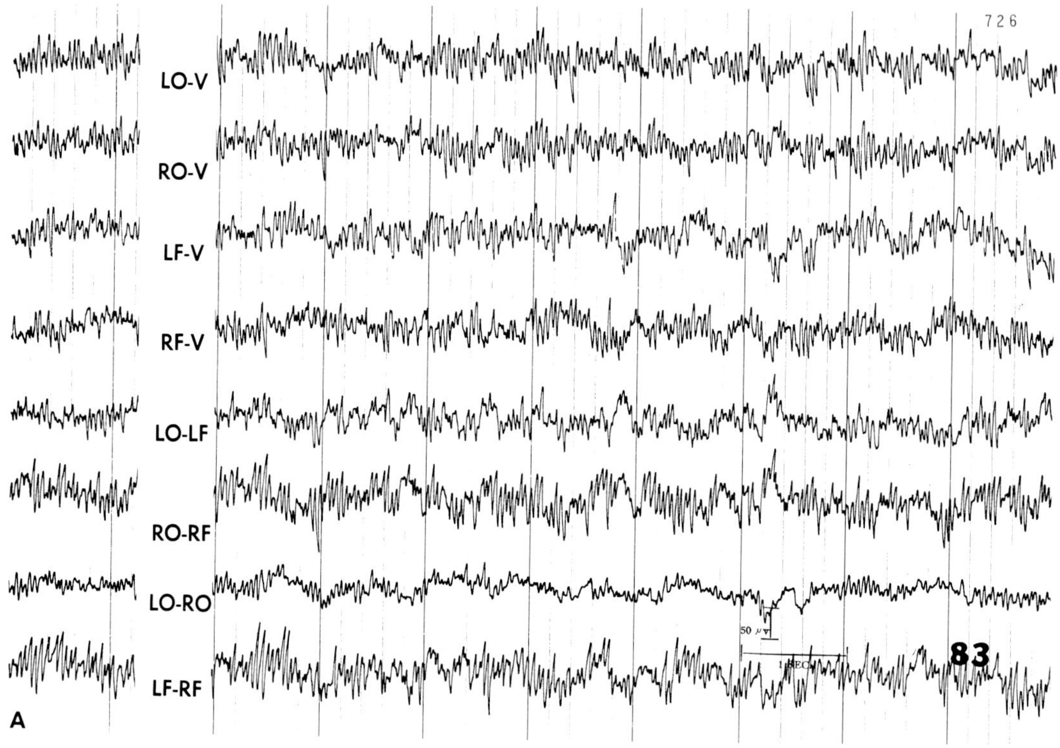

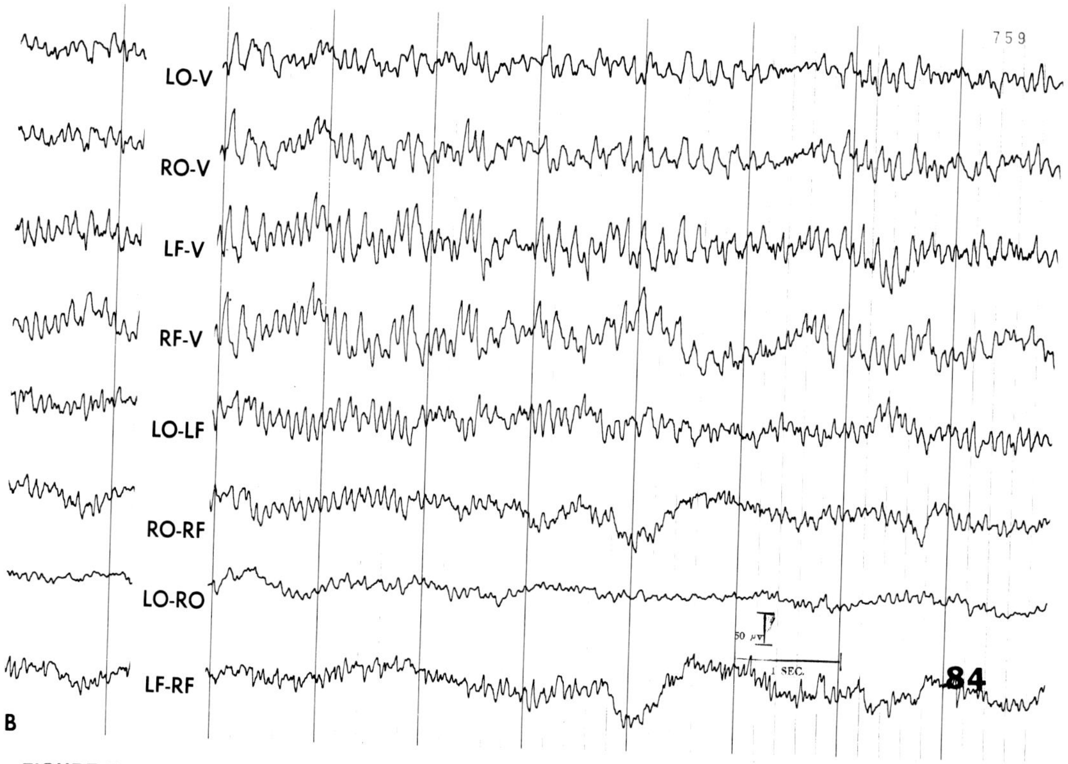

FIGURE 7–21 *A–D.* Electroencephalographic patterns seen in hydrocephalus. (From Redding, R. W., and Knecht, C. D.: Neurologic examination. *In* Ettinger, S. J. (ed.): *Textbook of Veterinary Internal Medicine.* W. B. Saunders Co., Philadelphia, 1975.)

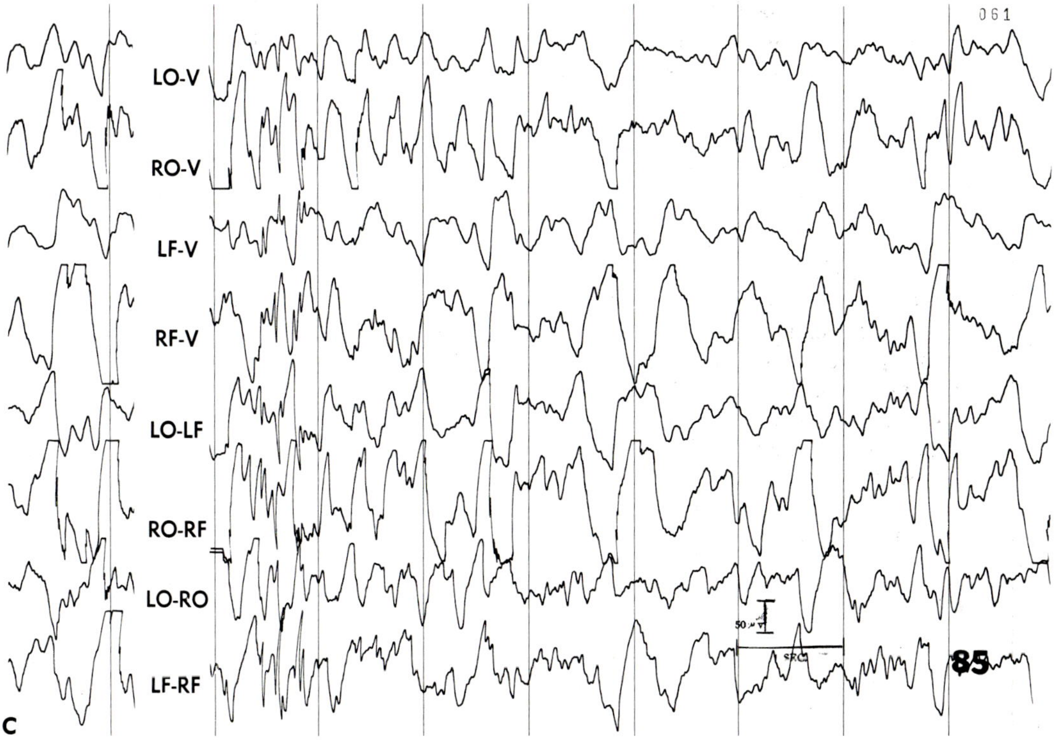

C

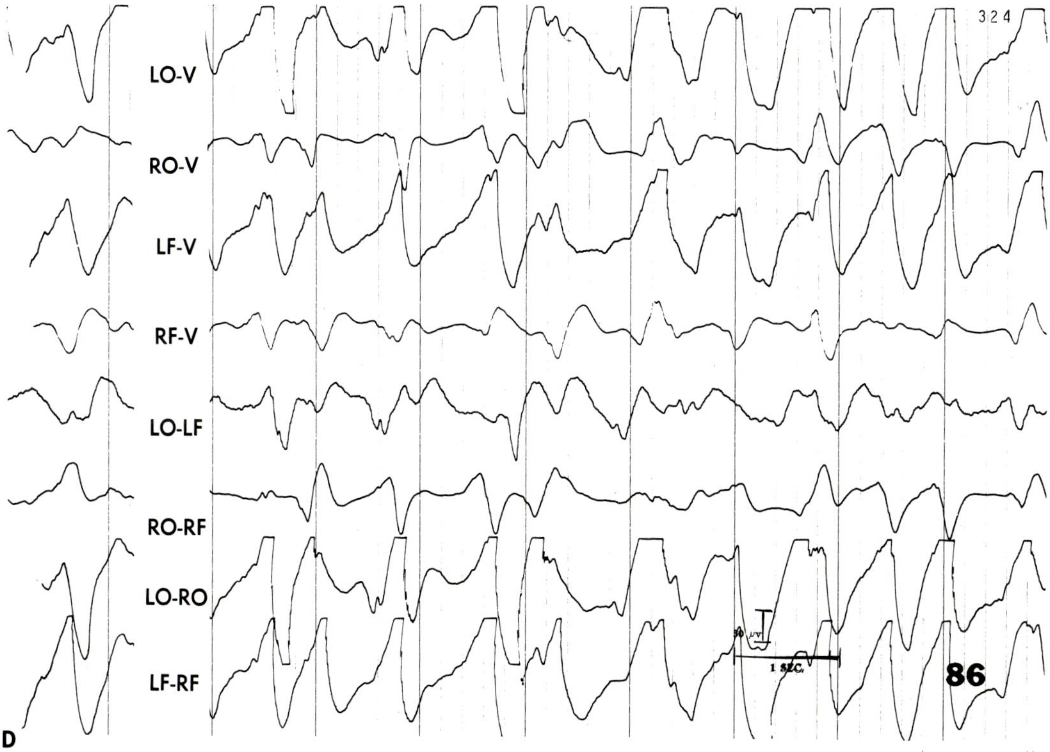

D

FIGURE 7–21 *Continued*

of hydrocephalus. Of all the abnormalities involving the cerebral cortex, hydrocephalus shows the greatest variety of changes in both frequency and amplitude. The spectrum ranges from high frequency–medium-to-high voltage to low frequency–high voltage. The electroencephalograms presented in Figure 7–21 demonstrate this wide range.

Hydrocephalus may be congenital or acquired and may be the result of cerebral injury. This is especially true of the toy breeds. The presence or absence of an open fontanel is not a good index for the diagnosis of hydrocephalus. Animals with a closed fontanel frequently show hydrocephalus-type patterns.

This author suspects that the different patterns seen in hydrocephalus may be related to the development of increased intraventricular pressure. In those EEG tracings that show high voltage, relatively fast activity (50 to 150 microvolts, 5 to 8 Hz), the early, rapid development of pressure is seen. Those tracings that show slower activity and even higher voltages (1 to 5 Hz, 100 to 200 microvolts) are related to cortical thinning as a result of a relatively long period of pressure development. There is also another pattern, consisting of higher frequencies and spike-like wave forms, that appears to be related to acquired hydrocephalus usually associated with previous cerebral trauma (Fig. 7–22).

VASCULAR DISORDERS

Vascular lesions of the cerebral hemispheres are relatively common in man and are accompanied by dramatic signs such as motor paralysis and sensory deficits. The signs of vascular disorders may occur in dogs and cats; however, the clinical signs are relatively less dramatic if they are superficial. It is probable that the so-called stroke-like syndrome seen in dogs in which there is a hemiparesis may be associated

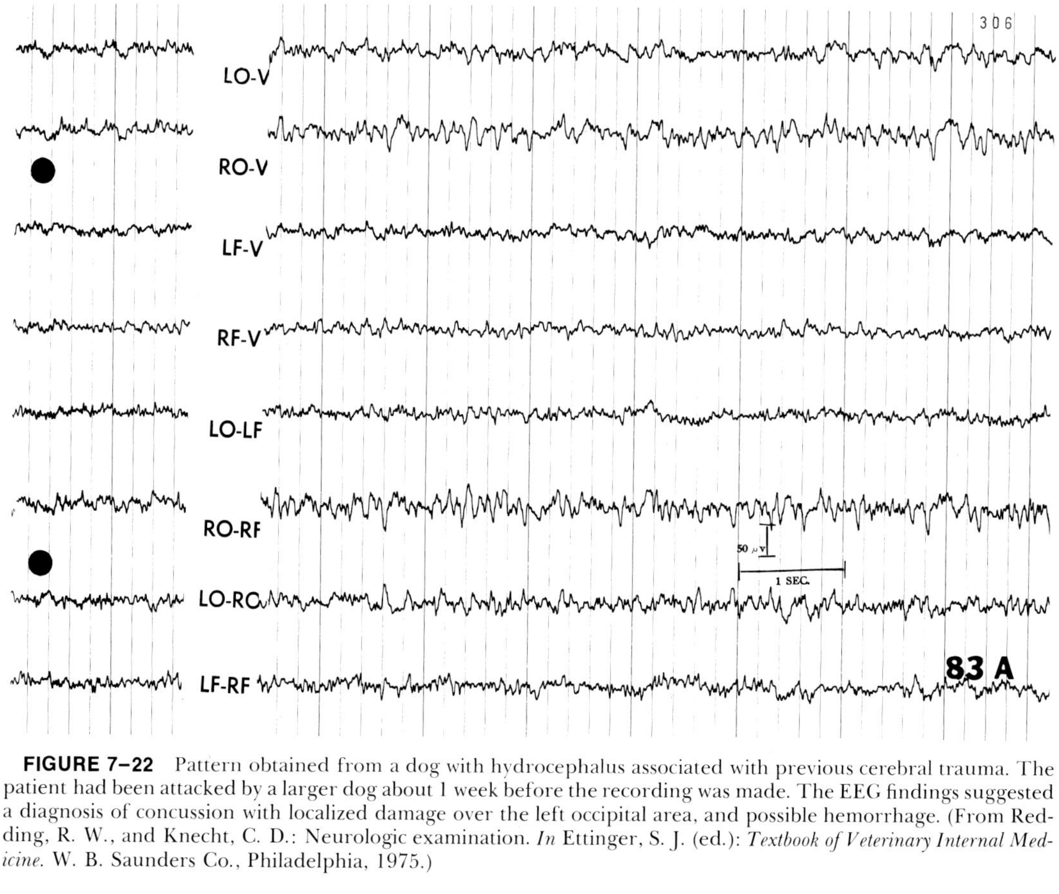

FIGURE 7–22 Pattern obtained from a dog with hydrocephalus associated with previous cerebral trauma. The patient had been attacked by a larger dog about 1 week before the recording was made. The EEG findings suggested a diagnosis of concussion with localized damage over the left occipital area, and possible hemorrhage. (From Redding, R. W., and Knecht, C. D.: Neurologic examination. *In* Ettinger, S. J. (ed.): *Textbook of Veterinary Internal Medicine.* W. B. Saunders Co., Philadelphia, 1975.)

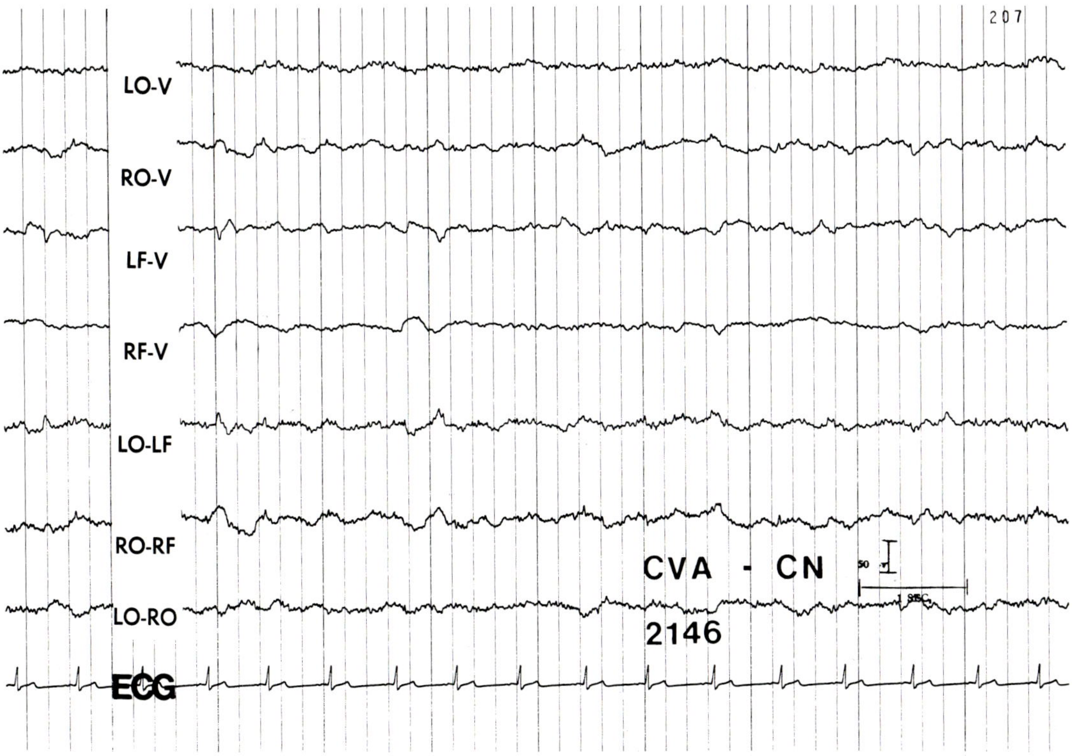

FIGURE 7–23 Tracing of an 8-year-old Labrador retriever that had a sudden onset of quadriplegia and depression. The wave forms are random and slow. An ECG artifact is confirmed by simultaneous recording of the electrocardiogram. Necropsy examination showed a rupture of the arteries with hemorrhage in the caudate nucleus.

with a vascular lesion of the basal nuclei. Electroencephalographic examinations of animals with hemiparesis and a stroke-like syndrome have been generally unremarkable. The brain waves appear to be relatively normal and have relatively good symmetry. In a few instances, abnormal low voltages may be seen in one hemispheric lead, but this is not the common observation. The use of the electroencephalogram in the diagnosis of cerebral vascular accidents (CVA) appears to be limited in veterinary medicine. In one confirmed case of a CVA of the caudate nucleus in a dog with quadriplegia and mental depression generalized random slow waves were visible (Fig. 7–23).

METABOLIC DISEASES

Hypothyroidism

In hypothyroidism, the electroencephalogram shows extremely low voltage–medium frequency activity (Fig. 7–24). The voltages are generally so low that they are difficult to measure when the standard recording technique of 50 microvolts per centimeter is used.

Other metabolic diseases have not been studied sufficiently in veterinary medicine to establish the EEG patterns.

TOXINS

Chlorinated Hydrocarbons

Chlorinated hydrocarbon intoxication (Fig. 7–25) frequently results in a high frequency–low voltage activity which is generalized in nature and not specifically diagnostic for a particular agent.

Organophosphate Poisoning

The electroencephalogram in organophosphate intoxication also shows high frequency–low voltage activity and is not specifically diagnostic.

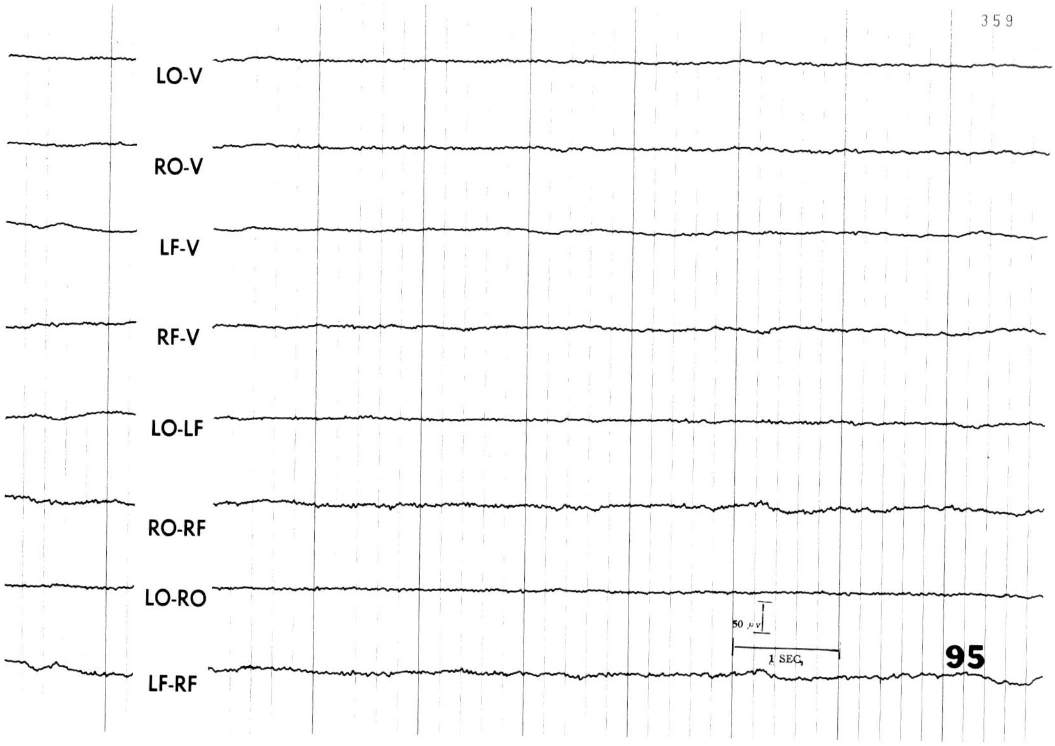

FIGURE 7–24 Tracing obtained from an animal suffering from hypothyroidism. (From Redding, R. W., and Knecht, C. D.: Neurologic examination. *In* Ettinger, S. J. (ed.): *Textbook of Veterinary Internal Medicine.* W. B. Saunders Co., Philadelphia, 1975.)

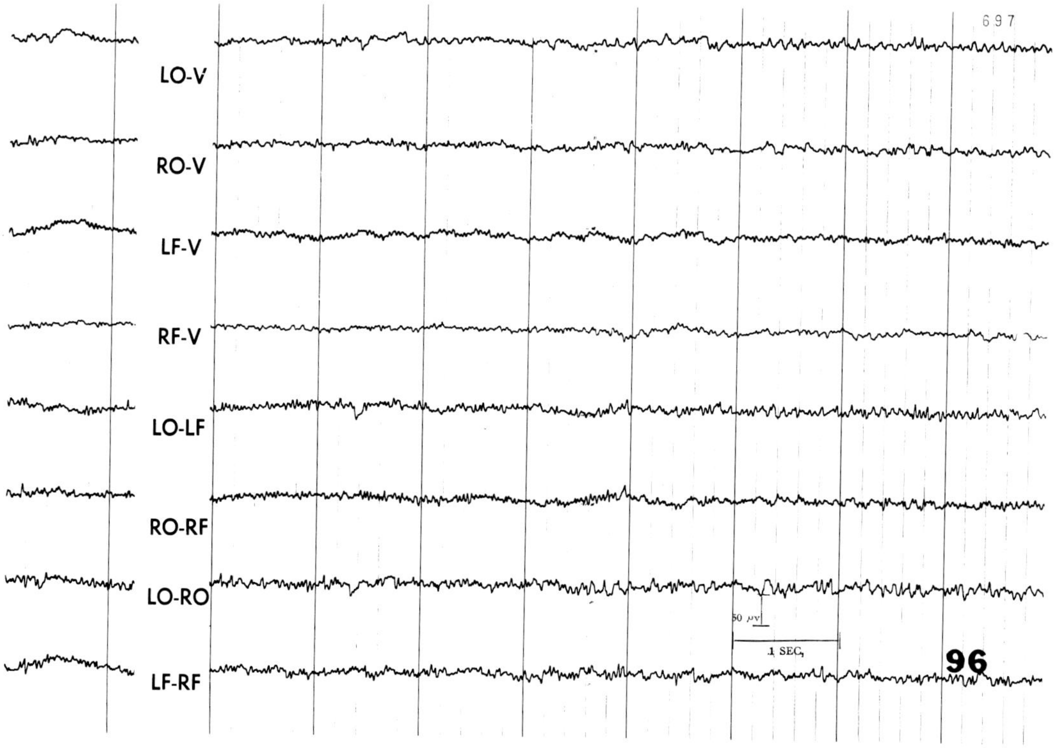

FIGURE 7–25 EEG taken from a patient with chlorinated hydrocarbon intoxication. (From Redding, R. W., and Knecht, C. D.: Neurologic examination. *In* Ettinger, S. J. (ed.): *Textbook of Veterinary Internal Medicine.* W. B. Saunders Co., Philadelphia, 1975.)

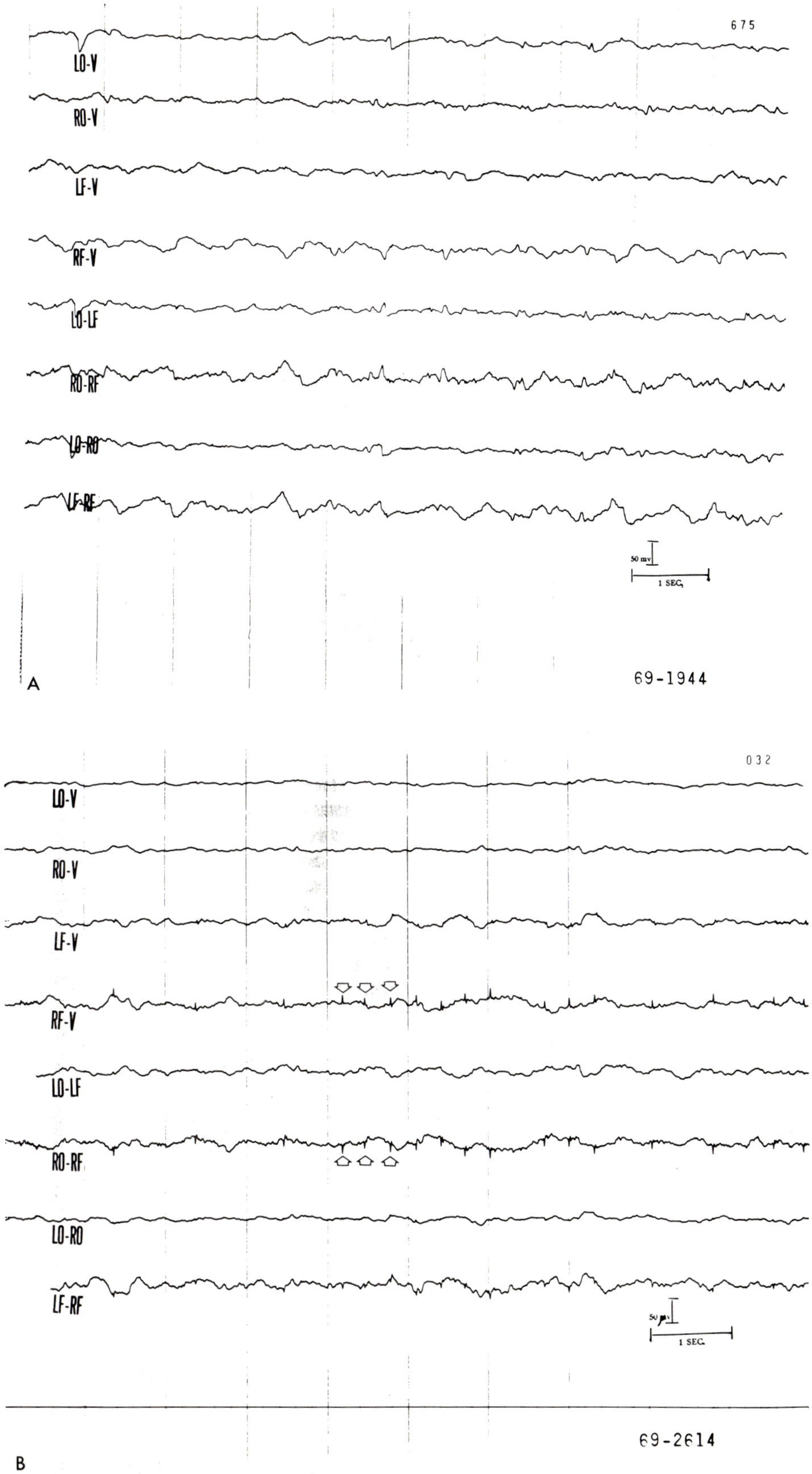

FIGURE 7–26 *A* and *B*. Recordings obtained from animals with brain abscesses. Generalized low-voltage slow wave present. Focal spike activity (arrows) seen in *B*. The brain abscess followed an infection of the right eye.

BRAIN ABSCESSES

Brain abscesses (Fig. 7–26 *A* and *B*) frequently show localized slow wave activity upon which there may be superimposed spikes indicating the focus of the infectious process.

Cerebral Edema

Generalized cerebral edema, usually associated with head trauma, results in generalized slow wave activity which gradually disappears and is replaced by normal patterns, if there is no residual brain damage. Localized cerebral edema is difficult to detect electroencephalographically. Experimental studies in which localized edema was produced failed to demonstrate any electroencephalographic abnormalities, although the local edema was as large as 3 cm in diameter and 2 to 3 cm deep.[63]

Space-Occupying Masses

The changes in the EEG associated with brain tumors are a result of the reaction of the electrically active brain tissue to the growing mass; the tumor itself is electrically silent. The site of the tumor influences the recording. If it is deep within the brain and remote from the recording electrodes, the abnormalities seen are minimal and tend to be diffuse; if it is near the surface, marked abnormalities may be seen; if it is deep and located on the midline, generalized abnormal slow waves are seen in both hemispheres (Fig. 7–27 *A-D*); if it is more superficial and unilateral, the record shows localized slowing of greater magnitude.

In general, tumors produce slow activity with high voltages. Occasionally, there are bursts of high frequency activity superimposed on the slow wave activity. In some cases, high frequency spiking is the pre-

Text continued on page 201

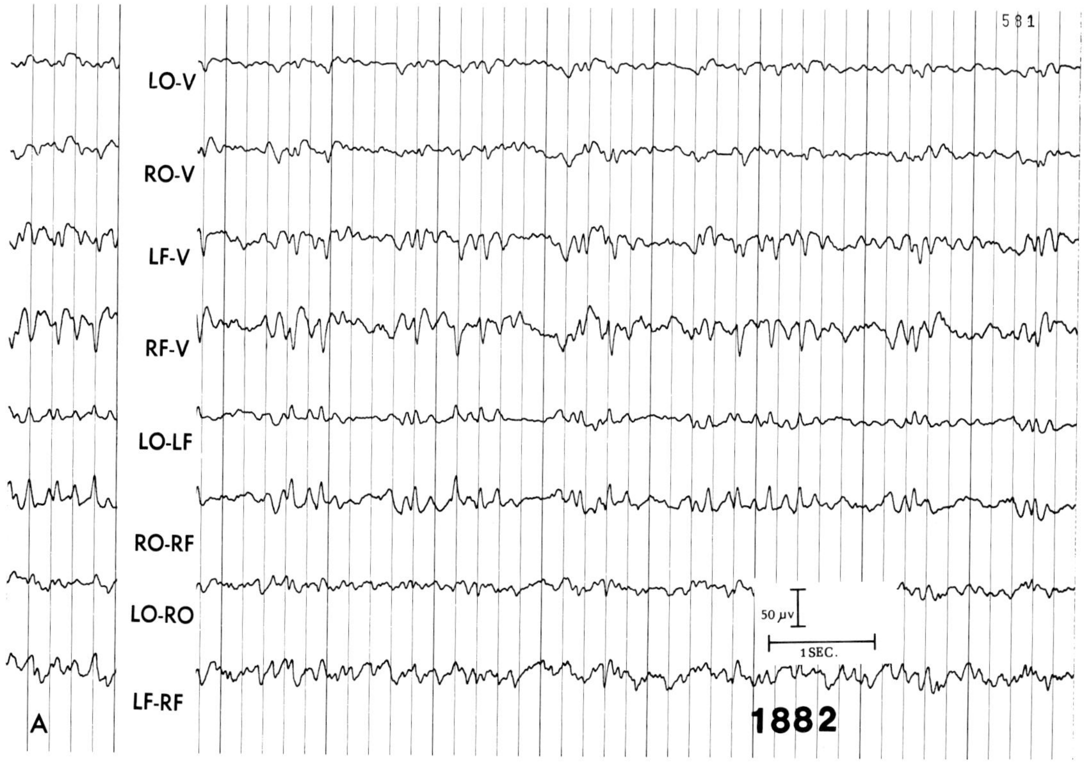

FIGURE 7–27 *A*. Tracing from a 10-year-old Boston terrier with a history of Jacksonian-type seizures starting on the left side and eventually including the entire body. Note the sharp wave originating in the right frontal region. An oligodendroglioma involving the right frontoparietal cortex was found at necropsy.

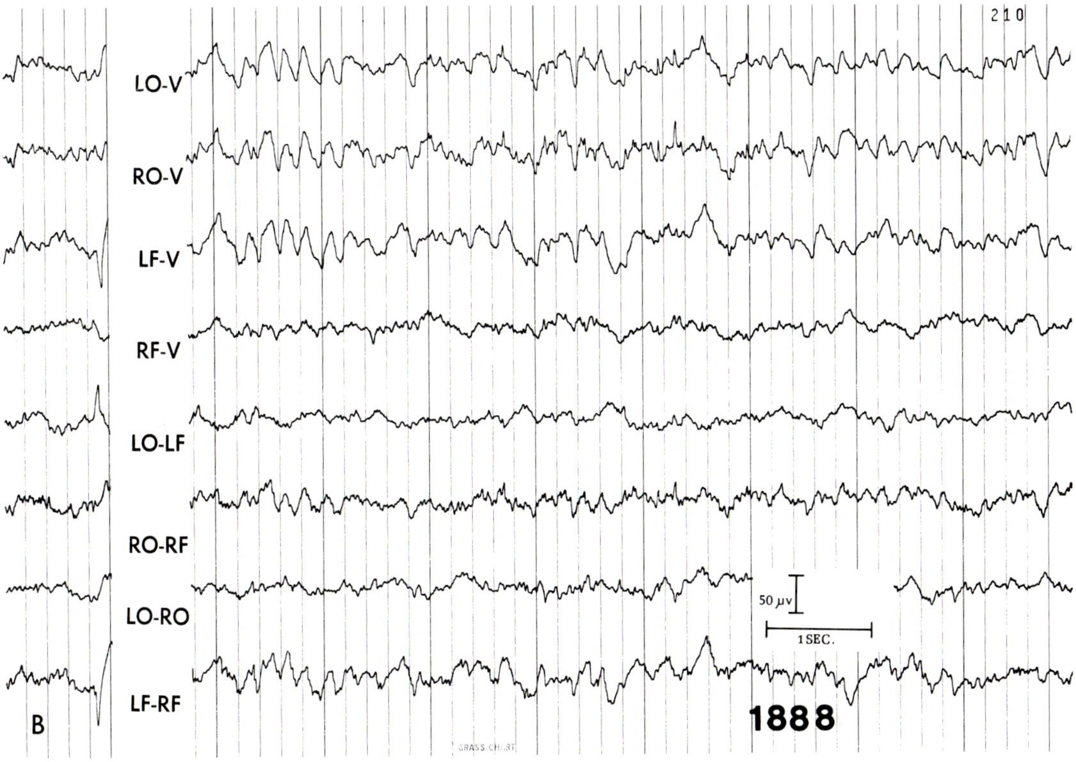

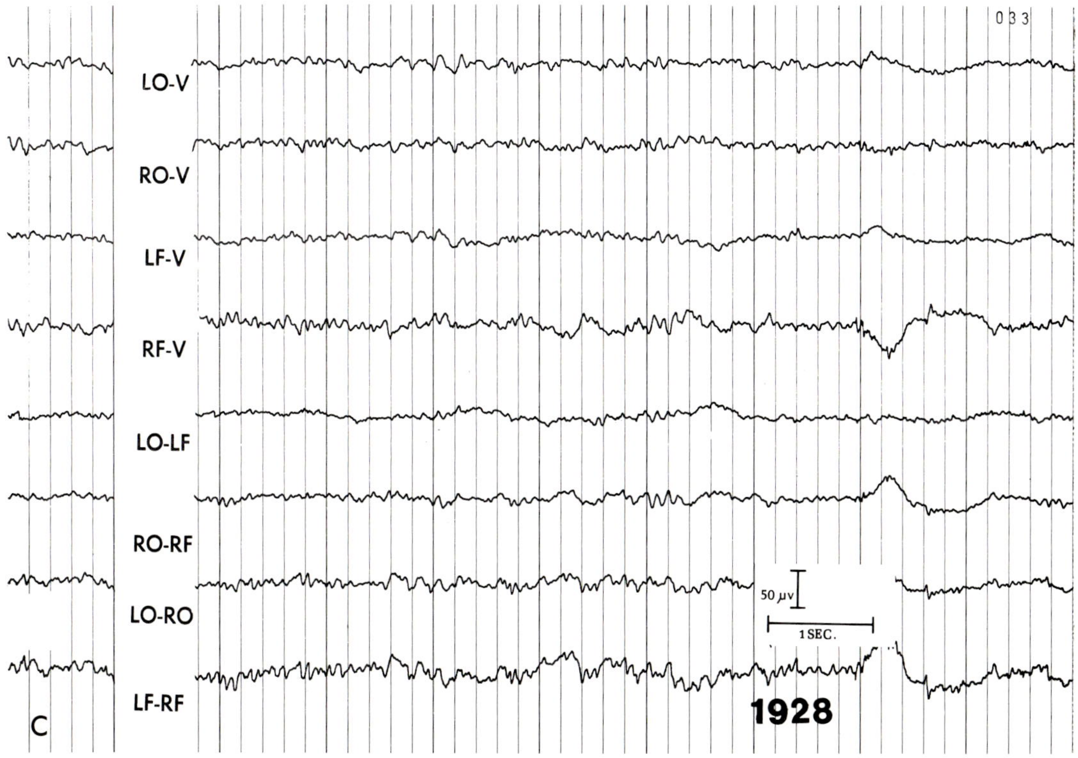

FIGURE 7–27 *Continued* *B.* Tracing from a 5-year-old Boston terrier that had become suddenly blind. Note the generalized slowing and paroxysmal 5-Hz discharges. Some spikes are also evident. An oligodendroglioma involving the left caudate nucleus and protruding into the lateral ventricle was found at necropsy. *C.* Tracing obtained from a 4-year-old poodle with grand mal type seizures. Note generalized, random, medium to slow waves, 5–12 Hz, 10–30 microvolts. A hemangioblastoma of the midbrain and upper medulla was found at necropsy.

Legend continued on the following page

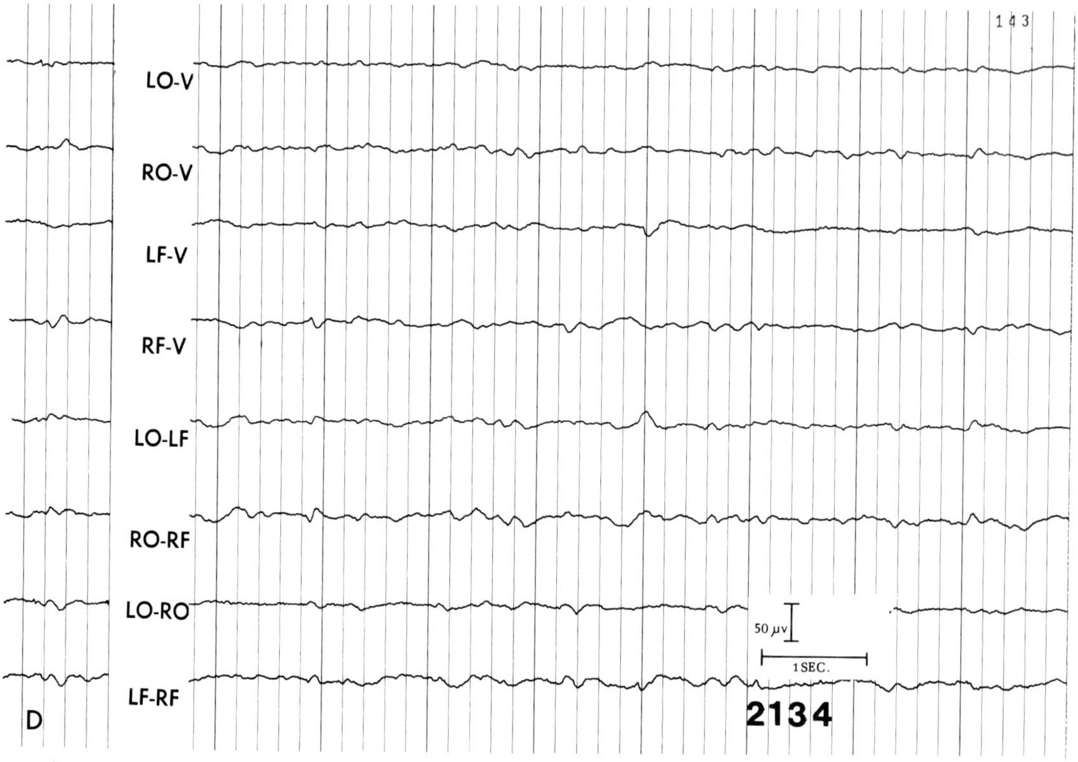

FIGURE 7–27 *Continued* *D.* Tracing obtained from a 6-year-old Great Dane with a history of blindness and ataxia. At the time of the EEG recording the animal was severely depressed. Note the generalized random slow waves in all leads. The animal did not respond to auditory or tactile stimulation. A diffuse cerebral astrocytoma was found at necropsy.

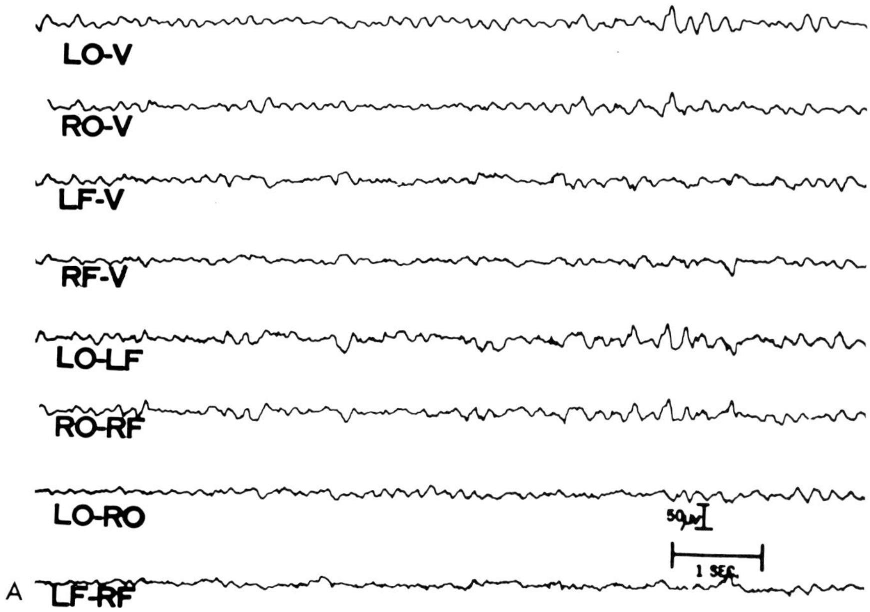

FIGURE 7–28 *A.* Tracing obtained from a dog with frequent seizures of the grand mal type. A diagnosis of infection with *Toxoplasma gondii* was made at necropsy.

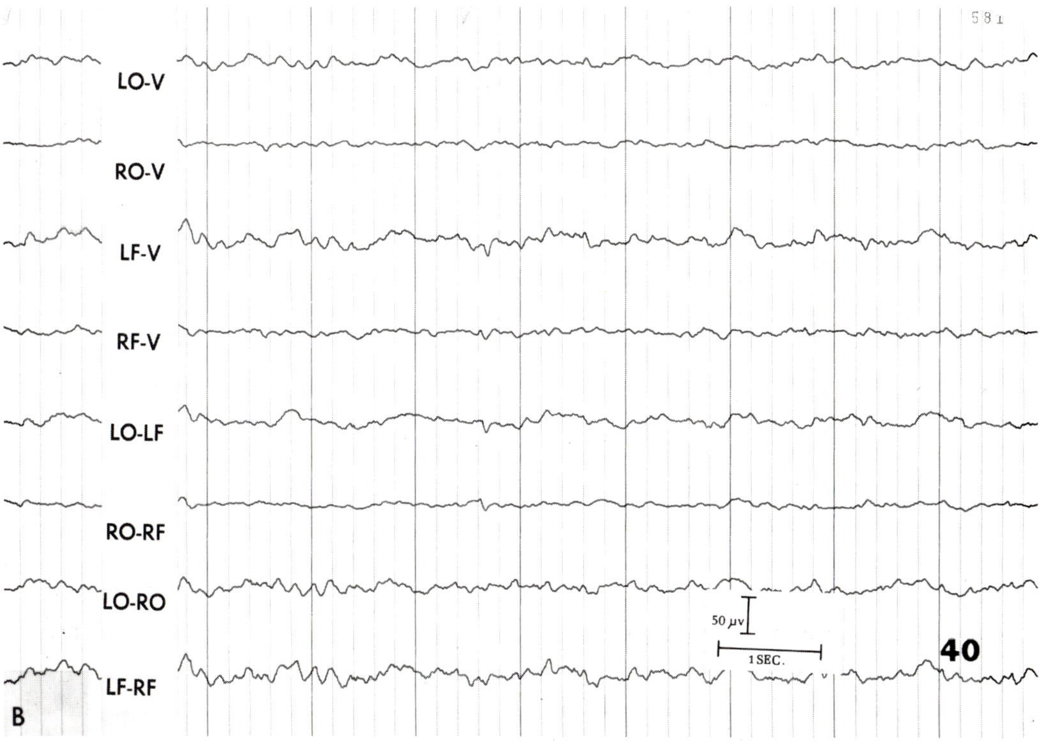

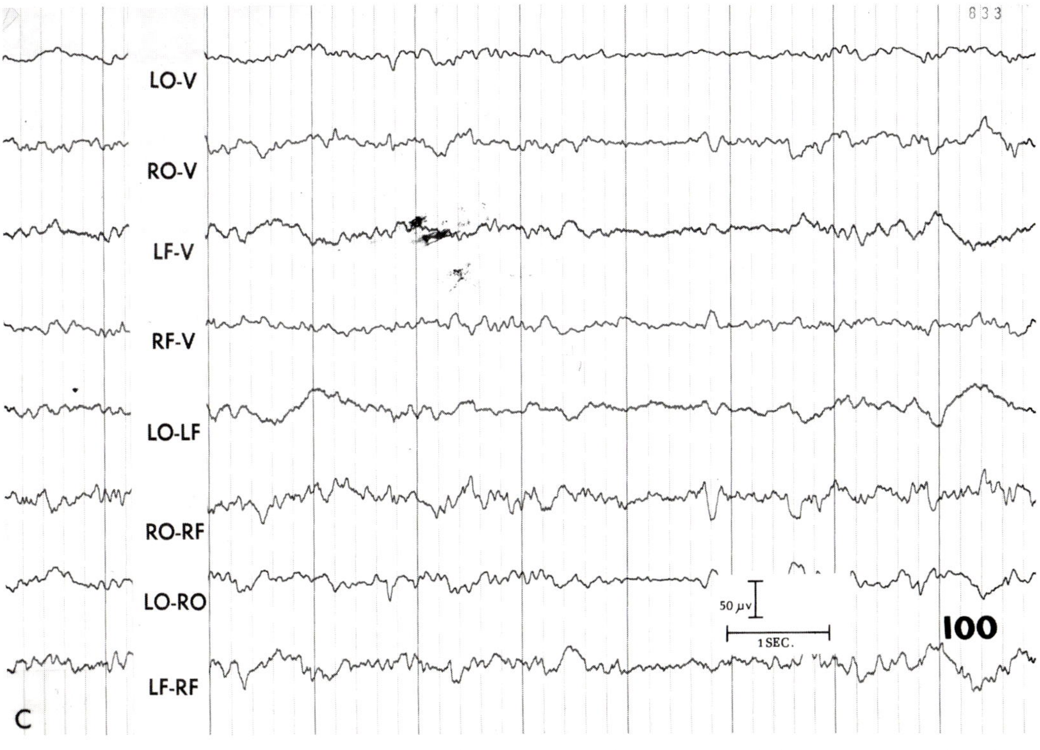

FIGURE 7–28 *Continued* *B*. Tracing obtained from a 3-year-old Afghan hound with a severe uveitis and post-orbital abscess of the left eye. The animal developed depression and seizures. Note the asymmetry of leads and slow waves in the left frontal area. A diagnosis of blastomycosis was made at necropsy. *C*. Tracing obtained from a dog with generalized seizures and depression. Note the irregular random wave forms. A diagnosis of cryptococcosis was made at necropsy.

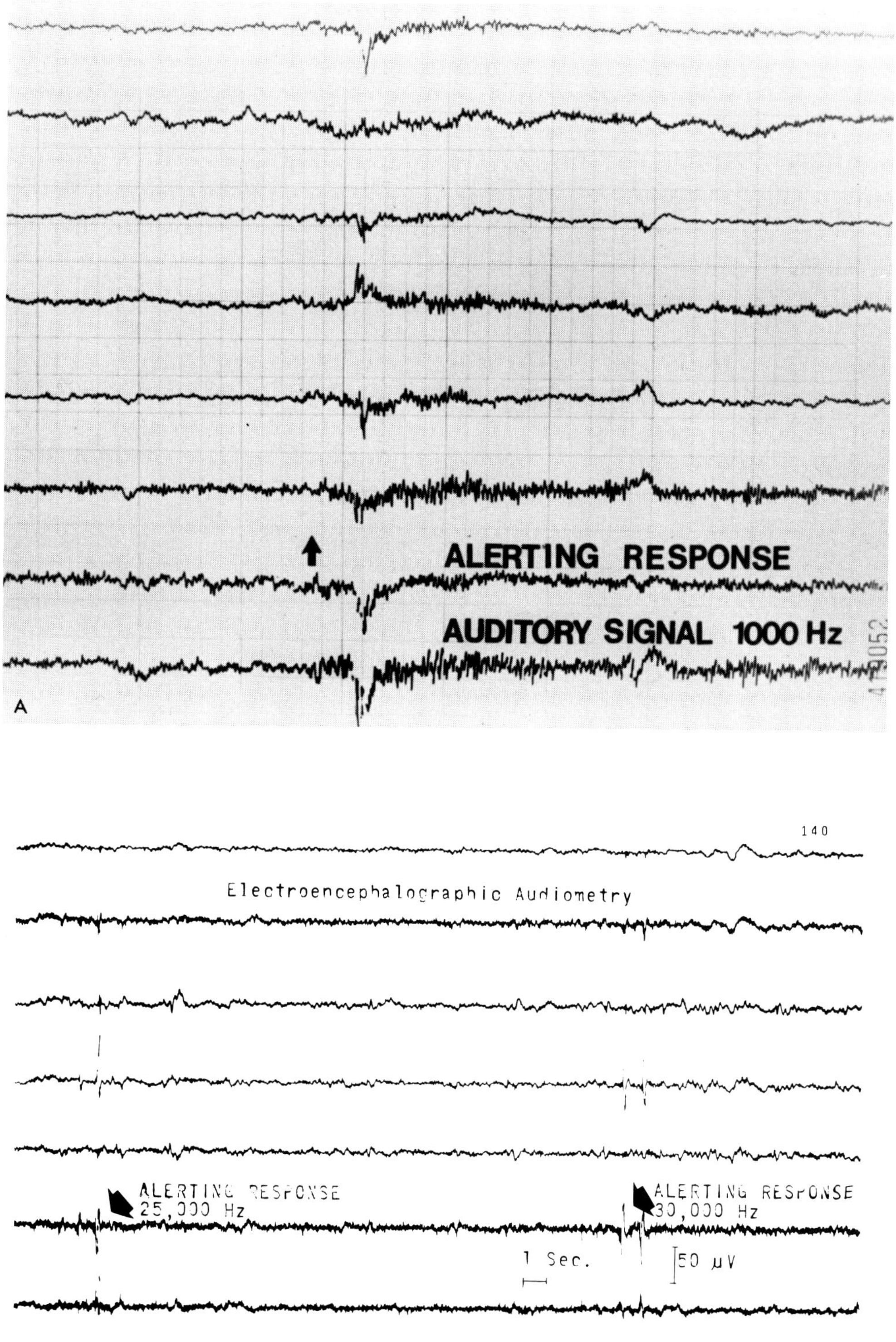

FIGURE 7–29 *A*. Typical arousal (alerting) response seen following an auditory signal. Paper speed 30 mm/sec. *B*. Alerting response seen at both 25 and 30 kilohertz (arrows) auditory signals. Paper speed 6 mm/sec.

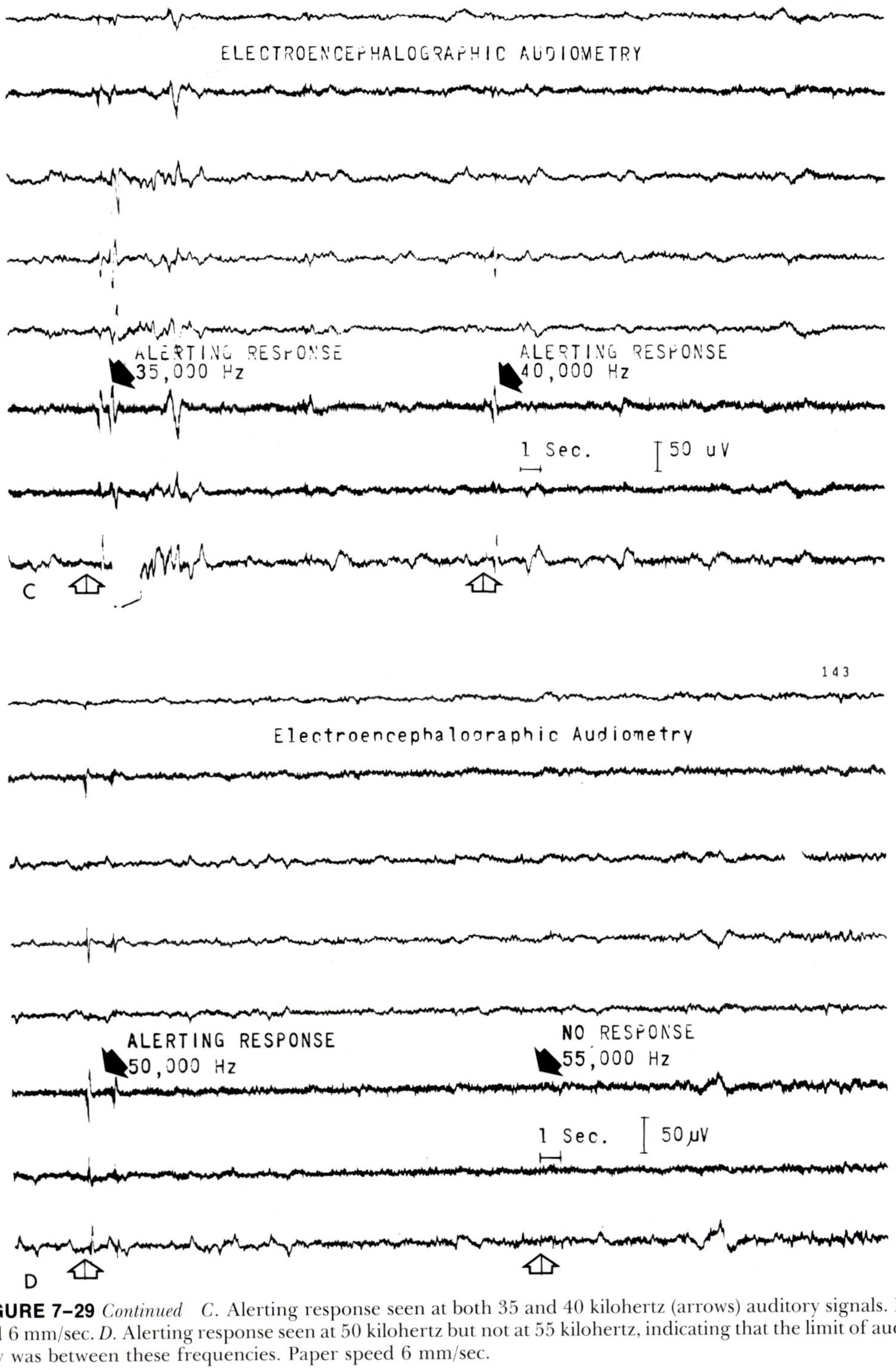

FIGURE 7–29 *Continued* *C*. Alerting response seen at both 35 and 40 kilohertz (arrows) auditory signals. Paper speed 6 mm/sec. *D*. Alerting response seen at 50 kilohertz but not at 55 kilohertz, indicating that the limit of auditory acuity was between these frequencies. Paper speed 6 mm/sec.

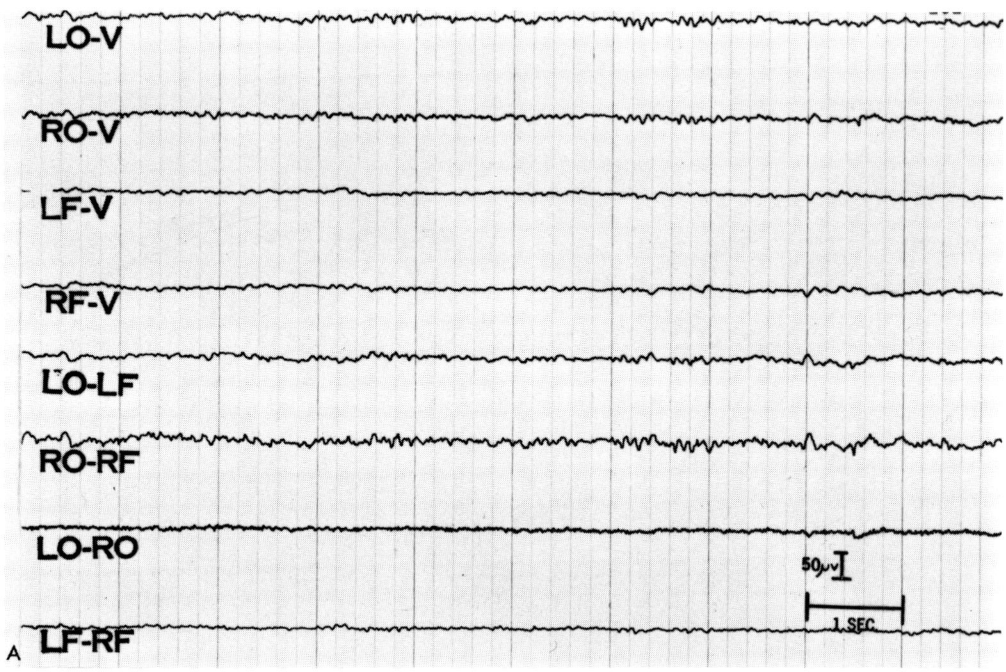

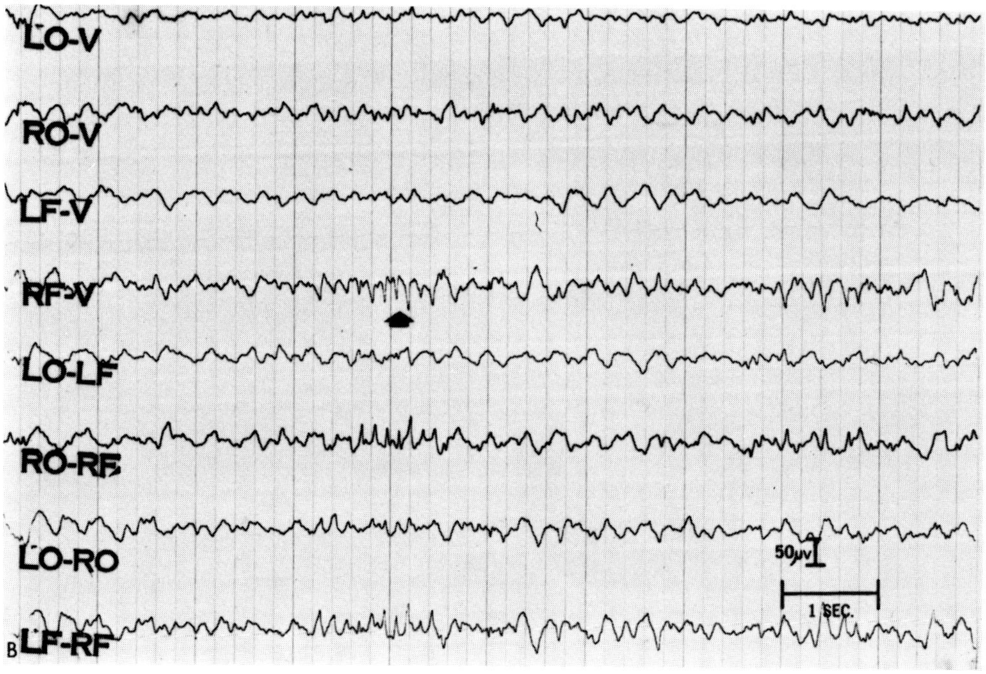

FIGURE 7–30 *A–D.* Depths of cortical depression induced by sodium pentobarbital in dogs. Left occipital (LO-V), right occipital (RO-V), left frontal (LF-V), and right frontal (RF-V) leads are paired against a common terminal, "V," vertex. Bipolar leads taken across the left hemisphere (LO-LF), right hemisphere (RO-RF), occipital (LO-RO), and frontal (LF-RL) regions. *A.* Electroencephalogram of healthy, awake, relaxed, mature dog. *B.* Dog in stage III, plane 3 surgical anesthesia; there is "barbiturate spiking" (arrow), especially in right frontal area. *C.* Burst suppression observed in dog in very deep anesthesia, stage III, plane 4. *D.* Complete suppression of cortical activity in dog due to excessive depression by sodium pentobarbital. Death due to medullary paralysis will follow soon.

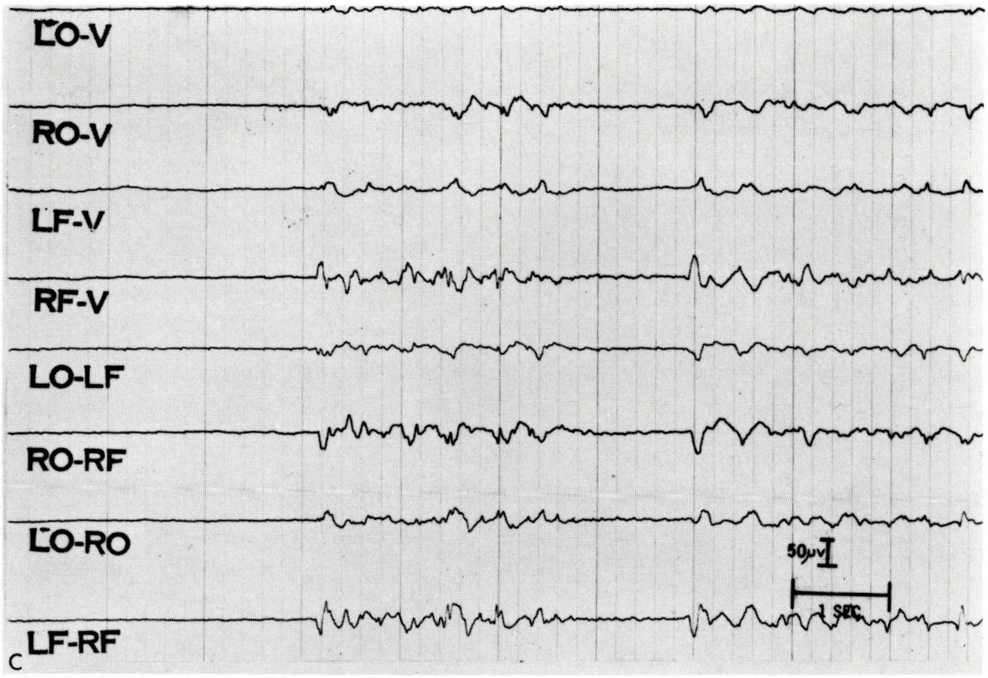

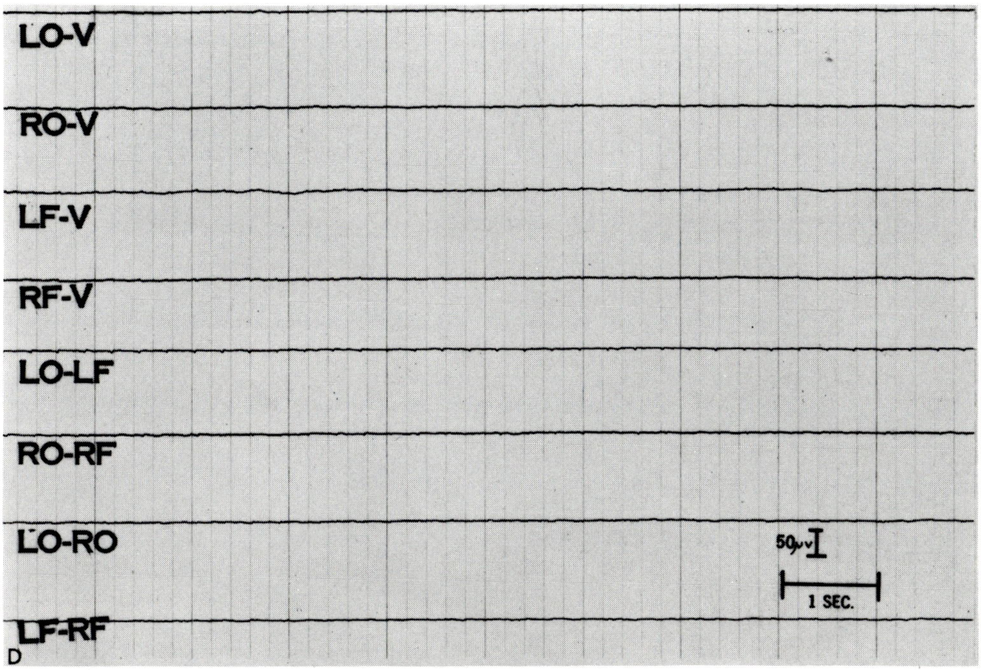

FIGURE 7–30 *Continued*

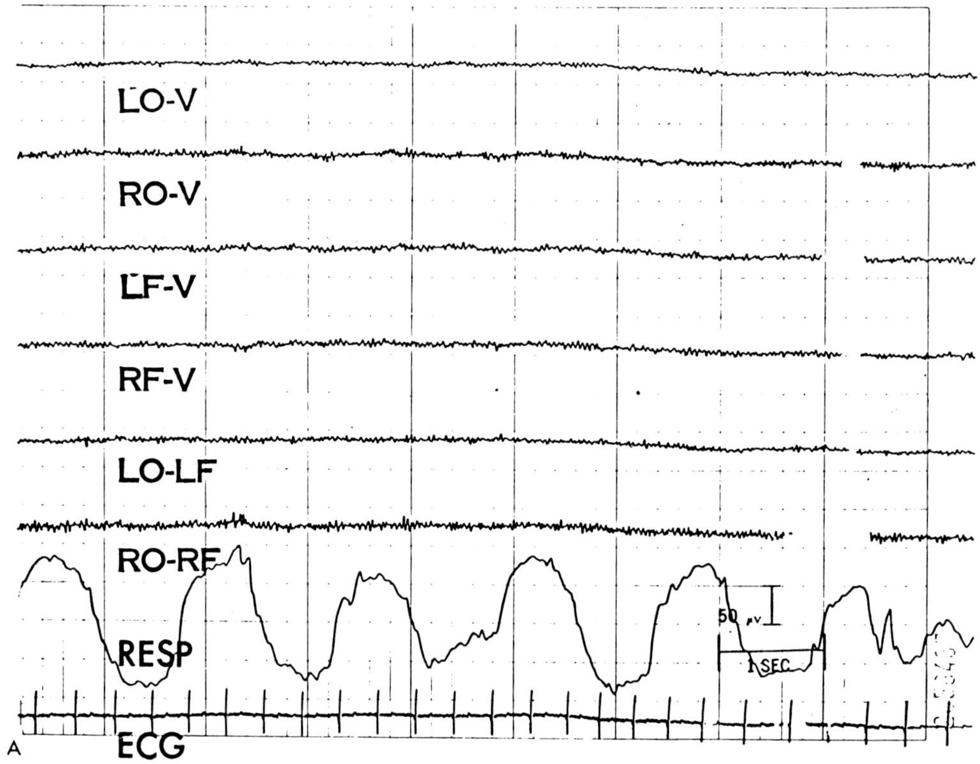

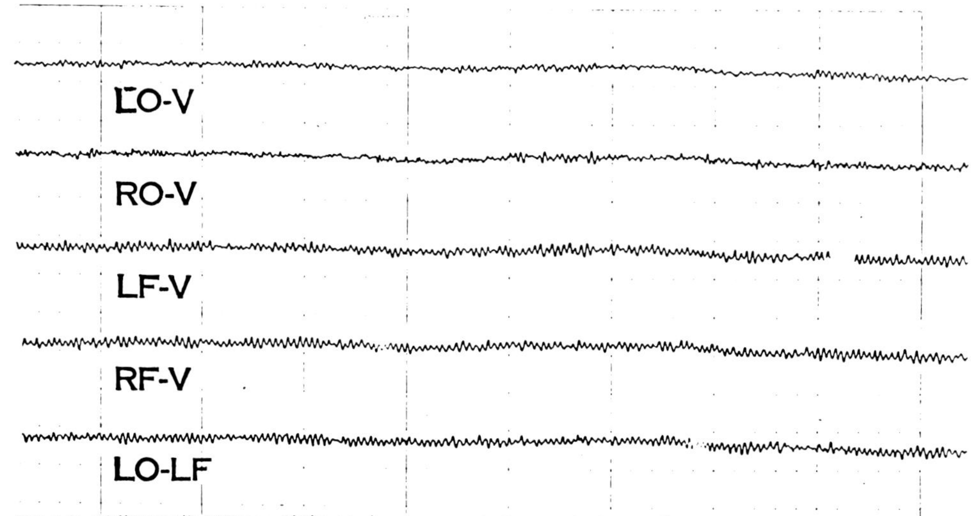

FIGURE 7–31 Depths of cortical depression induced by halothane. *A*. Electroencephalogram of a healthy, awake, attentive, mature dog. *B*. Halothane induction shows a 15–20 Hz pattern with spindling. *C*. Dog in stage III, plane 1. *D*. Dog in stage III, plane 2.

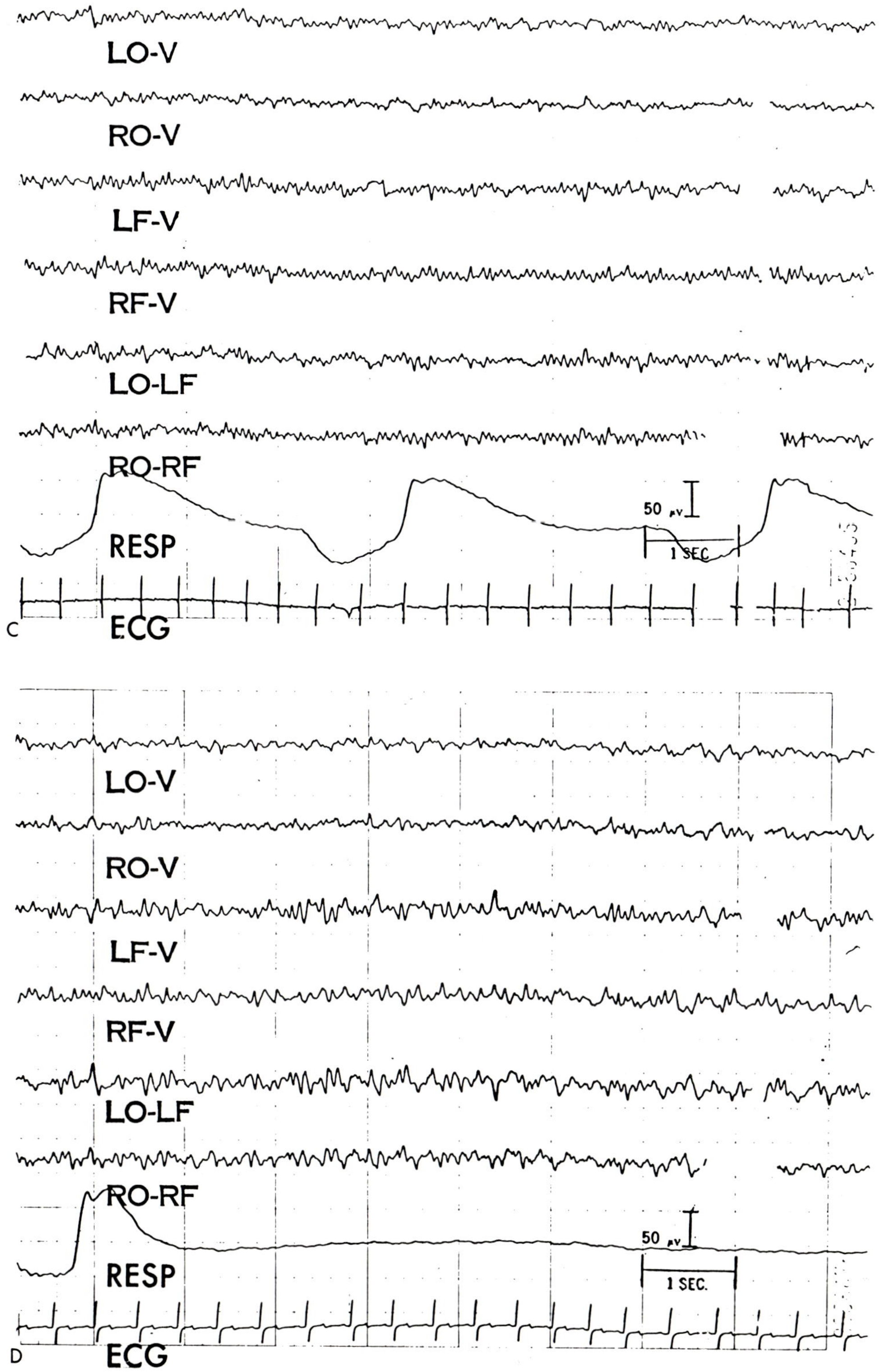

FIGURE 7–31 *Continued*

Figure 7–31 continued on following page

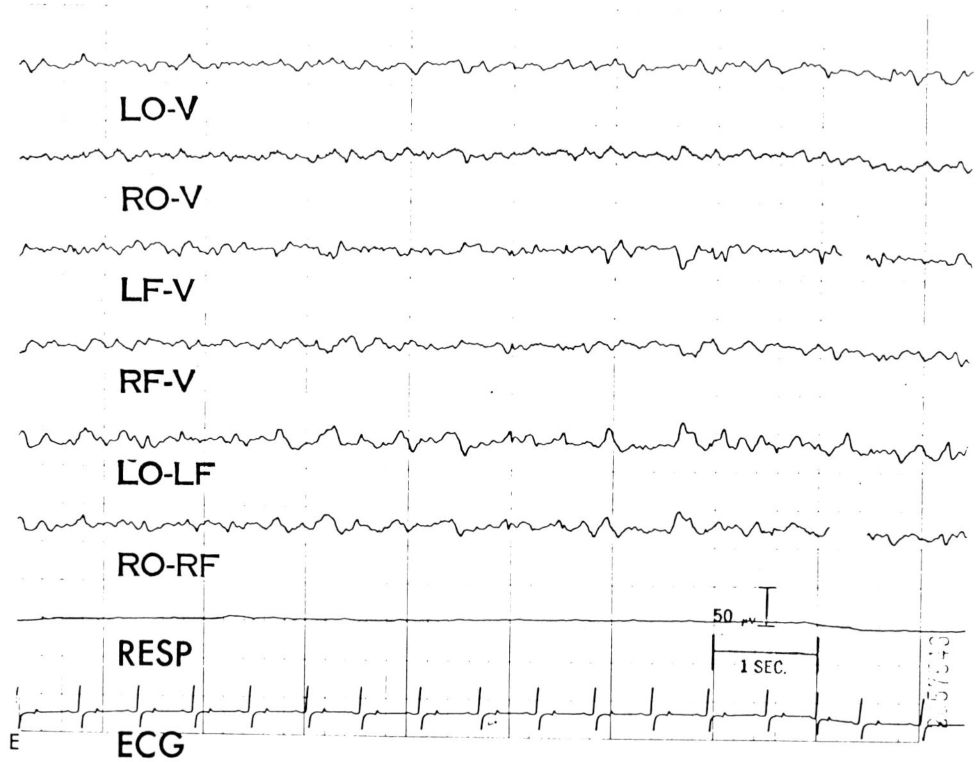

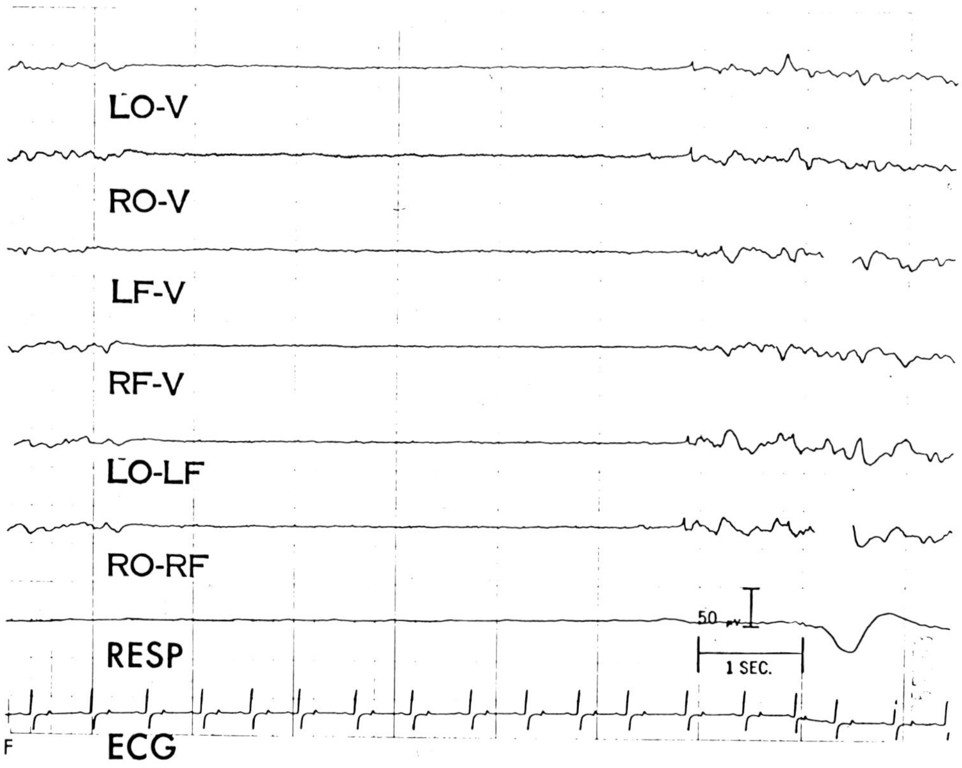

FIGURE 7–31 *Continued* *E.* Dog in plane III, stage 3–4. *F.* Dog in plane IV with burst suppression, indicating impending medullary paralysis.

dominant feature. In the dog, it is possible to demonstrate midline tumors that influence both hemispheres and to localize unilateral hemispheric tumors if they involve the occipital, parietal, or frontal areas. With the techniques now available, it is not possible to demonstrate temporal tumors unless they are large enough to produce abnormalities of other associated structures.

Other Infections

Invasion of the brain by organisms such as *Blastomyces dermatitidis, Toxoplasma gondii,* and *Cryptococcus neoformans* give rise to abnormal EEG patterns. The patterns are not diagnostic for the specific infection, but are suggestive of brain damage (Fig. 7–28).

ELECTROENCEPHALOGRAPHIC AUDIOMETRY

A dog's hearing ability is difficult to determine. Clinical tests used to determine whether a dog can hear consist of auditory stimuli produced by loud noises, high- and low-pitched whistles, and spoken words or commands familiar to the dog. If the dog hears these sounds, he may respond by changing his posture or by moving his head, eyes, and ears toward the direction of the sound. If the dog is unresponsive to these sound stimuli, it is assumed that he is deaf. However, disinterest, distraction, temperament, depression, pain, and other unrelated conditions can prevent the dog's reacting to the sounds and commands. The final decision as to whether a dog can hear or not is an arbitrary one at best.

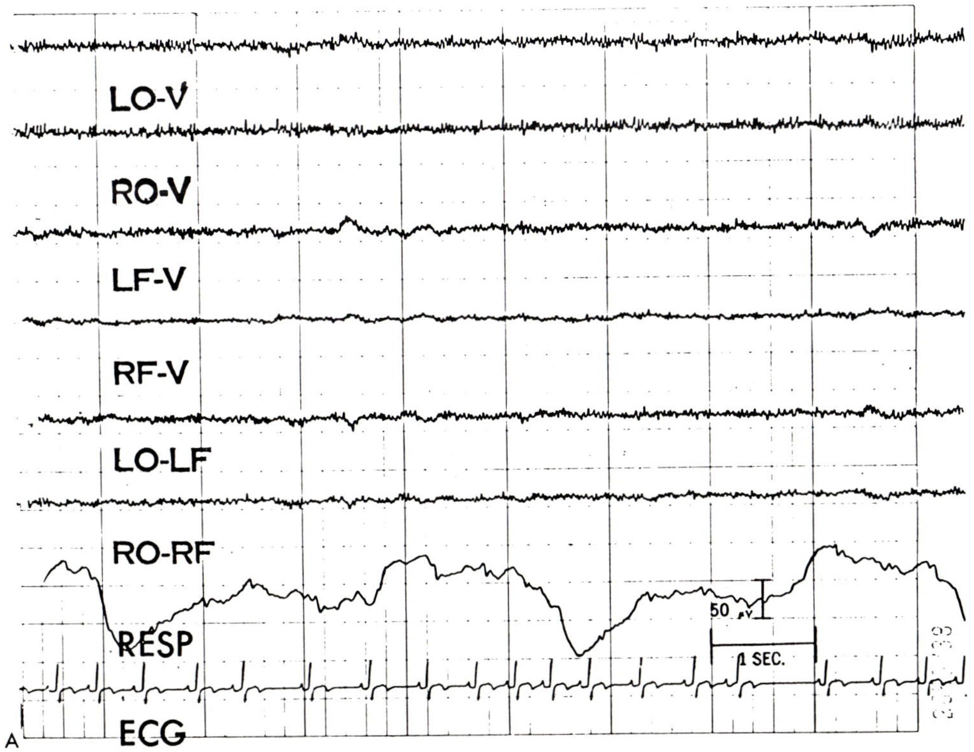

FIGURE 7–32 Depths of cortical depression induced by methoxyflurane. *A*. Electroencephalogram of a healthy, awake, attentive, mature dog.

Figure 7–32 continued on following page

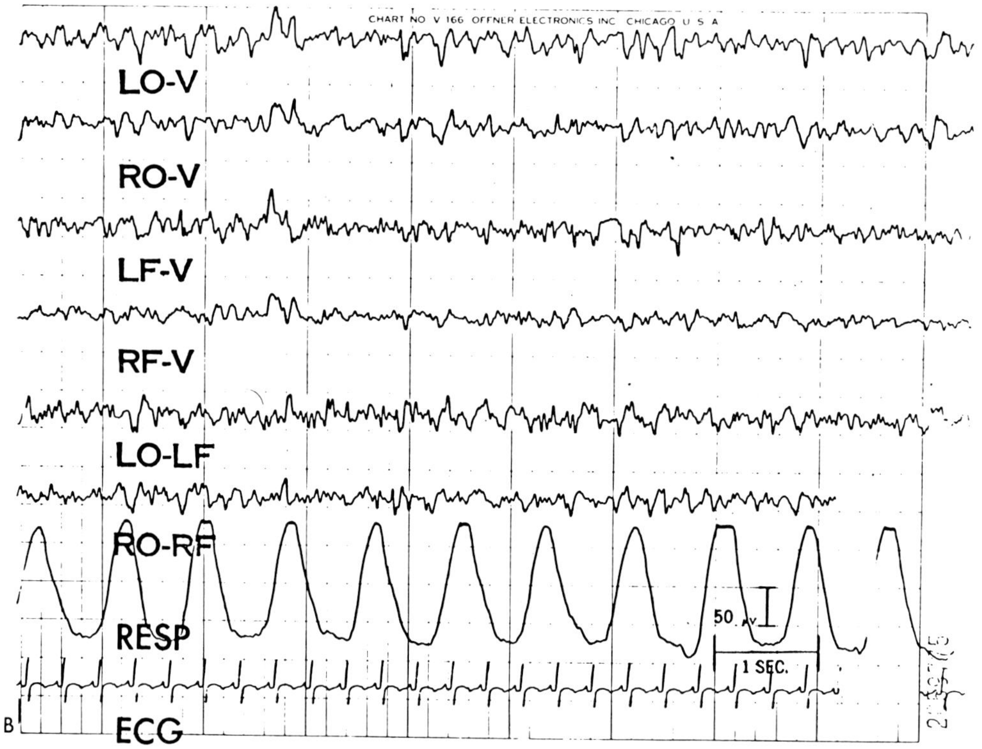

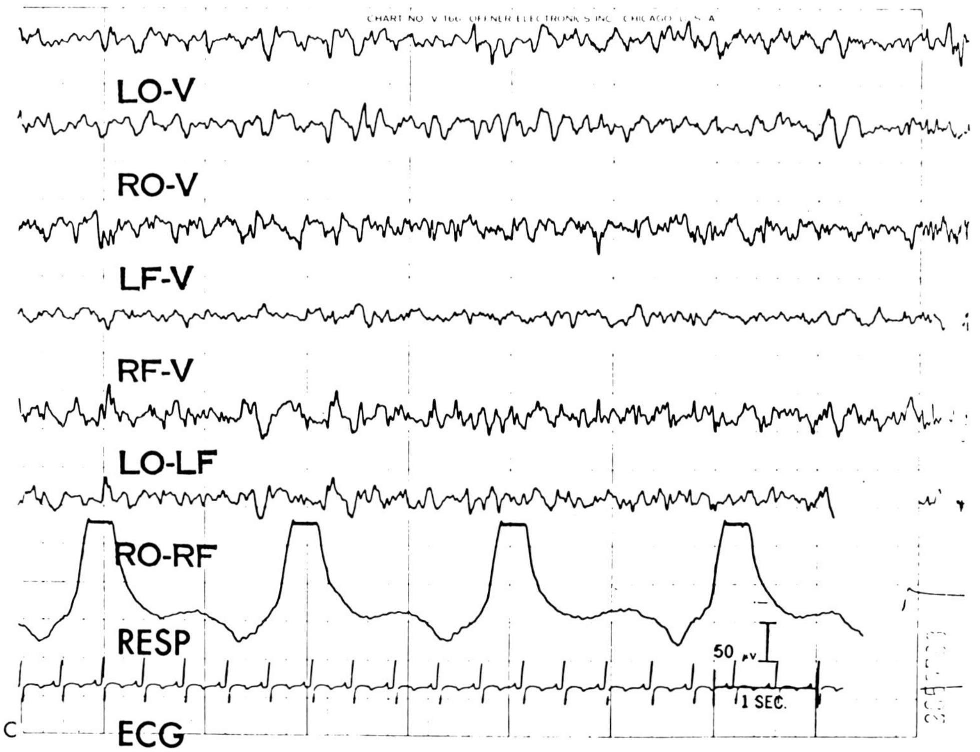

FIGURE 7–32 *Continued* *B*. Induction with methohexital and inhalation of methoxyflurane, 3 per cent. The pattern seen is a mixture of barbiturate random spiking and slow wave depression, *C*. Dog in stage III, plane 1, 30 minutes after methohexital induction. Cortical depression due to effects of methoxyflurane.

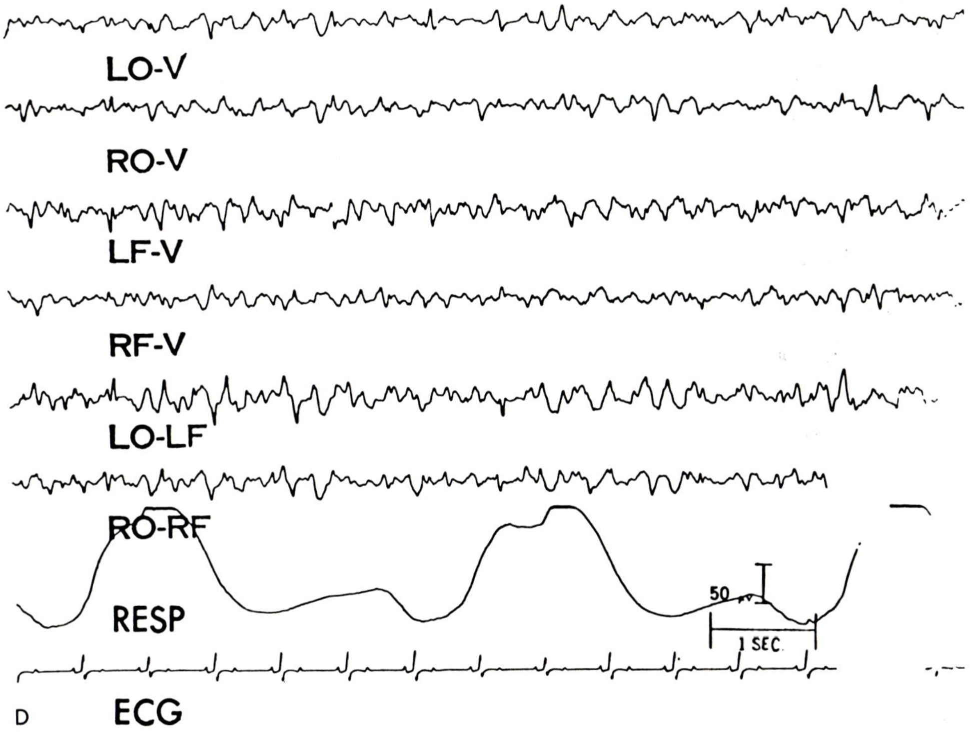

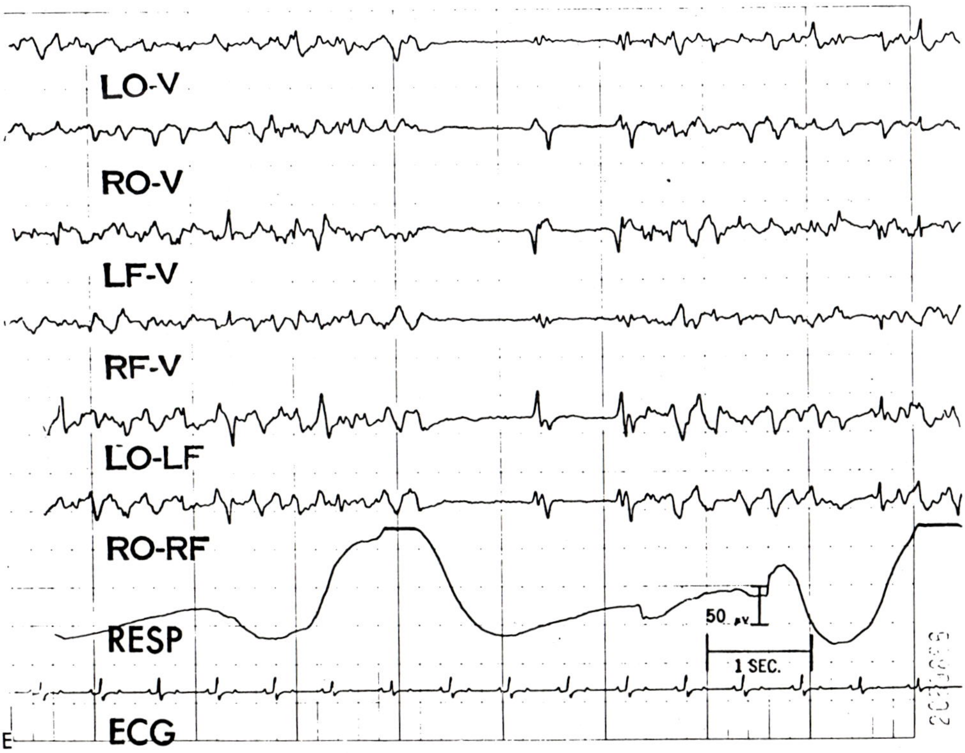

FIGURE 7–32 *Continued* *D.* Dog in stage III, plane 2. *E.* Dog in stage III, plane 4. Occasional burst suppression seen.

Figure 7–32 continued on following page

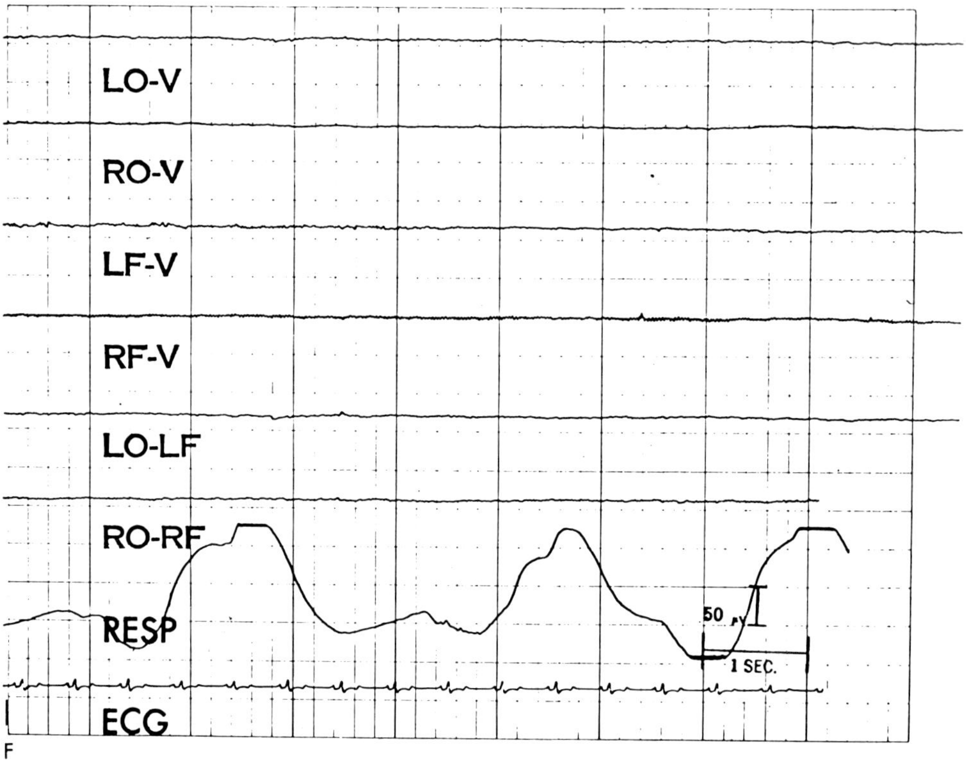

F

FIGURE 7–32 *Continued* *F.* Dog in stage IV, with severe cortical depression. This pattern could only be produced by forced respirations with methoxyflurane and a mixture of oxygen.

Electroencephalographic audiometry may be used to determine if the animal can hear and, if so, in what frequency range. This technique is based upon the *arousal (alerting) phenomenon,* a generalized response that is not specific for any type of stimulus. Auditory stimulation may act as a stimulus to alert the cerebral cortex and thereby make it possible to determine if the animal hears.

EEG tracings are obtained while the animal is in a relaxed state. During the recording period, sudden periodic auditory stimuli are elicited. The normal animal shows an increase in frequency and a decrease in voltage on the EEG. The most prominent feature of the recording is, however, a movement artifact at the time of the stimulus application. This movement artifact signals the reception of the sound by the animal. It is assumed that, if no change in the EEG and no movement artifact is seen, the animal cannot hear. The range of hearing can be determined if a variable-frequency audiogenerator and a high-frequency electrostatic loudspeaker are available. Using such equipment, the author has found an upper frequency range of hearing in a group of 25 dogs to be from 32 kilohertz to 52 kilohertz. In clinical cases of suspected deafness, the dogs either were found to be totally deaf or had an upper limit of hearing at 12 kilohertz. Figure 7–29 *A-D* shows a typical arousal response seen on EEG tracings.

ELECTROENCEPHALOGRAPHIC ANESTHESIA MONITORING

Electroencephalography is of value to an anesthesiologist and surgeon because the EEG correlates with the levels of depression produced by the anesthetics and the stages of anesthesia. In addition, it may serve as an indicator of generalized cerebral hypoxia and give evidence of localized impairment of cerebral blood supply.

Different anesthetic agents, both alone and in combinations, produce slightly different patterns; however, they all produce generalized slow wave activity and reduced voltages in deeper levels of anesthesia. Figures 7–30 through 7–32 show the patterns produced by three general anesthetic agents.

REFERENCES

1. Bagedda, G.: The electroencephalogram as an aid to the topographical diagnosis of a cerebral lesion in a puppy: neurosurgical treatment and the postoperative EEG: clinical course. J. Small Anim. Pract. *13*, 185, 1972.
2. Bagedda, G., and Arru, E.: Electroencephalography to assess brain damage before undertaking surgery on dogs. Clin. Vet. *94*, 373, 1971.
3. Bartels, K. E.: Surgical implantation of electroencephalographic electrodes in the dog. Am. J. Vet. Res. *37*, 83, 1976.
4. Beaver, B. V. G., and Klemm, W. R.: Electroencephalograms of normal anesthetized cats. Am. J. Vet. Res. *34*, 1441, 1973.
5. Blauch, B. S., and Cash, W. C.: A brief review of narcolepsy with presentation of two cases in dogs. J. Am. Anim. Hosp. Assoc. *11*, 467, 1975.
6. Brass, W.: Über electroencephalographische Untersuchungen beim Hund. Dtsch. Tieraerztl. p. 242, 1959.
7. Brechner, W. L., Walter, R. D., and Dillon, J. B.: *Practical Electroencephalography for the Anesthesiologist.* Charles C Thomas, Publishers, Springfield, Ill., 1962.
8. Charles, M. S., and Fuller, J. L.: Developmental study of the electroencephalogram of the dog. Electroencephalogr. Clin. Neurophysiol. *8*, 645, 1956.
9. Croft, P. G.: The EEG as an aid to diagnosis of nervous diseases in the dog and cat. J. Small Animal Pract. *3*, 205, 1962.
10. Croft, P. G.: Conditions affecting the central nervous system in small animals. J. Small Animal. Pract. *6*, 261, 1965.
11. Croft, P. G.: Use of the electroencephalogram in small animal medicine. Proc. Roy. Soc. Med. *58*, 548, 1965.
12. Croft, P. G.: Fits in dogs: a survey of 260 cases. Vet Rec. *77*, 438, 1965.
13. Croft, P. G.: The use of electroencephalographs in the detection of epilepsy as a hereditary condition in the dog. Vet. Rec. *80*, 712, 1968.
14. Croft, P. G.: Electroencephalography and space-occupying lesions in small animals. J. Small Anim. Pract. *13*, 175, 1972.
15. Cunningham, J. G.: Canine seizure disorders. J.A.V.M.A. *158*, 589, 1971.
16. deLahunta, A., and Cummings, J. F.: The clinical and electroencephalographic features of hydrocephalus in three dogs. J.A.V.M.A. *146*, 954, 1965.
17. Elsberry, D. D.: Computer processing of electroencephalographic data. Am. J. Vet. Res. *33*, 235, 1972.
18. Elul, R.: Specific site of generation of brain waves. Physiologist 7, 125, 1964.
19. Fletcher, T. F.: Electroencephalographic features of leukodystrophic disease in the dog. J.A.V.M.A. *157*, 190, 1970.
20. Florio, R., and Lapras, M.: Variations de l'électroencephalogramme dans l'épilepsie du chien: déductions cliniqués et thérapeutiques. Rev. Méd. Vét. *114*, 674, 1963.
21. Fox, M. W.: Postnatal development of the EEG in the dog. J. Small Anim. Pract. *8*, 71, 1967.
22. Fox, M. W., and Stone, A. G.: An electroencephalographic study of epilepsy in the dog. J. Small Anim. Pract. *8*, 703, 1967.
23. Fromm, G. H., and Bond, H. W.: The relationship between neuron activity and cortical steady potentials. Electroencephalogr. Clin. Neurophysiol. *22*, 159, 1967.
24. Gedoll, S. H.: Quantitative determination of hearing to audiometric frequencies in the electroencephalogram. Arch. Otol. *55*, 597, 1952.
25. Gibbs, F. A., and Gibbs, E. L.: *Atlas of Electroencephalography,* vols. 1–3. Addison-Wesley Pub. Co., Reading, Mass., 1958, 1959, 1964.
26. Hatch, R. D., Currie, R. B., and Grive, G. A.: Feline electroencephalograms and plasma thiopental concentrations associated with clinical states of anesthesia. Am. J. Vet. Res. *31*, 291, 1970.
27. Herin, R. A.: Induction technique changes and electroencephalographic body temperature, and pupillary light reflex studies in dogs anesthetized with electric current. Am. J. Vet. Res. *25*, 739, 1964.
28. Herin, R. A., Purinton, P. T., and Fletcher, T. F.: Electroencephalography in the unanesthetized dog. Am. J. Vet. Res. *29*, 329, 1968.
29. Hill, D., and Parr, G.: *Electroencephalography.* The MacMillan Co., New York, 1963.
30. Hughes, R. R.: *An Introduction to Clinical Electroencephalography.* John Wright and Sons, Ltd., Stonebridge Press, Bristol, 1961.
31. Kaleb, P., Rotztocil, V., and Kalab, Z.: Blockage of myopotentials by means of chlorpromazine during electroencephalographic examination of dogs. Acta Veterinaria Brno. *44*, 69, 1975.
32. Kiloh, I. G., and Osselton, J. W.: *Clinical Electroencephalography.* Butterworths, London, 1966.
33. Klemm, W. R.: Attempts to standardize veterinary electroencephalographic techniques. Am. J. Vet. Res. *29*, 1895, 1968.
34. Klemm, W. R.: Electroencephalograms of anesthetized dogs and cats with neurologic diseases. Am. J. Vet. Res. *29*, 337, 1968.
35. Klemm, W. R.: Subjective and quantitative analysis of the electro-encephalograms of anesthetized normal dogs—control data for clinical diagnosis. Am. J. Vet. Res. *29*, 1267, 1968.
36. Klemm, W. R.: *Animal Electroencephalography.* Academic Press, New York, 1969.
37. Klemm, W. R.: Electroencephalography in small animal medicine. Southwest. Vet. *22*, 92, 1969.
38. Klemm, W. R.: *Applied Electronics for Veterinary Medicine and Animal Physiology.* Charles C Thomas, Publishers, Springfield, Ill., 1976.
39. Klemm, W. R., and Hall, C. L.: Electroencephalographic "seizures" in anesthetized dogs with neurologic diseases. J.A.V.M.A. *157*, 1640, 1970.
40. Klemm, W. R., and Hall, C. L.: Electroencephalograms of anesthetized dogs with hydrocephalus. Am. J. Vet. Res. *32*, 1859, 1971.
41. Klemm, W. R., and Hall, C. L.: Electroencephalographic pattern abnormalities in dogs with neurologic disorders. Am. J. Vet. Res. *33*, 2011, 1972.
42. Klemm, W. R., and Hall, C. L.: Current status and trends in veterinary encephalography. J.A.V.M.A. *164*, 529, 1974.

43. Klemm, W. R., and Mallo, G. L.: Clinical electroencephalography in anesthetized small animals. J.A.V.M.A. *148*, 1038, 1966.
44. Laidlaw, J., and Stanton, J. B.: *The EEG in Clinical Practice.* E. and S. Livingstone, Ltd. Edinburgh, 1966.
45. Li, C. I, McLinnan, H., and Jasper, H. H.: Brain waves and unit discharges in cerebral cortex. Science *116*, 656, 1952.
46. Lucas, E. A., Powell, E. W, and Murphree, O. D.: Hippocampal theta in nervous pointer dogs. Physiol. Behav. *12*, 609, 1974.
47. Miller, M. H., and Polisor, L. A.: *Audiology Evaluation of the Pediatric Patient,* Charles C Thomas, Publishers, Springfield, Ill., 1964.
48. Pampiglione, G.: *Development of Cerebral Function in the Dog.* Butterworth, Inc., Washington, D. C., 1963.
49. Parker, A. J., Marshall, A. E., and Sharp, J. G.: Study of the use of evoked cortical activity for clinical evaluation of spinal cord sensory transmission. Am. J. Vet. Res. *35*, 673, 1974.
50. Prynn, R. B., and Redding, R. W.: The EEG continuum with methoxyflurane and halothane anesthesia. Am. J. Vet. Res. *29*, 1913, 1968.
51. Prynn, R. B., and Redding, R. W.: Electroencephalogram in occult canine hydrocephalus. J.A.V.M.A. *152*, 1651, 1968.
52. Redding, R. W.: A simple technique for obtaining an electroencephalogram of the dog. Am. J. Vet. Res. *25*, 854, 1964.
53. Redding, R. W.: Application of electroencephalography in small animal medicine. Proc. A.A.H.A. *230*, 1968.
54. Redding, R. W.: Diagnosis and therapy of seizures. J. Am. Anim. Hosp. Assoc. *5*, 79, 1969.
55. Redding, R. W., and Colwell, R. K.: Verification of the significance of canine electroencephalograms by comparison with electrocorticogram. Am. J. Vet. Res. *25*, 857, 1964.
56. Redding, R. W., Prynn, B., and Colwell, R. K.: The phenomenon of alternate sleep and wakefulness in the young dog. J.A.V.M.A. *144*, 605, 1964.
57. Redding, R. W., Prynn, B., and Wagner, J. L.: Clinical use of the electroencephalogram in canine encephalitis. J.A.V.M.A. *148*, 141, 1966.
58. Rogers, D.: Canine electroencephalographic audiometry. Senior seminar, Auburn University, Auburn, Alabama, 1970.
59. Rougier, G., and Faure, J.: Potentials bioélectriques du chien eveille et normal recueillie sur le crane. J. Physiol. (Paris) *12*, 716, 1950.
60. Ruckenbush, Y.: L'électroencephalogramme normal du chien. Rev. Méd. Vét. *114*, 119, 1963.
61. Sandove, M. S., Becka, D., and Gibbs, F. A.: *Electroencephalography for Anesthesiologists and Surgeons.* J. B. Lippincott Co., Philadelphia, 1967.
62. Schweingruker, R., Ketz, F., and Frankhauser, R.: Zu Frage der genuinen Epilepsie beim Hund. Psychiat. Neurol. *143*, 65, 1962.
63. Sims, M., and Redding, R. W.: The use of Dexamethasome in the prevention of cerebral edema in dogs. J. Am. Anim. Hosp. Assoc. *11*:439, 1975.
64. Tonuma, F.: Electroencephalography with barbiturate anesthesia in the dog. Can. Vet. J. *8*, 181, 1967.
65. Turbes, C. C., and Jobe, D.: EEG studies on emotional disorders of the cat and dog. Personal communication, 1973.
66. Ventruroli, M.: L'electroencefalogramma normale del cane. Clin. Veterinaria *85*, 252, 1962.
67. Weiderholt, W. C.: Electrophysiologic analysis of epileptic beagles. Neurology *24*, 149, 1974.

PART TWO

GENERAL NEUROSURGERY

CHAPTER 8

GENERAL CONSIDERATIONS IN NEUROSURGERY

GENERAL COMMENTS

Competence in neurosurgery is possible only if one has a thorough knowledge of anatomy, surgical physiology, pathology, and basic surgical techniques, as well as a complete understanding of the basic aspects of neurological diagnosis, which were discussed in Part I. Most veterinary neurologists, lacking additional competent staff, must currently either personally perform or directly supervise all aspects of the neurological examination (physical examination, electroencephalography [EEG], electromyography [EMG], x-ray, cerebrospinal fluid [CSF] pressures, and laboratory work) as well as the medication and any required surgery. This promotes patient welfare and a successful outcome and, eventually, real progress in the specialty of neurosurgery.

Because of its *anatomical* peculiarities and unique functions, the central nervous system (CNS) is markedly different from other systems and organs in the body. The brain and spinal cord are uniquely constructed of soft, friable tissue, supported by a relatively weak connective tissue called neuroglia. Both of these organs are surrounded with membranes called meninges, which help to support the organs and to maintain their general shape and conformation. The brain and cord, along with their meninges, are intimately housed in the bony cavities called the cranium and spinal column.

The CNS is highly *vascular.* In man, the brain represents only 2.2 per cent of the total body weight, but it receives 15 per cent of the total cardiac output.[11] In the dog, the brain is said to represent about 0.6 per cent of the body weight and the blood flow is 63 ml/min/100 gm of brain.[16] The brain also has the highest oxygen requirement of any tissue in the body—about 20 times that required for resting muscle[25]—and 20 per cent of the total body oxygen consumption.[18] Therefore, the CNS is highly sensitive to lack of blood or oxygen. Since venous return must be comparable to arterial supply of CNS tissue, trauma may cause congestion, edema, and swelling. Because of the cerebral bony encasement, a little swelling quickly produces pathologic changes.

Another peculiarity of the CNS is the modified lymph system known as the *cerebrospinal fluid.* The formation of CSF, its flow in the ventricles, its absorption, and its various functions are discussed in detail in Chapter 21. The CSF bathes and acts as a cushion to the delicate CNS tissues, and it is of special concern to the neurosurgeon.

Last, but not least, the special peculiarity of the CNS is its very complex *physiological functions,* which are extremely vital for the physical well-being of the patient. Improper handling or indiscriminate invasion or resection of these tissues can kill or severely incapacitate the patient. It is an established fact that the capacity of the CNS to regenerate is extremely limited, although compensatory function can develop. The peripheral nerves can generally regenerate in time if continuity is maintained.

From the aforementioned peculiarities of

CNS tissues, one must conclude that neurosurgery involves some special considerations. Because of generous blood supply, these tissues heal readily. However, because of the previously mentioned *barriers*, such as the blood-brain, CSF-brain, and CSF-blood barriers, antibiotics or chemotherapeutic agents may not reach the brain in high enough concentrations to combat infections properly. Therefore, very meticulous surgical manipulations and complete asepsis are mandatory when CNS tissue is surgically invaded. In addition to strict asepsis, broad spectrum antibiotics and occasionally adrenocortical steroids should be administered prior to and after surgery.

Since the brain is highly vascular, direct surgical invasion is generally accomplished by blunt dissection or low-grade cautery rather than by scalpel. Hemostasis must be maintained. These tissues cannot be sutured directly, but must be approximated indirectly by dural suturing or reconstruction. Appropriate fluid, medications, and nursing care must be prescribed judiciously [15,31]

ANESTHESIA[17, 27, 39, 41, 50]

Anesthesia is one of the most important considerations in the well-executed neurosurgical procedure. Unfortunately, the veterinary surgeon may not have an anesthesiologist or even a person with sufficient training to whom he can delegate all details of presurgical medication and the anesthetic procedure. The surgeon himself, then, will need to prescribe and supervise these considerations personally. He will be able to do this only after all data are evaluated from the physical, x-ray, EEG (if appropriate), and laboratory examinations.

LOCAL ANESTHESIA

Local or regional anesthesia in veterinary neurosurgery has limited application because of lack of patient cooperation and lack of the general muscle relaxation necessary for the procedures. On occasion, epidural anesthesia can be used in spinal operations in the posterior lumbar, sacral, or coccygeal areas. Sedatives are generally needed to maintain a quiet, motionless patient when local or regional anesthesia is employed. The use of sedatives, tranquilizers, or local anesthetics in the various diagnostic procedures, such as EEG, spinal taps, and radiographic examinations, has been discussed in Part I.

PREANESTHETIC THERAPY[27, 29]

Preanesthetic drugs are used to (1) allay apprehension and aid in restraint, (2) ease induction of anesthesia and recovery, (3) act as pharmacological adjuncts to general anesthesia, and (4) counteract the side effects and reflex responses evoked by some general anesthetic agents. The common preanesthetic agents are anticholinergics (e.g., atropine), narcotics, and tranquilizers. Generally, patients who have CNS injuries should not be given narcotics and tranquilizers while being monitored during medical therapy since they depress or obliterate the conscious state. Usually brain injuries do not cause mania or hysteria, and the use of such drugs is therefore not necessary. Restlessness due to discomfort can usually be controlled with proper nursing and medical care. Also, narcotics in general and morphine in particular promote nausea, salivation, and vomiting; loss of body temperature; depression of respiration and blood pressure; and depression of the conscious state. Tranquilizers other than diazepam (Valium) are epileptogenic, a hazard which could have serious consequences in CNS injury. Therefore, of the tranquilizers, diazepam is the preferred drug for sedation or as a preanesthetic. Among the narcotics, mild doses of oxymorphone hydrochloride (Numorphan) would be appropriate for sedation or preanesthesia in a fractious patient. Levallorphane (Lorfan), nalorphine (Nalline), and naloxone (Narcan) are specific antagonists for narcotics, and naloxone is also specific for reversing the effects of its parent compound, oxymorphone.[27, 29]

Atropine is the almost universal preanesthetic agent. Atropine blocks acetylcholine at the postganglionic terminations of cholinergic fibers in the autonomic nervous system. It inhibits salivation and production of mucus in air passages. It blocks bradycardia and hypotension following laryngeal stimulation produced by the endotracheal tube. Methoxyflurane or halothane is generally chosen as the anesthetic agent in CNS surgery, and atropine lessens the bradycardia that results from increased vagal tone associated with the use of these anesthetics. The main disadvantage of atropine is that it may increase tachycardia already present in young animals. In bronchiectasis, atropine may promote retention of secretions and diminish the elimination of them. The usual dose of atropine as a preanesthetic agent is 0.04 mg/kg (0.02 mg/lb) of body weight.[29]

GENERAL ANESTHESIA

General anesthesia is usually required for major neurosurgical procedures. Because the patient frequently is in a state of neurological depression or suffering from concomitant disorders of other organs, barbiturates should not be used as the primary anesthetic agent. Medium-acting barbiturates, such as sodium pentobarbital, should rarely be used, because of depression of vital functions (cardiovascular and respiratory) and lack of necessary elimination due to slow detoxification and elimination. One must have the capability of immediate control of the plane of anesthesia, especially in CNS surgery. This can be accomplished only by using inhalation anesthetic agents.[32, 33]

For decades, ether has been one of the safest inhalation agents, but for most operative facilities and methodologies it is hazardous because of its explosive properties. In more recent years, the availability of nonexplosive agents, such as halothane (Fluothane) and methoxyflurane (Metofane), and efficient equipment for administration of anesthetics has solved this problem. There seems to be little indication for any other method of general anesthesia in veterinary neurosurgery today.

Halothane and methoxyflurane are related agents and have similar metabolic effects. Both agents are effective anesthetics, but because of their respective physical properties, they must be administered in different types of vaporizers. Since they can be effectively used with oxygen in a semiclosed system, the unit cost per patient is not prohibitive in veterinary practice (Figs. 8–1 to 8–3).

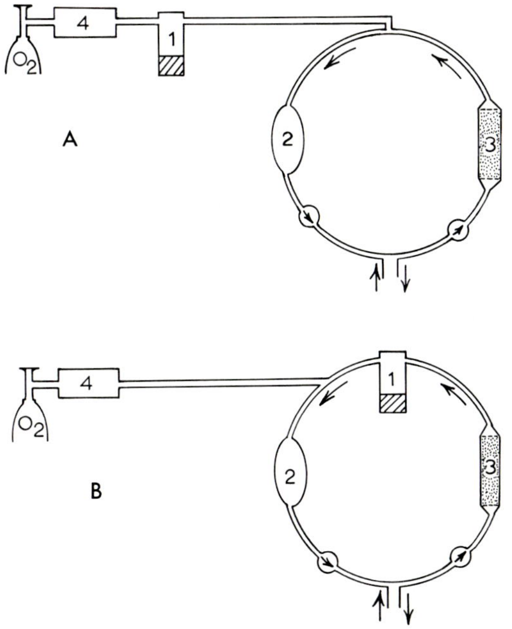

FIGURE 8–1 Schematic drawing for halothane and methoxyflurane circle system administrations. *A.* Out-of-circuit vaporizer used for halothane. *B.* In-circuit vaporizer used for methoxyflurane. (1) Vaporizer; (2) rebreathing bag: (3) CO_2 absorber; (4) flow meter.

Since halothane is a very potent agent that volatilizes more easily than methoxyflurane, it is mandatory that special vaporizers be used in the anesthetic circuit. Halothane has the advantage of producing a more prompt anesthetic effect and a quicker recovery. Since it is more volatile than methoxyflurane, it should be given with care and skill.

Methoxyflurane is considerably less volatile than halothane, so induction is slower. Since it is stored in body fat during anesthesia, it is less readily eliminated; hence recovery is somewhat slower than it is with halothane. However, recovery seems to be accomplished with less excitement. A special vaporizer is also needed for this agent.

Both methoxyflurane and halothane are stable and can be left in the vaporizer between operations. Since each agent is given with oxygen in a closed system, the level of anesthetic effect is easily and delicately controlled, and tissue oxygenation can be varied according to patient and surgical requirements. These two agents are effective in both diagnostic and surgical procedures involving the nervous system.

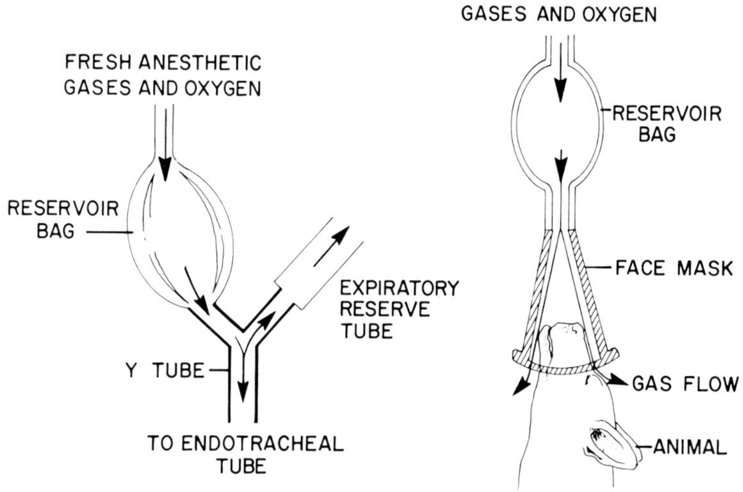

FIGURE 8–2 Examples of two types of semiopen (nonrebreathing) systems useful in dogs weighing less than 5 kilograms. The Ayre's Y system (left) is used when the animal is intubated. To prevent dilution of the anesthetic with room air, the expiratory reserve tube should be large enough to equal twice the tidal volume of the animal. When a mask is used (right), the mask should be applied loosely to allow continuous escape of gas. Carbon dioxide rebreathing will be prevented in both systems by fresh gas flow rates equal to twice the minute alveolar ventilation volume—i.e., 1 to 2 l/min. (From McDonell, W.: Principles of anesthesia. *In Canine Surgery*, 2nd Archibald ed. American Veterinary Publishers, Santa Barbara, Calif., 1974.)

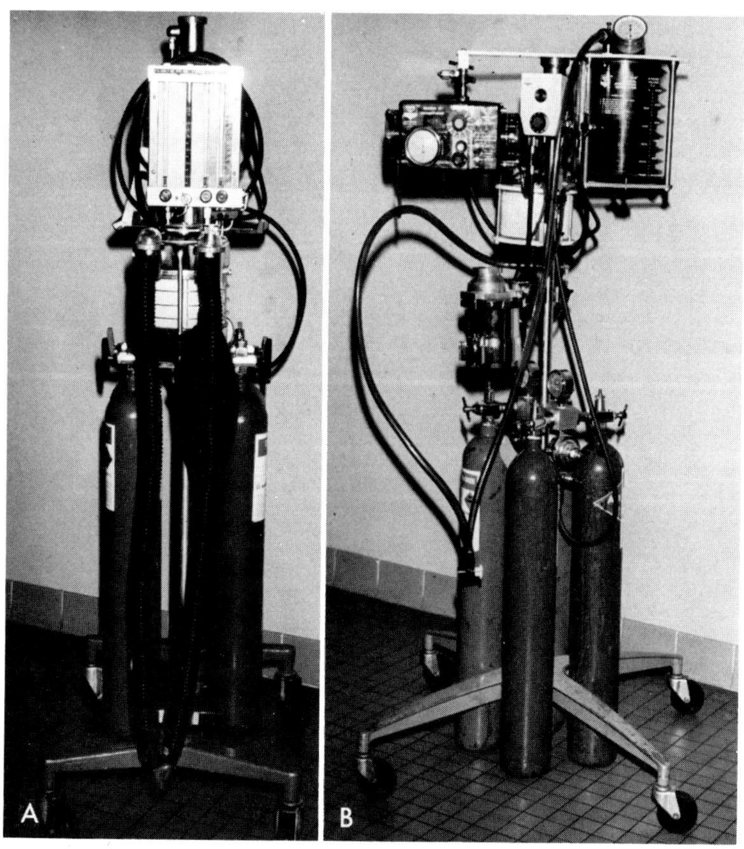

FIGURE 8–3 *A*. Example of modern gaseous anesthesia equipment. *B*. Resuscitative equipment.

In recent years nitrous oxide has been used as an adjunct in gaseous anesthesia. Nitrous oxide (N_2O) is nonexplosive, nonirritating, quickly absorbed, and eliminated without effect in most organs of the body, and is therefore considered one of the safest anesthetic agents. For optimal results, it should be mixed with an equal amount of oxygen in one of the halothane or methoxyflurane anesthetic machines. With care, a higher proportion of nitrous oxide to oxygen can be used, e.g., 70–30 or 60–40 per cent. Nitrous oxide promotes smooth induction and requires less maintenance anesthetic for surgical procedures.[27]

However, it is contraindicated in the initial stages of neurosurgery until hyperventilation has been established. Nitrous oxide can cause an increase in intracranial pressure because of vasodilatation unless hyperventilation has been previously established.[12] Nitrous oxide is also contraindicated when air has accumulated in the body, such as after diagnostic pneumoventriculography, pneumocystography, and pneumoperitoneal procedures, and in clinical cases of pneumothorax or emphysema. Such accumulations of gases in the body will be accentuated with nitrous oxide anesthesia.[27]

Adrenergic stimulants or analeptics are not recommended, since they tend to potentiate the occurrence of cardiac irregularities. In methoxyflurane and halothane anesthesia analeptics are seldom necessary because the anesthetic level can be effectively controlled. However, if a stimulant is needed, mephentermine (Wyamine, a vasoconstrictor) and pentylenotetrazole (Metrazole) or methetharimide (Mikedimide), both corticomedullary stimulants, can be employed.[13-15, 31]

Since inhalation agents such as halothane and methoxyflurane are most effectively and economically used in a closed or semiclosed system, tracheal intubation is necessary. The patient and necessary equipment are prepared so that intubation can be quickly performed. A light dose (8 to 12 mg/kg) of an ultrashort barbiturate anesthetic (sodium pentothal) is promptly and carefully administered intravenously. When the animal undergoes initial CNS depression, the tube is quickly positioned and secured in the mouth. The cuff is inflated moderately so that it will not produce a mucosal necrosis, and the volatile anesthetic is administered in maximum concentration. By the time the barbiturate wears off, the volatile agent has initiated its effect, and the entire induction phase of anesthesia has been efficient, smooth, and safe. If the patient's state is too critical for the very light administration of a barbiturate, either induction with halothane and nitrous oxide by means of a mask or local anesthesia (Pontocaine solution, 2 to 4 per cent) of the epiglottis and laryngeal orifice can facilitate the intubation procedure. In a severely depressed patient, the latter method works nicely.

As the patient starts to recover from anesthesia, the endotracheal tube should be removed. Careful observation for at least 5 minutes should then be routine in case laryngeal spasms occur. In such an event, a tracheostomy should be performed immediately. Introduction of the endotracheal tube by mouth after laryngeal spasms have developed is generally dangerous to the patient and frustrating to the surgeon, and the spasm may continue indefinitely.

Cerebral hypoxia is a prominent cause of edema and swelling. Therefore, any circumstance that would promote hypoxia should be corrected immediately.

MONITORING THE PATIENT

It was emphasized previously that a veterinary surgeon, in addition to performing the surgical procedure, must also supervise the anesthesia and monitor the patient's condition. In neurosurgery, one must generally have a semiskilled person available to regulate and administer the anesthetic and to keep accurate charts on the rate and quality of respiration and pulse and the presence of reflexes. Such assessments should be made continuously and recorded every 5 to 10 minutes. The surgeon should be constantly receiving such data from the anesthetist.

In monitoring during anesthesia, the reading of vital signs (pulse, respiration, and estimated blood pressure) should be recorded every 5 to 10 minutes, and body temperature should be recorded as the surgeon prescribes. The depth of anesthesia should be considered continuously. The reflex signs and responses to nervous stimuli in light and deep surgical anesthesia using methoxyflurane and halothane can be summarized as follows:

1. Atropine given as a preanesthetic agent makes pupillary changes inconsistent, but in general they should be constricted in light and dilated in deep anesthesia.

2. The oral reflex (spreading jaws forcibly) is present in light anesthesia and absent in deep anesthesia.

3. Respiration is irregular in rate and depth in light anesthesia and regular in deep anesthesia. In deep anesthesia, the chest moves inward on inspiration and outward on expiration owing to paralysis of the intercostal muscles.

4. The heart rate is fast in light anesthesia and slower and stronger in surgical anesthesia. Deep anesthesia produces a slow, weak heart rate.

5. The oral membrane in light halothane and methoxyflurane anesthesia are pink and slightly moist. Deep anesthesia produces dry, pink velvety, and warm mucosa.

Blood pressure can be estimated by palpating the femoral and lingual arteries. If the lingual artery is imperceptible, marked peripheral vasoconstriction and hypotension have occurred. In the lip mucosa, the rate of capillary filling after digital blanching should be almost instant. If it takes more than 2 seconds, hypotension or compensatory sympathetic vasoconstriction is surely present. In such a case, usually the membranes are pale before blanching.

Central venous pressure (CVP) is easily ascertained in critical surgery by passing the tip of the indwelling catheter into the anterior vena cava adjacent to the right atrium. This pressure indicates venous return to the heart in relation to cardiac output and normally ranges from 1 to 3 cm water. Values under 8 cm of water may be normal, while those over 8 cm indicate some degree of overload of the vascular system or heart failure. Jennings[20] has described a method of estimating CVP when a dog is in the dorsal recumbent position. With the head elevated 10 degrees, the jugular vein is filled by digital pressure, thus allowing the venous blood to seek its own level; the percentage of the vein that remains distended is noted. In normal or subnormal CVP no distension of the vein is evident, while a high CVP shows a fully distended vein. The distal jugular vein is occluded first, and then the anterior portion; the percentage of vein that remains distended when distal pressure is removed is recorded as the reading. Because of ease of observation, this method would probably be most reliable in a lean, long-necked dog. After such jugular distension the reading is compared with the CVP readings.[20]

One of the best physical means of monitoring cardiac function is an esophageal stethoscope. If the surgeon is working alone, a tube extension and ear piece can be assembled for him or he can attach the esophageal probe to an amplifier.

Electronic equipment has become available to aid in patient monitoring during actual surgery or in general intensive care. Solid state equipment that is economically feasible for the practicing surgeon can monitor EEG, EKG, pulse, and respiration by auditory (beep) and/or visual recording (oscilloscope screen and blinking light) (Fig. 8–4). Very inexpensive equipment, such as a whistle attachment in the circle flow tubes of the anesthesia machine, can demonstrate respiratory movements but may restrict the volume flow and increase the dead space. A photoelectric transducer auditory signal can be incorporated into the tubing of the machine to monitor the respiratory flow of air.* A pulse rate monitor and a "rough" indicator of peripheral circulation is available; it employs a photoelectric probe which is clipped on hairless tissue such as the tongue or lip.† An esophageal stethoscope can monitor the heartbeat as well as the respiratory flow (Figs. 8–5 and 8–6).

Equipment is now available to aid in monitoring that very important vital sign, blood pressure. Indirect blood pressure apparatus employs a cuff to the anterior tibial artery; serial recordings from it during surgery can provide a comparative monitoring of the patient's arterial blood pressure.‡ In acutely ill patients, arterial blood pressure can be recorded directly by cannulating an artery, such as the femoral artery, and connecting heparinized tubing di-

---

*Veterinary Precision Respiration Monitor, Industrial Scientific Research Corp., Anaheim, California.

† Pulse Rate Monitor, Equiquip Companies, Box 187, Newbury Park, California.

‡Arteriosonde 1010, Hoffman La Roche, Inc., Cranbury, New Jersey.

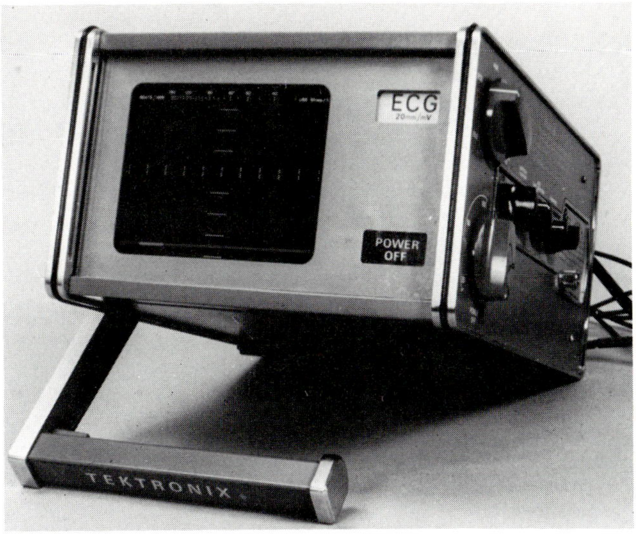

FIGURE 8–4 An electronic ECG, EEG, and pulse monitor.

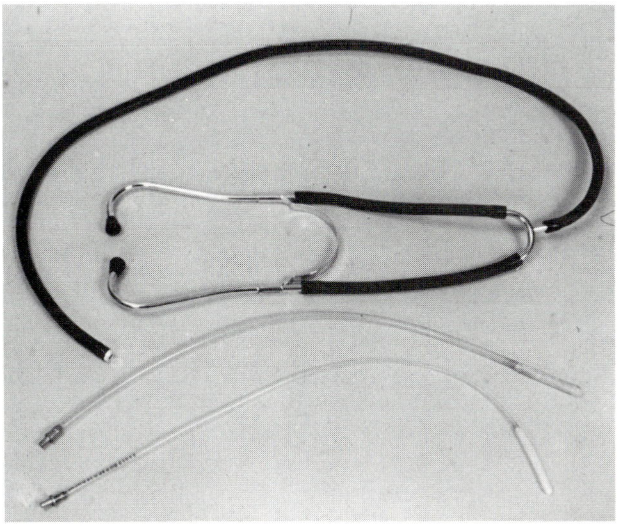

FIGURE 8–5 An effective and inexpensive means of monitoring pulse and respiration is the esophageal stethoscope.

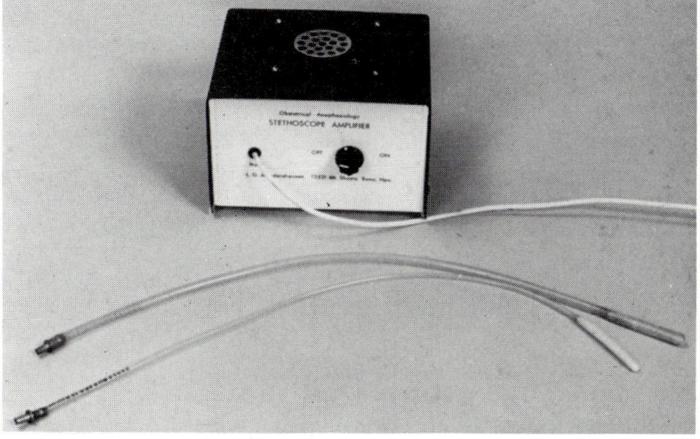

FIGURE 8–6 The heart sounds received by the probes can be amplified inexpensively so that audible monitoring is effected. The standard stethoscope is not needed.

rectly to a manometer or to a pressure transducer and recording device*[27] Evaluation of central venous pressure has been discussed. Blood pH, pCO_2, and pO_2 can be monitored if a blood gas analyzer is available.

At our clinic, routine monitoring in all major operations is performed by the esophageal stethoscope directly or by an amplifier† to demonstrate cardiac and pulmonary function, as well as the oscilloscope and/or EKG write-out recording, and general vital sign recordings. Critical cases are monitored with blood gas analyses. It is felt that this has been a major step in promoting patient well-being and that it is an extremely useful aid to the surgeon and other personnel in the understanding of physiological phenomena that occur during surgery.

SHOCK

Shock[42] is a difficult term to define in one sentence since it can be initiated by a multiplicity of insults that cause a body response to a disruption of physiological homeostasis and controlling mechanisms. One definition of shock would be that it is a clinical syndrome in which the cardiovascular system is incapable of perfusion of the animal in the normal physiological limits of pressure and flow. *Circulatory shock* is a condition in which tissue perfusion is not sustained, regardless of whether it was created by a reduction in cardiac output as in *hemorrhagic shock* or by the intense vasoconstriction that occurs during the early phase of *septic shock*. Cardiovascular compensation is an attempt to maintain adequate perfusion of two vascular beds immediately essential to life—the cerebral and coronary circulations—and the less critical vascular bed consisting of the splanchnic, cutaneous, and muscle systems. Once shock has occurred, it is rarely self-limiting. It may continue into the progressive phase even though the cause itself has not increased in severity. Other stages may be termed the "refractive phase," in which therapy sustains physiological mechanisms but is not capable of reversing the damage; and the "irreversible phase," in which no type of therapy can produce recovery.[42]

DYNAMICS OF SHOCK

The most common causes of the cardiovascular compensatory actions are hemorrhage, sepsis, trauma, and fluid loss. Reduction in blood pressure and cardiac output are compensated by tachycardia, which maintains cardiac output. The sympathetic nervous system and hormonal mechanisms increase peripheral vascular resistance and promote a redistribution of available intravascular fluid volume. Catecholamine release sustains perfusion of the coronary, cerebral, arterial hepatic, and adrenal vascular beds initially. These organs are more sensitive to blood-oxygen changes than the splanchnic and cutaneous structures. Systemic blood pressure maintained at 30 to 35 mm Hg for 2 hours will produce ischemic brain damage. Since the CNS has a major role in maintaining integration of homeostatic mechanisms in the body, reduction in blood-oxygen flow during shock can be deleterious to recovery. Changes in coronary blood flow are minimal when mean systemic pressure is maintained at 70 mm Hg or above; however, any pressure below this reduces coronary flow. In progressive shock, toxic materials developing from tissue ischemia at the capillary level contribute to cardiac depression and failure.[42]

As shock progresses, the depression of circulation of the splanchnic, mesenteric, muscular, and cutaneous tissues leads to changes in capillary perfusion and function. Loss in circulatory volume and endotoxin formulation in septic shock promote active changes at the microcirculatory levels distal to the metarterioles. Pre- and postcapillary sphincters contract, and blood is shunted away from the capillary beds. Hypotensive and endotoxic shock may produce severe ischemia of the gastrointestinal tract, causing continuous loss of plasma, fluids, and whole blood. If this occurs, shock has progressed to the irreversible stage.[42]

The pulmonary system can frequently be involved in shock, especially if traumatic injuries of the chest and upper abdomen

---

*Arterial Pressure Monitor, U.S. Catheter and Instrument Corp., Glen Falls, New York.

†Cardiopulmonary Sound Amplifier, L. G. Menderhausen, 13521 Mt. Shasta, Reno, Nevada.

have occurred. If surgery is necessary to remove a portion of liver, the stresses of anesthesia, surgery, shock, circulating materials from hepatic tissues, bile salts, toxins, and vasoactive substances may cause pulmonary involvement and death. Occasionally, pulmonary insufficiency develops a few hours or up to 5 days after trauma and apparently successful therapy. Death results from progressive hypoxemia and hypercarbia. If refractory shock continues for some time, pulmonary atelectasis, congestion, alveolar and parenchymal edema, and hemorrhage occur and death ensues. The mechanisms involved seem to be the release and absorption of toxins, vasoactive substances, metabolites from ischemic and damaged tissue, and the reinfusion of blood containing particulate debris and altered platelets. It is felt that infusion of stored blood containing platelet aggregates, microclots, and other particulate debris can contribute to pulmonary pathologic and physiologic changes, especially in shock.[42]

Although acute renal failure in shock is said to be uncommon in young animals, it can be a serious problem in an older animal or one with existing renal damage. Prolonged hypotension and poor renal perfusion seem to be the main factors; however, the activity of vasoactive hormones such as reninangiotensin and catecholamines contributes. If vasoconstriction persists for more than 12 to 24 hours, renal tubular damage occurs. Clinical signs are oliguria, glycosuria, renal tubular cells in urine sediment, and an increase in serum creatinine, potassium, and blood urea nitrogen.[42]

CLINICAL SIGNS

The classic signs of shock are tachycardia, hypotension as evidenced by a narrowing of pulse pressure or its absence in a small peripheral artery (e.g., dorsal pedal artery), weak pulse, mucous membranes that may be pale or muddy with a capillary refill time of more than 2 seconds, lowered rectal and extremity temperature (legs feel cold), hyperventilation (increased rate and effort), depressed mental status and mydriasis from cerebral hypoxia, general muscle weakness from inadequate muscle perfusion, and decreased urinary output. There are some exceptions to these signs—the mucous membranes may be hyperemic, and the temperature may be elevated in septic shock.[42]

TREATMENT

The characteristic signs of shock should be quickly determined, and treatment must be initiated as promptly as possible to hinder progression into an irreversible stage. Shock is seldom self-limiting. The initial and critical life-supporting procedures are (1) to ensure adequate ventilation and oxygen exchange, (2) to initiate resuscitative fluid therapy, and (3) to arrest major hemorrhage. Other procedures are considered when more details of the patient's condition are established. A summary of treatment of shock will be outlined.

1. Adequate ventilation is especially important in treatment of shock and in central nervous system injuries. Occasionally administration of oxygen by mask, intranasal catheter, or an oxygen cage is sufficient. If the animal is in marked distress an endotracheal tube, a tracheostomy catheter, or a tracheostomy tube is used. The endotracheal tube should be cuffed and moderately inflated to avoid aspiration of fluids; to facilitate removal of pulmonary secretions; and to administer oxygen or anesthesia.

2. Control of surface hemorrhage can be done by pressure bandage or ligation. An internal hemorrhage necessitates emergency surgical procedures.

3. Fluids providing balanced electrolytes such as lactated Ringers solution (or fluid with gluconate and acetate substituted for lactate) should be started rapidly. A vascular catheter with an appropriately large bore should be inserted in a leg vein, and fluids should be given at a rate of at least 80 ml/kg initially and up to 200 ml/kg in the first 12 hours in extreme cases. A large bore catheter should also be placed in the jugular vein so that the tip lies in the anterior vena cava for measurement of central venous pressure if needed. Appropriate blood samples are taken from the jugular catheter for monitoring the patient, and fluids are given through both catheters initially in the acute stage of therapy and as needed thereafter.[42]

Replacement with whole fresh blood may be indicated when in the judgment of the clinician the patient has suffered from severe blood loss, traumatic shock, or severe anemia, or if after proper initial replacement therapy the hematocrit falls to below 25 per cent. If blood is needed, it should be used in a ratio of 1 unit to every 3 to 4 units of fluid. In extreme blood loss (60 to 70 per cent), the ratio may be as high as six units of fluid to one unit of blood. If there is a history of previous transfusion, crossmatching is mandatory. To obviate the potentially dangerous phenomenon seen in the use of stored blood, fresh blood should be used or at least filtered through commercially available filters.[42]

4. Glucocorticosteroids should always be used in endotoxic and traumatic shock, such as intravenous administration of hydrocortisone sodium succinate (Solu-Cortef, 10–50 mg/kg) and dexamethasone (Azium, 2–6 mg/kg or more in cases of severe CNS trauma). These steroids are beneficial to the cardiovascular system because they decrease platelet adhesiveness and increase coronary blood flow, and they also block the myocardial depressant factor. They prevent the release of proteolytic enzymes and the swelling and bursting of lysosomes and release of lysosomal enzymes, increase lactic acid metabolism, prevent degranulation of mast cells, and increase phagocytic activity of leukocytes. Lillehei[23] terms corticosteroids the safest and most effective vasodilators. Their primary disadvantage is venular constriction that causes a bottleneck on the output side of the viscerocutaneous bed. Steroids also prevent capillary damage caused by bacterial endotoxin. Steroids are preferred over conventional vasodilators since phenoxybenzamine may expand venous capacity so rapidly that a severe hypovolemia results, and the effect of chlorpromazine does not last long enough.[23]

5. Broad spectrum antibiotics should be given intravenously.

6. Acid-base balance and need for sodium bicarbonate should be determined. If the equipment for such a determination is not available, 2 to 6 mEq/kg of sodium bicarbonate should be given partially as a bolus and the rest in intravenous fluids, since metabolic acidosis is a constant hazard.[42]

7. A urinary catheter should be inserted to monitor kidney function. If urine flow is less than 1.0 ml of urine per kg body weight per hour, mannitol can be given intravenously. A 25 per cent solution is diluted with equal parts of normal saline and given in a dose of 0.5 to 2 gm/kg. If diuresis is not evident within an hour, furosemide (Lasix) should be given in a dose of 2 mg/kg, and if this is not effective, the dose should be doubled.[42]

8. Vital signs should be evaluated at 15 to 20 minute intervals until they are stable. The syndrome of disseminated intravascular coagulation (DIC) can occur in shock; the signs are overt hemorrhage, prolonged clotting time, thrombocytopenia, and abnormal prothrombin and partial thromboplastin times. Heparin should be given when there is evidence of widespread coagulation of microcirculation; the dose is 250 IU/kg intravenously, repeated every 4 hours. Heparin should not be given routinely but only when there is evidence of DIC.[42]

9. Vasoactive drugs can be given when necessary if both the action of the drug and the condition of the patient are well understood. Otherwise they may cause damage. Isoproterenol (Isuprel) is a vasoactive drug which has been used in septic and traumatic shock. Its primary advantage over other vasopressors is its beta stimulatory effect. It increases myocardial contractility by its direct stimulatory effect on myocardial receptors, and it has a direct vasodilatory effect on peripheral receptors. The dual action of cardiac stimulation and peripheral vasodilation is beneficial. One should be aware of possible hypotension when using isoproterenol; preferably, adequate fluid replacement should take place before it is used. An alpha blocker, chlorpromazine (Thorazine) can be given in a total dose of 5.25 mg, depending on the size of the animal.[42]

10. All vital signs, laboratory results, monitoring data, and methods of therapy should be entered on the record for serial comparisons. Such record keeping promotes effective and intelligent therapy.[42]

GENERAL CONSIDERATIONS IN CLINICAL THERAPY

Some of the basic considerations in the body mechanisms of shock and its therapy have been described here. Textbooks should be consulted for details. It is the author's opinion that many clinicians overtreat with vasoactive drugs, some of which may be contraindicated. After airway, hemostasis, and hypovolemic measures have been initiated and steroids and antibiotics have been administered, patient monitoring and intensive care should be the rule rather than unrestrained use of other drugs. The patient should be handled as little as possible, and radical rapid changes of position should be avoided. Lifting, carrying, and rapid rotations of the patient cannot be tolerated by the stressed cardiovascular and pulmonary organs. Sedatives, analgesics, tranquilizers, and anesthesia should be avoided whenever possible. Anything that will disturb the neurological status is especially contraindicated in a CNS emergency.[42]

An important factor to be monitored in surgery and in shock is the patient's body temperature. If the patient's rectal temperature is below 37° C (or approximately 99° F), the body should be warmed, preferably by circulating warm water heating pads* or by blankets. Conventional heating pads or infra-red lamps should be used only with extreme caution, since the animal's skin can easily be burned, and cutaneous vasodilation and body fluid "shift" to the extremities or heat area may result. An electronic temperature probe or a continuous (nonconstricted mercury column) recording thermometer should be used.[42]

*Aqua-Pads, Gorman-Rupp Industries Division, Bellville, Ohio. Distributed by American Hospital Supply Corp., Chicago, Illinois.

POSITIONING OF PATIENT

Precise positioning of the patient as it relates to specific surgical procedures will be discussed with each procedure. Generally, the positioning of the patient in neurosurgery must be such that venous congestion, edema, and swelling of the brain will not be enhanced. The animal should not be stretched or secured to the table so that circulation or respiration is compromised. Frames over the body, especially the chest and head, make for easier visualization and also relieve these areas of heavy draping and pressure from other equipment. Cushions should always be used on the table for greater comfort of the patient, to alleviate pressure of bony prominences, and to conserve body temperature. In toy dogs and cats, a circulating warm water pad* may be used to maintain body temperature (Fig. 8–7). To promote natural surgical and venous drainage, the skull should be firmly immobilized in an elevated position for brain surgery. This position will provide for maintenance of an open air passage, direct oxygen administration, and ease of observation by the anesthetist, as well as patient comfort. Since neurosurgery is generally critical, positioning must provide for the maintenance of continuous intravenous administration and electronic monitoring. Neurosurgery is frequently time-consuming, so comfort to both the patient and the surgical team must be considered. The use

*Gorman-Rupp Industries Division, Bellville, Ohio.

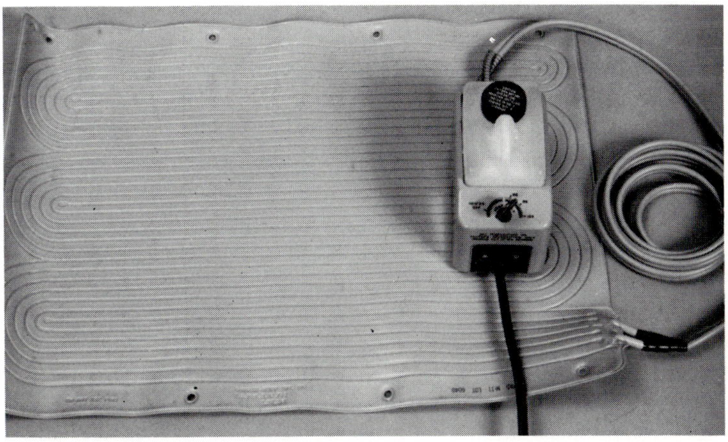

FIGURE 8–7 Circulating warm water pads are an effective means of combating loss of body temperature during and after general anesthesia and surgery.

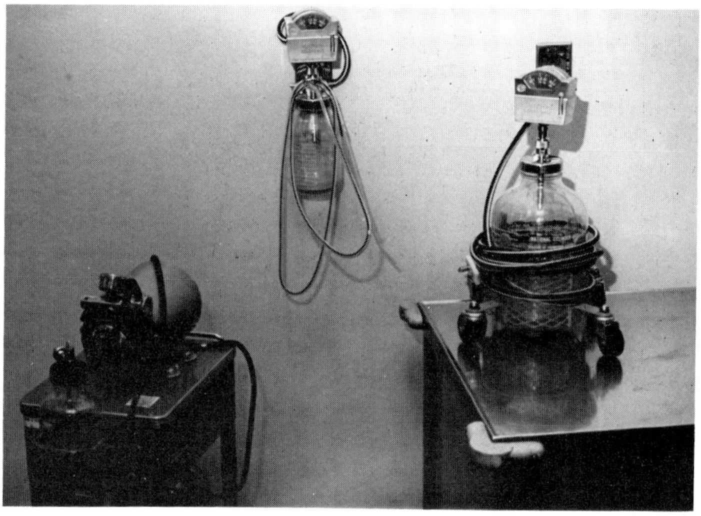

FIGURE 8–8 A variety of portable and stationary aspiration equipment.

of a table of the proper height and of standing platforms or comfortable operating stools makes for greater efficiency.[32, 33]

SURGICAL EQUIPMENT[13, 14, 32, 33]

Surgical equipment should, of course, include basic instrumentation used in general surgery. Special emphasis is placed on the need for copious quantities of warm isotonic saline and for aspiration equipment, since continuous bathing of CNS tissues is essential. Electrocautery equipment is most helpful, especially in cranial surgery. Use of gas anesthesia machines and physiological monitoring equipment has been emphasized. Naturally, it is necessary to have plenty of space to accommodate appropriate instrument tables and unusually large quantities of surgical equipment. In order to maintain strict asepsis, additional quantities of linen and diminished personnel traffic should be considered.

Special neurosurgical instruments and equipment are desirable. Some of this equipment is utilized in other surgical specialties. For example, ultra-high-speed drills,* rongeurs, and trephines are useful in orthopedics; and small scissors, forceps, needle holders, and fine suture material

*Hall Air Drill, Hall International Inc., Santa Barbara, California.

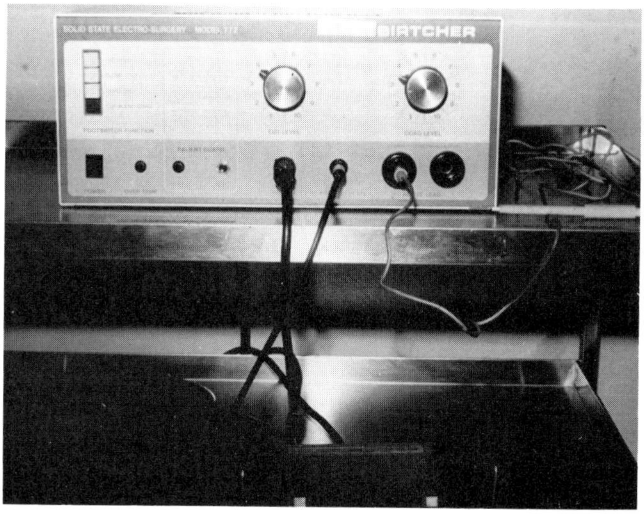

FIGURE 8–9 A surgical electrocautery machine is useful equipment in modern neurosurgery and surgery in general.

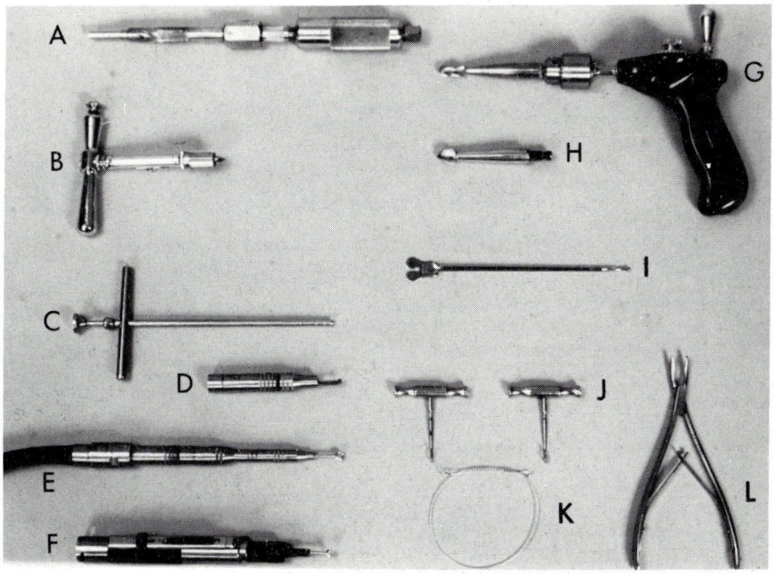

FIGURE 8–10 Various instruments useful in entering the calvarium in brain surgery: *A.* micrometer trephine; *B.* Galt trephine; *C.* Michelle laminectomy trephine; *D.* craniotome (Stryker); *E.* Stryker air drill; *F.* Hall air drill; *G.* hand drill and bur; *H.* pointed bur; *I.* grooved director; *J.* handles for wire saw; *K.* wire saw; *L.* Lampert rongeurs.

are routinely used in eye surgery. Items that are not generally used in other operations include brace and bur equipment in lieu of the high-speed drill, carded cotton flannel fiber pledgets or strips (Cottonoid) to control oozing and hemorrhage, absorbable gelatin sponges (Gelfoam) for permanent implantation on hemorrhaging surfaces, bone wax* for plugging bone surface

*Bone wax, Ethicon, Inc., Sommerville, New Jersey.

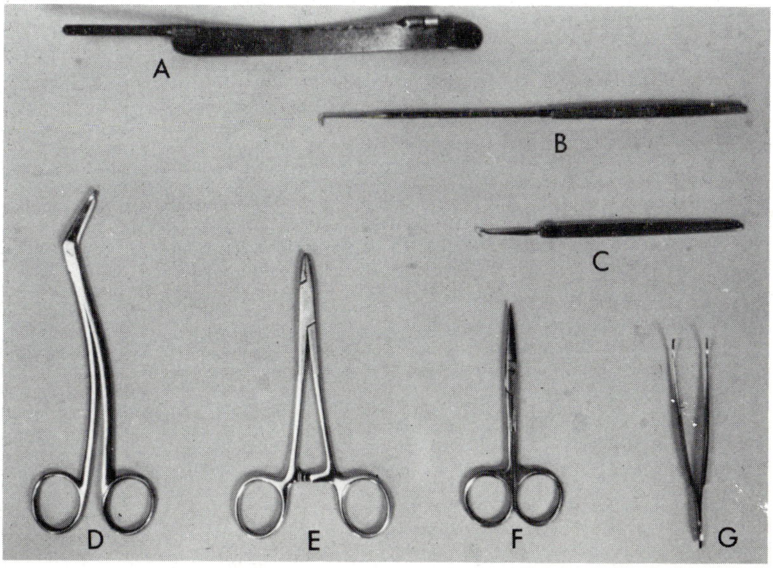

FIGURE 8–11 Various instruments useful in handling intracranial tissue: *A*, brain retractor; *B*, dural hook; *C*, dural hook; *D*, dural scissors; *E*, ophthalmic needle holder; *F*, iris scissors; *G*, iris forceps.

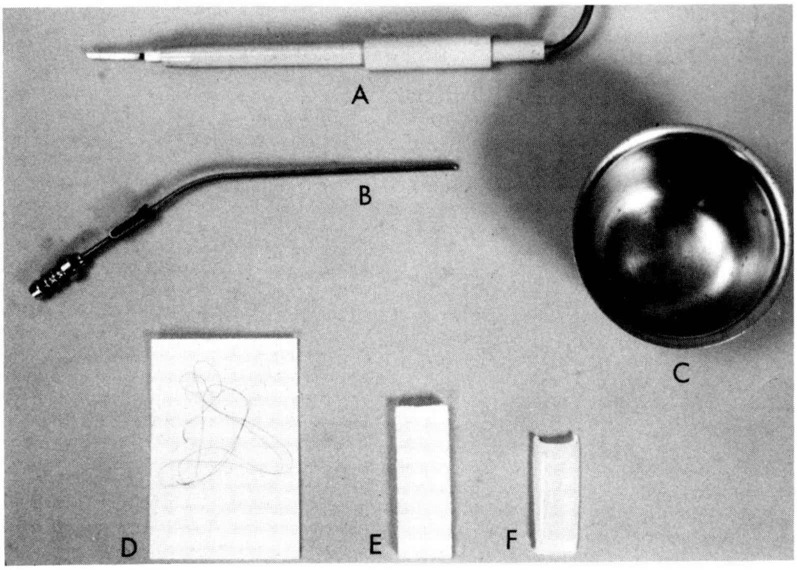

FIGURE 8–12 Means of controlling CNS hemorrhage: *A*, low tension cautery; *B*. aspirator tip; *C*. bowl for saline to bathe CNS tissue; *D*. cotton flannel patches (Cottonoid) with 6–0 ophthalmic silk suture for ligations; *E*. absorbable gelatin sponge (Gelfoam); *F*. bone wax. Silver clips and applicator forceps not shown.

hemorrhages, and silver clips for clamping meningeal vessels. Special endoscopic brain retractors and a surgical head lamp with or without magnification are useful items of equipment. In delicate operations, the surgical microscope is a valuable aid. These items are pictured here and are shown again in more detail under discussions for specific surgical procedures (Figs. 8–8 to 8–15).

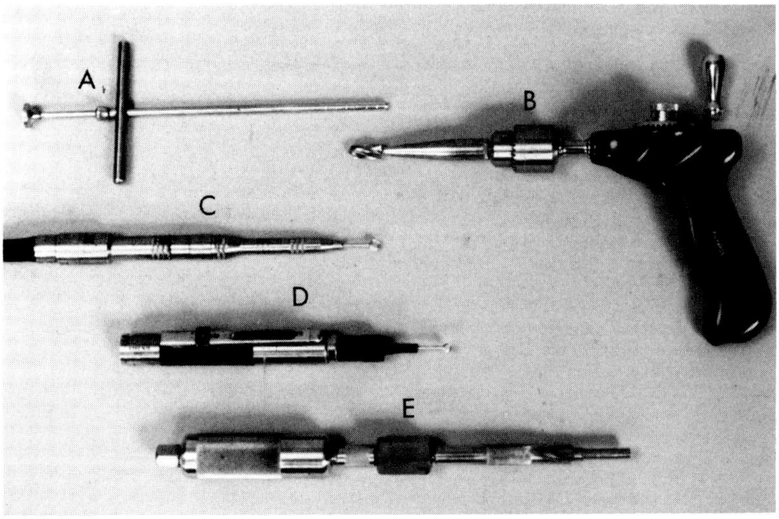

FIGURE 8–13 Instruments useful in laminectomies: *A*, Michelle laminectomy trephine, 7/32 inch diameter; *B*, orthopedic hand drill and bur, which may be used in lieu of trephination; *C*, Stryker high-speed air drill; *D*, Hall high-speed air drill; *E*, micrometer trephine with preset depth guard.

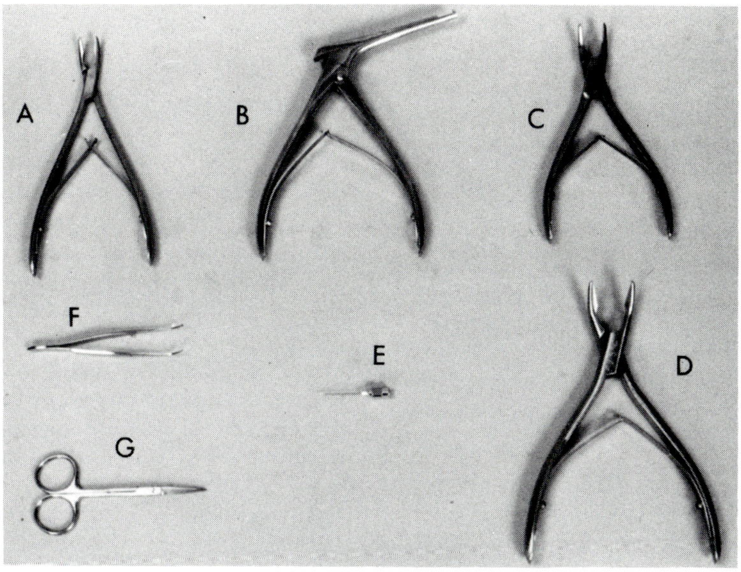

FIGURE 8-14 Instruments useful to laminectomies: *A*, Lampert rongeurs; *B*, Kerrison laminectomy rongeurs; *C*, Reiner rongeurs; *D*, mastoid rongeurs; *E*, 23-gauge intravenous needle that can be used to perform a durotomy or to elevate the dura while using an iris scissors for a durotomy; *F*, iris forceps for grasping the dura; *G*, iris scissors for durotomy.

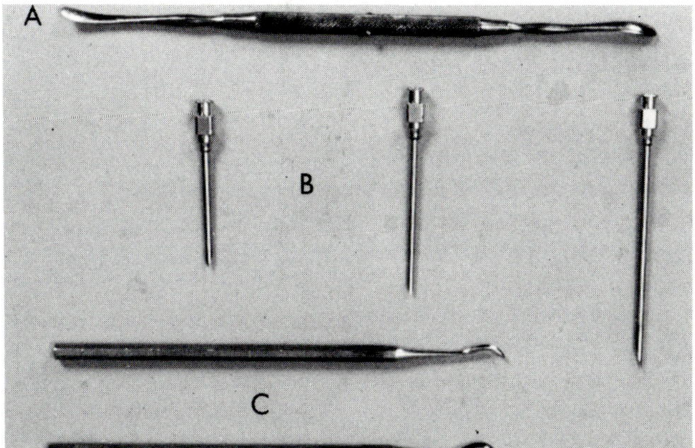

FIGURE 8-15 Instruments that are useful in disk fenestrations: *A*, periosteal elevator used for any disk or laminectomy approach; *B*, various lengths of 12–14 gauge intravenous needles; *C*, various widths and curvatures of dental claw-type tartar scrapers for removing disk and extradural deposits.

CONTROL OF HEMORRHAGE[13, 14, 31–33]

Proper positioning of the head at an elevated level will aid in preventing venous congension in brain surgery. Avoidance of major vessels during tissue invasion, copious use of warm saline in bathing CNS tissue, and much patience on the surgeon's part are fundamental to hemostasis. Systemic clotting agents have questionable efficacy, and we do not use them routinely. Low-current electrocautery is effective in controlling capillary bleeding in CNS tissue, in muscle, and in subcutaneous areas. Although use of ligatures is fundamental in control of hemorrhage, it is nearly impossible to apply ligatures in brain tissue. Bone wax can be rubbed on bone surfaces and in severed bone for hemorrhage arising from the diploic spaces. Silver clips or carefully placed 6–0 silk ligatures are effective in controlling meningeal hemorrhage.

Cotton flannel pledgets or strips are used along with copious saline irrigations to promote clotting of surface bleeding. This is a foreign material, and it should be marked by black thread or by some other means to distinguish it from the absorbable gelatin sponge material, which can be left in the surgical area. The aspirator tip should never be placed directly on CNS tissues but against the cotton strip or gelatin sponge material. Direct suction would traumatize nervous tissue. If there appears to be danger of a postoperative extradural hematoma, the dura or dural graft should be sutured to pericranial tissues to obliterate this space. If deemed necessary, a drain may be appropriately positioned to facilitate removal of fluid in such an event.

Occasionally, a subcutaneous accumulation of serum or blood may occur postsurgically, particularly after spinal surgery in large patients. This can generally be avoided if special care is used to assure absolute hemostasis in all tissues in closure of the surgical area. It is also routine practice to "dovetail" bandage spinal patients firmly with a 2- or 3-inch elastic material. This practice discourages accumulations of serum and aids in spinal immobilization and support. A patient that has undergone cranial surgery is bandaged similarly; however, care is exercised here not to restrict air passage.

Hypothermia is frequently employed as an aid in promoting hemostasis in elective neurosurgeries in humans. This procedure will be discussed in more detail later in this chapter.

CONTROL OF CNS EDEMA AND SWELLING

The danger of CNS edema and subsequent swelling will be emphasized throughout this text (see especially Chapter 12). Methods used to help control or prevent swelling are: (1) elevation of the head; (2) prevention of hypoxia, by promoting an open airway by means of endotracheal intubation, tracheostomy, and oxygen administration in a medical or postsurgical patient or by hyperventilation during surgery; (3) use of adrenal corticosteroids, particularly before and after surgery; (4) administration of hypertonic solutions; and (5) use of hypothermia.[14, 28, 31, 33]

Swelling can occur in cases of injury, hypoxia, ischemia, surgical manipulation, metabolic and toxemic disorders, and improper positioning. Hypoxia of brain tissue in general is a prominent cause of swelling. In veterinary practice, trauma to the head region of brachycephalic breeds is particularly dangerous with respect to proper ventilation. These breeds have difficulty normally, and heat or traumatic stress rapidly promotes an edema of the glottis and pharyngeal tissues so that ventilation is impeded. In such cases, prompt tracheostomy and oxygen administration is imperative.[33]

HYPERVENTILATION

In neurosurgical procedures, one can readily demonstrate the efficacy of controlled hyperventilation and continuous aspiration of CSF in the basal cisterns as a means of reducing brain volume. Fluid flows from the extracellular spaces into the CSF, and aspiration of it from basal cisterns is effective in reducing edema and swelling.[10, 28] Hyperventilation (increase of 25 to 50 per cent in rated minute volume—which can be produced in the 30 lb dog by 15 respirations/minute deep enough to slightly expand the chest) causes lower intracranial tension while maintaining normal arterial vascularity and blood pressure.[31] Manual manipulation of the breathing bag and a high concentration of oxygen for several minutes facilitates this procedure. Excessive hyperventilation, however, may cause vasoconstriction and resultant hypoxia as well as changes in blood pH. The importance of tracheostomy and a high atmospheric oxygen chamber for the patient cannot be overemphasized as an aid in controlling CNS swelling following surgery.[33]

CORTICOSTEROIDS

The administration of glucosteroids has been shown to actually reduce CNS tissue volume, particularly of the brain, in edema. That it restores the integrity of the abnormally permeable blood-brain barrier seen in trauma has been observed by studies conducted with the electron microscope.[24] Corticosteroids such as dexamethasone used as intravenous injections initially, followed by lower maintenance doses, should be routine in any case of CNS trauma or in elective surgery in which tissue manipulations encourage formation of edema. After relief has been obtained, oral steroids are gradually reduced for several more days so that adrenocortical depression doesn't develop.[7] See Chapter 12.

HYPERTONIC SOLUTIONS

Hypertonic solutions have been used in nonhemorrhaging brain trauma to decrease CSF pressure and intracranial mass. These solutions consisted of 50 per cent glucose, 50 per cent sucrose, 25 per cent saline, 50 per cent magnesium sulfate, concentrated human albumin, and concentrated human plasma.[28] More recently, urea and mannitol solutions have been used, particularly during or after surgical procedures on the central nervous system.[6]

Although urea is highly effective, more surgeons are currently recommending the use of a solution of 20 to 25 per cent mannitol given intravenously at a dose of 1 gm/kg body weight. Mannitol is nontoxic to the kidneys; in fact, it can be given to patients with nephritis.[13, 18, 19] It causes little or no secondary rise of CSF pressure, or "rebound" effect, such as that characteristically seen with urea or dextrose solutions.[38, 48, 49]

In addition to its use in reducing CNS fluid and volume, mannitol has been used effectively in oliguria from renal shut-down in shock and postoperative procedures. The principle mechanism of mannitol diuresis in these patients is acute expansion of blood volume, with a subsequent increase in glomerular filtration rate.

Mannitol has been effective in treatment of glaucoma.[46] Side-effects are infrequent when mannitol is properly used, but they can occur in cardiac and hepatic disease.[40] One report indicated that an anaphylactic reaction was seen in a person after mannitol administration; however, the patient responded promptly to epinephrine.[43] Parker has demonstrated experimentally that hemodynamic changes can be seen after mannitol administration in dogs suffering from severe vascular hypovolemia. Preferably, blood volume should be restored before mannitol is used.[34]

In our hands, mannitol has been considered along with corticosteroids for all types of nonhemorrhaging CNS trauma treated primarily by medical or surgical methods. Hypertonic solutions should not be given in cases of intracranial hemorrhage, which can be determined by visual examination of CSF or by cranial bur holes. Shrinking the brain would promote greater accumulation of hemorrhage in such cases.[19] However, mannitol has been used in conjunction with steroids in cases of hematomyelia (less danger of aggravating hemorrhage), in decompressive spinal surgery where marked damage to the cord was observed, and in craniotomies. It has been given intravenously in 25 per cent solution at a rate of 1 to 2 gm/kg body weight and repeated as often as two to four times daily for not longer than 24 to 36 hours. General severe dehydration should be avoided or uremia will result.[19] Marked clinical response is usually seen within 12 hours, at which time mannitol is either drastically reduced or stopped. Since severe distension of the bladder results from the diuresis, recumbent cases will require frequent catheterizations or an indwelling catheter. Replacement of body fluids should be initiated as promptly as deemed advisable.[8]

HYPOTHERMIA

In human neurology, hypothermia is frequently employed to aid in the control of cerebral edema and swelling in both medical and surgical patients. This technique reduces oxygen requirements for the brain and inflammatory and edematous reactions to infection and bleeding. In certain cases of hyperpyrexia secondary to neurological disorders, hypothermia is effective in promoting patient recovery.[2] Occasionally, hyperthermia will occur during anesthesia or in postoperative neurosurgery, especially if the procedure has involved areas close to the hypothalamus or the medulla, such as surgery on the anterior cervical cord or brain. The temperature rises at a fast pace, and serious CNS damage from dehydration, hypotension, hypoxia, acidosis, hyperkalemia, and tachycardia can occur. Such occurrences should be avoided by careful monitoring and, if necessary, treated medically or by physical hypothermia.[14, 36]

The chief value of hypothermia in neurosurgery is for elective surgery in CNS aneurysms or thrombosis and for tumor resections. Cold facilitates the surgical correction by reducing blood and metabolic needs, and it greatly reduces postsurgical inflammatory reactions such as edema. Hypothermia is used in certain cases of craniocerebral trauma to relieve critical neurological manifestations while specific therapy against the primary lesion is performed.[2, 30]

The methods of hypothermia employed in man for the CNS have been *total body* cooling (usually by blanket or occasionally by ice packs) and *regional* cooling of the brain. Moderate hypothermia of 28 to 30° C (82.4 to 86° F) is used primarily for surgery; temperatures of 32 to 33° C (89.6 to 91.4° F) are used for long-term periods, as in postsurgical or nonsurgical trauma. All hypothermia must be very carefully monitored and all physiological considerations must be fully understood by responsible personnel.[2]

The clinical use of hypothermia has been limited in the dog. Its chief use has been to treat hyperpyrexia that occurs in heat stroke or occasionally after CNS surgery, to treat cranial trauma, in neurosurgery, and occasionally in cardiovascular surgery.

Local or regional hypothermia is discussed in detail in Chapter 12. After Albin's[1] stimulating research in local hypothermic profusions in experimentally traumatized cords of monkeys, other researchers have continued to evaluate the use of local hypothermia in both clinical and experimental trauma. Lumb,[26] Brasmer,[5] Yturraspe,[51] Trotter,[45] and associates have advocated the use of lactated Ringers slush in prolonged and, in some cases, routine decompressive procedures involving the spinal cord. Tator and Deecke[44] concluded that both hypothermic and normothermic Elliott's B solution was effective in moderately traumatized spinal cords, while normothermic solutions seemed more effective in heavily traumatized cords. General agreement exists among neurosurgeons that isotonic perfusions are beneficial, but whether hypothermic or normothermic solutions are more effective is yet to be resolved. Possibly the mechanical dialysis of noxious, injury-related chemicals from the wounded cord by use of perfusion solutions is more important than the hypothermic temperature of the fluid.

General body hypothermia in the dog has usually been produced by immersion in a tub of ice water; however, some experimental work has been performed with extracorporeal or bypass cooling.[21, 22]

A relatively simple cooling-heating unit used by one veterinary investigator utilized an intragastric procedure. Following initial anesthesia to facilitate intratracheal tubation, an empty intragastric balloon was passed through the esophagus and into the stomach. In 2 hours the rectal temperature of a 60-lb dog was lowered to 25.5° C (78° F). Out of 23 dogs used, 10 were normal, 11 were used for experimental heart surgery, and 2 were patients with clinical abdominal procedures that had guarded prognoses. Two of the dogs that had heart operations died during the procedure, and two died 2 days later. Both clinical cases survived. Twenty-one out of 23 dogs were successfully rewarmed and a total of 19 survived.[37]

To the author, it appears that the clinical use of systemic and regional hypothermia in the dog looks promising and could, with the proper technique, be useful to the neurologist and neurosurgeon. Until more data are available, however, one should maintain normothermia or slight hypothermia in the CNS patient.[4]

POSTOPERATIVE CONSIDERATIONS

Most postoperative considerations have been mentioned earlier in this chapter. It was stressed that postsurgical observation must be intensive, particularly to maintain patient comfort and rest, adequate oxygenation, and normal body temperature.[47] Unrestricted postsurgical activity, such as aimless "thrashing," could jeopardize the results of the surgical procedure and effect a fatal outcome. Tranquilizers in general should not be used because of their hypotensive, vasodilatory, and nonalgesic effects. However, mild doses of diazepam (Valium) have been useful in quieting the animal and alleviating any tendencies toward seizure in postoperative neurosurgery. Pentazocine (Talwin) has been useful as a powerful postsurgical analgesic. Narcotics such as meperidine (Demerol) and oxymorphone (Numorphan) in mild doses continue to be effective.

Hyperthermia can be a serious event if it occurs during anesthesia or after cranial or spinal surgery near the cranium. So-called "malignant hyperthermia" is nonresponsive to therapy. In postsurgical hyperthermia ice in plastic bags should be placed around the body, or antipyretics such as methampyrone* should be used until normothermia has been established.[9, 27]

The airway must be kept open so that ventilation can be maintained. Tracheostomy may be necessary in post-traumatic cranial surgery. Placing the dog in an oxygen chamber for recovery is a customary procedure. Tracheostomy tubes must be checked hourly for a 6- to 12-hour period after surgery, and three to six times daily thereafter (see Chapter 12 for details).

Bandaging after CNS operations may be optional in most cases; however, bandaging of dogs, particularly larger dogs, that have had extensive spinal surgical procedures is beneficial. It is thought to be helpful also for most craniotomies. Bandaging helps prevent subcutaneous seroma formations, self-mutilation accidents, and enviornmental contamination of the surgical site.

Hypertonic solutions should be administered frequently to the postoperative patient. These should be reduced or stopped completely in at least 24 to 36 hours to prevent severe dehydration and kidney disorders.

Broad spectrum antibiotics should be given in postoperative cases. Frequently, corticosteroids should also be given for a few days after neurosurgery. Gradually decreasing the doses of steroids should be the standard procedure.

Postsurgical care after the first 24 hours must not be neglected if the outcome is to be satisfactory. The veterinary neurologist must supply well-planned *long-term* postoperative care and not lose interest in the patient or become too involved with other matters. The most exquisitely executed surgical procedure and correction can frequently be negated by postsurgical care that is administered in a slovenly fashion. Immediate postoperative care must provide for proper nutrition and hydration by use of intravenous fluids. Patients with cranial injuries must frequently be fed concentrated nutritious fluids or food by means of a stomach tube, pharyngostomy, or careful hand feeding on a more or less long-term basis (3–7 days) after surgery.[3]

Proper care of the urinary tract is particularly important in dogs with spinal injuries, and will be discussed in Chapters 13 and 14.

One must be alert to the possibility of decubital lesions and prevent their occurrence in recumbent animals. It should be routine practice to keep these animals on foam rubber cushions and to place paraplegics in carts or braces periodically throughout the day. Paraplegics are often liable to develop decubital lesions in the perineal area. Pulmonary sequelae, such as edema, congestion, or pneumonia, can occur. Frequent gentle rotation of recumbent patients and adequate ventilation of the respiratory tract aid in the prevention of these events.

Finally, one must successfully rehabilitate CNS patients. The first step in rehabilitation is interest and compassion for the patient. An animal that isn't handled and exercised properly will lose interest in life and will never respond successfully. Reha-

---

*Novin (Dipyrone), Haver-Lockhart Labs, Kansas City, Missouri.

bilitation is particularly necessary for dogs that have undergone spinal decompression. Details of rehabilitation are given in Chapter 14.

REFERENCES

1. Albin, M. S., White, R. J., Acosta-Rua, G., and Yashon, D.: Study of functional recovery produced by delayed localized cooling after spinal cord injury in primates. J. Neurosurg. *29*, 113, 1968.
2. Blair, F., *Clinical Hypothermia*, McGraw Hill Book Co., New York, 1964.
3. Bohning, R. H., Jr., De Hoff, W. D., McElhinney, A., and Hofstra, P. C.: Pharyngostomy for maintenance of the anorectic animal. J.A.V.M.A. *156*, 611, 1970.
4. Bouzarth, W. F., Kazi, K. H., Bubelin, J., and Shenkin, H. A.: Effect of temperature upon craniocerebral trauma. J.A.M.A. *199*, 567, 1967.
5. Brasmer, T. H., and Lumb, W. V.: Lumbar vertebral prosthesis in the dog. Am. J. Vet. Res. *33*, 493, 1972.
6. Clasen, R. A., Cooke, P. M., Pandolfi, S., Corneck, G., and Bryar, G.: Hypertonic urea in experimental cerebral edema. Arch. Neurol. *12*, 424, 1965.
7. Clasen, R. A., Cooke, P. M., Pandolfi, S., Cornecki, G., and Hass, G. M.: Steroid-antihistamine therapy in experimental cerebral edema. Arch. Neurol. *13*, 581, 1965.
8. Goldstein, S. L., Himwich, W. A., Knapp, F. M., and Rovine, B. W.: Effects of urea and other dehydrating agents upon dog brain. J. Neurosurg. *21*, 672, 1961.
9. Gordon, R. A., Britt, B. A., and Kalow, W.: International symposium on malignant hyperthermia. Charles C Thomas, Springfield, Illinois, 1973.
10. Gurdjian, E. S.: *Operative Neurosurgery*, 2d ed. The Williams and Wilkins Co., Baltimore, 1964.
11. Guyton, A. C.: Textbook of Medical Physiology, 5th ed., W. B. Saunders Co., Philadelphia, 1976.
12. Henriksen, H. T., and Jorgensen, P. B.: Effect of nitrous oxide on intracranial pressure in patients with intracranial disorders. *In Yearbook of Anesthesia.* Year Book Medical Publishers, Chicago, Illinois, 1974.
13. Hoerlein, B. F., and Few, A. B.: Brain surgery in the dog—preliminary studies. J.A.V.M.A. *143*, 21, 1963.
14. Hoerlein, B. F.: *Canine Neurology, Diagnosis and Treatment*, 2nd ed. W. B. Saunders Co., Philadelphia, 1971.
15. Hoerlein, B. F.: Surgical peculiarities of the nervous system. Presented at the Am. Anim. Hosp. Assoc., 33rd Annual Meeting, 1966.
16. Homburger, E., Himwich, W. A., Etstein, B., York, G., Maresca, R., and Himwich, H. E.: Effect of Pentothal anesthesia on canine cerebral cortex. Am. J. Physiol. *147*, 343, 1946.
17. Hunter, A. R.: Anesthesia for neurosurgical operations. *In* Gray, T. C., and Nunn, J. F. (ed.): *General Anesthesia*, 3rd ed., vol. 2. Appleton-Century-Crofts, New York, 1971.
18. Jackson, F. E.: The pathophysiology of head injuries. Clin. Symps. *18*, 67, 1946.
19. Jackson, F. E.: The treatment of head injuries. Clin. Symp. *19*, 4, 1966.
20. Jennings, P. B., and Coppinger, T. S.: Use of external jugular venous distention in the dog to estimate central venous pressure. J. Am. Anim. Hosp. Assoc., *11*, 668, 1975.
21. Kenyon, J. R.: Experimental deep hypothermia. Brit. Med. Bull. *17*, 43, 1961.
22. Knowles, R. P., and Wasman, S. C.: Hypothermia by cold temperature. Vet. Med. *51*, 26, 1956.
23. Lillehei, R. C.: Corticosteroids to dilate, drugs for emergency. Medicine 7, 109, 1975.
24. Long, D. M., Hartman, J. F., and French, D. A.: The response of human cerebral edema to glucosteroid administration. Neurology *16*, 521, 1966.
25. Luhan, J. A.: *Neurology, A Concise Clinical Textbook.* The Williams and Wilkins Co., Baltimore, 1968.
26. Lumb, W. V., and Brasmer, T. H.: Improved spinal plates and hypothermia as adjuncts to spinal surgery. J.A.V.M.A. *157*, 338, 1970.
27. Lumb, W. V., and Jones, E. W.: *Veterinary Anesthesia.* Lea and Febiger, Philadelphia, 1973.
28. Matson, D. D.: Treatment of cerebral swelling. N. Engl. J. Med. *272*, 626, 1965.
29. McDonnell, W.: *Principles of Anesthesia, Canine Surgery*, 2d Archibald ed. American Veterinary Publications, Inc., Santa Barbara, Calif., 1974.
30. McQueen, J. P., and Jeaves, L. D.: Hypothermia and intracranial hypertension. J. Neurosurg. *19*, 277, 1962.
31. Oliver, J. E., Jr.: *Canine Cranial Surgery.* Thesis, Auburn University, Auburn, Alabama, 1966.
32. Oliver, J. E., Jr.: Principles of canine brain surgery. Anim. Hosp. *2*, 73, 1966.
33. Oliver, J. E., Jr.: Surgical approaches to the canine brain. Am. J. Vet. Res. *29*, 353, 1968.
34. Parker, A. J.: Blood pressure changes and lethality of mannitol infusions in dogs. Am. J. Vet. Res. *34*, 1523, Dec. 1973.
35. Redding, R.: Unpublished data.
36. Saidman, I. J., Havard, E. S., and Eger, E. I.: Hyperthermia during anesthesia. J.A.M.A. *190*, 1029, 1961.
37. Schneider, H. P.: A cooling-heating unit for canine surgery. J.A.V.M.A. *117*, 828, 1965.
38. Shenkin, H. A., Goluboff, B., and Hoft, H.: The use of mannitol for the reduction of intracranial pressure in intracranial surgery. J. Neurosurg. *19*, 897, 1962.
39. Short, C. E.: *Clinical Veterinary Anesthesia, A Guide for the Practitioner.* C. V. Mosby Co., St. Louis, 1974.
40. Silverberg, D. S., and Johnson, W. J.: The use of mannitol in oliguric renal failure. Med. Clin. N. Amer. *50*, 1159, 1966.
41. Soma, L. R.: *Textbook of Veterinary Anesthesia.* The Williams and Williams Co., Baltimore, 1971.
42. Soma, L. R., Burrows, C. F., and Marshall, B. E.: Shock, etiology and management. *In* Kirk, R. W. (ed.): *Current Veterinary Therapy V*, W. B. Saunders Co., Philadelphia, 1974.
43. Spaeth, G. L., Spaeth, E. B., Spaeth, P. G., and Lucier, A. C.: Anaphylactic reaction to mannitol. Arch. Ophthal. *78*, 583, 1967.

44. Tator, C. H., and Deecke, L.: Value of normothermic perfusion, hypothermia perfusion, and durotomy in the treatment of experimental acute spinal trauma. J. Neurosurg. *39*, 52, 1973.
45. Trotter, E. J.: Modified dorsal laminectomy and selective regional spinal cord hypothermia in the treatment of thoracolumbar disk disease. *In* Bojrab, M. J. (ed.): *Current Technique in Small Animal Surgery I.* Lea and Febiger, Philadelphia, 1975.
46. Weiss, D. I., Shaffer, R. N., and Wise, B. L.: Mannitol infusion to reduce intraocular pressure. Arch. Ophthal. *68*, 341, 1962.
47. Wise, B. L.: Preoperative and postoperative care in neurological surgery. Charles C Thomas, Springfield, Illinois, 1972.
48. Wise, B. L., and Chater, N.: Use of hypertonic mannitol solutions to lower cerebrospinal fluid pressure and decrease brain bulk in man. Surg. Forum *12*, 398, 1961.
49. Wise, B. L., and Chater, N.: The value of hypertonic solution in decreasing brain mass and lowering cerebrospinal fluid pressure. J. Neurosurg. *19*, 1038, 1962.
50. Wylie, W. P., and Churchill-Davidson, H. C.: *A Practice of Anesthesia.* Lloyd-Luke Ltd., London, 1972.
51. Yturraspe, D. J., and Lumb, W. V.: Second lumbar spondylectomy and shortening of the spinal column of the dog. Am. J. Vet. Res. *34*, 521, 1973.

PART THREE

PERIPHERAL NERVES

CHAPTER 9

PERIPHERAL NERVOUS SYSTEM

SECTION 1
PERIPHERAL NERVE DISTRIBUTION AND FUNCTION*[10, 11]

B. F. Hoerlein, D.V.M., Ph.D.

The peripheral nervous system is composed of all the cranial and spinal nerves and their associated ganglia. There are 12 pairs of cranial nerves and 36 to 37 pairs of spinal nerves. These nerves are the means of communication between the brain and spinal cord and the rest of the body. Sensory (afferent) nerves carry impulses from their part of the body to the central nervous system, and motor (efferent) nerves return to the part. All spinal nerves have mixed sensory and motor fibers, whereas cranial nerves may be more specialized and may vary in type.[6]

At this point, we again briefly mention the lower and upper motor neurons (LMN, UMN). All fibers leaving the CNS are motor fibers, referred to as LMNs. The cell bodies of the spinal LMNs are in the gray matter of the ventral horn of the spinal cord. These LMNs innervate both voluntary and involuntary muscles. The LMNs receive many synapses from afferent components of the segmental spinal reflexes and from a variety of descending tract fibers in the spinal cord. The descending tracts, originating from such areas as the cerebral hemisphere, basal ganglia, and vestibular nuclei, are called upper motor neurons or UMNs.[8]

As a rule, the clinical manifestations of peripheral neuropathies in dogs are changes in sensations and varying degrees of motor dysfunction. Degrees of sensation vary from complete loss (anesthesia) to diminished sensation (hypesthesia) to increased sensation (hyperesthesia or pain). These degrees of sensation may be observed by palpation, by superficial pinching or pricking a part, or by an electronic recording of a cortical response to a noxious stimulus (evolved potential). Generalized pain is often indicated by the animal's reluctance to move and its whining or crying.

Motor dysfunction can be manifested by

*The author is indebted to Dr. Robert P. Worthman, Washington State University, Pullman, Washington, for furnishing ideas for drawings and actual materials used in this chapter, and to Dr. C. W. James (deceased), Auburn University, and Dr. Edward Robinson, Dothan, Alabama, for furnishing material on cutaneous sensation.

actual disturbances in locomotion, e.g., dragging and curling a paw, weakness or paresis, and lack of muscle reaction, or paralysis. Increased or abnormal muscle action is evidenced grossly by twitching, tremors, spasms, and such responses as clonus. The size and consistency of muscles indicate the state of motor function and can vary from complete atrophy, as in paralysis, to a large, firm, inflexible muscle, as in spasticity. Motor dysfunction as seen by electronic testing will be discussed in section 2 of this chapter.

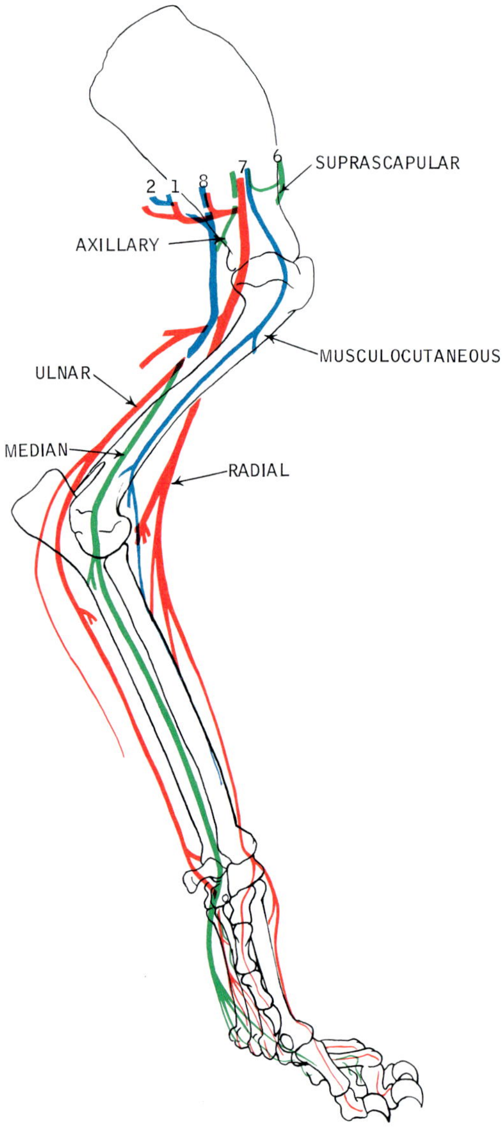

FIGURE 9–1 A medial view of the front limb illustrating the relative course and distribution of the major nerves to the front leg.

This chapter approaches the peripheral nervous system by discussing the distribution and function of the peripheral nerves in Section 1, the electronic diagnostics concerned with nerves and muscles in Section 2, and the clinical syndromes involving the peripheral nerves and muscles in Section 3. The distribution of peripheral nerves in individual animals of a species is constant enough that their dysfunction can generally be ascertained clinically by a set of clinical signs. The purpose of Section 1 is to aid in the clinical diagnosis of these mononeural injuries and neoplasia.

THE MAJOR NERVES OF THE PECTORAL LIMB

In the upcoming discussion of the functions of the peripheral nerves, the terms "motor" and "sensory" distribution will be used. In the academic sense, one must realize that even motor nerves contain sensory fibers, such as proprioceptors. On the other hand, a sensory nerve such as a cutaneous nerve contains autonomic fibers that are motor to blood vessels, sweat glands, and smooth muscle such as the erector pili. It is with these facts in mind that the reader should interpret the following discussions.

The nerves of the pectoral limb arise from the brachial plexus,[10, 11] which is formed by the ventral branches of the last three cervical nerves and the first two thoracic nerves (C6–8, T1–2) (Figs. 9–1 and 9–2).[11]

SUPRASCAPULAR NERVE – MOTOR (C6–7 COMPONENTS)

Motor. To supraspinatus and infraspinatus muscles (Fig. 9–3).

Signs of Paralysis. The loss of extensor action by these muscles on the shoulders is difficult to detect. The muscles serve largely as lateral ligaments for the shoulder joint. Atrophy is pronounced, and the spine of the scapula becomes prominent (Sweeny) (Fig. 9–4).

AXILLARY NERVE

Mixed (C7 primarily, fibers also from C6 and C8).

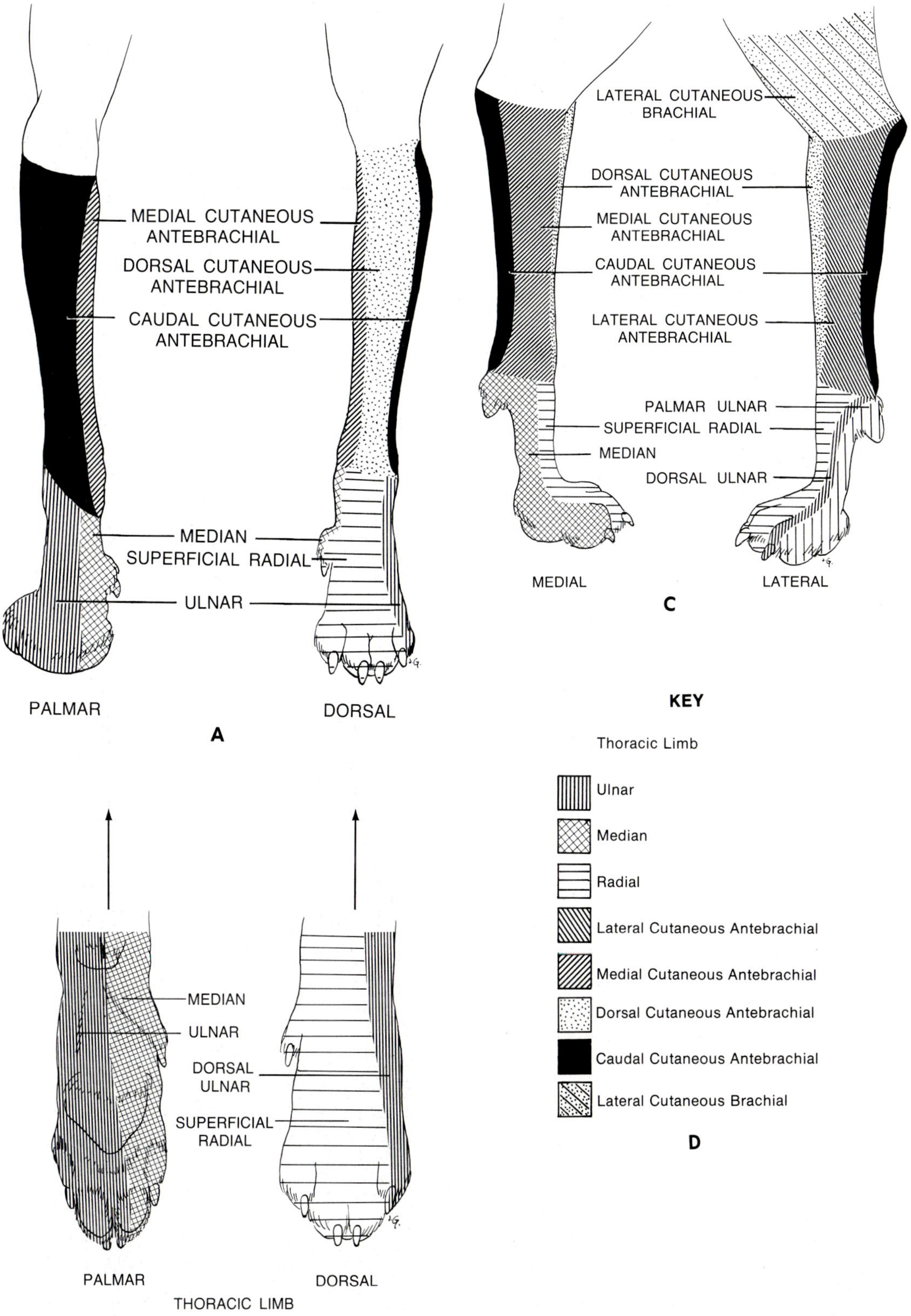

FIGURE 9–2 Cutaneous sensory distribution in the front limb. *A* and *B*. Dorsal and palmar (volar) views. *C*. Lateral and medial views. (Courtesy of Drs. Charles James and Edward Robinson. Sensory determinations were made by sectioning the nerve and testing the cutaneous sensation by needle prick, pinching the skin with a forceps, and by use of heat.)

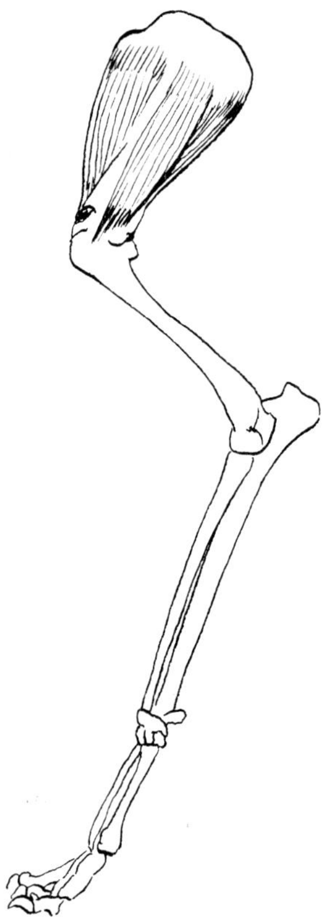

FIGURE 9–3 The suprascapular nerve supplies the supraspinatus and infraspinatus muscles.

MOTOR. Flexors of the shoulder (teres major, teres minor, deltoideus, part of subscapularis) (Fig. 9–5).

SENSORY. Skin of dorsolateral brachium (true arm).

SIGNS OF PARALYSIS. Small area of cutaneous desensitization on lateral side of arm. There is no pronounced motor dysfunction on sectioning the nerve.

TEST. Weakened shoulder flexor reflex.

RADIAL NERVE—MIXED (C7–8 AND T1–2 COMPONENTS)

The entire radial nerve may be injured by fractures of the first rib or by traumatic avulsion of its roots from the spinal cord.

MOTOR. To all the extensor muscles of the elbow, the carpus, and the digits (Fig. 9–6).

SENSORY. From the skin on the dorsal and lateral parts of the forearm and the dorsal aspect of the paw.

SIGNS OF PARALYSIS. The leg can bear no weight when the entire radial nerve is injured primarily because the extensors of the elbow are paralyzed (Fig. 9–7). This joint remains flexed when the animal walks. When the nerve is injured distal to the branches that supply the triceps muscle, the paralysis is much less marked. Fractures of the humerus may easily involve this part of the radial nerve. The elbow can be extended, but there is a tendency for the animal to knuckle over onto the dorsal side of the paw when walking (Fig. 9–8). After a time, the paralysis may be difficult to detect. Knecht demonstrated that in experimental sections of the radial and axillary nerves, the functional ability to compensate was considerably reduced.[5] Sectioning the radial and thoracodorsal nerves caused a permanent elbow drop.

Since the sensory branches of the radial nerve supply the dorsal and lateral parts of the forearm and the dorsal aspect of the paw, differentiation of high radial from brachial plexus paralysis can be made by examination of the sensory fields.

TEST. Extensor thrust reflex and supporting and placing reactions are absent in radial paralysis.

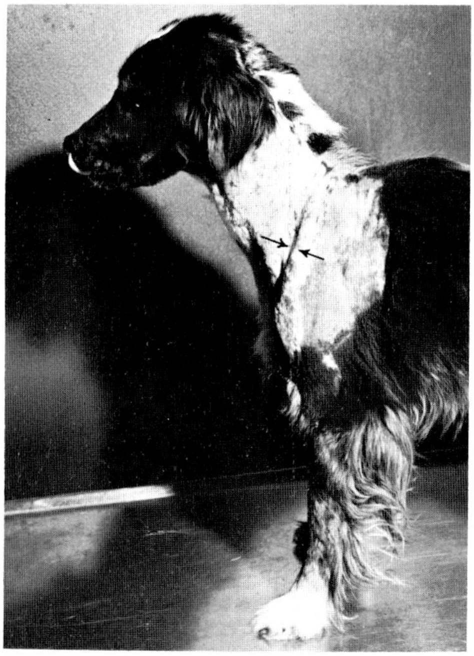

FIGURE 9–4 Left suprascapular nerve paralysis in a dog, 6 months after neurectomy. Notice the prominence of the suprascapular spine (arrows) due to muscle atrophy.

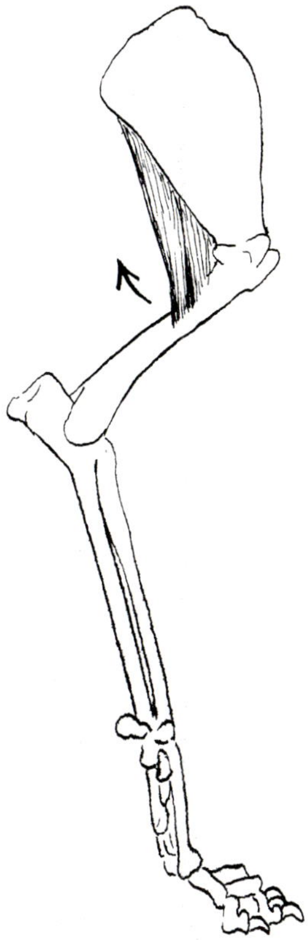

FIGURE 9–5 Medial view. The axillary nerve supplies motor fibers to the flexors of the shoulder (teres major, teres minor, deltoideus, and part of subscapularis).

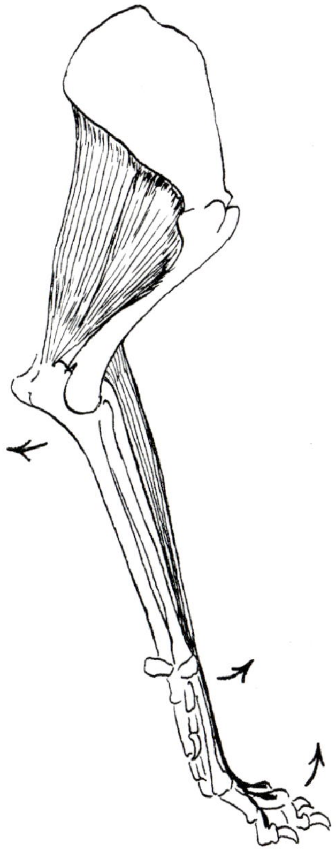

FIGURE 9–6 Medial view. The radial nerve supplies the extensor muscles of the elbow, the carpus, and the digits.

MUSCULOCUTANEOUS NERVE—MIXED (C7 COMPONENT)

MOTOR. To special flexors of the elbow joint (biceps and brachialis muscles) (Fig. 9-9).

SENSORY. It is sensory to the medial side of the forearm.

SIGNS OF PARALYSIS. Paralysis of this nerve causes little change in gait. There appears to be a slight straightening of the angle of the elbow joint. With some difficulty, the dog can still flex the elbow (as in raising the paw to the edge of the table) (Fig. 9–10). This ability is probably due to the flexor action on the elbow joint by the extensor muscles of the carpus and digits which originate on the humerus. Skin is desensitized on the medial side of the forearm.

TEST. Flexor reflex (elbow) weakened in musculocutaneous paralysis.

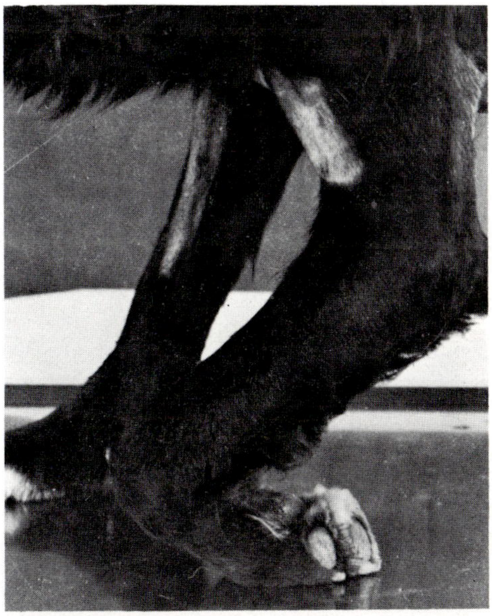

FIGURE 9–7 The entire left radial nerve of this dog is destroyed. All joints other than the shoulder remain flexed, and the leg can bear no weight.

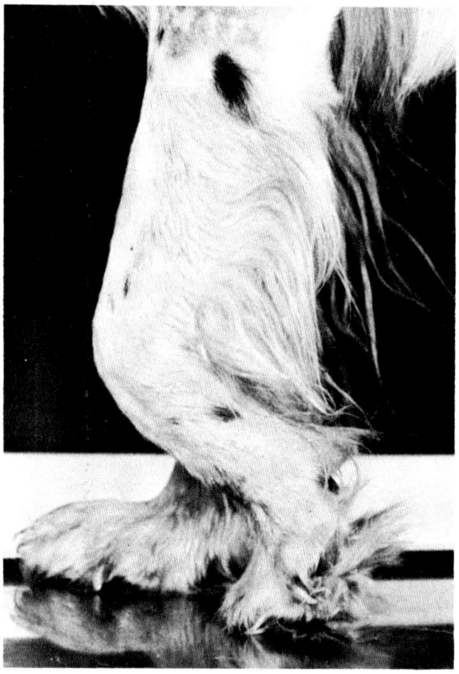

FIGURE 9–8 The left radial nerve has been transected distal to the branches which supply the extensors of the elbow; weight bearing can occur, but there is a tendency to knuckle over on the dorsal side of the paw.

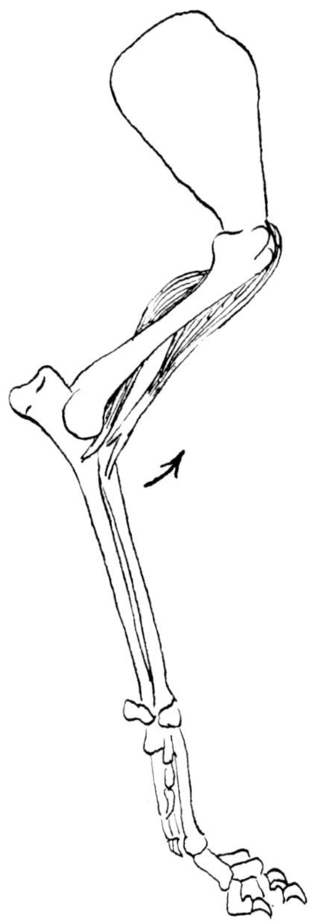

FIGURE 9–9 Medial view. The musculocutaneous nerve supplies the special flexors of the elbow (biceps and brachialis).

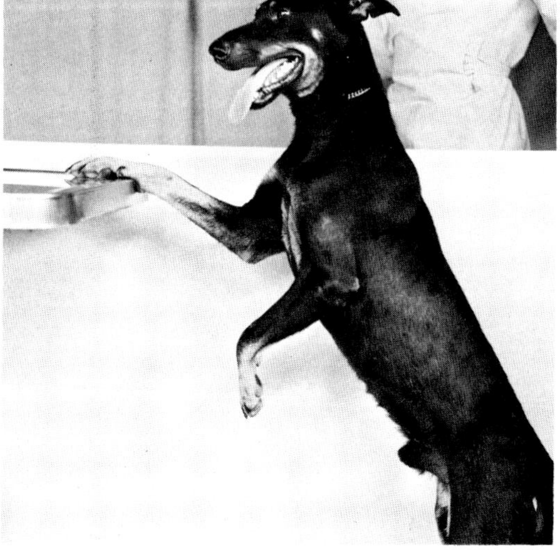

FIGURE 9–10 Some difficulty is experienced by the dog in elevating the left paw to the edge of the table due to paralysis of the special flexors of the elbow supplied by musculocutaneous nerve.

MEDIAN AND ULNAR NERVES—MIXED (C8 AND T1–2 COMPONENTS)

MOTOR. To all the flexor muscles of the carpus and digits (Fig. 9–11).

SENSORY. These two nerves together with the anastomotic branch of the musculocutaneous nerve transmit sensation from the palmar side of the paw. Sensation from the skin on the caudal side of the forearm and the dorsolateral aspect of the fifth digit is mediated solely by the ulnar nerve.

SIGNS OF PARALYSIS. Loss of both these nerves causes little alteration of gait. There is some sinking of the carpus and fetlock due to the loss of tone to the flexors of these joints (Fig. 9–12). Injury to the ulnar nerve does cause desensitization in the areas that are supplied solely by it. The palmar aspect of the paw is completely desensitized only when three nerves—the median, the ulnar, and the musculocutaneous—are injured.

TEST. Active flexion of carpus is lost.

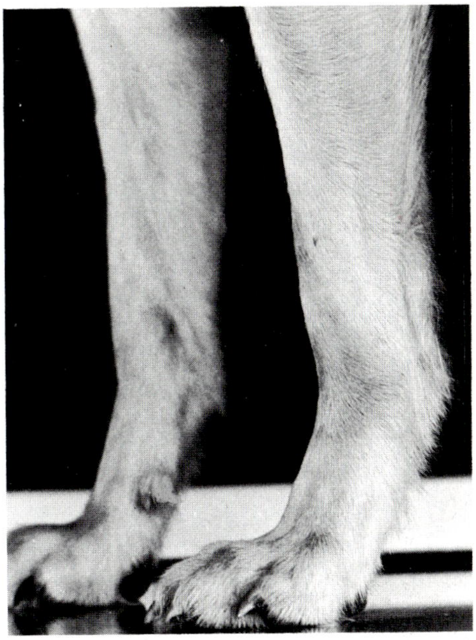

FIGURE 9–12 Left median and ulnar nerve paralysis in a dog. No lameness is evident other than a slight sinking of the left carpus and fetlock due to loss of tone in the flexors of these joints

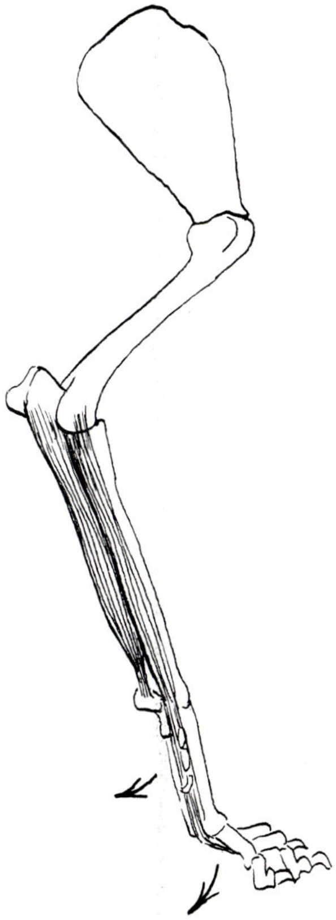

FIGURE 9–11 The muscles supplied by the median and ulnar nerves. These nerves supply all the flexor muscles of the carpus and digits.

THE MAJOR NERVES OF THE HIND LIMB AND PELVIS

The nerves of the hind limb arise from the lumbosacral plexus.[10, 11] This plexus is formed by the ventral branches of the last four lumbar and the three sacral nerves (L4–7, S1–3) (Figs. 9–13 and 9–14).

OBTURATOR NERVE—MOTOR (L4–6 COMPONENTS)

The nerve is vulnerable to trauma as it courses down the shaft of the ilium (Fig. 9–15).

MOTOR. To the muscles that adduct the thigh (external obturator, pectineus, adductor, and gracilis muscles).

SIGNS OF PARALYSIS. The pelvic appendage slides laterally on a smooth surface in a unilateral obturator nerve injury (Fig. 9–16). With a bilateral obturator nerve lesion, the animal literally "does the splits" on such a surface, but walks quite normally on a "nonskid" surface.

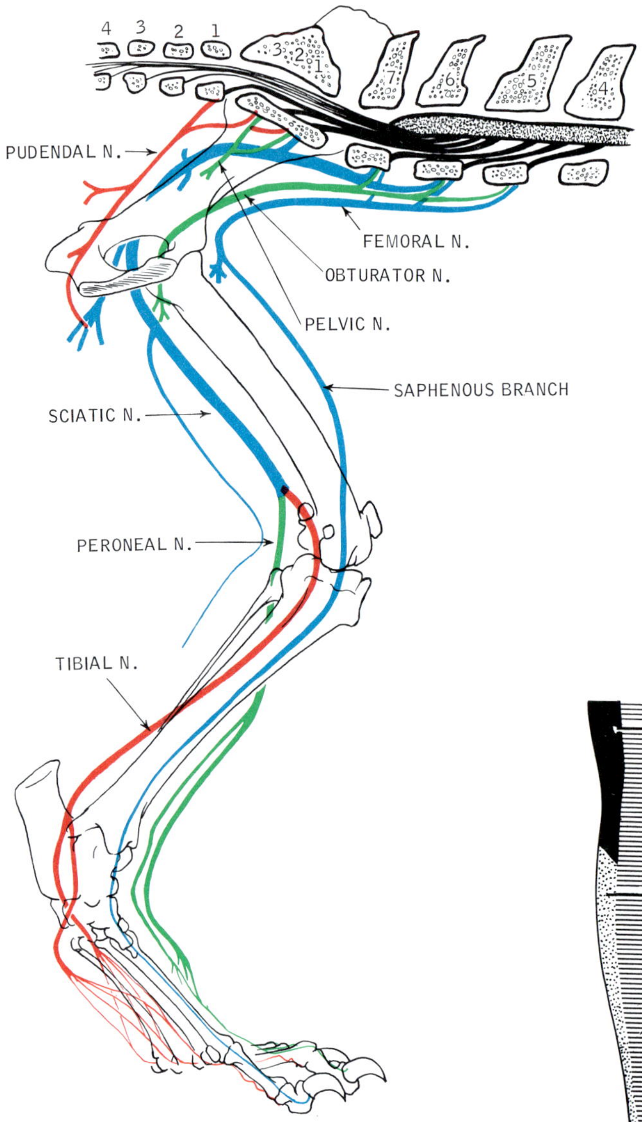

FIGURE 9–13 A medial view of the hind limb illustrating the relative course and distribution of the major nerves.

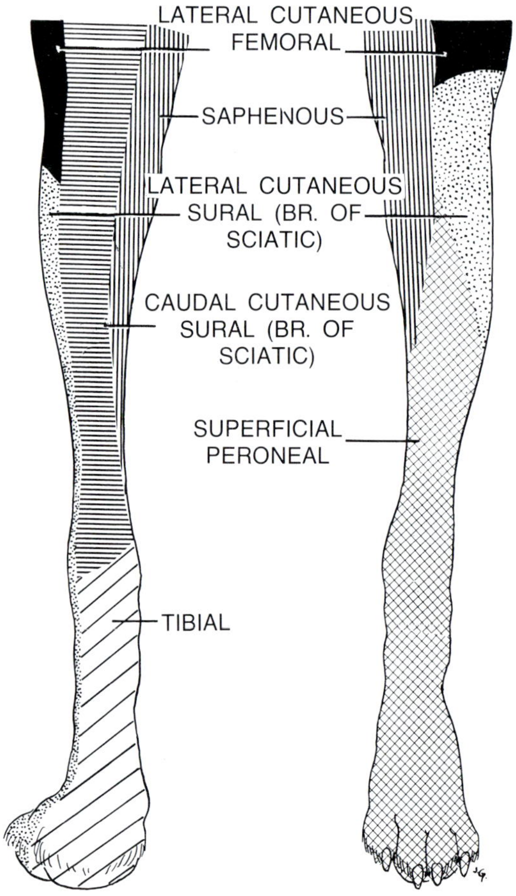

A

FIGURE 9–14 Cutaneous sensory distribution in the hind limb. *A* and *B*. Dorsal and plantar views.

Legend continued on the opposite page

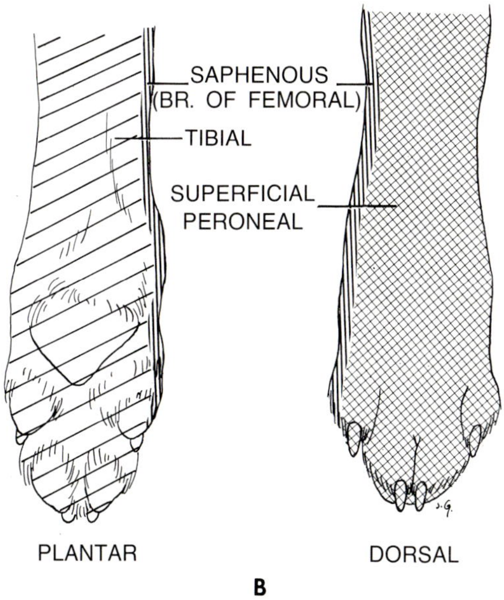

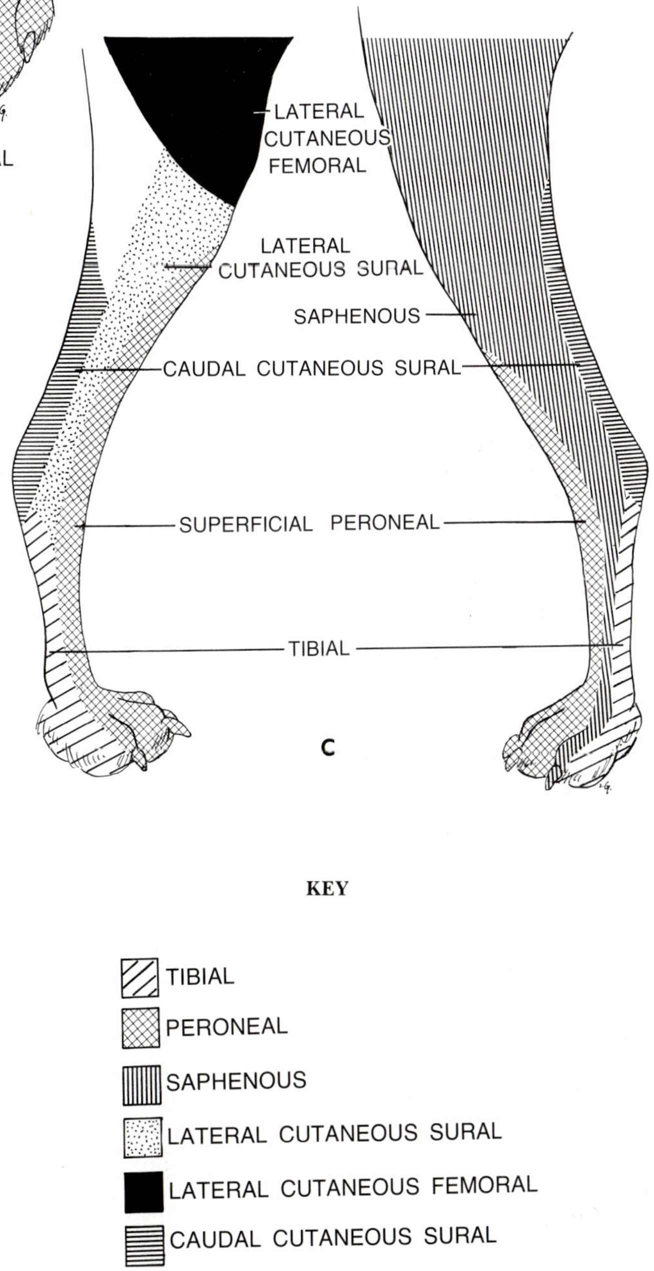

FIGURE 9–14 *Continued.* *C.* Lateral and medial views (see Fig. 9–2).

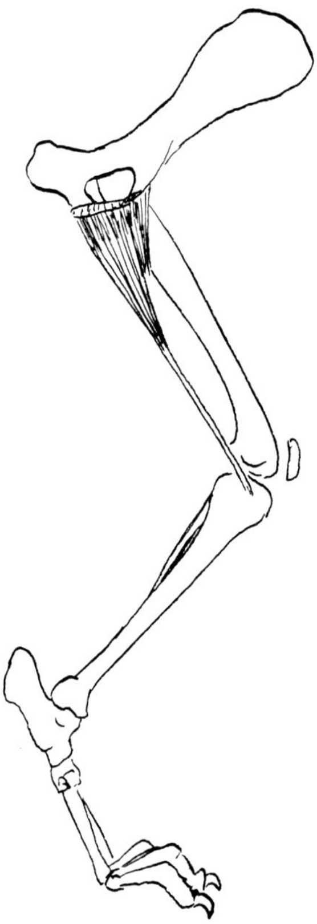

FIGURE 9–15 Medial view. The obturator nerve supplies the muscles that adduct the thigh (external obturator, pectineus, adductor, and gracilis muscles).

FEMORAL NERVE—MIXED (L4–6 COMPONENTS)

MOTOR. To the major extensors of the stifle joint (and proprioceptors concerned with the knee jerk reflex) and to the iliopsoas and sartorius muscles (Fig. 9–17).

SENSORY. Saphenous branch is sensory from the skin on the medial surface of the thigh, stifle, leg, and paw.

SIGNS OF PARALYSIS. The stifle joint can neither be extended nor fixed to prevent the collapse of the leg when bearing weight. (The stifle is the key joint of the hind limb.) When walking, the dog must take a quick step with the unaffected leg to prevent the complete collapse of the paralyzed leg while it is bearing weight (Fig. 9–18). Desensitization occurs in the area supplied by the saphenous branch of the femoral nerve.

TEST. Extensor thrust (stifle). Both afferent and efferent arms of the knee jerk reflex are in the femoral nerve.

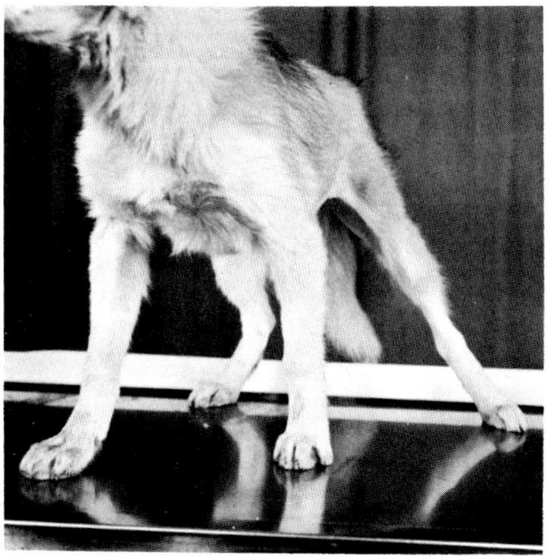

FIGURE 9–16 A dog in which the left obturator nerve is injured. Notice the abductor present since the adductor muscles are nonfunctional.

PERONEAL (FIBULAR) NERVE—MIXED

A terminal branch of the sciatic nerve, the peroneal or fibular nerve is vulnerable

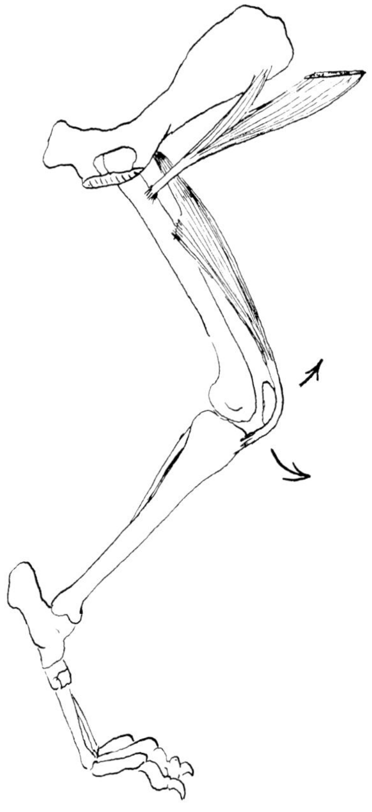

FIGURE 9–17 Medial view. The femoral nerve supplies the major extensors of the stifle joint (quadriceps femoris) and the iliopsoas and sartorius muscles.

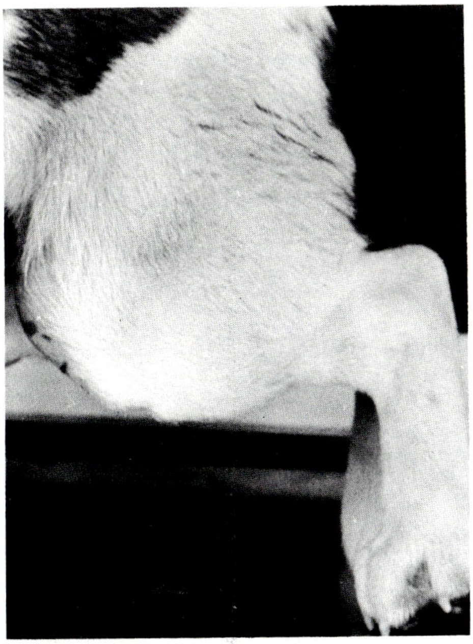

FIGURE 9–18 In left femoral nerve paralysis, the dog's leg collapses when a step is taken because the stifle can neither be extended nor fixed to bear the body weight.

to trauma as it crosses the lateral aspect of the stifle joint quite superficially.

MOTOR. To the muscles that flex the hock and extend the digits (Fig. 9–19).

SENSORY. From the dorsal aspect of the distal part of the true leg, the hock, and the paw.

SIGNS OF PARALYSIS. Lesions of this nerve result in a straightening of the hock and a tendency for the dog to knuckle over onto the dorsum of the fetlock and digits (Fig. 9–20). Although the hock cannot be flexed, the dog soon learns to place the foot properly by a greater flexion of the hip and extension of the stifle joints. The dorsal aspects of the paw, hock, and tibial areas are anesthetized in this paralysis.

Paralysis of the peroneal nerve has been frequently observed in this clinic. The chief cause has been intramuscular injections directed into the caudal thigh muscles, which envelop the peroneal and tibial nerves. No doubt the tibial nerve is also affected in many of these injections, but the clinical signs are primarily those of a peroneal deficit. All clinicians should dissect a specimen to review the locations of these nerves.

TEST. Flexor reflex (hock).

TIBIAL NERVE – MIXED

The tibial nerve, a terminal branch of the sciatic nerve, descends in contact with the caudal aspect of the stifle joint.

MOTOR. To the muscles that extend the hock and flex the digits (Fig. 9–21).

SENSORY. From the skin and pads on the plantar aspect of the paw.

SIGNS OF PARALYSIS. The hock joint remains flexed when the dog is walking, and, when weight is supported on the affected limb, this flexion is accentuated (Fig. 9–22). Sensation is lost from the plantar aspect of the hind paw.

TEST. Extensor thrust reflex (hock).

SCIATIC NERVE – MIXED (L5–7 AND S1–2 COMPONENTS)

The nerve is vulnerable within the pelvic cavity (pressure and fractures of the ilium),

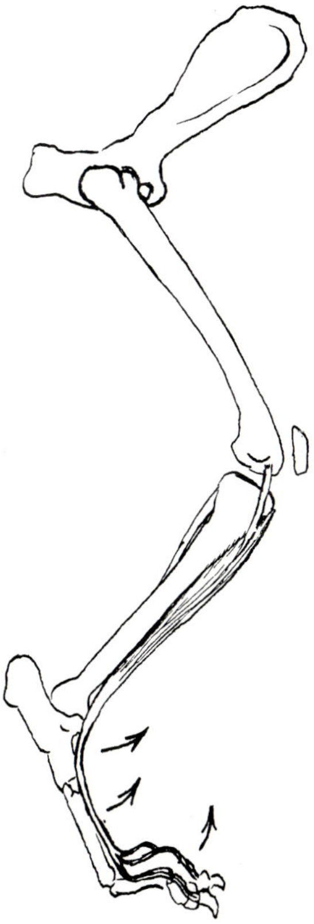

FIGURE 9–19 Medial view. The peroneal or fibular nerve supplies the muscles that flex the hock and extend the digits.

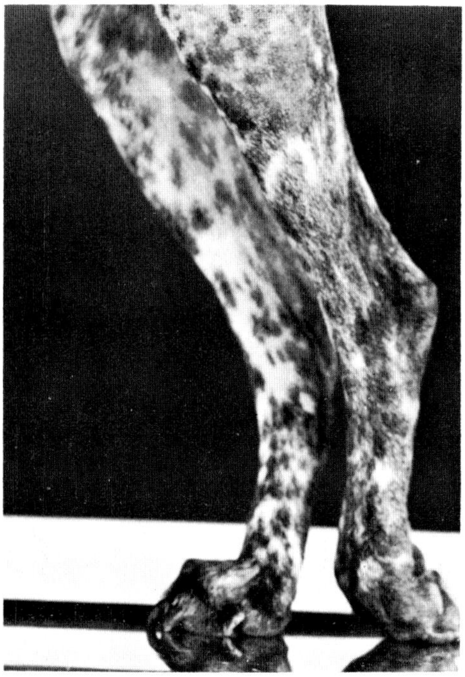

FIGURE 9–20 Peroneal or fibular nerve paralysis of the dog's left leg results in a straightening of the hocks and a tendency to knuckle over onto the dorsum of the fetlock and digits.

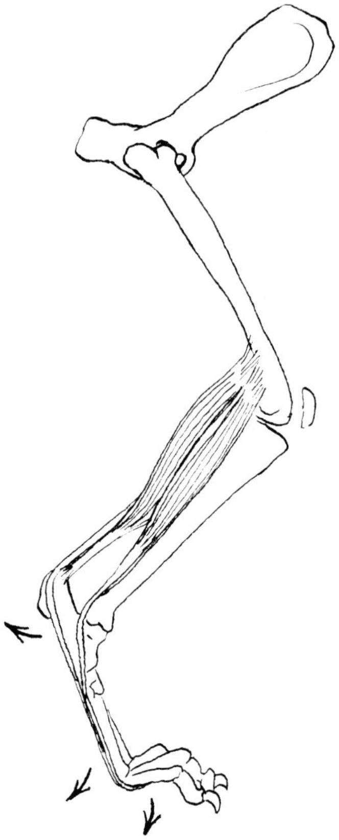

FIGURE 9–21 Medial view. The tibial nerve supplies the muscles that extend the hock and flex the digits.

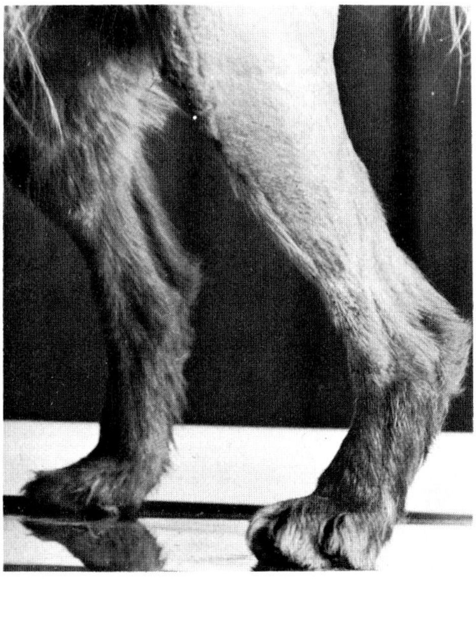

FIGURE 9–22 Left tibial nerve paralysis in the dog results in a permanent flexion of the left hock. When the dog bears weight this flexion is accentuated.

and it is endangered by trauma and surgical procedures near the proximal end of the femur. Irritating injections into the caudal thigh muscles may also involve this nerve.

MOTOR. The peroneal and tibial nerves, which have already been described, are the two terminal branches of the sciatic nerve. In addition, this large nerve supplies the massive caudal thigh muscles that help to extend the hip and flex the stifle joints. Branches given off within the pelvis supply the gluteal and other muscles that extend and abduct the hip (Fig. 9–23).

SENSORY. In addition to sensory components of the tibial and peroneal nerves, the sciatic nerve innervates the skin on the caudal and lateral sides of the true leg.

SIGNS OF PARALYSIS. Cutaneous desensitization exists below the stifle except for the medial side of the leg, hock, and paw (via the femoral nerve). The gait is markedly altered by paralysis of the muscles to all the joints below the stifle joint; only the extensors of this joint remain functional. When the sciatic nerve is injured at the level of the greater sciatic foramen, the hock of the affected leg aimlessly and passively flexes and extends as weight is shifted on the appendage. The leg does not collapse when bearing weight because the femoral nerve fixes the stifle joint. The animal stands "knuckled over" on the dorsal side of the paw. The hip joint remains functional, despite the paralysis of the caudal thigh muscles. The action of this joint is apparently maintained by the gluteal, obturator, and femoral nerves. Injury to the entire sciatic nerve within the pelvic cavity involves the branches to the gluteal muscles and to the small associated pelvic muscles. In addition to the symptoms just described, paralysis of these extensor and abductor muscles of the hip results in flexion of the hip joint and

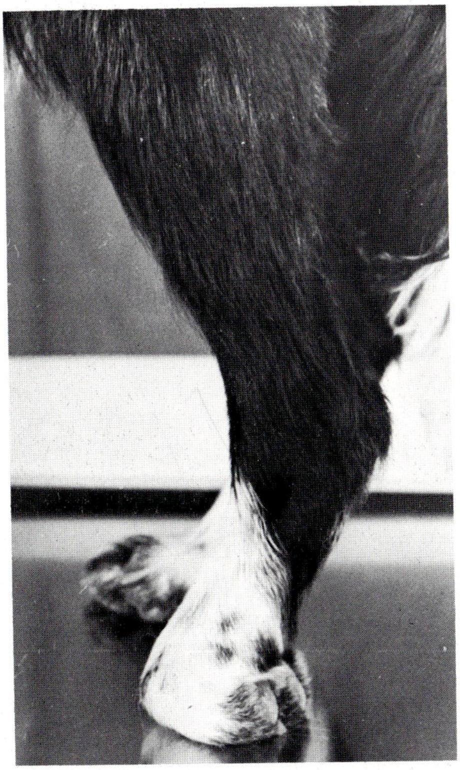

FIGURE 9–24 With left sciatic nerve paralysis, the animal stands "knuckled over" on the dorsal side of the paw, while the hock aimlessly and passively flexes and extends as weight is shifted on the appendage.

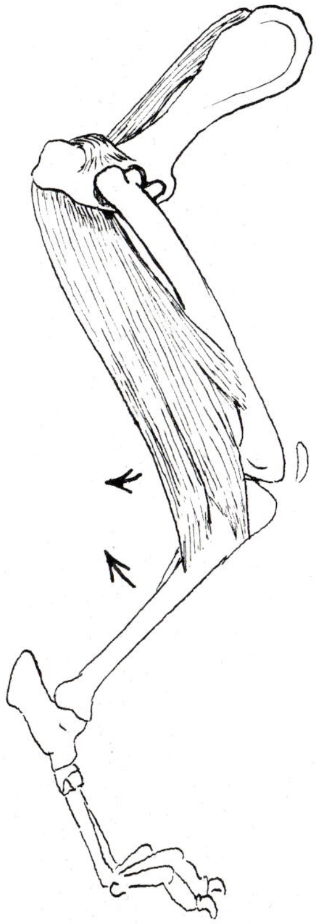

FIGURE 9–23 Medial view. The sciatic nerve supplies the massive caudal thigh muscles that help to extend the hip and flex the stifle joints. The peroneal and tibial nerves are terminal branches of the sciatic, and their function has been described (see Figures 9–19 and 9–21).

drawing of the affected limb toward the midline. Only the femoral and the obturator nerves remain functional (Fig. 9–24).

PUDENDAL NERVE—MIXED (S1–3 COMPONENTS)

MOTOR. To the external anal sphincter and the skeletal muscles associated with the penis, vulva, and urethra.

SENSORY. From the penis or clitoris, and the skin of the anal opening, the vulva, and part of the scrotum.

SIGNS OF PARLAYSIS. Anesthesia in the areas just indicated. Relaxed external anal sphincter.

TEST. Anal reflex. Touching the skin near the anal orifice normally results in visible contraction of the anal sphincter.

PELVIC NERVE—MIXED

Those fibers in first and second sacral components that are parasympathetic unite to form the pelvic nerve.

MOTOR. To the smooth muscle and glands of the pelvic cavity (rectum, bladder, etc.) which, upon contraction, cause urination, defecation, and erection.

SENSORY. From the pelvic viscera.

SIGNS OF PARALYSIS. Absence or alteration of pelvic visceral reflexes (urination, defecation, and erection). See also the discussion of disorders of micturition, Chapter 13, page 461.

SUMMARY OF NERVE LESIONS IN THE LIMBS

The most important signs of the various nerve injuries in the foreleg are:

1. Radial nerve. Entire nerve—dog can bear no weight. Below middle humerus—dorsal knuckling of the front paw; cutaneous hypesthesia of the dorsal aspect of the paw.
2. Median and ulnar nerves. Both injured—no active flexion of carpus (it is flexed largely by gravity when the elbow is flexed), and therefore the dog compensates for it when walking. There is a slight sagging of the carpus on standing. Hypesthesia of the palmar aspect of the paw.

In the hind leg, the most important signs of the various nerve injuries are:

1. Obturator—causes abduction or "splits" on a slick surface.
2. Femoral—collapse of leg when walking. Sensory deficit of the medial aspect of the thigh, leg, and paw.
3. Peroneal—the straight hock does not permit good elevation of the paw on rough surfaces, so that dorsal knuckling of the paw occurs only periodically. Cutaneous hypesthesia of the dorsal aspect of the true leg, hock, and paw.
4. Tibial—exaggerated flexion of the hock when standing or walking. Hypesthesia of the plantar surface of the paw.
5. Sciatic—straightening of the entire leg makes weight-bearing possible. Dorsal knuckling of the paw is constant, therefore the paw is dragged and mutilated. Hypesthesia of caudal and lateral aspects of the true leg.
6. Pelvic and pudendal—lack of anal reflex and the presence of urinary retention.

LUMBAR, SACRAL, AND COCCYGEAL TACTILE DERMATOMES[2]

Fletcher and Kitchell demonstrated the dorsal root dermatomes in the dog, using sophisticated electrophysiological equipment. In laminectomies on 35 dogs, each rootlet was isolated by blunt dissection, severed close to the cord, and placed across silver electrodes. Visualization of monophasic spike potentials on a cathode ray oscilloscope was obtained, along with an auditory response and photographic record. Tactile response was stimulated by rubbing a small brush or spatula on hairs of the body surface. Proprioceptive activity was elicited by movement of the joints and pressure applied to the sensory field. The tactile distribution boundaries of each rootlet were recorded.[2]

The dermatome distributions were summarized as follows: L1–2 supplied the flank; L3 and L4 supplied the cranial thigh as well as the flank. L5, L6, and L7 supplied the proximal and distal portions of the pelvic limb. S1 supplied the caudal aspect of the rump, thigh, and crus. S2 innervated the caudal rump and perineum, along with the genitalia, upon which the ventral midline overlap was greater than elsewhere. S3 encircled the base of the tail, adjacent trunk, and practically the whole anus owing to increased overlap there. The coccygeal dermatome formed serially overlapping bands around the tail (Figs. 9–25 and 9–26).[21]

This author feels that knowledge of these dermatomes will contribute to the veterinary clinician's ability to diagnose corresponding lesions of the lumbar and sacral cord, such as cord tumors, herniated disks, fractures, and other compressions.

CRANIAL NERVE INJURIES

Injuries to individual cranial nerves do not occur frequently, as these nerves are quite well protected from minor trauma. In some cases of cranial fracture, hemorrhage, and concussion, the nerves may be damaged within or close to their source. Neoplastic lesions in the brain will frequently cause a deficit in one or more cranial nerves. Such signs are most helpful in locating the lesion diagnostically. To understand the clinical signs of cranial nerve injuries, one must review their anatomical aspects and functions (Fig. 9–27).

THE CRANIAL NERVES

I. OLFACTORY NERVE—SENSORY

Rhinitis may involve the brain directly, because the subarachnoid space follows along the olfactory nerve fibers through the cribriform plate to the olfactory area of the nasal cavity. The olfactory and optic nerves are frequently considered tracts of the central nervous system rather than peripheral nerves.[4,7] The olfactory nerve brings the sensation of smell from the nasal cavity to the encephalon at the olfactory bulb. Hyposmia or anosmia is generally associated with rhinitis rather than trauma.

TEST. Cloves, lavender, anise, asafetida, benzol, and xylol appear to stimulate *only* the olfactory organs in the dog.

OCULAR NERVES

For a detailed discussion of cranial nerves II, III, IV, and VI, see Chapter 18, page 647.

II. OPTIC NERVE—SENSORY

The optic nerve can be examined directly with an ophthalmoscope (papilledema, optic atrophy, detached retina, and retinal atrophy). The cerebral dura and underlying arachnoid with its cerebrospinal fluid-filled space surround the optic nerve up to the sclera (CSF space is exposed during eye enucleation).

In the dog, approximately 70 to 80 per cent of the optic nerve fibers decussate at the optic chiasma. Some nerve fibers of each optic nerve thus proceed to both the right and left *lateral* geniculate bodies, the pretectal area, and the superior colliculi. Axons from the pretectal region and the superior colliculi then pass to the nuclei of the motor nerves of both eyes, and axons from the right and left lateral geniculate bodies of the thalamus pass to the visual cortex of their respective cerebral hemispheres. This *partial* decussation helps to explain such a phenomenon as the consensual reflex, and enables one to differentiate between blindness in one eye and a unilateral oculomotor nerve paralysis.

TESTS. Retinal reflex: Throw a cotton ball at a plastic sheet held before the eyes. (Air currents must be eliminated to exclude blinking caused by a corneal reflex.) Fixed dilated pupil: Disruption of the sensory path of the optic nerve or the motor path (parasympathetic) of the oculomotor nerves, which together form the pupillary reflex. The pupil remains dilated because of stimulation of the dilator muscles of the pupil by sympathetics in the absence of a parasympathetic constrictor effect (see Chapter 18).

III. OCULOMOTOR NERVE—MOTOR

The nerve is *motor* to most of the eye muscles (dorsal, medial, and ventral rectus; ventral oblique) and to the levator palpebrae muscle, which elevates the upper eyelid. This nerve also carries parasympathetic

Text continued on page 251

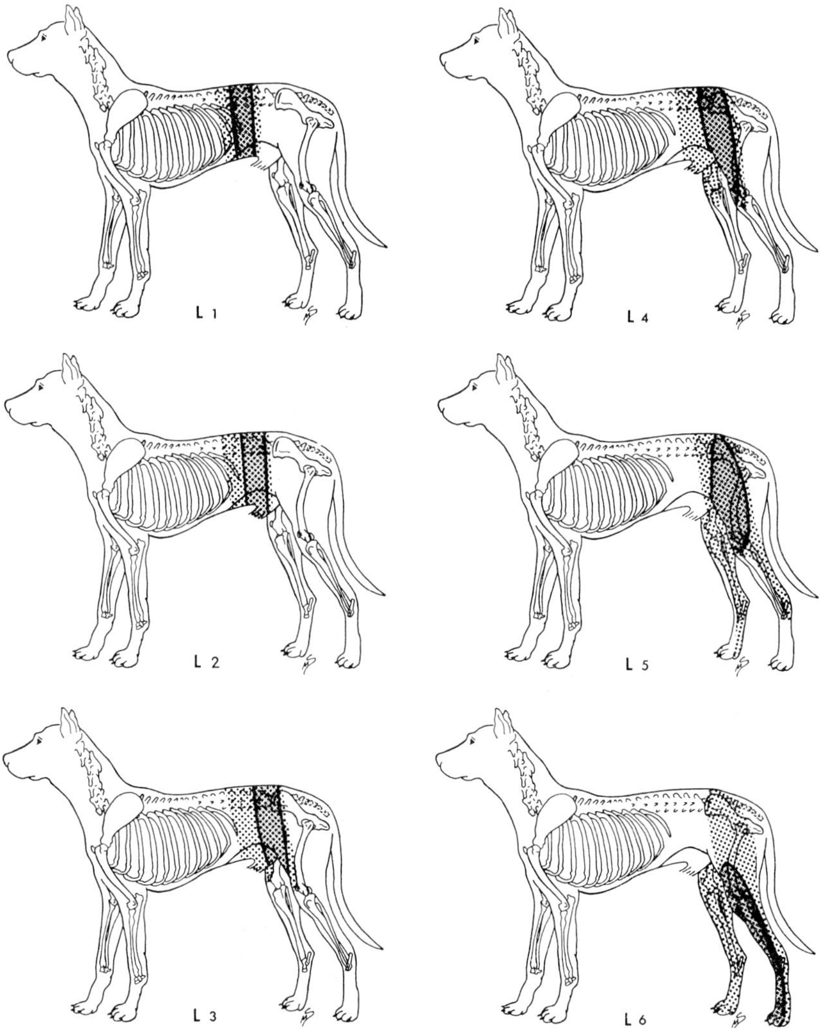

FIGURE 9–25 The tactile dermatomes are illustrated in relation to skeletal landmarks. Superimposed on the most common distribution for each dermatome is the region of maximal innervation (darker area) depicted on the lateral surface only, though it continued symmetrically to the ventral (or medial) surface. The maximal innervation zones were not prominent caudal to S_1. (From Fletcher, T. F., and Kitchell, R.: The lumbar, sacral, and coccygeal dermatomes of the dog. J. Comp. Neurol. *128*, 171, 1966.)

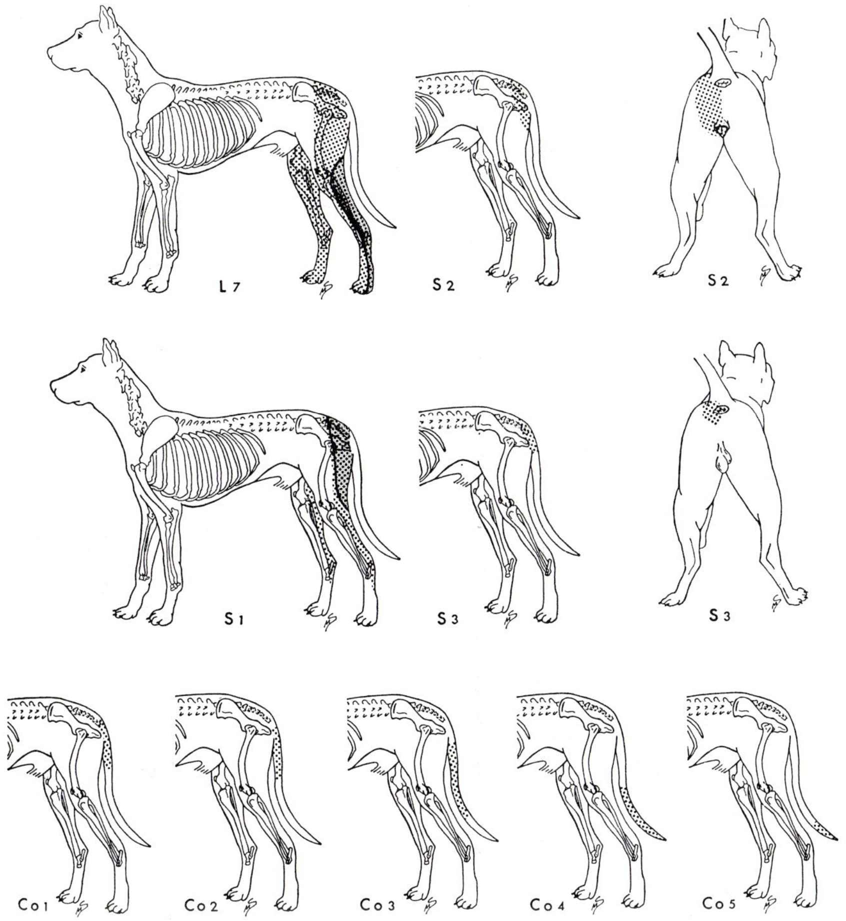

FIGURE 9–25 *Continued.*

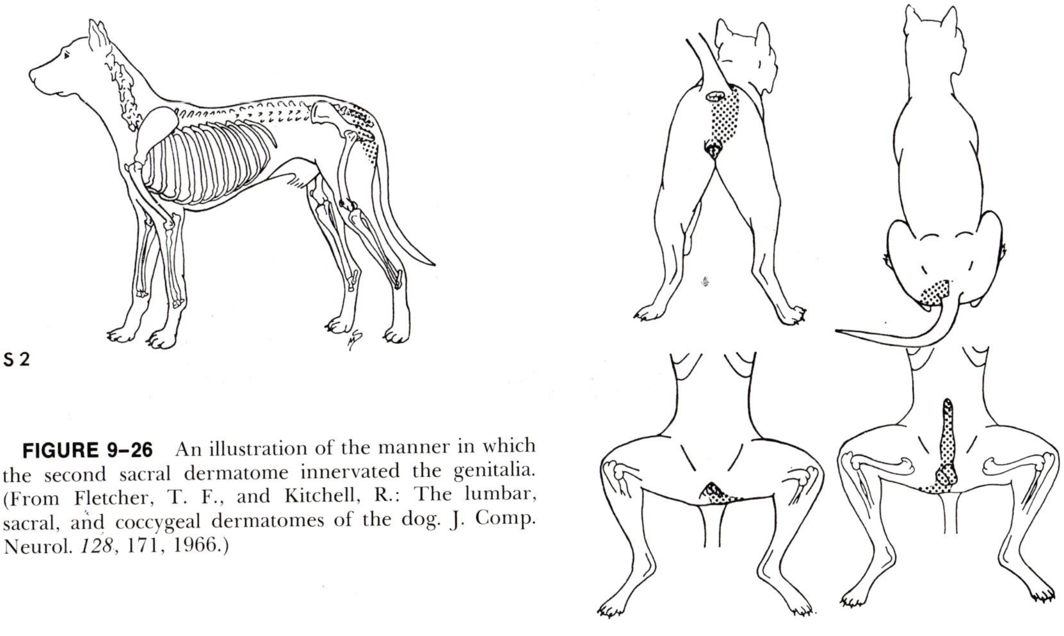

FIGURE 9–26 An illustration of the manner in which the second sacral dermatome innervated the genitalia. (From Fletcher, T. F., and Kitchell, R.: The lumbar, sacral, and coccygeal dermatomes of the dog. J. Comp. Neurol. *128*, 171, 1966.)

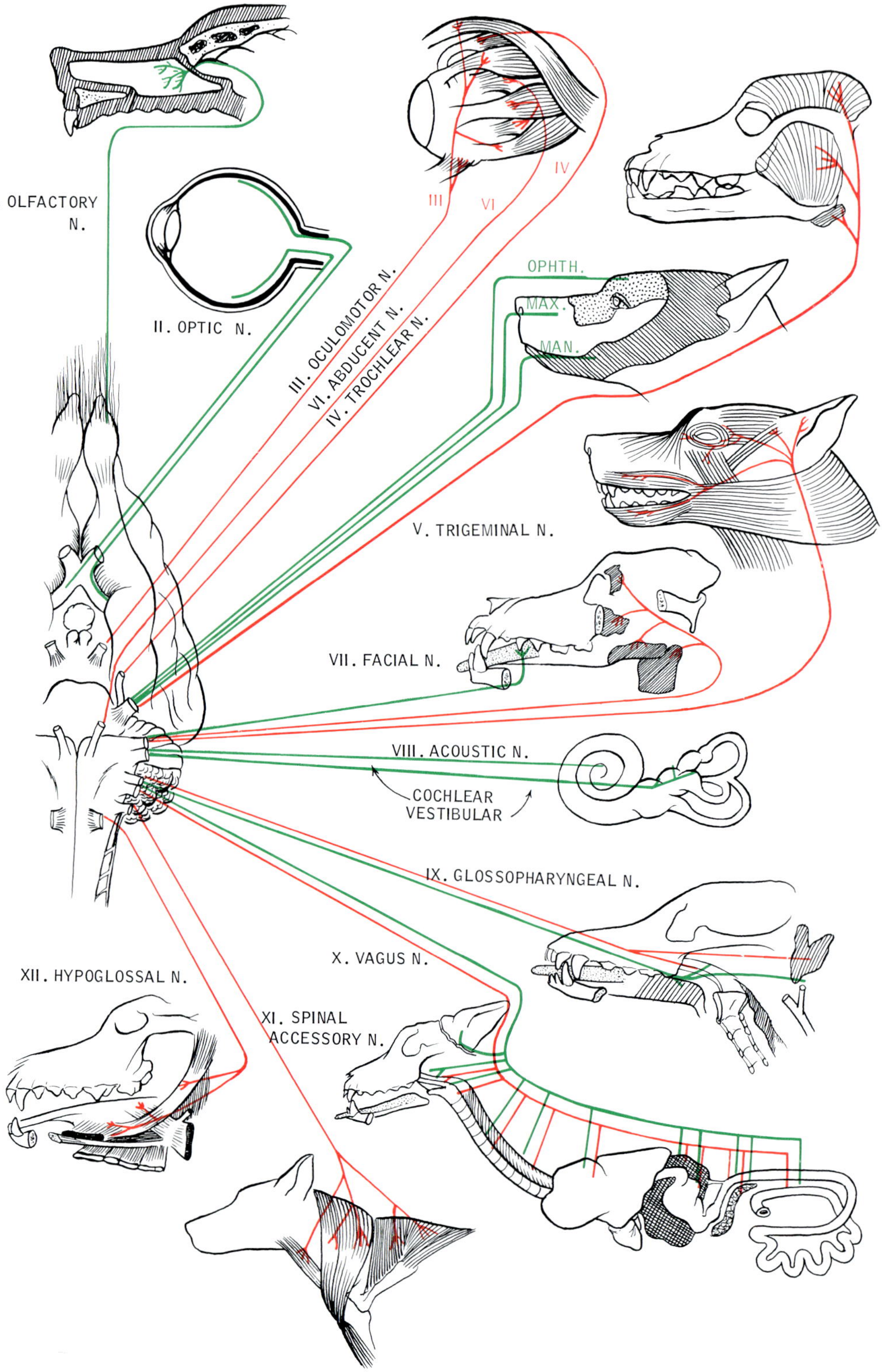

FIGURE 9–27 The origin and major distribution of the cranial nerves in the dog.

fibers to the ciliary ganglion for innervation of the ciliary muscle, which performs accommodation, and the sphincter pupillae, which promotes constriction of the pupil.

SIGNS OF PARALYSIS. Paralysis results in drooping of the upper eyelid, dilatation of the pupil, and deviation of the eyeball to the lateral side and downward.

TEST. Pupillary reflex: Normal pupil constricts in response to a light directed into same eye or opposite eye (consensual reflex).

IV. TROCHLEAR NERVE—MOTOR

The trochlear is motor to the dorsal oblique muscle. Paralysis moves the axis of vision upward and inward.

The oculomotor, trochlear, and abducent nerves control eyeball movements. Strabismus is an uncontrollable deviation of one or both eyeballs from the normal axis. Esotropia is an inward deviation which is referred to as convergent strabismus if it is bilateral, in which case it results in crossing axes. Siamese cats and some dogs may have congenital convergent strabismus. Exotropia is an outward deviation and, if bilateral, it is referred to as divergent strabismus. Some dogs, such as the Chihuahua and the pug, have congenital divergent strabismus.[1]

V. TRIGEMINAL NERVE—MIXED

In general, the nerve is *sensory* from the skin and most of the deeper structures of the head, and is *motor* to the muscles of mastication. The nerve is divided into three main branches, and the function of each will be discussed separately.

1. The maxillary nerve is sensory from the lower eyelid, roof of oral cavity, upper teeth, nasal cavity, skin of the nostrils, and upper lip.

TEST. Sensation by palpation, pinching, or pin-pricking.

2. The ophthalmic nerve is sensory from the upper eyelid, medial canthus, eyeball, posterior part of the nasal cavity, frontal region including sinus, and skin of the caudal part of the nose.

TEST. Corneal reflex: Direct air current from empty syringe to lateral canthus of eye (out of field of vision to eliminate retinal reflex). Test for sensation.

3. The mandibular nerve is sensory from the floor of the oral cavity, cheeks, lower lip, lower teeth, anterior two-thirds of the tongue, skin of the lateral cranium, and base of the ear. Taste functions result from the chorda tympani branch of the facial nerve, which joins the lingual branch of the mandibular nerve. It is the motor supply to the muscles of mastication.

SIGNS OF PARALYSIS AND TESTS. Loss of sensation. Ability to chew is impaired. Unilateral motor paralysis may result in a slight deviation of the mandible toward the normal side. Bilateral paralysis results in a dropped jaw, as seen in rabies. Masseter and temporal muscles may atrophy.[11] Taste—sugar, salt, quinine, or acetic acid on the anterior portion of the tongue.[6]

VI. ABDUCENT NERVE—MOTOR

The nerve is motor to the lateral rectus and retractor muscles of the eyeball. Paralysis results in rotation of the eyeball toward the medial canthus.

VII. FACIAL NERVE—MIXED

The nerve passes along the roof of the middle ear and is thus vulnerable in middle ear infections. It is *motor* to the muscles of facial expression (ears, lips, cheeks, and eyelids), and *sensory* (for taste) from the anterior two-thirds of the tongue. Parasympathetic fibers in the facial nerve supply the mandibular and sublingual salivary glands as well as the lacrimal and nasal glands.

SIGNS OF PARALYSIS. In a complete paralysis, all the superficial muscles of the head are flaccid. The ear droops, the eyelid remains open, the normal lines around the cheeks, muzzle, and face are smoothed out. The eyelid cannot close when the corneal or retinal reflexes are tested. Facial paralysis is essentially motor, and except for taste, there is no loss of sensation from the skin and mucous membranes (Fig. 9–28).

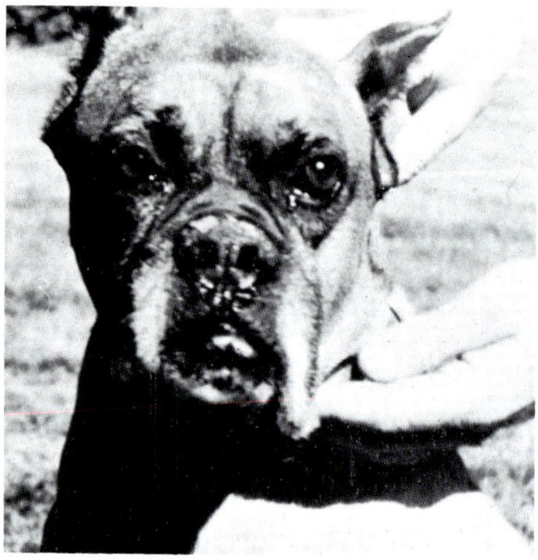

FIGURE 9–28 A 10-year-old boxer showing a paralysis of the left facial nerve. Notice the sagging lip particularly.

VIII. ACOUSTIC NERVE–SENSORY

The acoustic nerve is composed of two nerves, the cochlear and the vestibular.

The *cochlear nerve* transmits impulses that originate in the cochlea, a part of the inner ear that is a specialized receptor for sound.

SIGNS OF PARALYSIS AND TESTS. Deafness is rather easily tested by calling the dog's name or noting its reaction to various noises, e.g., holding a watch near the animal's ear, but out of its field of vision.

The *vestibular nerve* is closely associated with the cerebellum and has receptors in the utricle, the saccule, and the ampulla. It transmits proprioceptive impulses initiated by changes in position of the head. The entire vestibular mechanism is an important dynamic apparatus that is continually discharging stimuli into the nerves that supply skeletal musculature, e.g., the dog may display head tilt with inner ear infection. For further discussion of labyrinthitis and vestibular disease, see Chapters 11 and 16.

SIGNS OF PARALYSIS AND TESTS. Symptoms may include nystagmus, head tilt, rolling movements, circling, hypotonia or hypertonia, incoordination, and prostration. Postural and attitudinal reflexes are abnormal. The caloric test will be abnormal (see Chapter 3).

IX. GLOSSOPHARYNGEAL NERVE–MIXED

With the vagus nerve, the glossopharyngeal nerve is motor to muscles of the pharynx. It is sensory (including the sense of taste) from the root of the tongue, pharynx, tonsils, middle ear, and carotid sinus. Parasympathetic fibers in this nerve supply the parotid and zygomatic salivary glands.

SIGNS OF PARALYSIS AND TESTS. Loss of sensation from the pharynx and the root of the tongue. Pharyngeal (gag) reflex is lost on the affected side. Some difficulty in swallowing is noted. The carotid sinus reflex has its afferent arm in this nerve. Pressure over the sinus normally produces slowing of the heart and a fall in blood pressure. Taste responses should be tested on the posterior third of the tongue.

X. VAGUS NERVE–MIXED

The nerve is *motor* and *sensory* to the larynx and, with the glossopharyngeal nerve, supplies the pharynx and soft palate. It is sensory from part of the external ear canal and from the thoracic and abdominal viscera. Parasympathetic fibers in this nerve supply the thoracic and abdominal organs, causing slower heart rate, constricted bronchioles, increased bronchial secretion, increased peristalsis, relaxation of the pyloric sphincter, and stimulation of (digestive) glandular secretion.

SIGNS OF PARALYSIS. Loss or impairment of voice. Dyspnea due to flaccid vocal cords. Difficulty swallowing, associated with regurgitation of fluids through the nostrils. There may be a paralysis of the soft palate and loss of the gag reflex. Cough is a constant symptom of vagal *irritation.* Dilatation of stomach, tachycardia, etc. may result from vagal paralysis, while diarrhea may result from vagal irritation. (An interesting example of referred "pain" is the vomiting of the young dog with an ear inflammation. Since the vagus is sensory from both the external ear canal and the stomach, the dog may vomit because the brain fails to distinguish the true source of the irritation.) Pinprick testing of the external ear canal can be used to determine vagal sensory function to this area. Salivary taste reflex can be tested.[6]

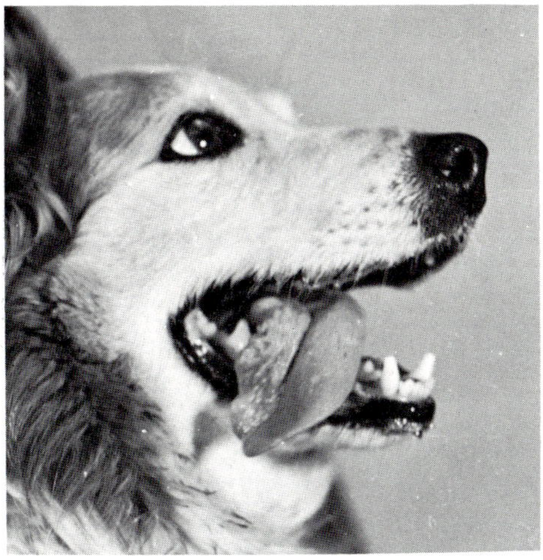

FIGURE 9–29 A right hypoglossal nerve injury in a dog hit by a car about 4 years previously. Notice the atrophy of the right side of the tongue. When it is protruded, the tongue draws toward the same side as the injury. The dog submerges his muzzle to lap water.

XI. (SPINAL) ACCESSORY NERVE–MOTOR

The bulbar part of the accessory nerve is distributed with the vagus; the spinal portion is *motor* to the trapezius and part of the sternocephalicus and brachiocephalicus muscles. Nerve injury is manifested by signs of weakness, paralysis, and atrophy of the involved muscles.

XII. HYPOGLOSSAL NERVE–MOTOR

The nerve is *motor* to the muscles of the tongue. Injury to the nerve causes paralysis of one-half of the tongue. When the tongue is protruded, it deviates toward the paralyzed side; the muscles on the affected side of the tongue atrophy (Fig. 9–29).

SUMMARY OF CRANIAL NERVE LESIONS

The most important conditions seen clinically that might result from lesions of the cranial nerves are:

Trigeminal nerve paralysis–drooping jaw, excessive salivation, difficulty in mastication (e.g., rabies).

Hemifacial nerve spasms, paralysis, and Horner's syndrome must be differentiated by careful examination, and are usually caused by middle ear infection or injuries.[9]

Partial vagus nerve paralysis (bulbar paralysis)–excessive salivation, dysphagia, difficulty in barking, fluid regurgitation through the nose.[6]

Oculomotor nerve paralysis–ptosis, dilated pupil, lateroventral deviation of the eyeball.[6]

Other disorders of the special senses, such as smell, sight, and hearing, involve the olfactory, optic, and acoustic nerves, respectively. Lesions in the vestibular portion of the acoustic nerve and its cerebellar associations may cause nystagmus, incoordination, and equilibrial deficits. Changes in the canine optic disks are difficult to determine unless they are marked and unilaterally located. Consult the foregoing discussion of the cutaneous distributions of the cranial nerves when skin testing reveals pronounced deficits.

Frequently, cerebral conditions produce a combination or variety of the conditions just outlined. The treatment of cranial nerve injuries is generally medical. Supportive treatment with vitamin therapy and good nursing care is important, but rest is probably the most essential factor in treatment. Surgical drainage of middle ear infections may be indicated in facial nerve disorders.[9]

REFERENCES

1. Chrisman, C. L.: Diseases of peripheral nerves and muscles. *In* Ettinger, S. J. (ed.): *Textbook of Veterinary Internal Medicine.* W. B. Saunders Co., Philadelphia, 1975.
2. Fletcher, T. F., and Kitchell, R. L.: The lumbar, sacral and coccygeal dermatomes of the dog. J. Comp. Neurol. *128,* 171, 1966.
3. Fox, J. G., and Gutnick, M. J.: Horner's syndrome and brachial paralysis due to lymphosarcoma in a cat. J.A.V.M.A. *160,* 977, 1972.
4. Gardner, E.: *Fundamentals of Neurology,* 6th ed. W. B. Saunders Co., Philadelphia, 1975.
5. Knecht, C. D., and St. Clair, L. E.: The radial-brachial paralysis syndrome in the dog. J.A.V.M.A. *154,* 653, 1969.
6. McGrath, J. T.: *Neurologic Examination of the Dog.* 2nd ed. Lea and Febiger, Philadelphia, 1960.
7. Miller, M. F., Christensen, G. C., and Evans, H. E.: *Anatomy of the Dog.* W. B. Saunders Co., Philadelphia, 1964.
8. Parker, A. J., and Small, E.: The nervous system. *In* Carcott, E. J. (ed.): *Feline Medicine and Surgery.* American Veterinary Publications, Santa Barbara, 1975, p. 364.
9. Roberts, S. R., and Vainisi, S. J.: Hemifacial spasm in dogs. J.A.V.M.A. *150,* 381, 1967.
10. Worthman, R. P.: Demonstration of specific nerve paralyses in the dog. J.A.V.M.A. *131,* 174, 1957.
11. Worthman, R. P.: The nerve of that dog. (Teaching brochure on peripheral nervous system of the dog.) Washington State University, 1960.

SECTION 2

PERIPHERAL NERVE ELECTRODIAGNOSTICS, ELECTROMYOGRAPHY, AND NERVE CONDUCTION VELOCITY

JOHN M. BOWEN, D.V.M., PH.D.*

The high incidence of peripheral nerve injuries in man during the First and Second World Wars promoted widespread application of electrodiagnostic testing. This procedure was recommended for veterinary use by Allam and co-workers in 1949. Owing to lack of refinements in instrumentation and the expense of the technique, electromyography did not begin to develop as an independent field until 1944 and was not introduced into veterinary medicine until 1967,[7] although it had been used previous to this time in animal research.[29] Interest in the clinical applications of peripheral nerve electrodiagnostics, electromyography, and nerve conduction velocity as diagnostic aids in veterinary neurology has expanded rapidly in recent years.[11, 18, 25]

*Professor, Dept. of Physiology and Pharmacology, College of Veterinary Medicine, University of Georgia, Athens, Georgia.

Muscles under voluntary control are innervated by nerve fibers arising from motoneuron cells in the ventral horns of the spinal cord and in certain cranial nerve nuclei. These neurons are called lower motoneurons and are excited or inhibited by impulses from upper motoneurons or sensory neurons (Fig. 9–30. See also Figs. 2–3 and 2–4). The sensory neurons of special importance are associated with muscle spindles, which are receptors that are sensitive to changes in muscle length (Fig. 9–30). The degree of sensitivity of a muscle spindle to stretch is influenced by the activity of small motoneurons (gamma efferents) supplying the muscle fibers within the spindle. When excitation exceeds a threshold value in the motoneuron cell, an impulse is initiated in the axon and is conducted peripherally to the nerve terminals at a velocity dependent upon the diameter of the axon. The nerve terminals are located on the surface of muscle fibers and constitute the prejunctional component of the neuromus-

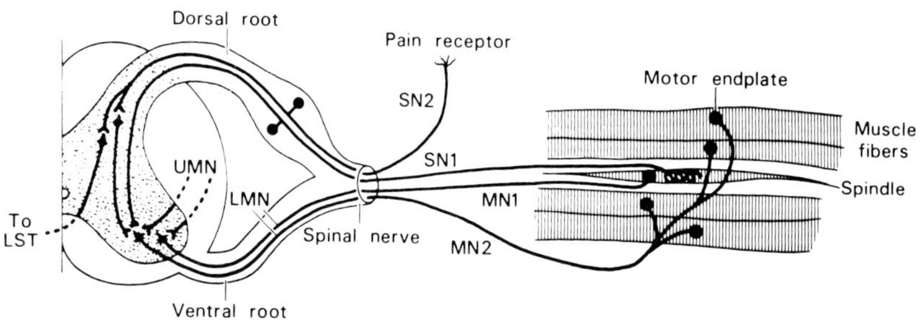

FIGURE 9–30 Inter-relationships between upper motor neurons (UMN), lower motor neurons (LMN), sensory neurons (SN), striated muscle fibers, and a muscle spindle. Understanding these inter-relationships is very important in the clinical applications of EDT and EMG. Input to MN1 comes from UMN, whereas input to MN2 comes from UMN and also from muscle spindles via SN1 and sensory receptors via SN2. Sensory input via SN2 also passes to higher centers via the lateral spinothalamic tract (LST). The motor unit size for MN2 is four.

cular junction. Each muscle fiber usually has only one neuromuscular junction. Entrance of the nerve impulse into the nerve terminal results in the release of acetylcholine (excitation-secretion coupling), which diffuses across the neuromuscular junction to the postjunctional or end-plate membrane, where it effects localized depolarization of the muscle cell. If this localized depolarization or end-plate potential is of suprathreshold magnitude, muscle action potentials are initiated and conducted from the end-plate region to the ends of the muscle fibers. In transit, the muscle action potential triggers the mechanical response (excitation-contraction coupling).

One lower motoneuron innervates a fixed number of muscle fibers. This neuron and the muscle fibers it supplies constitute a motor unit (Fig. 9–30). The size of a motor unit in terms of the number of muscle fibers innervated decreases as refinement of muscle movements increases in the various muscles of the body. Thus, the extraocular muscles have small motor units (about three muscle fibers) and antigravity muscles have large motor units (about 1000 muscle fibers). The size of a motor unit potential is influenced by the number of muscle fibers in a motor unit. Electromyographic activities of slow-contracting motor units (Type I fibers) and fast-contracting motor units (Type II fibers) differ,[53] firing of the former being better sustained than that of the latter.

A deficit in motor function can result from alterations in input to a lower motoneuron, as in upper motoneuron disease, or it can result from pathology at any of several points in the motor unit itself, i.e., the ventral horn cell, ventral root, peripheral nerve, nerve terminals, and muscle fibers (Fig. 9–30). When attempting diagnosis of a condition involving a deficit in motor function, it is important that the clinician determine the level at which the disorder arises. The first approach should always be a standard neurological examination, as described in another section in this book. It is the object of this section to describe electromyographic and electrodiagnostic testing procedures that can serve as valuable adjuncts to the neurological examination.

The purpose of electrodiagnostic testing (EDT) of peripheral nerves is to demonstrate the presence, absence, reduction, or abnormality of the contractile response of a muscle to electrical stimulation of either the muscle itself (direct stimulation method) or its motor nerve (indirect stimulation method). An important advantage is that subject cooperation is not necessary. The purpose of electromyography (EMG) is to demonstrate quantitative or qualitative alterations in the electrical activity of a muscle in the resting state, or following either direct or indirect electrical stimulation, or during either voluntary or reflex activation. In addition, EMG provides a means of evaluating nerve conduction velocity and nerve terminal conduction time. Since it is now possible to record the electrical activity of nerves in the intact animal, the term electroneuromyography is employed by some workers.[20] Review of 561 cases of neuropathies and myopathies in man indicated to the clinicians involved that EDT was of value in 60 per cent of their cases, whereas EMG was of value in 34 per cent.[2] No single method appeared satisfactory for all cases.

PERIPHERAL NERVE ELECTRODIAGNOSTICS

If the neurological examination indicates the need for further information on the state of innervation of a muscle or muscles, EDT or EMG should be employed. Firm guidelines have not been established for choosing between the two methods. Often a survey evaluation of peripheral nerves with EDT will aid the electromyographer in planning the EMG examination. When the individual performing the EDT or EMG does not also perform the neurological examination, the results of this examination should be reviewed, noting particularly the duration of the disorder and its location. Then volitional movement of the involved region should be observed, and the region should be palpated during movement to determine the degree of muscle tone, contractile activity, and atrophy present. If the disorder is not bilateral, the symmetrical, normal muscles can be examined from a comparative standpoint. Anesthetics or tranquilizers may be administered prior to EDT of peripheral nerves. Clinical concentrations of these agents will not influence electrically induced motor responses examined in EDT, but will suppress or abolish sensory responses that sometimes provide additional information that is helpful in reaching a final diagnosis. Equipment requirements for performance of peripheral nerve EDT include a source of electrical stimuli (stimulator) and the electrodes for application of the stimuli to a nerve or muscle.

STIMULATORS

A wide variety of stimulators are available commercially or can be constructed for use in EDT. An example is shown in Figure 9–31. Allam and co-workers modified an ordinary flashlight containing one 1.5 volt battery for peripheral nerve stimulation in dogs.[1] For direct current or galvanic stimulation of muscle in man, a 45-volt dry cell battery has been employed.[42]

The choice of stimulator depends upon the type of electrical pulses needed from the standpoint of pulse duration and repetition rate. The repetition rate of pulses used in EDT may be divided into three types: (1) single pulses of short duration, usually less than 1 millisecond (msec); (2) single pulses of long duration, ranging from 100 msec to several seconds (galvanic stimulation); and (3) repetitive pulses of short duration with repetition rate usually ranging between 3/sec and 200/sec (faradic stimulation). A simple dry cell battery can be used to provide the second type of pulse if approximation of the desired duration suffices. Electronic stimulators constructed from standard electronic parts[14] and commercially available stimulators for clinical use* usually provide the first and third types of pulses. To obtain all three types of pulses, a commercial laboratory stimulator is needed (Fig. 9–31). Such a unit provides calibrated dials for widely varying pulse intensity, duration, and repetition rate. Control of duration is essential for determination of chronaxy or evaluation of strength-duration curves.

The output pulse of a laboratory stimulator has a rectangular shape. Pulse amplitude should be variable from 0 to 100 volts (needle electrodes) or 0 to 300 volts (surface electrodes); duration or pulse width should be variable from 0.05 to 100 msec; and frequency should be variable from 0.5 to 30 pulses/sec. Ideally, the stimulator output should be isolated from the electrical ground by an isolation device (Fig. 9–31) to prevent stray electrical currents which could create a safety hazard to the animal. A constant current adapter (Fig. 9–31) is useful if electrode resistances are variable during an examination. Although the laboratory stimulator has greater clinical utility, the smaller, portable units provide excellent results. Batteries should be considered for emergency use only or for use by clinicians who rarely deal with neurological problems.

*Peripheral Nerve Stimulator NS-2, Professional Instruments Company, Houston, Texas.

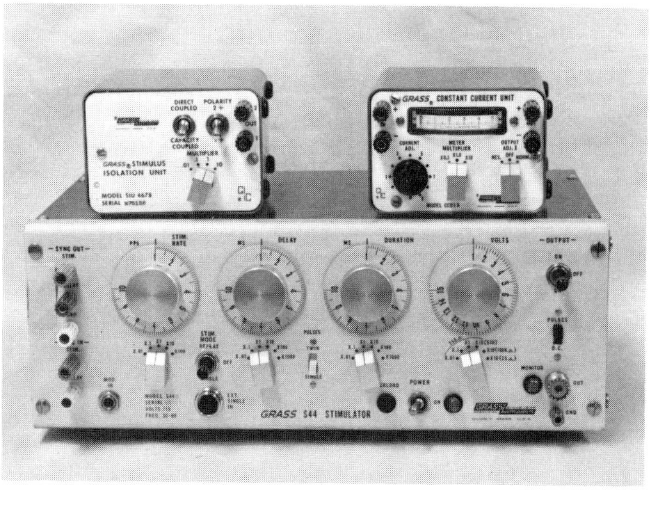

FIGURE 9–31 Stimulator for electrodiagnostic testing. Controls enable regulation of the amplitude, duration, and frequency of the rectangular stimulus pulses. Important accessories include a stimulus isolation unit (top left) and constant current unit (top right). When this stimulator is a component of an electromyograph, it is used also for inducing evoked potentials and in the determination of nerve conduction velocities.

ELECTRODES

Two electrodes are needed to effect stimulation of a nerve or muscle. One is referred to as the stimulating electrode and is connected to the cathode or negative terminal of the stimulator; the other, the indifferent electrode, is connected to the anode or positive terminal. When these electrodes are placed at different points along a peripheral nerve, excitation will occur first at the cathode as current flowing between the electrodes increases from zero. Several types of electrodes may be used. Surface electrodes consist of a metal disk or ball, about 1 cm in diameter with an insulated handle, as the stimulating electrode, and an 8 by 10 cm wire mesh or a metal plate as the indifferent electrode. Examples of surface electrodes are shown in Figure 9–32. These electrodes are particularly useful in the determination of chronaxy and in measurement of strength-duration curves.

Both electrodes and the skin must be dampened with saline solution or coated with a special electrode paste prior to application of a stimulus. Current flowing across the electrode-skin junction at a given voltage will vary with the resistance of this junction. Thus, the junction should be inspected frequently and more saline solution or paste applied to maintain good electrical contact. Surface electrodes consisting of alligator clips, as described for recording electroencephalograms (see Chapter 7), may also be used.

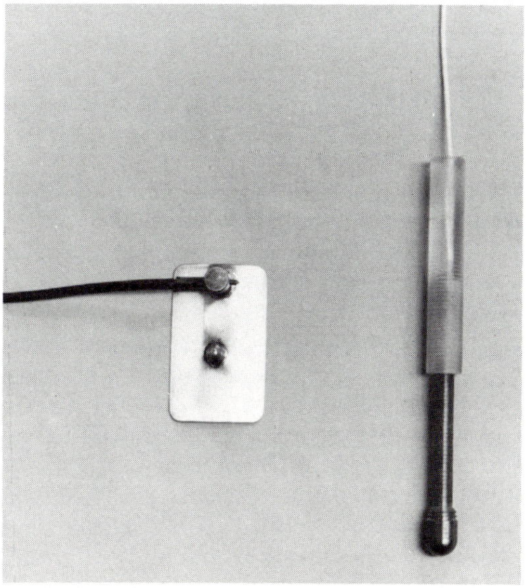

FIGURE 9–32 Surface electrodes for electrodiagnostic testing. The plate is the indifferent electrode, and the probe with the insulated handle and rounded tip (1 cm) is the stimulating electrode.

Needle electrodes may consist of standard 1-inch, 25-gauge stainless steel hypodermic needles. Bowen prefers to use a 1-inch, 28-gauge, Teflon-insulated, monopolar electromyographic electrode, with 5 to 8 mm of its tip scraped free of insulation with a razor blade for the stimulating electrode. This type of stimulating electrode provides excellent localization of motor nerves and even of their small branches. The indifferent electrode is prepared in a similar manner except that all of the insulation is removed from the needle shaft. These solid needle electrodes are well tolerated by most dogs and cats. The electrode tips should be sharpened as necessary.

PROCEDURE FOR ELECTRODIAGNOSTIC TESTING OF PERIPHERAL NERVES

Sites selected for application of EDT depend upon the nature of the deficit in motor function and its location. Commonly used sites of stimulation are shown in Figure 9–33. There are many others in addition to those shown. A suitable site is a motor point or any point along the course of a motor nerve that is accessible to a needle electrode.[1, 49] A motor point is located in the region of a muscle where its motor nerve enters or in a region that has a high density of nerve terminals. The nerve terminals are usually localized in a fairly narrow band which passes transversely across the muscle at about the midpoint of the muscle fibers. Potentials recorded from the end-plate region of a muscle differ in shape from those recorded from nonend-plate regions.

When the disorder is unilateral, the initial phase of EDT should be directed toward evaluation of the response of the symmetrical, normal muscle. The threshold voltage for minimal contractile response should be determined for the normal muscle and then for the suspect muscle as follows: The skin at the stimulation site is cleaned as if for a hypodermic injection. Ethyl alcohol (78 per cent v/v) is a satisfactory disinfectant. The indifferent electrode

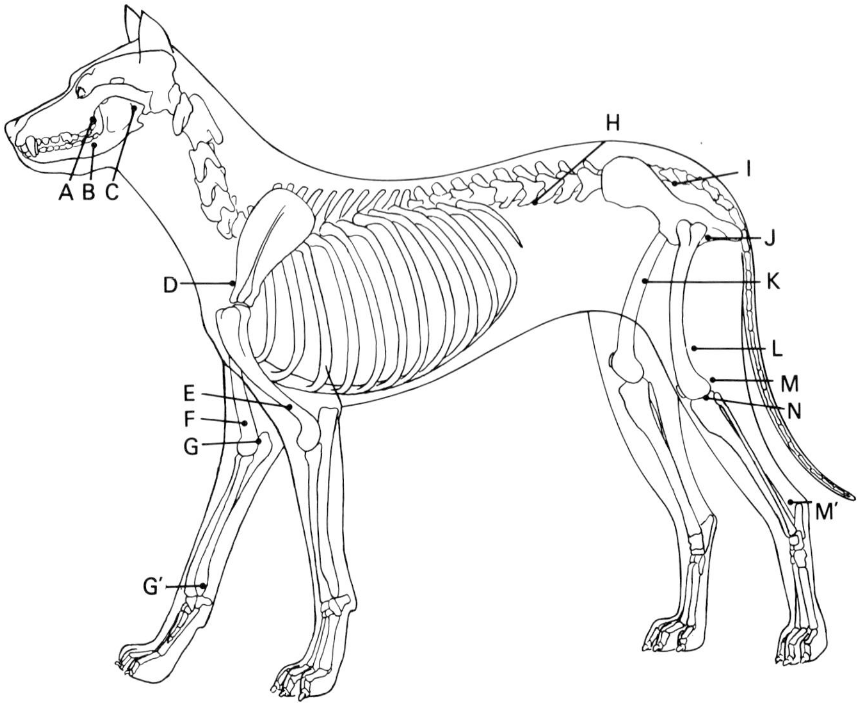

FIGURE 9–33 Anatomical localization of sites for stimulation of the principal nerves examined in electrodiagnostic testing. *A* and *B*. Dorsal and ventral buccal branches of the facial nerve—unilateral movement of the lips. *C*. Masseteric branch of the trigeminal nerve—masseter muscle contraction and closure of the mouth. *D*. Suprascapular nerve—contraction of the supraspinatus and infraspinatus muscles. *F*. Radial nerve—extension of the elbow, carpus, and digits. *F*. Median nerve—flexion of the carpus and digits. *G*. Ulnar nerve—flexion of the carpus and digits. *G*. Ulnar nerve—flexion of the digits. *H*. Spinal nerves—movements of the muscles of the chest and abdomen. *I*. Coccygeal nerves—movement of the tail. *J*. Ischiatic nerve—extension of the hip and flexion of the stifle joints and combined effects of tibial and peroneal nerve stimulation. *K*. Femoral nerve—extension of the stifle joint. *L*. Ischiatic nerve (use caudal approach)—combined effects of tibial and peroneal nerve stimulation. *M*. Tibial nerve (use caudal approach)—extension of the hock and flexion of the digits. *M'*. Tibial nerve—flexion of the digits. *N*. Peroneal (fibular) nerve—flexion of the hock and extension of the digits.

is inserted subcutaneously between the stimulating electrode, which is positioned over a motor nerve or at a motor point, and the brain or spinal column. The distance between the two electrodes is not critical, and several stimulation sites in a limb can be examined without moving the indifferent electrode. However, it is very important that the same procedure and electrode positions be used for comparison of responses of symmetrical muscles.

With the frequency of stimulation adjusted to 1/sec or slower and the voltage output set at zero, the voltage is gradually increased until a maximal contractile response is observed. The contractile response should be very brisk and should be followed by immediate and complete relaxation. A noninvasive myographic technique for quantitating force of contractions of some muscles in the dog has been described by Bowen.[8, 12] In unanesthetized animals, maximal contractile response usually cannot be evoked without concomitant sensory reaction on the part of the animal. This should be noted and also evaluated later on the suspect side. Then the voltage should be reduced until minimal contractile response is observed. Voltage at this point is called the threshold voltage or simply the threshold. In symmetrical muscles with normal innervation, threshold values will be very similar. Observation of the minimal contractile response is often difficult in animals because of the hair coat. If the hair has been removed, oblique lighting is helpful; if not, palpation of the muscle and its tendon must be used to determine minimal response. If the stimulating electrode has been inserted at the motor point, observation of the movement of the needle hub frequently will serve as a means of determining threshold.

Often the first point of insertion of the stimulating electrode is not the optimal one for determining threshold. Therefore, an attempt should be made to determine whether movement of the tip of the stimulating electrode reduces threshold. When the tip of the electrode is touching a normal motor nerve, threshold will be less than 2 volts, whereas it may be 20 volts or more when the electrode is 8 mm away from the nerve.[24]

When a muscle exhibits an abnormal reaction to stimulation of its motor point or motor nerve, the response to stimulation with single pulses of long duration (galvanic stimulation) and repetitive pulses of short duration (faradic stimulation) can be examined as described later to provide additional help in establishing a diagnosis. In addition, if a laboratory stimulator is available, chronaxy measurements and strength-duration curves can be determined.

Chronaxy is defined as the minimum pulse duration required to produce a just-minimal contraction of a muscle that is stimulated at its motor point with a pulse strength which is twice rheobase. Rheobase is the threshold voltage required to induce a response with pulse durations greater than 100 msec. For normally innervated muscles, chronaxy is about 0.1 msec. Values exceeding 1 msec are considered abnormal. Strength-duration (S-D) curves are prepared by plotting on one axis the strength of the stimulus required to induce a just-minimal contractile response to motor point stimulation at various pulse durations, and on the other axis the pulse duration, which is varied from 0.05 msec to 100 msec. Chronaxy is one point on the S-D curve. The S-D curve reflects the degree of innervation of a muscle. The curves differ characteristically for muscles that are fully innervated, partially denervated, or completely denervated because nerve fibers are excited by shorter duration pulses than muscle fibers. Serial S-D curve determinations are useful in following the progress of a neuropathy and in making an objective prognosis. Heckman[26] has recommended measurement of nerve action potentials for plotting excitability curves because of technical errors in standard S-D curve measurements. These errors include inconsistencies in defining the just-minimal contraction and incorrect localization of the motor point. However, determination of neural excitability curves requires electromyographic equipment, whereas S-D curve measurements require only the laboratory stimulator. Chronaxy values and S-D curves for muscles of dogs[51] and cats[39] have been reported.

INTERPRETATION OF RESULTS OF ELECTRODIAGNOSTIC TESTING OF PERIPHERAL NERVES

EDT has its greatest value in aiding diagnosis of disorders of lower motoneurons and in establishing functional integrity of nerves and muscles suitable for compensatory grafting in motor nerve disorders.[28, 35] When a lower motoneuron has been damaged to the extent that functional innervation of a muscle is no longer present, the following results will be obtained with EDT.

1. Absence of response to stimulation of the motor nerve normally supplying the muscle. This applies to all points proximal to the injury immediately after damage occurs. Since degeneration migrates peripherally following nerve damage, the nerve terminals and thus the motor point will retain their excitability for 3 to 21 days, depending upon the distance between site of nerve injury and affected muscle. At the time of nerve terminal degeneration, an abrupt reduction in excitability or increase in threshold occurs and the motor point disappears. Immediately after a motor nerve has been severed, the threshold of the distal segment may be lower than normal, a change that can also occur in the presence of inflammation of this tissue. An increase in threshold may occur in normally innervated muscles when edema is present and when the size and volume of a muscle have been reduced, as in disuse atrophy. The latter can readily be distinguished from denervation atrophy by EDT. Often trauma can disrupt normal anatomical relationships, resulting in displacement of motor points. This may result in an apparent discrepancy in the thresholds of symmetrical muscles.

2. Sustained contraction during galvanic stimulation. This is known as Erb's reaction.[15] After 2 or 3 weeks, the response of denervated muscle to this type of stimulation becomes sluggish and sometimes vermicular.

3. Absence of response to faradic stimulation at normal intensities. Positive results for galvanic stimulation and negative results for faradic stimulation are jointly referred to as the "reaction of degeneration."[36]

4. Chronaxy greater than 1 msec.

5. Strength-duration curves typical of denervated muscle. Strength-duration curves are not as sensitive a test as EMG for detecting early evidence of reinnervation, but they may give earlier evidence of denervation following nerve injury than EMG.

In muscles exhibiting partial denervation, intermediate changes will be present and are often difficult to evaluate without strength-duration curves or electromyograms.

In some cases, a deficit in motor function is caused by factors other than lower motoneuron disorders. In these cases, EDT demonstrates the presence of normal lower motoneuron function, and thus indirectly implies the presence of pathology at other sites, such as upper motoneurons or joints.

Disorders of muscle exhibit gross weakening of motor response in EDT. Chronaxy usually remains normal, whereas threshold tends to increase as fibrous tissue replaces muscle tissue. In myotonia, the most significant feature in EDT is the continuation of contraction or delayed relaxation after termination of stimulus. Erb's reaction and a decrease in rheobase may be present.[15]

In botulism and tick paralysis, a generalized depression or absence of induced contractile response is observed. Rapid recovery from tick paralysis following tick removal is noteworthy. In both of these conditions, the toxins do not appear to alter sensory perception of electrical stimulation. Polyradiculoneuritis (coon dog paralysis) is also characterized by generalized weakness and depression of contractile response.[21] Chronaxy and strength-duration curves indicate partial to complete denervation. This condition is often difficult to distinguish from botulism, but is probably the more common of the two in the dog. EMG may be of value in differential diagnosis since botulism does not affect nerve conduction velocity.[6]

Several cases of apparent myasthenia gravis in the dog have been reported.[40] Muscular weakness and a favorable therapeutic response to cholinesterase inhibitor drugs were common to these cases; however, EDT was employed in only one of these cases with results that were not as definitive as those seen in myasthenia gravis in humans.[56] The standard test in man involves comparison of contractile responses induced by stimulation at 1 to 3/sec and 30 to 50/sec. The responses to these two frequencies in the normal individual are stable and similar, whereas the response of the diseased individual fades markedly during high-frequency stimulation. This abnormal response is often completely antagonized when the subject has been pretreated with neostigmine or edrophonium.

In puerperal tetany resulting from hypocalcemia, threshold is significantly reduced. Localization of disease processes in the spinal cord, such as syringomyelia and compression, is aided by EDT.

OTHER APPLICATIONS FOR NERVE STIMULATORS

A nerve stimulator may be used to provide optimal positioning of the tip of a hypodermic needle (stimulating electrode) for injection of local anesthetics and agents for performing destructive blocks in painful or spastic conditions.[24, 34, 55] For this purpose it is best to use a 2- or 3-inch, Teflon-insulated (except at the tip), 22-gauge hypodermic needle.[34] Greenblatt and Denson reported on the successful use of this procedure in 17 different types of nerve blocks in human medicine.[24] A significant advantage was the reduction by 50 per cent or more in the amount of local anesthetic required to block several of the nerves tested.

The nerve stimulator is very useful in locating nerves during surgery. In open reduction of a fractured humerus, care must be taken not to damage the radial nerve or its branches. These can be identified with the stimulator shown in Figure

9–31 or with a sterile, disposable unit* designed specifically for this purpose. The latter cannot be used for EDT.

The action of muscle relaxant drugs such as succinylcholine can be monitored by use of a nerve stimulator.[33] The dosage is adjusted to provide the desired degree of depression of muscle contractile response induced by nerve stimulation.

Finally, electrical stimulation has been applied to denervated muscle in man in an attempt to delay irreversible changes in this tissue prior to reinnervation. Rate of recovery of motor function was significantly increased by this electrotherapeutic technique.[45] Sixty contractions per day induced through large surface electrodes have been recommended.[47]

ELECTROMYOGRAPHY

Electromyography (EMG) permits visual, graphic, and audio evaluation of the electrical activity of striated muscles. The evaluation may be qualitative or quantitative and provides information which, when combined with the results of the neurological examination, frequently is the determining factor in reaching a diagnosis. It is particularly helpful when clinical signs are modified by pain, upper motoneuron disease, and compensatory actions of synergistic muscles. In addition, the prognosis is aided by evaluation of results of serial electromyographic examinations. The instrument used to record the electrical activity of muscle is the electromyograph.

THE ELECTROMYOGRAPH

The electromyograph can be purchased commercially with all components installed in a single console (Fig. 9–34), or components can be purchased individually and arranged in a manner suitable to the electromyographer. The latter unit is termed a hybrid electromyograph and is often less expensive than the commercial electromyograph. However, operation of a hybrid electromyograph is often less convenient,

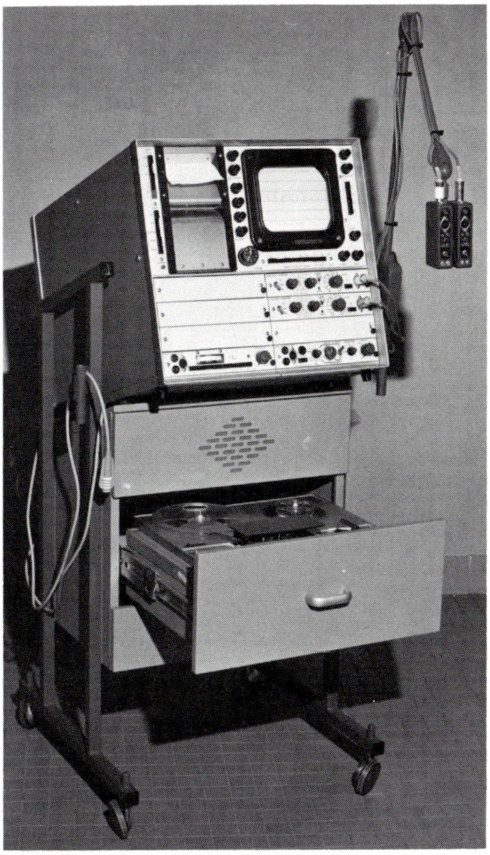

FIGURE 9–34 A two-channel direct recording electromyograph which includes a cathode ray tube display, fiberoptic graphic recorder, stimulator, and audio monitor. (Model TE-4, TECA Corporation, White Plains, New York).

although its performance characteristics may be excellent. Components of an electromyograph are shown in Figure 9–35. The essential components of an electromyograph are the electrodes, amplifier, oscilloscope, and the loudspeaker system. The electromyograph amplifier is a high impedance, high gain, and low noise differential amplifier which has three input terminals: positive, negative, and ground. A signal applied symmetrically to both positive and negative terminals is rejected. This is referred to as common mode rejection and is very useful in attenuating 60 cycle interference from nearby power lines. Since a motor unit potential is applied asymmetrically to the electrodes, a potential difference will exist between positive and negative input terminals. This potential difference will be amplified by the electromyograph amplifier at least 50,000 times as much as common mode interfering signals.

---

*Edward Weck & Co., Inc., New Brunswick, New Jersey.

A system of electrical filters should be included in the electromyograph amplifier. Two filters are needed, one to attenuate frequencies lower than electromyographic signals and one to attenuate frequencies higher than electromyographic signals. For good fidelity recording of electromyographic signals, the lower and upper cut-off frequencies should be 2 Hz and 10 kHz, respectively. In clinical EMG some signal distortion is acceptable. Thus, when low and high frequency interference is a problem, the low cut-off frequency may be raised to 15 Hz and the high cut-off frequency may be lowered to 3 kHz.

The electromyographic oscilloscope provides a visual display of electromyographic signals. Since a motor unit potential has a duration of only a few milliseconds, the low inertia of the electron beam of the oscilloscope can follow the rapid voltage variations, whereas the pen of a mechanical oscillograph (as in an electroencephalograph) cannot follow these rapid changes. Fiberoptic graphic recorders have frequency responses compatible with clinical evaluation of electromyographic signals (Fig. 9–34).

Electromyographic signals can be converted into sounds with the aid of an audio amplifier and loudspeaker. Audio monitoring of these signals is time saving to the electromyographer because it aids positioning of the electrodes without requiring observation of the oscilloscope display. In addition, sounds of different types of electromyographic signals are characteristic

TABLE 9–1 CHARACTERISTIC SOUNDS OF ELECTROMYOGRAPHIC ACTIVITY

EMG Activity	Sound
Normal Muscle	
Resting	
Electrode insertion	No added sounds when electrode is released
Non–end-plate region	Electrical "silence" (background low level hissing; amplifier noise)
End-plate region	Moderately loud hissing
Nerve activity	High pitched hissing
Contracting (minimal effort)	
Single motor unit potentials	Sharp, single cracking or popping which ceases with relaxation
Contracting (maximal effort)	
Many motor unit potentials	Loud blast without single sounds which decreases in intensity and then ceases with relaxation
Abnormal Muscle	
Resting (denervation > 5 days)	
Insertion activity	Loud crackling which decreases after 1 to several minutes
Fibrillation potential	Sound like rain on a tin roof or frying eggs
Positive potentials	Varies from a musical tone or a sound like an idling outboard motor to a dive bomber roar
Fasciculation potentials	Sharp crackling or popping not associated with effort
Bizarre high frequency discharge	Banjo-like twang
Contracting (immediate postdenervation effort)	
Complete denervation	
No motor unit potentials	No change with effort
Partial denervation	
A few motor unit potentials	Response similar to normal minimal effort pattern even though a maximal effort is attempted
Reinnervation	
Miniature motor unit potentials	Rough, rasping, cracking or popping sound that has a higher pitch than normal motor unit potential sound
Giant motor unit potential	Very loud rasping or popping sound
Myotonia (tap electrode)	Dive bomber roar
Interference	
ECG	Dull thumping that follows pulse rate
60 Hz	Hum or buzz

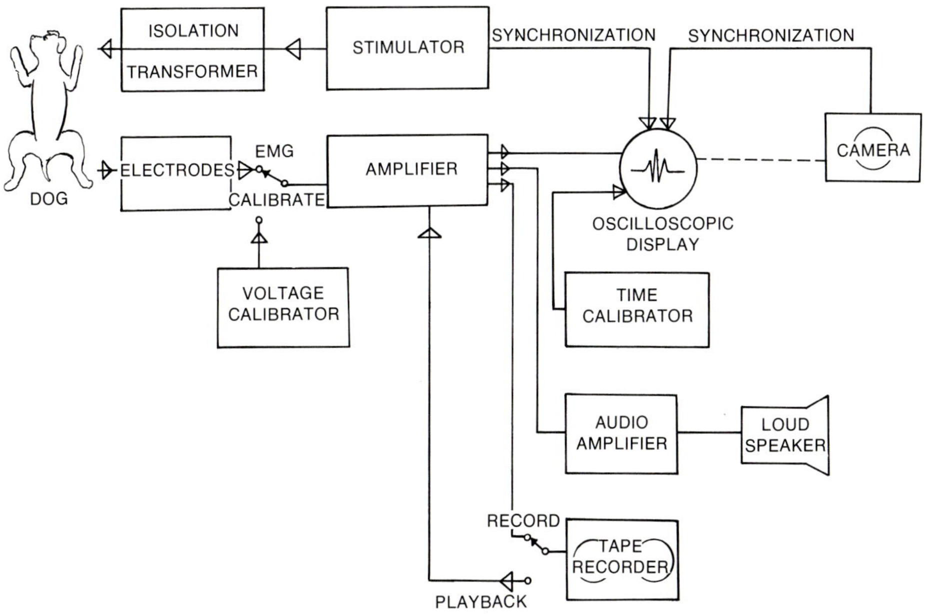

FIGURE 9–35 A schematic diagram of a complete instrumentation system for electromyography in the dog. (Adapted from Rogoff, J. B., and Reiner, S.: Electrodiagnostic apparatus. *In* Licht, S. (ed.): *Electrodiagnosis and Electromyography.* 2nd ed. Waverly Press, Baltimore, 1961.)

(Table 9–1), and often the signal is more readily identified by ear than by eye. The electromyophone is an inexpensive instrument designed specifically for audio evaluation of electromyographic signals (Fig. 9–36).

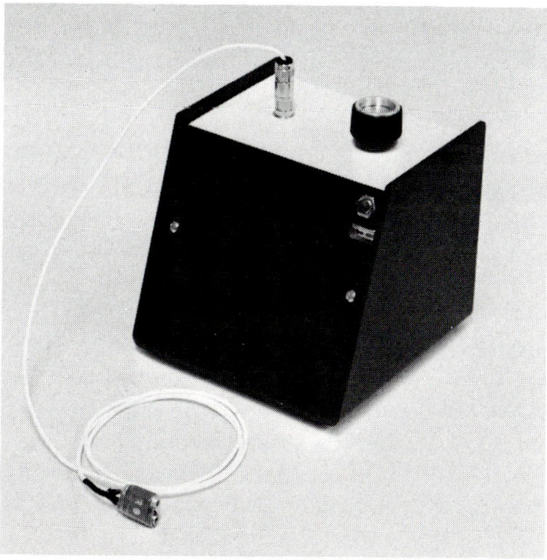

FIGURE 9–36 An electromyophone. Electromyographic activity is recorded with two needle electrodes and is converted to sound only. The unit is easy to operate, portable, and inexpensive; it is a clinically acceptable substitute for the electromyograph in many (but not all) neurological problems. Power is provided by batteries.

Permanent records of electromyograms can be prepared by photographing the oscilloscope display of the signal with a Polaroid or 35 mm camera synchronized with the oscilloscope sweep or by recording the signal on magnetic tape (Fig. 9–34). The development of the storage oscilloscope has been of great value in EMG since it permits retention of the display of single or multiple sweeps for many minutes. This procedure reduces photographic expenses. Inexpensive cassette magnetic tape recorders can be used to record the audio signal, but accurate recording of individual electromyographic potentials for detailed configurational analysis requires a high quality audio tape recorder or, preferably, an instrumentation quality tape recorder. Photographs and magnetic tape records are useful for comparison of the progression or regression of a disease process at subsequent examinations. Fiberoptic graphic recorders may also be used to obtain permanent records of electromyograms (Fig. 9–34).

For general clinical use, a single channel electromyograph is satisfactory, but two, three, and four channel units are also available (Fig. 9–34).

A stimulator and a stimulating electrode system must be added to the electromyograph if evoked potentials and nerve conduction velocities are to be evaluated. The stimulator should be the laboratory type (Fig. 9–31) and should have circuitry that triggers the oscilloscope sweep and, after a variable delay, the stimulus pulse, so that the display contains both the stimulus artifact and the evoked potential (Fig. 9–40). In addition, an external triggering input should be available for synchronizing the stimulator and thereby the oscilloscope with the action of a percussion hammer or a camera shutter.

Other electronic devices for use in electromyography include integrators, delay lines, telemetry systems, and digital computers. Details of their use in electromyography have been provided by Bowen[11] and Basmajian and co-workers.[5]

ELECTRODES

Three electrodes are required for recording electromyograms with a differential amplifier. These electrodes are referred to as the exploring, reference, and ground electrodes and are connected to the positive, negative, and ground input terminals, respectively. With this arrangement of electrode connections, an upward deflection on the oscilloscope display indicates that the exploring electrode is positive relative to the reference electrode, and a downward deflection indicates that the exploring electrode is negative relative to the reference electrode. Some electromyographers prefer the reverse of these connections. Under these conditions, a positive potential is a downward deflection. To serve as a stable reference, the reference electrode should be positioned over an electrically inactive tissue such as bone or tendon. In animal EMG, surface electrodes may be employed, but better results are obtained with needle electrodes. The monopolar and concentric needle electrodes are the most commonly used types of needle electrodes (Fig. 9–37). The monopolar needle electrode is an excellent choice for use in veterinary clinical EMG. A monopolar recording electrode consists of a 25 or 37 mm, 28-gauge needle,* insulated with Teflon except for the very tip (Fig. 9–37). Tips should be examined frequently and the electrode discarded (or used for EDT) when fraying of insulation is apparent and the exposed tip length exceeds about 0.5 mm. Teflon is an excellent material for insulation of the needle electrode because it lacks tissue toxicity and because it creates an extremely smooth, slippery surface which seems to minimize pain associated with passage of the needle through the skin and subcutaneous tissues. Such electrodes are very well tolerated by unanesthetized animals. A monopolar electrode of this design records evoked potential activity from a spherical volume of muscle tissue with a radius of about 2 cm from the electrode tip and fibrillation potential and motor unit potential activity from a volume of muscle having a radius of about 1 mm. A 12 mm, 26-gauge uninsulated needle electrode* serves as a reference electrode for combination with a monopolar exploring electrode. The ground electrode consists of either a needle electrode, the same as used for the reference electrode, or a large surface electrode coated with electrode paste.

*Type MF25 or MF37, Teca Corporation, White Plains, New York.

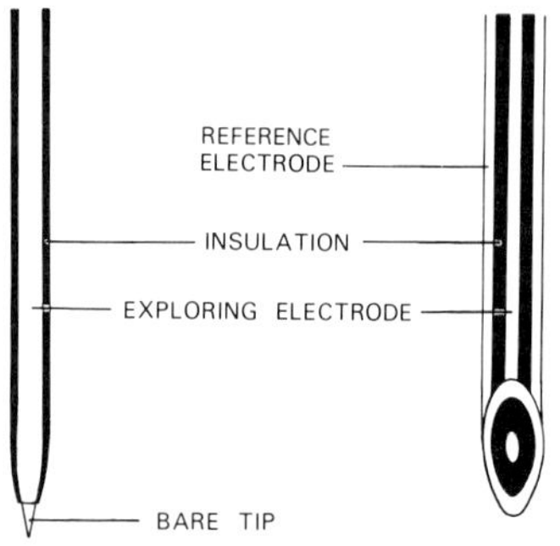

FIGURE 9–37 Diagrams of a monopolar needle electrode and a concentric needle electrode.

In a concentric needle electrode, the exploring and reference electrodes are combined into a single unit (Fig. 9–37). The exploring electrode is represented by the tip of an insulated wire sealed into the barrel of a 24- to 30-gauge hypodermic needle. The shaft of this needle electrode serves as the reference electrode. The concentric electrode samples the electrical activity of a much smaller volume of muscle tissue than

*Type RE12, Teca Corporation, White Plains, New York.

the monopolar electrode. Because of the proximity of the exploring and reference electrodes, interference (60 Hz) is better rejected by the differential amplifier with this electrode arrangement than that with monopolar electrodes. Bowen has found this arrangement most helpful when conducting electromyographic examinations on large animals under conditions conducive to electrical interference problems. The concentric electrode induces more pain upon insertion than the monopolar electrode.

Both monopolar and concentric electrodes will be displaced by muscle movement. To record activity associated with muscle contraction, manual fixation of the limb is desirable. An alternate approach that minimizes the problem of electrode displacement is to implant fine wire hook electrodes in the muscle.[4] The procedure for implantation is easy and requires a small gauge hypodermic needle. Fine wire electrodes are frequently used in kinesiological studies. Needle and wire EMG electrodes should be sterilized before use and the insertion sites should be cleansed with an antiseptic.

Stimulating needle electrodes used in EMG are identical to those previously described for use in EDT.

Focal myopathic changes produced by needle electrode insertion have no permanent effects, but can lead to misinterpretation of muscle histopathology when an insertion tract is present in a biopsy.[22] Therefore, biopsies should be obtained from areas not subjected to needle electrode insertion.

PROCEDURE FOR ELECTROMYOGRAPHIC EXAMINATION

Knowledge of both the anatomy of the skeletal muscles and peripheral nerves and the types of electrical activity associated with various nerve and muscle diseases is essential to performance of a diagnostically useful electromyographic examination. The results of a neurological examination, including EDT if performed, should be reviewed before application of EMG. It is very important that the history indicate as definitively as possible the time elapsed since onset of the neurological problem. Each examination must be tailored to the specific neurological problem. Thus, a routine examination procedure cannot be established for EMG as for ECG or EEG. Furthermore, interpretation of the results is influenced by a number of factors operative during the examination, so interpretation should be done at the time of the examination. The results of each step of an examination often determine the nature of subsequent steps.

Preparation of the animal for an electromyographic examination includes (1) warming of the region to be examined with a heat lamp or heating pad if the tissue temperature is subnormal, (2) application of an antiseptic to the skin overlying the muscle to be examined with needle electrodes, and (3) treatment with general anesthetics or tranquilizers if indicated. General anesthesia is usually required for determination of nerve conduction velocity and for identification of localized denervation activity in the paraspinal muscles when this is obscured by motor unit potential activity caused by tensing of these muscles. In other types of electromyographic examinations, general anesthesia is best avoided because it does suppress voluntary induction of motor unit potential activity. However, a light plane of general anesthesia will not suppress motor unit potential activity in flexor muscles that can be activated by withdrawal reflexes. Fractious or frightened animals may be tranquilized, but muscle tension or tremors noted when these animals are not treated with a tranquilizer may aid evaluation of motor unit potential activity. Selection of a recumbent or standing position for examination of the unanesthetized animal will depend upon whether resting or contracting muscle activity is to be evaluated.

Ground and reference electrodes are positioned first and then the exploring electrode is inserted into the belly of the muscle, care being taken to avoid nerves or vessels. To reposition the exploring electrode, the tip should be withdrawn to a subcutaneous level and then reinserted into the muscle at a new angle. Complete analysis of muscle can best be accomplished by dividing the region surrounding the point of insertion of the needle into quadrants.

Each quadrant is sampled at two or three different levels of insertion.[20] This procedure must be varied to conform with the dimensions of the muscle being tested. Large muscles are best divided into halves or thirds horizontally and/or vertically and each subdivision examined as described previously. Positioning of stimulating electrodes is described in the subsections on EDT and nerve conduction velocity.

The time required for an electromyographic examination varies from a few minutes for a single muscle to an hour or more for detailed evaluation of many muscles and determination of conduction velocities of several nerves. After-effects of needle electromyographic examinations are negligible, and signs of tenderness at insertion or stimulation sites are very rare in animals.

Various report forms have been devised for describing the results of an electromyographic examination. The Mayo Clinic form provides a suitable model.[27] The report should include a summary of the significant findings of the needle electrode examination, conduction velocity values, and the electromyographer's interpretation of these results. Johnson and co-workers[32] have summarized the types of errors which appear in electromyographic examination reports.

ELECTRICAL ACTIVITY OF SKELETAL MUSCLE

Electrical activity of muscle recorded with needle electrodes during an electromyographic examination can be divided into four types, as follows: (1) activity associated with electrode insertion or movement, (2) spontaneous activity of the resting muscle, (3) activity associated with voluntarily or reflexively induced muscle contractions, and (4) activity induced by electrical stimulation of motor nerves. Abnormality of the electrical activity is defined by its presence or absence, alterations in its configuration, and its repetition rate. A composite diagram of normal and abnormal electrical activity is presented in Figure 9–38, and the sounds associated with this activity are described in Table 9–1. No electromyographic waveform can be considered pathognomonic of a specific disease entity. The standard terminology* for human electromyograms is used in this discussion of animal electromyograms.

1. Activity Associated with Electrode Insertion or Movement. Insertion of a needle electrode into a normally innervated muscle initiates a brief burst of electrical activity that includes a large baseline deflection and monophasic and polyphasic potentials of variable amplitude and duration (Fig. 9–38*A*). The burst of activity ends very soon after cessation of needle movement. This response can be reinitiated after insertion by pressing or tapping on the electrode, but again it is of brief duration and terminates almost as soon as the needle stops moving. When needle insertion is followed by prolonged discharge of electrical activity (Fig. 9–38*A'*), response of the muscle fibers to mechanical injury by the electrode reflects cellular hyperirritability and is considered abnormal. In a denervated muscle, increased insertion activity becomes noticeable on the fourth or fifth day postdenervation (Fig. 9–39). This activity is especially prominent from the eighth to tenth days; thereafter it declines in duration and intensity (Fig. 9–39). The duration of insertion activity usually does not exceed 3 minutes in denervated muscle of the dog.[29] Increased insertion activity slightly precedes onset of fibrillation activity in a denervated muscle.

Potentials associated with insertion activity in denervated muscles usually measure 100 to 650 μV in amplitude, 1.9 to 4.1 msec in duration, and 50 to 200/sec in frequency.[29] Positive sharp waves (so named because of their characteristic shape) may be greater than 1 mV in amplitude in insertion activity. Sound associated with insertion activity is described in Table 9–1.

2. Spontaneous Activity of the Resting Muscle. Normal resting muscle lacks electrical activity once the electrode has attained a stable position in the muscle (Fig. 9–38*A*). Normal muscles are said to be "electrically silent" because of the absence of an audible signal from the loudspeaker of the

*Terminology of Electromyography. Subcommittee Report. J. A. Simpson, Chairman. Electroencephalogr. Clin. Neurophysiol. *26*, 224, 1969.

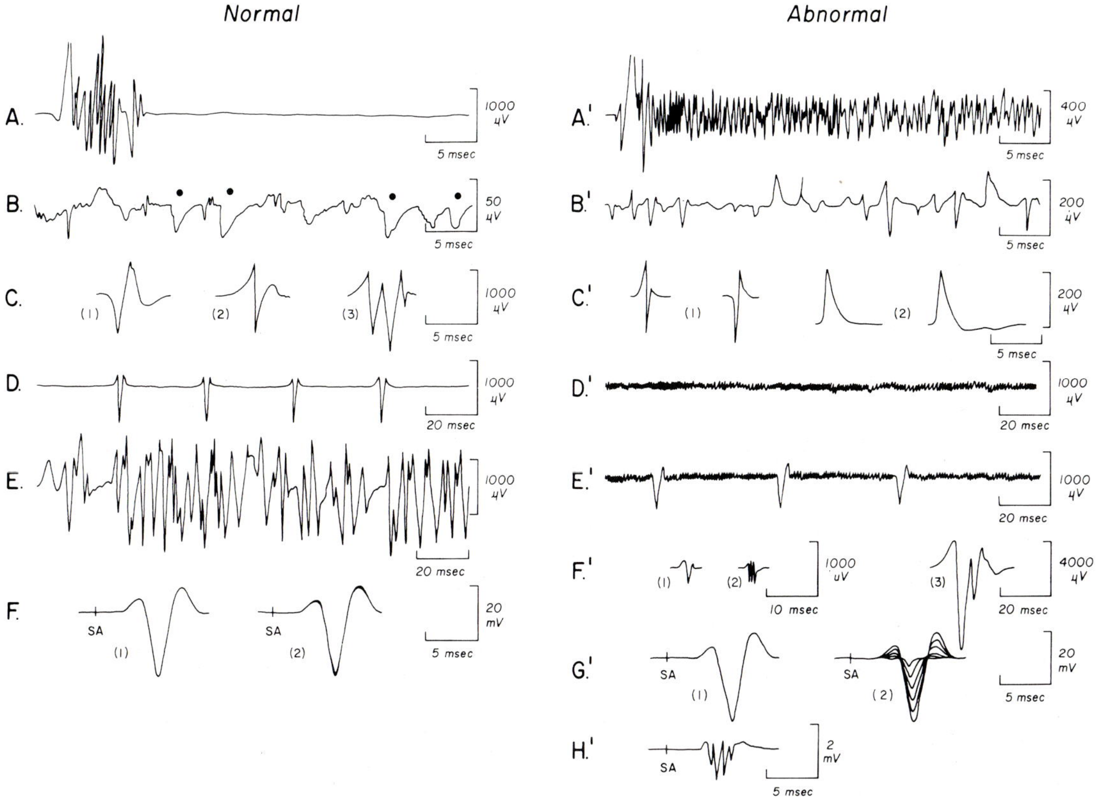

FIGURE 9–38 Composite diagram of major types of electromyograms encountered in clinical examinations. It is important to note the calibration values for each electromyogram.

Normal Activity: A. Brief burst of activity associated with needle electrode insertion, followed by electrical silence soon after electrode movement stops. *B.* End-plate noise encountered when the electrode tip is positioned in the end-plate region. The dots indicate probable individual miniature end-plate potentials. *C.* Motor unit potentials recorded from (1) the end-plate region, (2) the non–end-plate region of a muscle, and (3) a polyphasic motor unit potential. *D.* Repetitive firing of a single motor unit. *E.* Interference pattern associated with the high frequency discharge of several motor units during maximal sustained voluntary effort. *F.* Evoked potentials: (1) response to a single stimulus, and (2) superimposition of six responses induced at a frequency of 30/sec. (SA is the stimulus artifact.)

Abnormal Activity: A'. Prolonged burst of activity associated with needle electrode insertion into a muscle 8 days after denervation. *B'.* Denervation activity after disappearance of insertion activity. *C'.* (1) Fibrillation potentials recorded from non–end-plate and end-plate regions and (2) positive sharp waves without and with a slow terminal negative phase. *D'.* Attempted use of a completely denervated muscle reveals only background denervation activity. *E'.* Attempted use of a partially denervated muscle reveals the repetitive firing of a single motor unit in addition to the background denervation activity. *F'.* (1) Small and (2) polyphasic motor unit potentials that are noted during reinnervation and (3) a giant motor unit potential associated with a chronic neuronopathy. *G'.* Evoked potentials in a myasthenia gravis–like syndrome: (1) response to a single stimulus, and (2) lack of superimposition of six responses induced at a frequency of 30/sec because of a progressive reduction in amplitude. *H'.* Polyphasic evoked potential such as that frequently noted in polyradiculoneuritis.

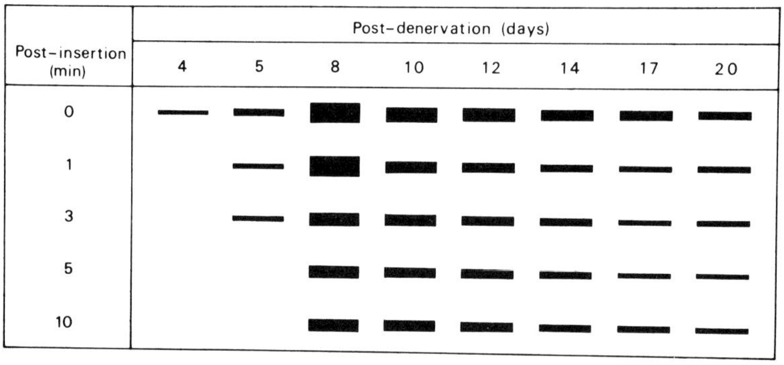

FIGURE 9-39 Variations of the relative magnitudes of insertion and denervation activities with time after neurectomy and after needle electrode insertion. (Adapted from Inada, S., Sugano, S., and Ibaraki, T.: Electromyographic study on denervated muscles in the dog. Jap. J. Vet. Sci. *25*, 327, 1963.)

electromyograph (Table 9-1). Exceptions are noted if the tip of the exploring electrode lies within the end-plate region from which end-plate noise is recorded (Fig. 9-38*B*) or adjacent to a nerve from which nerve action potentials are recorded. End-plate noise represents the summation of miniature end-plate potentials and consists of low amplitude (3-60 μV) negative discharges that are continuous at frequencies up to 600 to 1000 Hz.[54] This activity is normal and should not be confused with fibrillation activity. The sound associated with end-plate noise differs from that associated with fibrillation activity and nerve action potentials (Table 9-1).

Spontaneous activity, termed pre-innervation infantile activity, has been recorded from the muscles of human fetuses but not from muscles of canine fetuses.[7]

Several days after denervation of a striated muscle, spontaneous, randomly occurring potentials can be recorded (Fig. 9-38*B′*). These potentials are termed fibrillation potentials and represent the action potential of a single muscle fiber, or in some instances a few muscle fibers. They commonly arise in the end-plate region of the muscle fiber[30] as the result of an instability in the membrane potential. The time of onset of fibrillation potentials after denervation varies according to species. In the rat, onset takes 2 to 3 days, in the cat and the dog (Fig. 9-39), 5 days, and in man, 16 days.[23] As a general rule in mammals, the smaller the size of the animal, the earlier the onset and the greater the intensity of fibrillation activity. In addition, the shorter the distance along a nerve from the site of nerve injury to muscle, the earlier the onset of fibrillation activity.[41] Atrophy begins before fibrillation potentials can be recorded, and a 50 per cent reduction in muscle mass will occur within about 2 weeks after complete denervation.[48] Disuse atrophy such as occurs after tenotomy is characterized by an absence of fibrillation activity. However, a recent study on stroke victims indicates that some fibrillation activity may be present in upper motoneuron disease.[31]

Fibrillation potentials are monophasic (negative) or biphasic (usually positive-negative in nonend-plate regions and negative-positive in end-plate regions) but rarely triphasic in wave form (Fig. 9-38B′ and *C′*). Amplitude is usually 100 to 300 μV but may be less than 50 μV or greater that 600 μV. Duration has a range of 0.5 to 5 msec. The rhythm is random and sustained as long as viable muscle tissue is present, although amplitude and duration decrease with cicatrization. The sound associated with fibrillation potential activity is described in Table 9-1. A marked reduction in fibrillation potential activity signals onset of successful motor nerve reinnervation.[13, 23]

Fibrillation potential activity may be modified by physiological and pharmacological factors. Heat enhances fibrillation activity, and a heat lamp should be used to warm muscles to be examined in animals with subnormal body temperatures. Repeated passive stretching of a denervated muscle enhances fibrillation activity also. Neostigmine increases fibrillation activity, but a preanesthetic dose of atropine has no effect.

3. Activity Associated with Voluntarily or Reflexively Induced Muscle Contractions. Potentials recorded from a normal muscle during a voluntary or reflex contraction represent the summation of the electrical activity of the individual muscle fibers composing a motor unit. These po-

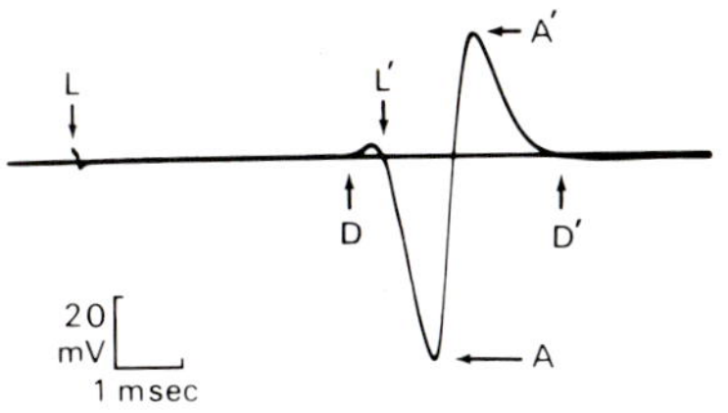

FIGURE 9–40 An evoked potential of a canine plantar interosseous muscle which has been superimposed on a tracing of the baseline or zero potential line. The stimulus artifact is the small deflection beneath *L*. Latency is the interval between *L* and *L′*; duration is the interval between *D* and *D′*; and amplitude is the difference between maximal negative (*A*) and maximal positive (*A′*) deflections. The potential has three phases. The stimulus was applied to the tibial nerve at a point slightly above the tuber calcis.

tentials are termed motor unit potentials (Fig. 9–38*C* and *D*). The contraction itself does not produce electrical activity. Motor unit potentials are characterized by their amplitude, duration, number of phases, and firing rate. The first three characteristics are determined as shown in Figure 9–40 for evoked potentials. The firing rate is the number of times a potential occurs each second. Amplitude is markedly influenced by electrode position. Shifting the electrode tip by 0.5 mm from the position of maximal amplitude of a motor unit potential may cause as much as a tenfold or greater reduction in the recorded potential. Thus, a maximal amplitude and also the shortest duration of a particular motor unit potential is recorded from a very small region. The potentials that arise in close proximity to the electrode tip produce a sharp cracking sound (Table 9–1), whereas potentials arising a short distance away from the tip produce soft thumping sounds because of their lower amplitude and longer duration. Sound is very helpful in positioning the tip of the exploring electrode correctly. Configuration will vary according to whether the electrode is in the end-plate or nonend-plate region of the muscle (Fig. 9–38*C*).

The motor unit potentials associated with the repetitive discharge of a single motor unit are remarkably similar in configuration (Fig. 9–38*D*) and are relatively easy to identify among the activity of two or three other motor units. Ideally, motor unit potential activity should be evaluated at various levels of tonic muscle contraction. In a normally innervated muscle, the smallest potentials appear with minimal contractile tension. As the force of contraction is increased by recruitment of additional motor units, the size of the potentials increases and the firing rate of the individual potentials increases. At maximal contraction, the number of motor units that are firing is so great that normally it is impossible to define the configuration of a single motor unit potential. Thus, this activity pattern is termed an interference pattern (Fig. 9–38*E*). In man, clinical electromyographic examinations include evaluation of the effort pattern associated with graded voluntary contractions. A similar approach in animal electromyography is desirable but is usually precluded by lack of subject cooperation. Therefore, activity associated with minimal contractions and that associated with maximal or near maximal contractions is evaluated in animal EMG.

Methods for inducing an effort pattern in the limb muscles in animals include use of flexor (pedal) reflexes for flexor muscles and increasing weight-bearing by placing the animal on an inclined plane or by lifting one to three of the other limbs. Such antigravity motor unit potential activity is most readily found in the gastrocnemius muscles. Stretching the pectineus muscle by abduction of the stifle will reflexively induce motor unit potentials in this muscle in a lightly anesthetized dog.[9] The mean firing rate for motor unit potentials is about 10 to 15/sec. Characteristics of motor unit potentials of muscles of dogs are summarized in Table 9–2.

The smaller the number of fibers in a motor unit, the smaller the motor unit potential. Muscles with highly refined movements have small motor units and thus small motor unit potentials. In young animals motor unit potentials gradually increase in duration as the animal grows. Aged animals may have potentials with larger amplitude and longer duration than those recorded during the intermediate years.

Fasciculation potentials have the characteristics of motor unit potentials but differ in that they occur spontaneously and sporadically rather than with voluntary effort. They reflect the presence of an irritative process at the motoneuron cell body or along its axon. They are not usually considered a significant abnormality when present alone. When fasciculation occurs in

TABLE 9–2 CHARACTERISTICS OF EVOKED POTENTIALS AND MOTOR UNIT POTENTIALS OF CANINE MUSCLE MOTOR POINTS[a]

Stimulation Sites	Recording Site (Muscle)	Potential	Latency (msec)[b]	Amplitude (mV)[b]	Duration (msec)[b]	Phases[b]
–	Supraspinatus	MUP	–	1.37 (0.14–4.82)	2.73 (1.40–4.78)	2.1 (1.0–2.6)
–	Deltoideus	MUP	–	1.03 (0.20–2.54)	2.95 (1.90–4.51)	2.3 (1.4–3.2)
–	Biceps	MUP	–	1.01 (0.33–2.04)	2.79 (2.08–4.05)	2.4 (2.0–3.5)
–	Triceps	MUP	–	0.93 (0.36–2.47)	2.72 (1.95–3.43)	2.4 (1.9–4.1)
Radial nerve where it crosses humerus	Extensor carpi radialis	EP	2.2 (1.4–4.8)	54 (28–92)	12 (8.0–20)	3 (2–5)
–	Extensor carpi radialis	MUP	–	0.85 (0.17–2.22)	2.62 (1.60–4.38)	2.3 (1.4–3.2)
Radial nerve	Extensor digitorum communis	EP	2.1 (1.4–3.1)	55 (29–106)	10 (4.0–16)	3 (2–5)
Radial nerve	Extensor digitorum lateralis	EP	2.0 (1.6–2.8)	78 (28–180)	9.3 (4.4–17)	3 (2–5)
Radial nerve	Extensor carpi ulnaris	EP	2.1 (1.4–2.6)	61 (14–154)	7.8 (5.0–13)	3 (2–4)
Ulnar nerve above medial epicondyle of humerus	Flexor carpi ulnaris	EP	2.2 (1.0–3.6)	92 (38–165)	10 (3.5–16)	4 (2–6)
–	Flexor carpi ulnaris	MUP	–	1.86 (0.75–4.47)	3.17 (1.76–4.68)	2.6 (2.0–3.3)
Ulnar nerve above accessory carpal bone	Interosseus	EP	2.6 (1.8–3.4)	54 (28–152)	5.0 (3.4–12)	2 (2–4)
Median nerve craniodorsal to medial epicondyle of humerus	Pronator teres	EP	2.1 (1.3–2.8)	53 (20–154)	9.0 (3.0–16)	4 (2–6)

[a]Evoked potential results from Bowen, J. M.: Electromyographic analysis of evoked potentials of canine muscle motor points. J.A.V.M.A. *164*, 509, 1974. Motor unit potential results from Bowen, J. M.: Unpublished data.
[b]Average and range.

a large number of motor units, the resultant involuntary muscle contraction is called a tonic or clonic spasm. Clonic spasms are relatively common in pectineus muscles of dogs.[9]

In chronic neuronopathies, nearby functional nerve fibers develop branches that innervate some of the denervated muscle fibers, thereby creating very large motor units. The potentials of these motor units may be ten times the amplitude usually associated with motor units in a particular muscle and are commonly termed giant motor unit potentials. Since the new nerve branches have a slow conduction velocity, giant motor unit potentials are usually polyphasic. During recovery from neuropathies, giant motor unit potentials may be present, but the more common type of potential is that of a motor unit with subnormal amplitude and frequently increased number of phases; it resembles a myopathic motor unit potential (Fig. 9–38*F′*).

A reduction in amplitude and duration of motor unit potentials is a characteristic of primary diseases of muscle and reflects a decrease in the number of active muscle fibers in the motor unit. These potentials are termed myopathic motor unit potentials. In human EMG, it has been reported

TABLE 9–2 CHARACTERISTICS OF EVOKED POTENTIALS AND MOTOR UNIT POTENTIALS OF CANINE MUSCLE MOTOR POINTS[a]—(*Continued*)

Stimulation Sites	Recording Site (Muscle)	Potential	Latency (msec)[b]	Amplitude (mV)[b]	Duration (msec)[b]	Phases[b]
Median nerve	Flexor carpi radialis	EP	1.8 (1.0–2.8)	60 (30–94)	8.4 (3.8–16)	3 (2–5)
—	Flexor carpi radialis	MUP	-	1.72 (0.27–5.27)	3.19 (1.69–4.45)	2.4 (1.0–2.9)
Median nerve	Flexor digitorum profundus	EP	2.0 (1.0–3.0)	67 (18–106)	8.5 (2.8–16)	3 (2–6)
—	Middle gluteal	MUP	-	0.89 (0.41–2.10)	2.31 (1.38–3.19)	2.1 (1.0–2.8)
—	Biceps femoris	MUP	-	0.75 (0.26–1.52)	2.69 (1.90–4.56)	2.2 (1.9–3.2)
—	Semitendinosus	MUP	-	0.63 (0.26–1.34)	2.74 (1.74–3.96)	2.3 (1.8–4.4)
—	Vastus lateralis	MUP	-	0.72 (0.35–1.63)	2.73 (1.94–3.86)	2.1 (1.5–2.6)
—	Gracilis	MUP	-	0.77 (0.32–1.78)	2.60 (1.77–4.24)	2.3 (2.0–3.0)
—	Pectineus	MUP	-	1.68 (0.54–4.73)	3.17 (1.46–4.53)	2.2 (1.5–3.1)
Peroneal nerve caudal to patella	Tibialis cranialis	EP	2.3 (1.4–4.0)	54 (29–90)	14 (8.0–22)	3 (2–5)
—	Tibialis cranialis	MUP	-	0.79 (0.26–1.88)	2.70 (1.51–4.06)	2.2 (1.4–3.0)
Tibial nerve caudal to distal end of femur	Gastrocnemius (lateral head)	EP	2.1 (1.2–3.2)	93 (40–140)	11 (7.0–18)	4 (2–5)
—	Gastrocnemius (lateral head)	MUP	-	1.88 (0.56–4.11)	3.36 (2.59–3.93)	2.7 (2.1–3.1)
Tibial nerve	Gastrocnemius (medial head)	EP	1.7 (1.0–3.0)	96 (30–160)	12 (6.0–17)	3 (2–5)
Tibial nerve at tuber calcis	Interosseus	EP	4.0 (3.4–4.8)	56 (22–112)	4.6 (2.8–8.0)	2 (2–4)

that the mean amplitude of 30 randomly recorded motor unit potentials should deviate by more than 40 per cent from the normal mean value to be considered abnormal.[16] Small motor unit potentials in myopathies have the appearance of fibrillation potentials but may be distinguished from the latter by their regular rhythm and association with voluntary contractions.

4. Activity Induced by Electrical Stimulation of Motor Nerves. Since most peripheral nerves contain both sensory and motor fibers, electrical stimulation of such mixed nerves activates both types of fibers. The presence of a sensory response to stimulation provides important electrodiagnostic information. The potentials recorded from a muscle following stimulation of the peripheral nerve innervating this muscle are termed the M, F, or H waves, depending on their onset latency and the stimulus intensity. Only the M wave is of significance in animal EMG. It is an evoked potential that results from the summation of one or many individual motor unit potentials. The actual number of motor unit potentials contributing to the M wave is a function of stimulus intensity. Usually a supramaximal stimulus intensity is used in order to evaluate the maximum size of the evoked potential of that muscle region. A major advantage of the evoked potential (M wave) is that it can be evaluated without any cooperation from the animal. Examples of processes altering evoked potentials are shown in Figure 9–41.

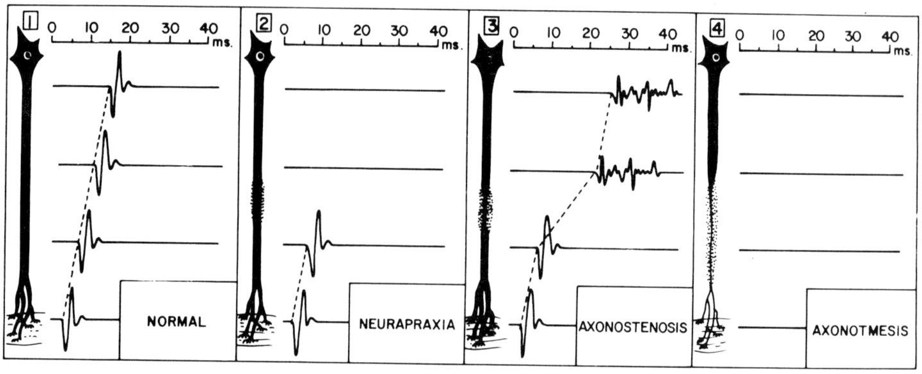

FIGURE 9–41 Muscle-evoked potentials induced by stimulation of the motor nerve at different levels. (1) The latency of the normal response increases progressively with very little change in potential configuration as the distance from the stimulating electrode to muscle increases. (2) Neurapraxia, or localized interruption of conduction as by compression, blocks nerve impulses initiated above but not below the level of the interruption. (3) Axonostenosis, or reduction in axon diameter, slows conduction velocity and increases asynchrony of motor unit potential discharge. Response to stimulation below the affected region is normal. (4) Axonotmesis, or axon discontinuity, is associated with an absence of an evoked potential. (Adapted from Bauwens, P.: Electrodiagnosis revisited: Tenth John Stanley Coulter Memorial Lecture. Arch Phys. Med. Rehabil. *42*, 6, 1961.)

The important characteristics of evoked potentials include latency, amplitude, duration, and number of phases (Fig. 9–40).[10] Mean values for the characteristics of evoked potentials are presented in Table 9–2. Latency represents the time for nerve impulse conduction from the stimulation site to the nerve terminal, neuromuscular delay (about 0.5 msec), and time for conduction from the end-plate region to the exploring electrode. It is best measured when the stimulating electrodes are applied to the nerve near the muscle and when they are positioned in the end-plate region. Under these conditions, latency may be termed the terminal conduction time. Some electromyographers consider single latency determinations to be a satisfactory clinical substitute for nerve conduction velocity determinations.[19] Since nerve fiber compression prolongs latency, latency can be used to determine the level of compression.

The amplitude of an evoked potential provides an approximate indication of the number of muscle fibers activated by nerve stimulation. Values for amplitude range from a few millivolts to over 100 millivolts (Table 9–2). During reinnervation the evoked potential amplitude increases but may never attain the control value if reinnervation is incomplete. The reduction in muscle fiber size associated with disuse atrophy also leads to a reduction in size of the evoked potential, but latency and number of phases are unaffected. Duration and number of phases of the evoked potential are a measure of the synchrony of discharge of the individual motor unit potentials and of the number of these units discharging. When synchrony decreases, as shown by increased terminal conduction time, the duration and number of phases increase. When the number of units responding decreases, the number of phases often increases and the duration may decrease. Normally the number of phases is less than 5 (Table 9–2). Demyelinating nerve diseases frequently cause an increase in the number of phases (Fig. 9–38*H'*).

When a motor nerve is severed, the distal segment undergoes wallerian degeneration. The degeneration begins at the site of severance and migrates peripherally. Thus, immediately after severance the entire distal segment responds well to electrical stimulation, but no response occurs when the proximal segment is stimulated. Over a period of several days the distal segment remains responsive to stimulation but only if the electrode is moved closer to the muscle each day. The evoked potential decreases in amplitude and latency increases, and, depending upon length of the distal segment, conduction ceases abruptly after about 5 to 8 days.[25]

In a normal muscle the evoked potentials can be superimposed on the oscilloscope display during stimulation at a frequency of 30/sec with very little evidence of fatigue being noted during a 5-second period of stimulation (Fig. 9–38*F*). In contrast, myasthenia gravis is characterized by a rapid decrease in evoked potential amplitude during stimulation at this frequency (Fig. 9–38G′). This response may be noted during reinnervation and occasionally in ventral horn cell disease and syringomyelia.

RECORDING ARTIFACTS

Electrical activity derived from sources other than those of electromyographic interest is considered an artifact. Included among recording artifacts are electrical activity of cardiac muscle (a biphasic wave of long duration) and brain (temporal muscle records), electrode movement, and electrical devices such as electric cautery, diathermy, electric motors, and fluorescent lighting. The source of interference should be identified and appropriate steps taken to exclude it from the electromyographic records. Incorrect electrode positioning, poor electrode-tissue contact, and proximity of the electronic interference generator are common causes of interference.

NERVE CONDUCTION VELOCITY

Passage of a nerve impulse along a nerve fiber requires a finite time that is characteristic of a particular diameter of nerve fiber. Demyelinating neuropathies are associated with a slowing of the conduction velocity of a nerve impulse. In contrast, slowing of conduction velocity is very rare in neuronopathies and does not occur at all in myopathies. Nerve conduction velocities of certain long peripheral nerves can be measured clinically in an anesthetized animal with the aid of an electromyograph, laboratory stimulator, and needle recording and stimulating electrodes.

PROCEDURE FOR DETERMINING NERVE CONDUCTION VELOCITY

Motor nerve conduction velocity is determined by inserting the exploring electrode into the most distal muscle supplied by the nerve being evaluated (Fig. 9–42). Single supramaximal stimuli are applied successively at two points along the course of the nerve, and the evoked potentials are photographed. Three evoked potentials for each site of stimulation should be superimposed on the photograph to ensure that the response is stable. Latency of each set of evoked potentials should be measured to the nearest 0.1 msec and the difference obtained. The latency difference represents the conduction time for impulses in the fastest conducting fibers of the nerve segment between the proximal and distal stimulation sites. When the length of the nerve segment (measured to the nearest mm) is divided by the latency difference or conduction time, the conduction velocity is given in meters per second (Fig. 9–42).

Normal values for conduction velocities for several nerves are given in Table 9–3. Impulse conduction to muscles in the proximal part of an extremity is faster than that to muscles in the distal part of the extremity. The limiting factor in determination of nerve conduction velocities is the length of nerve accessible to stimulation at two sites which should be separated by at least 100 mm. Thus, the accessible courses of the femoral and usually the radial nerves are too short for accurate determination of conduction velocities. Experimental errors arise primarily in the reading of the two latencies and the one conduction distance. Serial evaluations of the same nerve may normally be expected to vary by 4 to 6 meters per second. Conduction velocities for nerves on the right and left sides of the body do not differ significantly.[37] In the dog and cat, conduction velocities below 40 meters per second are abnormal, while those between 40 and 50 meters per second are suspect. Some electromyographers consider latency a satisfactory substitute for nerve conduction velocities in general clinical evaluations.[19]

A linear relationship exists between nerve conduction velocity and the temperature of tissues adjacent to the nerve down to 20° C.[38] For each degree centigrade below normal tissue temperature, a correction of 1.8 meters per second should be added to the measured conduction velocity. Alternatively, a heating pad or heat lamp can be used to restore the temperature of the tissue to a normal range. Very

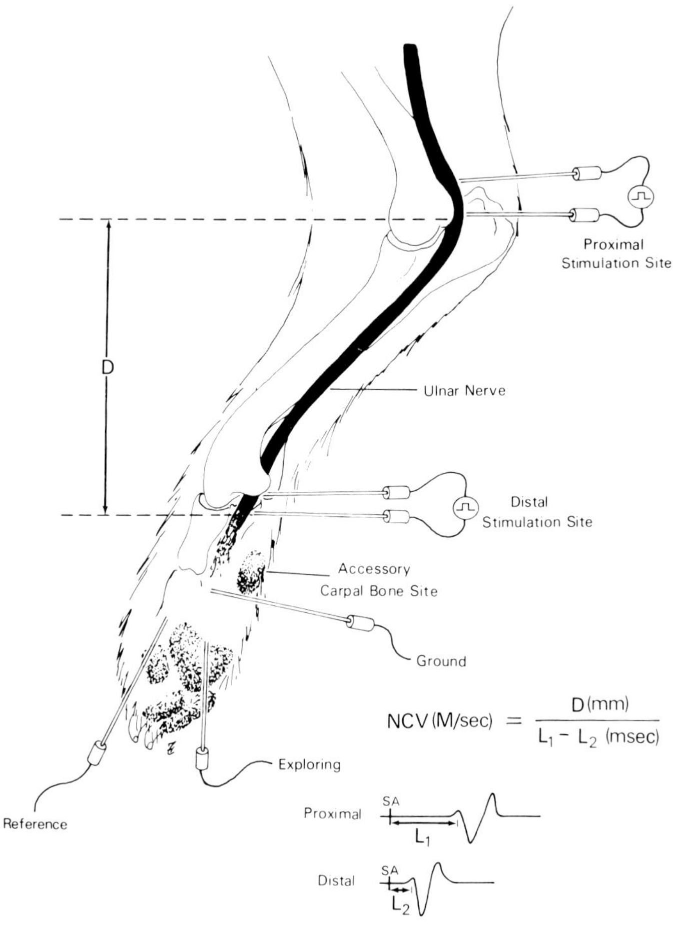

FIGURE 9–42 Schematic diagram of the latency technique for determination of ulnar motor nerve conduction velocity. Latency (L_2) of the evoked potential induced by stimulation at the level of the accessory carpal bone is subtracted from the latency (L_1) of the evoked potential induced by stimulation at the level of the olecranon. The difference represents the conduction time for impulses in the fastest conducting fibers of the nerve segment (D) between the stimulating electrodes. Conduction velocity is calculated with the formula given in the diagram. The exploring electrode tip was in an interosseous muscle.

young (less than 8 weeks) and very old (more than 12 years) animals have reduced nerve conduction velocities in comparison with those of animals in the intermediate age range. Protein malnutrition has been reported to reduce nerve conduction velocities reversibly in rhesus monkeys.[46]

Direct measurement of nerve conduction velocity can be accomplished by placing the tip of a needle-exploring electrode adjacent

TABLE 9–3 MOTOR NERVE CONDUCTION VELOCITIES[a] FOR THE DOG AND CAT

Nerve	Stimulation Sites[b]	Recording Site (Muscle)	Dog (msec)[c]	Cat (msec)[c]
Ulnar	G and G′	Interosseus	60 (53–68)	77 (66–89)
Ischiatic–tibial	J and M′	Interosseus	60 (52–67)	79 (64–85)
Ischiatic–tibial	J and M	Gastrocnemius	86 (76–100)	91 (73–103)
Ischiatic–peroneal	J and N	Cranial tibial	77 (62–92)	75 (60–90)

[a]Calculated using the onset latency difference method.
[b]Letters refer to Figure 9–33.
[c]Average and range.

to a nerve and then applying a supramaximal stimulus to the nerve either proximal or distal to the recording site. Conduction time is the interval between the stimulus artifact and the evoked nerve potential. While satisfactory results using a stimulus at only one site are possible, the small amplitude of the signal (< 50 μV) makes recording difficult unless an averaging electronic device is used. The added technical difficulties and equipment requirements of the direct method are distinct disadvantages to the use of this method for clinical determination of motor nerve conduction velocity. Since an alternate method for determination of sensory nerve conduction velocity is not available, the direct method must be used. To avoid activation of motor nerves, values should be determined for purely sensory nerves, or the stimulus should be applied at a region which has a high density of sensory fibers and a negligible density of motor fibers, e.g., the digits. Responses to 50 to 100 stimuli must be averaged to define the sensory nerve potential. Sensory nerve conduction velocities are faster by about 5 meters per second than motor nerve conduction velocities;[43] in aged animals they are also decreased. Combined measurement of sensory nerve potentials and somatosensory cerebral evoked potentials permits localization of a lesion in peripheral as well as central sensory pathways. Measurement of somatosensory cerebral evoked potentials involves stimulation of a peripheral nerve and recording of the evoked potential at a point over the contralateral hemisphere. The presence of normal peripheral sensory conduction velocity and absence of somatosensory cerebral evoked potentials indicates that the lesion lies between the dorsal root ganglion and the cerebral cortex. In neuropathies, records of sensory nerve potentials are difficult to obtain.

INTERPRETATION OF RESULTS OF ELECTROMYOGRAPHIC EXAMINATIONS

Diagnosis of diseases affecting nerves, muscles, or the neuromuscular junction is greatly aided by information derived from an electromyographic examination. When possible and where indicated, histologic and histochemical evaluations of muscle biopsies and serum muscle-enzymes should be integrated with electromyographic and neurologic information. The principal electromyographic differences between neuropathies and myopathies are presented in Table 9–4. The distinction between neuropathies and myopathies based on electromyographic findings is not easy to establish in animals, although difficulties are encountered in this area in human EMG also.[52] Electromyographic findings in specific neuropathies and myopathies are summarized in Table 9–5. Other aspects of diagnosis and therapy of the diseases mentioned are presented in the next section of this text and in other texts.[17]

TABLE 9–4 COMPARISON OF USUAL ELECTROMYOGRAPHIC FINDINGS IN NEUROPATHIES AND MYOPATHIES

Electromyographic Parameters	Neuropathy	Myopathy
Motor unit potentials		
Amplitude	Normal or increased	Decreased
Duration	Increased	Decreased
Phases	Increased	Increased
Effort pattern		
Number of motor unit potentials	Decreased	Normal
Firing frequency of motor unit potentials	Normal	Increased
Fibrillation potentials and positive sharp waves	Many	Few
Nerve conduction velocity	Decreased	Normal

KINESIOLOGY

Kinesiology utilizes EMG to define the role of a specific muscle or group of muscles in posture and in simple and complex body or limb movements. Tokuriki[50] has conducted extensive kinesiological studies on dogs during walking, trotting, and galloping.

TABLE 9–5 CHARACTERISTIC ELECTROMYOGRAPHIC FINDINGS IN DISEASES AFFECTING THE PERIPHERAL NERVOUS SYSTEM AND MUSCLE

Lesion or Disease	Insertion Activity	Fibrillation Potentials and Positive Sharp Waves	High Frequency Discharges	Motor Unit Potentials			Evoked Potential Amplitude	Nerve Conduction Velocity
				Amplitude	*Phases*	*Effort Pattern*		
Upper motoneuron lesion (cord compression)	Increased	Absent or few	None	Normal	Normal	Reduced	Reduced (disuse atrophy)	Normal
Neuropathy (spinal muscular atrophy)	Increased	Present	Bizarre	Sub- to supra-normal	Increased	Reduced	Reduced	Normal
Mononeuropathy (trigeminal nerve)	Increased	Present	Bizarre	Near normal if present	Near normal if present	Reduced if present	Absent or reduced	Decreased if measurable
Traumatic polyneuropathy (brachial plexus)	Increased	Present	Bizarre	Near normal to supra-normal if present	Near normal if present	Reduced if present	Absent or reduced	Normal if measurable
Hereditary polyneuropathy (neuronal abiotrophy)	Increased	Present	Bizarre	—[a]	—	—	Absent or reduced	Decreased
Allergic polyneuropathy	Increased	Present	Bizarre	Reduced	Increased	Reduced	Reduced	Decreased

Metabolic polyneuropathy (diabetes mellitus)	Increased	Present	Absent	Reduced	Increased	Reduced	Reduced	Decreased
Toxic polyneuropathy (lead poisoning)	Increased	Present	None	Reduced	Increased	Reduced	Reduced	Decreased
Botulism (botulinum toxin)	Increased	Absent or few	None	Reduced	Normal	Reduced	Reduced	Normal
Tick paralysis (Tick toxin)	Normal	Absent	None	Reduced	Normal	Reduced	Reduced	Normal to decreased
Myasthenia gravis	Normal	Absent or few	None	Reduced	Normal to increased	Normal to reduced	Reduced by 30/sec stimulation	Normal
Myositis	Increased	Present	Bizarre	Reduced	Increased	Increased	Reduced	Normal
Nutritional myopathy	Increased	Absent or few	Bizarre	–	–	–	–	Normal
Hereditary myopathy	Increased	Absent	Myotonic-like	–	–	–	–	Normal
Endocrine myopathy (Cushing's disease)	Increased	Absent	Myotonic-like	Reduced	Increased	Increased	Reduced	Normal
Myotonic dystrophy	Increased	Absent or few	Myotonic	–	–	–	–	Normal

[a]Response in affected dogs or cats has not been investigated.

REFERENCES

1. Allam, M. W., Nulsen, F. E., and Lewey, F. H.: Electrical intraneural bipolar stimulation of peripheral nerves in the dog. J.A.V.M.A. *114,* 87, 1949.
2. Arieff, A. J.; Dobin, N. B., and Tigay, E. L.: Comprehensive electrodiagnosis. J.A.M.A. *181,* 1140, 1962.
3. Bascuas, J. A., Bascuas, J. L., and Marin, M.: Electromyographic discoveries in dogs with distemper. Veterinaria (Madrid) *38,* 565, 1973.
4. Basmajian, J. V., and Stecko, G.: A new bipolar electrode for electromyography. J. Appl. Physiol. *17,* 849, 1962.
5. Basmajian, J. V., Clifford, H. C., McLeod, W. D., and Nunnally, H. N.: *Computers in Electromyography.* Butterworths & Co., Reading, Mass., 1975.
6. Bishop, G. H., and Bronfenbrenner, J. J.: The site of action of botulinus toxin. Am. J. Physiol. *117,* 393, 1936.
7. Botelho, S. Y., Steinberg, S. A., McGrath, J. T., and Zislis, J.: Electromyography in dogs with congenital spinal cord lesions. Am. J. Vet. Res. *28,* 205, 1967.
8. Bowen, J. M.: Monitoring neuromuscular function in intact animals. Am. J. Vet. Res. *30,* 857, 1969.
9. Bowen, J. M.: Electromyographic analysis of reflex and spastic activities of canine pectineus muscles in the presence and absence of hip dysplasia. Am. J. Vet. Res. *35,* 661, 1974.
10. Bowen, J. M.: Electromyographic analysis of evoked potentials of canine muscle motor points. J.A.V.M.A. *164* , 509, 1974.
11. Bowen, J. M.: Electromyography. *In* Klemm, W. R. (ed.): *Applied Electronics for Veterinary Medicine and Animal Physiology.* Charles C Thomas, Publisher, Springfield, Ill., 1976.
12. Bowen, J. M.: Electronic evaluation of motor function and dysfunction. *In* Klemm, W. R. (ed.): *Applied Electronics for Veterinary Medicine and Animal Physiology.* Charles C Thomas, Publisher, Springfield, Ill., 1976.
13. Bowen, J. M.: Quantitative EMG analysis of the time course of denervation in the canine pectineus muscle. Arch. Phys. Med. Rehabil. In press.
14. Breskend, S.: Build a solid state muscle stimulator. Radio-Electronics, June, 1965, p. 42.
15. Bryant, S. H., Lipicky, R. J., and Herzog, W. H.: Variability of myotonic signs in myotonic goats. Am. J. Vet. Res. *29,* 2371, 1968.
16. Buchthal, F., and Rosenfalck, P.: Electrophysiological aspects of myopathy with particular reference to progressive muscular dystrophy. *In* Bourne, G. H. (ed.): *Muscular Dystrophy in Man and Animals.* Hafner Publishing Company, Inc., New York, 1963.
17. Chrisman, C. L.: Diseases of peripheral nerves and muscles. *In* Ettinger, S. J. (ed.): *Textbook of Veterinary Internal Medicine.* W. B. Saunders Co., Philadelphia, 1975.
18. Chrisman, C. L., Burt, J. K., Wood, P. K., and Johnson, E. W.: Electromyography in small animal clinical neurology. J.A.V.M.A. *160,* 311, 1972.
19. Christie, B. G. B., and Coomes, E. N.: Normal variation of nerve conduction in three peripheral nerves. Ann. Phys. Med. *5,* 303, 1960.
20. Cohen, H. L., and Brumlik, J.: *A Manual of Electroneuromyography.* Harper and Row, New York, 1968.
21. Cummings, J. F., and Haas, D. C.: Coonhound paralysis: An acute idiopathic polyradiculoneuritis in dogs resembling the Landry-Guillain-Barré syndrome. J. Neurol. Sci. *4,* 51, 1967.
22. Engel, W. K.: Focal myopathic changes produced by electromyographic and hypodermic needles ("needle myopathy"). Arch. Neurol. *16,* 509, 1967.
23. Feinstein, B., Pattle, R. E., and Weddell, G.: Metabolic factors affecting fibrillation in denervated muscle. J. Neurol. Neurosurg. Psychiat. *8,* 1, 1945.
24. Greenblatt, G. M., and Denson, J. S.: Needle nerve stimulator-locator: Nerve blocks with a new instrument for locating nerves. Anesth. Analg. *41,* 599, 1962.
25. Griffiths, I. R., and Duncan, I. D.: Some studies of the clinical neurophysiology of denervation in the dog. Res. Vet. Sci. *17,* 377, 1974.
26. Heckman, J. R.: Excitability curve: A new technique for assessing human peripheral nerve excitability in vivo. Neurology *22,* 224, 1972.
27. Howard, F. M.: Electromyography and conduction studies in peripheral nerve injuries. Surg. Clin. N. Am. *52,* 1343, 1972.
28. Hussain, S., and Pettit, G. D.: Tendon transplantation to compensate for radial nerve paralysis in the dog. Am. J. Vet. Res. *28,* 335, 1967.
29. Inada, S., Sugano, S., and Ibaraki, T.: Electromyographic study on denervated muscles in the dog. Jap. J. Vet. Sci. *25,* 327, 1963.
30. Jarcho, L. W., Berman, B., Dowben, R. M., and Lilienthal, J. L.: Site of origin and velocity of conduction of fibrillary potentials in denervated skeletal muscle. Am. J. Physiol. *178,* 128, 1954.
31. Johnson, E. W., Denny, S. T., and Kelley, J. P.: Sequence of electromyographic abnormalities in stroke syndrome. Arch. Phys. Med. Rehabil. *56,* 468, 1975.
32. Johnson, E. W., Fallon, T. J., and Wolfe, C. V.: Errors in EMG reporting. Arch. Phys. Med. Rehabil. *57,* 30, 1976.
33. Katz, R. L.: Comparison of electrical and mechanical recording of spontaneous and evoked muscle activity. Anesthesiology *26,* 204, 1965.
34. Khalili, A. A., and Betts, H. B.: Isolated block of musculocutaneous and perineal nerves in the management of spasticity with special reference to the use of a nerve stimulator. Anesthesiology *28,* 219, 1967.
35. Knecht, C. D., and St. Clair, L. E.: The radial-brachial paralysis syndrome in the dog. J.A.V.M.A. *154,* 653, 1969.
36. LaFratta, C. W.: An appraisal of the more popular methods of electrodiagnostic testing. J. South. Med. Assoc. *57,* 649, 1964.
37. Lee, A. F., and Bowen, J. M.: Evaluation of motor nerve conduction velocity in the dog. Am. J. Vet. Res. *31,* 1361, 1970.
38. Lee, A. F., and Bowen, J. M.: Effect of tissue temperature on ulnar nerve conduction velocity in the dog. Am. J. Vet. Res. *36,* 1305, 1975.

39. Liu, C. T.: Effect of aspirin on strength-duration curve of the traumatized muscle in cats. J. Trauma *10*, 68, 1970.
40. Lorenz, M. D., deLahunta, A., and Alstrom, D. H.: Neostigmine-responsive weakness in the dog, similar to myasthenia gravis. J.A.V.M.A. *161*, 795, 1972.
41. Luco, J. V., and Eyzaguirre, C.: Fibrillation and hypersensitivity to ACh in denervated muscle: Effect of length of degenerating nerve fibers. J. Neurophysiol. *18*, 65, 1955.
42. Oester, Y. T., and Licht, S.: Routine electrodiagnosis. *In* Licht, S. (ed.): *Electrodiagnosis and Electromyography,* 2nd ed. Waverly Press, Baltimore, 1961.
43. Oester, Y. T., Zallis, A. W., and Rodriquez, A. A.: Possible diagnostic applications of sensory evoked potentials. Arch. Phys. Med. Rehabil. *53*, 21, 1972.
44. Pearson, R. B.: *Handbook on Clinical Electromyography.* The Meditron Company, El Monte, Calif., 1961.
45. Rosselle, N., Schellens, L., Ghesquiere, F., Diniz, P., Geerinckx, P., and De Meirsman, J.: Electromyographic evaluation of therapeutic methods in complete peripheral paralysis. Electromyogr. Clin. Neurophysiol. *14*, 549, 1974.
46. Roy, S., Singh, N., Deo, M. G., and Ramalingaswami, V.: Ultrastructure of skeletal muscle and peripheral nerve in experimental protein deficiency and its correlation with nerve conduction studies. J. Neurol. Sci. *17*, 399, 1972.
47. Scarff, J. E.: Peripheral nerve injuries: Principles and treatment. Med. Clin. N. Am. *42,* 611, 1958.
48. Solandt, D. Y., and Magladery, J. W.: The relation of atrophy to fibrillation in denervated muscle. Brain *63*, 255, 1940.
49. Thomson, F. K., and Bowen, J. M.: Electrodiagnostic testing: Mapping and clinical use of motor points in the dog. J.A.V.M.A. *159*, 1763, 1971.
50. Tokuriki, M.: Electromyographic and joint-mechanical studies in quadrupedal locomotion. III. Gallop. Jap. J. Vet. Sci. *36*, 121, 1974.
51. Tradati, F.: L'esame elettrodiagnostico nella patologia neuromuscolare del cane. Clinica Vet. (Milano) *86*, 347, 1963.
52. Warmolts, J. R., and Engel, W. K.: A critique of the "myopathic" electromyogram. Trans. Am. Neurol. Assoc. *95*, 173, 1970.
53. Warmolts, J. R., and Engel, W. K.: Open biopsy electromyography. I. Correlation of motor unit behavior with histochemical muscle fiber type in human limb muscle. Arch. Neurol. *27*, 512, 1972.
54. Wiederholt, W. C.: "End-plate noise" in electromyography. Neurology *20*, 214, 1970.
55. Wright, B. D.: A new use for the Block-Aid Monitor. Anesthesiology *30*, 236, 1969.
56. Zacks, S. I., Shields, D. R., and Steinberg, S. A.: A myasthenic syndrome in the dog: A case report with electron microscopic observations on motor end plates and comparison with the fine structure of end plates in myasthenia gravis. Ann. N.Y. Acad. Sci. *135*, 79, 1966.

SECTION 3
CLINICAL DISORDERS OF NERVES AND MUSCLES

B. F. Hoerlein, D.V.M., Ph.D.
J. M. Bowen, D.V.M., Ph.D.

This section on the various clinical disorders of peripheral nerves and muscles will include their respective neurological signs, the diagnostic significance of the testing procedures discussed in Section 2, the results of histological and histochemical evaluations of muscle biopsies, alterations in serum muscle enzymes, and appropriate therapy.

INTRODUCTION*

The neuromuscular system is a complex functional and interrelated organization of neural and muscular elements. The neural elements include motoneurons at cord and brain stem levels, primarily sensory neurons, and autonomic/mixed somatic peripheral nerves. The muscular component comprises both intrafusal (muscle spindle) and extrafusal fiber systems. The terms peripheral neuropathies and myopathies refer to injury or disease of these neuromuscular components.

Considerable progress has been made in understanding neuromuscular disorders in human medicine, especially over the past decade. This has resulted from detailed clinical examination in conjunction with biochemical, histochemical, and structural studies. Electrodiagnostic data (nerve conduction velocity and electromyographic studies) and examination of body fluids (cerebrospinal fluid, urine, and serum), as well as special studies in enzymology, have proved their value in the diagnosis of and differentiation between many human neuromuscular disorders. Accordingly, a comprehensive and workable classification of neuropathies and myopathies has evolved.

A comparable state does not currently exist in veterinary medicine. As in comparative studies of other body systems, it is probable that similar neuromuscular disorders occur in animals but are presently unrecognized. Those disorders which have been described and are reviewed in this section cannot be readily classified. A clearer understanding of the diagnosis of animal neuromuscular problems will eventually result from following the same methods of systematic, clinical, and pathological evaluation and correlation that have been used in human medicine.

The importance of the neuromuscular system in general and its relationship to other body systems in particular can no longer be ignored. Both clinical and applied research are warranted in order to expand the present knowledge in this area.

*Introduction furnished by Dr. K. Braund.

UPPER MOTONEURON DISEASE

Electromyography (EMG) cannot be used for direct evaluation of the functional integrity of upper motoneurons. When a motor dysfunction is present, elimination of lower motoneuron dysfunction indirectly implicates upper motoneuron pathology. Recent evidence indicates that in humans increased insertion activity, fibrillation potentials, and positive sharp waves occur in upper motoneuron diseases.[36] These responses have not been studied in animals; if present, they are quantitatively much less than those for lower motoneuron disease with a similar degree of motor dysfunction and atrophy. Although the effort pattern may be markedly reduced in upper motoneuron disease, the evoked potentials show only minor changes, which are primarily the result of the disuse atrophy. Motor unit potential firing rates are lower in muscular weakness associated with upper motoneuron disease than in a comparable weakness associated with a lower motoneuron disease.

Electromyography can be used to document the pattern of input of upper motoneurons to lower motoneurons. Motor unit potential bursts that recurred at a rate of 60 to 80 times per minute were noted in canine distemper myoclonus and chorea.[9] Evidence of lower motoneuron disease was not observed in these dogs, but in another study on canine distemper, fibrillation potentials and positive sharp waves were recorded.[5] The spontaneous activity tends to be localized rather than generalized in a particular muscle and may be found in many different muscles. Further study is needed to determine whether this activity is due to lower or upper motoneuron dysfunction. Synchronus bursts of motor unit potentials have been recorded from muscles of young swine affected by myoclonia congenita.[18] This disease involves a spinal cord abnormality. During episodes of progressive muscular hypertonicity in Scotch terriers, the interference patterns were of longer duration and of higher amplitude than patterns recorded prior to an episode.[53] This condition has been termed "Scottie cramp" and is not associated with a neuropathy or myopathy. The efficacy of drugs in suppressing the hyperkinetic episodes was monitored with EMG. Intervertebral disk protrusion produces upper motoneuron dysfunction as well as lower motoneuron dysfunction. Use of EMG in localizing disk protrusion is described later.

LOWER MOTONEURON DISEASE

NEURONOPATHIES

Trauma, infectious processes, and neoplasms of the spinal cord that damage the ventral (anterior) horn cells are associated with the appearance of fibrillation poten-

TABLE 9–6 INNERVATION OF MUSCLES OF THE THORACIC LIMBS

Root	Nerve	Muscles
C1–6	Spinal accessory (external branch)	Trapezius Brachiocephalicus
C7–8	Thoracodorsal	Latissimus dorsi
C6–7	Suprascapular	Supraspinatus Infraspinatus
C7 (C6, C8)[a]	Axillary	Deltoideus Teres minor
C7	Musculocutaneous	Biceps brachii
C6–8	Ventral thoracic	Superficial pectoral
C7–8, T1–2	Radial	Triceps Extensor carpi radialis Extensor digitorum communis Extensor digitorum lateralis Extensor carpi ulnaris Supinator
C8, T1–2	Median	Pronator teres Flexor carpi radialis Flexor digitorum superficialis Flexor digitorum profundus
C8, T1–2	Ulnar	Flexor carpi ulnaris Flexor digitorum profundus Interossei

[a]Sometimes involved.

TABLE 9–7 INNERVATION OF MUSCLES OF THE PELVIC LIMB

Root	Nerve	Muscle
L6–7	Cranial gluteal	Tensor fasciae latae Gluteus medius Gluteus profundus
L7, S1–2	Caudal gluteal	Gluteus superficialis
L4–6	Femoral	Sartorius Vastus lateralis Rectus femoris Vastus medialis
L5–7, S1–2	Ischiatic	Biceps femoris Semitendinosus Semimembranosus
L5–7, S1–2	Peroneal	Tibialis cranialis Extensor digitorum longus Peroneus longus
L5–7, S1–2	Tibial	Gastrocnemius Flexor digitorum superficialis Flexor digitorum profundus Interossei
L4–6	Obturator	Pectineus Gracilis Adductor
S1–3	Pudendal	External anal sphincter External urethral sphincter

tials in muscles innervated by the affected cord segments. Tables 9–6 and 9–7 aid in relating the damaged ventral horn cells with the muscles innervated by these cells. Often EMG indicates that the lesion is more widespread than was indicated by the neurological examination. A valuable electromyographic finding in neuronopathies is the presence of a normal or near normal motor nerve conduction velocity; neuropathies frequently have significantly reduced conduction velocities.

Progressive spinal muscular atrophy in man results from a pathologic process affecting the ventral horn cells. A similar condition in dogs affecting the ventral horn cells has been described; it differs from the human disorder in that it is not progressive.[26] Electromyographs revealed fibrillation potentials and positive sharp waves in many muscles of the fore and hind limbs, giant motor unit potentials (up to 8 mV) of normal duration in several hind limb muscles, fasciculation activity in the gastrocnemii muscles, and normal nerve conduction velocities.

A myelopathy is usually produced by dorsal herniation of an intervertebral disk. The production of ischemia in the cord seems to be more important in the pathogenesis than direct cord compression.[24] In thoracolumbar disk protrusions, the lesion may be localized to two, three, or four cord segments or it may involve many cord segments. Segmental electromyographic evidence for denervation aids greatly in determining the level of the lesion. The superficial and especially the deep dorsal cervical and paraspinal muscles should be examined carefully, and any unusual activity should be noted. The anal sphincter and coccygeal muscles should be examined when caudal cord lesions are suspected. If pain or nervousness causes an excessive effort pattern in the paraspinal muscles, general anesthesia or a tranquilizer should be used to produce muscle relaxation. Sometimes the electromyographic changes are very subtle and include only a repeated positive sharp wave, fasciculation potentials, or a bizarre high frequency discharge in a very localized area. When the abnormal activity is unilateral, surgical intervention on that side should be considered. Previous disk protrusions from which spontaneous recovery has occurred may have left residual spontaneous activity which can be misleading with regard to the present disk problem. If disk surgery has been performed, considerable denervation activity may be present and will probably prevent valid electromyographic evaluation of the present disk problem.

Congenital cord abnormalities such as spinal dysraphism in Weimaraner dogs may be associated with damage to motoneuron cells.[7]

MONONEUROPATHIES

Paralysis of the trigeminal nerve results in loss of control of the mandible and can be seen in a variety of disorders, including tumors, abscesses, trauma, encephalitis, and excessive and prolonged opening of the mouth.[63] Since the etiology of this condition is often not clear, it is frequently termed idiopathic mandibular paralysis. The onset of idiopathic trigeminal paralysis is abrupt, and after about 5 days fibrillation potentials and many positive sharp waves can be recorded from the masseter and pterygoid muscles. Temporal muscles are less markedly affected. Recovery occurs within 14 days after onset, suggesting that the lesion is located in the terminal portion of this cranial nerve. This condition may represent an allergic manifestation. Since trigeminal paralysis also occurs in rabies, cases of mandibular paralysis should be examined initially with caution.

Any peripheral nerve may be subjected to damage by traumatic injury. Causes of injury range from extrinsic problems such as automobile accidents to intrinsic problems such as dystocia. Traumatic injuries to an individual nerve will be manifested by lack of function to the muscle innervated by the nerve. The injury may be inflammatory and result in pain or a hyperactive response clinically, or it may result in reduced function (or none) and observable muscle atrophy. Initially, there is absence of an effort pattern or a reduced effort pattern on the EMG, and after about 5 days function will be much improved if the injury was a simple compressive one. If the injury was more severe and axonal degeneration has occurred, fibrillation potentials and positive sharp waves will appear. Reference to Tables 9–6 and 9–7 will help to determine which nerve or nerves are affected, based on distribution of the spontaneous muscle activity. Compressive injuries tend to produce a localized prolongation of terminal nerve conduction time which reverts to normal when the stimulus is applied below the site of injury.

Intramuscular injection of drugs often produces a localized neuropathy involving intramuscular nerve branches. Usually the effects are noted only electromyographically through the presence of fibrillation potentials and positive sharp waves several days after the injection, but if a large nerve such as the sciatic is affected, a severe lameness may occur. The neuropathy is produced by the physical trauma of the injection including a compression effect and, in some instances, by a toxic effect of the localized, high drug concentration. Great care must be observed in intramuscular injections, since these traumatic nerve or muscle reactions are serious clinical problems for the veterinarian.

The general treatment of injury to one or more nerves depends on the extent of the injury and the nature of the function involved. Frequently, patients will make at least a partial recovery from neuronal injuries of the limbs with rest alone. In general, clinical therapy of nerve injuries includes administration of low doses of steroids, splinting or immobilization of the area to reduce the effects of injury and tissue damage, and selective physical therapy. In some cases, nerve anastomosis, grafting, or transplantation can be considered. Tendon transplantation and arthrodesis in cases of radial paralysis have been proposed but are not widely used.[41]

SPINAL NERVE ROOT DISORDERS

Dysfunction of spinal nerve roots may be produced by herniation of intervertebral disks, spondylosis, trauma, and spinal neoplasms. Electromyography may be used to determine the early presence of the disorder and to localize it, since denervation will occur in muscles which are innervated by the damaged root. The limb muscles should be examined, and special attention should be directed toward the paraspinal muscles. Electromyographic findings and procedures are the same as those described for neuronopathies.

Polyradiculoneuritis (Coon Hound Paralysis, Acute Polyneuritis)

The disorder is usually found in dogs used for hunting raccoon, although it may be seen in other breeds or types of dogs. Cummings and de Lahunta[12, 14] have studied this disorder at length and agree with Kingma and Catcott[40] that it stems from a raccoon bite or scratch that precedes the onset of clinical signs by 7 to 14 days. Other workers have felt that the "treeing" of raccoons has caused spinal cord trauma.[34, 48] Others have felt that this or a similar syndrome may be due to the ingestion of *Clostridium botulinum* toxin.[8, 31, 33, 35, 56]

In past years, the Auburn clinic commonly observed a tetraplegia in hunting dogs and other breeds during the summer months. In 1975–1976, nine cases were seen in the Auburn clinic. These dogs may have a history of "roaming" the woods as well as being in the hunt, but most have a history indicating little chance of exposure to a raccoon. Cummings relates that in Great Britain, where there are no raccoons, this syndrome has not been reported.[12]

Specific evidence of etiology is lacking. It is theorized that the bite or scratch from the raccoon serves an an antigenic stimulus that triggers immunological disturbances that damage Schwann cells.[14]

This disease affects the ventral roots and spinal nerves symmetrically. Sensory neurons appear to be less susceptible than motoneurons. The lesions are characterized by (1) segmental demyelination with preservation of axonal continuity; (2) concomitant degeneration of myelin and axons; (3) leukocytic infiltration of varying type and amount; (4) secondary chromatolysis and swelling of the ventral horn cells; and (5) neurogenic muscle atrophy. This disorder appears to be clinically and pathologically identical to the Landry-Guillain-Barré syndrome in man.[14]

The clinical signs are manifested by a posterior weakness and hyporeflexia in the early stages, and a rapidly ascending weakness until all limbs are in a state of flaccid tetraplegia. The dog is alert, apprehensive, and afebrile. The spinal reflexes are greatly reduced or absent, and paralysis of the respiratory muscles may occur. Frequently, the voice is abnormally weak or of a different quality. At the peak of the illness (10 days), the extremities may be cool and body temperature may be subnormal.[12, 14]

Laboratory and radiographic results are essentially normal. Spinal fluid pressure may be increased even though the results of tests on cerebrospinal fluid taken from the cisterna are normal. Electromyographic examination about 1 week after onset reveals an increased insertion activity, fibrillation potentials, positive sharp waves, and occasional bizarre high frequency discharges. Evidence for denervation usually first appears in the interosseus muscles. Evoked potentials are reduced in amplitude and markedly polyphasic (Fig. 9–43), and during the most severe stage, no potentials can be evoked in some muscles. If the peripheral nerve fibers are also involved directly in the neuropathy, nerve conduction velocities will be reduced, but more in motor than in sensory fibers. Since limb temperatures tend to be subnormal in this disease, the effects of temperature should be considered before concluding that a nerve conduction velocity value is subnormal. Electromyography is useful in monitoring progression of recovery.

The length of the disease is usually 3 to 6

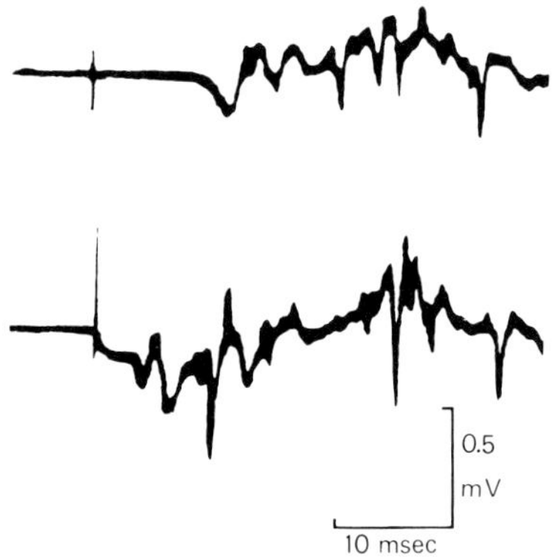

FIGURE 9–43 Effect of polyradiculoneuritis on an evoked potential of a canine interosseous muscle. The asynchronous discharge of the motor unit potentials including the evoked potential was caused by the reduced nerve conduction velocities (34 meters/sec for the fastest conducting fibers) and the reduced number of functional motor units.

weeks, and the prognosis is generally guarded to good. However, in extreme paralysis with resultant severe muscle atrophy, full recovery may not occur. Recurrences have been seen, and Cummings describes one case in which a dog suffered three separate attacks.

Treatment consists of maintaining urine and fecal eliminations, keeping the animal clean, avoiding formation of decubital lesions by keeping the dog on an air or water mattress or foam rubber cushion, and using physical and hydrotherapy to combat muscle atrophy after the acute phase. Adrenocortical steroid therapy in the initial stage may alleviate some of the severe neurological damage. Dexamethasone at a dose of 1.0–1.5 mg daily has been suggested. Supervised exercise will aid in rehabilitation. Urinary infections, particularly cystitis, must be combatted constantly (see Chapters 12 and 13).

POLYNEUROPATHIES

Avulsion of the Brachial Plexus

Avulsion of the brachial plexus is a common traumatic polyneuropathy in the dog. During severe abduction of the fore limb, nerve roots of the brachial plexus are stretched or torn from the spinal cord, causing dorsal and ventral root avulsion intradurally. In severe abduction the dorsal border of the scapula is displaced ventromedially so that severe tension is exerted on the brachial plexus. The primary clinical signs of damage to C6–T2 ventral nerve roots are complete inability to support weight on the affected limb, which drags during walking; absence of flexor or extensor thrust reflexes; absence of superficial or deep sensation in the limb; and a fast progressive atrophy. A flaccid diaphragm on the side of the lesion may be noted with fluoroscopy. Severe damage that affects the sympathetic innervation of the pupils and eyelids (C7–T2) will produce signs of Horner's syndrome, such as ptosis, miosis, and enophthalmus. In the affected limb, electromyographic changes show a lack of voluntary motor unit potentials beginning immediately after injury. Positive sharp waves and fibrillation potentials appear about 5 days after injury. Three to 7 days after the injury, no response to stimulation of the nerves of the limb will be noted.[11] The presence of some motor unit activity indicates that limb amputation should be delayed, and serial electromyographic examinations should be made for several months to determine whether reinnervation is occurring. Roots associated with functional recovery can be determined by relating electromyographic results to information presented in Table 9–6. The EMG is particularly useful when tendon transplantation is to be employed for treatment of partial brachial plexus paralysis.[41] Muscles used in this procedure include the flexor carpi radialis and the biceps brachii or brachialis muscles. These muscles should be free of fibrillation potential and positive sharp wave activities if they are to be used in tendon transplant surgery.

Griffiths noted that 55 per cent of a series of 18 dogs with brachial plexus avulsion showed partial Horner's syndrome with an ipsilateral miosis. Ipsilateral loss of the cutaneous reflex was seen; however, a contralateral response was present on the nonaffected side when the affected side was stimulated. The spinal cords and nerve roots were studied in six of these dogs, and intradural avulsion of the dorsal and ventral nerve roots contributing to the plexus was present in all cases. Retraction balls were present in axons of the motor neurons within the cord, and the ventral horn cells showed retrograde reactions.[27]

In complete avulsion of the plexus, treatment is unsuccessful. In incomplete avulsion, partial function of the limb may be possible. Surgery is generally not attempted in avulsion of the brachial plexus, with the exception of possible tendon transplantation when the plexus is partially damaged.[11, 41]

Brachial Plexus Neuropathy

Two reports of brachial plexus neuropathy in the dog resemble a well-defined syndrome in man which apparently is not related to trauma.[1, 13] The predominant sign in man is a sudden onset of pain associated with muscular weakness either simultaneously or after a variable period of time. Fibrillation potentials have been recorded from some of the muscles of the thoracic limbs on the twelfth and twentieth days after the onset of paresis. Evoked potentials could not be induced in the palmar interosseous muscles. The syndrome may involve the rostral, caudal, or entire brachial plexus; involvement may be complete or incomplete and can occur bilaterally. The disorder may be a manifestation of a systemic or localized infectious disorder, possibly viral, or the result of an allergic or hypersensitivity phenomenon. In man, the involvement may follow the administration of vaccines, antisera (especially tetanus antisera), horse serums, or other foreign proteins. In a 9-month-old Great Dane the reported signs included vomiting, facial edema, generalized urticaria, and later a neurological deficit in the thoracic limbs. Skin testing helped in identifying a horse meat diet as the specific allergen in this acute bilateral brachial plexus neuritis.[13]

In a 1½-year-old spayed female Doberman periods of pain were followed by pectoral limb motor deficits involving postural reactions and supraspinatus and infraspinatus muscle atrophy. The cause was undetermined in this case, as it often is in human patients also. This dog showed some improvement in the 4-month observation period. Human patients generally recover completely, although it sometimes takes 3 years or longer. Steroid therapy, analgesics, and physical therapy are often used, but there is little evidence that they alter the course of the disease.[1]

Metabolic and Toxic Polyneuropathies

Many metabolic and toxic diseases which can cause polyneuropathies are discussed in detail in Chapters 11 and 17.

DISORDERS PRODUCED BY NEUROTOXINS

The neurotoxins that are most frequently encountered clinically produce tetanus, botulism, and tick paralysis.

Tetanus

Tetanus is a disease caused by *Clostridium tetani.* This anaerobic bacterium is deposited in deep lacerations and puncture wounds and produces a neurotrophic exotoxin. It is said that signs of tetanus are usually seen within 5 to 8 days following the introduction of the organism into subcutaneous tissues. It is thought that the toxin spreads by means of the peripheral nerves. In the 1965–66 period, 507 cases of tetanus affecting man were reported in the United States, of which 68 per cent were fatal.[42] Even though it has been estimated that the dog is 300 times more resistant to tetanus toxin than the horse, the disease in dogs has been reported frequently in the literature.[20, 61] Twenty-one dogs with tetanus were reported in the Brisbane area of Queensland, Australia within a 6-year period.[16]

The initial signs of tetanus in the dogs are generalized muscle hyperexcitability and chronic spasms. We have observed tonic muscle contractions of the face that promote a "smiling" appearance as well as hypertonicity of the auricular muscles that cause dorsal retraction of ear flaps or, in prick-eared dogs, the ears touch each other over the top of the head. Diarrhea is frequently seen. Tonic spasms and opisthotonos occur in the terminal stages. In a clinical case, Zontine described in detail the signs, laboratory results, and the course of treatment over a period of several days.[74]

Treatment and Prevention. Routine immunization of dogs aganist tetanus is rarely performed; however, in enzootic areas or where dogs are in constant contact with horses, immunization with toxoid or antitoxin should be considered.

Since dogs are quite resistant to the effects of tetanus toxin, most veterinarians generally don't administer antitoxin to dogs with traumatic wounds. In endemic areas, where conditions favor the development of infection, antitoxin (500 to 1000 units) should be given. Proper débridement, cleansing, and use of hydrogen peroxide flushing of wounds is important. Sizeable doses of penicillin or other antibiotics should be given.[30]

When clinical signs have developed, antitoxin and penicillin or other antibiotics should be used immediately. Therapeutic doses of antitoxin will vary with the severity of the signs; reports of 2500 to 1000,000 units given intravenously appear in the literature. Sensitivity should be observed by injecting 0.1 to 0.2 ml subcutaneously one-half hour before giving a large dose.[30] Mason has stated that 30,000 u of antitoxin given to a 27- to 30-kg dog should be a maximum dose.[47] Penicillin doses of 500,000 to several million units have been given daily.

Supportive treatment with muscle relaxants such as mephenesin, chlorphenesin carbamate (Maolate), and *d*-tubocurarine, with tranquilizers or barbiturates is indicated to relieve muscle spasms. Oxygen should be administered in cases of respiratory impairment. Hyperbaric oxygen has been effective, but the necessary equipment is rarely available in veterinary clinics. Fluids and nutriment administrations and general good nursing care are mandatory. Zontine emphasizes that the owner must be aware of the cost of the antitoxin and intensive care required for proper treatment in advanced cases of tetanus.[16, 17, 20, 30, 32, 43, 47, 62, 74]

Botulism

Botulism as a disease in dogs has been a controversial subject. Dogs are most frequently affected by eating discarded, improperly canned vegetables and meats or by eating spoiled carcasses. Work by Graham and Erikson[23] in 1922, Jackson,[35] Brasmer and Shideler,[8] Mosier,[56] Howell,[33] and Hoerlein[31] suggests strongly that botulism exists as a clinical entity in dogs. Jackson[35] and Hoerlein[31] have seen limberneck in chickens and quadriplegia in dogs that were fed discarded, home-canned vegetables. The clinical signs include a general weakness or paresis resembling tick paralysis and polyradiculoneuritis (coon hound paralysis). Both autonomic and skeletal muscles are affected, and in humans swallowing and respiration are severely impaired.

Barsanti and workers[4] have recently reported an outbreak of clinical botulism in 19 of 20 foxhounds belonging to one owner and other dogs released on the same hunt by other owners. Forty dogs belonging to the same kennel who had not been hunted recently were unaffected. The day after the hunt, 3 dogs were unable to rise, 16 appeared weak, and 1 was not located. Two days later, six of the weak dogs had quadriplegia.

Three dogs hospitalized at the University of Georgia for botulism suffered from diffuse LMN dysfunction that affected both cranial and spinal neuromuscular systems. All dogs were mentally alert and showed the following signs: quadriplegia, deficient postural reactions, bilateral mydriasis with a sluggish direct and consensual light response, diminished jaw tone, diminished palpebral and gag reflexes, and deficient spinal reflexes. On EMG, motor unit potentials were markedly reduced in amplitude and nerve conduction velocities were decreased. The most severely affected dog died.[4]

The serum from the most severely affected dog and feces from all three hospitalized dogs were positive for botulinum toxin, type C. When three other dogs still at the kennel were tested, the sera of all three were negative, but the feces of the only one tested was positive for botulinum toxin, type C.[4]

All five dogs treated improved, two at the clinic and three at the kennel. At the end of 9 days, three were walking and two were mildly paretic. The two dogs at the clinic received parenteral fluids, antibiotics, and supportive treatment. One vial of trivalent botulism antitoxin (types A, B, and E) was given intramuscularly to four of the dogs.[4]

The clinical signs of these proven cases of botulism are similar to those described by clinicians in other reports.[8, 31, 35] It is felt that what has been described as experimental botulism[23] and suspected clinical botulism has now been documented as a clinical disease entity by the Georgia report of cases confirmed by laboratory examination.

Botulinum toxin blocks the release of acetylcholine from motor nerve terminals. The sensory nerves are not affected. In the acute stage, amplitudes of motor unit and evoked potentials are reduced in the EMG, but the nerve conduction velocity is normal. When the animal survives for 5 days or longer, fibrillation potentials appear and have characteristics comparable to those recorded from muscles denervated by severing their motor nerve supply.[33] Neostigmine therapy and repetitive stimulation may partially overcome the action of the toxin.

The diagnosis of botulism depends on identification of the toxin in serum or in the gastrointestinal contents (by injecting a sample into mice). In most clinical cases the animals have been afflicted for several days, and no doubt the toxin has been largely or totally absorbed. Botulism should be differentiated from so-called coon hound paralysis and tick paralysis. In veterinary medicine the treatment is supportive except in the initial stages of an acute case when there is an opportunity to administer polyvalent antitoxins. These are not readily available in most areas. Neostigmine therapy and repetitive stimulation may partially overcome the action of the toxin. A high percentage of cases recover in 3 to 4 weeks with good symptomatic treatment.[49]

Tick Paralysis

In the United States tick paralysis in the dog is generally caused by the neurotoxin released by the common female wood tick, *Dermacentor variabilis. Dermacentor venustus, Amblyomma maculatum*, and *A. americanum* have also been mentioned as possible vectors in this country. Vectors vary in different parts of the world.[61, 66] This disease is widely distributed and is universally recognized by practicing veterinarians. Tick paralysis has been transmitted experimentally, and develops at or about the time of full engorgement of the tick. The onset of symptoms is sudden.

Tick paralysis occurs in man in much the same manner. In North America, *Dermacentor andersoni* and *Dermacentor variabilis* have been the responsible vectors. Recovery usually takes place 1 to 2 days, and rarely, up to 8 days after removal of the tick, provided that the respiratory system has not been affected.

In dogs, the symptoms vary from a posterior weakness to a generalized flaccid paralysis of all skeletal muscles. Sensation may be present. The progression of paralysis may cover a period of 1 to 2 days. In advanced cases respiratory paralysis and death may ensue. In clinical practice, tick paralysis should be differentiated from botulism and polyradiculoneuritis.

Ticks may be vectors for many bloodborne and systemic diseases, some of which may affect the nervous system. There have been occasional reports of such transmitted disease which is not host-specific for the dog. A recent report from Switzerland described the death of a dog from acute disseminated leptomeningoencephalitis as a result of a tick-transmitted virus identified as the Central European tickborne encephalitis virus which usually affects man and wild animals.[69]

A case of louping ill transmitted by a tick was seen in a working collie in Scotland. This was the first case diagnosed in a dog; the disease is seen normally in cattle and sheep.[45]

A report from Australia indicates that the neurotoxin of the *Ixodes holocyclus* can cause autonomic as well as motor dysfunction; the former is manifested by a deficiency in bladder function which may last for as long as a week after motor recovery. One of four afflicted dogs ruptured a bladder. It was concluded that dogs with tick paralysis should be catheterized for at least 1 week after motor recovery.[21] This form of tick paralysis apparently is not a common disorder in the USA.

The mechanism of action of the toxin has not been completely explained, but it appears to slow and block transmission primarily in the terminal portion of motor nerve fibers and secondarily in large motor and sensory nerves.[64] Thus, the reduction in release of transmitter at the neuromuscular junction is not due to direct action at the junction. The major electromyographic change is a reduction in amplitudes of evoked potentials. Response to repetitive stimulation is not altered and direct stimulation of muscle produces a vigorous, normal contraction. Neostigmine-like drugs do not effect improvement in motor function. Evoked potential latencies are prolonged, and conduction velocities of large motor and sensory nerves are slightly reduced. Evoked potential amplitudes improve more rapidly than nerve conduction velocities after removal of the tick. The EMG changes described in idiopathic polyradiculoneuritis are markedly different from those seen in tick paralysis.[10]

Treatment

The ticks must be removed by dipping the dog in an insecticide solution in order to kill all of them, including hidden ones. In our experience, recovery varies according to the number of ticks involved, but usually occurs in 24 to 72 hours after their removal. If ticks are buried in the dermis and subcutaneous tissues, surgical removal is suggested. Administration of glucose and calcium preparations may be helpful.

In Australia, where the tick neurotoxin seems more lethal (50 per cent mortality in dogs) than in the USA, a hyperimmune serum has been developed. This is an effective means of treatment during certain stages of the disease.[6]

Myasthenia Gravis

Myasthenia gravis in man is a disorder of the neuromuscular junction characterized by a variable degree of weakness during use of various voluntary muscles. The disorder closely resembles a state associated with partial curarization. The cause of myasthenia gravis is unknown. An autoimmune reaction may play an important role. The nature of the defect in neuromuscular transmission is controversial. Some evidence supports a theory that the amount of transmitter released from the nerve terminal is reduced, while other evidence points toward a reduction in the number of available receptors at the motor end-plate.[15]

In man, the disease has been associated with thymic (primarily), thyroid, and other endocrine dysfunction. Marked improvement has been noted in most patients who have undergone thymectomy, and those who have not responded well have shown evidence of accessory thymus tissue that was not removed at the time of surgery. Myasthenic mothers have given birth to affected babies who become normal in a few weeks. This observation indicates that there is placental transfer of a humoral agent which inhibits neuromuscular transmission. Another worker has reported two familial cases of myasthenia gravis, including four sets of identical twins.

Palmer reviewed 16 cases of myasthenia gravis in animals that had been reported prior to 1974. However, the condition is frequent, and many cases are not reported in the literature. One of ten cases analyzed was a cat. Most of the animals affected were young; however, one was 6 and the other 11 years of age. Only one case had a thymoma. There was no sex predominance, and most dogs were of larger breeds.[57] Myasthenia has also been reported in springer spaniel littermates.[37]

The usual signs are posterior weakness, a swaggering gait, and inability to rise quickly from a recumbent position. In addition, confirmed and suspected cases in dogs have shown intermittent muscle spasms, difficulty in eating and drinking, weakness in the jaw and tongue muscles, and megaesophagus (the dog's esophagus is largely striated muscle). A high-pitched voice has also been noted. In man, the EMG shows a progressive reduction in amplitude of evoked potentials after repetitive nerve stimulation of 30/sec but not at 3/second. A decline is absent or reduced after administration of an anticholinesterase agent. Nerve conduction velocities are normal. In myasthenia gravis in man, miniature endplate potentials are reduced. In electron microscopy, the synaptic vesicles in the end-plate are normal in mean diameter and density, but there is a reduction in the length of both pre- and postsynaptic membranes.[57]

The clinical diagnosis is based on the dramatic improvement shown in motor and electromyographic responses with administration of an anticholinesterase drug. Normal radiographic and EMG findings will aid in differentiating possible CNS lesions. Clinical signs, however, are usually characteristic. The differential diagnosis should include rabies, hypoglycemia, adrenocortical insufficiency, hypokalemia, polyradiculoneuritis (coon hound paralysis), and polymyositis. The EMG will aid in the differential diagnosis.

The so-called Tensilon test in humans is performed by assessing the short-term improvement that results from injecting edrophonium chloride (Tensilon). Zacks injected 1 mg over a 15-second period to a 10-kg dog suffering from myasthenia. In 1 minute the dog could stand and walk normally, but after 12 minutes it could no longer stand. Zacks and co-workers studied this dog at length with periodic electromyographic examinations. Muscle biopsies were also studied with light and electron microscopy. This dog was given pyridostigmine therapy in a dose that varied from 45 mg to 180 mg/day. In time, the dose was reduced to 45 mg every 2 days, and finally treatment was discontinued after some 2 months. The disorder recurred about 10 months later.[73]

The drugs used for diagnosis and therapy are edrophonium chloride (Tensilon), neostigmine bromide (Prostigmin bromide), neostigmine methylsulfate (Prostigmin methylsulfate), pyridostigmine bromide (Mestinon bromide), and ambenonium chloride (Mytelase chloride). Pyridostigmine and neostigmine bromide are available in slow-release tablets, the release period lasting between 6 and 12 hours. Dosage should be adjusted for each dog on the basis of therapeutic response and undesirable side effects. The dog's health should be kept as normal as possible, stress and illness should be avoided, and neuromuscular blocking agents such as streptomycin, neomycin, and other antimicrobial agents with similar potential action should be avoided.[57] The dose can be gradually reduced according to the animal's progress and finally discontinued. Remissions are frequently seen, but not always; if one occurs, the course of therapy is repeated.

DISORDERS OF MUSCLE

Muscular disorders will be discussed very briefly, since they are not primarily neurogenic diseases but must be considered when arriving at neurological diagnoses. The term myositis denotes chiefly inflammatory disease, while myopathy denotes primarily atrophy or degeneration. In man, the predominant muscular disorders are polymyositis, muscular dystrophy, myotonia, chronic myopathy secondary to neoplasia or endocrine disease, and various other hypotonias and myopathies.[3] In the dog, the primary disorders are myasthenia gravis, myositis and polymyositis (from septic, parasitic, and idiopathic causes), muscular dystrophy, nutritional myopathy, myotonia, and greyhound cramp.[59]

MYOSITIS

Myositis is an inflammatory condition that involves muscle fibers and their associated connective tissue. The causes include trauma, strain, and infectious processes. Pain occurs in the acute, subacute, and chronic forms but is especially prominent in the acute form. Diagnosis is aided by determination of serum muscle enzymes, histologic evaluation of muscle biopsies, and cultures of associated abscesses. Electromyographic examination provides evidence of a myopathy (Table 9–4), particularly in the chronic form. Some fibrillation potential and positive sharp wave activities may be present also, probably because the inflammatory process has affected some intraumuscular nerve fibers.

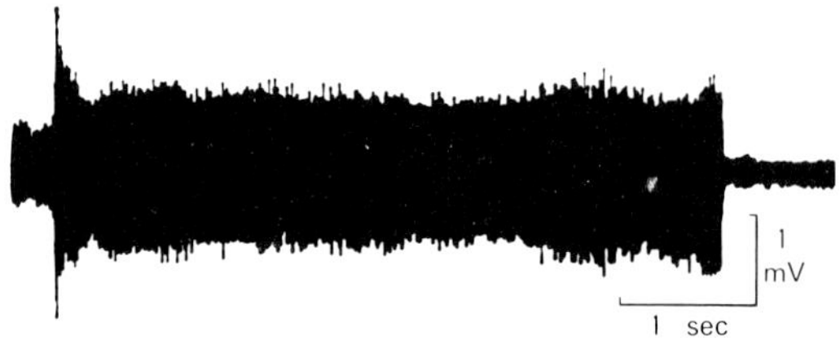

FIGURE 9–44 A bizarre high-frequency discharge recorded from the semitendinosus muscle of a dog with myotonia-like signs.

Myositis may also result from unknown causes. The principal examples are eosinophilic myositis and atrophic myositis. The muscles of mastication are affected primarily, although one case of eosinophilic myositis has been reported in which other than masticatory muscles were affected.[60] Both eosinophilic myositis and atrophic myositis have acute onsets and often affect bilaterally symmetrical muscles. In some cases insertion activity, fibrillation potential, and positive sharp wave activity are pronounced 5 to 7 days after onset, suggesting involvement of nerve fibers. Bizarre high frequency discharges (Fig. 9–44) may occur, and polyphasic evoked potentials of decreased amplitude have been noted. Slowing of nerve conduction velocity does not occur in myositis.

POLYMYOSITIS[2]

Polymyositis is an inflammatory disease of many muscles. The most common cause in the dog is *Toxoplasma gondii,* which produces a very severe necrotizing myositis. The eosinophilic myositis found predominantly in German shepherds and confined largely to the temporal and masseter muscles has been mentioned. The type discussed in this section is an *idiopathic type* of polymyositis which is seen in many breeds but affects German shepherds most commonly. Physical signs include a slightly stiff gait, weakness and collapse on exercise, vomiting shortly after eating, a hoarse bark, temporal muscular swelling or atrophy, difficulty in chewing and swallowing, and possibly pain in the proximal limb musculature.

The differential diagnosis includes myasthenia gravis primarily, polyneuritis, cervical cord disease, hyperadrenocorticism (corticism), and nutritional bone disease. Elevation of any one or all of the following enzymes is helpful in diagnosis: serum glutamic oxaloacetic transaminase (SGOT), lactic dehydrogenase (LDH), creatinine phosphokinase (CPK), and aldolase. Creatinine phosphokinase and aldolase are enzymes found only in skeletal muscle, and elevation of either is a most reliable sign. Occasionally, radiographic examination may reveal esophageal dilatation and impaired esophageal contractions on the barium swallow in cases of polymyositis. Muscle biopsies reveal characteristic inflammatory foci.[2]

Oral treatment with prednisolone at a dose of 0.25–0.5 mg/kg every 8 hours generally provides prompt relief. When the signs and serum enzymes are normal, the steroid should be withdrawn gradually over a 7- to 10-day period. The prognosis is guarded or favorable unless permanent damage to esophageal, laryngeal, and masticatory muscles has occurred.[2]

MYOTONIA

Myotonia is defined as increased muscular irritability and contractility with decreased power of relaxation, resulting in a tonic spasm. In man, these disorders are frequently congenital or hereditary. Griffiths recently described characteristic EMG findings in two canine myotonic cases and signs in two dogs which were classified as having atypical myotonia or pseudomyotonia.[25, 26]

Myotonia is characterized by delayed relaxation of skeletal muscles after voluntary movement or electrical stimulation. Electromyographically this response is associated with a high frequency, repetitive discharge (Fig. 9–45) which varies in intensity so that

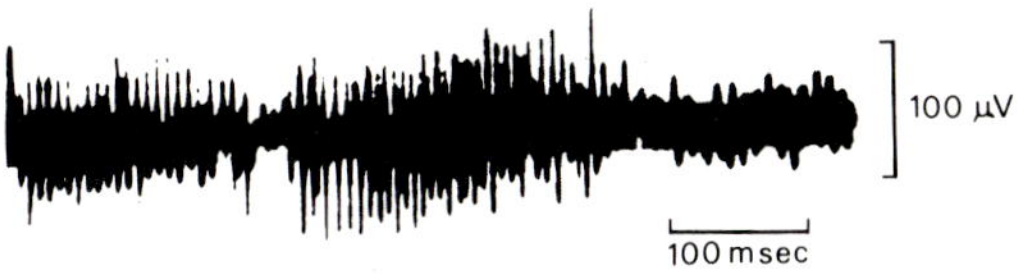

FIGURE 9–45 A myotonic discharge of a triceps muscle of an anesthetized Chow. It was myogenic in origin because neuromuscular transmission had been blocked by succinylcholine. The discharge was induced by muscle percussion. (From Griffiths, I. R., and Duncan, I. D.: Myotonia in the dog: A report of four cases. Vet. Rec. *93*, 184, 1973.)

the sound is comparable to that of an airplane during a bombing maneuver. Thus, the term "dive-bomber" has been applied to this response. Needle electrode movement and muscle percussion will also induce this response, which is probably the result of a process that creates muscle cell membrane hyperexcitability. The myotonic discharge is unaffected by neuromuscular blockade induced by either depolarizing (succinylcholine) or nondepolarizing (gallamine) muscle-relaxing drugs. Fibrillation potentials and positive sharp waves are absent usually, and nerve conduction velocities are generally normal. Although the electromyographic results are similar to those for myotonic disease in man, the lack of similar muscle pathology and systemic signs such as alopecia and cataracts indicates that the underlying disease process in dogs differs from that in myotonia dystrophica in man.[25] Stiffness, particularly of the hind limbs, is the most noteworthy sign in the dog. A pseudomyotonia associated with a myopathy has been noted in dogs also.[25] In this disease the myotonic discharge begins and terminates abruptly. A similar response has been noted in cases of human polymyositis. Myotonic discharges are occasionally recorded in canine polyradiculoneuritis, but these should probably be termed bizarre high frequency discharges[12] (Fig. 9–44).

Histological examination in Griffiths' two cases showed that both dogs had muscular dystrophy, and the striated muscles showed fibers of variable size, occasional necrosis, an increase of central nuclei, and an excess of connective tissue. Serum values of CPK, SGOT, and SGPT were all elevated. Percussion during anesthesia caused a depression (dimple) lasting about 30 seconds in the tongue, deltoid, and vastus lateralis muscles. This dimple was considered to be a diagnostic sign.[25]

The diagnosis is based on serum enzyme studies, histological and enzyme studies on muscle biopsies, and characteristic EMG and nerve conduction studies. In man the disease is generally treated by quinine or (more effectively) procainamide hydrochloride. The initial human adult dose is 0.25 gm four times daily; it can be increased to a maintenance level of 4 gm a day.[3] Griffiths found that phenylhydantoin and procainamide had little effect in his dogs.[26]

MUSCULAR DYSTROPHY

Muscular dystrophy is a true myopathy consisting of progressive atrophy and degeneration of muscle and fibrous infiltration. In man, true muscular dystrophy is a genetically determined, primary degenerative disease of muscle. In dogs, hereditary dystrophies have not been reported except possibly for one dog with dystonia.[26] However, cases of dystrophy in dogs with idiopathic etiology but characteristic histologic changes have been reported.[26, 34, 72]

Pseudohypertrophic muscular dystrophy has been observed in young dogs. The disease is progressive, and signs include weakness and a stilted gait. Electromyographic examination reveals evidence for both neuropathic and myopathic processes.

NUTRITIONAL MYOPATHY

A noninflammatory myopathy or type of muscular dystrophy due to a vitamin E–selenium deficiency has been seen in young dogs.[67] Van Vleet[68] has produced a vitamin E–selenium deficiency in dogs that could be prevented by adding vitamin E or selenium to the basic diet. Mild skeletal myopathy was present histologically when only selenium was added.[68] Manktelow[46] in 1963 reported a myopathy in dogs that resembled clinically and histologically white muscle disease in lambs in New Zealand.

Since the most active muscles are the most severely affected, the clinical signs include increasing inability to control the limbs, stiffness, dropping of the hock, and finally complete muscular failure. The neck muscles of nursing puppies frequently show a marked weakness. The muscles most frequently affected are the gastrocnemius, deltoideus, infraspinatus, and supraspinatus. Dogs are most frequently affected with the pseudohypertrophic form of the disease. Grossly, the muscles look white or resemble fish flesh. Histological examination demonstrates that the muscle fibers enlarge initially but progressively become degenerate and atrophic; fat and fibrous tissue infiltrate the fibers. In very advanced forms, the muscle tissue may be nearly unrecognizable.[46]

Nutritional myopathy or muscular dystrophy may be suspected if the dog presents progressive weakness associated with apparent hypertrophy or atrophy of muscles, particularly the muscles mentioned previously. Muscle biopsy and histological examination constitute a positive aid in diagnosis. Electromyography is characteristic of a myopathy.

The treatment has consisted largely of vitamin E–selenium combinations (Selectoc). There have been reports of favorable improvement; however, much depends on the stage of the disease.[46, 59]

HEREDITARY MYOPATHY

A recessive X-linked myopathy in male Irish terrier puppies has been reported.[70] Signs included a stiff gait, difficulty in swallowing, and muscle atrophy. Serum creatine-phosphokinase values were extremely high, but serum vitamin E levels were normal. Fibrillation potentials and positive sharp waves were absent, but high frequency myotonic-like discharges were present in all muscles examined. Muscle percussion did not induce dimpling or contraction. Administration of vitamin E, procainamide, and quinidine produced only transient improvement.[70, 71]

GREYHOUND CRAMP

This disorder has been seen exclusively in greyhounds during training or in an actual race. It is manifested by an acute muscle spasm of the hind limbs. The cause is unknown, except that it might be due to extreme muscular stress for which the animal is not in proper condition.

The clinical sequence of signs is as follows: the dog trails behind, his gait is stiff or wooden, he walks by dragging one hind leg after the other, his toes are curled under, his muscles are severely hardened and spastic, he is cyanotic, and he may fall down and may roll or struggle on the ground. After periods of rest and massage for 5 to 15 minutes, he usually recovers.[59]

Usually no treatment is necessary except proper conditioning, and rest and massage during an acute attack.

Gowing has reported a similar disorder in greyhounds that more closely resembles azoturia in horses.[22] It is more severe in that about 25 per cent of the victims die during the acute stage. Muscle atrophy is noted, particularly in the lumbar area several days after the acute attack. Muscle regeneration may occur, but generally the dogs are unsuitable for further use.

Other metabolic disorders that may be confused with possible brain disorders will be discussed in Chapter 17.

SCOTTIE CRAMP[39, 50–55]

Scottie cramp has in the past been considered a myopathy but currently is termed a CNS disorder. However, since it must be differentiated clinically from neuromuscular disorders, it is placed in this section for the clinician's convenience.

Scottie cramp is a descriptive term for a hyperkinetic disorder that has been observed for years in Scottish terriers by kennel owners and veterinarians. The disease is characterized by varying degrees and frequency of seemingly painless rigidity of limbs, back, and tail muscles or in some instances, rather generalized spasms. The episodes are short in duration and recovery is prompt. It has been shown to be inherited recessively, probably by an autosomal gene, since distribution of the disease is about equal between the sexes.[52] Muscle glycogen and phosphorylase levels have been found to be normal, as have calcium, blood lactic acid, and pyruvic acid clearance after exercise. No histopathological lesions have been noted. Biochemical and electromyographic evidence suggests that the cramping is of CNS origin and not primarily of muscular origin. Meyers and co-workers have more recently performed investigations on various drugs which affect the putative neurotransmitters dopamine, norepinephrine, and serotonin (5-HT). It has been concluded that serotonin is involved in the modulation of skeletal muscle tone. The current results of these works seem confusing, but future studies may determine the precise mechanism of serotonin in the cause of this disease.[54, 55]

The clinical signs usually appear when the puppy is 6 months old or older, possibly when the owner starts exercise on a leash. Episodes can be elicited by normal physical activity or by psychic changes. Excitement and fear facilitate the episodes, whereas anxiety and apprehension are often inhibitory. Amphetamine administrations induce a typical attack. The first signs of an attack are usually that a slight abduction develops in the front legs, the back becomes arched in the lumbar area, and the hind legs become overflexed and quickly hit the ground in a "stringhalt" gait. The dog hops on one leg and then the other as he flexes them in an effort to relieve the spasm. The head may be drawn between the front legs because of spasms of the ventral cervical musculature. In severe cases, the dog may somersault forward and curl into a ball: breathing appears to cease. After 15 seconds or so, the dog recovers, appears relaxed, and is panting. Dogs remain conscious and do not appear to be in pain. Affected animals seem to enjoy normal life expectancy. Episodes may be periodic or fairly consistent, and in some cases clinical signs worsen.

The treatment consists of largely avoiding the particular exciting influence. If exercise is the stimulating force, then it should be restricted. Since Meyers and coworkers found the CNS to be implicated in the cause of Scottie cramp, they evaluated various drugs known to counteract such episodes of muscle rigidity.[50, 51] They found that intramuscular injections of chlorpromazine (Thorazine, 1.0 to 1.75 mg/kg), acepromazine (Acepromazine, 0.075 to 0.1 mg/kg), and diazepam (Valium 0.50 to 1.50 mg/kg) were effective in suppressing signs of the disease. Oral diazepam in doses of 0.5 mg/kg given three times daily was highly effective in controlling episodes regardless of stimuli encountered. When the dose was reduced to twice daily, mornings and evenings, mild signs occurred before the evening administration. The EMG has been used to monitor response to therapy.

A case of Scotty cramp was treated at the Auburn clinic for some 2 years. The suggested dose of diazepam relieved clinical signs effectively for 1 year, after which the dose needed to be increased significantly. The incorporation of a muscle relaxant, chlorphenesin carbamate (Maolate), with diazepam controlled the episodes during the remainder of the observation period.

REFERENCES

1. Alexander, J. W., de Lahunta, A., and Scott, P. W.: A case of brachial plexus neuropathy in a dog. J. Am. Anim. Hosp. Assoc. *10,* 515, 1974.
2. Averill, D. R.: Polymyositis in the dog. *In* Kirk, R. W. (ed.): *Current Veterinary Therapy V.* W. B. Saunders Co., Philadelphia, 1974, p. 652.
3. Bannister, R.: *Brain's Clinical Neurology,* 4th ed. Oxford University Press, London, 1973.
4. Barsanti, J.: Unpublished data.
5. Bascuas, J. A., Bascuas, J. L., and Marin, M.: Electromyographic discoveries in dogs with distemper. Veterinaria (Madrid) *38,* 565, 1973.
6. Blood, D. C., and Henderson, J. A.: *Veterinary Medicine,* 3rd ed. The Williams and Wilkins Co., Baltimore, 1968, p. 841.
7. Botelho, S. Y., Steinberg, S. A., McGrath, J. T., and Zislis, J.: Electromyography in dogs with congenital spinal cord lesions. Am. J. Vet. Res. *28,* 205, 1967.
8. Brasmer, T. H., and Shideler, R. H.: Pseudobotulism in dogs. N. Am. Vet. *37,* 669, 1956.
9. Breazille, J. E., Blaugh, B. S., and Nail, N.: Experimental study of canine distemper myoclonus. Am. J. Vet. Res. *120,* 1375, 1966.
10. Chrisman, C. L.: Differentiation of tick paralysis and acute idiopathic-polyradiculoneuritis in the dog using electromyography. J. Am. Anim. Hosp. Assoc. *11,* 455, 1975.
11. Chrisman, C. L.: Diseases of peripheral nerves and muscles. *In* Ettinger, S. J. (ed.): *Textbook of Veterinary Internal Medicine, Diseases of the Dog and Cat.* W. B. Saunders Co., Philadelphia, 1975, p. 459.
12. Cummings, J. F., and Haas, D. C.: Coonhound paralysis: an acute idiopathic-polyradiculoneuritis in dogs resembling the Landry-Guillain-Barré syndrome. J. Neurol. Sci. *4,* 51, 1967.
13. Cummings, J. F., Lorenz, M. D., de Lahunta, A., and Washington, L. D.: Canine brachial plexus neuritis: a syndrome resembling serum neuritis in man. Cornell Vet. *63,* 589, 1973.
14. Cummings, J. F., and de Lahunta, A.: Canine polyneuritis. *In* Kirk, R. W. (ed.): *Current Veterinary Therapy V.* W. B. Saunders Co., Philadelphia, 1974, p. 655.
15. Drachman, D. B., Kao, I., Pestronk, A., and Toyha, K. V.: Myasthenia gravis as a receptor disorder. Ann N.Y. Acad. Sci. *274,* 226, 1976.
16. English, P. B., and Carlisle, C. H.: Tetanus in the dog. Aust. Vet. J. *37,* 62, 1961.
17. Eriksson, E., and Ullberg-Olsson, K.: Tetanus and dog bites. J. Small Anim. Pract. *3,* 137, 1962.
18. Fletcher, T. F.: Ablation and histopathologic studies on myoclonia congenita in swine. Am. J. Vet. Res. *29,* 2255, 1968.
19. Fox, J. G., and Gurmick, M. J.: Horner's syndrome and brachial paralysis due to lymphosarcoma in a cat. J.A.V.M.A. *160,* 977, 1972.
20. Ghaligi, S. B., and Jahagirdar, H. V.: Tetanus in a dog. Indian Vet. J. *41,* 604, 1964.
21. Gordon, R. N.: Bladder dysfunction in tick paralysis. Aust. Vet. Practitioner *2,* 13, 1972.
22. Gowing, G. M.: An azoturia-like condition in coursing greyhounds. Southwest. Vet. *17,* 183, 1964.
23. Graham, R., and Erikson, S.: Experimental botulism in dogs. J. Infect. Dis. *31,* 402, 1922.
24. Griffiths, I. A.: The extensive myelopathy of intervertebral disc protrusions in dogs ("the ascending syndrome"). J. Small Anim. Pract. *13,* 425, 1972.
25. Griffiths, I. R., and Duncan, I. D.: Myotonia: case reports. Vet. Res. *93,* 184–188, 1973.
26. Griffiths, I. R., Duncan, I. D., McQueen, A., Quirk, C., and Miller, R.: Neuromuscular disease in dogs: Some aspects of its investigation and diagnosis. J. Small Anim. Pract. *14,* 533, 1973.
27. Griffiths, I. R., Duncan, I. D., and Lawson, D. D.: Avulsion of the brachial plexus. 2. Clinical aspects. J. Small Anim. Pract. *15,* 177, 1974.
28. Griffiths, I. R.: Avulsion of the brachial plexus. 1. Neuropathology of the spinal cord and peripheral nerves. J. Small Anim. Pract. *15,* 165, 1974.
29. Hayhurst, E. E.: Outbreak of botulism poisoning in Solon, Ohio. Am. J. Pub. Health *16,* 228, 1926.
30. Hobson, H. P., and Ellett, E. W.: Bacterial diseases. *In* Catcott, E. J. (ed.): *Canine Medicine.* American Veterinary Publications, Inc., Santa Barbara, 1968, p. 150.
31. Hoerlein,iB. F.: *Canine Neurology.* 3rd ed. W. B. Saunders Co., Philadelphia, 1977.
32. Holmes, J. W. H., and Philpott, M.: Tetanus in the dog. Vet. Rec.*72,* 233, 1960.
33. Howell, H. W.: Observations on the relationship of botulism to coondog paralysis. Vet. Med. *58,* 799, 1963.
34. Inness, J. R. M.: Muscular dystrophy in dogs. Brit. Vet. J. *57,* 136, 1951.
35. Jackson, R. F.: Simultaneous occurrence of botulism in dogs and chickens. Vet. Med. *48,* 509, 1953.
36. Johnson, E. W., Denny, S. T., and Kelley, J. P.: Sequence of electromyographic abnormalities in stroke syndrome. Arch. Phys. Med. Rehab. *56,* 468, 1975.
37. Johnson, R. P., Watson, A. D. J., Smith, J., and Cooper, B. J.: Myasthenia in Springer spaniel littermates. J. Small Anim. Pract. *16,* 641, 1975.
38. Josefsson, J.: An electromyographic study of botulism intoxicated skeletal muscle. Acta Physiol. Scand. *50* (Suppl. 175), 79, 1960.
39. Joshua, J. O.: Scottie cramp. Vet. Rec. *68,* 411, 1956.
40. Kingma, J. T., and Catcott, E. J.: A paralytic syndrome in coonhounds. N. Am. Vet. *35,* 115, 1954.
41. Knecht, C. D.: Radial-brachial paralysis. *In* Kirk, R. W. (ed.): *Current Veterinary Therapy V.* W. B. Saunders Co., Philadelphia, 1974.

42. LaForce, F. M., Young, L. S., and Bennett, J. V.: Tetanus in the United States. N. Engl. J. Med. *280,* 569, 1969.
43. Lippincott, C. L., and Harter, W. L.: Oxygen saturation under pressure as a treatment for tetanus in a dog. J.A.V.M.A. *142,* 872, 1963.
44. Lorenz, M. D., de Lahunta, A., and Alstrom, D. H.: Neostigmine-responsive weakness in the dog, similar to myasthenia gravis. J.A.V.M.A. *161,* 795–800, 1972.
45. MacKenzie, C. P., Lewis, N. D., Smith, S. T., and Muir, R. W.: Louping ill in a working collie. Vet. Rec. *92,* 354, 1973.
46. Manktelow, B. W.: Myopathy of dogs resembling white muscle of sheep. N. Z. Vet. J. *11,* 52, 1963.
47. Mason, J. H.: Tetanus in the dog. J. S. Afr. Vet. Med. Assoc. *35,* 209, 1964.
48. McGrath, J. T.: *Neurologic Examination and Clinicopathologic Observations,* 2nd ed. Lea and Febiger, Philadelphia, 1960.
49. McNeil, E.: Food poisonings. *In* Catcott, E. J. (ed.): *Canine Medicine.* American Veterinary Publications, Inc., Santa Barbara, Calif., 1968,
50. Meyers, K. M., Lund, J. E., and Boyce, B. J.: Muscular cramping of central nervous origin in Scottish terrier dogs. Fed. Proc. *27,* 611, 1968.
51. Meyers, K. M., Lund, J. E., Padgett, G., and Dickson, W. M.: Hyperkinetic episodes in Scottish terrier dogs. J.A.V.M.A. *155,* 129, 1969.
52. Meyers, K. M., Padgett, G. A., and Dickson, W. M.: Genetic basis of scottie cramp. J. Hered. *61,* 189, 1970.
53. Meyers, K. M., Dickson, W. M., Lund, J. E., and Padgett, G. A.: Muscular hypertonicity: Episodes in Scottish terrier dogs. Arch. Neurol. *25,* 61, 1971.
54. Meyers, K. M., Dickson, W. M., and Schaub, R. G.: Serotonin involvement in a motor disorder of Scottish terrier dogs. Life Sci. *13,* 1261, 1973.
55. Meyers, K. M., and Schaub, R. G.: The relationship of seratonin to a motor disorder in Scottish terrier dogs. Life Sci. *14,* 1895, 1974.
56. Mosier, J. E.: Some clinical problems in small animal practice. Vet. Med. *52,* 445, 1957.
57. Palmer, A. C., and Barker, J.: Myasthenia in the dog. Vet. Rec. *95,* 452–454, 1974.
58. Parker, A. J., Cusick, P. K., Park, R. D., and Small, E.: Hemifacial spasms in a dog. Vet. Rec. *93,* 514, 1973.
59. Putman, R. W., and Archibald, J.: Diseases of the locomotor system. *In* Catcott, E. J. (ed.): *Canine Medicine.* American Veterinary Publications, Inc., Santa Barbara, Calif., 1968, p. 685.
60. Scott, D. W., and de Lahunta, A.: Eosinophilic polymyositis in a dog. Cornell Vet. *64,* 47, 1974.
61. Siegmund, O. H., and Eaton, L. G. (eds.): *The Merck Veterinary Manual,* 3rd ed. Merck and Co., Rahway, N.J., 1967.
62. Slesinger, L.: Treatment of tetanus with chlorpromazine. Veterinarstvi *14,* 319, 1964.
63. Srivastava, H. N.: A case of trigeminal paralysis in dog. Indian Vet. J. *47,* 271, 1970.
64. Swift, T. R., and Ignacio, O. J.: Tick paralysis: Electrophysiological studies. Neurology *25,* 1130, 1975.
65. Thom, C., Edmondson, R. B., and Giltner, L. T.: Botulism from canned asparagus. J.A.M.A. *73,* 907, 1919.
66. Tick paralysis. *In* Siegmond, O. H., and Eaton, L. G. (eds.): *The Merck Veterinary Manual,* 4th ed. Merck and Co., Rahway, N.J., 1973, p. 721.
67. Tvedten, H. W., and Trapp, A. L.: Myopathy in three dogs. Vet. Med. Small Anim. Clin. *70,* 63, 1975.
68. Van Vleet, J. F.: Experimentally induced vitamin E-selenium deficiency in the growing dog. J.A.V.M.A. *166,* 769, 1975.
69. Wandeler, A., Steck, F., Fankhauser, R., Kammermann, B., Gresikova, M., and Blascovic, D.: Isolierung des Virus der zentraleuropäischen Zeckenenzephalitis in der Schweiz. Path. Microbial. *38,* 258, 1972.
70. Wentink, G. H., van der Linde-Sipmay, J. S., Meijer, A. E., Kamphuisen, H. A. C., van Vorstenbosch, C. J., Hartman, W., and Hendricks, H. J.: Myopathy with a possible recessive x-linked inheritance in a litter of Irish terriers. Vet. Path. *9,* 328, 1972.
71. Wentink, G. H., *et al.:* Myopathy in an Irish setter with a metabolic defect of the isolated mitochondria. Zentralbl. Vet. Med. *A21,* 62–74, 1974.
72. Whitney, J. C.: Progressive muscular dystrophy in the dog. Vet. Rec. *70,* 611, 1958.
73. Zack, S. I., Shields, D. R., and Steinberg, S. A.: A myosthenic syndrome in the dog. A case report with electron microscopic observations on motor end plates and comparison with the fine structure of end plates in myasthenia gravis. Ann. N.Y. Acad. Sci. *135,* 79, 1966.
74. Zontine, W. J., and Uno, T.: Tetanus in a dog (a case report). Vet. Med. Small Anim. Clin. *63,* 341, 1968.

CHAPTER 10

PERIPHERAL NERVE SURGERY

Steven F. Swaim, D.V.M., M.S.

GENERAL CONSIDERATIONS

Neuritis, neuralgia, and total nerve dysfunction are frequently encountered in traumatic injuries of the dog, especially in accidents which involve the limbs. Trauma may vary according to whether the injuries are chronic or acute, intermittent or exceptional, external or internal. Most injuries due to violent external pressure, traction, laceration, or gunshots can cause severe damage or severance of the nerve. Neglected fractures can injure a nerve owing to the internal movement of fragments and jagged ends of bone. In some instances, medical personnel may induce injury by injecting a chemical or therapeutic agent in or around a nerve. Extremely high or prolonged administration of x-rays can produce thickening and scarring of the nerve sheath and endoneurium. From the history and clinical examination, one must determine the location and extent of injury in order to recommend the most efficient mode of repair.[5]

Two classifications have been advocated for evaluating nerve damage. Both classify structural damage within the nerve; however, one technique uses specific terms as a means of classification and the other uses degrees of damage. The former includes the terms neurotmesis, axonotmesis, and neurapraxia;[8, 10, 12, 62, 104] the latter classifies nerve damage from first degree (least severe) to fifth degree (most severe)[85] (Table 10–1).

Lesions of peripheral nerves in which the nerve is damaged but not severed are termed "lesions in continuity."[104] The most important factor about such lesions is the ability of the nerve to regenerate. In general, it may be stated that neurapraxic lesions will regenerate better than either axonotmesic or neurotmesic lesions, and axonotmesic lesions will regenerate better than neurotmesic lesions. The regenerative ability of a nerve is directly proportional to the amount of continuity present in the nerve's connective tissue structure. In neurapraxia and axonotmesis, when the endoneurial and Schwann sheaths remain intact, axonal regeneration is comparatively better. In neurotmesis, some axons never regenerate owing to blockage of their growth by external scar tissue at the anastomotic site.[57]

Recent studies on the effects of cryosurgery on peripheral nerves have shown that nerves subjected to this procedure undergo wallerian degeneration followed by regeneration through intact perineurial and epineurial channels. This fact could be important in surgical resection of tumors in which normal nerves must usually be sacrificed. In such instances, cryosurgery may destroy the tumor, and nerve function may be spared.[6]

TABLE 10–1 CLASSIFICATION OF NERVE DAMAGE

By Terms[8, 10, 12, 62, 104]

1. Neurotmesis: Complete severance of all structures of the nerve with wallerian degeneration of the distal stump.
2. Axonotmesis: Separation or damage of axons with wallerian degeneration occurring distal to the lesion. The endoneurial and Schwann sheaths remain intact.
3. Neuropraxia: Interruption in function and conduction of the nerve. Usually associated with a lesion of the myelin with no accompanying wallerian degeneration.

By Degrees[85]

1. First degree: Conduction is blocked at the site of injury, but all nerve components are intact.
2. Second degree: Axon is disrupted, and there is wallerian degeneration. All other nerve structures remain intact.
3. Third degree: Axon and endoneurial tube associated with it are disrupted, but individual fasciculi remain intact.
4. Fourth degree: Axons, endoneurial tubes, and fasciculi are disrupted, but the epineurium remains intact.
5. Fifth degree: Complete severance of all nerve structures.

One of the main causes of peripheral nerve injury—one that can result in severe damage—is nerve traction. Traction injuries can result in lesions in continuity in which the damage extends for great distances along the nerve.[5, 8, 40] Within the nerve there may be complete division of the axons, rupture of the connective tissue sheaths within the nerve, much internal scarring, and rupture of blood vessels with intraneural hemorrhage.[40, 97, 104]

Studies have been conducted to determine how much stretch a nerve can withstand before damage occurs. A human nerve can be stretched up to 6 per cent of its mobilized length without causing internal damage within the nerve. Further stretching (up to 10 to 11 per cent of its mobilized length) causes interruption of nerve fibers, rupture of Schwann tubes and blood vessels, and the appearance of connective tissue in the nerve stumps. Rupture of the endoneurium and perineurium has been noted after 20 to 30 per cent extension.[23, 41, 53] Studies in cats showed that the peroneal nerves may be stretched 100 per cent of their length, yet functional recovery will be complete 14 days later.[11, 53] Further studies on dogs must be conducted on this problem to determine more accurately the amount of stretch that can be withstood by the peripheral nerve of a dog.

One of the main sources of peripheral nerve damage in veterinary medicine is damage to the brachial plexus resulting from traction and avulsion of the nerves from the spinal cord. In humans, studies have been done on the meningeal-neural relations in the intervertebral foramen. These studies have shown the mobility of the neural structures and their meningeal sleeves and fibrous sheaths in the intervertebral foramen. This system allows free movement in the foramen as the vertebral column moves. However, the nerve complex does not have unlimited freedom of movement through the foramen. The continuity of the nerve sheath with the dural sac and the plugging action of the dural funnel at the foramen limit the extent of any lateral movement when lateral traction is applied (Fig. 10–1). In the lower cervical area, where there is a wide range of movement between the cervical spine, shoulder girdle, and shoulder joint, an additional protective device is provided in the form of strong attachments that bind the spinal nerves securely to the transverse processes of the vertebrae.[87] The nature of this type of injury in veterinary medicine needs to be investigated. Diagnosing and treating this

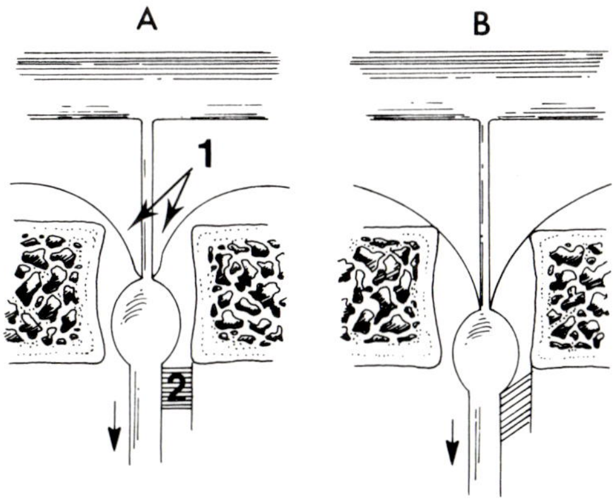

FIGURE 10–1 *A.* Mobility of the neural structures and their related connective tissues at the intervertebral foramen. Mobility of the nerve complex has limitations resulting from the continuity of the nerve sheath with the dural sac and the plugging action of the dural funnel (1). *B.* Additional limitation comes from attachments of the nerves to the transverse processes of the vertebrae (2). (Adapted from Sunderland, S.: Meningeal-neural relations in the intervertebral foramen. J. Neurosurg. *40,* 756, 1974.)

type of injury and determining the prognosis present a real challenge.

In humans, myelography is believed to be a satisfactory method of demonstrating avulsion of the roots of the brachial plexus from the spinal cord or separation of these roots within the intervertebral foramina. Two myelographic abnormalities have been reported. First, a pseudomeningocele or diverticulum-like structure extending through the intervertebral foramen into the soft tissues of the neck may indicate a complete or incomplete avulsion of the nerve roots with a concomitant tear of the arachnoid and dura. The second abnormality is a blunting or distorting of the normal nerve root sheath which indicates a complete separation of the nerve root at the intervertebral foramen.[60, 69]

One of the most practical means of determining the location and extent of an injury is to test various reflexes (Chapters 1 and 3). If the toe pinch and knee jerk or other tendon reflexes are absent, gross injury to the appropriate nerve or segment of the spinal cord has occurred. Lesser damage may be determined by observing the cutaneous sensations and responses and by electrical testing. Allam[1] has reported practical methods of faradic stimulation of the peripheral nerves of the limbs in dogs. If there is a failure of response, significant nerve damage has occurred, and surgical repair is indicated. If faradic current elicits a response but voluntary paralysis is present, the patient is likely to recover without surgical intervention. Allam used injection needles as electrodes and DC or AC current of 3 to 5 milliamperes, such as might be obtained with a 1½ volt flashlight battery.[1] Electrodiagnostic testing and electromyography is discussed in depth in Chapter 9, Section 2.

When peripheral nerve damage has occurred and other diagnostic methods have failed to yield definitive information about the nerve's function, exploratory surgery may be necessary to evaluate the nerve damage. There are three main reasons for performing exploratory surgery: (1) to establish an accurate diagnosis, and in particular, to determine how much of a nerve has been divided; (2) to establish a reasonably accurate prognosis; and (3) to improve the function of the nerve.[104]

The technique for surgical exploration of an injured nerve involves certain principles. The nerve must be freely isolated in all areas of possible injury and positively identified as the nerve in question. All points of possible compression and abnormal adhesion should be relieved. The nerve should be examined by three methods: (1) inspection, noting the size of the neuroma; (2) palpation, noting the neuroma's consistency; and (3) stimulation, observing the reaction which occurs. If the nerve sheath is thickened, it may be split along the longitudinal axis of the nerve; this will expose the nerve bundles adequately to prove their condition.[2, 104]

The neuroma is of particular interest during exploratory nerve surgery. Usually, a normal or almost normal nerve indicates axonotmesis or intact fibers. A fusiform neuroma indicates a combination of axonotmesis and neurotmesis or axonotmesis mainly with some intact fibers. It may also indicate intraneural bleeding. If a fusiform neuroma is soft it indicates relatively good axonal regeneration across the lesion, and the prognosis for spontaneous recovery is better. However, intraneural scarring may be manifest by a palpable induration in this type of neuroma. Intraneural fibrosis with a large, firm, bulbous neuroma usually indicates widespread neurotmesis with poor regeneration of axons across the lesion.[5, 68, 75, 81, 104] The presence of blood vessels within a neuroma is associated with a better prognosis for nerve regeneration.[5] A lateral neuroma indicates partial division of a nerve or partial neurotmesis with the remainder of the nerve containing normal fibers or fibers that have undergone axonotmesis.[68, 104] These lateral neuromas may recover spontaneously, and it is probably best not to excise them.[59, 68, 75] However, nerves that have been cut one-half to three-fourths of the way through often require resection and repair. A neuroma with a dumbbell configuration suggests that the nerve has been completely transected and the ends are being held in approximation only by scar tissue[81] (Fig. 10–2).

A surgeon may elect to perform external or internal neurolysis of a damaged nerve in an attempt to improve its function. External neurolysis is accomplished by freeing the nerve and laying it in a bed free of scar tissue (Fig. 10–3*A*). Internal neurolysis involves incising the epineurium longitudinally in the involved area and beyond, separating the nerve fibers with a sharp

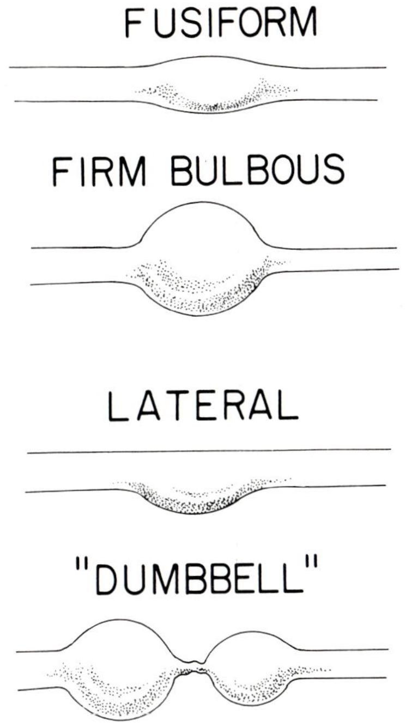

FIGURE 10–2 Various shaped neuromas that may be formed on traumatized peripheral nerves. (Adapted from Smith, J. W.: Microneurosurgery of peripheral nerves. *In* Rand, R. W. (ed.): *Microneurosurgery.* C. V. Mosby Co., St. Louis, 1969.)

tenotome.[2, 12, 68, 104] In cases of traumatic fibrous neuroma of the nerve, internal neurolysis is of questionable value, and resection and anastomosis should be considered[2] (Fig. 10–3*B*).

A final diagnostic procedure that may be performed at the time of surgery is trial section of the damaged area of the nerve. A transverse incision is made at the point of greatest induration and deepened not more than ½ millimeter at a time until normal nerve bundles are encountered. The fibrous tissue springs apart so that the nerve bundles are seen before they are cut. As a general rule, if the trial section is carried across more than one-half to three-fourths of the diameter of the nerve, complete resection and anastomosis are indicated[74, 75, 81, 104] (Fig. 10–3*C*).

Another method for evaluating the amount of intraneural fibrosis is the injection of saline tinted with a harmless dye into the nerve near the lesion. The diffusion of the saline will be arrested if scar tissue is present; otherwise, the liquid will spread freely between the funiculi and beneath the sheath.[75]

NERVE DEGENERATION

After a nerve has been severed or damaged, nerve degeneration followed by regeneration occurs. The most widely accepted theory of degeneration is that of Waller, who suggested that the portion of the nerve which has been severed and completely separated from the central trophic area degenerates completely, while regeneration occurs from the undegenerated proximal stump connected to the trophic center.

Immediately after severance there is hemorrhage and projection of a clot from the severed nerve ends. Within an hour there is marked swelling about 0.5–1 cm on either side of the point of severance. This is due to the accumulation of acid mucopolysaccharide, which has an affinity for water. The accumulation of blood, plasma and serum also adds to the swelling of the nerve.[17, 28]

Nerve degeneration occurs in the proximal nerve stump, but it is not as extensive as that in the distal nerve stump. It has been called "traumatic degeneration" and extends no further than the second or third node of Ranvier from the point of severance.[9, 12, 17]

Wallerian degeneration takes place in the entire distal nerve stump. In this process, the axons and their myelin coatings undergo degeneration. The axons at the proximal end of the distal nerve stump tend to enlarge and isolate themselves from the rest of the distal stump, forming a unit that survives for approximately 2 weeks.[9, 28] The remaining parts of the distal axons break down more rapidly, and 48 hours after severance there is evidence of axon and myelin degeneration at all levels of the distal stump.[17, 28] In the early stages of degeneration, the myelin first disappears from the outer surface of the coating surrounding the axon. This may be due to enzymatic activity of the Schwann cells surrounding the myelin.[43]

Following degeneration of the axons and myelin, their degenerated products are removed, leaving only the connective tissue framework of the distal nerve stump. This removal is accomplished by macrophages which originate from histiocytes present in the connective tissue and blood vessel walls of the nerve.[43] Macrophages also orig-

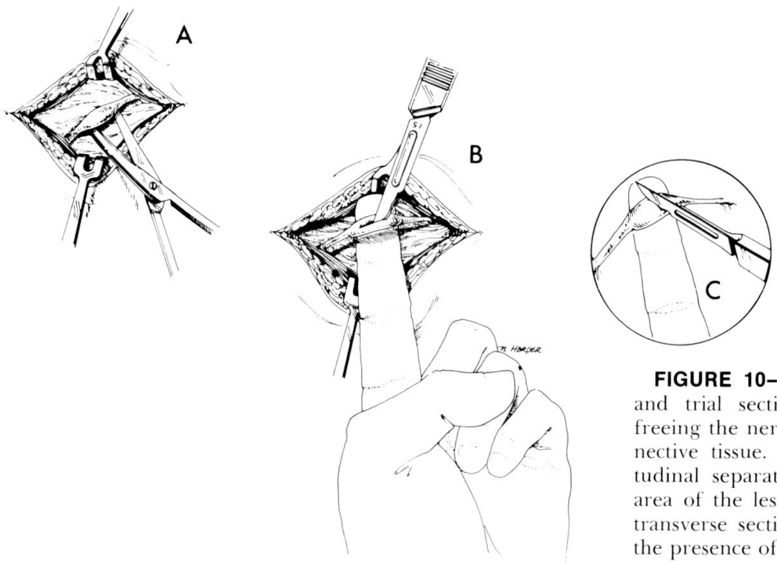

FIGURE 10–3 Techniques for neurolysis and trial section. *A.* External neurolysis—freeing the nerve from the surrounding connective tissue. *B.* Internal neurolysis—longitudinal separation of nerve bundles in the area of the lesion. *C.* Trial section—gradual transverse sectioning of a nerve to ascertain the presence of viable nerve bundles.

inate from converted blood monocytes.[97] Schwann cells also play a role in phagocytizing axonal and myelin waste products.[5, 31, 97] These cells appear at about the seventh day after injury and reach the height of invasive activity during the third week.[43] The phagocytic process may last for as long as 32 days after injury, during which time the nerve stump becomes less swollen, phagocytic activity subsides, and an orderly realignment of neurilemmal bands occurs.[16, 17]

The neuromuscular junctions are also involved in the degenerative process. The motor end-plates disappear as early as 3 to 5 days after severance. Experiments have shown that the neuromuscular elements of a nerve degenerate simultaneously with or even prior to degeneration of the nerve itself[84] (Figs. 10–4 and 10–5).

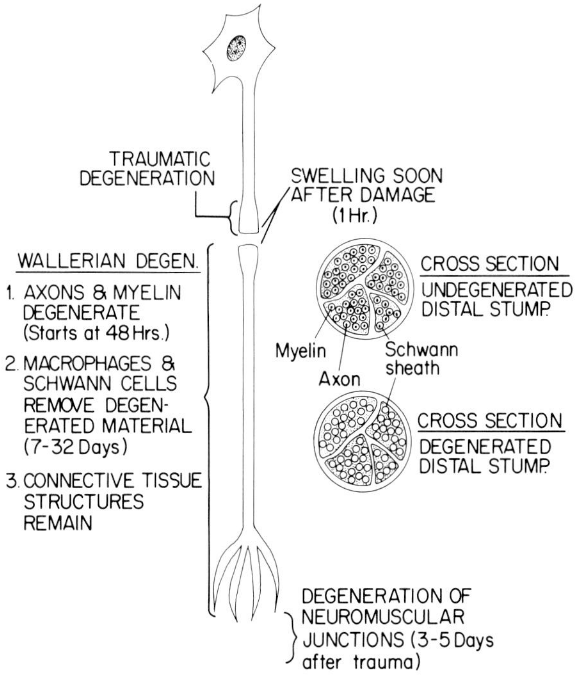

FIGURE 10–4 Process of nerve degeneration.

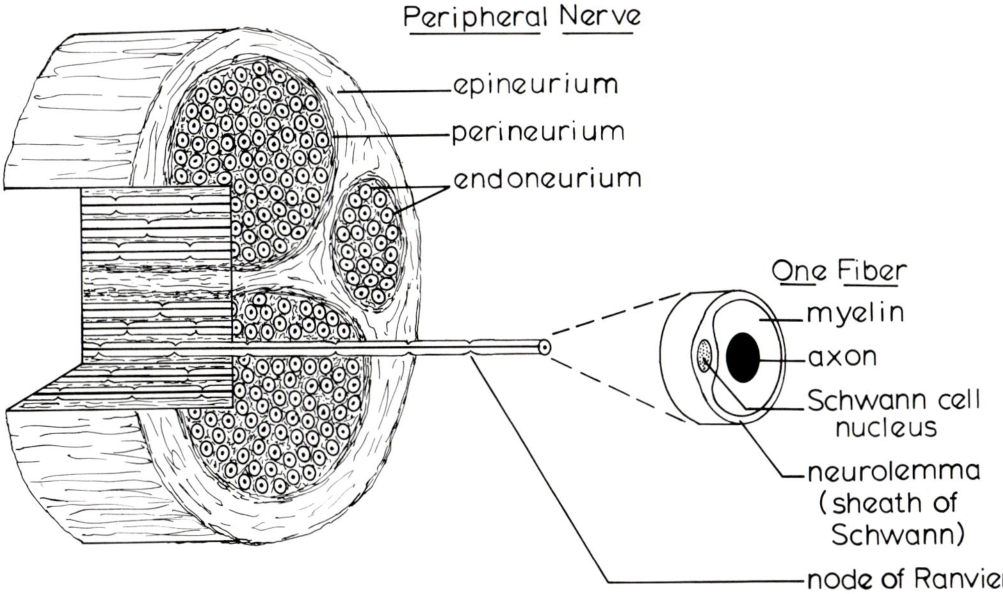

FIGURE 10–5 Schematic drawing of the structure of a peripheral nerve. (Adapted from Ham, A. W.: *Histology*, 5th ed. J. B. Lippincott Co., Philadelphia, 1965.)

NERVE REGENERATION

Nerve regeneration consists of several processes; however, regeneration of the degenerated portion of a peripheral nerve is based upon the downgrowth of new axons from the central nondegenerated portion of the nerve.[12, 44] The process begins within the cell bodies of the severed axons. The cell body becomes progressively larger for about 10 to 20 days, remains enlarged during active regeneration, and then returns to normal size as it matures. During this time there is an increase in both RNA and DNA activity within the cell. The increased enzymatic activity and incorporation of amino acids within the cell body reflect the increased metabolic activity. These changes within the cell body are more pronounced the nearer the cell body is to the place of nerve severance.[5, 21, 28]

After the nerve cell body has synthesized the new protoplasm, it migrates from the cell body along the axon. The flow of newly synthesized cellular protein occurs at a rate of about 1 mm per day and advances in a semisolid column, which has a consistency similar to that of molten lava or toothpaste. The protoplasm is moved by microperistaltic waves of the nerve sheath.[98, 100]

Following severance of a nerve, the changes that occur at and between the proximal and distal nerve stumps strongly influence nerve regeneration. The regeneration of axons between nerve stumps involves the proliferation of epineurial and endoneurial connective tissue, Schwann cells, capillaries, and axons. Fibroblasts of epineurial origin, the endoneurial connective tissue within the nerve, and capillaries begin to proliferate at the proximal and distal nerve stumps. These tissues migrate toward each other, forming a bridge and capillary bed between the nerve stumps along which regenerating axons may grow to reach the distal nerve stump. This bridge is subject to distortion by invading extraneural connective tissue.[17, 62]

The Schwann cells of the proximal and distal nerve stumps probably play the most important role in axonal regeneration between stumps. As early as the second day, electron microscopy reveals a cellular proliferation of Schwann cells, which greatly outnumber the connective tissue cells of endoneurial and perivascular origin. The examination may also reveal sprouting of axons at the level of the most distal node of Ranvier of the proximal stump.[20] The Schwann cells of the proximal stump grow toward the distal nerve stump's Schwann cell protrusions and eventually connect with them. The proliferating Schwann cells of the proximal stump have a little headstart on the axons within the Schwann tubes. As a result, the advancing Schwann cells serve as guides for the regenerating axons that follow.[97]

The deposition of myelin around regenerated axons in the distal stump is an integral part of nerve regeneration. Alkaline phosphatase plays an important part in the myelinization procedure. Pinner and Campbell found that within 24 hours after transection, alkaline phosphatase activity was present in the proximal and distal stumps and was concentrated at the incisures and nodes. Capillary budding was largely responsible for this early increase in alkaline phosphatase, which persisted through the thirtieth day. This response is apparently due to the metabolic demand imposed by nerve regeneration. As degeneration progressed in the distal stump, the amount of alkaline phosphatase decreased. This enzyme is most likely associated with the neurilemmal cell membrane.[63, 64] The myelinization process begins almost as soon as an axon makes contact with the distal Schwann cell tubes.[17]

Growth or regeneration in the marginal zone of realignment is a lengthy process that takes place at the rate of 0.25 mm a day. Beyond this marginal zone, however, regeneration occurs at an average rate of 1 mm a day or 1 inch a month. Bateman explained that in experimental investigations regeneration of axon tips occurred at the rate of 3 to 4 mm a day, whereas the average rate of functional return is not more than 1 or 2 mm a day. These figures are approximate; growth is rapid in proximal areas and slow in fine terminal branches. At the periphery, the state of the motor end-plate and health of the muscle fibers are controlling factors. The amount of function recovered varies from 80 per cent of normal in a purely motor nerve to 50 to 60 per cent in a mixed nerve.[5, 59]

The final stage of regeneration is the terminal adjustment of motor and sensory elements. When a motor fiber approaches its termination, it undergoes rapid division, each new branch retaining a myelin sheath until it is in contact with the muscle fiber. At this point the neurilemma fuses with the sarcolemma. The new branches may stimulate the reappearance of the old end-plate structure, or new contact areas may be formed. Voluntary function appears a considerable time after returned function can be demonstrated by faradic stimulation[5] (Fig. 10–6).

The process of nerve regeneration is not complete until new nerve fibers have been produced comparable in number and size to those seen in a normal nerve.[71] Consequently, attention has been directed at the diameter attained by a nerve fiber and the factors that may limit its dimension. If a nerve fiber does not make connection with a terminal end-plate, the fiber will atrophy and have a smaller diameter; however, if the nerve fiber does make terminal connection with an end-plate, the diameter increases throughout its length.[8, 77, 99] There are two other factors that govern the diameter of a nerve fiber in the regenerating nerve. First, the caliber of the parent fiber in the proximal stump affects the diameter of the nerve fiber in the distal stump. Second, the diameter of the particular Schwann tube into which the fiber penetrates governs the final diameter of the nerve fiber.[39, 71]

In man, it is felt that some degree of function will be possible if the nerve is regenerated within a 20-month period, but that if this period is exceeded, irreversible atrophy may occur.[59] In the dog, if it is assumed that regeneration can take place at the rate of 1 inch per month, it follows that most nerves could regenerate fast enough, since few of them would be longer than 20 inches. However, the dog's inability to cooperate and difficulties in preventing crippling muscle atrophy during the period of regeneration must be considered.

One of the major deterrent factors in nerve regeneration is the formation of a neuroma at the end of the proximal stump and a smaller glioma or schwannoma at the end of the distal stump. These occur most often when the nerve ends have not been approximated surgically and remain separated by a gap. Neuromas start to form soon after a nerve has been severed. A blood clot forms at the end of the proximal nerve stump. As the clot organizes, a mass of randomly oriented fibrin strands is left at the end of the nerve stump. The Schwann cells proliferate toward the end of the nerve stump, encounter the tangled scaffolding of fibrin, and follow it. The regenerating axons following the Schwann

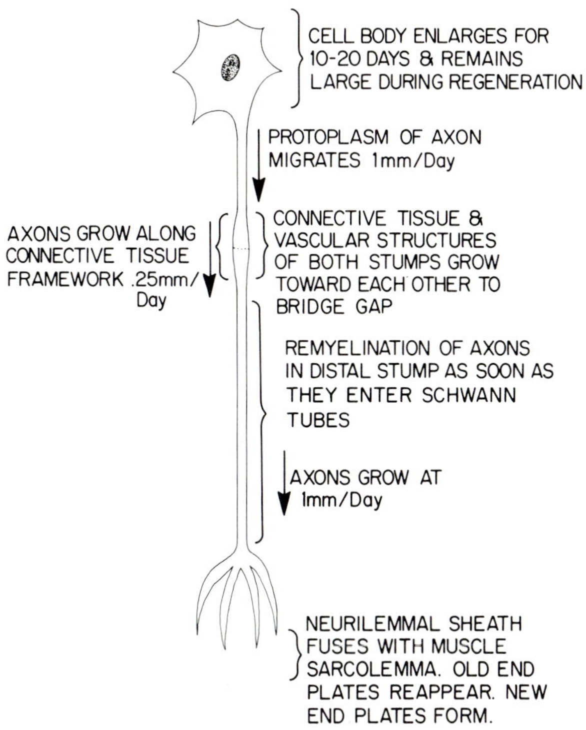

FIGURE 10–6 Process of nerve regeneration.

tubes also are guided by this pre-established random pattern. The distortion and blockage of axonal regeneration is further complicated by invasion of extraneural connective tissue into the area between the nerve stumps (Fig. 10–7). A third factor contributing to axonal blockage and disarray is the proliferation of connective tissue elements (endoneurium, perineurium, and epineurium) within the nerve. As regenerating axons approach neuromas, they undergo much branching; the more extensive the neuroma, the more branches are formed. The tangled mass of axons soon becomes enveloped by Schwann cells and becomes myelinated. In well-oriented, unobstructed nerve structures axons advance without branching. Since so many axons are blocked by neuromas, this branching may be a compensatory measure that ensures production of enough axons so that some will be able to find their way through the neuroma and penetrate the distal nerve stump.[4, 17, 18, 23, 29, 47, 49, 52, 54, 91, 97]

The schwannoma or "peripheral glioma" is formed in the same way as a neuroma. The main difference is a lack of axons in the schwannoma.

The problem of neuromas has been acute in many species of mammals, especially in man and in horses. In amputations or neurectomies, neuromas or severed nerves have been the source of severe pain. In 25 per cent of the neurectomies performed in the horse, painful neuromas resulted.[29] Most small animal surgeons

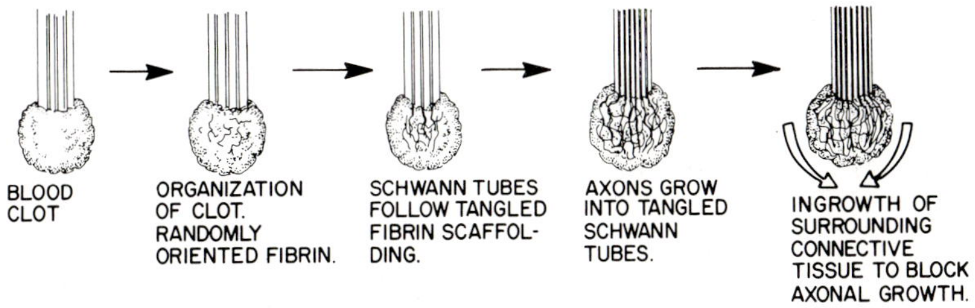

FIGURE 10–7 Pathogenesis of a neuroma.

agree that clinical evidence of postsurgical neuromas in the dog are rarely encountered. However, Poth consistently saw neuromas in the dog after experimental nerve transections.[67] Perhaps they are small and do not cause the distressing pain noted in other species.

The prevention of neuromas following neurectomies and nerve anastomosis and grafting is a problem for the neurosurgeon. At least 150 different methods have been suggested for the treatment and prevention of neuromas. These methods include ligation; the use of 95 per cent alcohol, cellophane tubes, glass tubes, silver tubes, arterial sleeves, tannic acid, or gentian violet; and crushing of the nerve stump.[29, 66] Recently the use of a silicone rubber cap* has been suggested. Evans reported successful results in 97 per cent of 178 neurectomies involving 52 horses.[29] Midgley, Ducker, Tauras, and others have reported good results in humans.[26, 57, 94] Evans has described epineurial capping as a means of preventing neuromas in horses.[29] Fackelman and Clodius have described a technique utilizing electrocoagulation, ligation, and folding of the nerve end back on itself to prevent neuromas following posterior digital neurectomy in horses.[30] The prevention of neuromas following anastomosis and grafting will be discussed later in this chapter.

In summary, the process of regeneration is preceded by a period of dynamic degeneration and phagocytosis, especially in the entire distal stump and in the proximal stump up to the most distal one or two nodes of Ranvier. The biggest problem associated with localized nerve trauma (severance) is neuroma formation at the ends of the nerve stumps.

GENERAL SURGICAL PRINCIPLES

It has been shown that methods of repair should vary with types of injury. Lacerations produce a localized and well-confined response. A sharply localized injury, such as a glass or knife cut, is most apt to be treated surgically.[69] Stretching elongates the zone of reaction, while burns and radiation kill large areas or blocks of tissue. Massive damage to surrounding tissue by infection, widespread hemorrhage, or hematoma formation incites extensive fibrosis. In such cases, technical repair, regeneration, and return of function will all be hampered.[5] Injuries that cause nerve damage over a considerable distance or trauma to adjacent tissues, particularly blood vessels, are much less apt to be amenable to surgical intervention.[69]

The time at which repair of peripheral nerve injuries should be done depends on the type of injury. Two types of nerve repair may be used depending on the time at which repair is done.[35] In primary (immediate or emergency) repair, the ends of the severed nerves are sutured together within 8 to 12 hours after the time of injury. In secondary (deferred or early secondary) repair, the ends of the severed nerves are sutured together within 3 to 4 weeks after injury and certainly within 6 months after injury.

Primary nerve repair should be done when there is evidence of partial laceration of a major nerve,[51] and when there has been little soft tissue trauma and no contamination.[12, 74, 102] Secondary repair of a nerve should be done when trauma and contamination are associated with the nerve damage. The extent of the zone of interstitial damage and degeneration within the proximal and distal segments can be seen more readily a short time after such surgery; the damaged area can be accurately trimmed away to provide viable nerve tissue for repair.[28, 69, 74, 102] When nerve severance has been associated with trauma or infection, it is advisable to anastomose the ends of the severed nerve to prevent retraction. Such sutures also help mark the nerve for identification at a later date.[12] Approximately 21 days after suturing, the nerve should be re-exposed, examined, and the degenerated nerve tissue removed so that definitive nerve repair may be undertaken.

The instruments needed for peripheral nerve surgery are not elaborate. Instruments should include small ophthalmic needle holders; jewelers' forceps; 1 vs 2 toothed Adson forceps; small, curved, blunt-pointed scissors; sharp scalpel blades;

---

*Silastic Nerve Cuffs, Medical Products Division, Dow Corning Corporation, Midland, Michigan.

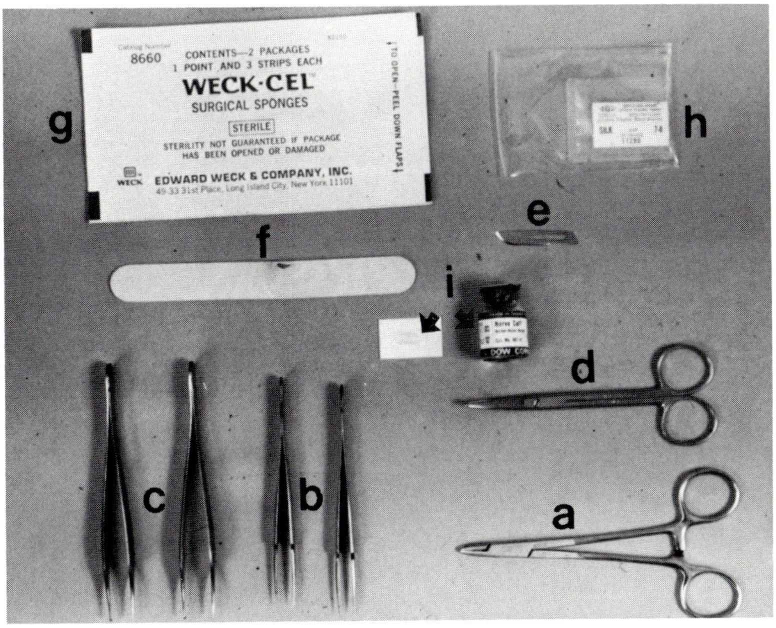

FIGURE 10–8 Instrumentation for peripheral nerve surgery. a, Small ophthalmic needle holders; b, jewelers' forceps; c, 1 over 2 teeth Adson forceps; d, small curved, blunt-pointed scissors; e, sharp scalpel blade; f, wooden tongue depressor; g, lint-free surgical sponges; h, fine (5–0 to 7–0) suture material with a swaged needle; i, silicone rubber sleeves.

wooden tongue depressors; some lint-free material for surgical sponges*; 5–0 to 7–0 suture material with a swaged needle; and various sizes of silicone rubber sleeves (Fig. 10–8). The use of such sleeves will be discussed later.

Preparation of the surgical instruments prior to surgery is important. Campbell has found from microscopic examination of experimental preparations than an inflammatory response and subsequent scarring may result from dust, lint, grease from fingers, desquamated cells, blood, and tissue residue left on instruments from previous use. To avoid such problems he advocates that instruments be cleaned with a detergent-free soap, since detergents are irritating substances. Instruments should be cleaned with an ultrasonic apparatus and baked for 2 hours at 160° C in containers wrapped in heat-resistant paper. This avoids contamination by the "fillers" used in institutional textiles and by detergents and bleaches used in laundries, which would be disseminated by autoclaving.[17] Such measures may seem extreme, but it should be borne in mind that the slightest microscopic debris (coagulated blood, cells from the instruments, or lint from the linen) may result in a connective tissue reaction at the suture site which could block axonal regeneration.[4, 17]

The entire limb should be prepared for aseptic surgery, since it may be necessary to expose a nerve maximally to do an effective neurorrhaphy. The surgeon may need to flex or position the limb during surgery.[5, 68, 69]

A nerve should be approached through the fascial planes; however, if a muscle must be penetrated it should be done parallel to its fibers. If a muscle must be divided to expose a nerve, it should be severed at a point of attachment so that it can be sutured.[76]

After the nerve is exposed it must be freed from the surrounding tissues for some distance proximal and distal to the site of injury. The nerve should be grasped only by its epineurium[61] or by mechanical holders whose edges are protected by sponge rubber.[5] This helps give the additional length that will be necessary in apposing the nerve stump after the nerve has been trimmed. This procedure has been called "getting rope."[12] Mobilization of a

---

*Weck-cel. Edward Weck & Co., Inc., Long Island City, New York.

nerve will usually supply enough slack to overcome a 2 to 3 cm gap.[2, 68, 76] The amount of nerve that can be freed from the surrounding tissue without damaging the nerve's blood supply is controversial. Smith states that dependence on longitudinal blood vessels within a nerve for more than 6 to 8 cm is not advisable.[79] Terzis *et al.* have found that nerve regeneration across mildly stretched repair sites is the same as regeneration across a properly tailored nerve graft.[95] Poor nerve regeneration was noted when the repair sites were moderately stretched or when a graft that was excessively long was used, and only minimal functional recovery was noted in nerves that had a severely stretched repair site.[95]

The most commonly used techniques in overcoming a gap are mobilization of the nerve stumps and placing the limb in flexion.[102] However, these techniques are not without problems. After the leg has been immobilized in flexion for a few weeks it is slowly extended, and at this time damage can occur in the nerve both proximal and distal to the anastomotic site.[5, 40, 41, 42, 55, 73, 81, 93] The strength of a nerve suture line increases to its maximim point during the first 3 weeks after suturing.[40] Part of this strength is attributed to the adhesions that form around the nerve. These may be sufficient to immobilize the nerve stumps so that tension will not separate the anastomotic site.[2] No method of union will hold if traction on the nerve is present during its regeneration. Excess tension favors fibrosis, separation of nerve ends, large neuromatosis formation, and ultimately poor regeneration. However, nerve ends that are joined too closely may have edges that are crumpled and folded, and this favors the formation of a large neuroma.[5]

Some forethought is required before cutting a nerve to remove a neuroma. After removal of a neuroma, there will be two nerve stumps to be sutured together. It is imperative that these stumps be sutured together without rotation of either stump. Small blood vessels or prominent nerve fiber bundles may serve as landmarks to prevent rotation when suturing the nerve. Another technique for preventing nerve rotation is to place a single fine silk suture through the epineurium of the proximal and distal nerve stumps before resecting the neuroma. These sutures are placed exactly in line with each other and are lined up the same way when the nerve is sutured.[23, 51, 61]

Damaged nerve tissue must be removed from a nerve before any form of repair may be done. The neuroma on a nerve should be cut in its center, perpendicular to the long axis of the nerve. A sharp scalpel blade should be used to cut the nerve, which is laid across a sterile wooden tongue blade. The proximal nerve stump is laid on the tongue blade and sliced perpendicularly in serial sections with the scalpel blade (Fig. 10–9 *A*, *B*). When viable nerve tissue (normal fasciculi without excessive connective tissue between them) is exposed, the neuromatous tissue is excised and discarded. The same procedure is undertaken on the distal nerve stump.[88, 89] Another procedure for trimming nerve ends involves wrapping the end of the nerve in a collar of Surgicel and Vi-drape, and snugging this collar around the nerve with a pair of right angle forceps. A razor blade or dermatome blade is used to make trans-

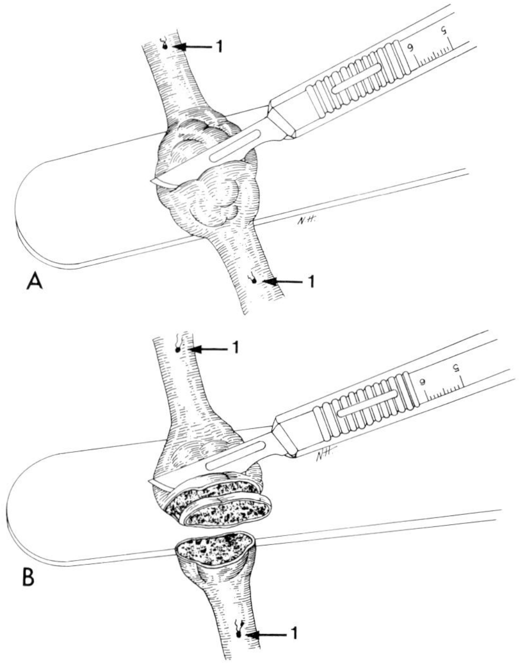

FIGURE 10–9 Removal of a neuroma. *A.* The neuroma is laid on a sterile wooden tongue blade and cut in its center perpendicular to its long axis. *B.* Serial sections are sliced from the neuroma to expose viable nerve tissue. Epineurial marking sutures for nerve alignment (1). (From Swaim, S. F.: Isolated peripheral nerves. *In* Bojrab, M. J. (ed.): *Current Techniques in Small Animal Surgery I.* Lea & Febiger, Philadelphia, 1975.)

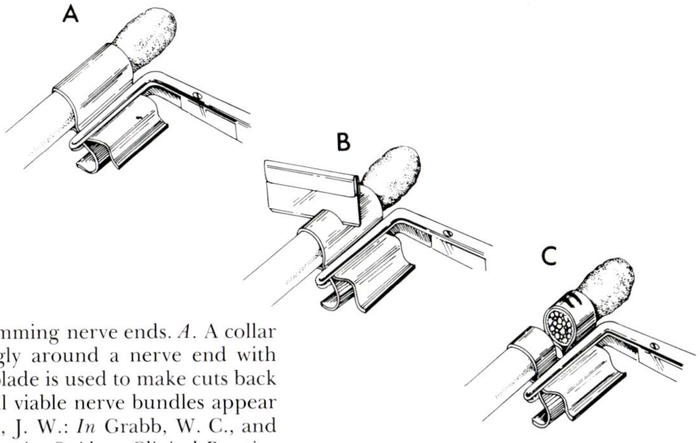

FIGURE 10–10 A technique for trimming nerve ends. *A*. A collar of Surgicel and Vi-drape is held snugly around a nerve end with right angle forceps. *B* and *C*. A sharp blade is used to make cuts back along the nerve at 1 mm intervals until viable nerve bundles appear on cross section. (Adapted from Smith, J. W.: *In* Grabb, W. C., and Smith, J. W. (eds.) *Plastic Surgery: A Concise Guide to Clinical Practice*. Little, Brown and Co., Boston, 1968.)

verse cuts back along the nerve at 1 mm intervals until an interface that appears healthy is seen[80] (Fig. 10–10). Because of the likelihood of excessive fibrosis and absence of identifiable nerve tissue in the distal stump, the distal neuroma must be trimmed generously to assure that there will be patent Schwann tubes for regenerating axons from the proximal stump to grow into.[5, 40, 43, 68]

Hemostasis is vital during peripheral nerve surgery because a surgical field containing excess blood promotes scar formation at the nerve suture site.[5] The use of cotton and gauze sponges at the ends of the nerve stumps should be avoided so that lint will not contaminate the anastomotic area. Lint-free ophthalmic sponges or gelatin sponges should be used for blotting the ends of the nerve.[88, 89, 90] The use of tourniquets is controversial; some say they should not be used[68, 76] and others say that they may be used with caution.[69]

Placing and tying sutures to anastomose nerve stumps or nerve stumps and grafts requires much attention. As a general rule the suture material should pass only through the epineurium and not into the neural tissue[5, 7] (Fig. 10–11). Suture materials that invade the neural elements of a nerve result in scar tissue formation in an amount directly proportional to the amount of invasion.[7] The suture tension should be such that the bundles barely contact each other, and all knots should be tied with equal tension.[61] An operating microscope with a magnification of 25 is most helpful in the procedure.[59]

Recently, the use of an operating microscope has been found to be advantageous in nerve surgery. Such microsurgery has been found to enhance the ease of dissection and aids in differentiating normal neural patterns from those altered by neuroma and scar formation. Microsurgery also increases the accuracy of funicular alignment through better placement of epineurial sutures, and it reduces rotational errors in surgery. Operating microscopes are also beneficial in visualization of small nerves,[78] and in suturing individual funiculi.[58] Stay sutures or transfixion needles placed in the nerve trunks themselves should be used only when approximation would otherwise be very difficult. Stay sutures should include only the epineurium.[5, 14, 66] Other techniques have been described for nerve anastomosis and will be described later. After repair, radiography and metallic sutures have proved beneficial as a

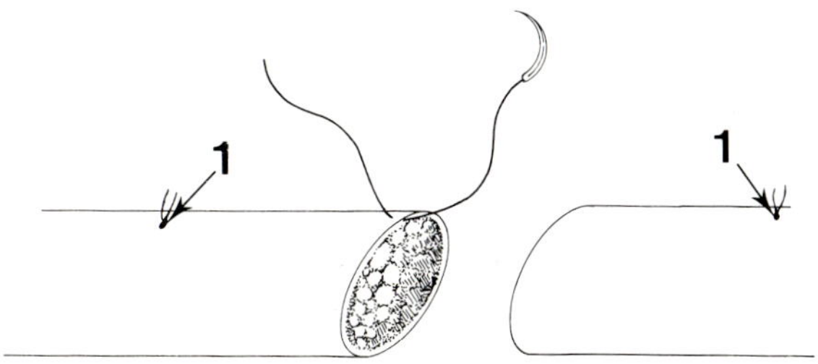

FIGURE 10–11 Anastomosing sutures are placed through the epineurium only. Epineurial marking sutures for alignment (1). (Adapted from Swaim, S. F.: Isolated peripheral nerves. *In* Bojrab, M. J. (ed.): *Current Techniques in Small Animal Surgery I*. Lea & Febiger, Philadelphia, 1975.)

means of periodically examining the unity of the suture site. Following suturing of the nerve, a radiopaque suture is placed in the epineurium of both stumps near the anastomotic site. Radiographs taken periodically of the nerve and the recorded distance between the metallic marking sutures determine the unity of the anastomotic site.[5, 26, 68]

NERVE ANASTOMOSIS

The best means of nerve repair is careful end-to-end anastomosis of the nerve stumps.[76, 88, 90] This form of repair should be used when there has been little or no loss of nerve tissue, either at the time of original injury or at the time of trimming degenerated nerve tissue at secondary repair.

Simple interrupted sutures placed through the epineurium of nerves have been extensively used as a means of nerve anastomosis. Many types of small diameter (5–0 to 8–0) suture materials have been used. Silicone-coated silk[17, 88, 89, 90] and monofilament nylon[13] have been found useful. The silicone coating helps eliminate connective tissue reaction to the silk within the nerve. The surgeon should avoid placement of too many sutures when anastomosing a nerve because the connective tissue reaction within the nerve increases with the number of sutures. Four sutures placed equidistant around a nerve will give a stable anastomosis[69, 88, 89, 90] (Fig. 10–12). When suturing several peripheral branches to one parent nerve trunk, it is necessary to unite the peripheral branches with a single epineurial suture so they are grouped together as one nerve. The anastomosis is then completed in the usual manner.[5, 15]

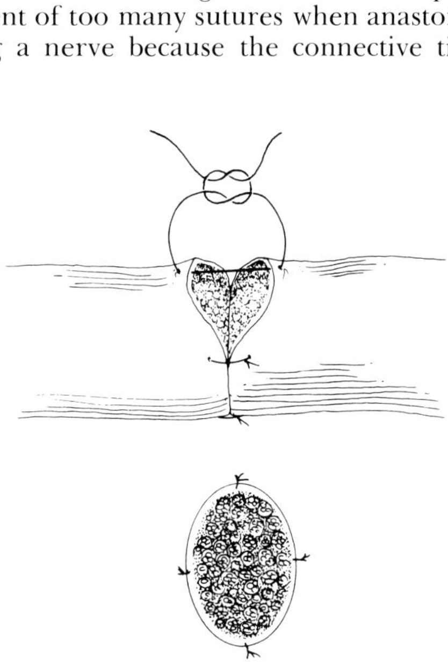

FIGURE 10–12 Four anastomosing sutures are placed equidistant around the nerve. (Adapted from Swaim, S. F.: Isolated peripheral nerves. *In* Bojrab, M. J. (ed.): *Current Techniques in Small Animal Surgery I.* Lea & Febiger, Philadelphia, 1975.)

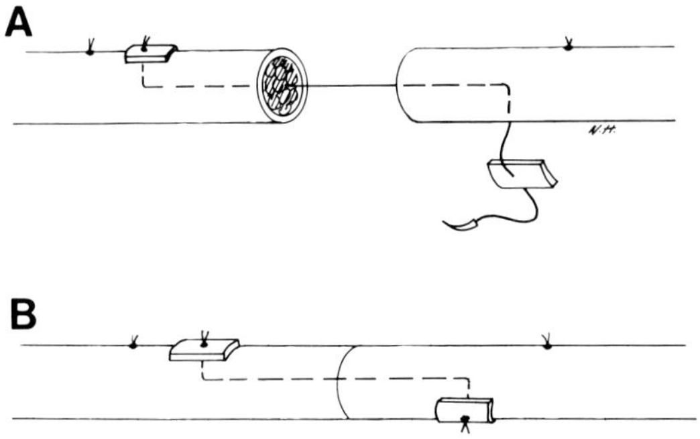

FIGURE 10–13 Technique for intraneural nerve anastomosis. *A.* Placement of the suture. *B.* Completed suture. (Adapted from Swaim, S. F.: Peripheral nerves. *In* Archibald, J. (ed.): *Canine Surgery,* 2nd Archibald ed. American Veterinary Publications, Santa Barbara, Calif., 1974.)

Other techniques of anastomosis have been described, including intraneural nerve anastomosis.[82] A swaged needle and small diameter monofilament nylon are inserted into the proximal nerve stump 7 to 8 mm proximal to the transection site and directed along the nerve parallel to its long axis. The needle is reinserted between the corresponding fibers of the distal stump and retrieved through the epineurium 7 to 8 mm from the transection site. Two small sections of fascia[82] or silicone rubber patches[88, 89, 90] are used as anchor plates, over which the ends of the suture are tied. These patches serve to stabilize the suture within the nerve and hold the nerve stumps in apposition[82] (Fig. 10–13). Such anastomoses have the disadvantage of connective tissue invasion at the anastomotic site. Rotational movement of the nerve stumps on the single suture also may interfere with nerve regeneration across the anastomotic site.[88, 90]

Funicular suturing may also be used as a means of nerve anastomosis. This involves the suturing of individual funiculi of a nerve.[86] Grabb *et al.* describe such a technique using one or two 10–0 nylon su-

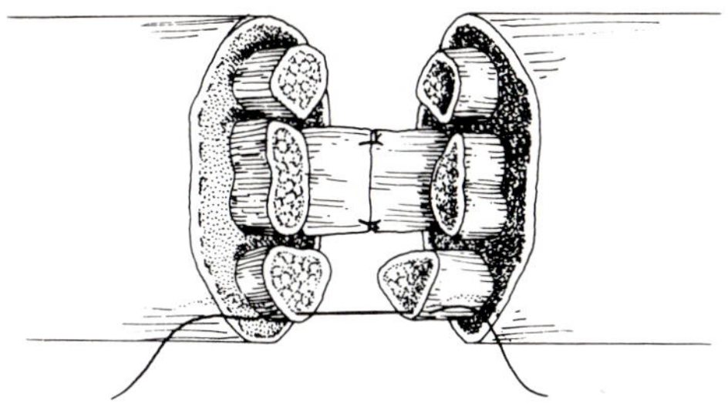

FIGURE 10–14 A technique for funicular nerve suture using 10-0 nylon. Technique requires an operating microscope. (Adapted from Grabb, W. C., Bement, S. L., Koepke, G. H., and Green, R. A.: Comparison of methods of peripheral nerve suturing in monkeys. Plast. Reconstr. Surg., *46*, 31, 1970.)

tures in each funiculus (Fig. 10–14). Microsurgery instruments and an operating microscope were used. Grabb *et al.* concluded that the funicular suture technique gives a closer to normal range of restored motor function than does the epineurial suture technique. No significant difference in return of function was noticed whether funiculi were aligned according to like size or similar predominant function (sensory or motor).[36] Milleri has described the use of pieces of a smaller nerve (sural nerve) to graft between individual funiculi of larger nerves.[58] Tsuge *et al.* have developed the "anchor funicular suture" technique, which is intermediate between the epineurial suture technique and the funicular suture technique[96] (Fig. 10–15). This technique involves placement of two or three 5–0 to 7–0 nylon loop sutures in the epineurium of the nerve. If there is inadequate coaptation between the funiculi, 10–0 nylon sutures may be used to appose the individual funiculi.

It has been shown histologically that the quality of nerve regeneration is not as good if attention is not given to the alignment of individual funiculi. If funiculi are not aligned, regenerating axons grow into the epineurial tissue and are not available for good regeneration.[46]

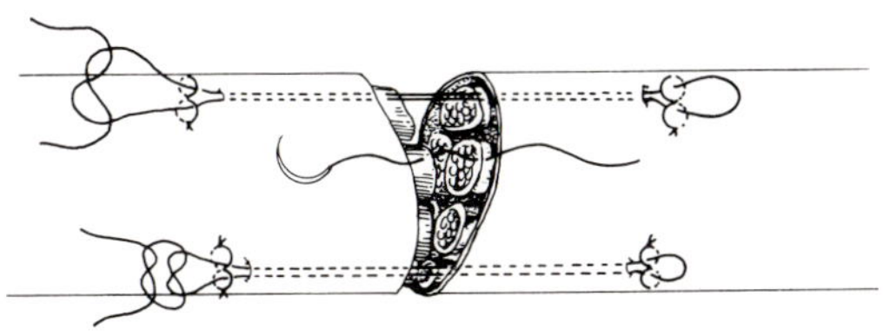

FIGURE 10–15 The anchor funicular suture technique for nerve anastomosis. The technique employs funicular sutures as well as epineurial anchor sutures. (Adapted from Tsuge, K., Yoshikazu, I. and Sukaue, M.: A new technique for nerve suture: The anchor funicular suture. Plast. Reconstr. Surg. *56*, 496, 1975.)

Various nonsuture techniques have been used for anastomosing peripheral nerves. Freeman and co-workers have reported the use of a nonsuture technique for anastomosing nerves that are small in diameter.[34] A surgical adhesive tape (Micropore, Steri-Strip) of a nonwoven fabric of viscous rayon is used; it is coated on one side with an adhesive copolymer of iso-octylacrylate and acrylic acid and is porous, permeable to tissue fluids, and readily available. The nerve stumps are aligned and sandwiched between two pieces of tape. A tubular sheath is formed around the nerve by crimping the tapes together 2 mm on either side of the nerve.[33] Freeman reported more favorable results in micropore anastomosed nerves than in sutured nerves and control nerves of mice. He also reported that the tape prevented the ingrowth of connective tissue at the neural suture line and permitted healing with minimal neuroma formation.[34]

Another study by Freeman, largely in dogs, revealed that the micropore tape caused a minimal inflammatory reaction, which resulted in a film of fibrous tissue lining a sac of adhesive globules that slowly disappeared. Although the tape was apparently removed by macrophages, a few macrophages were seen after 3 weeks. When examined grossly the anastomoses were intact. The main disadvantage of this technique is the danger of "slippage," in which the nerve ends become separated within the cuff as a result of slight prolonged tension on the nerve.[33]

Based on this work of Freeman, it appears that prevention of tension on the approximated area is a necessity. The use of micropore tape as a cuff around anastomotic sites will be discussed later.

Other methods of nerve anastomosis include plasma clot suture, rapid polymerizing tissue adhesives, and tubular splicing.

SHIELDING THE ANASTOMOTIC AREA

The critical step in any nerve anastomosis is inhibition of the formation of connective tissue or scar encroachment at the point of nerve juncture. The anastomotic area must be insulated from the surrounding connective tissue. The technique currently used to accomplish this is sheathing, which prevents axonal escape, stimulates axonal regrowth in a longitudinal direction, and prevents the ingrowth of juxtaposed extraneural connective tissue into the wound at the site of nerve juncture.[54] Former methods include encircling the nerve with soft dry tissue such as muscle and use of such materials as autogenous arterial segments, plastic and rubber tubing, tantalum, gold, absorbable gelatin mesh, liquid plastics such as tissue glue (Eastman 910 Monomer), and plasma clots. The plasma clot was the most satisfactory of these substances.[5, 23, 48, 76, 92]

Campbell and workers have used an inert porous plastic sheathing material called Millipore. This material, as its name suggests, has minute pores with a maximum diameter of 0.45 microns. The pores permit extracellular fluids to pass through and across the surface, and these fluids help meet the nutritional requirements of proliferating epineurial cells. Epineurial continuity is reestablished before regeneration of the stroma is appreciably advanced. This allows a linear pattern of regeneration in the more deeply seated stroma through this outer layer "contact guidance" phenomenon. However, Millipore has the same disadvantage as tantalum, which undergoes fragmentation with subsequent scar formation. Millipore calcifies and breaks up into small pieces after about 2 months in the body.[3, 19] Micropore is reported to be absorbed by the body in approximately 3 weeks and therefore appears to be preferable for shielding the anastomotic area.[32]

Studies have been done on nerve anastomoses and grafts to evaluate micropore tape cuffs placed around anastomotic sites on the radial nerves of dogs. After 6 months in the animal it was found that the tape was still present but no longer formed a cuff. The tapes had separated at their edges, leaving a nerve anastomotic site sandwiched between two pieces of tape. More connective tissue reaction was present around the anastomotic sites than when silicone rubber cuffs were used. The neuromas that were present were at the anastomotic sites rather than at the edges of the cuff as occurred with silicone rubber cuffs. There had been connective tissue invasion under the edges and through the pores of the tape as shown by adhesions of the tape to the underlying nerve by connective tissue. Microscopic examination of the neuromas on these nerves revealed the invasion of extraneural connective tissue into the anastomotic sites.[90]

An ideal shield currently available is made of a silicone rubber material called Silastic. It is a flexible, thin-walled, tubular sheath designed to provide uniform, nonconstricing nerve encasement. It is tissue-inert, evoking a thin pseudosynovial membrane response around the sheath, which is free of giant cells. This material is available in assorted diameters and lengths, packaged in vials and ready for use.[26, 29, 57]

Certain factors must be considered when selecting the proper size of nerve cuff, the most important being the diameter of the nerve cuff. It has been found that a silicone rubber cuff should have an internal cross-sectional area that is two or three times the size of the cross-sectional area of the nerve on which it is used.[25, 26, 27, 28] This is necessary to allow for the swelling that occurs in the nerve immediately after the operation.[25, 28] It has been found that an injured regenerating axon will increase in diameter from its normal size of 1 to 2 microns to 7 microns.[27] Cuffs that are too small in diameter tend to constrict the nerve and cause neuroma formation proximal and distal to the cuff. If a cuff is larger than three times the cross-sectional area of the nerve, connective tissue will invade the nerve under the cuff and at the anastomotic site, blocking axonal regeneration.[26, 97]

Length and thickness are important factors to be considered when selecting a nerve cuff. Nerve cuffs should be no longer than 8 to 10 mm.[17, 26] Nerve cuffs that are too long interfere with the blood supply to the nerve at the center of the cuff. If the cuff is too short, it will tend to slip and give inadequate protection to the anastomotic site. Thin-walled cuffs should be used, since thick-walled cuffs result in increased neuroma formation proximal and distal to the cuff.[26]

The cuff can be placed on a thin-nosed closed hemostat and transferred to the proximal stump[57] (Fig. 10–16*A*), or the proximal stump can be pulled through the cuff by means of epineurially placed sutures[29] (Fig. 10–16*B*). A third technique involves placing the cuff on a pair of jewelers' forceps, grasping the epineurium at the tip

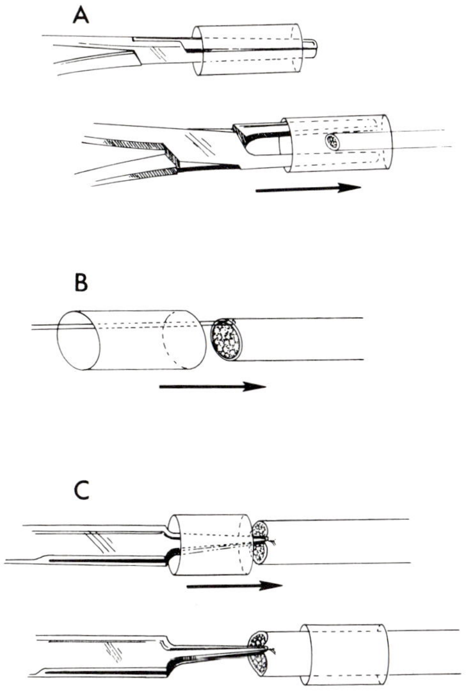

FIGURE 10–16 Techniques for transferring cuffs onto nerve stumps. The cuff is transferred onto the nerve (*A*) from a pair of hemostats, (*B*) by means of an epineurial guide suture, (*C*) from a pair of jewelers' forceps.

of the nerve stump with the forceps, and sliding the cuff onto the nerve stump[88, 89, 90] (Fig. 10–16*C*).

The nerve stumps are approximated with four interrupted sutures of 7–0 silicone-coated silk placed in the epineurium and equidistant around the nerve (Fig. 10–12). The cuff is placed over the anastomotic area and anchored in the epineurium at both extremities with interrupted sutures to avoid slippage (Fig. 10–17*A*). A thin-walled cuff with a diameter greater than that of the nerve will undergo distortion (folding over on itself, invagination, or both) if it is not properly anchored (Fig. 10–17*B-D*). Such distortions may result in nerve constriction that impairs regeneration. Nerve cuffs that are too small in diameter may constrict the nerve (Fig. 10–17*E*). This results in poorly myelinated nerve fibers as they pass through the area of nerve surrounded by the cuff.[88, 89, 90]

NERVE GRAFTS

It has been emphasized that a considerable gap in nerve ends is difficult to counteract, since any tension at the surgical site will disrupt healing. A lengthy tissue incision and an anatomical relocation of the nerve may be successful in compensating for the defect. The techniques used to overcome large gaps in nerves are too numerous to be discussed in detail; however, they include nerve stretching, bone resection to shorten a limb, nerve pedicle flaps, tubulization, implantation of various foreign materials in the nerve gap, and direct neurotization of muscles. Further references to these techniques are available.[90] Various forms of nerve grafts have also been used to overcome gaps in nerves, including heterografts, homografts, and

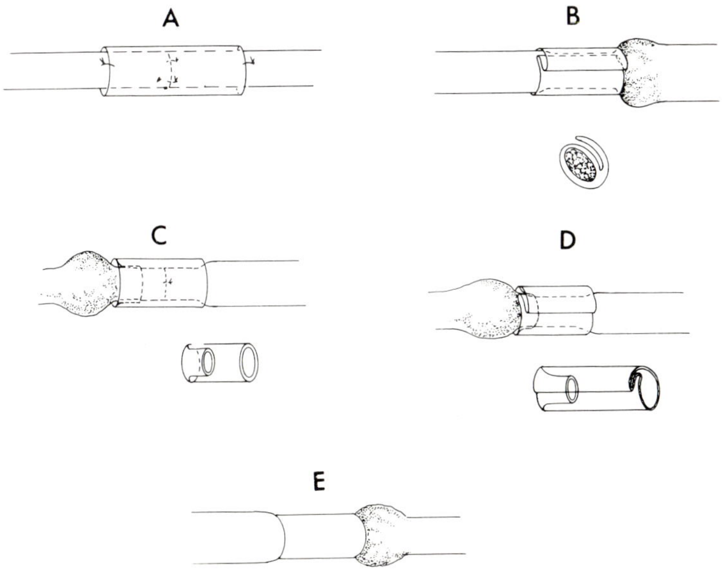

FIGURE 10–17 Proper and improper cuffing of a nerve anastomotic site. *A*. A cuff placed over an anastomotic site and anchored at *both* ends. *B*. Folding over a cuff with resultant neuroma at proximal end of the cuff. *C*. Invagination of cuff with resultant proximal neuroma. *D*. Folding over and invagination of a cuff with resultant proximal neuroma. *E*. Cuff that is too small in diameter with resultant proximal neuroma. (Adapted from Swaim, S. F.: Peripheral nerves. *In* Archibald, J. (ed.): *Canine Surgery*, 2nd Archibald ed. American Veterinary Publications, Santa Barbara, Calif., 1974.)

autografts, usually in the form of cable grafts.

Some stretching of peripheral nerve stumps to accomplish anastomosis over a gap may be done; however, as mentioned previously, there is a limit to the amount of stretch a nerve can withstand before damage occurs. In a recent study Terzis found that axonal regeneration was optimal when end-to-end sutures were made without tension. Regeneration through a mildly stretched repair site was equivalent to regeneration after a properly tailored graft was placed in the defect. Poor nerve regeneration occurred when either excessively long grafts were used or when the nerves were moderately stretched to accomplish anastomosis. Severely stretched nerves exhibited minimal functional recovery.[95]

It has been shown that nerve stumps anchored to a common and adjacent structure such as muscle can occasionally bridge small gaps of 1 to 2 cm sufficiently to maintain some function[55, 88, 89, 90] (Fig. 10–18). This bridging can be facilitated by use of a tubulated bridge such as a vein. Gaps of three to seven times the diameter of the nerve have been bridged in monkeys by use of a vein sheath. Weight recovery in the gastrocnemius muscle supplied by the posterior tibial nerve in animals studied varied from 50 to 93 per cent compared to 30 per cent in controls.[56]

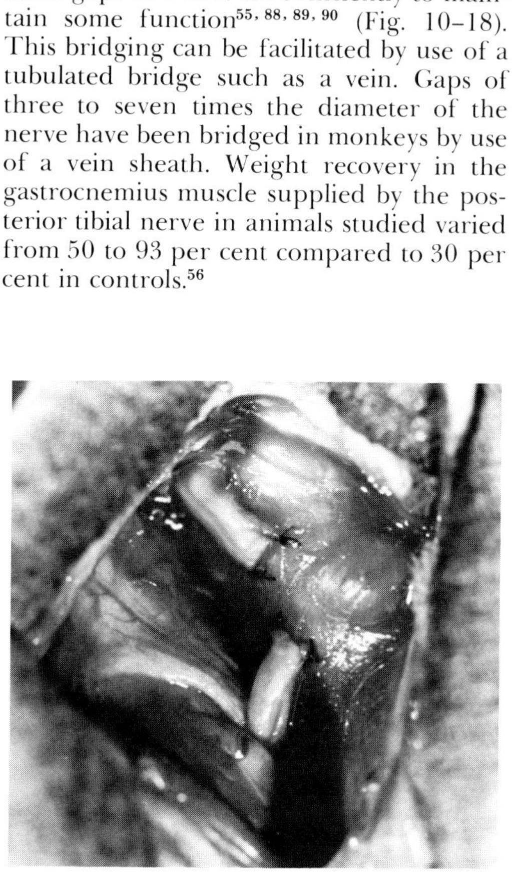

FIGURE 10–18 Two nerve ends have been sutured in line with each other on a smooth muscle surface. Gap between the nerve ends is about 2 cm. (From Swaim, S. F.: Peripheral nerves. *In* Archibald, J. (ed.): *Canine Surgery*, 2nd Archibald ed. American Veterinary Publications, Santa Barbara, Calif., 1974.)

Partial or complete autogenous cross-grafting of one nerve to another has been successfully performed in many disorders. In the human, function has been maintained in the facial nerve by cross-grafting another nerve such as the spinal accessory[17, 37, 38] Occasional autogenous grafting has been done in clinical conditions in the dog. Knecht has described techniques for connecting the musculocutaneous nerve to the radial nerve. In one technique the viable proximal stump of the musculocutaneous nerve was anastomosed by end-to-end suturing to the distal stump of the radial nerve. In another technique the proximal musculocutaneous stump was sutured into a pie-shaped incision that had been made in the radial nerve.[50]

Other donor nerves that could be used in the dog are the lateral cutaneous nerve of the thigh and the median nerve of the fore limb. Autogenous grafts are more successful than either heterogenous or homologous grafts owing to the lack of tissue rejection and the rapidity with which regenerating axons traverse this type of graft.[7]

Ideally, a homograft or a heterograft could be used in bridging a large nerve defect (Fig. 10–19). In the past such attempts have been discouraging. However, exciting results have recently been obtained in dogs with the use of frozen electron-irradiated homografts and heterografts. Irradiation has an immunosuppressive effect on such transplants.[54, 55] A study by Comtet *et al.* in 1972 compared irradiated nerve homografts with nerve homografts stored in merthiolate. The grafts were compared functionally by measuring the excitability of the homografts and that of the reinnervated muscles and by histological examinations. The grafts were taken from the posterior tibial nerves of 32 dogs and stored by one of the two methods for 12 months. Segments of the sciatic nerve were then excised and replaced by one of the grafts. The grafts were sutured in place with 6–0 atraumatic silk, and the anastomotic sites were protected with silicone foil. Evaluation of the grafts revealed some muscle reinnervation, as noted by clinical examination. There were also swellings at the anastomotic sites with atrophy of the midportion of both types of grafts. Impulse transmission was a little slower in the merthiolate-stored grafts than in the irradiated grafts, and both were slower than normal. Histologic

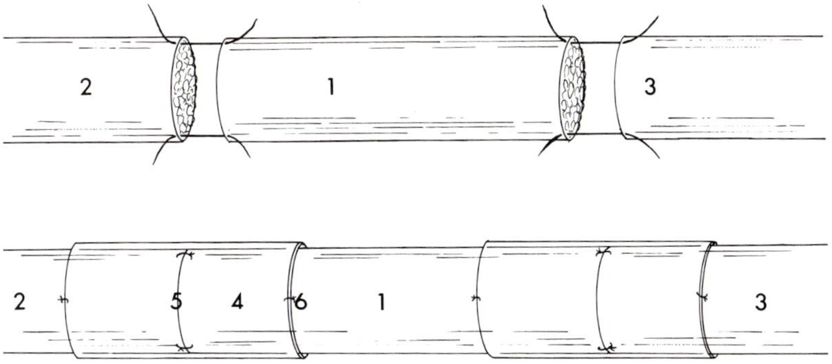

FIGURE 10–19 The use of silicone rubber sheaths with nerve homografts. 1, Homograft; 2, proximal nerve stump; 3, distal nerve stump; 4, silicone rubber sheath; 5, anastomosis of proximal nerve stump to homograft; 6, anchor sutures of sheath to the epineurium of the graft. (Adapted from Pinner-Poole, B.: *Nerve Suture and Nerve Grafts.* Dixieme Congress de la Soc. Intern. de Chir. Orthop. et de Traum, September, 1966.)

examination revealed dead tissue without wallerian degeneration or homograft rejection, minimal myelinization, and neurotization in both types of grafts. Owing to poor histologic findings, the authors did not advocate the use of either type of graft.[22]

Fresh, nonirradiated nerve grafts have also been found effective in dogs.[88, 89, 90] In a series of 12 dogs in which different cuff material was used around anastomotic sites of nerve grafts, all dogs demonstrated return of nerve function.[90]

When obtaining a nerve graft, it is necessary to keep certain factors and techniques in mind. The graft and the recipient nerve should be as similar in diameter as possible. Nerve grafts of inadequate diameter provide an insufficient number of Schwann tubes for the regenerating axons of the proximal stump to follow.[7, 74] If the diameter of thc graft is excessive, blood vessels will be unable to penetrate it sufficiently.[74, 81]

The success of a nerve graft also depends on its length. Since grafts have a tendency to shrink, a graft should be 15 to 25 per cent longer than the gap to be spanned. As the length of the graft increases, the danger of ischemic necrosis at the center of the graft also increases, especially when the graft is laid in a relatively avascular bed.[42] The length of a graft is closely related to the axonal regeneration time and the development of immune response to the graft. Nerve homografts and heterografts evoke an immune response in the host. This eventually leads to rejection of the graft. Regenerating axons will advance through a graft as long as Schwann tubes remain patent. To be successful, the axons must traverse the graft and penetrate the empty Schwann tubes of the distal stump before the graft is destroyed by the inflammatory immune response. Thus, an increase in length of the graft may decrease the chance that regenerating axons will reach the distal nerve stump before the graft has been rejected by the immune reaction of the host.[55, 102]

Predegenerated nerve grafts (grafts taken from the distal stumps of nerves that have been severed and have undergone wallerian degeneration have been used to insure faster regeneration of axons across a gap. However, studies have shown that nerve regeneration across a nerve gap is no faster through a predegenerated graft than through an undegenerated graft.[7, 44, 45, 70, 92, 101, 103]

Freezing and irradiation of nerve grafts reduce the antigenicity of nerve homografts.[54, 55, 81] When irradiation is used in preparation of a nerve graft, the graft must be obtained within 4 to 6 hours after the death of the donor. If refrigeration is employed, the material may be obtained up to 24 hours after death. The specimen is taken under clean but not necessarily aseptic conditions, all extraneous material is removed, and the graft is placed in a polyethylene bag which is sealed in a heat press. Two additional bags are placed around the first for additional protection. Cultures may be taken prior to and after irradiation as a safety precaution. The specimen is frozen and maintained at −12° C. The specimen is electron-irradiated with 2 million r.e.p. (or 1.66 megarads) with a Van de Graff generator or a linear accelerator for 10 seconds at the temperature of dry ice. Grafts may be stored up to 6 months but should be used shortly after irradiation.[54, 55]

A 3-cm length of peroneal nerve was removed from the main branch of the sciatic nerve and replaced with a 3.5 cm irradiated homograft. Normal gait returned in 5 to 6 months in all three experimental dogs. Some functional return was demonstrated by electromyography as early as 3 weeks after surgery. The graft sites were reexplored surgically 7 months after surgery. Slight to moderate scar tissue was seen around the grafts; however, all grafts produced vigorous contractions upon electrical stimulation. The grafts were removed surgically and studied histopathologically while another irradiated graft was substituted in the resulting defect in the same dogs. Normal function returned the second time.[55]

The use of irradiated homografts in man has been encouraging, but not completely successful.[55]

The experiments with irradiated heterografts in dogs showed more inflammatory reactions than those with homografts. However, when 3-cm irradiated heterografts from calves (two cases) and from humans (two cases) were placed in 2-cm peroneal nerve defects in the dog, all were successful. Results in rats were not as successful. Heterografts have been evaluated when an immunosuppressive drug, 6- (1 methyl-4-nitro-5-imidayolyl) thiopurine, commonly called Imuran, was given. Imuran given preoperatively was effective in protecting nonirradiated heterografts from destruction; however, none of the group that received Imuran regained function. Animals with irradiated heterografts who were given Imuran showed a 60 per cent recovery rate despite a severe inflammatory response. Immune rejection to nonirradiated nerve homografts can be prevented in animals by administration of Imuran in nontoxic doses. Therefore, it is possible that in future studies in man, preoperative and postoperative administration of Imuran may enhance nerve regeneration through the use of homografts and heterografts, whether irradiated or not.[55]

In a recent study of nerve anastomosis, fresh, nonirradiated nerve grafts, and nerve gaps were evaluated clinically, electrically, and histopathologically. With respect to nerve grafts, it was found that fresh, nonirradiated homografts resulted in functional return of the radial nerve in 12 dogs when these grafts were placed in a 2-cm nerve gap. Functional return was verified by electrical stimulation of the radial nerve proximal to the graft and by noting the dog's ability to extend the carpus and digits, using a modification of the conventional sight-placing reaction. The average time for the first appearance of functional recovery (12.7 weeks) was longer than that in dogs which had undergone nerve anastomosis (9.5 weeks). Histopathologically, some of the grafts showed marked evidence of mononuclear reaction within and around them and others did not. In spite of this reaction, the grafted nerves still gave evidence of functional recovery.[90]

In two separate studies nerve gaps 2 cm in length have been created in peripheral nerves and the nerve stumps sutured to the adjacent musculature. In one of these studies,[55] the gap was created in the peroneal nerve of three dogs. Two of the three dogs showed partial return of function in 7 months; however, the bridged nerve fibers were difficult to identify in the surrounding scar tissue. Electrical stimulation showed that some proximal fibrils had reached the distal stump.[55] Similar histopathologic results were obtained in the second study in which a 2 cm gap was made in one radial nerve of three dogs.[90] In this study all three dogs showed evidence of functional recovery at an average of 10.3 weeks following surgery. Six months postoperatively, electrical stimulation of the affected radial nerves proximal to the gap resulted in evidence of nerve fiber regeneration across the gap.

There is a question whether the use of Silastic shields would enhance the regeneration of homografts and heterografts. Poole studied cats that had frozen irradiated homografts, 1 cm in length, which were then shielded in Silastic or Millipore, or both. In unshielded grafts, edema, swelling, and connective tissue proliferation occurred around the grafts until they were completely "bound down" in the surrounding tissue within 6 to 12 months. In shielded grafts, there was no edematous swelling or collagen build-up on the outer surface of the nerves. In fact, suture lines were difficult to locate in some specimens within 14 days. As stated previously, Millipore became calcified and fragmented and had to be removed.[17, 65]

A nerve graft should never be completely surrounded by an impermeable membrane, since this would prevent blood vessels from entering the graft and thus lead to necrosis. Revascularization of nerve grafts occurs by invasion of vessels from tissue as well as from the host stumps. Thus the bed of the graft should be in a well-vascularized area that is free of scar tissue and hematomas.[9, 81, 90, 92]

Since Millipore allows the transport of extracellular fluids to the graft and anastomotic sites, it should be used initially and subsequently replaced by Silastic shields in grafts of considerable length. Campbell feels that Silastic shields should not exceed 8 to 9 mm in length, whereas Midgley used shields up to 15 mm long.[17, 65]

Results of research indicate that nerve anastomosis is the best form of nerve repair. Several techniques are available for the veterinarian, and the surgeon can use the technique for which he feels best equipped and qualified to perform. In general, nerve anastomosis using silicone-coated silk suture for meticulous approximation of the epineurium and Silastic insulation for the anastomotic site is the most highly recommended technique. The bridging of a large defect may be done by means of a fresh, nonirradiated or a frozen, irradiated homologous graft. Another alternative is the use of immunosuppressive drugs with either type of graft.

When a small gap of 1 to 2 cm remains in a nerve and provisions have not been made for placing a graft in the gap, partial function may return if the gap is bridged by carefully securing the proximal and distal stumps to a common structure such as a muscle. However, anastomosis and Silastic cuffs insure a more complete recovery.

POSTOPERATIVE CARE

After meticulous repair of the nerve ends has been accomplished, the wound is closed routinely. If there is reason to believe that tension exists on the nerve anastomosis or graft, the part should be splinted in a relaxed position for at least 2 weeks.[23] If a limb has been immobilized in flexion to relieve tension on the nerve, slow extension should be started in the second week after surgery and completed in the fifth week.[83]

Much thought must be given to the maintenance of normal limb position and the avoidance of gross muscle atrophy while regeneration occurs and function returns. It is important that the joints, muscles, tendons, and skin of an affected limb be maintained in good condition during this time.[72, 73] This may be done by gentle massage, passive exercise, and the application of moist and dry heat after the initial wound has healed.[12, 47, 59, 61, 76, 83, 93] In addition, good health, good nutrition, and vigorous activity aid healthy nerve grafts and result in a greater degree of functional recovery than when the dog is emaciated and inactive.[93] During nerve regeneration, it is important that the desensitized part be protected from injury and overstretching of muscles.[102] The prevention of self-mutilation is particularly important in dogs.

REFERENCES

1. Allam, M. W.: Electrical intraneural bipolar stimulation of peripheral nerves in the dog. J.A.V.M.A. *114*, 87, 1949.
2. Babcock, W. W.: A standard technique for operations on peripheral nerves. With special reference to the closure of large gaps. Surg. Gynec. Obstet. *45*, 364, 1927.
3. Bassett, C. A. L., and Campbell, J. B.: Calcification of Millipore in vivo. Transplant. Bull. *26*, 132, 1960.
4. Bassett, C. A. L., Campbell, J. B., and Husby, J.: Peripheral nerve and spinal cord regeneration: Factors leading to success of a tubulation technique employing Millipore. Exp. Neurol. *1*, 386, 1959.
5. Bateman, J. E.: *Trauma to Nerves in Limbs.* W. B. Saunders Co., Philadelphia, 1962.
6. Beazley, R. M., Bagley, D. H., and Ketcham, A. S.: The effect of cryosurgery on peripheral nerves. J. Surg. Res. *16*, 231, 1974.
7. Bentley, F. H., and Hill, M.: Nerve grafting. Brit. J. Surg. *24*, 368, 1936.
8. Blackwood, W., and Holmes, W.: *Histopathology of Nerve Injury,* Part I. Medical Research Council, Special Report Series *282*, 88, 1954.
9. Blumke, S., Niedorf, H. R., and Rode, J.: Axoplasmic alterations in the proximal and distal stumps of transected nerves. Acta Neuropathol. 7, 44, 1966.

10. Bowden, R. E. M., and Gutmann, E.: Denervation and re-innervation of human voluntary muscle. Brain *67*, 273, 1944.
11. Brown, D. D., and Doherty, M. M.: Effects of transient stretching of peripheral nerve. Arch. Neurol. Psychiat. *54*, 116, 1945.
12. Brown, H. A., and Brown, B. A.: Treatment of peripheral nerve injuries. Rev. Surg. *24*, 1, 1967.
13. Brown, P. W.: Factors influencing the success of the surgical repair of peripheral nerves. Surg. Clin. N. Amer. *52*, 1137, 1972.
14. Brugghen, A.: *Neurosurgery in General Practice.* Charles C Thomas, Springfield, Ill., 1952.
15. Bunnell, A.: Surgery of the peripheral nerves of the hand. Surg. Gynec. Obstet. *44*, 145, 1927.
16. Cajal, S. R.: *Degeneration and Regeneration of the Nervous System.* Oxford University Press, Oxford, 1928.
17. Campbell, J. B., and Luzio, J.: Facial nerve repair: New surgical techniques. Symposium on facial nerve rehabilitation. Acad. Ophthal. Otolaryngol. *68*, 1068, 1964.
18. Campbell, J. B.: Phantom limb pain: A new surgical approach. Neurology *15*, 272, 1965.
19. Campbell, J. B., Bassett, C. A. L., Husby, J., Nhulin, C. A., and Feringa, E. R.: Microfilter sheaths in peripheral nerve surgery: A laboratory report and preliminary clinical study. J. Trauma *1*, 139, 1961.
20. Causey, G.: *The Cell of Schwann.* E. and S. Livingstone, London, 1960.
21. Causey, G., and Stratmann, C. J.: Changes in the nucleic acid content of ganglion cells during chromatolysis and after stimulation. Biochem. J. *64*, 29, 1956.
22. Comtet, J. J., Deliry, P., Faure, A., Tommasi, M., Mallet-Guy, Y., and Transy, M. J.: Comparative study of two series of preserved nerve grafts in dogs. Lyon Chir. *68*, 352, 1972.
23. Davis, L. E.: *Principles of Neurological Surgery*, 4th ed. Lea & Febiger, Philadelphia, 1953.
24. Davis, L., and Ruge, D.: Functional recovery following the use of homogeneous nerve grafts. Surgery *27*, 102, 1950.
25. Dow Corning: Silastic nerve cuff (Ducker-Hayes design). Bull. 14–367, Aug., 1968.
26. Ducker, T. B., and Hayes, G. J.: Experimental improvements in the use of Silastic cuffs for peripheral nerve repair. J. Neurosurg. *28*, 582, 1968.
27. Ducker, T. B., and Hayes, G. J.: Peripheral nerve injuries: A comparative study of the anatomical and functional results following primary nerve repair in chimpanzees. Milit. Med. *133*, 298, 1968.
28. Ducker, T. B., Kempe, L. G., and Hayes, G. J.: The metabolic background for peripheral nerve surgery. J. Neurosurg. *30*, 270, 1969.
29. Evans, L. H., Campbell, J. B., Pinner-Poole, B., and Jenny, J.: Prevention of painful neuromas in horses. J.A.V.M.A. *153*, 313, 1968.
30. Fackelman, G. E., and Clodius, L.: New techniques for posterior digital neurectomy in the horse. Vet. Med. Small Anim. Clin. *67*, 1339, 1972.
31. Fisher, E. R., and Turano, A.: Schwann cells in wallerian degeneration. Arch. Pathol. *75*, 517, 1963.
32. Freeman, B. S.: Adhesive anastomosis techniques for fine nerves, experimental and clinical techniques. Amer. J. Surg. *108*, 529, 1964.
33. Freeman, B. S.: Adhesive neural anastomosis. Plast. Reconstr. Surg. *35*, 167, 1965.
34. Freeman, B. S., Perry, J., and Brown, D.: Experimental study of adhesive surgical tape for nerve anastomosis. Plast. Reconstr. Surg. *43*, 174, 1969.
35. Grabb, W. C.: Median and ulnar nerve suture, an experimental study comparing primary and secondary repair in monkeys. J. Bone Joint Surg. *50A*, 964, 1968.
36. Grabb, W. C., Bement, S. L., Koepke, G. H., and Green, R. A.: Comparison of methods of peripheral nerve suturing in monkeys, Plast. Reconstr. Surg. *46*, 31, 1970.
37. Gurdjian, E. S.: *Operative Neurosurgery*, 2nd ed. The Williams and Wilkins Co., Baltimore, 1964.
38. Guth, L.: Regeneration in the mammalian peripheral nervous system. Physiol. Rev. *36*, 4, 1956.
39. Guttmann, L., and Sanders, F. K.: Recovery of fibre numbers and diameters in the regeneration of peripheral nerves. J. Physiol. *101*, 489, 1943.
40. Highet, W. B., and Holmes, W.: Traction injuries to the lateral popliteal nerve and traction to peripheral nerves after suture. Brit. J. Surg. *30*, 212, 1943.
41. Highet, W. B., and Sanders, F. K.: The effects of stretching nerves after suture. Brit. J. Surg. *30*, 355, 1943.
42. Hoen, T. I., and Brackett, C. E.: Peripheral nerve lengthening. I. Experimental. J. Neurosurg. *13*, 43, 1956.
43. Holmes, W., and Young, J. Z.: Nerve regeneration after immediate and delayed suture. J. Anat. *77*, 63, 1942.
44. Huber, G. C.: Transplantation of peripheral nerves. Arch. Neurol. Psychiat. *2*, 466, 1919.
45. Huber, G. C.: Repair of peripheral nerve injuries. Surg. Gynec. Obstet. *30*, 464, 1920.
46. Hudson, A. R., Morris, J., Weddell, G., and Drury, A.: Peripheral nerve autografts. J. Surg. Res. *12*, 267, 1972.
47. Klemme, R. M., Woolsey, R. D., and DeRezende, N. T.: Autopsy nerve grafts in peripheral nerve surgery. Clinical application: "Glue" suture technique. J.A.M.A. *123*, 393, 1943.
48. Kline, D. G., and Hayes, G. J.: An experimental evaluation of the effect of a plastic adhesive, methyl 2-cyanoacrylate, on neural tissue. J. Neurosurg. *20*, 647, 1963.
49. Kline, D. G., and Hayes, G. J.: The use of a resorbable wrapper for peripheral nerve repair. J. Neurosurg. *21*, 737, 1964.
50. Knecht, C. D., and St. Clair, L. E.: The radial brachial paralysis syndrome in the dog. J.A.V.M.A. *154*, 653, 1969.
51. Larsen, R. D., and Posch, J. L.: Nerve injuries in the upper extremity. Arch. Surg. *77*, 469, 1958.
52. Lehman, R. A. W., and Hayes, G. J.: Degeneration and regeneration in peripheral nerves. Brain *90*, 285, 1967.
53. Liu, C. T., Benda, C. E., and Lewey, F. H.: Tensile strength of human nerves. Arch. Neurol. Psychiat. *59*, 322, 1948.
54. Marmor, L.: Regeneration of peripheral nerves

by irradiated homografts. J. Bone Joint Surg. *46A*, 383, 1964.
55. Marmor, L.: *Peripheral Nerve Regeneration Using Nerve Grafts.* Charles C Thomas, Springfield, Ill., 1967.
56. Matson, D. B., Alexander, E., Jr., and Weiss, P.: Experiments on the bridging of gaps in severed peripheral nerves of monkeys. J. Neurosurg. *5*, 230, 1948.
57. Midgley, R. D., and Woolhouse, F. M.: Silicone rubber sheathing as an adjunct to neural anastomosis. Surg. Clin. N. Amer. *48*, 1149, 1968.
58. Millesi, H.: Microsurgery of peripheral nerves. Hand *5*, 157, 1973.
59. Mullen, S.: *Essentials of Neurosurgery.* Springer Publishing Co., New York, 1961.
60. Murphey, F., and Kirklin, J.: Myelographic demonstration of avulsing injuries of the nerve roots of the brachial plexus: A method of determining the point of injury and the possibility of repair. Clin. Neurosurg. *20*, 18–28, 1973.
61. Naffziger, H. C.: Methods of secure end-to-end suture of peripheral nerves. Surg. Gynec. Obstet. *32*, 1921.
62. University of Michigan Medical Center, Department of Pathology: *Neuropathology.* Feb., 1964.
63. Pinner, B., and Campbell, J. B.: Identification of alkaline phosphatase at the node of Ranvier and incisures of Schmidt-Lantermann in normal and regenerating peripheral nerves. Proc. 5th Int. Congr. Neuropathol. Zurich, Sept. 1965. Excerpta Medica Int. Congr. Series *100*, Amsterdam, p. 871.
64. Pinner, B., Davison, J. F., and Campbell, J. B.: Alkaline phosphatase in peripheral nerves. Science *145*, 936, 1964.
65. Pinner-Poole, B., Tomasula, J. J., and Campbell, J. B.: Nerve suture and nerve grafts. Dixième Congres Soc. Intern. Chin. Orthop. Traum. Paris, Sept. 4, 1966, p. 782.
66. Poppen, J. L.: *An Atlas of Neurosurgical Techniques.* W. B. Saunders Co., Philadelphia, 1960.
67. Poth, E. J., Fernandez, E. B., and Drager, G. A.: Prevention of formation of end-bulb neuromata. Proc. Soc. Biol. Med. *60*, 200, 1945.
68. Rizzoli, H. V.: Treatment of peripheral nerve injuries. *In Neurological Surgery of Trauma.* U.S. Govt. Print. Off., Washington, D.C., 1965, p. 565.
69. Rowe, S. N.: The surgical treatment of nerve lesions. *In* Vinken, P. J., and Bruyn, G. W. (eds.): *Handbook of Clinical Neurology.* American Elsevier Publishing Co., Inc., New York, 1970, p. 513.
70. Saunders, F. K., and Young, J. Z.: The degeneration and reinnervation of grafted nerves. J. Anat. *76*, 143, 1942.
71. Saunders, F. K., and Young, J. Z.: The role of the peripheral stump in the control of fibre diameter in regenerating nerves. J. Physiol. *103*, 119, 1944.
72. Seddon, H. J.: The use of autogenous grafts for the repair of large gaps in peripheral nerves. Brit. J. Surg. *35*, 151, 1947.
73. Seddon, H. J.: Nerve grafting and other unusual forms of nerve repair. Medical Research Council Special Report Series, *282*, 389, 1954.
74. Seddon, H. J.: Nerve injuries. J. Univ. Mich. Med. Cen. *31*, 4, 1965.
75. Seddon, H. J.: *Surgical Disorders of the Peripheral Nerves.* The Williams and Wilkins Co., Baltimore, 1972.
76. Seletz, E.: *Surgery of Peripheral Nerves.* Charles C Thomas, Springfield, Ill., 1951.
77. Simpson, S. A., and Young, J. Z.: Regeneration of fibre diameter after cross unions of visceral and somatic nerves. J. Anat. *79*, 48, 1945.
78. Smith, J. W.: Microsurgery of peripheral nerves. Plast. Reconstr. Surg. *33*, 317, 1964.
79. Smith, J. W.: Factors influencing nerve repair. I. Blood supply of peripheral nerves. Arch. Surg. *93*, 335, 1966.
80. Smith, J. W., and Grabb, W. C. (eds.): *Plastic Surgery: A Concise Guide to Clinical Practice.* Little, Brown and Co., Boston, 1968, p. 716.
81. Smith, J. W.: Microsurgery of peripheral nerves. *In* Rand, R. W. (ed.): Microneurosurgery. C. V. Mosby Co., St. Louis, 1969, p. 64.
82. Snyder, C. C., Webster, H. D., Pickens, J. E., Hines, W. A., and Warden, G.: Intraneural neurorrhaphy: A preliminary clinical and histological evaluation. Ann. Surg. *167*, 691, 1968.
83. Spurling, R. G., and Woodhall, B.: Experiences with early nerve surgery in peripheral nerve injuries. Ann. Surg. *123*, 731, 1946.
84. Steindler, A.: Direct neurotization of paralyzed muscles: Further study of the question of direct nerve implantation. Amer. J. Orthop. Surg. *14*, 707, 1916.
85. Sunderland, S.: A classification of peripheral nerve injuries producing loss of function. Brain *74*, 491, 1951.
86. Sunderland, S.: Funicular suture and funicular exclusion in the repair of severed nerves. Brit. J. Surg. *40*, 580, 1953.
87. Sunderland, S.: Meningeal-neural relations in the intervertebral foramen. J. Neurosurg. *40*, 756, 1974.
88. Swaim, S. F.: Peripheral nerve surgery in the dog. J.A.V.M.A. *161*, 905, 1972.
89. Swaim, S. F.: Peripheral nervous system: Isolated peripheral nerves. *In* Bojrab, M. J. (ed.): *Current Techniques in Small Animal Surgery I.* Lea and Febiger, Philadelphia, 1975, p. 10.
90. Swaim, S. F.: Peripheral nerve surgery in the dog. Thesis (M.S.), Auburn University, Auburn, Ala., 1971.
91. Sweet, P. W.: The alcoholized nerve graft: An experimental study. Ann. Surg. *89*, 191, 1929.
92. Tarlov, I. M.: *Plasma Clot Suture of Peripheral Nerves and Nerve Roots.* Charles C Thomas, Springfield, Ill., 1950.
93. Tarlov, I. M., and Epstein, J. A.: Nerve grafts: The importance of an adequate blood supply. J. Neurosurg. *2*, 49, 1945.
94. Taurus, K., and Frackelton, W.: Silicone capping of nerve stumps in the problems of painful neuromas. Surg. Forum *18*, 504, 1967.
95. Terzis, J., Faibisoff, B., and Williams, H. B.: The nerve gap, suture under tension vs. graft. Plast. Reconstr. Surg. *56*, 1975.
96. Tsuge, K., Yoshikazu, I., and Sakaue, M.: A new technique for nerve suture: The anchoring funicular suture. Plast. Reconstr. Surg. *56*, 496, 1975.
97. Weiss, P.: The technology of nerve regeneration: a review. Sutureless tubulation and related

methods of nerve repair. J. Neurosurg. *1*, 400, 1944.
98. Weiss, P.: "Panta rhei"—and so flow our nerves. Amer. Sci. *57*, 287, 1969.
99. Weiss, P., Edds, M. V., and Cavanaugh, M.: The effect of terminal connections on the caliber of nerve fibers. Anat. Rec. *92*, 215, 1945.
100. Weiss, P., and Hiscoe, H. B.: Experiments on the mechanism of nerve growth. J. Exp. Zool. *107*, 315, 1948.
101. Weiss, P., and Taylor, A. C.: Repair of peripheral nerves by grafts of frozen-dried nerve. Proc. Soc. Exp. Biol. Med. *52*, 326, 1943.
102. Woodruff, M. F. A.: *The Transplantation of Tissues and Organs.* Charles C Thomas, Springfield, Ill., 1960.
103. Young, J. Z., Holmes, W., and Saunders, F. K.: Nerve regeneration: Importance of the peripheral stump and the value of nerve grafts. Lancet, *239*, 128, 1940.
104. Zacnary, R. B., and Roaf, R.: Lesions in continuity. Medical Research Council Special Report Series *282*, 57, 1954.

PART FOUR

THE CENTRAL NERVOUS SYSTEM IN GENERAL

In this part, an effort will be made to deal with those disorders that do or can involve both the spinal cord and the brain. Chapter 11 deals with the infectious diseases caused by viruses, bacteria, and parasitic, protozoan, and mycotic microorganisms. In addition, the cerebrovascular, neoplastic, congenital-hereditary and degenerative disorders, and those disorders caused by toxic agents are also presented. Chapter 12 deals with CNS injuries or trauma. The various CNS disorders involving the spinal column and skull abnormalities, compressions, epilepsy, hydrocephalus, and other CNS diseases are dealt with elsewhere in the text.

CHAPTER 11

PRIMARY DISORDERS OF THE CENTRAL NERVOUS SYSTEM

B. F. HOERLEIN, D.V.M., PH.D.*
MARC VANDEVELDE, D.V.M.

MICROBIAL INFECTIOUS DISEASES

Infectious diseases involving the central nervous system can constitute a sizable portion of a total small animal practice. Statistics from the 1974–75 annual report of the Small Animal Teaching Hospital at Auburn University show that, of a total of 15,012 sick animals, 1156 (7.7 per cent) had disorders that involved the nervous system. Of 2234 cases of infection involving all systems 214, or 9.6 per cent, involved the nervous system; there were disorders caused by infectious microorganisms such as viruses, bacteria, protozoan, and mycotic organisms. Of all sick animals admitted (15,012), 214, or 1.4 per cent, had infectious diseases of the nervous system. During 1975–76, 24 per cent of those dogs with CNS disorders who died or were destroyed were affected with infectious diseases involving primarily the brain.

VIRAL DISEASES

There has been a tremendous recent interest in the relationship between the acute and the chronic, slow, or latent virus infections. The most important contributions in human medicine in this area have been the experimental transmission of Kurn disease and Creutzfeldt-Jakob disease to subhuman primates and the isolation of measles virus from brain biopsy specimens of patients with subacute sclerosing panencephalitis.[108] Since measles and distemper viruses are related immunologically, there may be many zoonotic implications from the developments.

The well-established "slow" virus diseases in animals are scrapie and visna in sheep, lymphocytic choriomeningitis in mice, Aleutian disease in mink, and transmissible mink encephalopathy which can infect numerous animals.[108] Recent evidence has established that canine distemper can appear as a slow virus in old dog encephalitis.[141, 233] In the future the etiology of many diseases in the chronic neuropathies may have to be revised.[152, 168, 237]

Canine Distemper

Canine distemper is beyond a doubt the most common disease of dogs. In the Au-

*Ocular fundic photos courtesy of Dr. R. A. Albert.

burn annual diagnostic report for 1968–69, 127 cases of distemper were seen in approximately 16,000 accessions. The same report showed that distemper vaccines were administered in 1873 cases. In contrast, in the year 1975–76, 90 cases of distemper were seen among a total of 16,152 nonsurgical accessions (0.6 per cent). Distemper is caused by a pantropic paramyxovirus that affects all body tissues. It is a highly contagious disease, and can be spread via air or infective excretions. The incubation period is 4 to 6 days. So-called hard pad disease, which is characterized by a persistent fever, hyperkeratosis, sloughing of the foot pads, and convulsions, is considered to be another manifestation of the virus of Carré. Clinically, distemper affects the respiratory, ocular, and nervous systems most frequently. Nervous symptoms may follow respiratory signs.[4] However, in dogs who have been vaccinated but have inadequate immunity, respiratory signs may be very transient or imperceptible to the owner; nervous signs predominate.[223]

Neurological signs can appear as: neuritis; weakness; posterior incoordination; choreiform muscle spasms; rolling, circling, and falling to one side; tilting the head; and convulsions. These may be either acute or latent manifestations and may appear months to years later. Distemper myelitis should be suspected in any dog, young or old, vaccinated or nonvaccinated, when signs of posterior weakness and a swaggering gait are seen. Choreiform muscle spasms or myoclonus are nearly pathognomonic for the clinical diagnosis of distemper. The cause of distemper myoclonus has experimentally been shown to be primarily a disease of the spinal cord. The maintenance of myoclonus is not dependent upon higher centers, but it can be modified by their activity.[24] The establishment of a diagnosis of nervous distemper necessitates securing a careful history and considering the possible presence of hepatitis, mycoses, toxoplasmosis, ticks, or mild compressions.

The clinical diagnosis may be aided by a careful ocular fundic examination. The presence of diffuse or "patchy" areas of hyperreflectivity and bright colored "medallion" lesions indicative of chorioretinitis is characteristic of viral infections, especially distemper. These lesions may indicate a past or latent infection[121] (Fig. 11–1). (See also Chapter 18.)

The electroencephalographic (EEG) tracing of a viral disease such as distemper may be characteristic in some phases or stages of the disease (see Chapter 7). Positive fundic lesions coupled with a characteristic EEG tracing (if such equipment is available) can

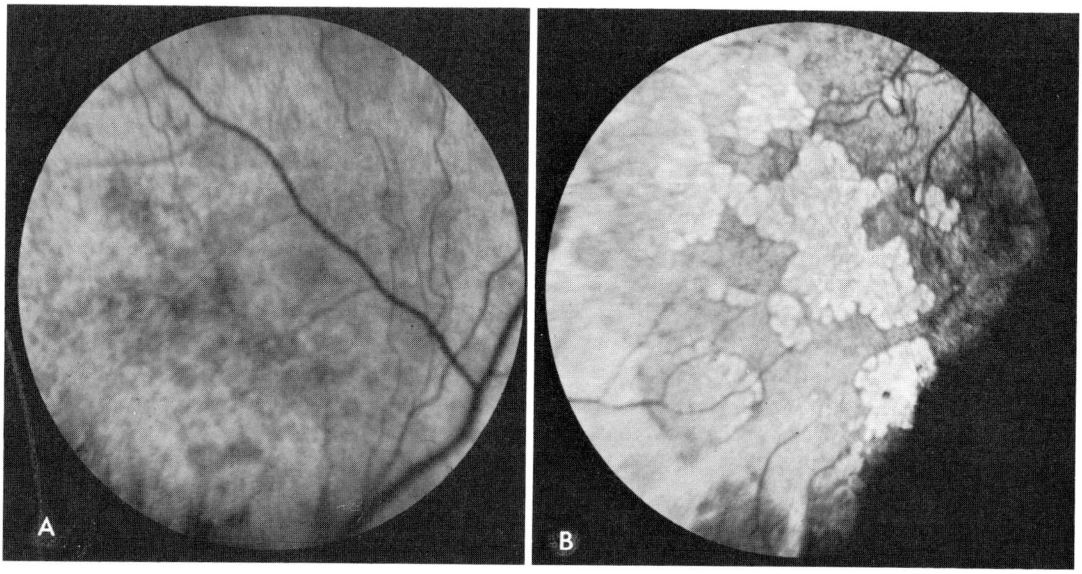

FIGURE 11–1 *A*, This is a confirmed case of active distemper retinitis. Note the irregular borders of the lesions that are characteristic of the early stages of distemper. *B*, Chronic chorioretinitis in a dog that had had respiratory distemper 4 months previously. The predominant clinical sign at that time was a posterior weakness. Note the hyperreflective lesions that have smooth and slightly pigmented borders.

be practical aids in the clinical diagnosis of distemper. Radiographic examinations are helpful in establishing the absence of some compressive lesions, especially in the spine, that could account for the clinical signs.[103]

Routine hemogram, kidney and liver function tests, and cerebrospinal fluid examinations may also be helpful in establishing a diagnosis of distemper. Laboratory aids in diagnosis may depend on the in vivo demonstration of inclusion bodies in nasal, tracheal, bronchial, conjunctival, tongue, vaginal, or urethral epithelial cells. Cello has demonstrated eosinophilic bodies in circulating neutrophils up to 6 weeks after the onset of signs. Since the life span of a neutrophil is only 8 to 9 days, there must be a continuous source of virus.[34]

Since inclusion bodies may occur in animals which have had subclinical or latent distemper and in recently vaccinated animals, the clinical picture must be evaluated as a whole before a positive diagnosis is established. Elevated serum antibody titers can be expected 2 to 3 weeks after onset of disease and are therefore of little use in the diagnosis of the acute case. The use of the immunofluorescence test for the presence of viral antigen (FA test) in many types of tissue cells is an important clinical diagnostic aid. The FA test is positive in recently vaccinated animals.[88] Necropsy diagnosis is made upon demonstration of intracytoplasmic inclusion bodies in the visceral epithelium or either intracytoplasmic or intranuclear inclusions in the central nervous system and demyelinization of the brain and spinal cord.[116]

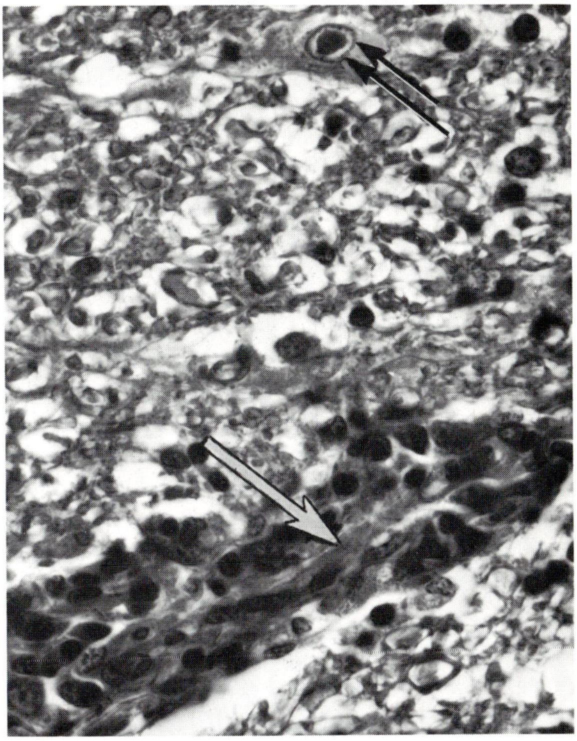

FIGURE 11–3 Acute canine distemper encephalitis. White matter in the spinal cord shows a disorganized appearance of the myelin. Note the perivascular mononuclear infiltrate (arrow) and intranuclear inclusion body (double arrow). Hematoxylin and eosin, high power.

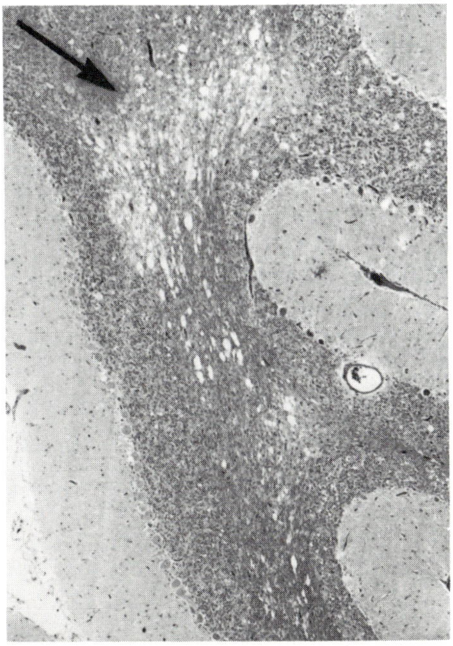

FIGURE 11–2 Canine distemper encephalitis produces this typical lesion in the cerebellum. Note the area of necrosis in the white matter (arrow). Hematoxylin and eosin, low power magnification.

Pathologically, the distemper encephalitis has many variations.[58] The majority of the cases, however, are characterized by multifocal lesions, especially those involving the white matter of the brain and spinal cord, that result in demyelination. Lesions are most consistently found in the cerebellopontine angle, the cerebral peduncles, optic tracts, and the spinal cord. The demyelinating lesions are accompanied by inflammatory infiltrates and progressive changes of the glial cells. Intranuclear and intracytoplasmic viral inclusion bodies are seen in nearly all cases (Figs. 11–2 and 11–3).

Treatment

There is no specific treatment for nervous distemper. Most treatments that have been proposed have in time been discredited. Some clinicians feel that the intravenous administration of the tissue culture–modified, live virus distemper or distemper, hepatitis vaccine in the viremic stage of the disease is effective. Most clinicians routinely use injectable B-complex and C vitamins coupled with a broad spectrum antibiotic such as chloramphenicol. An additional intravenous injection of sulfadimethoxine (Symbio) has been advocated.[214] When encephalitis is evident clinically or is suggested by the EEG, it is recommended that anticonvulsants be started immediately in an effort to prevent a convulsive syndrome. Anticonvulsants should be continued for several months after apparent recovery.[103]

Prevention

The accepted methods of vaccination of puppies against distemper are more firmly established now than at any time in the history of veterinary medicine. Since maternal passive antibodies are acquired by the puppy from an immune bitch, active immunizing agents will be partially or completely ineffective if used at an early age. Ideally, the normogram of the pregnant bitch before whelping will indicate the ideal time for active immunization of the puppy. When a normogram is not possible, opinions still vary as to the proper time for vaccination during the nursing stage or shortly thereafter.

The use of measles vaccine in the nursing puppy or in the presence of maternal antibody interference has been proposed. However, the efficacy of measles vaccine has been questioned, and the possible occurrence of measles virus in slow viral diseases of man and animals makes one reluctant to recommend its widespread use. The American Veterinary Medical Association panel on immunization procedures recommends the use of modified live virus (MLV) vaccine of chick embryo or tissue cell culture origins for best results.[228, 229] It should be given as soon after weaning as possible and repeated between 12 and 16 weeks of age. An alternate and probably the most effective method is to administer the vaccine every 2 weeks until the puppy is 16 weeks of age. Most veterinarians suggest a booster shot annually or anytime the dog is taken into a high exposure situation.

CHRONIC PROGRESSIVE FORMS OF DISTEMPER

In the dog, encephalitides with an atypical and protracted clinical course have been recognized by most investigators of canine distemper. The clinical signs in such cases often include gradual loss of mentality, paresis, incoordination, blindness, convulsions, and myoclonic seizures. The clinical course extends usually over several weeks and months. Cordy[40] described the so-called old dog encephalitis (ODE) in mature animals, which is clinically and pathologically different from common distemper encephalitis. Recently (1972), Lincoln and coworkers demonstrated distemper virus antigen in the brain of two ODE cases by means of immunofluorescence techniques.[141, 142] Van Bogaert and Innes[116] described diffuse subacute sclerosing panencephalitis (SSPE) in the dog, which probably is the same entity as old dog encephalitis. Chronic progressive forms of distemper encephalitis with massive necrosis and sclerosis of the cerebrum were observed by Vandevelde *et al.*[223] These authors also found evidence that protracted distemper infection in the CNS might be related to the inflammatory reticulosis (Fig. 11–4).

Since both clinical and pathological findings in all these forms of chronic progressive distemper encephalitis are very different from the classical form of distemper, it is reasonable to postulate a different type of pathogenesis in these cases. One might assume that particular strains of distemper virus could be responsible for chronic progressive encephalitis. This appears possible in view of findings that different laboratory strains of distemper show considerable differences in their behavior in cell culture and their ultrastructural characteristics.[38] However, attempts to isolate virus from cases of old dog encephalitis have been unsuccessful so far. It is possible that once the special techniques used in isolation of the human SSPE virus are applied, a virus will be isolated. Transmission experiments could then demonstrate whether the virus

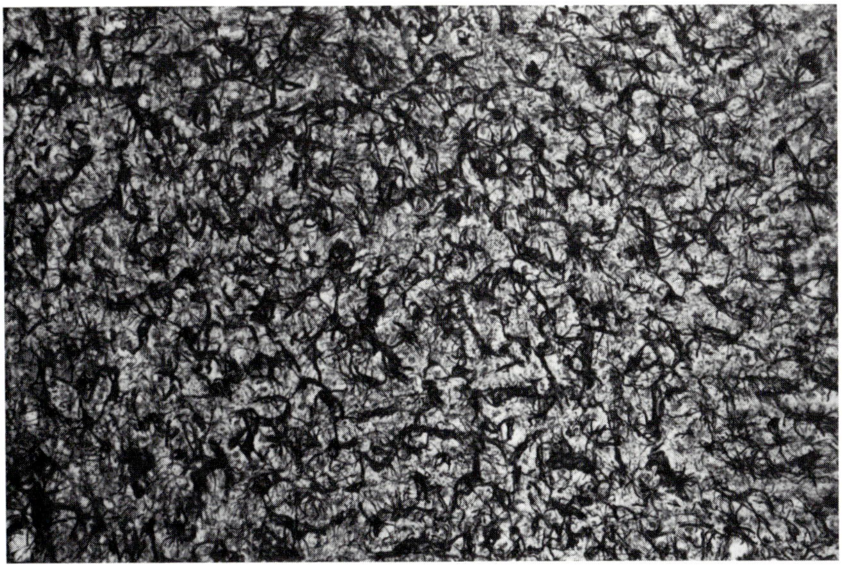

FIGURE 11–4 Chronic progressive distemper encephalitis. Note the diffuse fibrillary astrogliosis in the cerebral cortex. (Maurer stain for astrocytes, medium power.)

itself could produce chronic progressive lesions in a normal animal. On the other hand, it is very possible that special aberrations of the reactive mechanisms in the individual animal infected with a common distemper strain result in an atypical encephalitis.

The relationship between chronic distemper and SSPE in man is a pertinent and important possible zoonotic consideration. Subacute sclerosing panencephalitis is a lethal disease in man caused by a measles-like paramyxovirus.[108] Since the distemper virus is antigenetically related to the measles virus,[114, 238] it is logical to speculate on the possible similarities in pathogenesis of human SSPE and chronic progressive distemper encephalitis. Clinical points of similarity are the protracted clinical course, the progression of the neurological signs, and the demonstration of exceedingly high antibody titers in the blood and CSF. Pathologically, the lesions in the brain (especially the excessive proliferation of astrocytes) are similar in some cases of chronic distemper to those in human SSPE. In neither disease can the virus be isolated by conventional techniques. The pathogenesis of SSPE is largely unknown. Transmission experiments with SSPE virus in a range of animal species have provided useful information on the nature of the virus but failed to reproduce the typical clinical as well as the pathological features of spontaneous human SSPE. It is obvious therefore that the study of the chronic progressive distemper encephalitis might be extremely useful for the comparative study of SSPE in man.

Rabies

Rabies is a disease caused by a neurotropic rhabdovirus that affects all mammals. It is said that 90 per cent of human rabies is acquired from the dog. The disease causes an acute encephalomyelitis and is characterized by intracytoplasmic inclusions called Negri bodies found predominantly in neurons of the hippocampus. Clinically, rabies is typically divided into dumb and furious forms. Besides changes in temperament, it involves bulbar and spinal paralysis that affects the jaw and limb musculature, respectively. Death generally occurs within 10 days of the first symptoms.[213]

Through effective vaccination programs in dogs, human rabies from dogs has in recent years been largely eliminated. However, the incidence of rabies in wild animals and in bats in certain areas of the country has been considerable and a cause of great concern for animal and human health. In Greene County, Tennessee, a rabies out-

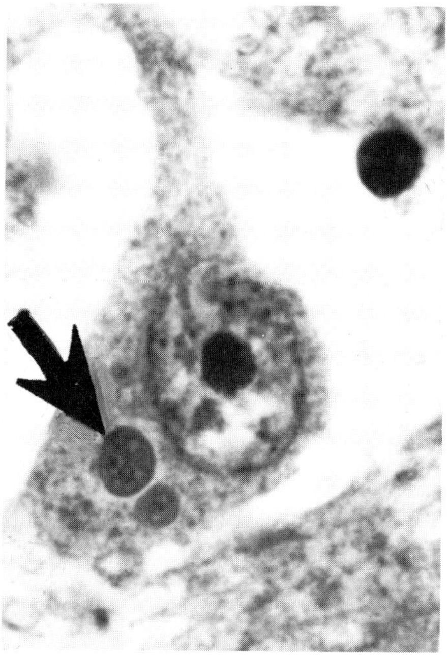

FIGURE 11–5 Rabies. The neuron in the Ammon's horn shows intracytoplasmic viral inclusions, or Negri bodies (arrow). Hematoxylin and eosin, high power.

break in 1964 forced grammar schools to convene late in the morning so that the children would not be so vulnerable to attacks by rabid wild animals while waiting for buses. According to the U.S. Public Health Communicable Disease Center, the incidence of rabies in dogs has dropped from 5688 cases in 1953 to 296 cases in 1968. During the same period, the cases in skunks increased from 319 to 1400 and in bats from 8 in 1953 to 291 in 1968. In man, 14 cases were seen in 1953 and 1 in 1968.[208]

Rabies encephalitis in the dog is characterized by inflammatory lesions, mainly localized in the brain stem, and massive degenerative lesions in the neurons, such as neuronophagia, nodular and diffuse gliosis, and perivascular mononuclear infiltrations. Characteristic intracytoplasmic viral inclusion bodies (Negri bodies) are found especially in the neurons of the Ammon's horn and the Purkinje cells of the cerebellum.[58] Negri bodies, however, are not present in all cases, and the most reliable diagnostic methods depend on immunofluorescence techniques (Fig. 11–5).

Treatment

Treatment is generally not attempted in the dog because of the possible consequences to public health. Rabies is usually considered to be a fatal disease in man, but there is some evidence that animals may sometimes recover.[26, 216] Prophylaxis after exposure usually consists of inoculations of serum or vaccine, or both.

Prevention in Animals

Because of the availability of the various modified live virus (MLV) vaccines, the use of the old inactivated tissue vaccines has largely been discontinued. The MLV tissue culture or chick embryo vaccines are highly effective in control, and there is little or no chance of postvaccinal reactions. Chick embryo origin vaccine occasionally has produced allergic reactions in animals that are sensitive to egg products. Of 500,000 dogs vaccinated with chick embryo origin antirabies vaccine in the state of New York, anaphylactic shock was seen in nine cases. Recovery usually occurred without treatment or after treatment with epinephrine or antihistamines.[11] Other reports of reactions have been rare.[136]

The World Health Organization in 1960 recommended the use of low egg passage (LEP) vaccines (Flury) for dogs and of high egg passage (HEP) (Flurry) or inactivated vaccines for cats. Cabasso found HEP vaccines effective in cats.[29] Recently, modified live viral high and low passage tissue culture vaccines have been introduced, and some of these are recommended for dogs and cats alike. It is suggested that manufacturers' recommendations be used carefully in administration of the tissue culture vaccines.

Aujeszky's Disease (Pseudorabies, "Mad Itch")

Aujeszky's disease is caused by a DNA virus of the herpes group. It occurs naturally in cattle, sheep, dogs, cats, rats, and swine. In all but adult swine, it is a highly fatal disease. Affected cattle, dogs, or cats usually develop intense pruritus in localized areas of skin. Bouts of frenzy and self-mutilation occur as the infection ascends the nervous system via the peripheral nerves, ganglia, spinal cord, medulla oblongata, and brain. The course of the disease is short, and death occurs within 24 to 48 hours after the appearance of paralysis. The signs that tend to distinguish Aujeszky's disease from rabies are the shorter course of disease, the presence of pruritus, and the lack of aggressive attacks on man or on other animals.[88, 116]

On several occasions, this disease has occurred in dogs that have been around infected cattle. In one necropsy series of 900 animals, 39 dogs and 8 cats were infected with the disease. In a kennel of dogs in Sweden which were fed swine offal, 14 of 45 dogs died of pseudorabies.[113] Consumption of dead suckling pigs or diseased porcine or bovine organs and the presence of the brown rat in the infected areas have been the means of spreading the infection.[26, 53, 101, 205] In dogs and cats the Aujeszky virus causes an acute polioencephalitis which is located in the lower brain stem and involves especially the nuclei of the fifth to the seventh and eighth nerves. The lesions are characterized by perivascular mononuclear infiltrations, nodular gliosis with microabscess formation, and intranuclear eosinophilic viral inclusion bodies.[56]

Treatment and Prevention

There is no commercial vaccine available in this country. Isolation of infected animals, proper handling of dead animals, and destruction of the rat population constitute a means of control. No fatalities in humans have been reported, but several human cases have been reported in Europe. Precautions should be used in handling diseased animals or tissues.

In a reported outbreak in Russia, ten dogs died within 7 days. The remaining seven dogs in the kennel, who were treated with immune serum, methenamine, and a vaccine, remained healthy.[26, 101]

Herpes Canis

The canine herpesvirus causes a fatal septicemic disease of infant puppies, most commonly between the first and third weeks of life. Six-week-old puppies are remarkedly resistant to various modes of experimental infection.[254] The syndrome causes crying, diarrhea, dyspnea, colic, depression, and death in 1 to 3 days. Congestion and focal necrosis in the lung, liver, kidney, and brain are characteristic necropsy lesions. When suckling puppies were artificially infected via the nose and mouth, CNS lesions were seen within 72 hours. Disseminated nonsuppurative encephalomyelitis and ganglioneuritis with destruction of gray and white matter were prominent. British workers have associated the virus with abortions, stillbirths, and infertility in a kennel of Alsatians.[187] Death is so rapid that no mode of treatment other than supportive has been suggested.[32, 184, 253]

Feline Infectious Peritonitis in Cats

Recently several reports have been published on CNS lesions in cats suffering from feline infectious peritonitis.[61, 211] In the clinical brain and eye form of this disease, nonspecific gastrointestinal signs were observed in most cases. However, abundant peritoneal effusion typical of conventional feline infectious peritonitis is usually lacking.[211] The combination of encephalitic signs with bilateral endogenous granulomatous uveitis is indicative of this disease.

Pathologically, severe inflammatory lesions associated with the CSF pathways are present. A pyogranulomatous meningitis and ependymitis are characteristic, and hydrocephalus can result from obstructive lesions[61] (Fig. 11–6).

Other Viruses

Stone[221] has recently concluded that, based on serological evidence, herpes simplex is a possible cause of encephalitis in the adult dog. Based on the study of 11 cases of varied CNS disorders, he also felt that a clinical degenerative encephalitic process "with or without hemorrhage and vascular changes" occurs in the aged dog. Of ten cases involving CNS disturbance, Stone and Fox[222] demonstrated serological evidence of mumps in two cases. In random examination of 42 clinically normal dogs, two showed elevated serum titers for mumps virus. Four other dogs with various clinical disorders had elevated titers for mumps, which receded when the dogs recovered. It was postulated that mumps or

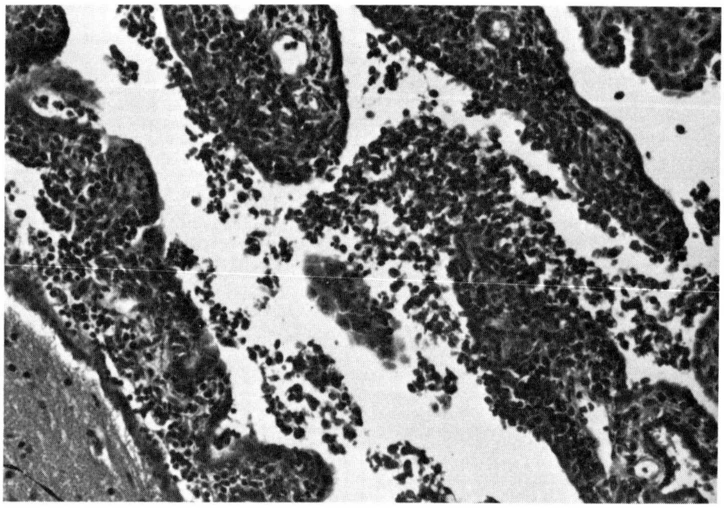

FIGURE 11-6 Feline infectious peritonitis. Note the marked infiltration of inflammatory cells in the choroid plexus of the fourth ventricle. Hematoxylin and eosin, medium power.

related myxoviruses may be implicated in some cases of atypical encephalitis. It is most likely, in view of these observations, that there is a variety of unknown infectious agents which are responsible for sporadically occurring cases of encephalomyelitis. Of all cases diagnosed pathologically as encephalomyelitis in the Auburn small animal hospital, approximately 15 per cent cannot be classified in one of the known etiological categories.

Postvaccination Reactions

Postvaccination rabies paralysis is a disseminated encephalomyelitis of the demyelinating type. It is a marked allergic reaction caused by phenolized brain tissue vaccine and has been reproduced experimentally.[118] This disorder is now of mainly historical interest, because the use of this vaccine has been largely replaced by the chick embryo or tissue culture–modified live virus (MLV) vaccine. Mass inoculation clinics may still use the killed tissue vaccine since it does not need reconstituting and is therefore more convenient. However, MLV vaccines, which have not caused this disorder and provide more effective immunity, should be used for the dog.

The onset of signs generally occurs 2 to 3 weeks after inoculation. Posterior weakness and incoordination may ascend the cord until a total tetraplegia and death finally result.

The treatment is symptomatic. Frequent drainage of the urinary bladder is necessary. Antibiotics to prevent secondary infections and anti-inflammatory agents such as the adrenocorticoid hormones are indicated. Antihistamines have been used.[138] Many workers feel that the disease is an allergic encephalopathy and that antiallergic agents might be indicated. Vandevelde[232] reported three dogs with severe disseminated polioencephalitis which was localized largely to the caudal portion of the brain stem, where tissue culture live rabies vaccine had been given. Severe clinical disease was produced. This number of cases is very small considering the large number inoculated; however, the authors felt that the disease might have been caused by the vaccine virus.[232]

Fankhauser and co-workers[57] have reported atrophy of the Purkinje cells in three of six puppies given tissue culture measles vaccine for protection against distemper at 6 weeks of age. The dogs became clinically ill with ataxia, intention tremors, and characteristic signs of cerebellar dysfunction 5 days after immunization. No evidence of distemper infection was seen histologically.[57]

Other vaccine reactions of various kinds have been reported in the literature. The postvaccination rabies paralysis has been the most serious clinical syndrome in the past. If a live vaccine is used, there is always a chance that it will become an active pathogen.

Feline Panleukopenia and Other Viral Cerebellar Atrophies

Cerebellar atrophy hypoplasia, or agenesis, can be caused by one of a group of parvoviruses, such as feline panleukopenia virus, rat virus, and porcine parvovirus, all of which induce natural infections. The panleukopenia virus apparently causes a usually mild infection in mother cats, but the virus passes through the placenta and destroys the external germinal layer of the developing cerebellum so effectively that the kittens develop severe ataxia at 3 to 4 weeks of age. These kittens can become carriers of the virus for weeks or even months after birth. The intrauterine infection generally occurs in the third trimester but can also occur shortly after the birth of the kittens. The rat virus also affects rat fetuses late in pregnancy, and ataxia is evident later in life. Experimental inoculation of rat virus into intrauterine or newborn kittens, hamster, and ferrets produces the same disorder. Damage from the panleukopenia virus is thought to be caused by a selective affinity of the virus for cells with active deoxyribonucleic acid (DNA) synthesis affecting mitosis. Eosinophilic nuclear inclusions have been seen by the eighth day, and cytopathic effects progressed to necrotic foci, particularly in the Purkinje cells, in 14 to 21 days. Virus titers were present only in the cerebellum[127] (Fig. 11–7).

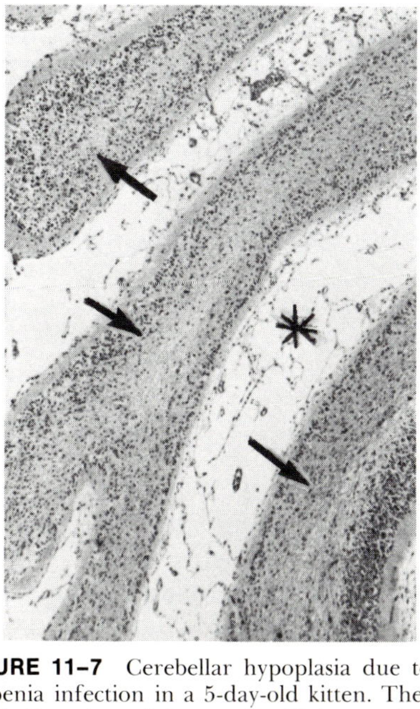

FIGURE 11–7 Cerebellar hypoplasia due to panleukopenia infection in a 5-day-old kitten. There is a marked distention of the arachnoidal space (asterisk) due to atrophy of the cerebellar folia. Note the absence of an external granular cell layer and the extreme hypocellularity of the internal granular cell layer (arrows). Hematoxylin and eosin, low power.

Clinically, these observations are confirmed when a whole litter of kittens or most of its members show ataxia at an early age. The necropsy data and histopathological signs of this illness are similar to those reported by Kilham. Therefore, it is felt that cerebellar hypoplasia is generally caused by an intrauterine or neonatal infection from panleukopenia virus and is not always a hereditary disease as thought formerly.[127]

BACTERIAL DISEASES

Bacterial Meningitis

Meningitis very frequently accompanies any traumatic or septic condition of the central nervous system. This discussion will be confined to the septic inflammation of the leptomeninges. There are three principal ways in which the leptomeninges may become infected. They are (1) traumatic injury and penetrating wounds, (2) extension of a pre-existing pyogenic infection from a focus close to or continuous with the CNS, and (3) infection through the blood stream.[14] Since dogs and cats are not subject to contagious bacterial meningeal disease such as the meningococcus that affects humans, the third method of infection is not frequently encountered. Meningitis resulting from fulminating or neglected otitis, sinusitis, rhinitis, and panophthalmitis occurs. Traumatic injuries and the resulting septic contamination of the CNS are frequently encountered. Contamination during surgery of the CNS and careless spinal taps or tail docks can also cause septic meningitis. Almost any pathogenic bacterium or mycotic organism may be involved.[134]

A recent case report of meningitis in a cat stated that the isolated organism resembled *Flavobacterium meningosepticum.* The cat was 9 months of age and was suddenly afflicted with hyperesthesia, incoordination, partial blindness, and depressed photomotor reflexes. There was no pyrexia. The cat recovered after treatment with chloramphenicol and diligent supportive care.[210]

The clinical signs of septic meningitis in cats may not be as dramatic as those commonly seen in humans. Pyrexia is generally moderate. Hyperesthesia, pain, muscular rigidity and periodic spasms, and occasional pupillary or optic disk changes occur. Acute meningitis may cause vomiting and convulsions.

The diagnosis is based on a history of trauma or existing septic disorder and the examination and culture of spinal fluid. The treatment consists of proper management of the cause of the sepsis, such as repair of a traumatic defect, appropriate treatment of the focus of infection. The appropriate antibiotic or antibacterial agent should be used, based on the identification of the causative organism.

Inflammatory meningitis resulting from the use of radiographic contrast media was discussed in Chapters 5 and 14.

CNS Abscesses

Brain abscesses occur in dogs but are frequently undiagnosed. The Auburn clinic diagnosed two clinical cases during 1968 by means of electroencephalography and radiography. During 1975, four brain abscesses were diagnosed on necropsy out of 300 cases of CNS disease examined pathologically. These can develop from extensions of infections in septic meningitis, or from metastases through blood or lymph channels. Allen, reporting on 38 brain abscesses in man, indicated that the reason 37 per cent died was that there was a delay in diagnosis and proper treatment. Twenty-five per cent of the patients had paresis or seizures as associated symptoms.[5]

The diagnosis of brain abscesses may depend on physical signs correlated with the history, increased cerebrospinal fluid (CSF) pressure, increased CSF cell counts (particularly neutrophils), and protein present in CSF. Contrast radiography and EEG findings have been helpful in some cases.

Treatment consists of surgical drainage, antibiotic therapy, or both. In dogs, the ears, eyes, and sinuses should be examined as possible foci of infection and should be treated accordingly.[5]

Tuberculosis

Canine tuberculosis is infrequently seen in the United States, but necropsy data from Europe show an incidence of 0.83 to 5.6 per cent.[116] Dogs are susceptible to both human and bovine types of infections.

The alimentary tract is most frequently affected; however, cases with dissemination have been seen. Hjärre found only four cases of meningitis in a series of 175 necropsies.[100]

Osteomyelitis, Septic Spondylitis, Discospondylitis

Osteomyelitis of the vertebrae is seen occasionally in the dog. Metastatic infections to the vertebrae most frequently are blood-borne, and some have developed from urinary infections.[126] Metastatic infections are frequently seen subsequent to vertebral trauma that has caused tissue devitalization. In dogs, osteomyelitis is generally encountered in a fight wound or in an infection carried into the area by a grass awn or other foreign body. The presence of a fistula or recurrent abscess is typical. Neurological signs characteristic of meningitis or local compression myelitis are frequent encountered. The most useful means of diagnosis is radiography.

The radiological signs of osteomyelitis vary not only in degree of infection and individual tissue response to it, but also according to the etiological agent or organism involved. Evidence of cortical destruction may be present. New bone production overlying and surrounding the area of infection produces a "moth-eaten" appearance. This process is fairly smooth, and lacks the usual rough, irregular, and wild appearance of a neoplasm. Surrounding the area of cortical destruction is a zone of increased density called sclerosis, which is probably comparable to the abscess wall in soft tissues and which results from the attempt to confine the infection.[31]

It should be emphasized that numerous

organisms can be incriminated as causes of osteomyelitis. The usual bacteria that cause suppuration are frequently encountered; mycotic organisms such as coccidioides, blastomycoses, and cryptococci may invade the bone either through a wound or by other means; tuberculosis of the spine has been reported in the dog.[166] Any one of these infections is capable of invading vertebral or cranial bone, causing a compression and subsequent pathologic lesions of the CNS (Figs. 11-8 to 11-12).

Specific infections in other species have been described as causes of vertebral diseases. Brucella and erysipelas infections in swine have caused septic spondylitis. Grabel and workers[78] gave the term "discospondylitis" to the lesion caused by erysipelas, and Schnelle[203] has used this term in disorders with similar radiographic signs in dogs. The author of this book has seen septic lesions of the disk, cartilaginous plates, and epiphyses occur when surgical disk fenestrations were accompanied by contamination. Sclerosis of the epiphyses of adjoining bodies, perarticular exostosis, and collapsed intervertebral spaces were present.

Canine brucellosis caused by *Brucella canis* has been recognized in recent years as an infection associated largely with abortion, lymphadenitis, epididymitis, and testicular atrophy. It is a highly contagious genital disease, especially in breeding kennels. A recent report by Henderson and coworkers[97] presents evidence that discospondylitis with spinal cord compression can be caused by *Brucella canis.* Three cases were reported and several others have been seen since the report was published. Two of the three dogs were treated surgically by cord decompression and curettage of the lesion, followed by 30 days of tetracycline therapy. Both dogs regained normal health and displayed receding *Brucella canis* titers after therapy. All three dogs were males, and in two the organism was cultured from the testes as well as from the vertebral lesions.[97] Ampicillin and streptomycin have also been advocated as treatment. Since *Brucella canis* infection has been reported in five persons up to 1973, the human health aspects should be considered in these dogs[139, 140] (Figs. 11-13 to 11-15).

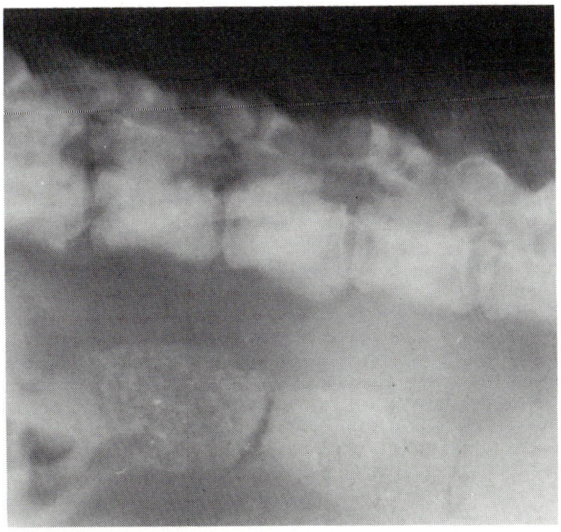

FIGURE 11-8 The osteomyelitis of the lumbar vertebrae in this dog was due to *Actinomyces* organisms. Bilateral fistulae in the flanks were observed, as well as a paraplegia. (Hoerlein, B. F.: Clinical spinal conditions in the dog. Vet. Med. *51*, 576, 1956.)

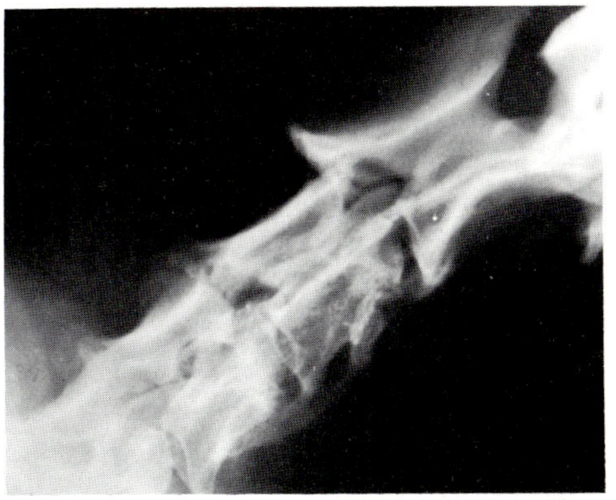

FIGURE 11-9 Osteomyelitis of the third and fourth cervical vertebrae was caused by pyogenic bacteria. The infection was introduced by a large stick which had lodged in the area and was not recognized as the source of the infection.

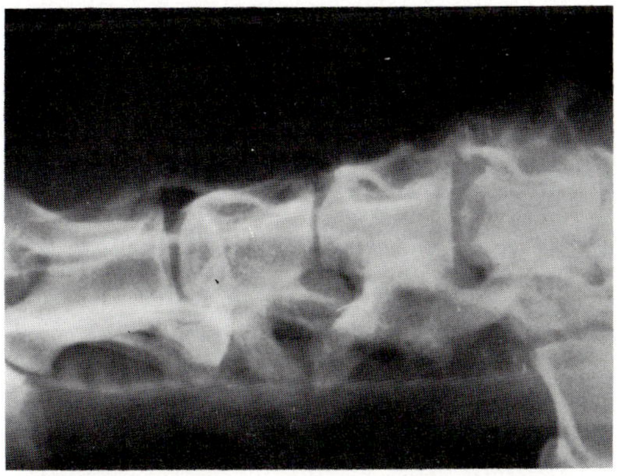

FIGURE 11-10 A ventrodorsal view of the case shown in Figure 11-9. Notice the proliferation of bone.

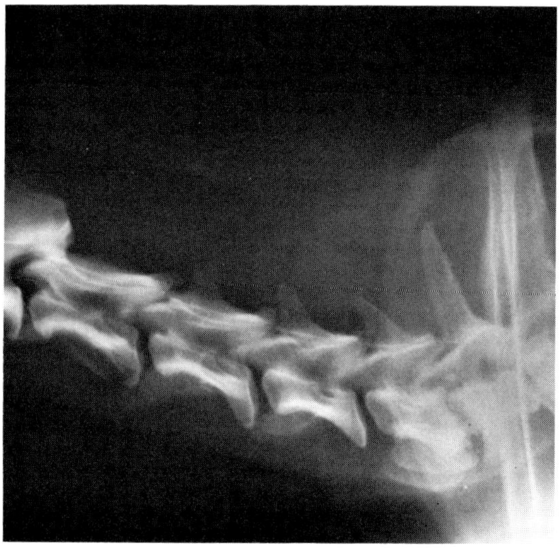

FIGURE 11–11 An osteomyelitis of the sixth and seventh cervical vertebrae. Notice the proliferation of bone on the vertebral bodies and in the spinal canal.

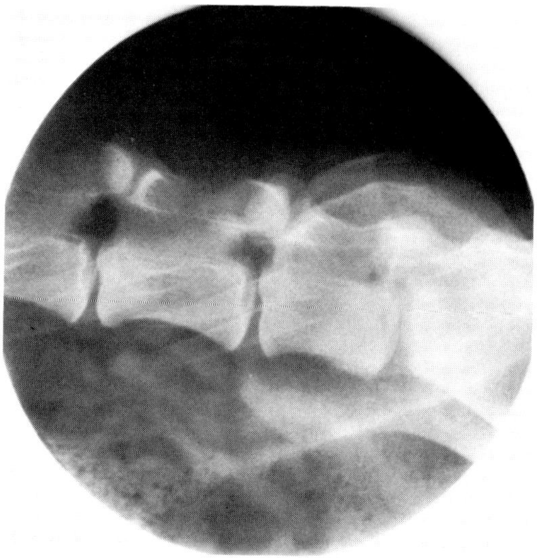

FIGURE 11–13 A case of confirmed canine brucellosis causing spinal pain and a posterior paresis. Notice the diskospondylitis at L7–S1 and the massive proliferation and destruction of tissue. A dorsal laminectomy was performed, the compressive mass was removed, and curettage of the lesion was done. *Brucella canis* was isolated in pure culture from the spinal lesion and a testicle. The titer (agglutination) was 1:200.

In *Spirocerra lupi* infection, a localized spondylitic exostosis occurs adjacent to the esophageal and other visceral lesions. There is evidence that larval migration in the vertebral periosteum may result in deformative ossifying inflammation of the vertebrae in this area.

Treatment

The basis of treatment is bone curettage and antibiotic therapy. Bacteriological cultures of the infected tissue and antibiotic sensitivity of determinations are useful in the selection of an antibiotic. The surgeon should remove as much pathologic tissue as possible and endeavor to promote fusion or arthrodesis. However, in advanced cases of vertebral osteomyelitis, the need to preserve neurological function may mean that only partial curettage of affected tissue can

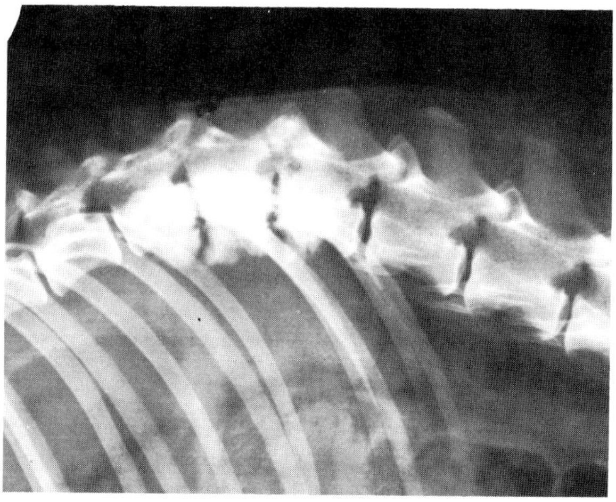

FIGURE 11–12 Diskospondylitis of T12, T13, and L1 vertebrae. This infection resulted from surgical disk curettage with unproperly sterilized instruments. (Hoerlein, B. F.: Clinical spinal radiography in the dog. J.A.V.M.A. *134*, 343, 1959.)

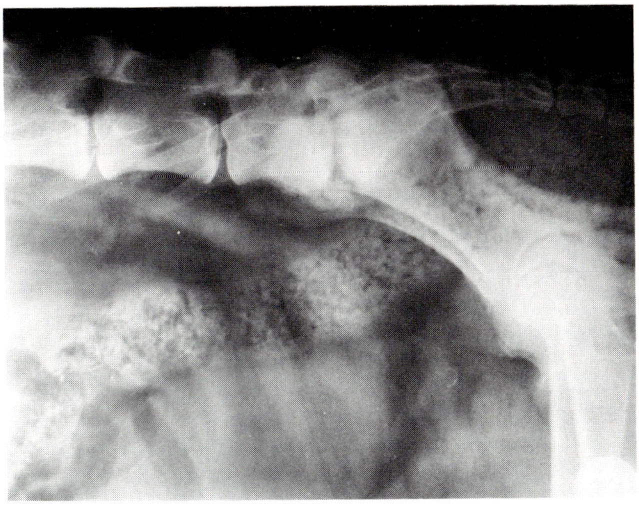

FIGURE 11–14 Same case as Figure 11–13. The radiograph was taken 2½ months after surgery. Tetracycline had been given for 30 days after surgery. The titer at this time was 1:50 and the dog had made a clinical recovery. Note the fusion taking place between L7 and S1 and the lack of tissue destruction.

be done. Additional support to the spine by means of internal fixation of involved vertebrae and/or coaptation casts or splints to the trunk of the animal may be needed.

Gage has recently published results of discospondylitis in 30 dogs. Negative cultures were obtained from 25 per cent of the involved dogs, but bacteria were present in the others. Diagnosis was based largely on characteristic radiographic findings. Treatment consisted of spinal cord decompression and curettage of the lesion, internal vertebral fixation, and antibiotics. Recovery occurred in seven of nine cervical cases and in all 21 of the patients with lumbar lesions.[73]

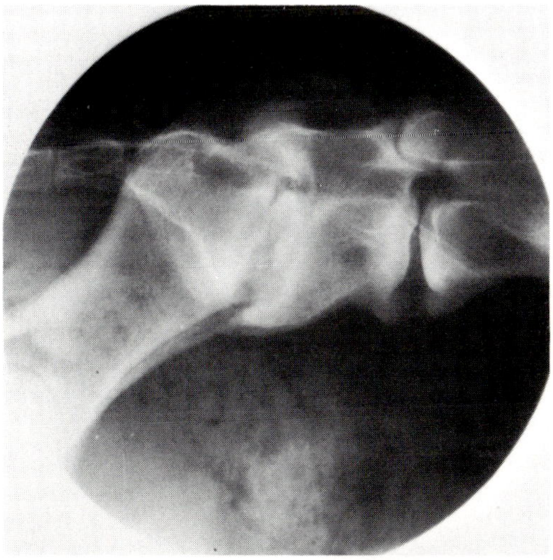

FIGURE 11–15 Same case as Figure 11–13. This radiograph was taken 34 months after surgery. The dog was clinically normal, and the titer was 1:50. Note the lack of tissue destruction, the osseous hypertrophic bridging of L7–S1, and the ventral spondylotic bridging at L6–7.

Toxoplasmosis

Toxoplasmosis is a protozoan disease caused by *Toxoplasma gondii.* This disease affects various mammals, birds, reptiles, and man. Toxoplasma antibodies have been found in 40 to 60 per cent of cats in the Kansas-Iowa area, and in 24 per cent of the dogs and 6 to 56 per cent of the sheep in the United States.[71] The organisms appear singly as round or ovoid bodies or as cyst-like structures in almost all body tissues. The disease is particularly vicious in the newborn infected in utero and in relatively young animals. In puppies, it may resemble distemper, and it has occurred concomitantly with distemper.

The respiratory and digestive systems are commonly affected. Chorioretinitis lesions on ocular fundic examinations are frequently seen, especially in cats (Fig. 11–16). Invasion of the central nervous system is frequently seen and signs depend on the area(s) affected. Encephalitis patterns on EEG may help in arriving at a diagnosis.[9] Moller,[162] Fankhauser,[55] Koestner,[129] Averill,[9] and others have investigated the pathology of the CNS. Koestner examined 63 proven cases of toxoplasmosis in dogs and found the CNS involved in 47 (74 per cent). Neuronal vascular damage and local necrosis were seen in acute cases, and glial nodules and scarring were seen in chronic cases. Ruptured cysts and hyperergic responses were characteristic of reactivated latent toxoplasmosis. Congenital cases were the most severe and were found in two consecutive litters whelped by the same bitch.[129]

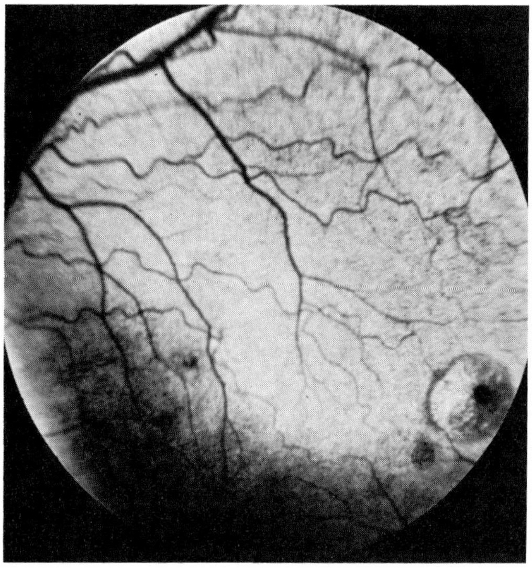

FIGURE 11–16 Fundic lesion from a confirmed case of toxoplasmosis. Note the hyperreflective area with a pigmented border and dark center at the 4 o'clock position.

Hartley[90] reported an interesting variation of toxoplasmosis in dogs. He described several cases in puppies in which encephalitis, myelitis, radiculoneuritis, and myositis were observed with minimal or no involvement of the extraneural tissues. Of the three cases of toxoplasmosis diagnosed pathologically in dogs in the Auburn clinic during 1975, two were affected with the syndrome described by Hartley[90] (Figs. 11–17 to 11–19).

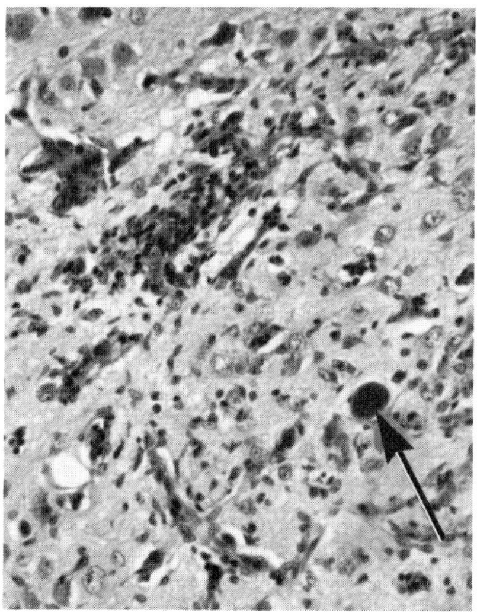

FIGURE 11–17 Toxoplasma encephalitis in a dog. Note the perivascular cuffing, vascular proliferation, and gliosis in the cerebral cortex. Arrow points to a toxoplasma pseudocyst.

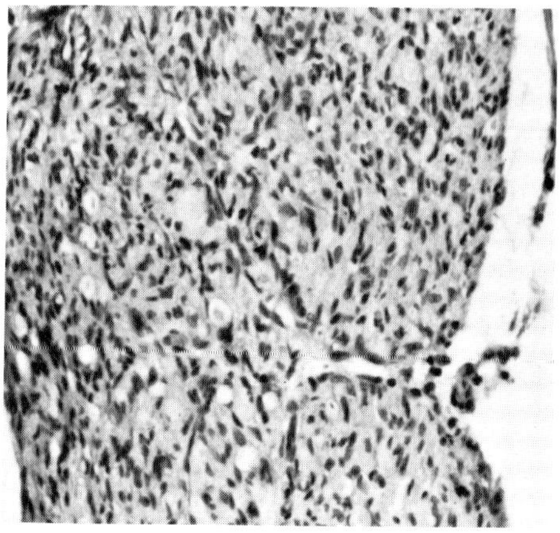

FIGURE 11–18 Toxoplasmosis. Note the radiculitis in the spinal nerve root, infiltration with inflammatory cells, and Schwann cell proliferation. Hematoxylin and eosin, medium power.

As mentioned, in dogs the most common clinical signs are pneumonia, hepatitis, and encephalitis. In cats the most prevalent signs are fever, bilirubinemia, mesenteric adenitis, dyspnea, diffuse pneumonia, leukopenia, anemia, iritis, retinitis, encephalitis, and intestinal obstruction due to granuloma. From present available studies, only Felidae can reasonably be expected to shed toxoplasma oocysts. After primary infection, cats and kittens may shed thousands to millions of oocysts over a period of 10 to 14 days. After sporulation in 1 to 5 days, these oocysts are highly infectious to other animals and man. Oocysts in cat feces remain viable for a prolonged period of time—several months in moist soil, sand, or water.[71, 242] From the life cycle of *T. gondii* the public health significance of toxoplasmosis is evident, especially in cats.

The clinical diagnosis is aided by a history of previous infections in a geographical area or in the household or kennel situation. The clinical signs, the characteristic EEG pattern, and the presence of ocular fundic lesions help in making a tentative diagnosis. The identification of oocysts in the feces of cats, a rising antibody titer, and isolation of the organism establish the diagnosis. Serologic examination should consist of taking at least two serum samples at weekly intervals for the Sabin-Feldman dye test or complement-fixation (CF) test. A five- to tenfold rise in dye test titer and a fourfold rise in CF titer indicate infection. The indirect fluorescent antibody test and the indirect hemagglutination test give sim-

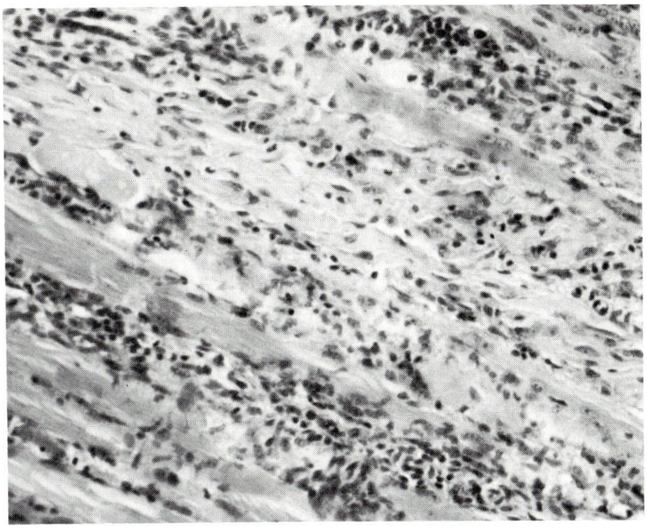

FIGURE 11–19 Myositis in toxoplasmosis. There is a marked necrosis of muscle fibers and dense inflammatory reaction. Hematoxylin and eosin, medium power.

ilar information. Identification or cultures of the organism in biopsy specimens or spinal fluid sediment or in necropsy is the most positive and usually most practical diagnostic means for the clinician. Animal inoculation of infectious material is best done in the mouse.[71]

Treatment

Because of public health factors, especially in cats, and because most canine patients are in the terminal stages of disease, treatment is infrequently attempted. Pyrimethamine (Daraprim) and sulfonamides seem to be the most effective treatment. Pyrimethamine is given in 0.5 to 1 mg/kg doses for 1 to 2 days and then in doses of 0.025 mg/kg daily for at least 2 weeks after signs regress or until toxicity develops. Sulfadiazine or trisulfopyrimidines are the preferred sulfonamides, given in 60 mg/kg divided doses four to six times daily. Folinic acid (calcium leucovorin) and yeast or B-complex vitamins are given concurrently, since folic acid deficiency and depression of bone marrow can occur with this therapy.[154,185]

If cats are treated, strict sanitation and frequent fecal tests for oocysts must be performed afterward. Infected litter must not be placed in the garbage, but should be put in the toilet or burned. Pregnant women and small children are especially susceptible to infection.

SYSTEMIC MYCOSES

Almost any of the mycoses can invade all tissues of the body, including the nervous system. Those most frequently causing damage to the CNS in the dog are histoplasmosis, blastomycosis, mucormycosis, cryptococcosis, and coccidioidomycosis. Two cases of encephalitis due to *Coccidioides immitis* in dogs have been reported. Granulomas were present in the brain in both, with organisms morphologically characteristic of *C. immitis.*[189] Meningoencephalitis due to *Cryptococcus neoformans* infections has been reported in dogs and cats.[17,39,239] Pathologically, granulomatous meningitis with enormous amounts of cryptococcus organisms is characteristic of this disease.

Involvement of the central nervous system in clinical blastomycosis has not been reported frequently in dogs.[135] However, Higgins[99] studied experimentally produced *Blastomyces dermatitidis* in dogs and found that 25 per cent of dogs with systemic organ involvement and all dogs with eye lesions also had lesions in the central nervous system. Disseminated pyogranulomatous encephalitis or, in some cases, large single granulomas involving the ventricles and choroid plexus were the pathological findings in this study[99] (Figs. 11–20 to 11–22).

Since the organisms causing these diseases are present in the vegetation and the soil of endemic areas, the anamnesis of the animal having lived in such an area pre-

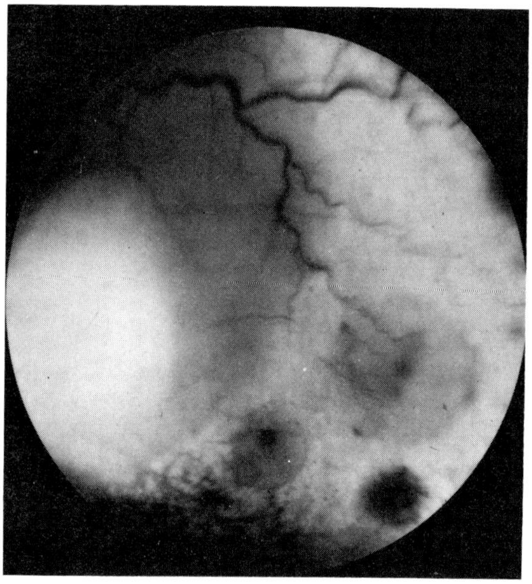

FIGURE 11-20 A confirmed case of cryptococcosis showing an uveitis. In the 8 to 12 o'clock position a large granulomatous lesion is visible. There is engorgement and increased tortuosity of the retinal vessels, and small target-like lesions with dark centers are visible on the right side of the photograph.

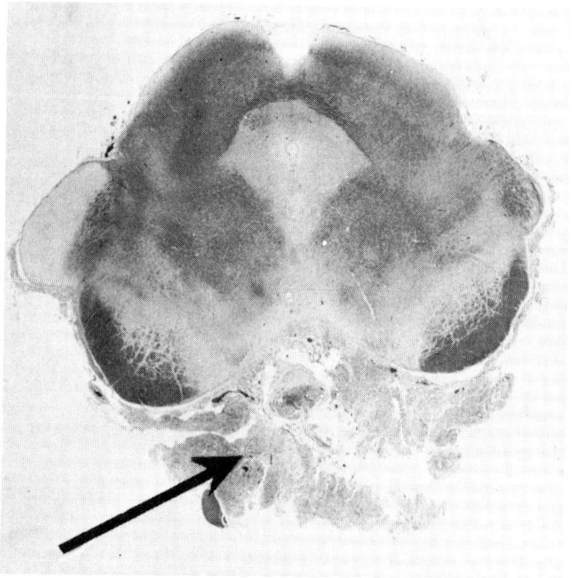

FIGURE 11-22 Blastomycosis in a dog, showing an extensive meningeal granuloma (arrow) on the base of the midbrain. Luxol fast blue-cresylecht violet stain, low power.

viously will help in differentiating other conditions of similar clinical appearance.[193]

In recent years, there has been a marked increase in the incidence of mycoses in humans particularly candidiasis, aspergillosis, phycomycosis, and cryptococcosis. Mycoses have occurred in patients with

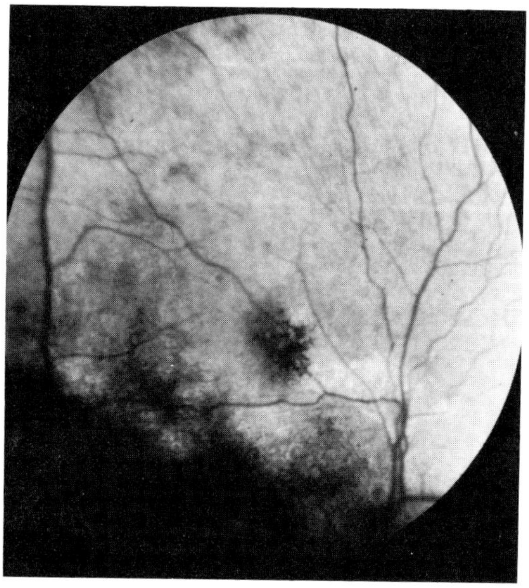

FIGURE 11-21 A confirmed case of blastomycosis. A hyperreflective area is visible near the center of the fundus. There is destruction of the tapetal cells and an increased pigmentation. Previous photographs had shown a vitreous opacity in this area.

various debilitating diseases, such as leukemia, lymphomas, aplastic anemia, carcinoma, and diabetes mellitus. Increase in fungal infections clearly parallels the use of antibiotics, corticosteroids, antimetabolites, and other cytotoxic drugs. Mycotic diseases of the brain are invariably secondary to infection elsewhere in the body by hematogenous dissemination.[63, 239]

Most mycotic infections involving the CNS in dogs produce characteristic signs of a septic encephalitis, such as moderate fever, pupillary or ocular fundic abnormalities, and motor signs consistent with any possible localization of the infection. If the encephalitis is general, general hyperesthesia, muscle tremors, weakness, or convulsions may occur. The EEG pattern may be characteristic for an encephalitis and the specific stage of disease (early, acute, chronic, compensating, or recovery). A careful ocular fundic examination is frequently most helpful in diagnosing the chronic or recurrent forms of granulomatous and degenerative chorioretinitis (see Chapter 18 for specific descriptions). The examination of spinal fluid sediment and culture is frequently rewarding. Radiologic examinations of the abdominal viscera and lungs can be helpful in establishing a clinical diagnosis.[103]

The laboratory diagnosis depends on identification or culture of the organism in tissue fluid such as spinal fluid, surgical biopsy, bronchial or tracheal washings, endoscopic biopsy of the respiratory or gastrointestinal tract, or necropsy specimens. Serological tests in patients with histoplasmosis, blastomycosis, or coccidioidomycosis can be diagnostic. The immunofluorescent (FA) tests are particularly helpful when, as frequently happens, the serum is termed anticomplementary. Recently, a double electroimmunodiffusion test for coccidiodes has been proposed. It takes 30 minutes to run and requires only one microliter each of antigen and antibody.[209]

Treatment

Generally, treatment of systemic mycosis is fruitless once the organism has invaded the nervous system. Hydroxystilbamadine, sulfonamides, and iodides have been used in the past in mycoses, especially blastomycosis. In actinomycosis and nocardiosis, surgical excision and drainage combined with administration of penicillin and sulfadiazine has been used.[212] In localized infections such as aspergillosis in the sinuses or nasal passages, local application of nystatin has been used. In mycoses such as histoplasmosis, blastomycosis, coccidioidomycosis, and cryptococcosis, amphotericin B is the agent of choice.[211] Ausherman[7] reported a treatment regimen for histoplasmosis and blastomycosis that had been used with gratifying results for 11 years. Good supportive therapy and frequent monitoring of the kidney function by blood urea nitrogen (BUN) tests is essential. The schedule is as follows:

1. Dissolve a 50 mg vial of amphotericin B in 10 ml of sterile water and add 5 per cent dextrose and water solution to a final volume of 250 ml.
2. Before each administration a BUN test is done, and if it rises to more than 1½ times the pretreatment figure, the drug is discontinued until it returns to normal.
3. The initial outpatient dose of amphotericin B is 0.5 ml/lb body weight intravenously in a 3 to 5 minute period.
4. After a day's rest at home, a second IV administration is given at 0.75 ml/lb.
5. After a day's rest, the dose is increased to 1.0 ml/lb, and this dose is continued three times weekly until 12 doses have been given.[7]

If the disease should have remissions, the treatment is repeated.

PARASITIC INVASION OF CNS TISSUES

Parasitic invasion of the nervous system has been reported for years in the horse, sheep, and other species. Some of these are host-specific and merely constitute a CNS form of the disease. However, foreign host parasites seem to find refuge in the CNS and migrate in these tissues, causing much mechanical damage and subsequent inflammatory response. These two types of CNS parasitic disorders will be discussed briefly so that the clinician can consider them when dealing with an unusual neurological case.

The cerebral form of *babesiosis* in dogs has been reported on occasion, and it bears a striking resemblance to cerebral malaria in man. Some dogs that have it go into sudden coma and die. Convulsions are seen in other cases.[15] In a case history by Botha in South Africa, a 2-year-old cross-bred ridgeback dog showed a series of convulsions.[22] Babesiosis was diagnosed, but the dog failed to respond to treatment. Necropsy examination showed thrombosis of small arteries and areas of necrosis in the brain. Histological examination revealed liquefaction necrosis with extensive hemorrhages in the cerebrum.[15, 18]

Granulomas caused by migrating larvae of the genus *Toxocara* have been observed histologically in the brain as well as in other tissues.[15] A 2½-year-old Great Dane suffered from a severe granulomatous inflammation of the hypothalamus and adjacent neurohypophysis caused by *Toxocara canis* larvae. The clinical syndrome included a severe diabetes insipidus.[196] Visceral larval migrans from various nonhuman ascarids have produced neurological lesions in children.[15, 195]

Georgi described a case of *cerebral coenurosis* in a cat showing vestibular disturbances. Improvement was noted after treatment, but the animal died in a few days. A

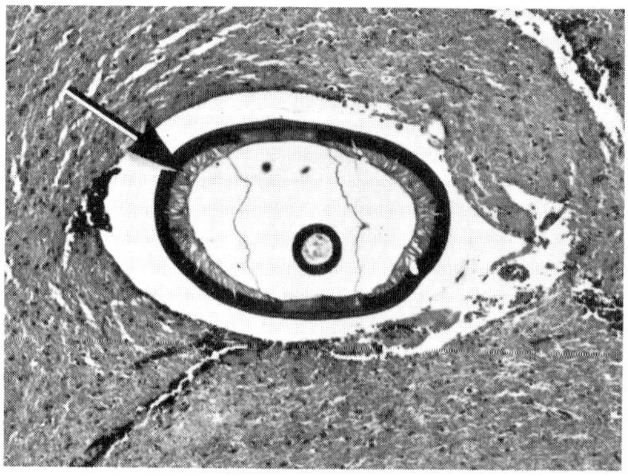

FIGURE 11–23 This demonstrates heartworm invasion in a dog's brain. Note the cross section of adult *Dirofilaria immitis* (arrow) in malacic brain tissue. Hematoxylin and eosin, low power.

coenurus cyst was seen in the left cerebral hemisphere.[76]

Heavner and Few reported finding numerous microfilariae of *Dirofilaria immitis* within the meningeal arteries, deep arteries, and capillaries of the brain and extravascularly within the brain.[95] The dog was showing periodic convulsions. Taguchi found adult *Dirofilaria immitis* in the lateral ventricles of the brain of a dog who showed signs of epilepsy and posterior paralysis and who was a rabies suspect.[224] Very recently, there have been at least three more reports of adult heartworms in the brains of dogs. All dogs had serious neurological signs[50, 151, 183] (Fig. 11–23).

Cuterebra larvae have been found in the brains of a dog[92] and a cat.[93] The cat was "acting peculiarly"—growling, clawing, irritable to sounds, and periodically making wild aggressive movements. The larva was found in the left cerebral hemisphere. The dog was having locomotor difficulties and finally progressed to quadriplegia and prostration. A cuterebra larva was seen in the mesencephalon and many pathologic changes from possible larval migration were seen in other areas of the brain in the dog. Both the cat and dog were examined for rabies, but no Negri bodies were seen, and animal inoculations were negative. Since cystic tapeworm and other parasitic invasions from normal and nonhost-specific organisms occur frequently in other animals, it is logical to assume that such invasions in the CNS of dogs will be diagnosed more frequently.

VASCULAR DISORDERS

CEREBROVASCULAR DISEASE

It has been mentioned repeatedly that secondary CNS vascular disorders that follow inflammations, infections, and trauma account for severe damage to the nervous system. In man, primary cerebrovascular problems account for considerable CNS dysfunction. Cerebrovascular disorders in animals have been thought to be much less frequent than in man. This may prove not to be entirely true as more emphasis is placed on comparative neuropathology.

In a recent study, Fankhauser, Luginbühl, and McGrath[59] attempted to clarify some aspects of cerebrovascular disease of various animal species by examining some 10,000 animals neuropathologically. Generally, cerebrovascular anomalies were infrequently observed in animals. Several cases of telangiectatic hamartomas and cavernous hemangiomas were found in dogs. Fibrosis of the intima, media, and adventitia, individually or combined, was observed with some frequency in all types and calibers of cerebrospinal vessels in the dog. They were most frequently seen in older dogs. According to Fankhauser, Detweiler, and coworkers, generalized atherosclerosis or arterial xanthomatosis is a very rare disease in the dog.[47, 59] However, in experimental work it has been observed that swine can replace nonhuman primates as subjects for studies of atherosclerotic vascular disease. Intracranial atherosclerosis is advanced in swine which are fed garbage, and the stages of development are identical to those in man.[193] In two out of three dogs with systemic atherosclerosis, the major cerebral arteries were severely involved. It was concluded that from the few cases of generalized atherosclerosis studied in the dog, the arteries of the dog could react similarly to those of man and swine under certain circumstances, such as hypothyroidism.

Calcification of cerebrospinal vessels occurred frequently in man and the horse but very infrequently in the dog and cat. The occurrences of CNS malacias and necrosis from presumably hypoxic, hypometabolic, or dysmetabolic changes were frequently encountered in a number of animal species. In several dogs with chronic congestive heart failure, cerebral malacias were observed. Edema and congestion were obvious findings in cases of cerebral necrosis in the dog. Thrombosis was infrequent in dogs, as expected, considering the rarity of generalized atherosclerosis. Naturally occurring intracerebral and intrameningeal hemorrhages from spontaneous rupture of vessels were common in man but appeared to be rare in animals. However, hematomyelia was fairly common in dogs with ruptured intervertebral disks or other spinal cord trauma. Hemorrhages into primary and secondary brain tumors were frequently observed in dogs; however, true vascular neoplasms were rarely found as primary tumors of the CNS in man or animals.[59]

McGrath discussed clinical vascular disease in dogs under the headings of cerebral vasospasm, cerebral arteriosclerosis, and apoplexy.[136]

CEREBRAL VASOSPASM

Cerebral vasospasm may occur more frequently in the dog than is commonly realized. In the literature on man, it appears that few neurologists of the past recognized the role of vasospasm in causing stroke-like symptoms. Westphal and Bär maintained that hypertension and spastic or arteriosclerotic functional disorders of the cerebral blood vessels caused sudden ischemia of the circumscribed parts of the brain.[245] If the arteries were subsequently dilated, a rush of blood would result, and rupture might follow. This is the concept of spastic ischemia or angiospasm.

Cerebral vasospasm differs from other forms of vascular accident in the short duration of symptoms and the complete recovery. The physician frequently refers to "little" strokes in older patients, which may cause a disturbance in personality for a few hours or a day or so. Perhaps this is angiospasm.

In man, transient paralytic apoplectic episodes without clinical evidence of residual infarction or cerebral vascular crises were formerly ascribed to vasospasm. Although vasospasm plays some role in cerebrovascular disease, current concepts of transient cerebral ischemia stress atheroma as the basic substrate, and dispersible emboli that become detached from a platelet fibrin thrombus at the atheromatous site or transient systemic hypotension that critically reduces blood flow through marginally adequate cerebral circulatory channels as more important causes.[218]

It has been shown that vasospasms accompany intracranial hemorrhage, mechanisms of which are still unknown. Catecholamines and serotonin have been incriminated as the cause of vasospasms that frequently occur with subarachnoid hemorrhage. However, serotonin and histamine levels were measured in 17 human patients with intracranial hemorrhage and no consistent differences were found from the levels of controls. Further studies are needed to determine the cause of this phenomenon.[199, 216, 249]

It is possible that cerebral vasospasms are associated with the clinical syndrome of old dogs that collapse for a few minutes and recover completely in a day or so. It is also possible that heart disease or cerebral emboli or thrombi may be involved. There may be vestibular disturbances, nystagmus, weakness, and even temporary hemiplegia. These attacks may be followed by recovery within several days.

Careful examination of the heart with electrocardiograms must be done. Cardiac disorders often cause such symptoms.

The treatment of primary CNS vasospasms includes rest and tranquilization if necessary, but, as almost all these subjects recovery promptly, little treatment is necessary. Cardiac disorders should be treated appropriately and monitored frequently for signs of remission or toxicity from drug therapy. Avoidance of conditions that seemed to stimulate the attack is desirable.

CEREBRAL ARTERIOSCLEROSIS

Sclerosis of the large intracerebral arteries in the dog is only rarely observed. Fibrosis of the intima is occasionally observed but does not cause changes in the nervous parenchyma. Atherosclerosis is a very rare condition in the dog, and only a few reports are available on generalized atherosclerosis in dogs who were afflicted with deficient function of the thyroid glands. Cerebral infarcts, however, were not observed in these cases.[150] An 8-year-old Labrador was brought to the Auburn clinic with sudden onset of mental deterioration, unilateral postural deficits, intention tremors, and a slight head tilt. A large infarct in the anterior midbrain resulted from atherosclerotic changes in several branches of the arteria media (Figs. 11–24 and 11–25).

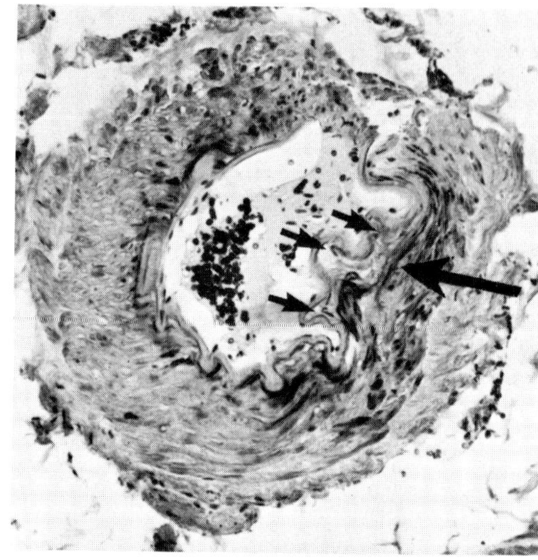

FIGURE 11–25 Same case as in Figure 11–24. A branch of the arteria media shows deposits of atheromatous material (dark staining material at large arrow) in the vessel wall. The irregular bulging of the intima (small arrows) produces a narrowing of the vascular lumen. Gomori's trichrome stain, medium power.

VASCULAR ACCIDENTS

Vascular accident is loosely termed apoplexy or stroke. The term apoplexy originally meant hemorrhage into the brain tissue, but now appears to include embolism and thrombosis as well.[52] Statistics published in 1963 listed 170,000 deaths in the United States from cerebral vascular accidents.[240] It was formerly believed that most "strokes" were the result of intracerebral hemorrhage. However, 70 per cent of cerebral vascular accidents are due to ischemia (50 per cent thrombotic, 20 per cent embolic), 20 per cent to intracerebral hemorrhage, and 8 per cent to subarachnoid hemorrhage. Spontaneous intracranial hemorrhage does not include traumatic hemorrhage.[240]

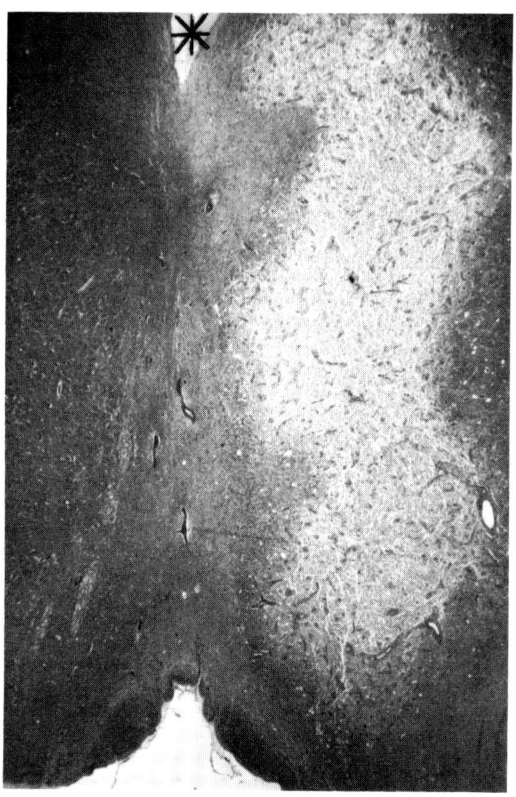

FIGURE 11–24 A large infarct is located in the midbrain on the right side of an 8-year-old Labrador. The asterisk shows the sylvian aqueduct. Hematoxylin and eosin, low power.

There are few discussions in veterinary literature of cerebral vascular accidents. Parker discusses the disorders in dogs and cats and refers to several case histories. He states that spontaneous intracranial hemorrhage occurs infrequently but that thrombotic and embolic occlusions of intracranial vessels occur occasionally.[181]

Almost any cerebral vascular disorder that affects circulation of blood will produce an ischemia of brain tissue involved. In most instances, this is transient in a localized occlusion because collateral circulation is established rapidly. In generalized cerebral ischemia, it has been established that learning and retention in the dog can be impaired. Six minutes of total cerebral ischemia produced no detectable change in learning, retention, or psychomotor performance. Eight minutes of complete ischemia produced severe impairment of learning, but had no effect on retention or psychomotor performance. There was no difference in the EEG recovery pattern between six and eight minutes of circulatory occlusion.[262]

Cerebral Hemorrhage

This is usually due to rupture of a vessel whose wall has undergone local or diffuse pathologic changes of a longstanding nature. The rupture may follow exertion or other stimulating influence, but frequently has no known cause. Hemorrhage may follow the formation of aneurysms. Mycotic or fat emboli may weaken a vessel wall and provoke a rupture.[244, 247] The onset of hemorrhage is sudden, the course is rapid, and loss of consciousness occurs quickly.[25]

In intracranial hemorrhage, as the mass of blood expands within the intracranial space, there is reduction in volume of the normal intracranial contents in order to accommodate the mass. As long as the volume of the mass does not exceed this replaceable intracranial volume, intracranial pressure will be normal. However, as the replaceable volume diminishes with continued expansion of the mass, there is a progressive rise in intracranial pressure. When the intracranial pressure reaches the vasopressor threshold, there is an increase in arterial pressure, following which an enormous rise in arterial and intracranial pressures is seen. Following a succession of pressure waves, the vasopressor mechanism begins to fail. Cerebral ischemia occurs as the differences between the arterial and intracranial pressures decline. Increased intracranial pressure causes cerebral vasodilation and an increase of brain blood volume. A further pressure increase beyond the maximal compensated intracranial volume leads to progressive ischemia and cerebral vasomotor paralysis. Finally, the intracranial and arterial pressures are the same, cerebral blood flow is nil, and death results.[137]

It is not known for certain whether massive hemorrhage following rupture of diseased vessels occurs in animals. Most intracerebral hematomas observed in small animals were caused by rupture of vascular malformations such as telangiectases, cavernous hemangiomas, and saccular aneurysms.[59]

Cerebral Embolism

Cerebral emboli occur most frequently in young persons, and the emboli usually develop from vegetative endocarditis. Air or fat emboli may be responsible, e.g., marrow fat dislodged in fractures.

Cerebral Thrombosis

Cerebral thrombosis is the most frequent form of vascular accident in man. This is usually due to atherosclerosis, slow rate of blood flow, and blood alterations. Syphilis, typhoid fever, tuberculosis, diphtheria, pneumonia, and other diseases may stimulate the development of cerebral thrombosis. The onset is slower than hemorrhage, and consciousness is lost more slowly.[25]

Cerebral Infarctions

All complete or incomplete necrotizing lesions in the central nervous system which are caused by cerebrovascular or cardiac disease and result in encephalomalacia, cavitation, sclerosis, and atrophy are called infarcts. Anemic infarcts of the brain in the dog have been described by Fankhauser *et al.*[59] These infarcts were often related to cardiac malformations and were located in the caudate nucleus and adjacent capsula interna and externa. Hemorrhagic infarcts are mainly caused by emboli in bacterial infections and are usually located in the cerebral cortex on the border of gray and white matter (Figs. 11–24 and 11–25).

Clinical Signs and Treatment of Vascular Accidents

The clinical signs and course of disease depend upon the severity of the lesion and its location. Generally, loss of consciousness occurs, and there is some degree of paralysis, which is usually one-sided and rarely bilateral. Disturbances of mentality and locomotion, hysteria, and depression may precede unconsciousness. In cerebral hemorrhage, the spinal fluid often is bloody, whereas in thrombosis it is not.

Common sense is called for in the *treatment* of a *vascular accident*. Control of convulsions or hysteria is essential. Administration of glucocorticosteroids such as dexamethasone is routinely performed to relieve inflammation and inhibit edema.

The head should be elevated if a rapid hemorrhage is suspected. In case of hemorrhage, ice packs applied to the head may be of value. Intravenous administration of vitamin K, calcium gluconate, and systemic coagulants (Klot) may also be helpful. Intravenous mannitol solutions would be helpful in combating cerebral edema but could be deleterious in cases of intracranial hemorrhage, since rapid shrinking of the brain will stimulate further hemorrhage. The use of dicumarol or heparin is indicated in cases of cerebral thrombosis, but this is difficult to diagnose in animal patients without a time-consuming angiogram. These should be given according to the dosage schedule for human use, based on the clotting time. General nursing practices must include care of the urinary bladder and the administration of antibiotics.

Most intracranial hemorrhages, other than intracerebral, are subdural. In the dog, spontaneous subdural hemorrhages can probably occur about as frequently as intracerebral hemorrhages. Schlotthauer reported two such cases in three dogs observed.[202]

Although the diagnosis of spontaneous subdural hemorrhage is difficult, the rapid development of signs and a history of trauma are helpful in making a tentative diagnosis. Exploratory calvarial bur holes should be used to diagnose intracranial hemorrhage. A craniotomy may be necessary for proper correction.

VASCULAR DISORDERS OF THE SPINAL CORD

Primary vascular disorders of the spinal cord were formerly thought to be rare. However, as research and technology progress, more vascular disorders will be demonstrated.

Anatomical Variations

It has been shown that the distribution of the spinal branches of the thoracolumbar segmental arteries in the dog is highly irregular and unpredictable. In a study of 20 dogs, many intervertebral foramina had two spinal arteries, and many did not have bilateral arteries from T10–11 through L5–6. Only five dogs had at least one artery to each spinal segment in this area. Four dogs had only two to four arteries in this span of seven vertebrae. One can conclude that with this precariously deficient blood supply, trauma and disease can easily create serious cord ischemia.[179]

Vascular Malformations

Vertebral angiomas are said to occur in about 10 per cent of human vertebral columns examined at autopsy. Out of 100 cases of extradural hemorrhage from hemangiomas with neurologic complications in man, 11 occurred in the last trimester of pregnancy.[165] It is our opinion that similar vascular pathologic changes probably occur in the dog also.

Vascular malformations of the cord itself are frequently described in man, and we have reported their occurrence in a dog. Oliver and Geary reported a cervical cord compression in a 6-year-old basset resulting from a left venous sinus aneurysm.[170] An iodized oil myelogram utilizing fluoroscopy and a spot-filming technique established the location of the lesion at C5. The dog had suffered incoordination and motor deficiency in the front limbs for approximately 4 months, and it was especially difficult for him to climb stairs. A dorsal laminectomy revealed an aneurysm measuring approximately 3 by 2 by 2 cm that anastomosed with the right venous sinus. No ligations or ablations were attempted, since the cord manipulation involved with ligations would have resulted in serious neurological consequences. The decompression afforded by surgery enabled the dog to make a gradual improvement postsurgically, with nearly complete return of normal function within a 6-month period.[170]

Many such malformations have been described in man. McGrath reported four cases of angiomas occurring intracranially in the dog.[156] Lawson, in the discussion of another paper, mentioned multiple cord compressions from enlarged venous sinuses in the dog.[143] Vandevelde and Fankhauser[231] described two cases in which the hemorrhage in the cord resulted from angiomatous malformations of the meningeal vasculature.

The diagnosis of these lesions is accomplished by arteriography, venography, and (usually) myelography. A worm-like configuration is frequently seen in myelography. A flow defect was observed in Oliver's case, and surgical exploration revealed the cause of the compression.

Total excision or ligation, or both, is common surgical procedure. As there is evidence that vascular malformations occur in dogs, clinicians and radiologists should strive for effective diagnostic procedures and should not hesitate to perform surgical correction.[51, 109, 133, 148, 170]

Hematomyelia

Hematomyelia can result from necrotizing changes in the spinal cord vasculature or from vascular malformations.[231] However, the majority of hematomyelia cases are related to intervertebral disk disease (ascending hemorrhagic myelomalacia) and will be discussed in detail later.

Vascular Occlusions

In the spinal cord, disorders such as general anemia, local anemia, ischemia, arterial thrombosis, and hyperemia are difficult to recognize clinically. Vascular occlusions may result from *spinal cord compression.*

In surgical intervention for protruding disks, thrombosis of venous sinuses in the compression area is frequently seen. This could contribute to the local cord edema associated with compressions of the spinal cord Lindblad and co-workers performed sinus venography and found a high incidence of venous sinus thromboses in cases of disk protrusion; they therefore propose this as a diagnostic procedure for disk protrusions.[143]

Spinal cord arteriosclerosis is apparently seen infrequently in dogs. In a survey of the various pathological findings in the spinal cords of 500 clinical and experimental dogs at Auburn University, Vandevelde[230] found only one dog with arteriosclerotic changes in the ventral spinal artery and its branches. However, no associated ischemic cord lesions were seen. Cord ischemia due to arteriosclerosis has been seen in man.[112]

Fibrocartilaginous Emboli

In recent years there have been reports of spinal cord infarctions in dogs (and one cat) which have resulted from apparent obstruction of meningeal and intramedullary arteries or veins by fibrocartilaginous emboli. Zaki reported the disorder in one cat and five Great Danes, two females and three males, ranging in age from 2 to 5 years.[259, 261] Griffiths reported fibrocartilaginous emboli in a total of five cases—a 4-year-old Labrador, a 3-year-old wire-haired fox terrier, and three other dogs.[81, 82] De Lahunta[144] reported five necropsy cases of ischemic myelopathy from presumed fibrocartilaginous embolism and four clinical cases that recovered. Greene[79] reported a case in a 6-year-old Labrador with right-sided hemiplegia and Horner's syndrome. In addition, the Auburn clinic has seen five cases during 1975–76, two in Great Danes and three in schnauzers.[230]

The clinical signs are predominantly acute, one-sided or bilateral motor deficit, usually paresis or paralysis that occurs without a history of trauma. The signs are dependent on the site of the lesion. Initial pain may be followed by a progressive paresis and paralysis within a few hours. The clinical signs are fairly characteristic of an acute spinal compression, such as a fracture, luxation, or disk protrusion. However, lateralization of signs is more frequently characteristic of a vascular lesion that causes a focal or localized pathological lesion on one side of the cord. Lateralization is generally not seen in cord compressions except in the early stages. Plain film spinography is generally negative but may show minor disk pathology. Myelography generally does not show major extradural compressions.

Laboratory and electrodiagnostic findings are not usually conclusive in establishing a definitive diagnosis. Pathologically, swelling, malacia with cavitation, and hemorrhage may be observed on gross examination. Histologically, there is extensive necrosis of parts of the gray and white matter and edema and hemorrhage in the surrounding areas. Several meningeal and intramedullary vessels are obstructed by fibrocartilaginous emboli. The emboli are present in arteries or veins of any caliber and often in both. Zaki[259, 260] reported em-

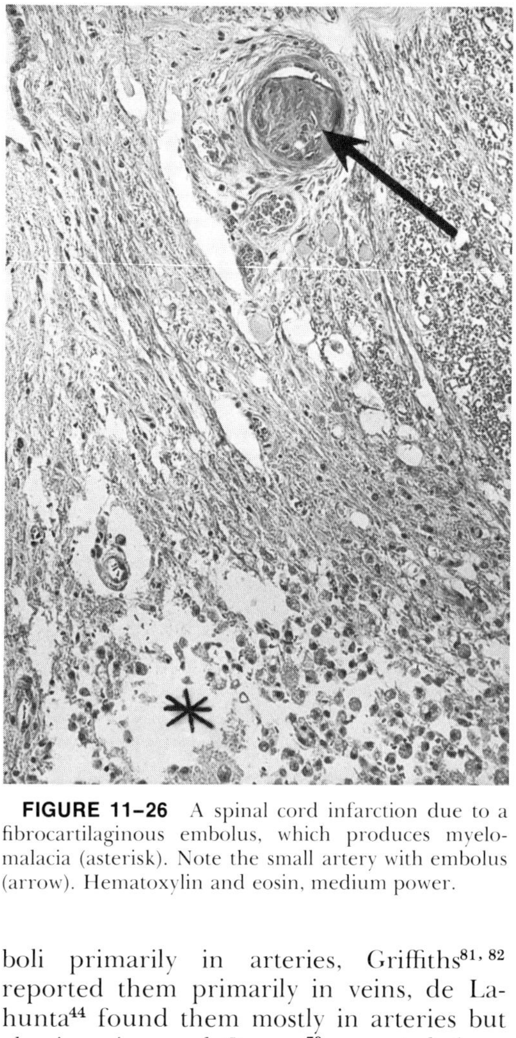

FIGURE 11–26 A spinal cord infarction due to a fibrocartilaginous embolus, which produces myelomalacia (asterisk). Note the small artery with embolus (arrow). Hematoxylin and eosin, medium power.

boli primarily in arteries, Griffiths[81, 82] reported them primarily in veins, de Lahunta[44] found them mostly in arteries but also in veins, and Greene[79] reported them in the arteries (Fig. 11–26).

In cases in which survival time is prolonged, mesenchymal scar formation, cholesterol deposits, and multinucleated giant cells have been observed in the infarcts. The fibrocartilaginous emboli are transformed to fibrillary masses covered by endothelial cells.[82]

The pathogenesis of this condition is largely unknown. The histochemical staining affinity of the emboli suggest their intervertebral disk origin. It is not likely, however, that spinal cord infarcts are related to disk pathology. In several hundred cases of severe disk pathology examined at Auburn University, no fibrocartilaginous emboli were observed. However, in the Labrador retriever described by Griffiths,[81] bulging of the dorsal annulus at T12–13 and L2–3 without complete rupture was observed. At L3–4 a small mass originated from the right annulus, and emboli were also present in the peridiscal artery. Emboli may originate from cartilaginous herniations from the intervertebral disk into the vertebral bodies (Schmorl's nodules).[259–261] The material could reach the cord by retrograde venous flow.

To explain the presence of emboli in arteries, arteriovenous malformations have been suggested. The emboli could then enter the arterial circulation during conditions of raised pressure such as straining or coughing. The presence of emboli in both arteries and veins in some cases substantiates this theory.[122]

The treatment is nonsurgical and consists of good nursing care, use of glucocorticosteroids, and antibiotics. The dog should be given complete rest for probably 1 to 2 weeks, and then physical therapy and supervised exercise until recovery progresses. In de Lahunta's four animals that recovered, improvement started within a few days, and the patients were nearly normal in most cases within a few months.[44]

Traumatic Occlusion of Spinal Arteries

In an experimental study of external trauma applied to the lumbar spinal areas of six anesthetized dogs, occlusion of two to eight of the segmental aortic branches to the spinal cord occurred. The occlusions occurred approximately 2.5 cm from the aorta. The trauma was sufficient to fracture the lumbar laminae in only two of the six dogs, so it was concluded that damage to segmental areas did not depend on fractures. The occluded arteries were isolated and examined, and it was found that half were thrombosed and half were ruptured and thrombosed. It was concluded that trauma in the lumbar spinal area could leave large areas of the spinal cord deficient in segmental blood supply. This ischemia combined with traumatic edema and other vascular damage to the cord can cause marked pathological effects.[180]

Aortic Occlusions

In an experimental study on dogs, it was shown that the complete cord ischemia that results from occlusion of the aorta for approximately 35 minutes produced irreversible paraplegia. Periods of less than 35 minutes produced transient neurological changes. Histologically, this mild cord ischemia produced loss of neurons in the dorsal horns, followed by separation of interstitial neural elements and cavity formation. In severe cases of ischemia, there is necrosis of long white tracts as well as neuron loss, which produces myelomalacia with cavitation. Cavitation involves primarily the central gray matter dorsal to the central canal and may extend into adjacent white matter.[252]

A more frequent *vascular* disorder that does *not* affect the spine primarily but causes a similar motor dysfunction is aortic thrombosis, which has been seen occasionally in our clinic[102] and has been reported by others.[117, 123, 138, 204] In the past few years, several dogs have suffered partial or complete aortic occlusion at the bifurcation of the iliac arteries due to masses of adult heartworms. In one such case there also were bilateral partial occlusions of the femoral arteries due to heartworms.[104] Aortic thrombosis or embolism has been reported frequently in cats.[10, 27, 70, 147, 204] It is felt that the terms embolus and thrombus may be used loosely clinically and that most cases involve emboli.

Occlusions of the terminal aorta probably result largely from emboli arising from vegetative growths seen in bacterial endocarditis in the left heart. It has been reported that in 27 dogs and 13 cats having acute vegetative endocarditis, 23 animals (14 dogs and 9 cats) developed emboli that caused severe pain and shock. In 11 of them, sudden tenderness of a limb, "sagging" gait, or intermittent paraplegia or paralysis followed partial or complete occlusion of the posterior aorta, femoral, or brachial arteries.[204] The primary symptoms are pain, posterior paresis, an effort to walk on the front legs, and urinary retention. The most diagnostic features are the presence of reflexes but the absence of diminution of the femoral pulse. Positive diagnosis can be made by a contrast aortogram. Twenty to 30 ml of Urokon, Hypaque, or any other widely used vascular contrast medium can be injected into the arterial circulation. In the first case reported in the dog, however, the contrast was given in the

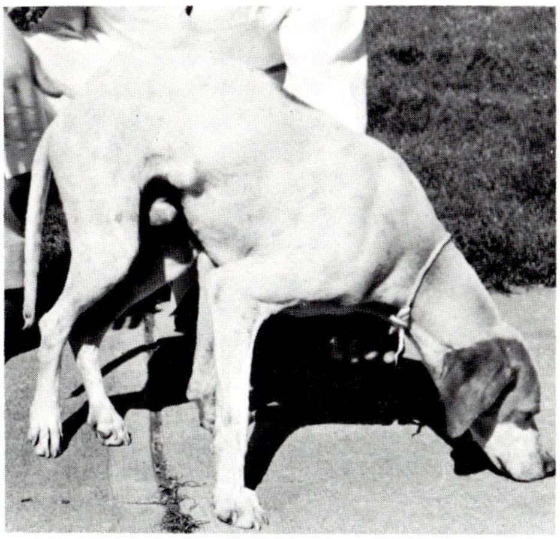

FIGURE 11–27 A 4-year-old pointer was suffering from a partial paraplegia. Notice that weight-bearing is largely accomplished on the pectoral limbs. The pelvic limbs were warm and painful. No femoral pulse could be detected in either limb.

cephalic vein. Impaired flow can be demonstrated 2 to 6 seconds after administration, depending on the site (Figs. 11–27 to 11–30).[102]

According to experimental work done in cats, the formation of a clot or thrombus is very important in reproducing the aortic paralytic syndrome. Ligation of the aorta at the level of the iliac bifurcation did *not* produce paralysis within a month's time. When a clot was produced by injecting thrombin between a permanent ligature and a proximally placed temporary one, paralysis resulted in 24 hours. The limbs were cold in the latter procedure, whereas they were warm in simple ligation. Collateral circulation was impaired following clot formation.[115]

In more recent work, Butler[28] performed single or double ligations of the aorta at the iliac bifurcations in 49 cats with no paralysis. When histamine was injected between the ligatures, no paralysis was seen. However, when 5-hydroxytryptamine (S-HT), a substance produced by the platelets in a thrombus, was injected between the ligatures, the paralytic syndrome occurred in 80 per cent of the cats. 5-Hydroxytryptamine interferes with the collateral circulation, but its mechanism of action is unknown.[28]

TREATMENT. A few spontaneous recoveries have been seen in cats. In mild cases, such recoveries can occur. In severe occlusions, surgical removal should be per-

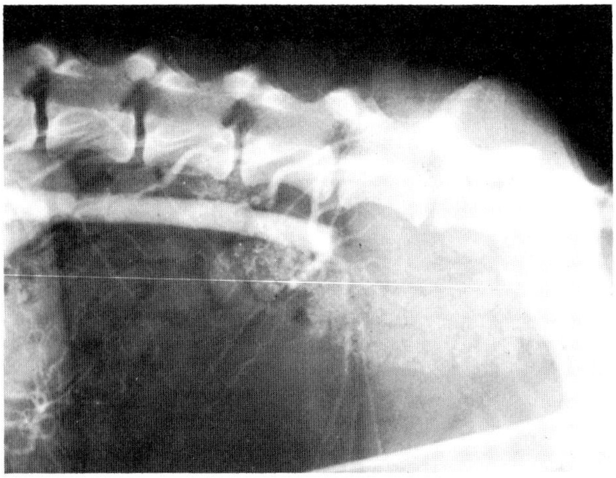

FIGURE 11–28 Same case as in Figure 11–27. An aortic occlusion was seen in this lateral aortogram, which was taken 6 seconds after injection of 20 ml of Urokon in the cephalic vein.

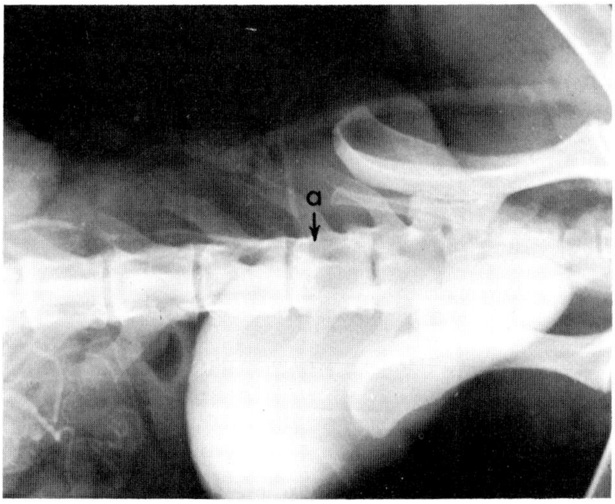

FIGURE 11–29 A VD aortogram of the case shown in Figures 11–27 and 11–28. (a) shows a point of occlusion. (Figures 11–28 and 11–29 from Hoerlein, B. F.: Clinical spinal conditions in the dog. Vet. Med. *51*, 575, 1956.)

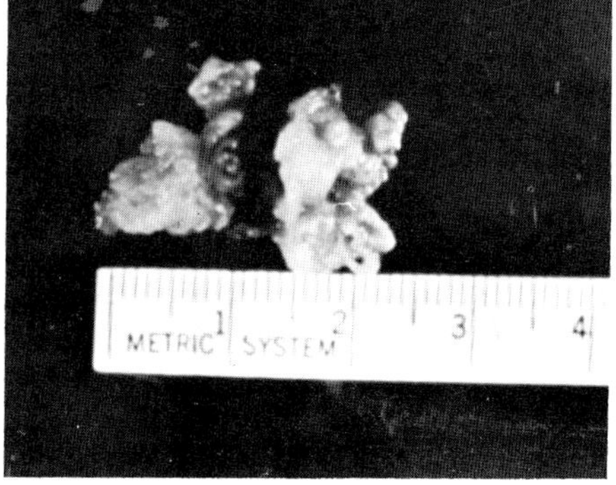

FIGURE 11–30 Aortic thrombus removed from the terminal aorta of the case shown in Figures 11–27 to 11–29.

formed if other assessments of physical condition may be favorable.[78] Saddle or aortic emboli in man are removed by means of a balloon catheter. The deflated catheter is passed up through a femoral artery well beyond the emboli. It is inflated appropriately and withdrawn, thereby forcing extraction of intermediate emboli. Severe vascular damage will necessitate a prosthesis, which would rarely be indicated in a clinical veterinary practice.[153, 227]

Fibrinolytic enzymes such as streptokinase, streptodornase, and plasminogen have not been widely used in veterinary medicine for treatment of aortic emboli. Postsurgical use of anticoagulants such as heparin or dicumarol might prevent a recurrence, but constant laboratory assessment of blood clotting times would be necessary for proper dosage. Long-term antibiotic therapy should be used to combat bacterial endocarditis.[27, 153]

CNS NEOPLASIA

BRAIN TUMORS

It is inappropriate to discuss the histopathology of brain tumors here, as most clinicians are more interested in the clinical signs, the location and removal of the lesion, and the clinical prognosis than in the pathologic characteristics of the tumors.

McGrath has effectively contributed to both the clinical and research aspects of veterinary medicine by correlating the neurological examination with the necropsy diagnosis.[156] He classified these intracranial tumors as primary and secondary. Primary intracranial tumors are those that develop from brain or meningeal stem cells, and secondary tumors are those that develop from other structures of the head and affect the brain by compression and destruction. Hematogenous metastasis from structures of the head or other parts of the body is included in secondary tumors.[156] Eighty per cent of the secondary tumors have metastasized from the blood stream.

Incidence

The incidence of brain neoplasia in the dog and cat has not been fully determined. Other tumors have been more thoroughly investigated because they can easily be seen clinically or at necropsy. Routine exposure of the brain and cord is not usually done by veterinary pathologists, who may already be overtaxed with work. Fixing and slicing the specimens is time-consuming and, unless it is done carefully, produces poor results. More work must be done along the lines suggested by Innes,[86] McGrath,[156] and Schlotthauer[202] to provide a better understanding of neoplasms of the central nervous system.

There is no reason to believe that such neoplasms occur less frequently than tumors affecting other systems. Dahme has reported an incidence of 0.98 per cent (24 of 2258 necropsies) primary intracranial tumors in animals.[43] The majority were found in short-skulled breeds of dogs. Luginbühl studied 155 cat brains and found eight tumors.[149] Schiefer[201] reported that out of 8013 dogs in necropsies over a 12-year period, 62 or 0.8 per cent had CNS tumors. Twenty-six were seen in boxers, whose risk incidence was estimated to be about 6.5 per cent.[201] McGrath reported on 136 intracranial neoplasms, of which 88 were primary, 10 secondary from other parts of the head, and 38 metastatic from other areas.[156] Of the primary tumors, 20 were astrocytomas and 10 were pituitary adenomas. Schlotthauer found six brain tumors in 130 cases of organic brain disease that were examined at necropsy.[202] Four were primary and two were metastatic.

Koestner reported that of 24 primary tumors of the central nervous ssytem, six were primary reticuloses.[130] Of these six, two were of possible inflammatory origin and four were definitely neoplastic. These lesions originated from undifferentiated perithelial cells, were confined to the central nervous system, were space-occupying masses, and were of unknown origin.

Few has diagnosed six brain tumors in 93 dogs whose clinical signs indicated the presence of a brain disorder—an incidence of about 6.4 per cent.[64] According to Innes and Saunders, the incidence of intracranial tumors in man is 2 to 5 per cent of all tumors.

The *breeds* most frequently affected in McGrath's series of 88 *primary* tumors are as follows: boxers, 42; Bostons, 18; mongrels, 7; German shepherds, 5; and miscellaneous, 16. The age incidence varied from seven months to 17 years, with 73 of 88 (83 per cent) occurring between the ages of 5 and 11 years. There were 57 males and 31 females.[156]

In McGrath's series of 48 *secondary* brain tumors, 38 were metastatic tumors, including primary adenocarcinomas seen most frequently in the mammary gland, the thyroid, the nasal sinus, and the bronchus. Other metastatic tumors included melanomas, hemangiosarcomas, osteosarcomas of mammary origin, and neurogenic sarcomas.

Luginbühl, Fankhauser, and McGrath[150] have recently published a most comprehensive study on spontaneous neoplasms of the nervous system in animals. Their findings add much to the knowledge of animal tumors, and those of interest to the author of this text are summarized in the following statements: Tumors of neuroectodermal (neuroepithelial) origin comprise about 30 per cent of the total number of nervous system tumors, and all except the plexus papilloma appear most frequently in boxers, Boston terriers, and other brachycephalic breeds. Oligodendrogliomas in the dog are the most frequently observed neuroectodermal tumors. Eighty-five per cent were seen in brachycephalic breeds, generally in frontal, olfactory, and temporal lobes. Most were in 5- to 11-year-old dogs, and two-thirds of them were males.

Astrocytomas were also seen largely in Bostons and boxers, and the majority were seen in the pyriform area of the brain. Of 20 glioblastomas, 17 were seen in brachycephalic breeds. Ependymomas appear most frequently in boxers that are 6 to 12 years of age. However, plexus papillomas appeared most frequently in nonbrachycephalic breeds, and only one of 15 appeared in the boxer. The fourth ventricle housed nine of the 15 plexus papillomas.[150]

Of the mesodermal tumors, 40 meningiomas were studied from the dog and 70 from cats. Meningiomas appeared most frequently in the dolichocephalic breeds, mainly in shepherds and collies. The usual location was parasagittally over the convexity of the cerebral hemispheres. They occurred less frequently in the cerebellum, and the least frequent site was the tentorium. Six were seen in the area of the spinal meninges. Neoplastic reticuloses may be among the most frequent tumors seen in the brain of the dog from 3 to 14 years of age, and show little breed predilection. Of the ectodermal tumors, pituitary adenomas occur in the dog with a frequency similar to that in man.[150]

From these data, one might conclude that CNS tumors are frequently seen in the dog, and no doubt an increased incidence will be reported as neurologists and pathologists make more careful clinical, gross, and histological examinations.

The most recent statistics on nervous tissue tumors in animals have been reported by Hayes *et al.*[94] from diagnoses reported by 11 veterinary teaching hospitals from March 1964 through December 1972. Of 248 animals, 199 cases of nervous tissue tumors were seen in dogs, 14 in cats, 7 in cattle, and 28 in horses. They were divided for purposes of analysis into three categories: glial, meningeal, and peripheral nerve tumors. In cats, the tumors were equally distributed among the three categories, whereas in dogs, twice as many

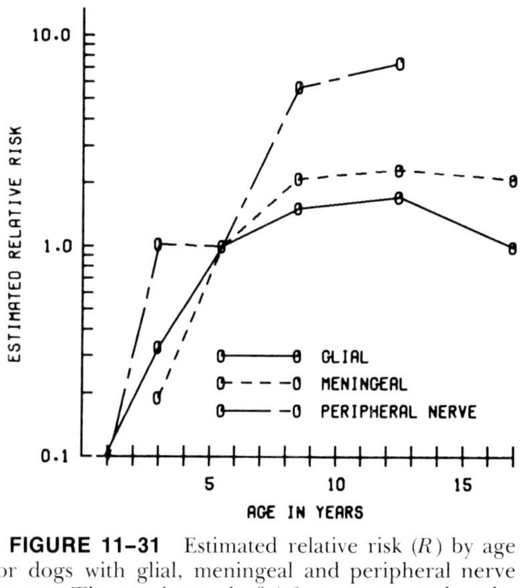

FIGURE 11–31 Estimated relative risk (R) by age for dogs with glial, meningeal and peripheral nerve tumors. The age interval of 4-6 years was used as the standard reference ($R = 1$). R values for the age intervals ≤ 1, 2-3, 4-6, 7-9, and 10-14 years were plotted at the midpoint of each interval. Adjustment was made for breed and sex in R calculations. (From Hayes, H. M., Priester, W. A., and Pendergrass, T. W.: Occurrence of nervous tissue tumors in cattle, horses, cats, and dogs. Int. J. Cancer *15*, 39, 1975.)

TABLE 11–1 ESTIMATED RELATIVE RISK[a] *(R)* OF CANINE NERVOUS-TISSUE TUMORS FOR ALL BREEDS WITH ≧4 TUMORS OBSERVED, BY BREED AND BY SEX WITHIN TUMOR CATEGORY*

Tumor Category	Risk Category	Cases Observed	R
Glial (96)	Breed		
	Boxer	33	23.3[b]
	Boston terrier	6	5.2[b]
	All breeds combined	96	1
	Poodle, miniature or toy	6	0.7
	All other purebred	38	0.7[b]
	Mixed breed	13	0.5[c]
	Sex		
	Female	42	0.8
	Male	54	1
Meningeal (50)	Breed		
	German shepherd	6	1.4
	Poodle, miniature or toy	5	1.1
	All breeds combined	50	1
	All other purebred	32	0.9
	Mixed breed	7	0.6
	Sex		
	Female	26	1.0
	Male	24	1
Peripheral nerve (53)	Breed		
	Beagle hound	4	2.4
	German shepherd	5	1.1
	Mixed breed	14	1.0
	All breeds combined	53	1
	All other purebred	30	0.9
	Sex		
	Female	31	1.3
	Male	22	1

*Hayes, H. M., Priester, W. A., and Pendergrass, T. W.: Occurrence of nervous tissue tumors in cattle, horses, cats, and dogs. Int. J. Cancer *15*, 39, 1975.
[a]Adjustment made for age and sex in determining breed *R* and for age and breed in determining sex *R*.
[b]Significantly different ($p < 0.05$) from *R* 1.
[c]Significantly different ($p < 0.01$) from *R* 1.

glial tumors as meningeal and peripheral nerve tumors were found. The risk for glial tumors in dogs reached a peak at 10 to 14 years of age, for meningeal tumors at 7 to 9 years, and for peripheral nerve tumors at 2 to 3 and 7 to 9 years. Three breeds—English bulldog, boxer, and Boston terrier—had an especially high risk of glial tumors. There was no detectable predisposition by sex for any nerve tumors among the four species. Among glial tumors in brachycephalic breeds 28 of 40 were astrocytomas. The highest relative risks among canine nervous tissue tumors were for glial tumors: in the boxer, 23.3 per cent, and in the Boston terrier, 5.2 per cent; the risk of meningeal tumors in the German shepherd was 1.4 per cent; and the risk of peripheral nerve tumors in the beagle was 2.4 per cent[94] (Figs. 11–31 and Tables 11–1 to 11–3).

TABLE 11–2 GLIAL TUMORS IN ALL DOGS BY CELL TYPE AND SITE*

	Site	
Cell Type	*Brain*	*Spinal Cord*
Astrocytoma	49	9
Ependymoma	14	8
Plexus-papilloma	8	
Oligodendroglioma	2	1
Medulloblastoma	3	
Glioma, undifferentiated	2	

*Hayes, H. M., Priester, W. A., and Pendergrass, T. W.: Occurrence of nervous tissue tumors in cattle, horses, cats, and dogs. Int. J. Cancer *15*, 39, 1975.

TABLE 11–3 GLIAL TUMORS IN BRACHYCEPHALIC DOGS BY CELL TYPE AND SITE*

Breed/Cell Type	Site: Brain	Site: Spinal Cord
Boxer		
Astrocytoma	22	2
Ependymoma	3	
Plexus-papilloma	2	
Oligodendroglioma	2	
Medulloblastoma	1	
Glioma, undifferentiated	1	
Boston terrier		
Astrocytoma	4	
Oligodendroglioma		1
Glioma, undifferentiated	1	
English bulldog		
Astrocytoma	1	
Ependymoma	2	
Pug		
Astrocytoma	1	

*Hayes, H. M., Priester, W. A., and Pendergrass, T. W.: Occurrence of nervous tissue tumors in cattle, horses, cats, and dogs. Int. J. Cancer *15*, 39, 1975.

Clinical Signs

The preceding discussion can be summarized to better comprehend the complexities of the clinical signs accompanying brain tumors.

It appears that those tumors of neuroectodermal origin, such as oligodendrogliomas, astrocytomas, and ependymomas, occur almost entirely in brachycephalic breeds, especially the boxer and Boston terrier. However, the plexus papillomas do not seem to have a predilection for any breed. The mesodermal tumors, such as meningiomas, appear most frequently in dolichocephalic breeds, and the neoplastic reticuloses have no breed predilection. The dog is most frequently affected between the ages of 4 and 11 years.[94] Deficiencies in cranial nerve function, general sensory and motor function, behavioral abnormalities, and convulsive disorders can be caused by brain tumors. The signs of cord tumors can be attributed largely to destruction or compression of the cord, which causes sensory and motor dysfunction. The signs can determine localization of the lesion.

Palmer and co-workers[176] studied 21 dogs afflicted with intracranial neoplasia. Useful localizing signs were seen when the tumor was small. Multiple brain changes complicated the early signs during spread and growth of the tumor. Common clinical signs included change in temperament, locomotor deficits, visual disturbance, papilledema, circling, turning and tilting of the head, hemiplegia, hemianopia, and sensory loss. Visual defects and abnormal pupillary responses were seen in 15 out of 21 animals, and papilledema occurred in 10 of 21 animals. The authors differentiate papilledema, papillitis, and pseudopapilledema. Papilledema is a passive edema of the optic disk, usually associated with increased intracranial pressure rather than primary inflammatory change; it does not usually result in loss of vision. It is an important clinical sign and must be interpreted carefully in the dog because of many normal variables. Papillitis is an inflammatory swelling of the disk associated with blindness, whereas pseudopapilledema is a congenital anomaly due to an excess of glial tissue and is considered a normal variant. Palmer noted that the various gliomas appeared to originate in tissue adjacent to the anterior part of the lateral ventricles, perhaps from subependymal plate, and appeared to cause destruction of similar areas of the brain.[176]

The principal works in English dealing with brain tumor in the dog are those of Innes,[116] McGrath,[156] and Palmer.[174] A tumor is chiefly evident by increased intracranial pressure caused by its growth, collateral inflammation, edema, hemorrhage, obstruction in the flow of cerebrospinal fluid, and focal tissue destruction of the tumor that causes dysfunction of the part affected.[116] The increase in intracranial pressure frequently masks or confuses the neurological signs; therefore, many signs are difficult to explain when based on necropsy findings.

It must be emphasized that the signs of neoplastic disease depend upon the location of the lesion or tumor. Some of the more common locations include (1) the cribriform plate, (2) the pituitary fossa, (3) the ventrolateral posterior fossa, and (4) the cerebellopontine angle. Besides the neurological, laboratory, radiographic, and brain scan examinations, EEG procedures are frequently diagnostic for space-occupying masses. Contrast cerebral angiography

Text continued on page 354

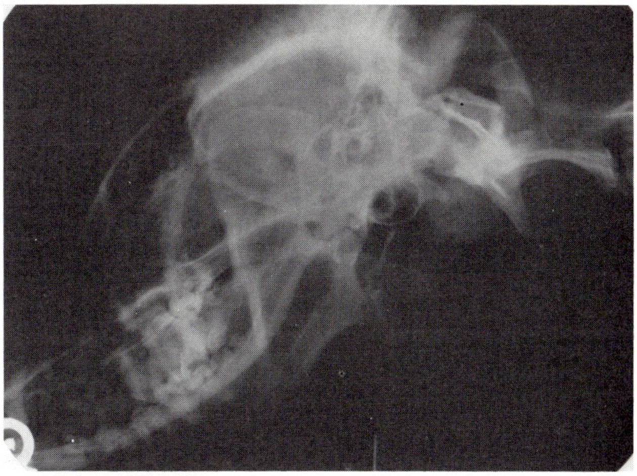

FIGURE 11–32 An osteogenic sarcoma involving the calvarium of a 7-year-old pointer, who was showing encephalitic clinical signs. Notice the typical "sunburst" osseous rays.

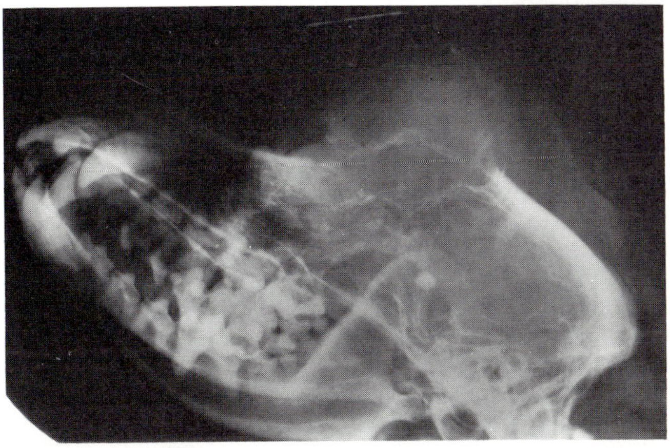

FIGURE 11–33 A malignant bone tumor involving the frontal bones and sinuses. The cranial bone shows necrosis and tumorous invasion into the prefrontal areas of the brain.

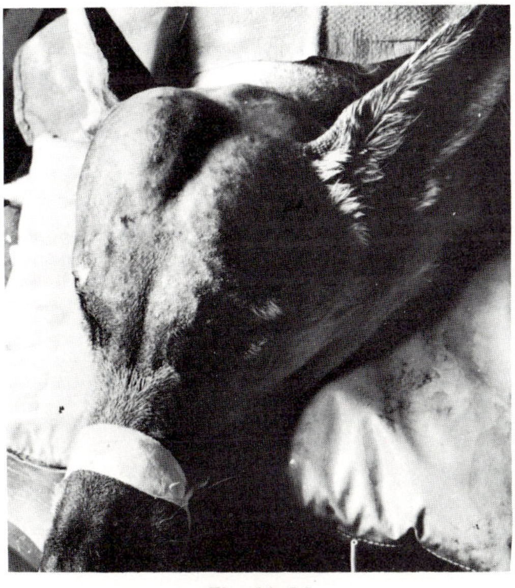

Fig. 11–34

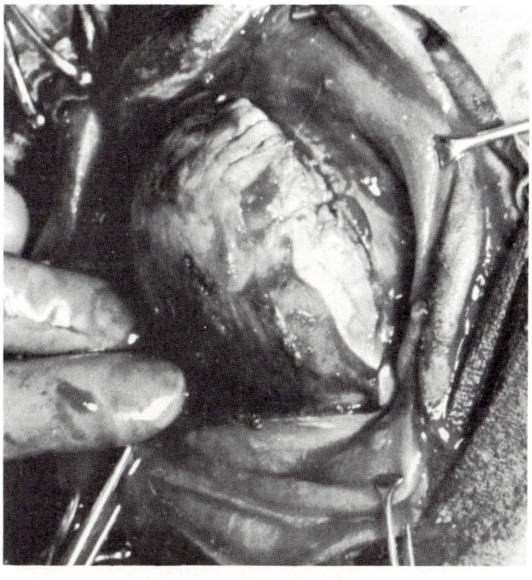

Fig. 11–35

FIGURE 11–34 A large, hard swelling had been developing on the right calvarium of this 8-year-old German shepherd for 2 to 3 months. The dog was beginning to become depressed and mentally dull.
FIGURE 11–35 At surgery, the tumor mass was found to be well encapsulated.

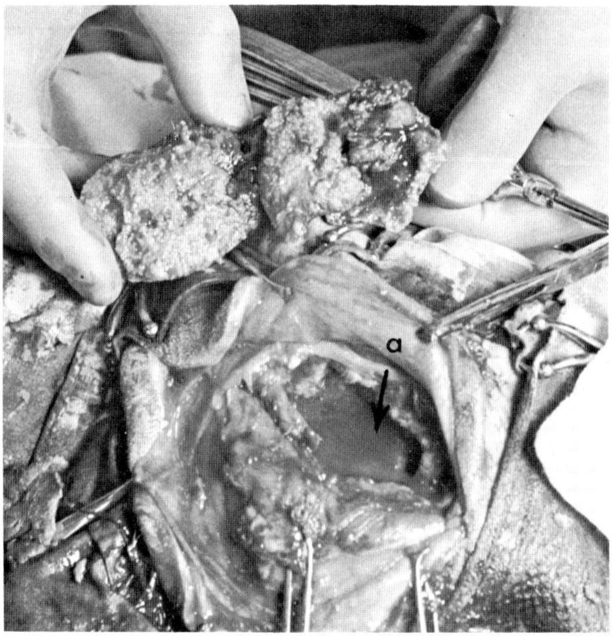

FIGURE 11–36 The mass of tissue was carefully removed and was found to have invaded the cranium in an area of approximately 3 cm in diameter (a). The bone defect seemed to be due to pressure necrosis, and the surrounding bone was normal. The tumor was a chrondrosarcoma. No recurrence has been seen during an 8-month followup postoperative period.

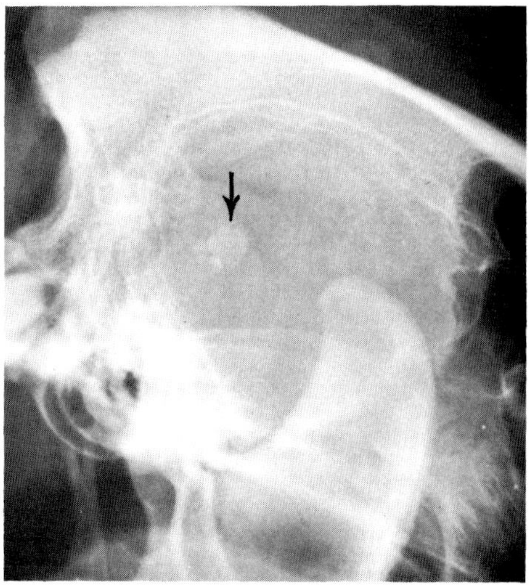

FIGURE 11–37 A lateral radiograph demonstrates calcification of the dura on the posterior cerebrum. This finding may be asymptomatic.

A

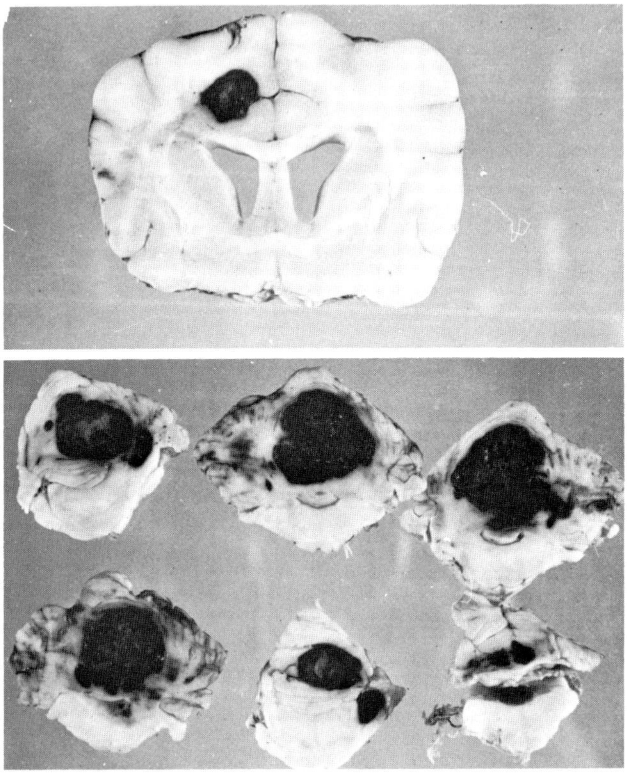

B

FIGURE 11–38 An 8-year-old pointer had metastatic hemangiosarcomas affecting the mediastinum, diaphragm, kidneys, ovary, brain, and spinal cord. The dog seemed to be normal until she became incoordinate and paralytic (spastic) and developed nystagmus. These signs all occurred within a period of 2 weeks. *A*, Brain cross section. *B*, Brain stem cross-section.

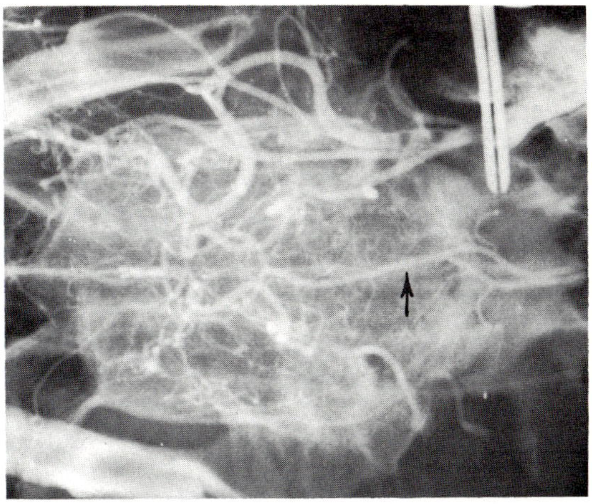

FIGURE 11–39 A VD cerebral arteriogram demonstrates a "sweeping curve" to the basilar artery. This is frequently seen in apparently normal dogs, but in this case a sizeable medullary tumor was observed pushing the artery laterally.

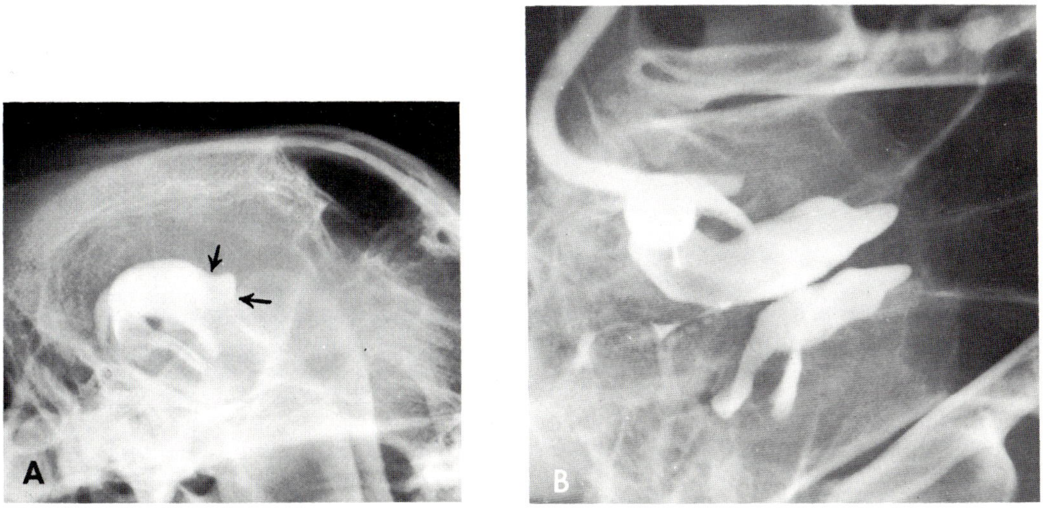

FIGURE 11–40 Pantopaque ventriculograms of a 7-year-old boxer that had an astrocytoma approximately 10 by 15 cm in the right olfactory and prefrontal lobes of the brain. Because of the tumor, the left ventricle was small (*A*) and the right ventricle was dilated posterior to the mass (*B*). It had pressed the midline to the left and caused a partially occluded left lateral ventricle. Notice the indentation in *A*. *A*, Lateral view. *B*, Ventrodorsal view.

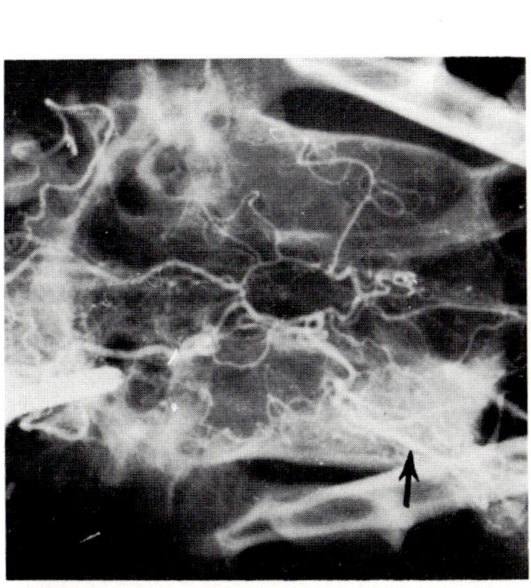

Fig. 11–41

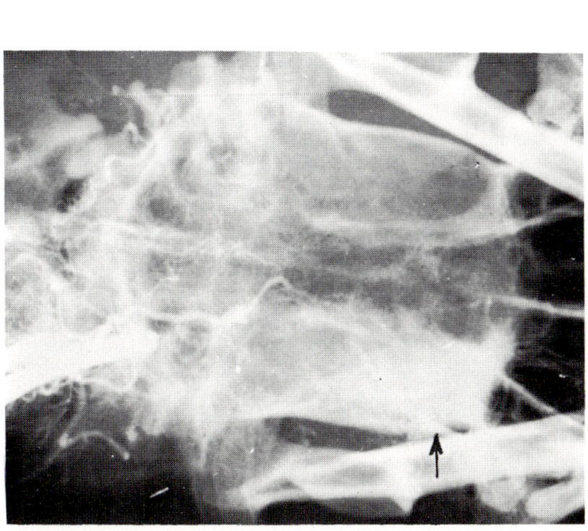

Fig. 11–42

FIGURE 11–41 A cerebral arteriogram shows unilateral "pooling" of vascular contrast medium in the frontal area. (From James, C. W., and Hoerlein, B. F.: Cerebral angiography in the dog. Vet. Med. *55*, 1960.)

FIGURE 11–42 Same case as shown in Figure 11–41. The contrast medium is still present in the cerebral venogram. Notice that the rest of the brain is almost clear of the venous medium. (From James, C. W., and Hoerlein, B. F.: Cerebral angiography in the dog. Vet. Med. *55*, 1960.)

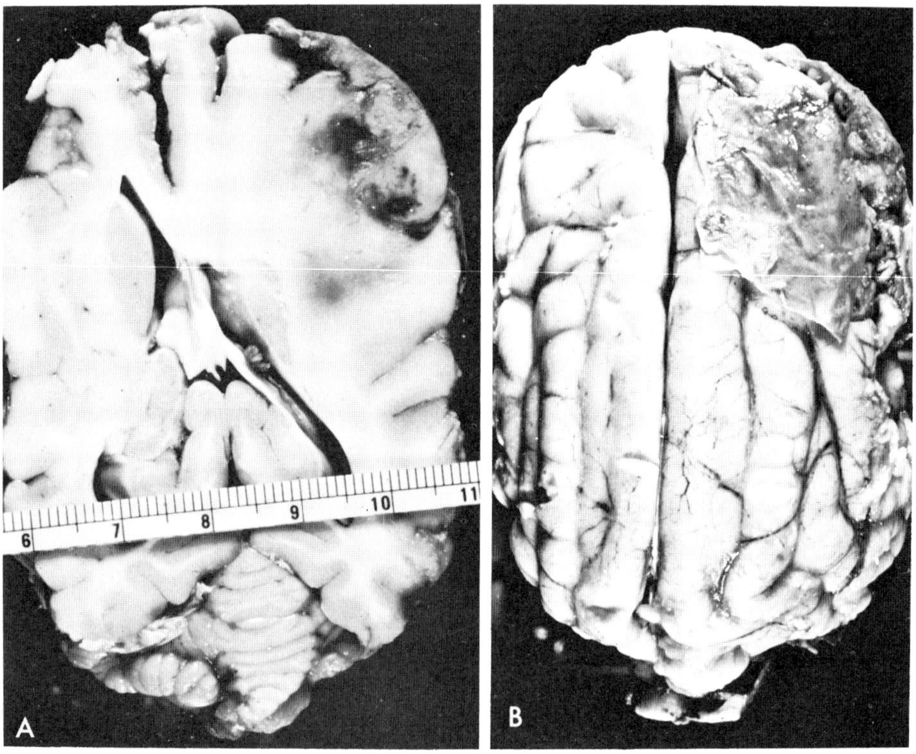

FIGURE 11–43 Same case as shown in Figures 11–41 and 11–42. The tumor was a meningioma. Predominant clinical signs were convulsions. (From James, C. W., and Hoerlein, B. F.: Cerebral angiography in the dog. Vet. Med. 55, Nov., 1960.)

and ventriculography may be indicated (Figs. 11–32 to 11–43).

Differential Diagnosis

The following conditions must be considered: distemper, encephalitis, meningitis, subdural hematoma, cerebral vascular disease and accidents, and epilepsy.

Even though neurologists in human medicine have gained a high degree of competence in diagnosis, errors can be expected. One report indicated that 34 tumors were found unexpectedly at necropsy. Twelve of these were incidental, but in 22 instances there were clinical histories of neurological disorders erroneously diagnosed during life. Confusion with cerebrovascular disease was most common.[159]

Treatment

Central nervous system tumors are treated chiefly by surgery and in some cases by radiation. Surgery is most likely to be successful in treating meningeal tumors. McGrath reported eight such tumors among 88 primary brain tumors.[156] Other surface tumors of the cerebral cortex may be removed surgically with a fair possibility of eventual return to a clinically normal state. It is doubtful that many deep-seated tumors are operable; those in the medulla and near the pituitary area are very difficult to explore. Successful brain surgery involves early and accurate diagnosis of the site of the lesion.

McClelland has reported that a combination of cytotoxic agents and x-ray therapy has been encouraging in treating reticulum cell sarcomas in dogs and cats. Cyclophosphamide, vinblastine, and steroids (methylprednisolone) were the primary drugs used. Four cases were completely cured, three were cured for up to 2 years, two for up to 1 year, and one for less than a year.[155] Fewer and co-workers reported on use of carmustine and vincristine in 81 human patients with recurrent primary or metastatic brain tumors. The overall response of clear clinical improvement was 48 per cent with carmustine and 30 per cent with the combination of carmustine and vincristine. In patients with glioblastoma, the response rates were 53 per cent and 25 per cent respectively. Two patients were still alive and leading normal lives at 13 and 14 months after initial therapy. These patients were selected because they had pronounced signs that could be evaluated by comparable periodic brain scans, radiography, and laboratory tests as well as by clinical response during the course of therapy.[65]

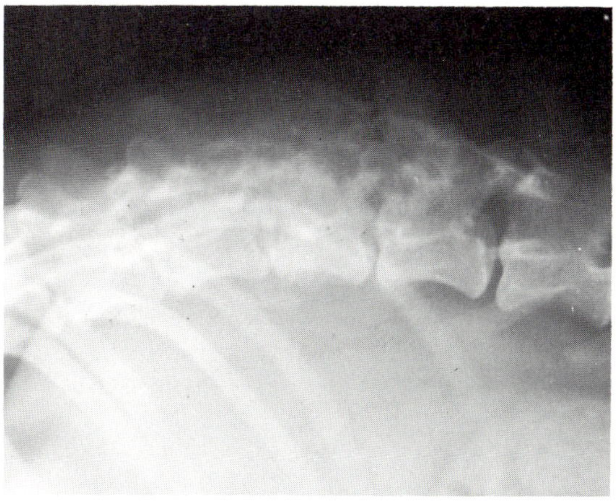

FIGURE 11–44 Lateral radiograph showing pathologic changes of L1–3 vertebrae characteristic of a malignant bone tumor. This 6-year-old Boston terrier was paraplegic.

VERTEBRAL AND SPINAL CORD TUMORS

Vertebral Neoplasms

Vertebral neoplasms generally cause a compression of the spinal cord because of their invasive growth patterns. They may occur as primary tumors in the spine or as metastases. An osteosarcoma has been reported in an 8-year-old dog that had metastasized from the leg to the fourth thoracic vertebra and the lungs. Vertebra T4 suffered a pathologic fracture, and a compression myelitis resulted.[36] Another recent report dealt with a cord compression secondary to a pancreatic carcinoma. The third lumbar vertebra had been invaded and weakened until a fracture occurred, causing paraplegia.[35] There was a more recent report of a malignant round cell tumor resembling a reticulum cell sarcoma that caused a compression myelitis at T2–3. The clinical signs were characteristic of compression in this area and also included a left-sided Horner's syndrome (miosis, ptosis, and enophthalmus).[218] In our clinic, we have seen malignant lymphomas, spinal cord schwannomas, meningiomas, and spinal bone tumors that cause a compression myelitis and subsequent motor dysfunction.

The signs of spinal bone tumors are characteristic of a compression myelitis, which is described on page 454. The diagnosis is suggested by the history of an insidious onset and a slow progression of symptoms, and the appearance of the disorder usually in middle-aged and older dogs. Other compression syndromes that should be considered are dural ossification, spondylosis, spinal cord tumors, and disk

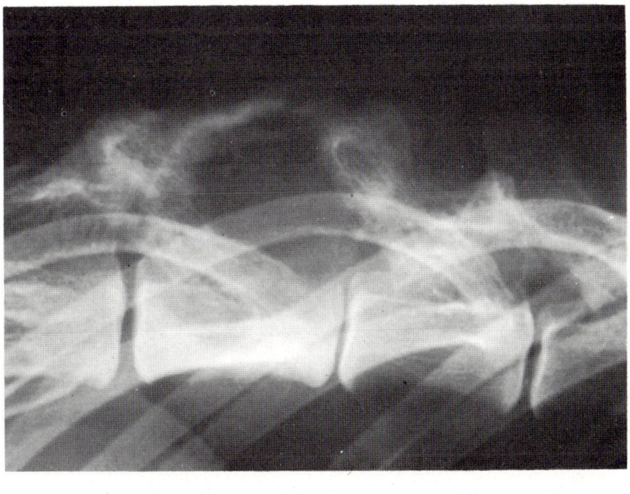

FIGURE 11–45 Malignant bone tumor of a thoracic vertebra characterized by massive bone destruction.

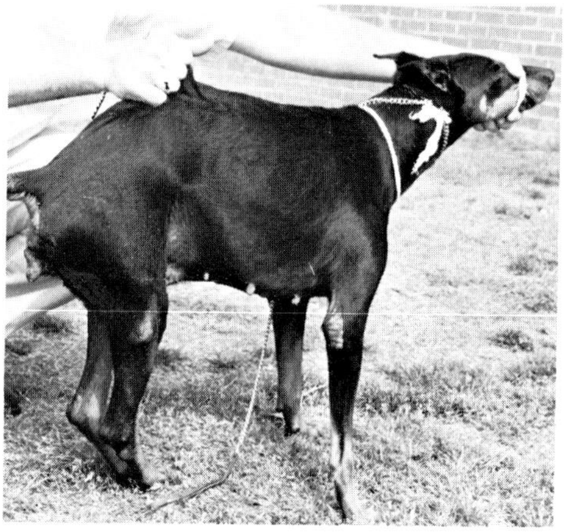

FIGURE 11–46 This 9-year-old Doberman was suffering from progressive paraplegia. Relief of neurologic signs was obtained by injecting large doses of adrenocortical steroids at 7-day intervals over a period of several months.

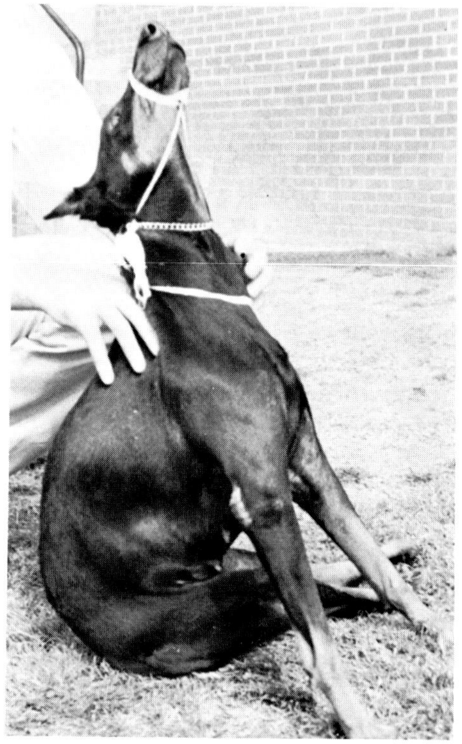

FIGURE 11–47 The same dog as shown in Figure 11–46. The dog was totally paraplegic and was becoming vicious because of the pain.

disease. A positive diagnosis can frequently be made by radiographic examination.

The radiographic changes in malignant vertebral neoplasms are characteristic; areas of destruction and proliferation are seen. Malignant bone tumors generally do not invade or cross a joint. Rarely is a zone of increased density at the junction between the affected and normal bone seen, because of the speed of progression. This is helpful in distinguishing a tumor from osteomyelitis.[31] We have, however, observed several cases in which the primary neoplasm affected more than one vertebra. The radiating appearance of new bone growth, so characteristic of osteogenic sarcomas of other bones, has not been seen frequently in the spine nor does the tumor look wild. Clinically, however, tumors of the spine may be seen in a medical clinic more frequently than are tumors of long bones because of the associated neurological disorders (Figs. 11–44 to 11–58).

Treatment

The treatment of vertebral malignancies is difficult in animals and usually impractical. Life might be prolonged by very early

Text continued on page 360

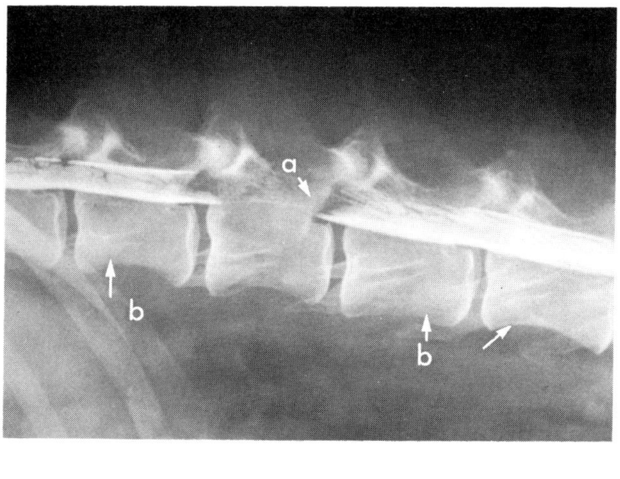

FIGURE 11–48 A lateral myelogram of the case shown in Figures 11–46 and 11–47: (a) subarachnoid filling defect; (b) osteoporosis of all the vertebrae—a general radiographic observation of the entire skeleton. The paralysis was due to a sarcoma, and the general demineralization was thought to be due to prolonged usage and large doses of adrenocorticoid steroids.

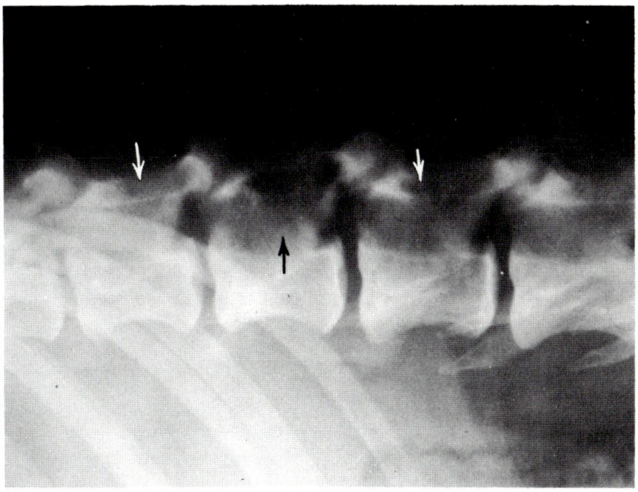

FIGURE 11–49 A multiple myeloma in the first three lumbar vertebrae caused a paraplegia from compression of the cord.

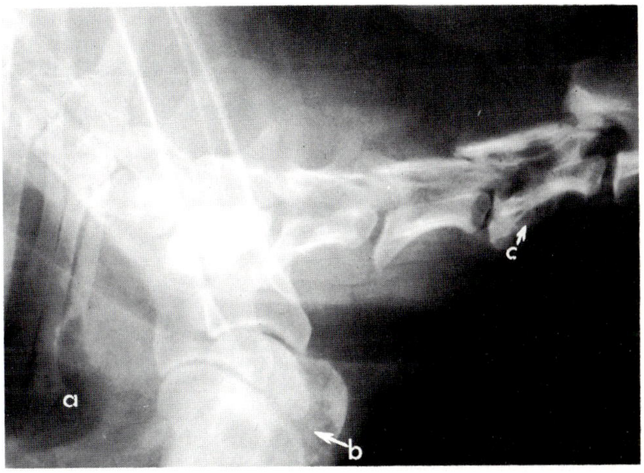

FIGURE 11–50 Metastatic hemangiosarcoma affecting numerous visceral organs, as well as the ribs, humerus, and third cervical vertebra: (a) rib tumor, (b) proximal humeral tumor, (c) cervical tumor.

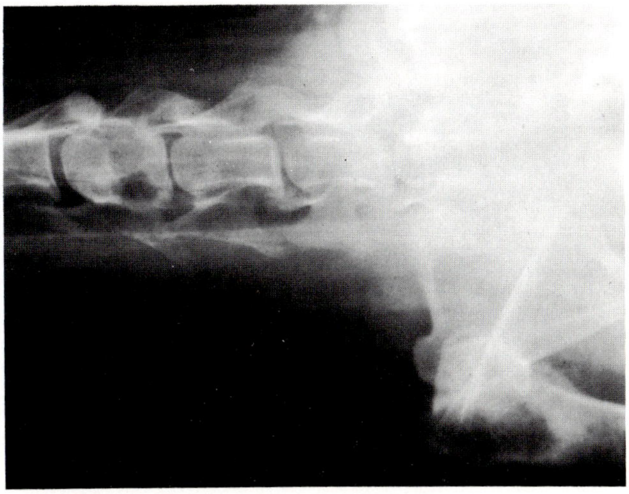

FIGURE 11–51 A ventrodorsal view of the case shown in Figure 11–50.

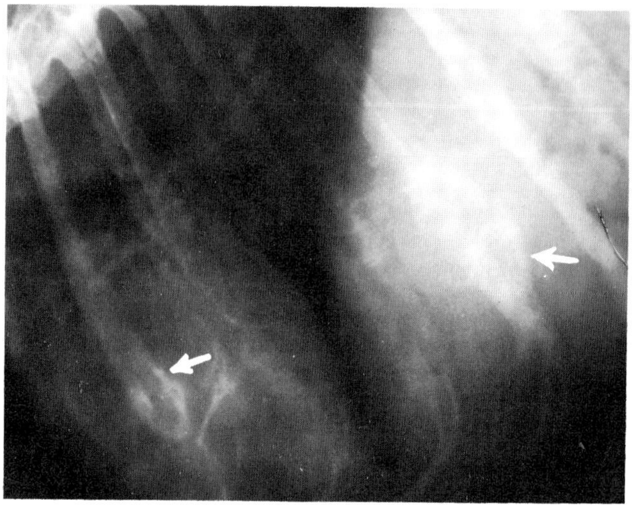

FIGURE 11–52 The rib tumors in the case described in Figures 11–50 and 11–51. The dog suffered primarily from neurological signs, which were tetraparesis and pain.

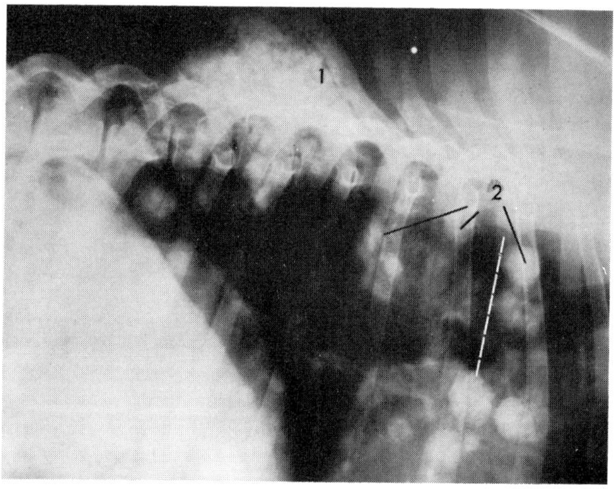

FIGURE 11–53 A primary osteogenic sarcoma in a 6-year-old male pointer affecting T6–9 with metastasis to the lungs. (1) primary tumor; (2) lung tumors.

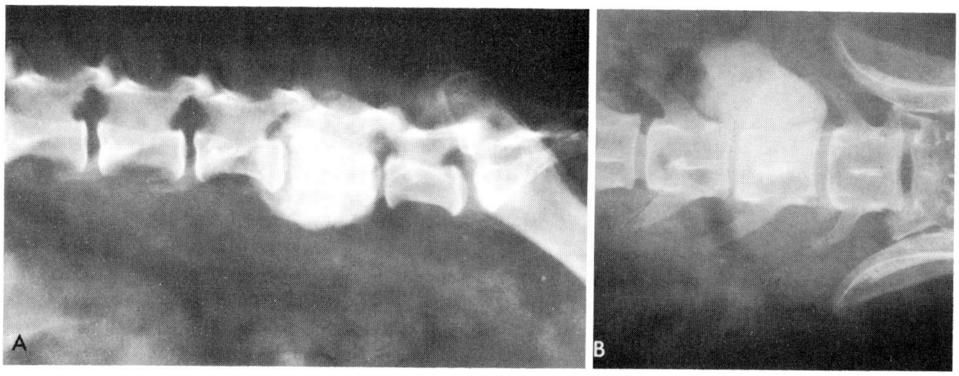

FIGURE 11–54 An osteosarcoma of L6 vertebra. *A*, Lateral view. *B*, Ventrodorsal view.

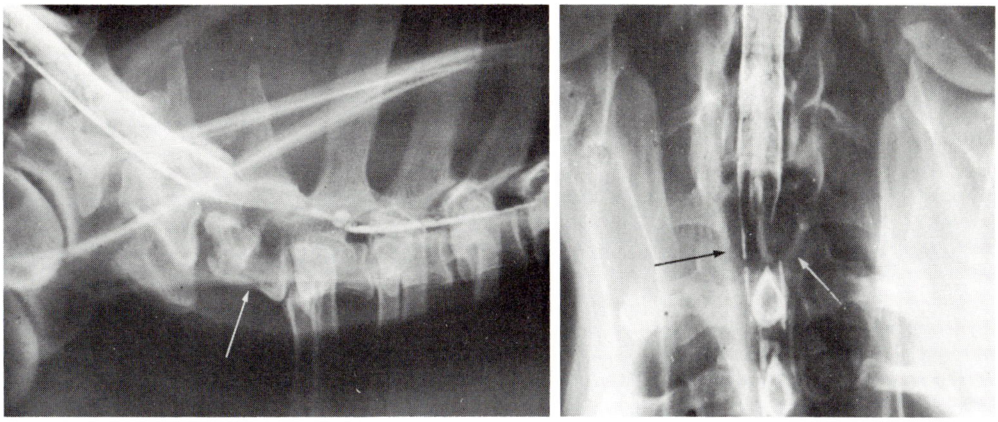

A B

FIGURE 11–55 A myelogram showing tumor metastasis to the vertebral column. Notice the destruction of C7 and the spinal cord compression. The primary lesion was an osteosarcoma of the distal radius. *A,* Lateral view. *B,* Ventrodorsal view.

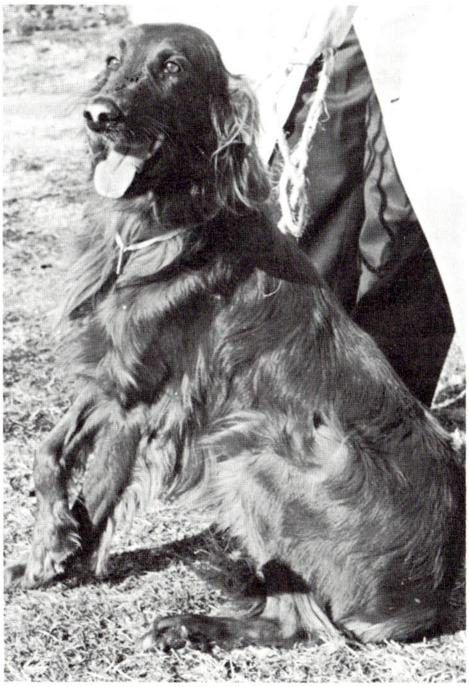

FIGURE 11–56 Five-year-old Irish setter was suffering from bilateral front leg weakness. Notice the muscle atrophy.

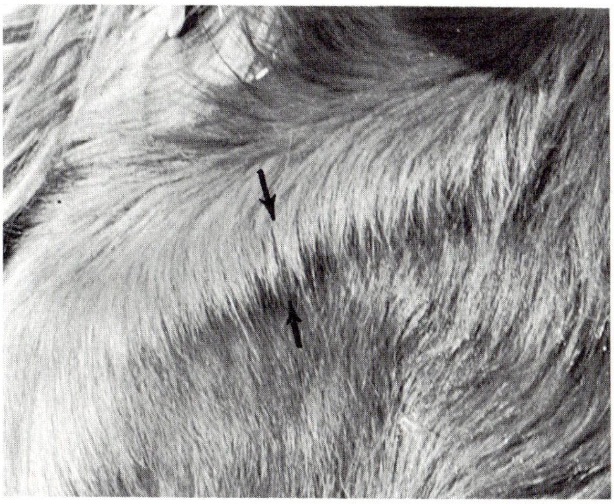

FIGURE 11–57 A close-up of supra- and infraspinatus muscle atrophy present in the case shown in Figure 11–56.

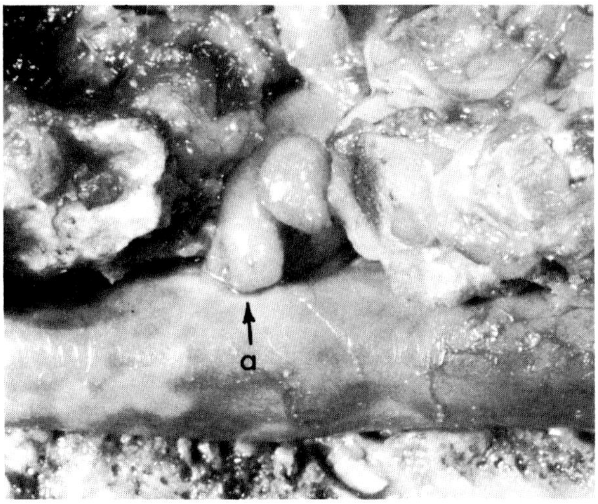

FIGURE 11–58 A neurofibrosarcoma was demonstrated on necropsy: (a) tumor of spinal nerve and spinal cord.

surgical removal of the tumor and if necessary a spondylectomy and immobilization of adjacent vertebrae with spinal plates or by implantation of a vertebral prosthesis.[23, 256] Benign neoplasia of spinal bone would be more amenable to such surgical procedures.

Osteocartilaginous Exostoses of the Spine

Multiple cartilaginous exostoses have been reported in humans, dogs, cats, and horses.[188] In man a definite hereditary basis has been established, and the disorder has also been seen in a litter of dogs.[75] Two cases seen by Prata and one case in the Auburn clinic involved the spine and caused spinal cord compressions and neurological deficits. One of Prata's cases was a 4-month-old mixed breed who had a cystic bony lesion at T_7 that was causing progressive neurological deficits until partial tetraplegia occurred. The other case of Prata was a 1-year-old Alaskan malamute who had multiple bony cysts at L3–4, T1, T2, and T4 dorsal spinous processes; T4–5 facets; and the dorsal lamina and right pedicle of T4. Signs of a UMN lesion consisted primarily of proprioceptive deficits, hyperreflexia, and clonus. Surgical decompression of both patients resulted in definite clinical improvement, and no progression of signs in the surgical areas has been noted in the postoperative observation periods of one-half year and 9 months respectively.

The case of spinal compression seen in the Auburn clinic was massive at the terminal cervical areas but less damaging in two other cranial thoracic areas. The patient was a 1-year-old Great Dane puppy.

In man, solitary osteocartilaginous exostosis is the most common benign neoplasm of bone, and less than 1 per cent of solitary lesions undergo malignant transformation. However, there is a 20 per cent risk for development of chondrosarcomas in multiple osteocartilaginous exostoses in man.[188]

Based on Prata's apparently successful experience with surgery, surgery should be considered in select cases as a possible temporary or semipermanent therapeutic measure.

Epidural Tumors

Tumors that occur in the spinal canal but are not of vertebral or meningeal origin frequently are reticuloendothelial tumors. These tumors frequently grow in the spinal canal of the cat and occasionally in the dog, causing a characteristic compressive myelomalacia. Frequently, adjacent abdominal lymph node enlargements can be palpated or demonstrated radiographically. The diagnosis can be suspected from other signs of malignant lymphoma and contrast myelography.[198]

Tumors of the Spinal Nerve Roots

Mulligan reported an incidence of 14 neurofibromas and 27 neurofibrosarcomas in 1000 canine tumors (4.1 per cent), chiefly among animals 7 to 14 years of age.[164] Lombardi[144] reported a series of 249 spinal tumors in man: 57 per cent were intradural, 17 per cent were extradural, 15 per cent were intramedullary, 11 per cent were intra- and extradural, and 4 per cent were malignant.[144] Most tumors were located in the thoracic spinal cord. Love reported that in 514 surgically treated intraspinal tumors in man, the clinical symptoms of the extramedullary intradural neurofibroma closely resembled those of the protruding disk.[145]

Meningioma

A meningioma produces a compression syndrome, since it presses progressively upon the neuronal tissues in the spinal cord. Depending upon the rate of growth, the course may be either slow or rapid. Meningiomas are seen more frequently than medullary tumors. We have noticed that one of the chief clinical differences between meningiomas and disk compression or other progressive spinal compressions is the rapid deterioration in the animal's neural state after the pain has become acute.

Medullary Tumors of the Spinal Cord

Medullary tumors appear to be encountered less frequently than meningiomas, judging from the few reports in the literature.

Regardless of the types of intramedullary tumor, the symptoms are indicative of the location of the tumor rather than the type. Since these tumors are generally localized, the characteristic symptoms may be a segmental weakness, reflex abnormalities, and muscle atrophy, progressing to final paralysis. In man, 80 per cent of the symptoms are usually unilateral initially, but as the tumor grows they may affect both sides.[156] In the dog, the absence of reflexes is thought to be a cardinal sign.

Leptomeningeal Cysts

This disorder is occasionally seen in man and may occur more frequently in dogs than clinicians think. Gage reported on an extensive cervical leptomeningeal cyst

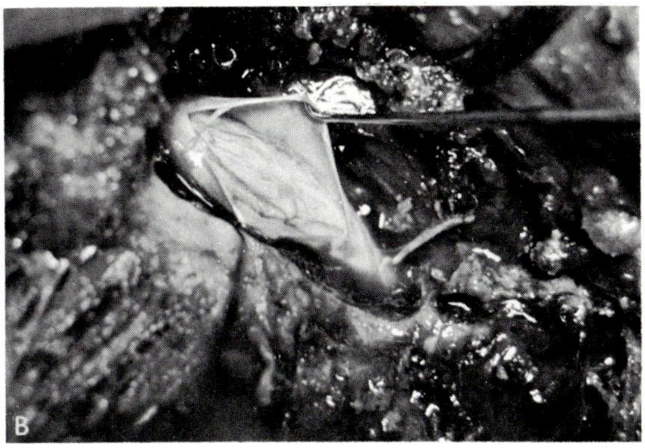

FIGURE 11–59 At surgery, a leptomeningeal cyst was seen. The dura was sutured to muscle fascia to maintain drainage. Clinical recovery resulted. (Courtesy of Gage, E. D., Hoerlein, B. F., and Bartels, J. E.: J.A.V.M.A. *152*, 1664, 1968.)

which occurred in a 10-year-old Weimaraner.[72] Neurological signs were characteristic of compression or cord neoplasia. A laminectomy revealed the cyst which could not be removed in toto but was incised and drained, and the dura was sutured to the adjacent musculature to maintain a constant draining fistula. Clinical recovery occurred.

The cyst formation was thought to be due to localized traumatic arachnoiditis associated with long-term, repeated efforts to open a heavy sliding glass door with his head and neck in order to gain access to the outside yard. The abnormal myelographic findings prompted the laminectomy (Fig. 11–59).[72]

A 4-year-old female beagle with paraparesis was reported to have a meningeal cyst within a hemivertebra that was connected to the subarachnoid space. The cord compression caused considerable dorsal columnar deformation, but the pial vasculature and dura were normal.[182]

Diagnosis and Treatment of Intraspinal Tumors and Cysts

The diagnosis of intraspinal tumors and cysts is based on clinical signs that should have localized the lesion generally. Occasionally CSF sediment will reveal an abnormal cytology, and a tumor can be suspected. Since flat film radiography is usually normal unless the tumor has produced some bony tissue destruction or laid down dense fibrous or calcific material, myelography will generally reveal the precise location. The use of the EMG may help in localization of the lesion.

The treatment consists of surgical exploration by means of a hemilaminectomy or dorsal laminectomy, and removal if feasible. These procedures have been discussed in Chapter 14.

CONGENITAL, DEGENERATIVE, AND HEREDITARY CNS DISORDERS

INHERITED METABOLIC DISORDERS

Metabolic Storage Diseases[12]

In the new concept of inherited diseases as "inborn errors of metabolism" (Sir Archibald Garrod),[12] certain diseases are thought to result from a mutation of a single gene that causes defective production of an enzyme dependent on it. As a result, cells lose their ability to carry out the specific metabolic reactions that are normally governed by this enzyme. In several instances the biochemical substrate normally metabolized by the deficient enzyme accumulates in the cells—therefore, the term "storage diseases." The central nervous system is frequently involved or even selectively affected. Several inherited metabolic storage diseases of man have been reported, and Baker has presented the most significant inherited metabolic diseases of dogs and cats in Table 11–4. These are all progressive degenerative disorders characterized by the usual clinical signs of tremors progressing to generalized locomotor disease. All these disorders are characterized by an absence or a severe deficiency of a specific enzyme which leads to an abnormal accumulation of the biochemical substrate normally hydrolyzed by that enzyme. Frequently, the name of the disease is derived from the nature of the accumulated material, such as GM_1 gangliosidosis. The mode of the inheritance is recessive, so only homozygous recessive individuals develop clinical signs of disease. Therefore, heterozygous carriers are the key to the perpetuation and extension of these traits. Carriers can be recognized by enzyme testing in special laboratories or by breeding trials. It is obvious that clinically affected animals should not be bred.[12] The majority of these storage diseases in small animals are due to errors in sphingolipid or glycolipid metabolism.

GM_1 and GM_2 Gangliosidosis in Cats

Baker and co-workers[73] have identified GM_1 gangliosidosis in Siamese cats with B galactosidase deficiency. This disease has been studied in detail using varied procedures of reproducing it in breeding. Clinically it is characterized by tremors progressing to generalized locomotor deficiency in the young kitten. Transmission is autosomal recessive and is strikingly similar to that of juvenile GM_1 (type 2) gangliosidosis of children.[73] A GM_2 gangliosidosis was recently discovered in a family of Siamese cats.[41] This condition is most similar to Tay-Sachs disease in man (Fig. 11–60).

GM_2 Gangliosidosis in German Short-Haired Pointers[16, 74, 125, 158]

GM_2 gangliosidosis has been described several times; however, a specific enzyme defect has not yet been confirmed. The dogs show the first neurological signs—nervousness and inability to learn—at 6 months of age. Later ataxia, blindness, deafness, psychic changes, and convulsions occur.

Globoid Cell Leukodystrophy (Krabbe's Disease)

Globoid cell leukodystrophy is a sphingolipidosis or lipid storage disease characterized by a deficiency of the enzyme cerebroside β galactosidase associated with degeneration of myelin. The activity of β galactocerebrosidase which normally splits galactose from galactocerebroside to yield ceramide is reduced. The destruction of myelin sheaths and axons and the accumulation of globoid macrophages in peripheral nerves and CNS white matter are common histological findings. The ultrastructural features of the globoid cells[67, 68] in this disease have also been studied carefully (Fig. 11–61).

The disease has been seen in this country

TABLE 11–4 INHERITED METABOLIC DISORDERS OF THE NERVOUS SYSTEM IN DOGS AND CATS*

Diseases	Breeds Affected	Lesions	Age of Onset	Signs	Biochemical Lesion
Canine globoid cell leukodystrophy (Krabbe's disease)	Cairn terriers; West Highland white terriers; mixed breeds	Demyelination; globoid cells	4 to 5 months	Progressive motor disability	Cerebroside accumulates; β-galactosidase deficiency
Feline globoid cell leukodystrophy	Domestic cat	Same as canine GLD	5 to 6 weeks	Same	Unknown
Feline sphingomyelin lipidosis (Niemann-Pick disease)	Siamese cat	Vacuolation of neurons and macrophages in liver, spleen, etc.	2 to 4 months	Same	Sphingomyelin accumulates; sphingomyelinase deficiency?
Feline metachromatic leukodystrophy	Domestic cat	Demyelination, gliosis	2 weeks	Same; rapidly progressing to convulsions; opisthotonus	Sulfatid accumulates arylsulfatase deficiency
Feline CNS glycogenosis (Pompe's disease)	Domestic cat	Neuronal accumulation of glycogen	Young adult	Unknown	Glycogen accumulates; α-glucosidase deficiency?
Canine GM_2 gangliosidosis (Tay-Sachs disease)	German shorthair pointers	Vacuolation of neurons	9 to 12 months	Ataxia; blindness; seizures	GM_2 ganglioside accumulates; hexosaminidase deficiency?
Feline GM_1 gangliosidosis	Siamese cats; domestic cat	Vacuolation of neurons	10 to 16 weeks	Tremors; incoordination; paraplegia	GM_1 ganglioside accumulates; β-galactosidase deficiency

Terms in parentheses refer to eponyms used for analogous human disorders.
*From Baker, H. J.: Inherited metabolic disorders of the nervous system in dogs and cats. *In* Kirk, R. W. (ed.) *Current Veterinary Therapy V*. W. B. Saunders Co., Philadelphia, 1974.

and in Europe, predominantly in Cairn terriers and West Highland white terriers. More recently, it has been diagnosed in a miniature poodle,[257] two female kittens,[120] and a beagle.[119] Most cases have been related to heredity. The signs appear when the animal is a few weeks to a few months old; coordination and locomotion are affected primarily. Motor deficits may progress to paralysis. Visual deficiency may be seen. Tremors and loss of spinal and postural reflexes are common. Fletcher[67] studied EEG changes as the disease progressed into generalized hemispheric asymmetrical spindling and spiking, excessive high voltage activity, and a decrease of EEG arousal to sound stimuli. As the disease progressed, the EEG revealed a generalized decrease in voltage and a static pattern regardless of the behavior state of the animal.[67]

The differential diagnosis should include other progressive CNS diseases such as distemper, syringomyelia, toxoplasmosis, and spinal anomalies. Hip dysplasia and myasthenia gravis might also be considered. The history of breed incidence, the characteristic clinical picture, and the absence of radiographic lesions will be helpful in the diagnosis. Histological examination and possible enzyme studies must confirm the diagnosis.

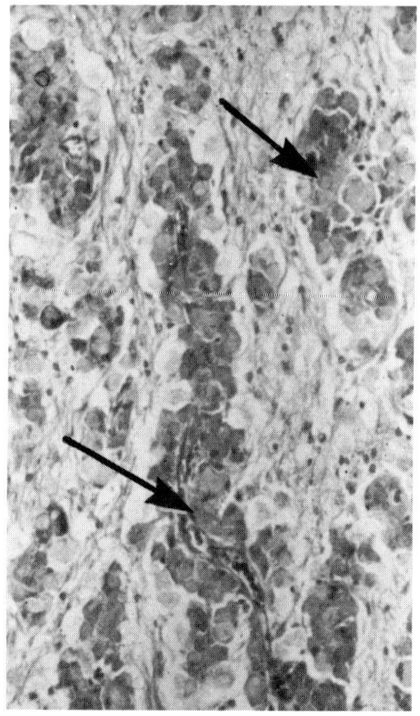

FIGURE 11–61 In this case of Krabbe's leukodystrophy in a West Highland terrier there is a demyelinating lesion in the cerebellum with a perivascular accumulation of globoid cells (arrows). Medium power.

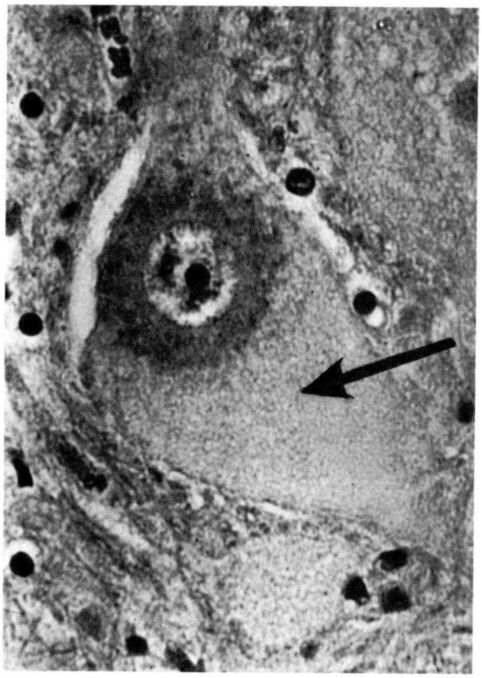

FIGURE 11–60. GM_1 gangliosidosis in a Siamese cat. A neuron contains a large amount of storage material (arrow). Hematoxylin and eosin, high power.

There is no effective treatment.

Canine Neuronal Glycoproteinosis (Lafora's Disease)

As in man, this disease appears to be inherited as an autosomal recessive trait. It is rarely diagnosed, and seems to be caused by an undefined metabolic disturbance. In dogs, the disorder has been seen in a basset hound, a miniature poodle, a group of beagles, a mixed breed dog, and a standard poodle. Clinical signs include depression, hyporeflexia, somnolence, and progressively severe seizures. The age of onset varies, and the disease has occurred in puppies as well as in one 12-year-old dog. The diagnosis is based on the presence of intraneuronal inclusions (Lafora's bodies) in the cerebellum within the Purkinje cells and their dendritic processes as well as neurons in the thalamic region. The inclusion is composed of an insoluble, complex, glycoprotein material. Treatment is basically symptomatic. If seizures occur, anticonvulsants are indicated. Neurologically affected animals should not be used for breeding until inherited disease has been eliminated as the cause.[42, 105, 106, 110, 173, 226]

Ceroid Lipofuscinosis in English Setters

Several cases of a storage disease that appears similar if not identical to *amaurotic familial idiocy* in man have been reported in English setters.[49, 87, 131, 132] Koppang[131, 132] reported a study of more than 100 English setters which have proved to have recessive inheritance of this disease in breeding trials. Clinical signs usually begin at 12 to 15 months of age and include reduced vision, dullness, disorientation, and aggressiveness. Ataxia, muscle spasms, and convulsions may develop. Necropsy lesions reveal a small brain of about two-thirds the normal weight and enlarged lymph nodes; the size of liver and spleen are normal. There is generalized deposition of lipid granules in the CNS and even in autonomic neurons in the heart, lungs, and gastrointestinal tract. The retinal lipid granules occur in ganglion cells. English setter disease is nearly identical to that described as juvenile amaurotic idiocy in man. Lipid bodies share many if not all of the same characteristics as ceroid and lipofuscin granules. Until the enzymatic nature of the disease is more firmly established, the proposed name of the disorder is neuronal ceroid-lipofuscinosis.[132]

Neuronal Lipidosis in Cocker Spaniels

A lipid storage disease of unknown biochemical nature has been described in five cocker spaniels or part cocker spaniels.[54,195] The clinical signs are similar to those previously described for other neuronal storage diseases.

Neuroaxonal Dystrophy in Cats

A newly recognized feline neurological disorder, characterized clinically by an abnormal coat color and development of ataxia during infancy, is caused by an inherited error of metabolism. Breeding experiments indicate that this neuroaxonal dystrophy is inherited in an autosomal recessive manner.[251]

Hereditary Ataxia in Smooth-Haired Fox Terriers

Bjorck *et al.*[18, 19] reported a hereditary neurological syndrome in smooth-haired fox terriers. Signs of ataxia began at the age of 2½ to 4 months and progressed slowly over a period of 4 to 10 months before the animals were destroyed. Pathologically, focal absence of myelin in the spinal cord was noted.

Hartley[91] saw a similar syndrome in Jack Russell terriers (a short-legged, smooth-haired terrier), but in addition to the spinal cord lesions there were widespread wallerian degeneration in the CNS and degenerative changes in the central auditory pathway and peripheral nerves.

Quadriplegia and Amblyopia in Irish Setters

Palmer[177] reported a study of 18 congenitally diseased Irish setter pups from nine litters. The clinical signs were inability to stand or walk, tremors, nystagmus, uncontrolled movements, and seizures. Two pups died at 5 to 6 weeks of age, and the rest were put to sleep later. Histological loss of the Purkinje cells, proliferation of astrocytes, and wallerian-type degeneration were seen in the white matter. Chromosome pattern, chemical analysis of brain lipids, and blood, urine, and CSF tests were normal. A fully penetrant autosomal recessive gene, postnatally lethal in the homozygote, was determined to be the cause of transmission.[177]

Hereditary Cerebellar Cortical and Extrapyramidal Nuclear Abiotrophy in Kerry Blue Terriers

A hereditary neurological disease in Kerry blue terriers was reported by de Lahunta and Averill.[45] After the onset of the disease, between 9 and 16 weeks of age, the animals showed pelvic limb stiffness and mild head tremors. The signs progressed within 3 weeks to marked cerebellar ataxia with spasticity. After 3 to 6 months of illness, muscle atrophy was apparent, and the animals became so severely incapacitated that they had difficulty eating. Pathologically, there was progressive degeneration of the Purkinje cells in the cerebellar cortex and the olivary nuclei, and in later stages there was bilateral degeneration of the substantia nigra and the caudate nuclei.

Hereditary Neuronal Abiotrophy in the Swedish Lapland Dog

This disorder has been observed since 1951, and a total of 26 cases are currently on record. The disease affects puppies 5 to 7 weeks of age without preference to sex. Progression of weakness results in tetraplegia and atrophy of distal limb musculature and joint fixation. Neurological and electrodiagnostic examinations furnish evidence of lower motor neuron disease. Fibrillation potentials and positive sharp waves are recorded from the pelvic limb musculature, and tibial and peroneal conduction values are reduced. Histological changes include central and peripheral chromatolysis, cell body shrinkage, neuronophagia, and axonal and myelin degeneration in both central and peripheral nervous tissues. The disease is hereditary, and its transmission is autosomal recessive. The disease is comparable with abiotrophies in man, such as spinal muscular atrophies and hereditary ataxias.[197]

Stockard's Paralysis

Stockard's paralysis has been produced in large breeds of dogs by cross-breeding. Great Dane–bloodhound and St. Bernard–Great Dane cross-matings have caused posterior paresis and paralysis in the pups at an average age of about 3 months. The disease was transmitted through an inheritable multiple factor and at least three dominant genes. The pathologic changes were due to degeneration and death of certain motor and preganglionic sympathetic neurons in the ventral and lateral gray horns respectively.[220]

It is possible that the condition could develop in certain families of large nonregistered dogs.

OTHER DEGENERATIVE DISEASES

Encephalomalacia in Dogs and Cats

Hartley[90] described necrotizing lesions in the cerebral cortex of 15 dogs. In most cases no cause could be established. In two cases the lesions probably resulted from cyanide poisoning. Clinical signs were dominated by acute onset of epileptiform convulsions that occurred with increasing frequency, myoclonic twitches, and occasionally severe mental deterioration. Similar observations were made by Fischer,[66] who found idiopathic symmetrical necrosis in the rhinencephalon and Ammon's horn in ten dogs. The dogs showed severe convulsive signs, and most had a history of gastroenteritis of diverse origin before the onset of the epileptiform convulsions.[29] Fankhauser[58] described Ammons horn necrosis in dogs who ingested iodochinoline preparations. The disease also occurs in cats.[62] The predominant clinical signs are sudden onset of aggressiveness and epileptiform attacks.

Neurofibrillary Accumulations

De Lahunta and Shively[46] reported widespread CNS damage due to accumulation of neurofilaments in the neurons of a puppy with generalized neurological dysfunction and weakness. Vandevelde *et al.*[236] observed a similar condition in a 6-week-old cat in which the motor neurons of the spinal cord were selectively affected. Clinically progressive weakness of the limbs, muscle atrophy, and finally tetraplegia were noted.

Leukodystrophy in Cats

Hegreberg[96] described a leukodystrophy in young kittens with progressive neurological deterioration, convulsions, and loss of motor reflexes. Pathologically, severe demyelinating lesions, gliosis, and intracytoplasmic inclusions were found. The disease appears to be familial.

Fatzer[60] reported five cases of a leukodystrophic disease in young kittens. Severe ataxia, abnormal postural reactions, head tremors, blindness, and abnormal behavior were clinically evident as soon as the animals were able to walk. Pathologically severe defects were found in the cerebral white matter. In addition, in four of the five cases, lesions consistent with cerebellar hypoplasia were observed, similar to those seen in infectious panleukopenia. It was concluded that the lesions were caused by a noxious effect upon the fetus.

Dysmyelination in Dogs

The term dysmyelination is used to define diseases of the CNS in which there is a congenital insufficient synthesis of myelin. Abnormal myelination in the CNS of the newborn has been reported in a variety of animal species. The best-known examples are congenital tremors in piglets and so-called jumpy mice. A similar syndrome was observed in three dogs at Auburn University during the period 1975–76. One animal was a male, 6-week-old Dalmatian who had been showing strong tremors since birth. On clinical examination the animal had trouble in supporting itself and appeared disoriented. The head continuously rocked back and forth, and the animal was shaking all over. The signs disappeared during sleep. Pathologically, there was almost complete lack of myelin in the central nervous system, whereas the peripheral nerves were perfectly well myelinated. On histological and ultrastructural examination only very few poorly developed myelin sheaths could be seen. The disease was thought to be due to a congenital malfunction of the oligodendroglial cells.

In a litter of chow dogs, two puppies had been showing similar signs. One animal was destroyed, and defective myelination was found on pathological examination. The other puppy was kept alive and gradually recovered, although it was still ataxic after several months and showed marked tremors, especially when excited.[230]

Demyelination in Miniature Poodles

A demyelinating disease of the brain and spinal cord in miniature poodles has been reported by several authors.[156, 217] The age of onset is from 9 weeks to 5 months. Cerebellar signs (ataxia, dysmetria, incoordination) are often predominant. In McGrath's cases,[156] posterior paresis progressing to tetraplegia with marked spasticity was noted. Postural reflexes are mostly abnormal, and the condition progresses, eventually leading to death.

Necrotizing Myelopathy in Afghan Hounds

A demyelinating malacic disease involving largely the thoracic spinal cord has been reported in seven Afghan hounds.[37] The age of onset varied from 3 to 13 months, and the course of the disease varied from 2 to 6 weeks before complete lack of function and death occurred. Clinical signs varied from ataxia, flaccid or spastic paraplegia, complete tetraplegia, respiratory distress, and intercostal paralysis to death. Four of the seven dogs were littermates, and another dog among the seven also had an affected littermate. Vascular studies demonstrated abnormal arterial and venous blood supply to the affected cord areas in some of the dogs. It is assumed that some interference with blood flow produced ischemia, softening, and necrosis in the affected sections of spinal cord.

Histological studies revealed no sign of infectious disease or similarity to previously described disorders of the canine spine or spinal cord. The occurrence of the disease in only one breed and in several littermates suggests that it could be hereditary.[37]

Diffuse Degenerative Myelopathy in Aging German Shepherds[8, 84]

This disorder is similar to other degenerative CNS disorders discussed previously. However, the disorder is confined to the spinal cord and shows no sign of an infectious viral or microbial origin.

Averill[8] reported on 22 dogs with progressive, ataxic, spastic paraparesis, 20 of which were German shepherds. The mean age was 9.6 years and there was no sex predominance. The clinical signs progressed over a 1 to 3 month period prior to elective termination. Necropsies on each of seven showed diffuse degeneration of the spinal cord myelin and axons in all funiculi

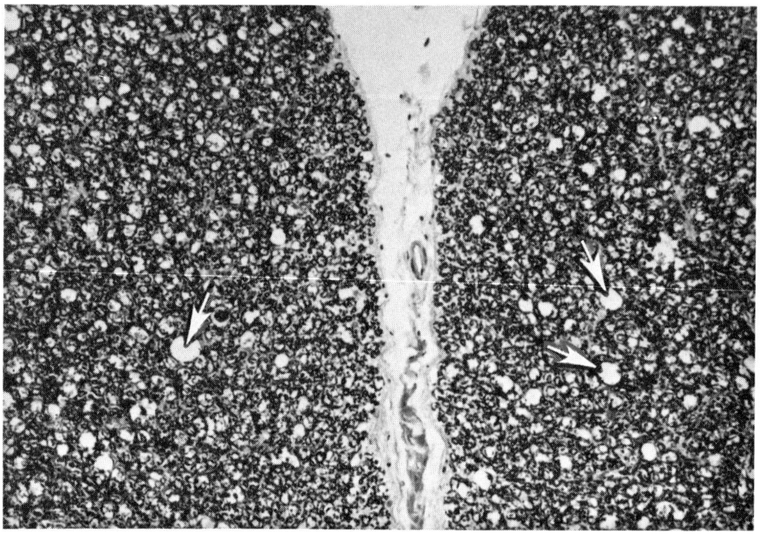

FIGURE 11–62 A case of ataxia in an aging German shepherd showing a few distended myelin sheaths (arrows) in the ventromedial columns of the spinal cord. Luxol fast blue-cresylecht violet stain, medium power.

with subsequent astrogliosis. The degenerative changes were not associated with intervertebral disk herniations, spondylosis deformans, or osseous metaplasia of the dura. The condition was regarded as a primary spinal cord degeneration of unknown cause (Fig. 11–62).

The clinical signs are initially confined to the pelvic limbs and consist of various degrees of posterior paresis, exaggerated segmental reflexes, crossed extensor reflexes, and proprioceptive deficiencies. Deep pain and sphincter reflexes are present in the early stages. The onset of the disease is usually so insidious that the owners are not alarmed and often do not present the dog for examination until 6 to 8 months after the first signs appear. As the disease progresses, the animal becomes unable to rise or walk with the pelvic limbs. Disuse atrophy of the caudal trunk and hindquarter muscles is evident. The front limbs may become involved late in the course of the disease. Spondylosis deformans and osseous metaplasia of the spinal dura were also seen in the dogs studied, but there was no correlation of these disorders either as to clinical signs or to microscopic lesions.[8]

Histological changes of disseminated demyelination were present in the cervical, thoracic, and lumbar cord segments but were most extensive in the middle to distal middle thoracic area. There are similarities between this myelopathy and that associated with vitamin B_{12} deficiency in man. The chief difference is that in vitamin B_{12} deficiency the lesions usually have a multifocal pattern instead of the topographically continuous pattern seen in the dog.[8] Griffiths and Duncan[84] reported another series of dogs affected with the same condition; these had lesions in the dorsal spinal nerve roots in addition to the changes reported by Averill. In Auburn, approximately ten cases a year appear at the Small Animal Clinic. The pathological changes found in these animals are consistent with those reported by Averill[8] and Griffiths and Duncan.[84] However, we feel that the lesions in some cases are so minimal that their relationship to the most severe clinical signs is questionable. Ultrastructural and biochemical studies of the CNS, particularly the myelin, in those animals will be necessary to establish the true nature of the disease.

The diagnosis should be based on neurological signs of a UMN disorder of the hind limbs, with no laboratory evidence of inflammatory disease in the CSF specimens. The differential radiographic examination should be based on evidence of a compression from disk protrusion, fracture, luxation, or neoplasia. Evidence of spondylosis or dural ossification may not be significant.

The treatment is palliative with steroids, phenylbutazone, indomethacin, salicylates, or high B complex vitamins. Steroids may be effective as long as they are maintained until the inflammatory neurological changes have caused permanent cord damage.

CONGENITAL MALFORMATIONS

Hydrocephalus

This entity is discussed in Chapter 21.

Lissencephaly in Lhasa Apso Dogs

This peculiar congenital malformation was detected in two Lhasa apso dogs presented at Auburn University. The dogs were approximately 1 year of age at the time of clinical examination and were having seizures of the grand mal type for several weeks prior to presentation. The behavior of both dogs had been abnormal since birth: inability to learn or to recognize objects and owner and unpredictable attacks of aggressiveness were observed. Visual perception seemed to be impaired in both animals, since they collided with stationary objects while running fast. Pathologically, the cerebral neocortex lacked fissuration (smooth cortex), and its histological configuration was severely abnormal, suggesting an arrest in neuronal migration during fetal development. The dogs were not directly related. Although it was not possible to trace the ancestry back in one animal, it was felt that hereditary factors could be involved.[80]

Cerebellar Hypoplasia and Cerebellar Vestibular Syndrome

Cerebellar hypoplasia is the most frequently reported developmental defect of the brain in cats and the second most frequent in dogs (hydrocephalus is first).[189] In dogs the defect is usually a malformation of the vermis of the cerebellum and is generally described as agenesis.[33, 52, 53, 171] Miniature poodles are affected on occasion with cerebellar demyelination.[217] Innes and Saunders cite case reports on congenital cerebellar disorders in two Boston terrier littermates and in airedales, as well as references by many different workers.[116] Cases of congenital cerebellar hypoplasia have been reported in sheep and calves.[116, 124] White found that 23 of 62 members of a family (five generations) were affected with periodic nystagmus, vertigo, and ataxia with onset in early childhood. The pattern of inheritance seems to be a single autosomal dominant trait.[248]

The clinical signs usually start as soon as the animal begins to move around. The most common findings are dysmetria, truncal ataxia, occasional circling, and intention tremor. The syndrome is usually not progressive, and the animal may improve with time as he learns to compensate. Dogs with agenesis of the vermis may have a flattened occipital bone and increased space in the posterior fossa which can be outlined by pneumoencephalography. Cats with a grossly hypoplastic cerebellum may have a reduced posterior fossa which may be visualized on a lateral radiograph of the skull.[171]

The vestibular or cerebellar-vestibular syndrome generally refers to disorders of one or more portions of the vestibular system. Broadly speaking, in veterinary terminology at least, the vestibular system includes the structures of the inner ear, the vestibular portion of the eighth cranial nerve, the vestibular nuclei in the medulla, and the various connections of the vestibular nuclei to the cerebellum, reticular formation, lower motor neurons via the vestibulospinal tract, and eye muscles. Primary cerebellar manifestations have been discussed in this chapter under drugs, encephalitides, and viral hypoplasia; primary vestibular manifestations have been covered under otitis interna, hemorrhage, tumors, and trauma with or without eighth nerve involvement. Prominent signs of vestibular disease include (1) circular walking in the direction of the affected ear, (2) head tilt with the affected ear down, (3) falling toward the ispilateral side, (4) ipsilateral foreleg hypotonia, (5) trunk curvature with the concavity toward the affected side, (6) reluctance to lie on the affected side, (7) spontaneous nystagmus with a slow component toward the side of the lesion, (8) downward ocular deviation of the ipsilateral eye and upward deviation of contralateral eye, and (9) occasional concomitant facial paralysis.[175]

Blauch and Martin[20] recently have reported a benign vestibular syndrome of old dogs characterized by horizontal directional nystgmus, head tilt, and ataxia. The fast component of the nystgmus is contralateral to head tilt and the affected side, and the patient spontaneously improves within 7 to 10 days, except that head tilt may persist for several weeks. Some reports have suggested that this syndrome may be due to strokes or vasospasms that indicate an unfavorable prognosis. Spontaneous recoveries or improvement occurs in these old dogs; however, recurrences in the same ear or side do occur. Although the cause is obscure, Blauch feels that it is probably a labyrinthitis that is either transitory or compensated for.[20]

The diagnosis of the cerebellovestibular syndrome demands a careful analysis of the history, neurological examination, laboratory and radiographic findings, and occasionally EEG examination when distemper or infectious encephalitis is involved. The treatment depends on the cause. Surgical therapy of middle and inner ear disorders is described in Chapter 16.

Congenital Deafness

Acquired deafness can result from many disorders, including infections in the brain or ear, traumatic injuries, toxic drugs, and neoplasia. However, congenital deafness is a well-known entity in several breeds of dog, particularly Dalmatians. Bull terriers, Sealyhams, Scotch terriers, border collies, and fox terriers have also been affected.[2, 111] Predominance of white in hair color appears to be a related characteristic. The ear structures appear normal on physical and radiographic examination. Definitive diagnosis of deafness is aided by electroencephalographic audiometry.

Spinal Dysraphism

Spinal dysraphism is an incomplete closure of the primary neural tube and was studied by McGrath in 78 purebred Weimaraners.[157] The classic clinical sign is an abnormal gait in the hind limbs in which the animal hops symmetrically like a rabbit. The dog stands peculiarly in a crouching position (Fig. 11–63). Signs in the hind limbs include a wide stance, hyperextension during standing, and unilateral abduction. Unilateral stimulation usually induces bilateral flexor and scratch reflexes in the hind limbs. Once the clinical signs are established, there is typically no progression or retrogression.[157]

Pathologic changes in the cord primarily

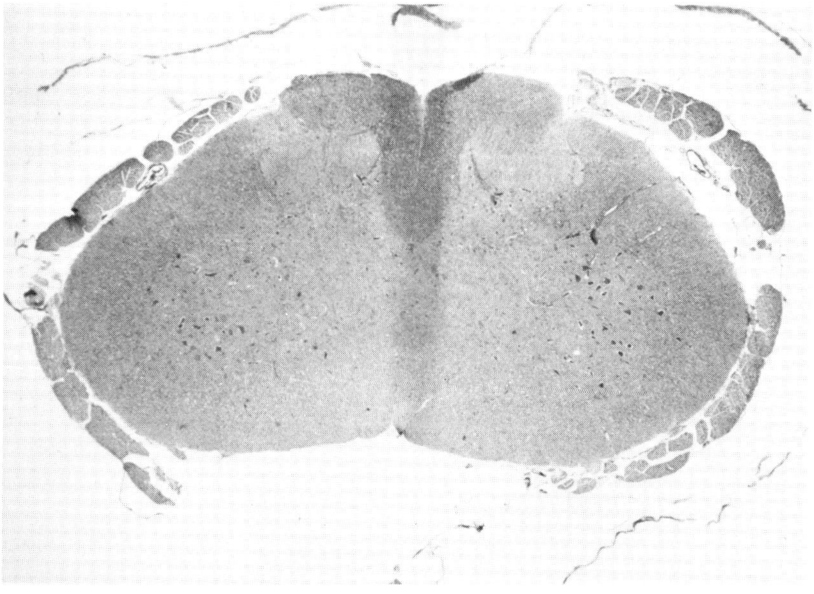

FIGURE 11–63 Dysraphism in a Weimaraner, lumbar spinal cord. Note the complete lack of the central canal. Hematoxylin and eosin, low power.

involve a hydromyelia, from which is a distension, a duplication, or an absence of the central canal. The ventral medial fissure may be absent and the ventral horns may be narrowed.[157]

A case of spinal dysraphism was seen in a 3-month-old Dalmatian who showed characteristic signs of synchronous hind limb hopping. At necropsy, the C2–T5 cord appeared syringomyelic—it had fluid-filled cavities covered by a thin layer of neuropil. The central canal was duplicated around C7 and absent between T12 and L2. There was a deviation of the ventral median fissure caudal to L2, with no dorsal sulcus and partially fused ventral horns.[167] At the Auburn clinic during the last 2 years six cases of dysraphism have been diagnosed in breeds other than the Weimaraner. These purebred breeds vary in size and type from the Chihuahua to the Labrador.[230]

This spinal anomaly in the Weimaraner is not a sex-linked inherited defect, since both sexes are equally involved. Dysraphic lesions occur during the last third of gestation.[157] Establishment of a diagnosis can probably be aided by careful radiography, considering the age and breed, and typical history. There is no treatment.

Syringomyelia

Syringomyelia is a chronic progressive disease that primarily affects the spinal cord. It can be congenital or acquired. The congenital form is infrequently seen and occurs in any breed, but is most common in the Weimaraner. According to McGrath, it is heritable in this breed.[156] Syringomyelia can occur at a few weeks of age, or it may go unnoticed for 1 to 3 years. There appears to be a relationship between spinal dysraphism and syringomyelia.[156] At 4 to 6 weeks of age, when the clinical signs of dysraphism appear, no macroscopic or microscopic syringomyelic cavities are found. But syringomyelia will frequently appear later, although the original clinical signs caused by dysraphism do not progress.

Syringomyelia is characterized by cavitation and gliosis of the spinal cord. The thoracic area is most commonly affected. The acquired type may be due to trauma, vascular occlusion, and disk protrusions, or it may be seen after viral myelitis, tumors, and meningitis. Occasionally a disk protrusion of long duration will cause a soft fluid-filled cord to appear adjacent to the compression. Microscopically, it is a characteristic lesion of syringomyelia. The congenital form is due to an anomalous vascular pattern leading to a low-grade ischemia and resulting degeneration, rarefaction, edema, and cavity formation.

The clinical signs vary as to location of the lesion. Peculiar crouching of the hind legs, abnormal postural reactions, bizarre reflex patterns, falling, weakness, cocking of the head, and a hopping gait have been described.[156]

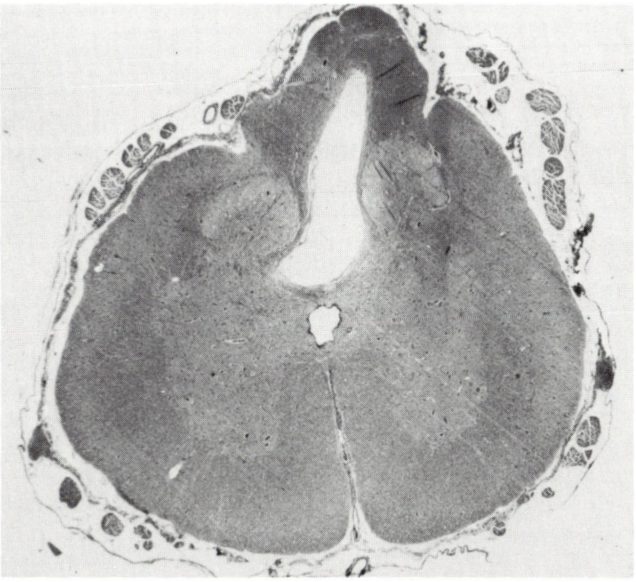

FIGURE 11–64 Syringomyelia in a Labrador puppy. Note the fluid cavity in the dorsal midline of the spinal cord. Hematoxylin and eosin, low power.

The differential diagnosis includes consideration of hip dysplasia in puppies and myasthenia gravis, spondylosis, distemper myelitis, and neoplasia in older animals. Syringomyelia is likely if the affected animal is a Weimaraner. Spinal radiography generally produces negative findings[156, 157] (Fig. 11–64).

Treatment

There is no known treatment for syringomyelia. Because of its chronicity and progressiveness, it is doubtful if anything other than symptomatic care can be given.

TOXICANTS

It has been estimated that there are more than 500,000 different household trade name toxic substances currently on the market, and about 1500 new products are being added each month. A large proportion of these products can be classified as neurologically important. The rational procedures that can be employed in treating a case of poisoning, even when the poisonous agent is not identified, are (1) prevent further absorption, (2) enhance the removal of the absorbed poison, and (3) use supportive therapy to combat the effects of the absorbed poison. Textbooks dealing with poisons should be consulted for specific details on therapy.[6]

INSECTICIDE POISONING

Poisoning with insecticides may be confused with the clinical appearance of a primary neurologic disorder. Most modern insecticides cause varying degrees of muscle tremor, weakness, and convulsion, and frequently apparent blindness and hysteria or other mental disturbances occur. The diagnosis is established chiefly by securing a careful history. Examination of the label on the container is necessary to determine the ingredients responsible so that treatment can be initiated. It is very important to remember that consideration of toxicity from insecticides, rodenticides, herbicides, or other pesticides should be a prominent part of the history in any neurological disorder.

OTHER CHEMICAL POISONS

Among other chemicals that may cause neurological disorders are *strychnine*, *lead*, *barium carbonate*, and *arsenic*. Lead and arsenic cause acute gastrointestinal disturbances, and chronic poisoning with these agents may lead to neurological disorders such as weakness, blindness, and tremor. The nature of the neuropathy produced by lead varies with the level and period of lead exposure. High levels over short periods of time produce demyelination, whereas lower levels over prolonged time periods produce axonal degeneration.[169] Prolongation of terminal conduction times, slowing of motor and sensory nerve conduction velocities, and marked reduction in amplitudes of evoked potentials occur. Fibrillation potentials, an increased number of polyphasic motor unit potentials, and a reduced interference pattern are present in a number of muscles. In the chronic form motor unit potentials may be absent in some muscles, and giant motor unit potentials may be found in other muscles.

Hexachlorophene toxicity causing acute CNS swelling and edema and caudal cerebellar herniation has been reported.[241] In 3-week-old puppies Scott found that half a bar of 0.75 per cent hexachlorophene soap could kill a medium size dog if ingested.[206]

Poisoning from consumption of spoiled garbage is attributable to toxins produced by staphylococci and clostridia. Both types of toxins produce neurological signs.[192]

Strychnine poisoning is usually severe, and dogs that have ingested strychnine have often been intentionally poisoned. Restlessness, anxiety, momentary muscular twitching, and violent generalized convulsions lasting from 1 to several minutes are common. The convulsions are triggered by the slightest external stimulus.

The treatment of strychnine poisoning is well known. Generally, emetics are of little value in the advanced case, but can be used at the onset of symptoms. The use of pentobarbital sodium or phenobarbital intravenously as a relaxant is a common practice. If anesthesia is needed for a prolonged period, inhalation anesthetics administered in a closed or semiclosed system can be used. Muscle relaxants such as methocarbamol (Roboxin) or chlorphenesin carbamate (Maolate) will help maintain relaxation. These agents must be administered as often as necessary until detoxification occurs, which may take from 1 to several days. Tranquilizers given by injection may be substituted for barbiturates in very mild cases. Good nursing care and stimulation of urination are very important aspects of therapy.

TOAD AND LIZARD POISONING

Neurotoxemia from exposure to or ingestion of toads or lizards has been reported in several countries. The marine toad, *Bufo marinus Linn,* is one of nine species of toads that are poisonous to dogs. This toad is native to the Caribbean islands and Latin America and has been introduced to other countries with tropical or subtropical climates to help control garden insects. When the dog plays with or attacks the toad, it sprays into the dog's mouth the toxic secretion of its parotid and dorsal glands, which are located posterior to the eye. The powerful cardiac glycoside possesses a digitaloid and emetic action. The clinical signs vary from profuse salivation and severe cardiac distress to nervous irritation, depression, and convulsions. Convulsive seizures can occur as soon as 30 minutes after exposure. The treatment must be prompt. The toxin should be irrigated from the dog's mouth, and salivation can be controlled with atropine, seizures with barbituates. Tracheal intubation may be necessary to maintain an open airway. Oxygen, steroids, and broad spectrum antibiotics may also be used, and good nursing care is a necessity.[172, 184]

The blue-tailed lizard and Gila monster[1] are reported to be poisonous to cats.

Drug Toxicity

In man, prolonged use of an antimalarial drug called chloroquine diphosphate may cause a myopathic and neuropathic disorder that can be confused with myasthenia gravis. The effect appears to be somewhat reversible with discontinuance of the drug.[246] Chlorpromazine has been reported to worsen symptoms of muscle weakness in cases of myasthenia gravis, and the administration of neostigmine did not completely overcome the effect of this tranquilizer.[160]

Peripheral neuropathies have been observed in man with long-term diphenylhydantoin therapy. One report studied 26 cases of weakness and loss of tendon reflexes in patients in whom this drug was the only one incriminated—most of them had been on therapy more than 10 years.[146] Diphenylhydantoin caused cerebellar atrophy and irreversible dysfunction in two persons receiving large amounts for 28 or more months.[207] Cases of peripheral neuropathy have been reported in man following a dosage of 300 to 400 mg/day of nitrofurantoin. The signs included pain, paresthesia, weakness, and muscle atrophy.[163] Motor nerve conduction velocities are subnormal, and in some muscles evolved potentials are absent.[107] When iodochlorhydroxyquin was given internally for diarrhea, it produced seizures, foaming at the mouth, tonic-clonic spasms, stiffness of the limbs, and other non-neurological signs in ten dogs and one cat. Sedatives and antibiotics had a beneficial effect; however, the cat died.[89, 191]

In man, there have been frequent reports of central neuropathies attributable to the phenothiazine tranquilizers. Persistent dyskinesia has frequently been observed. Even though phenylbutazone does not cause a primary neuropathy, it is used so widely in relief of spinal pain that it is desirable for the clinican to be cognizant of possible adverse effects. Several reports of toxicity have appeared in the veterinary literature, all associated with moderate to high dosages for extended periods of time. Blood dyscrasia promotes signs of submucosal hemorrhages, agranulocytosis, blood destruction, and icterus.[30, 225]

Neuromuscular blockade is a recognized complication of several antimicrobial drugs such as streptomycin, kanamycin, gentamicin, neomycin, polymyxin B, and perhaps the tetracyclines and sulfonamides.[3] Three days of therapy with ampicillin, erythromycin, or tetracycline reduced nerve conduction velocity significantly in human subjects. Nerve conduction velocities were normal 3 days after termination of therapy.[98] Neomycin therapy, when combined with muscle relaxants, has been shown to produce profound neuromuscular blockade. Neomycin has been shown to be one one-hundredth as potent as d-tubocurarine in inducing neuromuscular blockage. The two drugs act synergistically. Like curare, neomycin reduces the sensitivity of the postjunctional membrane to acetylcholine. In addition, neomycin has a prejunctional effect similar to that of a low calcium or high magnesium ion concentration manifested by inhibition of release of acetylcholine. Use of a sodium bicarbonate—calcium gluconate combination is a useful clinical method of reversing neomycin-induced paralysis.[215] Neomycin is also considered an ototoxic drug that attacks the auditory nerve directly, causing deafness.[69]

Gentamicin is a recent antibiotic which is very effective against some resistant infections and has also been reported to have a neuromuscular blocking potential. Respiratory failure which occurred in a man receiving gentamicin was partially reversed with calcium therapy.[243]

REFERENCES

1. Adair, H. S.: Blue tail lizard. Auburn Vet. *9*, 75, 1953.
2. Adams, E. W.: Hereditary deafness in a family of foxhounds. J.A.V.M.A. *128*, 302, 1956.
3. Adams, H. R.: Acute adverse effects of antibiotics. J.A.V.M.A *166*, 983, 1975.
4. Alexander, J. E., and Pettit, G. D.: Spinal osteochondrosis in a dog. Can. Vet. J. *8*, 47, 1967.
5. Allen, R., and Speakman, T. J.: Brain abscess and evaluation of current treatment. Canad. Med. Assoc. J. *86*, 852, 1962.
6. Aronson, A. L.: Emergency and general treatment of poisonings. *In* Kirk, R. W. (ed.): *Current Veterinary Therapy V*. W. B. Saunders Co., Philadelphia, 1974.
7. Ausherman, R. J.: Treatment of blastomycosis and histoplasmosis in the dog. J.A.V.M.A. *163*, 1048, 1973.
8. Averill, D. R.: Degenerative myelopathy in the aging German shepherd dog: Clinical and pathologic findings. J.A.V.M.A *162*, 1045, 1973.
9. Averill, D. R., and de Lahunta, A.: Toxoplasmosis of the canine nervous system: Clinicopathologic findings in four cases. J.A.V.M.A. *159*, 1134, 1971.
10. Axelson, R. D., Secord, A. C., and Weber, L. G.: Aortic embolism. Case report. J. Am. Anim. Hosp. Assoc. *4*, 183, 1968.
11. Baer, G. M., Goodrich, W. O., and Dean, D. J.: Anaphylactic shock following vaccination with CEO antirabies vaccine. J.A.V.M.A. *111*, 1018, 1962.
12. Baker, H. J.: Inherited metabolic disorders of the nervous system in dogs and cats. *In* Kirk, R. W. (ed.): *Current Veterinary Therapy V*. W. B. Saunders Co., Philadelphia, 1974, p. 700.
13. Baker, H. J. Lindsey, J. R., McKlann, G. M., and Farrell, D. F.: Neuronal GM, Gangliosidosis in a Siamese cat with β-galactosidose deficiency. Science *174*, 838–839, 1971.
14. Bannister, R.: *Brain's Clinical Neurology*, 4th ed. Oxford University Press, London, 1973.
15. Barron, C. N., and Saunders, I. Z.: Visceral larva migrans. Path. Vet. *3*, 315, 1966.
16. Bernheimer, H., and Karbe, E.: Morphological and neuro-chemical investigations into two forms of amaurotic idiocy in dogs: Data on GM-gangliosidosis. Acta. Neuropathol. *16*, 243, 1970.
17. Bistner, S., de Lahunta, A., and Lorenz, M.: Generalized cryptococcosis: Case report. Cornell Vet. *61*, 440, 1971.
18. Bjorck, G., Dyrendahl, S , and Olsson, S. E.: Hereditary ataxia in smooth-haired fox terriers. Vet. Rec *69*, 87–92, 1957.
19. Bjorck, G., Mair, W., Olsson, S. E., and Sourander, P.: Hereditary ataxia in fox terriers. Acta. Neuropathol. Suppl. I, 45–48, 1962.
20 Blauch, B , and Martin, C. L.: A vestibular syndrome in aged dogs. J. Am. Anim. Hosp. Assn. *10*, 37, 1974.
21. Boring, J. G., and Swaim, S. F.: Malignant schwannoma (neurilemmoma): An extramedullary intradural tumor causing cervical compression in a dog J. Am. Anim. Hosp. Assoc. *9*, 342–345, 1973.
22. Botha, H.: The cerebral form of babesiosis in dogs. J. So. Afr. Vet. Med. Assoc. *35*, 27, 1964.
23 Brasmer, T. H., and Lumb, W. V.: Lumbar vertebral prosthesis in the dog Am. J. Vet. Res. *33*, 493, 1972
24. Breazile, J. E., Blaugh, B. S , and Nail, N.: Experimental study of canine distemper myoclonus. Am. J. Vet. Res. *27*, 1375, 1966.
25. Brugghen, A.: *Neurosurgery in General Practice*. Charles C Thomas, Publishers, Springfield, Ill., 1952.
26. Bruner, D. W., and Gillespie, J. H.: *Hagan's Infectious Diseases of Domestic Animals*, 5th ed. Cornell University Press, Ithaca, N.Y., 1966.
27. Buchanan, J. W., Baker G. J., and Hill, J. D.: Aortic embolism in cats: Prevalence, surgical treatment and electrocardiography. Vet. Rec. *79*, 496, 1966.
28. Butler, H. C.: An investigation into the relationship of an aortic embolism to posterior paralysis in the cat. J. Small Anim. Pract. *12*, 141–158, 1971.
29. Cabasso, V. J., Sharpless, G. R., and Douglas, A.: Rabies vaccination of cats with HEP Flury vaccine Am. J. Vet. Res. *26*, 33, 1965.
30 Campbell, J. R., and Lawson, D. D.: A fatal syndrome in a dog following administration of phenylbutazone. Vet. Rec *81*, 469, 1967.
31. Carlson, W. D.: *Veterinary Radiology*. Lea and Febiger, Philadelphia, 1961.
32. Carmichael, L. E.: Canine herpesvirus infection in puppies. *In* Kirk, R. W. (ed.): *Current Veterinary Therapy V*. W. B. Saunders Co., Philadelphia, 1974, p. 959.
33. Carpenter, M. B.: A study of congenital feline cerebellar malformations. J. Comp. Neurol. *105*, 51, 1956.
34. Cello, R. M., Moulton, J. E., and McFarland, S.: The occurrence of inclusion bodies in the cir-

culating neutrophils of dogs with canine distemper. Cornell Vet, *49,* 127, 1959.
35. Cello, R. M., and Olander, H.: Cord compression and paraplegia secondary to pancreatic carcinoma. J.A.V.M.A *142,* 1407, 1963
36. Clinical pathology conference. J.A.V.M.A. *139,* 1340, 1961.
37. Cockrell, B. Y., Herigstad, R. R., Flo, G. L., and Legendre, A. M.: Myelomalacia in Afghan hounds. J.A.V.M.A. *162,* 1973.
38. Confer, A. W., Kahn, D. E., Krestner, A., and Krakawka, S.: Comparison of canine distemper viral strains: An electron microscopic study. Am. J. Vet. Res. *36,* 741, 1975.
39. Cordes, D. O., and Royal, W. A.: Cryptococcosis in a cat. N.Z. Vet. J. *15,* 117–121, 1967.
40 Cordy, D. R., and Snelbaker, H. A.: Cerebellar hypoplasia and degeneration in a family of Airedale dogs. J. Neuropathol. Exp. Neurol. *11,* 324, 1952
41. Cork, L. C.: Personal communication, 1976.
42 Cusick, P. K., Cameron, A. M., and Parker, A. J.: Canine neuronal glycoproteinosis: Lafora disease in the dog. J. Am. Anim. Hosp. Assoc. *12,* 518, 1976.
43. Dahme, E., and Schiefer, B.: Intracranielle Geschwulste bei Tieren. Zentralbl. Veterinaermed 7, 341, 1960.
44. de Lahunta, A., and Alexander, J. W.: Ischemia myelopathy secondary to presumed fibrocartilaginous embolism in nine dogs. J. Am. Anim. Hosp. Assoc. *12,* 37, 1976.
45. de Lahunta, A., and Averill, D. R.: Hereditary cerebellar cortical and extrapyramidal nuclear abiotrophy in Kerry blue terriers. J.A.V.M.A. *168,* 1119–1124, 1976.
46. de Lahunta, A., and Shively, G. N.: Neurofibrillary accumulation in a puppy. Cornell Vet. *65,* 240–247, 1975.
47. Detweiler, K. K , Ratcliffe, H. L , and Luginbühl, H.: Significance of naturally occurring coronary and cerebral arterial disease in animals. Ann. N.Y. Acad. Sci *149,* 868, 1968.
48. Dickson, E. C.: Botulism. Monograph 48, Rockefeller Institute, 1918.
49. Diezel, P. B., Rossner, J. A., Koppang. N., Ritzhaupt, P., and Bartling, D.: *In* Aronson, S. M., and Volk, B. W. (eds.): *Inborn Disorders of Sphingolipid Metabolism.* Pergamon Press, New York, 1967.
50 Donahoe, J. M. R., and Holzinger, E. A.: Dirofilaria in the brain. J.A.V.M.A. *164,* 518–519, 1974.
51. Doppman, J. L., DiChiro, G., and Morton, D. L.: Arteriographic identification of spinal cord blood supply prior to aortic surgery. J.A.M.A. *204,* 174, 1968.
52 Dorland Illustrated Medical Dictionary, 25th ed., W. B. Saunders Co., Philadelphia, 1965.
53. Dow, C., and McFerran, J. B.: Aujeszky disease. Vet. Rec *75,* 1099, 1963.
54. Fankhauser, R.: Degenerative, lipoidotische Erkrankung des Zentralnervensystems bei zwei Hunden. Schweiz. Arch. Tierheilkd. *107,* 73–87, 1965.
55. Fankhauser, R.: Polymyositis und Encephalomyelitis granulomatosa toxoplasmica beim Hund. Schweiz. Arch. Tierheilkd. *105,* 688, 1963
56. Fankhauser, R., Fatzer, R., Steck, F., and Zendali, J. P.: Morbus Aujeszky bei Hund und Katze in der Schweiz Schweiz. Arch. Tierheilkd. *117,* 623–629, 1975.
57. Fankhauser, R., Freudiger, U., Vandelvelde, M., and Fatzer, R.: Purkinje Zellatrophie nach Masernivirus-Vakzinierung beim Hund. Schweiz Arch. Neurol. Neurochir. Psychiat. *112,* 353–356, 1973
58. Fankhauser, R., and Luginbühl, H.: *Pathologische Anatomie des Zentralen und peripheren Nervensystems der Haustiere.* Paul Parey, Berlin and Hamburg, 1968.
59. Fankhauser, R., Luginbühl, H., and McGrath, J. T.: Cerebrovascular disease in various animal species. Ann. N.Y. Acad. Sci. *127,* 817, 1965.
60. Fatzer, R.: Leukodystrophische Erkrankungen im Gehirn junger Katzen. Schweiz. Arch. Tierheilkd. *117,* 641–648, 1975.
61. Fatzer, R.: Meningitis und Chorio-ependymitis granulomatosa bei Katzen. Schweiz. Arch. Tierheilkd. *117,* 633–640, 1975.
62. Fatzer, R.: Personal communication.
63. Fetter, B. F., Klintworth, G. K., and Hendry, W. S.: *Mycoses of the Central Nervous System.* Williams and Wilkins Co., Baltimore, 1967.
64. Few, A. B.: The study of the clinical signs and necropsy findings resulting from experimentally produced intracranial lesions in the dog Thesis, Auburn University, Auburn, Alabama, 1964.
65. Fewer, D., Wilson, C. B., Boldrey, E. B., Enot, K. J., and Powell, M. R.: The chemotherapy of brain tumors, clinical experience with carmustine (BCNU) and vincristine J.A.M.A. *222,* 549, 1972.
66. Fischer, K.: Herdformige symmetrische Hirngewebs-nekrosen bei Hunden mit epileptiformen Krampfen. Path. Vet. *1,* 133–160, 1964.
67. Fletcher, T. F.: Electroencephalographic features of leukodystrophic disease in the dog J.A.V.M.A. *157,* 190–198, 1970.
68. Fletcher, T. F., Zee, D. G., and Hammer. R. F.: Ultrastructural features of globoid-cell leukodystrophy in the dog. Am. J. Vet. Res. *32*:177–181, 1971.
69. Fowler, N. C.: The ototoxicity of neomycin in the dog. Vet. Rec. *82,* 267, 1968.
70. Freak, M. J.: Symposium on thrombosis. I. Arterial thrombosis (embolism) in the cat. J. Small Anim. Pract. *7,* 711, 1966.
71. Frenkel, J. K.: Toxoplasmosis. *In* Kirk, R. W. (eds.): *Current Veterinary Therapy V.* W. B. Saunders Co., Philadelphia 1974, p. 775.
72. Gage, E. D., Hoerlein, B. F., and Bartels, J. E.: Spinal cord compression resulting from a leptomeningeal cyst in the dog. J.A.V.M.A. *152,* 1664, 1968.
73. Gage, E. D.: Treatment of discospondylitis in the dog. J.A.V.M.A. *166,* 1164–1169, 1975.
74. Gambetti, L. A., Kelly, A. M., and Steinberg, S. A.: Biochemical studies in a canine gangliosidosis. J. Neuropathol. Exp. Neurol. *29,* 137, 1970.
75. Gee, B. R., and Doige, C. E.: Multiple carti-

laginous exostoses in a litter of dogs. J.A.V.M.A. *156*, 53, 1970.
76. Georgi, J. R., de Lahunta, A., and Percy, D. H.: Cerebral coenurosis in a cat. Report of a case. Cornell Vet. *59*, 127, 1969.
77. Gould, G. M.: *Blakiston's New Gould Medical Dictionary*. Blakiston Co., Inc., New York, 1953.
78. Grabel, I., Hansen, H. J., Olsson, S. E., Orstdicus, K., and Thal, E.: Dyscospondylitis and arthritis in swine erysipelas. Acta. Vet. Scand. *3*, 33, 1962.
79. Greene, C. E., and Higgins, R. J.: Fibrocartilaginous emboli as the cause of ischemia myelopathy in a dog. Cornell Vet. *66*, 131, 1976.
80. Greene, C. E., Vandevelde, M., and Braund, K.: Lissencephaly in two Lhasa Apso dogs. J.A.V.M.A *169*, 405, 1976.
81. Griffiths, I. R.: Spinal cord infarction due to emboli arising from intervertebral disc in the dog. J. Comp. Pathol. *83*, 225, 1973.
82 Griffiths, I. R., Barker, J., and Palmer, A. C.: Cholesterol masses in association with spinal cord infarction due to intervertebral disc emboli Acta. Neuropathol. *33*, 85, 1975.
83 Griffiths, I. R., Duncan, I. D., McQueen, A., Quirk, C., and Miller, R.: Neuromuscular disease in dogs: some aspects of its investigation and diagnosis. J. Small Anim. Pract. *14*, 533–554, 1973.
84. Griffiths, I. R., and Duncan, I. D.: Chronic degenerative radicular myelopathy in the dog. J. Small Anim. Pract. *16*, 461, 1975.
85. Gupta, B. N., Flo, G. L., and Whitcomb, D. L.: Malignant lymphoma with posterior paralysis. J.A.V.M.A. *156*, 1898–1902. 1970.
86. Habluetzel, J. E., Grimes, J. E., and Pigott, M. B.: Venezuelan equine encephalomyelitis virus infection. J.A.V.M.A. *162*, 462, 1973
87. Hagan, L. O.: Lipid dystrophic changes in the central nervous system of dogs. Acta. Path. Microbiol. Scand. *33*, 22, 1953.
88. Hagan, W. A., Bruner, D. W., and Gillespie, J. H.: *Hagan's Infectious Diseases of Domestic Animals*, 6th ed. Cornell University Press, Ithaca, N.Y., 1973
89. Hangarten, P.: Nervous disturbances after misuse of an enteric drug Schweiz. Arch. Tierheilkd. *107*, 43, 1965.
90 Hartley, W. J.: Polioencephalomalacia in dogs. Acta. Neuropathol. *2*, 271–281, 1963.
91. Hartley, W. J., and Palmer, A. C.: Ataxia in Jack Russell terriers. Acta. Neuropathol. *26*, 71–74, 1973.
92 Hatziolos, B. C.: Cuterebra larva causing paralysis in a dog. Cornell Vet. *57*, 129, 1967.
93. Hatziolos, B. C.: Cuterebra larva in the brain of a cat. J.A.V.M.A. *148*, 787, 1966.
94. Hayes, H. M., Priester, W. A , and Pendergrass, T. W.: Occurrence of nervous-tissue tumors in cattle, horses, cats, and dogs. Int. J. Cancer. *15*, 39, 1975.
95. Heavner, J. E., and Few, A. B.: Microfilariae of *Dirofilaria immitis* in the canine brain. South. Vet. *5*, 6, 1968.
96. Hegreberg, G. A., Thuline, H. C., and Francis, B. H.: Morphologic changes in feline leucodystrophy. Fed. Proc. *30*, 341, 1971.
97. Henderson, R. A., Hoerlein, B. F., Kramer, T. T., and Meyer, M. E.: Discospondylitis in three dogs infected with *Brucella canis*. J.A.V.M.A. *165*, 451, 1974.
98. Herishanu, Y., and Taustein, Y.: The antibiotics and the peripheral nerves. Confin. Neurol. *33*, 146, 1971.
99. Higgins, R. J.: Experimental blastomycosis in dogs with reference to lesions in the central nervous system and eye. Thesis (M.S.), Auburn University, Auburn, Alabama, 1976.
100. Hjarre, A.: Über Tuberkulose bei Hunden und Katzen. Acta. Tuberc Scand. *13*, 125, 1939.
101. Hobson, H. D., and Ellett, E. W.: Other viral diseases. *In* Catcott, E. J. (ed.): *Canine Medicine*. American Veterinary Publications, Inc , Santa Barbara, Cal., 1968. p. 144.
102. Hoerlein, B. F.: Aortic thrombosis. A case report. Vet. Med. *54*, 608, 1959.
103 Hoerlein, B. F.: *Canine Neurology*, 3rd ed. W. B. Saunders Co., Philadelphia, 1971.
104. Hoerlein, B. F., Horne, R. D., Wood, J. P., Bartels, J. E., and Hoff, E. J.: Aortic occlusion caused by dirofilariasis in a dog: Case report. Auburn Vet. *28*, 71, 1972.
105. Holland, J. M., and Davis, W. C.: Neuronal glycoproteinosis. Comp. Path. Bull. *4*, 1972.
106. Holland, J. M., Davis, W. C., Prieur, D. J., and Collins, G. H.: Lafora's disease in the dog Am. J. Pathol. *58*, 509, 1970
107. Honet, J. C.: Electrodiagnostic study of a patient with peripheral neuropathy after nitrofurantoin therapy. Arch. Phys. Med. Rehab. *48*, 209, 1967
108. Horta-Barbosa, L., Fucillo, D. A , and Sever, J. L.: Chronic viral infections of the central nervous system. J.A.M.A. *218*, 1185, 1971.
109. Houdart, R., Djindjian, R., and Hurth, M.: Vascular malformations of the spinal cord. The anatomic and therapeutic significance of arteriography. J. Neurosurg *24*, 583, 1966.
110. Hubert, J. P., Ectors, M., Ketalbant-Balasses, P., and Flament-Durant, J.: Fibrocartilaginous venous and arterial emboli from the nucleus pulposus in the anterior spinal system. Eur. Neurol. *11*, 164, 1974.
111. Hudson, W. R., and Ruben, R. V.: Hereditary deafness in Dalmatian dogs. Arch. Otolaryngol. *75*, 213, 1962.
112 Hughes, J. T., and Brownell, B.: Spinal cord ischemia due to arteriosclerosis. Arch. Neurol. *15*, 189, 1966.
113. Hugoson, G., and Rockborn, G.: On the occurrence of pseudorabies in Sweden, II. An outbreak in dogs caused by feeding abattoir offal. Zentralbl. Veterinaermed. [B] *19*, 64, 1972
114. Imagawa, D. T.: Relationship among measles, canine distemper and rinderpest viruses. Progr. Med. Virol. *10*, 160–193, 1968.
115. Imhoff, R. K.: Production of arotic occlusion resembling acute aortic embolism syndrome in cats. Nature *192*, 979, 1961.
116. Innes, J. R. M., and Saunders, L. Z.: *Comparative Neuropathology*. Academic Press, New York, 1962
117. Ishmael, J., and Ndall, N. D.: A case of aortic thrombosis in the dog. Vet. Rec. *79*, 570, 1966.
118. Jarvis, C. A., Burkhart, R. L., and Koprowski, H.: Demyelinating encephalomyelitis in the

dog associated with antirabies vaccination. Am. J. Hyg. *50*, 14, 1949.
119. Johnson, G. R., Oliver, J. E., and Seker, R.: Globoid cell leukodystrophy in a beagle. J.A.V.M.A. *167*, 380–384, 1975.
120. Johnson, K. H.: Globoid leukodystrophy in the cat. J.A.V.M.A *157*, 2057–2063, 1970
121. Jubb, K. V., Saunders, L. Z., and Coates, H. V.: The intraocular lesions in canine distemper. J. Comp. Pathol. *67*, 21, 1957.
122. Jurkovic, I., and Eiben, E.: Fatal myelomalacia caused by massive fibrocartilaginous venous emboli from nucleus pulposus. Acta. Neuropathol. *15*, 284, 1976.
123. Kabohm, C., and Riedel, W.: Thrombosis in the abdominal aorta. Kleintier-Prax *8*, 108, 1963
124. Kahrs, R. F., Scott, F. W., and de Lahunta, A.: Bovine viral diarrhea-mucosal disease, abortion, and congenital cerebellar hypoplasia in a dairy herd. J.A.V.M.A. *156*, 85, 1970.
125. Karbe, E., and Schiefer, B.: Familial amaurotic idiocy in male German short hair pointers. Path. Vet. *4*, 223, 1967.
126. Kendrick, J. L , and Hartman, J. T.: Infections metastatic to the vertebral column. J.A.M.A. *186*, 1093, 1963.
127. Kilham, L., Margolis, G., and Colby, E. D.: Cerebellar ataxia and its congenital transmission in cats by feline panleukopenia virus. J.A.V.M.A *158*, 888, 1971.
128. Kirk, R. W. (ed.): *Current Veterinary Therapy V.* W. B. Saunders Co., Philadelphia, 1974.
129. Koestner, A., and Cole, C. R.: Neuropathology of canine toxoplasmosis. Am. J. Vet. Res. *31*, 831, 1960.
130 Koestner, A , and Zeman, W.: Primary reticuloses of the central nervous system in dogs. Am. J. Vet. Res. *23*, 381, 1962
131. Koppang, N.: Familiare Glykosphingolipoidose des Hundes (juvenile amaurotische Idiotie). Ergeb. Path. *47*, 1–43, 1966.
132 Koppang, N.: Neuronal ceroid-lipofuscinosis in English setters. Juvenile amaurotic idiocy (AFI) in English setters. J. Small Anim. Pract. *10*, 639, 1970
133. Krayenbühl, H., Ysargil, M. G., and McClintoch, H. G.: Treatment of spinal cord vascular malformations by surgical excision. J. Neurosurg *30*, 427, 1969.
134. Kronevi, T., Nordstrom, M., Moreno, W., and Nilsson, P. O.: Feline ataxia due to nonsuppurative meningoencephalomyelitis of unknown etiology. Nord. Vet. Med. *26*, 720, 1974.
135. Kurtz, H. J., and Sharpnack, S.: Blastomycotic meningoencephalitis: Case report. Path. Vet. *6*, 375, 1969.
136. Lackermeier, S.: Neural postvaccinal complications following the inoculation of dogs with live rabies vaccines. Schweiz Arch. Tierheilkd. *108*, 581, 1966.
137. Langfitt, T. W., Weinstein, J. D., and Kassell, N. F.: Cerebral vasomotor paralysis produced by intracranial hypertension. Neurology *15*, 622, 1965.
138. Lefevre, A. B.: Antihistamine treatment of myelopathy following rabies vaccination. J.A.M.A *151*, 491, 1953.
139. Lewis, G. E., and Anderson, J. K.: *Brucella canis* antibodies in healthy persons. Am. J. Publ. Health *63*, 204, 1973.
140. Lewis, G. E., Crumrine, M. H., Jennings, P. B., and Fariss, B. L.: Therapeutic value of tetracycline and ampicillin in dogs infected with *Brucella canis.* J.A.V.M.A. *163*, 239, 1973.
141. Lincoln, S. D., Gorham, J. R., Davis, W. C., and Ott, R. L.: Studies of old dog encephalitis. II. Electron microscopic and immunohistologic findings. Vet. Path. *10*, 124–129, 1972.
142. Lincoln, S. D., Gorham, J. R., Ott, R. L., and Hegreberg, G. A.: Etiologic studies of old dog encephalitis. I. Demonstration of canine distemper viral antigen in the brain of two cases. Vet. Path. *8*, 1–8, 1971.
143. Lindblad, G., Ljunggren, G., and Olsson, S. E.: On spinal compression in the dog, an angiographic study. Adv. Small Anim. Pract. *3*, 121, 1962.
144. Lombardi, G., and Passerini, A.: Spinal cord tumors. Radiology *76*, 381, 1961.
145. Love, J. G., and Rivers, M. H.: Spinal cord tumors simulating protruding intervertebral discs. J.A.M.A. *179*, 138, 1962
146. Lovelace, R. E., and Horwitz, S. J.: Peripheral neuropathy in long-term diphenylhydantoin therapy. Arch. Neurol. *18*, 69, 1968.
147. Lucke, V. M., and Sumner-Smith, G.: Aortic embolism in the cat. Vet. Rec. *79*:236, 1966.
148. Luessenhop, A. J., and Cruz, T. D.: The surgical excision of spinal intradural vascular malformations. J. Neurosurg. *30*, 552, 1969.
149. Luginbühl, H.: Study of meningiomas in cats. Am. J. Vet. Res. *22*, 1031, 1961.
150. Luginbühl, H., Frankhauser, R., and McGrath, J. T.: Spontaneous neoplasms of the nervous system in animals. Progr. Neurol. Surg. *2*, 85, 1968.
151. Mandelker, L., and Brutus, R. L.: Heartworm encephalitis: Case report. J.A.V.M.A. *159*, 776, 1971.
152. Marsh, R. F.: Slow virus diseases of the central nervous system. *In* Brandly, C. A., and Cornelius, C. E. (eds.): *Advances in Veterinary Science and Comparative Medicine.* Vol. 18. Academic Press, New York, 1974, p. 155.
153. Martin, P.: Symposium on thrombosis. III. Surgical treatment. J. Small Anim. Pract. *7*, 721, 1966.
154. Martin, S. L., and Donovan, E. F.: Toxoplasmosis and hemobartonellosis. *In* Catcott, E. J. (ed.): *Canine Medicine.* American Veterinary Publications, Inc., Santa Barbara, Cal., 1968, p. 227.
155. McClelland, R. B.: Chemotherapy in reticulum cell sarcoma. Cornell Vet. *61*, 477, 1971.
156. McGrath, J. T.: *Neurologic Examination of the Dog with Clinicopathologic Observations,* 2d ed. Lea and Febiger, Philadelphia, 1960.
157. McGrath, J. T.: Spinal dysraphism in Weimaraners. Path. Vet. Suppl. *2*, 1965.
158. McGrath, J. T., Kelly, A. M., and Steinberg, S. A.: Cerebral lipidosis in the dog. J. Neuropathol. Exp. Neurol. *27*, 141, 1968.
159. McLaurin, R. L., and Helmer, F. A.: Errors in diagnosis of intracranial tumors. J.A.M.A. *180*, 1011, 1962
160. McQuillen, M. P , Gross, M., and Johns, R. J.: Chlorpromazine induced weakness in myasthenia gravis. Arch. Neurol. *8*, 286, 1963.

161. Mitten, R. W.: Vertebral osteomyelitis in the dog due to nocardia-like organisms. J. Small Anim. Pract. *15*, 563–570, 1974.
162. Moller, T.: Central nervous system changes in canine toxoplasmosis. Acta. Neuropathol. Suppl. *1*, 20, 1962.
163 Morris, J. S.: Nitrofurantoin and peripheral neuropathy with megaloblastic anemia. J. Neurol. Neurosurg. Psychiat. *29*, 224, 1966.
164. Mulligan, R. M.: *Neoplasms of the Dog*. The Williams and Wilkins Co., Baltimore, 1949.
165. Nelson, D. A.: Spinal cord compression due to vertebral angiomas during pregnancy Arch. Neurol. *11*, 408, 1964.
166. Nestel, B. L., and Nestel, H. M.: Spinal tuberculosis in the dog. J.A.V.M.A. *131*, 234, 1957.
167 Neufeld, J. L., and Little, P. B.: Spinal dysraphism in a Dalmatian dog. Case report. Cand. Vet. J. *15*, 335, 1974.
168. Notermans, S. L. H., Tijl, W. F. J., Willems, F. T. C., and Sloof, J. L.: Experimentally induced subacute sclerosing panencephalitis in young dogs. Neurology *23*, 543–555, 1973.
169. Oh, S. J.: Lead neuropathy: Case report. Arch. Phys. Med. Rehab. *56*, 312, 1975.
170 Oliver, J. E., and Geary, J. C.: Venous aneurysm in the spinal canal of a dog. J. Small Anim. Pract. *7*, 523, 1966.
171. Oliver, J. E., Jr., and Knecht, C. D.: Diseases of the brain. *In* Ettinger, S. J. (ed.): *Textbook of Veterinary Internal Medicine*. W. B. Saunders Co., Philadelphia, 1975, p. 370.
172 Otani, A., Palumbo, H., and Read, G.: Treatment of toad poisoning. Am. J. Vet. Res. *30*, 1865, 1969.
173. Padgett, G. A., and Hegreberg, G. A.: Myoclonic epilepsy (Lafora's disease) in man and dog J.A.V.M.A *165*, 745, 1974.
174. Palmer, A. C.: Clinical and pathological features of some tumors of the central nervous system in dogs. Res. Vet. Sci. *1*, 36, 1960.
175. Palmer, A. C.: Pathogenesis and pathology of the cerebellovestibular syndrome. J. Small Anim. Pract. *11*, 167, 1970.
176. Palmer, A. C., Malinowski, W., and Barnett, K. C.: Clinical signs including papilloedema associated with brain tumors in twenty-one dogs. J. Small Anim. Pract. *15*, 359, 1974.
177. Palmer, A. C., Payne, J. E., and Wallace, M. E.: Hereditary quadriplegia and amblyopia in the Irish setter. J. Small Anim. Pract. *14*, 343, 1973.
178. Palumbo, N. E., and Hubbard, R. E.: Surgical treatment of aortic embolism. J.A.V.M.A. *148*, 26, 1966.
179. Parker, A. J.: Distribution of spinal branches of the thoracolumbar segmental arteries in dogs. Am. J. Vet. Res. *34*, 1351, 1973.
180. Parker, A. J.: Clinical significance of traumatic occlusion of segmental spinal arteries. J.A.V.M.A. *162*, 1041, 1973.
181. Parker, A. J.: Do strokes occur in dogs and cats? Illinois Vet. *17*, 5, 1974.
182. Parker, A. J., and Smith, C. W.: Meningeal cyst in a dog J. Am. Anim. Hosp. Assoc. *10*, 595, 1974.
183. Patton, C. S., and Garner, F. M.: Cerebral infarction caused by heartworms. J.A.V.M.A. *156*, 600–605, 1970.
184. Peneyra, R. S.: Toad poisoning *In* Kirk, R. W. (ed.): *Current Veterinary Therapy V*. W. B. Saunders Co., Philadelphia, 1974, p. 160.
185. Percy, D. H., Munnel, J. F., Olander, H. J., and Carmichael, L. E.: Pathogenesis of canine herpesvirus encephalitis. Am. J. Vet. Res. *31*, 145, 1970.
186. Piper, R. C.: Toxoplasmosis. *In* Kirk, R. W. (ed.): *Current Veterinary Therapy III*. W. B. Saunders Co., Philadelphia, 1968, p. 613.
187. Poste, G., and King, N.: Isolation of a herpesvirus from the canine genital tract: Association with infertility, abortion, and stillbirths. Vet. Rec. *88*, 229, 1971.
188. Prata, R. G., Stall, S. G., and Yaki, F. A.: Spinal cord compression caused by osteocartilaginous exostoses of the spine in two dogs. J.A.V.M.A *166*, 371, 1975.
189. Priester, W. A., Glass, A. G., and Waggoner, N. S.: Congenital defects in domestic animals. General consideration. Am. J. Vet. Res. *31*, 1871, 1970
190 Pryor, W. H., Huizenga, C. G., Splitter, G. A., and Harwell, J. F.: *Coccidioides immitis* encephalitis in two dogs. J.A.V.M.A. *161*, 1108, 1972.
191. Puschner, H., and Fankhauser, R.: Neuropathologishe Befunde bei experimenteller vioform-Vergiftung der weissen Maus. Schweiz. Arch. Tierheilkd. *111*, 371–379, 1969.
192 Ramsey, F. K., Buck, W. B., and Duncan, J. R.: Diagnosis of garbage intoxication. Mod. Vet. Pract. *48*, 50, 1967.
193. Ratcliffe, H. L., Luginbuhl, H., and Pionik, L.: Coronary aortic and cerebral atherosclerosis in swine of three age groups: Implications. Bull. W. H. O. *42*, 225, 1970.
194. Rhoades, H. E., Reynolds, H. A., Rahn, D. P., and Small, E.: Nocardiosis in a dog with multiple lesions of the central nervous system. J.A.V.M.A. *142*, 278, 1963.
195. Ribelin, W. E., and Kintner, L. D.: Lipodystrophy of the central nervous system in a dog. A disease with similarities to Tay-Sachs disease of man. Cornell Vet. *46*, 532, 1956.
196. Richards, M. A., and Sloper, J. C.: Hypothalamic involvement by visceral larva migrans in a dog suffering from diabetes insipidus. Vet. Rec. *76*, 449, 1964.
197. Sandefeldt, E., Cummings, J. F., de Lahunta, A., Bjorck, G., and Krook, L.: Hereditary neuronal abiotrophy in the Swedish Lapland dog. Cornell Vet. *63*, Suppl. 3, Jan. 1973.
198. Schappert, H. R., and Geib, L. W.: Reticuloendothelial neoplasms involving the spinal canal of cats. J.A.V.M.A. *150*, 753, 1967.
199. Schaub, R. G., and Meyers, K. M.: Evidence for a small functional pool of serotonin in neurohumoral transmission. Res. Commun. Chem. Pathol. Pharmacol. *10*, 29, 1975.
200. Schiefer, B.: Über Keilwirbel beim Hund. Berl. Münch. Tierärztl. Wochenschr. *81*, 149, 1968.
201. Schiefer, *et al.*: Incidence of central nervous system tumors. Tierärztl. Umschau, *25*, 297–299, 1970. (Abst. Med. Vet. Pract. Inst. Vet., Ref. Serv., F4–146.)
202. Schlotthauer, C. F.: The nervous system, diseases of the brain. *In Canine Medicine*, 2nd ed. American Veterinary Publications, Inc., Santa Barbara, Cal., 1959, Chap. 15.

203. Schnelle, G.: Radiography of the canine intervertebral disc. Proceedings of the 100th American Veterinary Medicine Association Convention, July 28–Aug. 1, 1963.
204. Schouse, C. L., and Meier, H.: Acute vegetative endocarditis in the dog and cat. J.A.V.M.A. *129,* 278, 1956.
205. Schulz, W.: Aujeszky's disease. Monatschr. Vet. Med. *22,* 688, 1967 (Abstr. Mod. Vet. Pract. Int. Vet. Ref. Serv., F-1-288, 1968).
206. Scott, D. W., Bolton, G. R., and Lorenz, M. D.: Hexachlorophene toxicosis. J.A.V.M.A. *162,* 979–949, 1973.
207. Selhorst, J. B., Kaufman, B., and Horwitz, S. J.: Diphenylhydantoin-induced cerebellar degeneration. Arch. Neurol. *27,* 453, 1972.
208. Sencer, D. J.: National Communicable Disease Center Zoonoses Surveillance: Annual Rabies Summary, 1968.
209. Shrifrine, M., Poppagianis, D., and Neves, J.: Double electro-immunodiffusion: A rapid diagnostic test for canine coccidioidomycosis. Am. J. Vet. Res., *36,* 819, 1975.
210. Sims, M. A.: Flavabasterium meningosepticum: A probable cause of meningitis in a cat. Vet. Rec. *95,* 567, 1974.
211. Slauson, D. O., and Finn, J. P.: Meningoencephalitis and panophthalmitis in feline infectious peritonitis. J. Am. Vet. Med. Assoc. *160,* 729–734, 1972.
212. Small, E.: Systemic mycoses. *In* Kirk, R. W. (ed.): *Current Veterinary Therapy V.,* W. B. Saunders Co., Philadelphia, 1974, p. 980.
213. Smith, H. A., and Jones, T. C.: *Veterinary Pathology,* 2d ed. Lea and Febiger, Philadelphia, 1961.
214. Stallings, E. D.: Canine distemper therapy. *In* Kirk, R. W. (ed.): *Current Veterinary Therapy V.* W. B. Saunders Co., Philadelphia, 1974, p. 969.
215. Stanley, V. F.: Neuromuscular blockade probed. Antibiotic News, *6,* 6, 1969. (Abstr. Vet. Med. Small Anim. Clin. *64,* 280, 1969.)
216. Starr, L. E., Sellars, T. F., and Sunkes, E. J.: Apparent recovery of a dog from rabies. J.A.V.M.A. *121,* 296, 1953.
217. Steinberg, S. A.: Idiopathic or primary demyelination of the brain stem and spinal cord. Clinicopathologic conference. J.A.V.M.A. *143,* 404, 1963.
218. Steinberg, S. A., and Kelly, A. M.: Clinicopathologic conference. J.A.V.M.A. *148,* 170, 1966.
219. Stephenko, M. F.: An outbreak of Aujeszky's disease. Veterinariya *39,* 61, 1962.
220. Stockard, C. R.: The genetic and endocrine basis for differences and behavior. Am. Anat. Mem. No. 19, Wistar Institute Anat. Biol, 1941.
221. Stone, A. B.: Variant lesions in the central nervous system of dogs and cats. J. Small Animal Pract. *10,* 287, 1969.
222. Stone, A. B., and Fox, M. W.: Clinico-pathological studies of an encephalitic syndrome in dogs. J. Small Animal Pract. *8,* 709, 1967.
223. Storts, R. W., Boenig, D. M., and Johnson, W. D.: Pathogenesis of distemper. Southwest. Vet. *27,* 37–44, 1974.
224. Taguchi, M., Takehara, B., and Uriu, I.: A case report on a dog with aberrant *Dirofilaria immitis* in the lateral ventricles of its brain. J. Japan Vet. Med. Assoc. *12,* 432, 1959.
225. Tandy, J., and Thorpe, E.: A fatal syndrome in a dog following administration of phenylbutazone. Vet. Rec. *81,* 398, 1967.
226. Tomchick, T. L.: Familial Lafora's disease in the beagle dog. Fed. Proc. *32,* 821, 1973.
227. Turk, K. A. D.: Symposium on thrombosis II. The pathology of aortic-iliac embolism in man. J. Small Animal Pract. *7,* 719, 1966.
228. Vaccination, recommended procedures. Report of A.V.M.A. Panel on Canine Infectious Diseases. J.A.V.M.A. *156,* 1661–1668, 1970.
229. Vaccination, synopsis of procedures for dogs. A.V.M.A. Council on Biological and Therapeutic Agents. J.A.V.M.A. *162,* 228, 1973.
230. Vandevelde, M.: Personal communication, 1976.
231. Vandevelde, M., and Fankhauser, R.: Zur Pathologie der Ruckenmarks—Blutungen beim Hund. Schweiz. Arch. Tierheilkd. *114,* 463–475, 1972.
232. Vandevelde, M., and Fatzer, R.: Neurologische komplicaties by drie honden ma vaccinatie met een rabiesweefselkultuurvaccin. Vlaams Diergeneeskundig Tijdschrift. *43,* 253–259, 1974.
233. Vandevelde, M., Fatzer, R., and Fankhauser, R.: Chronisch-progressive Formen der Staupeenzephalitis des Hundes. Schweiz. Arch. Tierheilkd. *116,* 391–404, 1974.
234. Vandevelde, M., Higgins, R. J., and Greene, C. E.: Neoplasms of mesenchymal origin in the spinal cord and nerve roots of three dogs. Vet. Pathol. *13,* 47, 1976.
235. Vandevelde, M., Braund, K. G., and Hoff, E. J.: Central neurofibromas in the dog: A study of two cases. In press.
236. Vandevelde, M., Greene, C. E., and Hoff, E. J.: Lower motor neuron disease with accumulation of neurofilaments in a cat. Vet. Pathol. *13,* 428–435, 1976.
237. Vandevelde, M., and Hoerlein, B. F.: Subacute diffuse inflammatory degenerative disease and sclerosis in the dog's brain associated with canine distemper. Unpublished manuscript.
238. Vandick, B., and Degre, M.: Measles virus antibodies in serum and cerebrospinal fluid in patients with multiple sclerosis and other neurological disorders, with special reference to measles antibody synthesis within the central nervous system. Neurol. Sci. *24,* 201, 1975.
239. Wagner, J. L., Pick, J. R., and Krigman, M. R.: *Cryptococcus neoformans* infection in a dog. J.A.V.M.A. *153*:945, 1968.
240. Walton, J. N.: *Essentials of Neurology.* J. B. Lippincott, Philadelphia, 1961.
241. Ward, B. C., James, B. D., and Rubin, G. J.: Hexachlorophene toxicity. J. Am. Anim. Hosp. Assoc. *9,* 167–169, 1973.
242. Ward, J. M., Nelson, N., Wright, J. F., and Berman, E.: Chronic nonclinical cerebral toxoplasmosis in cats. J.A.V.M.A. *159,* 1012, 1971.
243. Warner, W. A., and Sanders, E.: Neuromuscular blockade associated with gentamicin therapy. J.A.M.A. *215,* 1153–1154, 1971.
244. Wechsler, I. S.: *Clinical Neurology,* 9th ed. W. B. Saunders Co., Philadelphia, 1963.
245. Westphal, K., and Bar, R.: Ueber die Entstehung des Schlogenfalles. Deutsche Arch. Klin. Med. *151,* 31, 1926.
246. Whisnant, J. P., Espinasa, R. E., Kierland, R. R., and Lambert, E. H.: Chloroquine neuromyopathy. Proc. Staff Meet. Mayo Clin. *38,* 501, 1963.

247. Whisnant, J. P., Sayre, G. P., and Millikan, C. H.: Experimental intracerebral hematoma. Arch. Neurol. *9*, 586, 1963.
248. White, J. C.: Familial periodic nystagmus, vertigo, and ataxia. Arch. Neurol. *20*, 276, 1969.
249. Wilkins, R. H., Silver, D., and Odom, G. L.: The role of circulating substances in intracranial arterial spasm. I. Serotonin and histamine. Neurology *16*, 482, 1966.
250. Winans, S. S.: Visual form discrimination after removal of the visual cortex in cats. Science *158*, 944–946, 1967.
251. Woodard, J. C., Collins, G. H., and Hessler, J. R.: Feline hereditary neuroaxonal dystrophy. Am. J. Path. *74*:551, 1974.
252. Woodard, J. S., and Freeman, L. W.: Ischemia of the spinal cord, an experimental study. J. Neurosurg. *13*, 63, 1956.
253. Wright, N. G., and Cornwell, H. J.: Symposium: Neonatal diseases of the dog. I. Viral-induced neonatal disease in puppies. J. Small Anim. Pract. *9*, 449, 1968.
254. Wright, N. G., and Cornwell, H. J. C.: The susceptibility of six-week old puppies to canine herpes virus. J. Small Anim. Pract. *10*, 669, 1970.
255. Young, G. B.: Inherited defects in dogs. Vet. Rec. *67*, 15, 1955.
256. Yturraspe, D. J., and Lumb, W. V.: Second lumbar spondylectomy and shortening of the spinal column of the dog. Am. J. Vet. Res. *34*, 521, 1973.
257. Zaki, F. A., and Kay, W. J.: Globoid cell leukodystrophy in a minature poodle. J.A.V.M.A. *163*, 248–250, 1973.
258. Zaki, F. A., Prata, R. C., Hurvitz, A. I., and Kay, W. J.: Primary tumors of the spinal cord and meninges in six dogs. J.A.V.M.A. *166*, 511–517, 1975.
259. Zaki, F. A., Prata, R. C., and Kay, W. J.: Necrotizing myelopathy in five Great Danes. J.A.V.M.A. *165*, 1080, 1974.
260. Zaki, F. A., and Prata, R. C.: Necrotizing myelopathy secondary to embolization of herniated intervertebral disk material in the dog. J.A.V.M.A. *169*, 222, 1976.
261. Zaki, F. A., Prata, R. C., and Werner, L. L.: Necrotizing myelopathy in a cat. J.A.V.M.A. *169*, 228, 1976.
262. Zimmerman, J. M., Nielson, H. C., King, T. C., and Colliver, J. C.: The effect of cerebral ischemia on learning and retention in dogs. J.A.M.A. *197*, 166, 1966.

CHAPTER 12

ACUTE TRAUMA TO THE CENTRAL NERVOUS SYSTEM

GENERAL COMMENTS

One of the greatest challenges to the veterinary practitioner is the effective management of acute central nervous system (CNS) injuries. The traditional method of relieving pain by use of narcotics and maintaining complete rest and quiet in the confines of a compartment is effective in some routine CNS trauma cases. The remainder are destined to die or spend the rest of their lives as hopeless cripples. The modern efficient clinician will seek to maintain life until an accurate diagnosis and prognosis can be presented to the client, and a course of action can then be established by mutual agreement of the clinician and the owner.

It is important that the clinician be knowledgeable about the anatomical and physiological peculiarities of the CNS to manage these disorders effectively. The skull encloses and protects a most delicate, complicated, and vital organ—the brain. The brain is said to be composed of some 14 billion neurons and a network of afferent, efferent, and interconnecting nerve fibers. The brain and spinal cord are uniquely constructed of soft, friable tissue, supported by a relatively weak connective tissue called neuroglia. Both of these organs are surrounded with membranes called meninges, which help to support the organs and to maintain their general shape and conformation. The brain and cord, along with their meninges, are intimately housed in the bony cavities called the cranium and spinal column.

The CNS is highly *vascular*. In man, the brain represents only 2.2 per cent of the total body weight, but it receives 15 per cent of the total cardiac output.[30] In the dog, the brain is said to represent about 0.6 per cent of the body weight[36] and the blood flow is 63 ml/min/100 gm of brain.[35] The brain also has the highest oxygen requirement of any tissue in the body—about 20 times that required for resting muscle[52]—and 20 per cent of the total body oxygen consumption.[36] Therefore, the CNS is highly sensitive to lack of blood or oxygen. Since venous return must be comparable to arterial supply of CNS tissue, trauma may cause congestion, edema, and swelling. Because of the cerebral bony encasement, a CNS swelling quickly produces pathologic changes.

The meninges also provide considerable protection to the brain. The dura mater particularly is a tough, semitranslucent, inelastic membrane that acts as a microbial barrier. Together with the arachnoidea, it forms a watertight container for cerebrospinal fluid and protects the cerebrum from the cranial bone so that adhesions and cicatrix formations don't occur. The cerebrospinal fluid contained within the meningeal and ventricular cavities is an important aid in the protection of vital CNS tissues from trauma because of its cushioning effect.[36]

It has been stated that the brain is extremely susceptible to injury because of its delicate metabolic needs. The neuron can only utilize glucose (and related sugars) and oxygen for energy, both of which depend on the competency of the respiratory and circulatory systems. The brain's needs for these agents is tremendous when compared to that of many other body tissues. Since the CNS utilizes 20 per cent of the total oxygen uptake and 15 per cent of the cardiac output in blood, the brain must extract more oxygen from the blood it receives than do other body tissues. This makes the oxygen-carbon dioxide balance much more critical in the brain. The brain tissue is highly susceptible to abnormal increases in pCO_2; therefore the metabolic disturbance caused by inadequate pulmonary ventilation, hypotension from shock, or both may far exceed the primary effects of the trauma.[36]

In addition to the blood, oxygen, and nutritional needs of the CNS, the previously mentioned blood-brain, CSF-brain, and CSF-blood barriers are unique factors in consideration of CNS trauma. If damage is so severe that the blood-brain barriers are destroyed, toxic substances will produce irreversible damage to the brain tissues. Also, these barriers inhibit proper CNS tissue concentration of antibiotics and chemotherapeutic agents when there is contamination and sepsis in acute CNS trauma. Therefore, hemorrhage, ischemia, sepsis, the blood-brain barrier, the vital and delicate nature of CNS tissues and special CNS physiological requirements, and the far-reaching effects of CNS trauma all contribute to making the proper care of the CNS trauma patient a complicated procedure.

TYPES OF CNS INJURY

BRAIN INJURY

The types of head injuries that are seen most frequently in the dog are skin and superficial lacerations and contusions, concussions, cranial fractures, and intracranial hemorrhage. Skin lacerations in the head region may bleed profusely, but they heal readily when they are properly cared for.[32]

Concussion is a widely used term that has no universally accepted definition and may cloak a multitude of diagnostic and therapeutic uncertainties. Originally it referred to the short-lived, stunning effect of a mild injury, with recovery and without sequelae. It also has acquired a meaning of a diffuse functional neuronal disturbance without recognizable morbid changes in the brain. It seems logical that even the mildest of brain injuries will cause some neuronal damage. Severe manifestations will be caused by the usual effects of trauma, such as vascular changes, edema, swelling hemorrhage, and death of tissue. Therefore, concussion will not be discussed as a separate entity (Fig. 12–1).[13, 22]

Cranial fractures can be extracranial or cranial. They are further classified as linear and depressed, comminuted, simple, or compound. Practically all extradural and many subdural hemorrhages are due to cranial fractures.

Intracranial hemorrhage may be extradural, subdural, or intracerebral. Hemorrhage into the cranial vault is common because there is such a copious arterial supply, and because the venous drainage involves many venous sinuses that may be surrounded by bone and are easily torn in skull fractures. Some arteries, such as the middle menin-

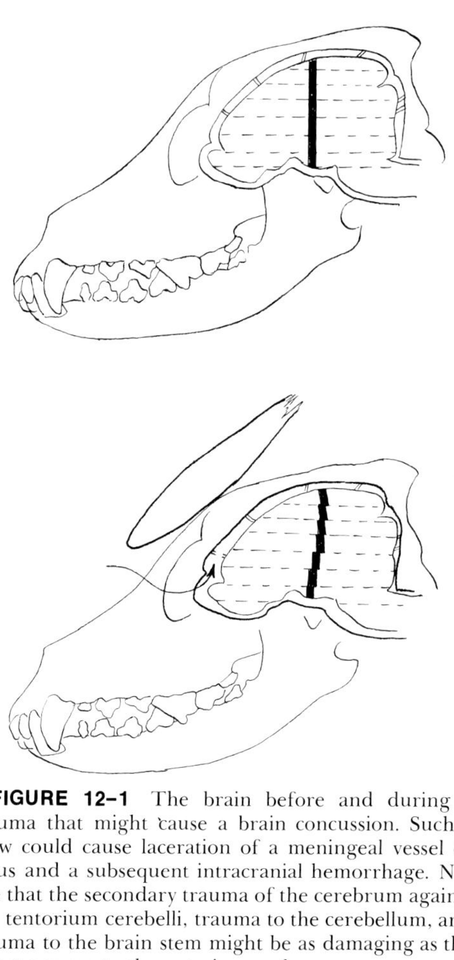

FIGURE 12–1 The brain before and during a trauma that might cause a brain concussion. Such a blow could cause laceration of a meningeal vessel or sinus and a subsequent intracranial hemorrhage. Notice that the secondary trauma of the cerebrum against the tentorium cerebelli, trauma to the cerebellum, and trauma to the brain stem might be as damaging as the direct trauma to the anterior cerebrum.

geal, are partially encased in bone, which makes them more susceptible to laceration in case of skull fractures. Intracranial hemorrhage will be discussed in detail during the course of the chapter.

SPINAL INJURY

Spinal injuries in acute CNS trauma generally include fractures, luxations and subluxations of the spinal column with varying degrees of cord compression, contusion, laceration, hemorrhages, and other vascular disorders. Occasionally, acute spinal trauma will produce an explosive ruptured disk with acute compression and traumatic sequelae.

FIRST AID

The management of a CNS injury from the time of the accident to its presentation in the clinic frequently determines the ultimate outcome. It is imperative that a clinician understand neurological anatomy, physiology, and therapy so that he may properly advise the client as to how the animal should be handled initially: an injured dog, since he is frequently hysterical, is difficult to handle.

RESTRAINT

Many animals should be handled with heavy gloves and should be carefully muzzled if they are hysterical and aggressive. Muzzling has psychological value in that the dog frequently knows his main defense mechanism is his jaws and teeth. If his jaws are immobilized, he may put up less resistance. One person may restrain the dog's head while another aids in transporting him. A flat appliance such as a door, section of wallboard or a blanket sling between poles or rods should be used to transport the dog. Every effort must be made to minimize twisting, extension, or flexion of the patient's spine or head.

CLEAR AIRWAY

A clear airway is a critical need which can be facilitated by forward traction on the tongue and swabbing blood, mucus, vomitus, or fluids out of the mouth and nostrils. Careful extension of the neck tends to furnish an easier passage for air; however, the normal relation of the neck to the rest of the body should be maintained so as not to aggravate any cervical cord compression resulting from cervical spinal fractures. If vomiting is occurring, every effort should be made to prevent aspiration by keeping the head at a lower level. Pressure should be applied to bleeding areas to prevent blood loss.[32, 61, 62]

The animal should be taken into the hospital on a mobile stretcher table, cart, or portable stretcher. The vital functions of the body must be evaluated. A prime consideration is the patency of the air passage and the ability of the patient to breathe. If the patient is having respiratory problems, an open airway must be established immediately. If the animal is unconscious, an endotracheal tube can be inserted and a resuscitative oxygen mixture can be administered. This is preferable to a tracheostomy, particularly if it is obvious that surgery must be done and cuffed tracheostomy tubes are not available. If the animal is conscious but the airway is not patent, a tracheostomy should be performed. A tracheostomy is preferable in the conscious patient, since a transient general anesthesia can be induced with halothane administered by means of a mask and/or by a local anesthetic infiltration of the surgical area. This allows for later evaluation of the neurological status of the animal, as he will be awake a few minutes after tracheostomy (Fig. 12–2).[32, 61, 62]

The tracheostomy procedure is easily accomplished by placing the animal in the dorsal recumbent position with his legs retracted caudally and cross-tied to the table under his body (Fig. 12–3).[32] The ventral surface of the neck is prepared for surgery in the usual manner. The skin incision (4 to 8 cm long) is made on the ventral midline while one hand stabilizes the trachea in a superficial position. The ventral cervical musculature is divided, the midcervical trachea is exposed, an incision is made between any two of the tracheal rings caudal to the larynx and the thyroid gland, and a cuff-type (if available) tracheostomy tube is inserted in proper intratracheal position. The skin incision is closed with 3–0 stainless steel wire. The flange of the tube is su-

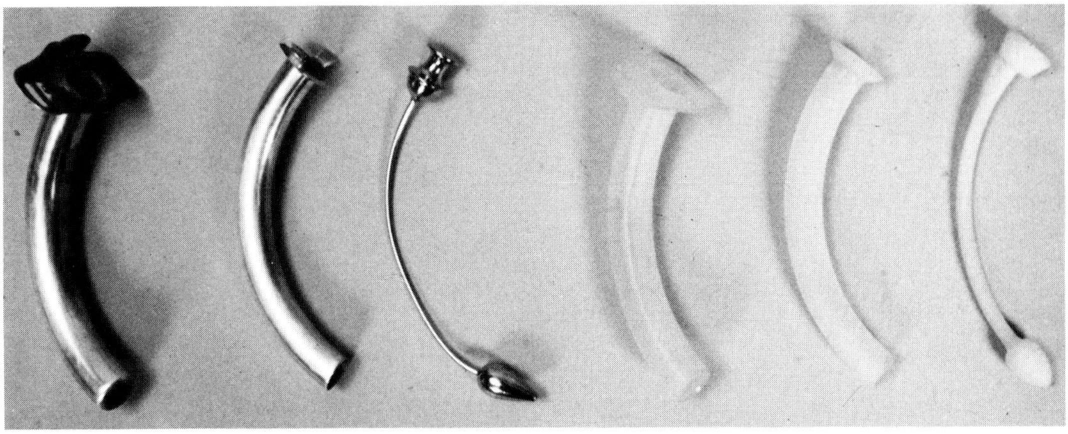

FIGURE 12–2 Standard plastic and silver tracheostomy tubes.

tured to the skin with dermal wire suture and, if possible, is also anchored in place with gauze around the neck of the animal.

The cuff of the tube is inflated moderately to limit aspiration of blood, mucus, or vomitus. Extreme inflation and distension of the cuff will cause pressure necrosis of the mucosa, particularly if it is left in place for a prolonged period of time. Accumulations of fluid in the trachea and main bronchi should be aspirated to provide better aeration. Resuscitative air, oxygen, or oxygen-anesthetic gas mixtures can be given when necessary if the cuffed tube is used.[32, 61]

The value of a tracheostomy is aptly summarized by the dictum: "The time to do a tracheostomy is the first time you think it may become necessary." Inadequate pulmonary aeration causing cerebral hypoxia is one of the chief causes of cerebral edema and brain swelling, as discussed in this chapter and in Chapter 20. Prompt tracheostomy can save the life of the dog with a head injury.[37]

EMERGENCY MEDICAL TREATMENT

Emergency therapy for shock is the second consideration in head injury. It has been discussed previously in Chapter 8. The use of broad spectrum antibiotics is always indicated in shock, particularly when CNS injury is involved. It must be emphasized that adequate tissue perfusion is as important as oxygenation if brain damage and death are to be avoided.

Adrenal corticoids are extremely worthwhile in the treatment of shock and in the control of cerebral edema. The immediate intravenous administration of prednisolone sodium succinate (10–40 mg/kg) is followed by 1–10 mg/kg dexamethasone, which should be given as often as needed. As the circulatory and neurogenic crisis subsides,

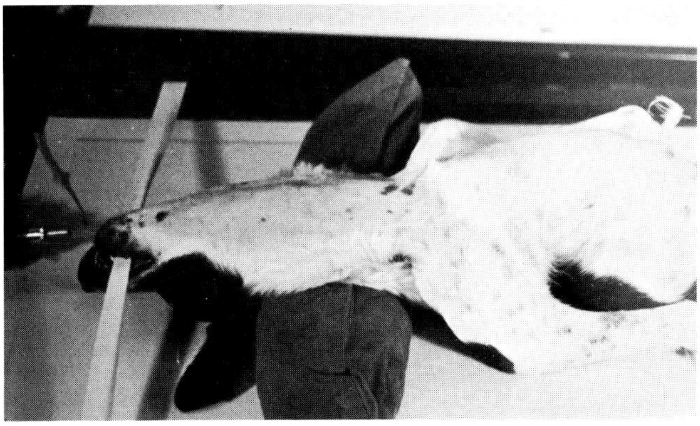

FIGURE 12–3 The dorsal recumbent position is appropriate for a tracheostomy.

the drug is used in diminishing quantities until it is discontinued completely.

Oxygen should always be administered in acute CNS trauma and use of hypertonic fluids should be considered as soon as brain hemorrhage has been eliminated as the primary diagnosis. Other medical considerations will be discussed later.

PHYSICAL EXAMINATION[45, 61]

Pizzi *et al.*[80] have divided the management of CNS trauma in man into three phases. In Phase I treatment is given for pathological conditions likely to cause rapid death, such as cardiovascular and respiratory disorders and space-occupying masses such as hematomas and focal contusions. In Phase II acute brain injuries are diagnosed by monitoring cerebral blood flow, the cerebral metabolic rate of oxygen, and intracranial and CSF pressures. In Phase III the patient is cared for in the intensive care unit.[80]

In the dog, the general physical examination must determine the status of vital signs, such as pulse, respiration, and blood pressure. Injuries that threaten life must be cared for before or during more detailed neurological examination. Hemorrhages, whether external or in a body cavity, must be stopped, and blood volume must be replaced or maintained. Acute chest injuries and occasional acute abdominal injuries demand immediate emergency care. Systemic shock must be treated before or during more detailed examinations. Systemic shock is infrequently encountered in uncomplicated head trauma; if it occurs 30 to 60 minutes after onset of trauma it is generally due to other body injuries. Severe fractures should not be manipulated excessively to satisfy curiosity, since pain resulting from such action promotes additional shock. Temporary splinting can be performed when time permits.

NEUROLOGICAL EXAMINATION

The importance of a prompt and careful neurological examination followed by immediate therapy can be illustrated by these statistics. Jamieson reported on 167 cases of extradural hematomas observed in man over an 11-year period. The overall mortality was 15.6 per cent, including a decline from 26.7 per cent in the first 60 cases to only 8 per cent in the last 60. He concluded that the outstanding avoidable cause of death was undue delay in diagnosis and treatment. He emphasized clinical assessment rather than special investigation and simple rather than more complex surgical procedures.[38]

Head Injuries[32, 61, 62]

All findings in a neurological examination must be recorded, as discussed in Chapter 3. Repeat or progressive examinations must also be recorded, and degrees of abnormalities should be graded or evaluated on a standard basis so that the improvement or worsening of the patient's status can be properly determined. The initial evaluation is the state of *consciousness*. The patient should be alert to people and objects and respond to standard painful stimuli such as the pinch of the base of the toenail by means of a forceps. The levels of consciousness are coma (unconscious with no response to painful stimuli), semicoma (unconscious but responsive to painful stimuli), delirium, confusion, depression, and alertness.[61]

The size and response of the pupil and nature of nystagmus are important in a neurological assessment. Posture, motor function, and vision should be evaluated. If convulsions or seizural disorders are present they also should be evaluated.[61]

Transient unconsciousness with rapid recovery is termed a concussion; a dog with such an injury should be observed for 24 to 48 hours for any signs of progressive CNS deterioration. Coma that lasts more than a few minutes, especially after an initial period of consciousness, usually indicates serve brain stem injury in the rostral reticular formation. Dogs are subject to hemorrhages and damage in the midbrain and pons; the usual signs are coma and decerebrate rigidity (extensor hypertonus in all four limbs). Brain stem compressions are seen in skull fractures, extrasubdural hematomas, and cerebral edema (Fig. 12–4).[61]

Bilateral miotic, bilateral mydriatic, and asymmetrical pupils are all suggestive of midbrain contusion. A favorable prognosis

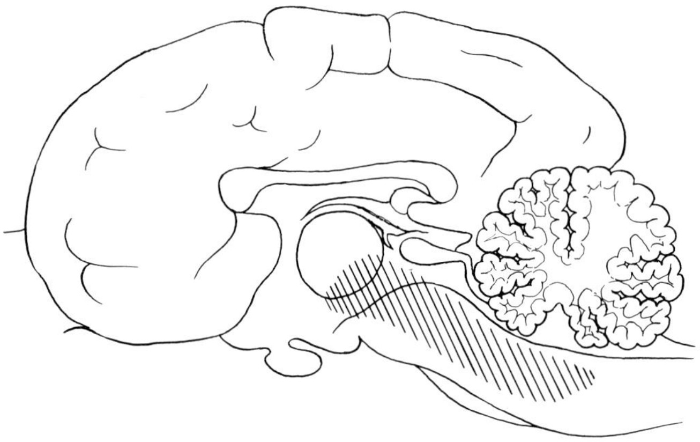

FIGURE 12–4 Traumatic lesions in the rostral portion of the reticular formation of the brain stem (hatched area) frequently cause coma.

is indicated if pupillary abnormalities disappear. In early damage to the midbrain and pons, the pupils are bilaterally constricted, but as the oculomotor nucleus is affected, the pupils become dilated. The oculocephalic responses may be altered so that the eyes remain fixed in the center of the orbit. No eyeball movements are seen as the head is turned in different directions (doll's head). Unilateral dilation of the pupil and later progression to ventrolateral strabismus and bilateral dilation indicate tentorial herniation. Progressively dilating pupils may indicate generalized cerebral hypoxia. Severe nystagmus (quick phase away from the affected side of the labyrinth) may indicate a petrous temporal bone fracture or a lateral cerebellopontine contusion.[61]

Decerebrate rigidity may occur with severe brain stem lesions caudal to the red nucleus. Severe vestibular disturbance peripherally or centrally in the pons and medulla will cause a head tilt or neck and body flexion. Head tilt, vestibular disorientation with rolling movements, and nystagmus usually are associated with injury to the membranous labyrinth from a fractured petrosal bone Paralysis or weakness of the body following head injury can result from laceration or contusion of the opposite side of the brain.[61]

Convulsions following head injury may be associated with intracranial hemorrhage and an expanding intracranial mass. A rapid rise in intracranial pressure may be indicated by a slower pulse and respirations and elevated temperature. If the intracranial pressure continues to rise and reduced cerebral circulation leads to progressive hypoxia, the vital signs may become reversed; in this case the pulse and respirations are rapid and the elevated temperature is maintained.[61]

Similar clinical signs may develop at different times in the course of the disease, indicating thereby the presence of brain stem hemorrhage or tentorial herniation. These differences are portrayed in Figure 12–5 and Table 12–1.[61]

Special Examinations of Head Injuries

Radiography of the skull for evidence of skull fracture is the most important special examination warranted in a patient with a severe head injury. If the patient is fractious and cannot be examined radiographically without sedation or anesthesia (which may be contraindicated), radiographs should be delayed if medically feasible. In cooperative patients when time is not a critical factor, an EEG examination can be helpful in ter-

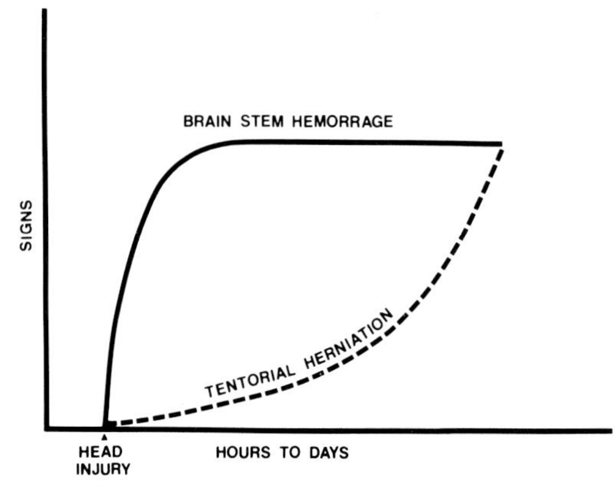

FIGURE 12–5 The sign-time graft illustrates the difference in the progression of signs in tentorial herniation and brain stem hemorrhage. (From Oliver, J. E., Jr.: Vet. Clin. N. Am. *2*, 341, 1972.)

TABLE 12–1*

	Brain Stem Hemorrhage	Tentorial Herniation
Onset	Early	Delayed
Course	Static to progressive	Progressive
Pupils	Constricted early, dilated late	Unilateral dilation; progression to bilateral dilation
Consciousness	Stuporous to comatose	Alert or apathetic, progressing to coma
Muscle tone	Decerebrate rigidity or flaccid paralysis	Normal or weak, progressing to decerebrate rigidity to flaccid paralysis
Reflexes	Usually symmetrical	Often unilateral asymmetry

*From Oliver, J. E., Jr.: Neurologic emergencies in small animals. Vet. Clin. N. Amer. *2*(2):341, 1972.

minating generalized cerebral edema or swelling. Echoencephalography may in the future become a diagnostic procedure in institutional clinics to determine midline shift of brain tissue due to space-occupying hemorrhage or swelling. Radioactive isotopes and brain scans may be diagnostic for cerebral trauma as well as neoplastic masses in the future. These procedures must be used only when surgical decompression is not urgent and time is available. Manipulation of the patient should be minimized.

Spinal Cord Injuries[32, 61, 64]

A traumatic injury to the spinal cord is not likely to be as fatal as a head injury; however, spinal cord injuries are more likely to produce permanent severe neurologic deficits such as paraplegia or tetraplegia. These injuries are devastating for the desirability of maintaining such an animal for a pet. Most injuries are the result of spinal fractures, luxations, and subluxations and occasionally an acutely ruptured disk. Since the cord damage is usually due to skeletal compressions and bony fragmentations, the spinal column must be kept immobile during the diagnostic procedures. Neurological localization of injury is based on the responses of the nonanesthetized animal to pain, segmental reflexes, and motor capabilities caudal to the lesion. Localization of sensory innervation is performed by palpation and needle prick of the skin of the trunk and limbs and is manifest as hyperesthesia of a segment due to nerve root irritation or anesthesia caudal to a segment due to severe compression or transection. Evaluation of the segmental nerve supply to a muscle or group of muscles, the myotome, is less effective in localization than sensory evaluation but is helpful in general sectional spinal segments. For example, a lesion in the L4–6 segments would abolish the knee jerk reflex that is mediated through the femoral nerve.

The prognosis of a spinal cord injury depends on the extent and reversibility of the injury. A sensory response to a noxious stimulus is a good criterion for a favorable prognosis. Firm pressure on a toe joint or the base of the toenail using a hemostatic forceps is considered an adequate stimulus for an alerting or aversive response such as turning the head, crying, or biting. Flexion of the leg alone is not an adequate response for a favorable prognosis since it is only a spinal reflex. Absence of the perpetual pain reflex is a very unfavorable sign. The presence of a crossed extensor thrust response indicates severe spinal cord damage and a poor prognosis. Persistent Schiff-Sherrington phenomenon (spastic paralysis of the fore limbs with flaccid paralysis of the hind limbs) is generally not accompanied by a pain response and presents a poor prognostic picture. This situation is generally seen in fracture or luxations in the middle to caudal thoracic region of the spinal column (Table 12–2).[61]

Special Examinations in Spinal Injuries

Radiographic examinations of the spine are necessary for more definitive localization of the injury and for information on the type of skeletal lesion and the most effective means of surgical correction. Detailed radiographs can usually be obtained only by means of anesthesia, which can be continued for appropriate surgical correction. Myelography is a necessary procedure

TABLE 12–2*

Spinal Cord	Signs Caudal to Lesion		
Segments	*Motor*	*Sensory*	*Autonomic*
C1–4	Tetraplegic with hyperreflexia	Anesthesia	Apnea, no micturition
C5–6	Tetraplegia with hyper reflexia, LMN suprascapular nerve	Anesthesia, hyperesthesia, midcervical	Apnea, phrenic nerve LMN, no micturition
C7–T1	Tetraplegia or paraplegia, with hyperreflexia, LMN brachial plexus	Anesthesia, hyperesthesia, brachial plexus	Diaphragmatic breathing only, no micturition
T2–L3	Paraplegia with hyperreflexia; Schiff-Sherrington syndrome	Anesthesia, hyperesthesia, segmental	Diaphragmatic, some intercostal and abdominal respiration, depending on level; no micturition
L4–S1	Paraplegia with LMN lumbrosacral plexus	Anesthesia, hyperesthesia, segmental	No micturition; S1-anal sphincter may be atonic
S1–S3	Knuckling hind foot, paralysis of tail	Anesthesia, hyperesthesia, segmental	No micturition, sphincters atonic
Cy1–Cy	Paralysis of tail	Anesthesia, hyper esthesia, segmental	None

*From Oliver, J. E., Jr.: Neurologic emergencies in small animals. Vet. Clin. N. Amer. *2*(2):341, 1972.
C = Cervical
T = Thoracic
L = Lumbar
S = Sacral
Cy = Coccygeal
LMN = Lower motor neuron

when skeletal lesions are not present or do not correlate with the neurological findings. Paraspinal EMG examinations may be helpful in localizing spinal compressions in more chronic spinal injuries.[45, 61]

PATHOGENESIS OF CNS INJURY

BRAIN INJURIES

The foregoing discussions of the consequences of brain injury in the dog have centered around the direct effects of hemorrhage, cerebral oligemia, and hypoxia. Since the brain requires extremely large amounts of blood and oxygen for its small size, derangements of blood and oxygen supplies are of prime importance.

One of the most devastating effects of trauma, outside of intracranial hemorrhage, is cerebral edema and swelling. The brain's allowance for such swelling is very limited because of the intimate presence of the cranial vault. The pressure of the cerebral mass against the nonelastic and nonexpandable vault soon leads to severe neuronal damage and clinical neurological deficits. It has been shown that 5 to 10 minutes of cerebral ischemia due to cardiac arrest will cause irreversible cortical dysfunction and microscopic ischemic necrosis, cerebral cortical hemorrhage, edema, and microcavitation of white matter. If cardiac function is restored, the dog may experience return of motor function but retain ocular, hearing, and smelling deficits.[70]

Another factor in brain injuries is the presence of cerebral vascular spasms which are usually associated with intracranial hemorrhage. Such spasms contribute to ischemia and brain swelling and edema with all the resultant histological changes. There is experimental evidence that the serotonin present in intracranial hemorrhage causes vasospasms in the brain. It was shown that when serotonin and blood containing appropriate amounts of serotonin were injected into the cisterna magna, cerebral arterial spasms resulted and lasted at least 3 hours. Phenoxybenzamine reversed the spasms produced by serotonin and blood containing serotonin.[5–7] Nagai showed that papaverine and isoxsuprine injections in the vertebral artery caused both early and late spasms, whereas methysergide and phentolamine released early but not late spasms.[59] It has also been shown that in uncomplicated head injuries, lactate was elevated initially in blood and CSF and decreased by the third day after injury. Arterial alkalosis continued after injury, and arterial pO_2 was below normal at all times. The fact that lactic acidosis in CSF continued for several days after injury suggests continued cerebral ischemia and hypoxia.[44]

Recent research has revealed the possible role of catecholamines in CNS damage. The term catecholamines applies to three naturally occurring compounds—dopamine, norepinephrine, and epinephrine. All three compounds contain a catechol nucleus and a single amine group. These substances can be synthesized in several tissues outside the brain, such as postganglionic sympathetic neurons, interneurons within sympathetic ganglia, and adrenal medullary chromaffin cells. Dopamine compounds occur in various areas in the brain and can ascend to terminate within the limbic cortex or descend to the spinal cord. Brain stem neurons convert dopamine to norepinephrine, which can terminate throughout most of the brain and spinal cord. The natural metabolic synthesis of catecholamines is diagrammed in Figure 12–6.[81]

There is growing evidence that catecholamines are related to neurological diseases because of changes of the levels of these substances in the brain, CSF, plasma, and urine and because of the responses of drugs acting at catecholamine synapses. Additional evidence has been substantiated in animal models. Human diseases which show altered catecholamine levels include Parkinson's disease (which responds to administration of L-Dopa), Huntington's disease, hepatic coma, cerebrovascular diseases ("stroke"), and spinal cord trauma. The effects of catecholamines in spinal injuries will be discussed in more detail later.[101]

SPINAL CORD INJURIES

It has been observed clinically that some cases of severe spinal cord trauma do not respond to prompt decompressive surgery and that total spinal cord destruction and dissolution may follow the injury within 24 to 48 hours. In these cases there seems to be an inherent autodestructive process in the cord in addition to the immediate physical disruption of cord elements from trauma.[65]

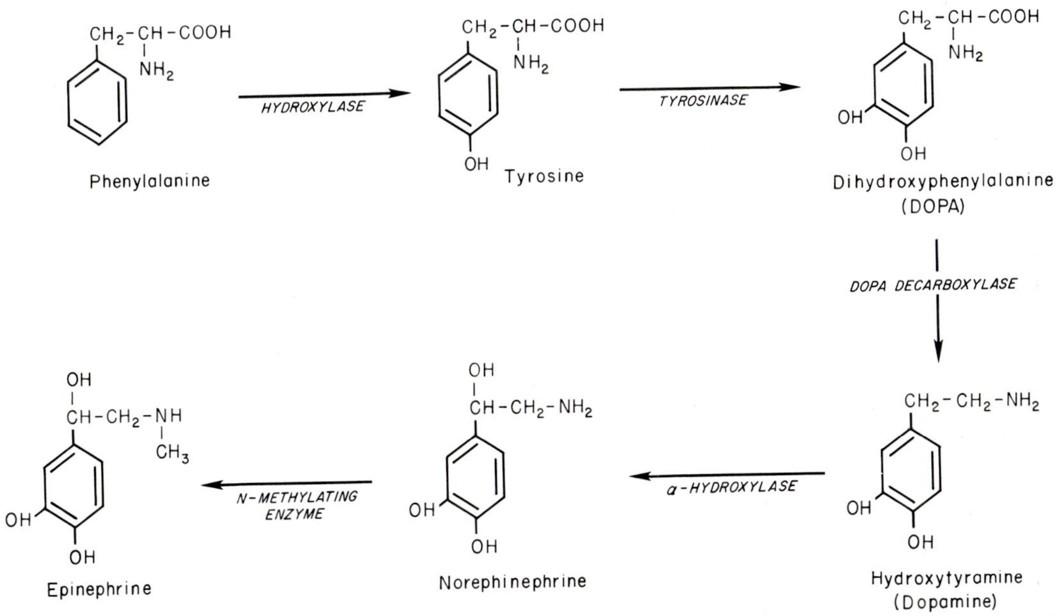

FIGURE 12–6 Biosynthesis of norepinephrine.

Vascular Effects

The spinal cord in man and particularly the dog apparently does not have a rich segmental arterial supply. In man, the cord is supplied by a variable number of anterior arteries (6 to 10) and posterior radicular arteries (10 to 28). Parker[73] demonstrated that out of 20 dogs studied only five had at least one spinal branch artery to each segment from T10 to L5. In four dogs the segmental arterial supply for as many as seven cord segments was apparently precarious, as it depended on only two to four spinal branch arteries.[73] Although it was noted that damage also occurred in segmental spinal veins, rapid collateral venous drainage was established.

Parker[72, 76] has also shown that paralumbar trauma does in fact occlude spinal arteries by thrombosis and rupture and that the spinal cord of the dog can suffer serious ischemia from traumatic injuries. Therefore, surgeons must be cognizant of this situation as well as the variable segmental blood flow to the spinal cord, and take care not to further endanger spinal arterial blood supply by careless surgical manipulations in cases of trauma.[74, 76]

In more detail, the blood supply to the cord can be divided basically into extrinsic and intrinsic vessels. The major extrinsic vessels, such as the aortic segmental, radicular, ventral spinal, and dorsolateral spinal arteries, provide a rich anastomotic source of nourishment. The pial–meningeal arterial plexus is a network of interlacing extrinsic vessels which connect these major vessels. For this reason segmental compression, ligation, or embolization of vessels outside the spinal cord may not be of primary clinical importance.[28]

The intrinsic spinal cord vessels consist of the central (sulcal) branches of the ventral spinal artery and arterioles from the superficial arterial plexus that radially penetrate the white matter. When hemorrhage or edema from traumatic spinal cord insult causes a rise in intramedullary pressure, the intrinsic vessels are compromised and the blood flow is diminished. An autodestructive process of ischemia that causes further spinal cord injury occurs.[28]

Terminal arterioles within the cord do not interconnect but give rise to interlocking capillary networks which are more numerous in the gray matter than in the white matter.[28] However, Griffiths[29] has shown that the white matter of the cord, in contrast to the cerebral cortex, has a higher proportion of blood flow than the gray matter. He further established that, even though the spinal cord exhibited autoregulation of blood flow similar to that of the cerebral cortex, the regional spinal blood flow was independent of the cerebrocortical circulation but dependent on metabolic changes of local and systemic origin.[29]

Light microscopic studies of experimentally traumatized cords revealed a few hemorrhages in the central gray matter within 30 minutes after injury; these resulted from delayed rupture of thin-walled vessels with red blood cell leakage into perivascular spaces. Within 2 hours, these hemorrhages enlarge when polymorphonuclear and microglial reactions become apparent. Ghost cells, eosinophilic nerve cells with indistinct nuclei, "smudged" cytoplasm, and loss of Nissl bodies are seen. Vascular congestion and blood extravasation emphasize traumatic vascular reactivity. At 4 hours, this process has advanced to a coagulation necrosis of up to 40 per cent of the central gray and adjacent white matter. In 24 hours, the spinal cord structures have been mainly replaced by amorphous necrotic tissue and aggregated red blood cells with only a small rim of identifiable white matter remaining. Hemorrhagic necrosis (HN) occupied 23.3 per cent of the total cord area at 2 hours and 69.4 per cent at 24 hours. Traumatic lesions spread in a longitudinal as well as a radial direction, extending several millimeters on either side of the traumatic site, and simulate dissecting hematomyelia.[65]

Ultramicroscopic studies with the electron microscope have shown the microvasculature to be the tissue in the cord that is most sensitive to trauma. In 5 minutes, postcapillary venules are distended with red blood cells and in 15 minutes vessel walls are ruptured. The white matter shows progressive changes until at 4 hours, 25 per cent of the axons have broken myelin sheaths or have been denuded or degenerated.[65]

Wilson and co-workers ligated multiple radicular arteries and produced hemorrhagic central cord lesions that closely paralleled those seen in traumatized cords.

Other workers have found a dramatic fall that continued for hours in tissue pO_2 within 1 hour after injury and a concomitant rise in tissue lactate.[65]

From these vascular studies it was concluded that trauma provokes a microvascular response that causes significant localized retardation of blood flow, and lethal tissue hypoxia develops within hours. This traumatic cord autodestruction can proceed without axial tissue distortion from physical compression. There are two theories of the mechanism of this failure: (1) that the traumatized vasculature is directly responsible, and (2) that spinal cord catecholamines are responsible for the vascular changes.[65]

Biochemical Changes in Traumatized Spinal Cords

In experimental cord trauma, there is a marked increase in protein, clots, and xanthochromia in the CSF. Marked reductions in spinal cord oxygen tension and a transient accumulation of spinal cord lactic acid occur following trauma.[46, 51] Eidelberg *et al.*[24] reported a massive flow of potassium into the CSF surrounding the cord after impact injury in cats. This was probably caused by membrane damage or failure of the potassium pump due to anoxia and local biochemical alterations. Artificial solutions could block spinal cord conduction as measured by cortical evoked potentials.

Release of intracellular lysosomal enzymes following spinal cord injury from acute impact may be related to delayed pathological processes. Lysosomal enzyme elevations first begin at 5 days and are maximal 2 to 3 weeks after injury, while nonlysosomal enzymes are not changed. In these studies maximum post-traumatic edema occurred between 6 hours and 11 days, and therefore it was deduced that edema was not related to the release of lysosomal enzyme.[102]

Catecholamines in Spinal Injuries

A great influx of experimental data accumulated from various catecholamine research efforts in the spinal cord is currently confusing the practicing clinician. The conflicting results have stemmed probably from differences in methods of producing experimental cord trauma, inadequate controls, and the use of several different species of animals. Pinpoint trauma produces different results from more expansive blunt trauma or annular constricitve trauma.[28]

Osterholm found a marked increase in norepinephrine (NE) levels in traumatized cat cord tissue. Introduction of norepinephrine in nontraumatized cords produced identical microscopic lesions.[66, 67] Naftchi *et al.* reported normal levels of NE in traumatized cat cords but marked *increases* in dopamine (DA) levels.[58] Bingham *et al.* found a progressive *decrease* in NE activity in traumatized monkey cords, whereas DA remained unchanged.[10] The various workers found that administration of the pharmacologic antagonist specific for an elevated catecholamine reduced or eliminated the noxious effect of that specific catecholamine. Epsilon aminocaproic acid (EACA) and methylprednisolone sodium succinate protected the traumatized cord from hemorrhage and edema.[14] Naftchi used the same anticatecholamines as Campbell and found that histamine and dopamine levels in the cord were dramatically reduced after treatment (both were elevated in controls).[58]

Although these and other findings present some conflicting data, the preponderance of evidence supports the concept that catecholamines are associated with traumatized hemorrhagic necrosis. Ablation injury experiments demonstrate the necessity for intact afferent–efferent spinal cord and root pathways in traumatic spinal cord autodestruction. A theory of a neurotransmitter-vascular alteration seems more likely than the concept of direct traumatic vascular disruption. Osterholm resolves the differences in NE and DA levels by stating that DA is a metabolic precursor, that the cord has no DA receptors but numerous NE receptors, and that NE is 20 to 100 times more efficient in activating the NE receptors and subsequent hemorrhagic syndrome. Catecholamine fibers terminate on small vessels in the cord and on gray neurons and originate from the posterior brain. Brain and spinal cord vessels regulate themselves in essentially the same manner and probably both are controlled from a single brain stem center.[65] Since Vise and others[97] feel that the rise in catecholamine levels within the damaged spinal cord may be derived from extravasation and hemorrhage, it must be concluded that the mechanism of action is still not definitely known.

Experimental Treatment of Cord Injuries

Although many of the so-called experimental treatments for spinal injuries are purely experimental, some have been used for a few years in clinical practice. Those that warrant clinical use will be discussed further in the section on clinical treatment (see p. 396).

Myelotomy

Myelotomy techniques were described as early as 1908 by Allen,[4] who had demonstrated the effects of calibrated weight-force experimental trauma to the spinal cord. These experiments subsequently led to myelotomy incisions, 1 to 1.5 cm in length, through the cord substance of the mid-dorsal column of the injured spinal cord. All five of the dogs so treated made uneventful recoveries, although some were reported to be slightly spastic Allen felt that the laminectomy should be done at the earliest possible moment, and if the cord was not severed, the median longitudinal incision should be made through the area of impact by means of a fine canaliculus knife in order to drain the injured tissue of the products of edema and hemorrhage (Fig 12–7).[2–4]

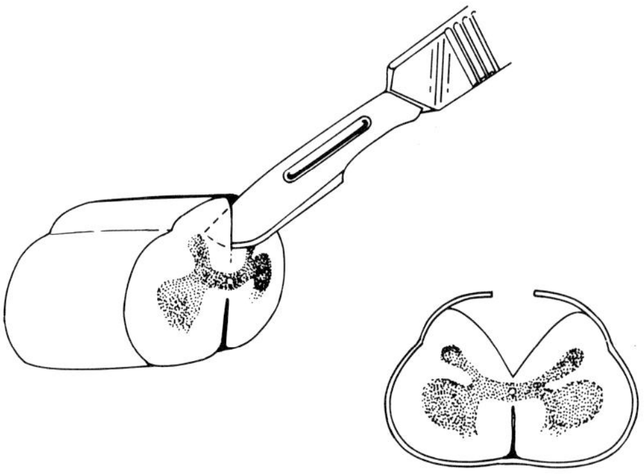

FIGURE 12–7 A myelotomy involves a dorsal midline incision through the dura and the dorsal median sulcus to the level of the central canal, extending 1 to 3 vertebral lengths.

The method remained largely untried for several years until reproposed by McVeigh in 1923,[55] Freeman and Wright in 1953,[26] and Campbell in 1972 [15] In veterinary medicine, Mendenhall and coworkers[56] established a spinal trauma unit at Colorado State University Veterinary College and carried out extensive anticatecholamine and antifibrinolytic treatments combined with immediate dorsal laminectomy on a minimum of three vertebral lengths, plus durotomy and myelotomy. This work will be discussed in more detail later.

Based largely on this work, a few veterinary surgeons have used myelotomy in a select number of cases. It has been shown that careful myelotomy on the precise midline in the dorsal median sulcus down to the central canal using a very sharp instrument such as a razor blade will cause minimal to moderate neurological deficits in normal dogs. Varying degrees and permanence of proprioceptive deficits may be seen, especially if the incision is off the midline.[9] Osterholm has found that a myelotomy above the injured cord area produced a reduction in norepinephrine levels in the injured cord and helped prevent resultant hemorrhage and necrosis. He felt that the value of myelotomy might rest with the chemical response to injury rather than solely with mechanical decompression of the injured area.[65]

Rhizotomy

It has been shown by Osterholm[65, 66] that a dorsal root–dorsal column system appears to be the afferent loop for traumatic hemorrhagic necrosis. A bilateral two-segment section of the dorsal root on either side of a future injury protects against traumatic lesion necrosis. He concludes that, until medical therapy against hemorrhagic necrosis can be developed, both myelotomy and dorsal root sectioning are appropriate methods of management of acute spinal cord injures.[65] The author of this text believes that there are no data on dorsal root sectioning in clinical spinal trauma in the veterinary literature at the present time. However, if the clinical case warrants this rather radical neurological procedure and if the owner is aware of all prognostic ramifications, extensive myelotomy and rhizotomy at and above the site of injury should be used occasionally in neurosurgery.

Durotomy

Durotomy in human neurosurgery has usually involved the use of either hypothermic or normothermic perfusion techniques. It was felt that perfusion may be more effective with an incised dura and exposed cord than with an intact dura, but recent work leads one to doubt this conclusion (Fig. 12–8).[92]

The original report of Albin stated that regional hypothermic perfusions can reduce spinal edema and swelling because hypothermia will diminish the metabolic needs of cord tissue in trauma.[1] It was felt that a longitudinal incision of the dura mater would lessen the compressive action of the dura on the swollen cord and thereby have a beneficial effect. The blood supply to the cord would then be at least partially restored and should reduce hypoxia in the cord.

Parker and Smith reported that longitudinal dorsolateral incisions of the normal canine spinal cord would yield only mild temporary neurological deficits. Conscious proprioception was impaired in 10 of 11 dogs when the incision was made through a hemilaminectomy defect at L1–3, but only three of eight dogs showed deficits when the incision was made at L4–6. Deficits were present up to 4 days after surgery.[74] These clinical observations agree with work by Swaim and Belcher[9] when durotomies were performed on the dorsolateral and dorsal aspects of the lumbar cord. However, microscopic cord demyelinization and pathology was seen adjacent to the incised area.

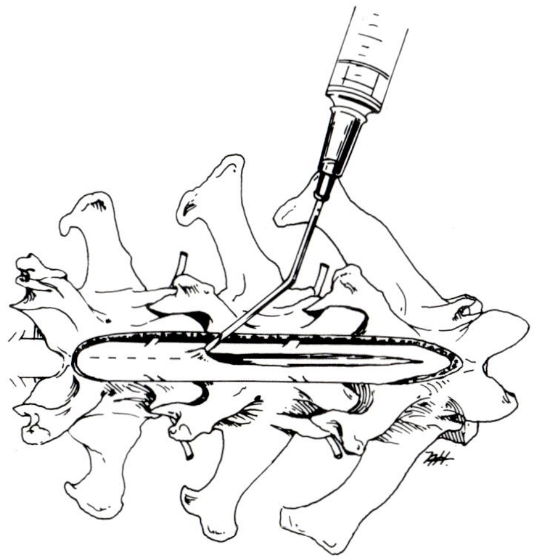

FIGURE 12–8 A durotomy can be performed through a dorsal or a hemilaminectomy approach for proposed maximal cord decompression. In questionable cases of malacia, the durotomy is of prognostic value. The dural incision can easily be performed with minimal cord trauma by bending a 23-gauge injection needle and using the cutting edge of the bevel for incising the dura.

Parker showed that when durotomies were performed immediately after experimental spinal cord trauma, the animals recovered more quickly than those in the control group.[78, 79] However, after a delay of 2 hours following trauma, durotomy incisions produced little benefit to dogs.[77] Recent work on monkeys has shown that durotomy is ineffective in treatment of experimental compressive spinal cord trauma, but hypothermic and normothermic perfusions are effective.[92]

In clinical work, Brasmer and Trotter have reported the value of durotomy and hypothermic perfusions in spinal surgery.[12, 94, 95] Other surgeons have continued to use the method of perfusion of the spinal cord and surgical area with room temperature saline, reserving durotomy largely for establishment of a more accurate prognosis. If the cord substance flows out of the dural incision, it is evident that malacia has taken place, and the prognosis is unfavorable. Such animals should be destroyed immediately.[90] Parker agrees that durotomy is clinically inappropriate except as an aid in prognosis.[77]

Hyperbaric Oxygenation

It has been noted that hyperoxygenation has a beneficial effect on spinal cord function in primates subjected to acute impact injuries. These experiments led to the conclusion that increased oxygenation of cord tissue decreased edema through local vasoconstriction.[31] Kelly found that hyperbaric oxygenation (100 per cent O_2 at two atmospheres) had a beneficial effect on clinical recovery whether it was delayed for 1 or 4 hours or serially administered at 1, 4, 24, and 48 hours.[43] However, when rats were exposed to 60 pounds per square inch gravity of oxygen on consecutive days, segmental foci of central necrosis of the spinal gray matter resulted. It was concluded that hyperbaric-administered oxygen on a long-term basis could be detrimental to spinal cord tissue.[8]

Local or Regional Hypothermia

Albin revived interest in spinal cord injury when he demonstrated encouraging results in the use of local hypothermic perfusion in experimentally traumatized spinal cords in monkeys.[1] Several investigators have used various traumatic forces, various perfusion procedures and different kinds of perfusates, and have worked with more than one species of animals. They have thereby proposed some confirmative and some conflicting results. Ducker and Hamit,[23] Osterholm,[65] and White[98] agreed that hypothermic perfusions seemed to be valuable. Osterholm found that norepinephrine levels in traumatized cords were significantly lower in hypothermic treated animals.[65] Black and Markowitz[11] found a somewhat slower recovery rate in hypothermia than in untreated controls. Tator and Deeke[92] concluded that both hypothermic and normothermic Elliott's B solution were effective in mildly traumatized cords, while normothermic solutions seemed more effective in heavily traumatized cords. Smith and Parker[88] demonstrated a beneficial effect from normothermic perfusion without a durotomy in a controlled experiment. Thus, there is general agreement that perfusion is beneficial in lessening the hemorrhagic necrosis that develops in traumatized spinal cords. Possibly the mechanism is a dialytic action of the injury-related chemical material from the wounded cord. Whether or not perfusion is best accomplished with hypothermic or normothermic perfusate is yet to be definitely established.

In small animal practice, Lumb,[53] Brasmer,[12] and Yturraspe and co-workers[103, 104] felt that hypothermic perfusions of lactated Ringer's "slush" and in some cases adjunctive systemic hypothermia were very beneficial in spondylectomy and vertebral prosthetic surgery. Trotter uses slush routinely in dorsal decompressive disk and vertebral fracture surgery.[94] It is not reported that these workers have used normothermic perfusion controls. Until more definitive work is done, veterinary surgeons should consider using prescribed perfusions in spinal surgery and select the temperature themselves until a definitive recommendation on the temperature of perfusate can be established.

Antifibrinolytic Therapy

The CSF has fibrinolytic mechanisms similar to those of plasma except that it lacks intrinsic activators. When hemorrhage occurs in the CNS, plasminogen is activated to degrade formed clots. Epsilon aminocaproic acid (EACA), which is structurally similar to lysine, acts as a competitive fibrinolytic inhibitor.[89] When EACA is used in conjunction with methylprednisolone, effective reduction of central gray matter hemorrhage and necrosis in injured spinal cords of cats has been noted.[14] Mendenhall *et al.* used EACA in their clinical study and felt that it was a helpful clinical drug.[56] The synergistic effect of EACA and steroids may help to preserve membrane integrity and promote clinical and electrophysiological recovery.[14]

Anticatecholamines

The influence of the catecholamines in the hemorrhagic necrosis that takes place in cord trauma, which seems to be independent of compressive effects on the cord, has been discussed in the previous section on pathogenesis of spinal cord trauma. Several agents that have an antagonistic action against these amines were mentioned. Although it is much too early to recommend clinical use of these agents, the most effective ones are discussed here briefly.

Osterholm and co-workers[65-68] tested 18 drugs or drug combinations known to promote anti-NE synthesis, storage site depletion, or receptor site blockage in standard injuries. They are listed here in descending order of effectiveness. Reserpine administered intramuscularly 15 minutes after injury and 12 hours later in doses of 2.5–5 mg/kg was most effective in preventing hemorrhagic necrosis. Levodopa in doses of 75 mg/kg was surprisingly effective against hemorrhagic necrosis in cord trauma. Alpha methyl dopa (AMT) given intravenously in doses of 40–800 mg/kg, which is commonly used as an antihypertensive agent, was also effective. A combination of AMT (50 mg/kg LD form) and phenoxybenzamine 20 mg/kg was superior to either drug given alone. If the AMT dose can be decreased 75 per cent by using this combination, the renal toxicity seen with AMT alone can be avoided.

Disulfiram administered in 7.2 mg/kg doses was effective in that it saved 53 per cent more cord area than saline alone. 6-hydroxydopamine administered by continuous epidural infusions of 10–50 mg/kg first depleted catecholamines and then selectively destroyed the cord fibers. Other drugs that were effective against hemorrhagic necrosis were fusaric acid, Fla-63, guanethidine, and bretylium tasylate. The degree of protection of all 88 drugs tested varied from 11.4 per cent to 62.4 per cent. Based on the analysis of all drug data, 75 per cent of all anti-NE treated animals (66 of 88) retained sufficient cord substance 24 hours after injury to predict future walking ability.[65]

Mendenhall *et al.* used reserpine in clinically damaged spinal cords along with other pharmacological and surgical therapy. Intensive care for several days was necessary in many instances owing to the nature of trauma, surgery, and drug therapy. Reserpine shows promise if administered in carefully monitored and special care clinical situations.[56]

DMSO (Dimethyl Sulfoxide)

DMSO has been proposed as an anti-inflammatory agent for many muscular and joint disorders. It is a dipolar aprotic solvent which crosses the dermal barrier rapidly in high concentrations with little or no permanent tissue damage. It has therefore also been used as a vehicle for dermal application of other medicines such as steroids. It can also cross the blood-brain barrier and assists the penetration of certain compounds such as C-pemoline, L-dopa, and epinephrine and norepinephrine.[21] In theory DMSO counteracts tissue anoxia by aiding diffusion of blood gases into tissue.[42]

DMSO was chosen as a possible therapeutic agent in experimental head and spinal cord injuries because of two considerations: (1) its ability to pick up water in tissue and thus act as an anti-inflammatory and diuretic agent, and (2) its protective properties in some cells subjected to mechanical or chemical damage. Forty rhesus monkeys were subjected to acute experimental head injury by extradural balloon compression of the brain. At the critical endpoint in the compression, saline, urea, or DMSO was injected. All saline-treated animals died, 10 of 15 urea-treated animals survived, and 14 of the 15 DMSO-treated monkeys survived. Among the survivors, neurological deficits appeared in four of the urea-treated group and one of the DMSO-treated animals.[20,21] The dose of DMSO was 2.2 gm/kg body wieght. Mild reactions from DMSO injections included increased respiratory rate and some skeletal muscle fasciculations that may result from anticholinesterase activity.[19-21]

Kajihara *et al.*[42] and de la Torre and co-workers[19-21] also used DMSO in experimental acute spinal injury in dogs. The DMSO-treated dogs did significantly better than untreated controls or animals treated by urea or glucocorticoids. The recovery rate was related to the initial dose and the time interval between the injury and the initial dose. High doses and earlier treatment resulted in much faster recovery. The combination of DMSO and dexamethasone produced no better results than DMSO alone. The reactions in dogs given DMSO included extension spasms of the hind limbs with muscle fasciculations immediately after injection, increased respiratory rate with a garlic odor in the breath, voluminous diuresis for the first 1 to 2 hours after injection, dark urine but no blood cells, and anorexia persisting for a few days after injection. DMSO-treated dogs had fewer microscopic cord changes than the other animals.[21] In another study, de la Torre treated 32 dogs with saline, mannitol, DMSO, and dexamethasone 1 hour after traumatizing the cord with a 500 gram centimeter force. After 90 days of observation, no animals treated with saline or mannitol recovered motor function. Those receiving DMSO or dexamethasone showed better recovery. DMSO produced the best results.[19]

The use of DMSO appears to be very promising according to the work by de la Torre and co-workers.[19-21] The prevention of hemorrhagic necrosis in the traumatized cord seems less spectacular than the use of anticatecholamine preparations. Future investigation will determine the clinical application of all these experimental drugs and methods.

MEDICAL TREATMENT OF CNS INJURY

In the earlier discussion of the emergency care of an animal with an acute CNS injury, we emphasized the necessity for careful handling, transport, and initial examination procedures that would minimize further CNS damage by manipulation. It was also emphasized that because an animal in extreme pain may be excitable and fractious two persons may be necessary to handle him. Muzzling will help minimize self-injury by improper movement. Quiet surroundings and gentle nursing will frequently reassure the patient so that use of sedatives will not be necessary. Any patient with possible brain damage should receive no narcotics, barbiturates, or long-acting profound tranquilizers that will disturb monitoring of the conscious state. Injectable anodyne preparations such as methampyrone (Pyrodyne) may be effective in reducing pain and will not interfere appreciably with neurological assessment. If general sedation is mandatory, diazepam would be the preferred drug.

The presence of arterial or substantial venous hemorrhage must be diagnosed and treated promptly. Blood volume and tissue perfusion must be maintained, shock must be treated, and the patent airway must be maintained by tracheostomy or pharyngeal endotracheal tube. The animal must be stabilized in a normothermic or slightly hypothermic state; hyperthermia must be treated vigorously by ice packs and antipyretics. Kidney function must be maintained. Broad spectrum antibiotics such as chloramphenicol should be started promptly. All methods of preventing CNS edema and swelling should be used, such as elevating the skull, administering oxygen, steroids, hypertonic solutions, and possibly systemic or regional hypothermia. The importance of monitoring and recording vital and neurological signs every 15 to 30 minutes for changes in physical status cannot be overemphasized.

We have previously discussed some methods of treating CNS injury that are still largely experimental. Now we will describe some procedures that many would feel are experimental but have rather wide clinical acceptance. Among these methods are the administration of oxygen, glucocorticosteroids, hypothermia, and hypertonic solutions as well as cranial burring, craniotomy, and spinal decompressive surgery.

OXYGEN AND HYPERVENTILATION

Few clinicians will argue the need to establish a patent airway and to use oxygen as an aid in preventing CNS hypoxia, edema, and swelling. Oxygen therapy is a basic mode of treatment in CNS injury. Moreover, it has been established that forced administration of oxygen by resuscitation or "bagging" will actively shrink edematous brain tissue during intracranial surgery. Hyperbaric oxygenation may gain widespread clinical use in the future. The effect of prolonged hyperventilation is not fully understood; possibly hyperventilation could cause damage by promoting irreversible cerebral hypoxia.[85] However, short-term hyperventilation of the critical patient can be a life-preserving procedure. Use of the oxygen compartment or tent should always be considered in the patient with acute CNS distress.

STEROIDS

Cerebral edema is characterized by a swollen brain with flattening of the gyri and narrowing of the sulci. Microscopically, the white matter seems to show more structural and chemical changes than the adjacent gray matter. The primary distinction seems to be that the excess fluid in white matter is largely extracellular, whereas in the gray matter it is intracellular. It has been shown that the deeper white matter is generally more involved than the superficial areas. The mechanism whereby brain edema is established is still in doubt. In experimental production of brain edema, edematous white matter shows a significant rise in sodium and total proteins and a decrease in potassium.[16, 69]

The causes of cerebral edema are many and varied and include injuries, hypoxia, ischemia, surgical manipulation, metabolic and toxic disorders, neoplasia, and head down positioning in a recumbent animal. Many investigators have tried to establish a standard method of producing edema experimentally so that therapeutic evaluation can be performed. These experimental methods include focal freezing, extradural balloons, exposure, anoxia, radiographic contrast media, and psyllium seed implantation. In the last-named method, Sims established that intramuscular injections of 2 mg/kg total daily dose of dexamethasone at 8 hour intervals appreciably reduced the sodium and water content of tissue around the implanted psyllium seed. Dexamethasone therapy was started the afternoon following the morning of surgical implantation and was continued for 5 days, at the end of which time the animal was killed.[87]

Other workers have found that the various steroids have beneficial effects in controlling CNS edema in experimental models.[82] Lewin[50] produced impact injury to the spinal cord in cats and found that there was a decrease in the percentage of dry weight and potassium level and an increase in the sodium concentration in injured tissue one day after injury. Edema was maximal between the third and sixth days and began to recede on the ninth day. Administration of dexamethasone started 48 hours before injury or 5 or 24 hours after injury had minimal effect on edema but prevented loss of potassium. All treated cats showed significantly better functional recovery than untreated animals. It was felt that the steroid maintained the structural integrity of the cellular elements in traumatized tissue.[50] Ducker and Hamit[23] initiated steroid treatment 3 hours after experimental cord trauma and found that even with this delayed therapy, 4 of 12 dogs regained nearly normal function. Administration of dexamethasone was continued for 1 week. Sato[84] found that intravenously injected dexamethasone reduced the production rate of CSF, reaching its maximal effect of 50 per cent reduction in 50 minutes. As mentioned previously, corticosteroids were shown to be effective in controlling the hemorrhagic necrosis and cord destruction in traumatized cords when given alone or in combination with anticatecholamines.[58] Steroids given in combination with hypothermic and normothermic perfusions in experimental cord trauma were also thought to be effective.[11, 12, 56]

In clinical evaluations, glucocorticosteroids have proved to be beneficial in cases of CNS trauma. Steroids apparently maintain vascular integrity after injury, protect cellular membranes during hypoperfusion states, and support lysosomes.[65] Most veterinary neurosurgeons administer 1 to 10 mg/kg of dexamethasone initially, repeated in lesser doses every 6 to 12 hours as needed. When the patient's condition has stabilized, the dose is cut in half each day for 4 to 10 days, when it is discontinued. Dexamethasone is also the agent of choice in systemic shock, along with antibiotics. Steroids are almost universally used in veterinary neurology in the patient with acute CNS trauma and also in surgical disk cases. In the latter cases the postoperative dose rarely exceeds 1 to 2 mg of dexamethasone daily per patient.[12, 53, 61, 62, 90]

Even though glucocorticosteroids are used extensively, their possible clinical sequelae must be kept in mind. In man long-term or high doses of steroids can cause gastrointestinal ulcerations, bleeding, pancreatitis, colonic ulcerations and perforations, and nephrosis. Hoerlein and Spano[33] reported a series of five cases involving routine intervertebral disk or spinal surgery in which pancreatitis, duodenal ulcers, colonic ulcers and perforations, and gastric ulcers occurred after surgery. Steroid therapy had been given in all cases prior to and following surgery. The doses were relatively small (1–4 mg dexamethasone daily for 4 to 5 days after surgery). However, anemia and elevation of serum alkaline phosphatase and serum glutamic pyruvic transaminase (SGPT) were prominent findings in another series of 14 postoperative spinal patients. It is routine in some clinics to give antacids and gastrointestinal protective agents when administering steroids in CNS patients. It was concluded that prior administrations of steroids, the presence of borderline clinical nephrosis, and the stress of surgery all contributed to the observed sequelae.[33]

HYPOTHERMIA

Hypothermia was discussed as an experimental procedure in acute CNS injury;

however, it has been used clinically for some time. Local hypothermia in spinal trauma, although of apparent benefit in prolonged and radical spinal surgery, may not be more beneficial than normothermic perfusion of the operative area. The usual durotomy performed in conjunction with local hypothermia may not be of added therapeutic value. However, *systemic* hypothermia may have a beneficial effect in CNS trauma and in brain surgery. Theoretically the principal value of hypothermia is the reduction of cerebral and spinal cord metabolic need for oxygen and glucose, but it is a complex, intensive care type of procedure that involves monitoring of blood gases and electrolytes which few veterinary practices can properly perform.

Again, it is emphasized that hyperthermia or hyperpyrexia is a continuous threat to the patient with acute CNS injury and surgical neurological disorders. Hyperthermia causes an increase in demand in cerebral blood flow, which in turn increases the intracranial volume and ultimately the intracranial pressure. Moderate hypothermia must be used in such patients until the normothermic or slightly hypothermic state can be established.[80]

HYPERTONIC SOLUTIONS

Hypertonic solutions have been used in nonhemorrhaging brain trauma to decrease CSF pressure and intracranial mass. These solutions consisted of 50 per cent glucose, 50 per cent sucrose, 25 per cent saline, 50 per cent magnesium sulfate, concentrated human albumin, and concentrated human plasma given intravenously.[54] Glycerin has been given orally for the control of glaucoma and dehydration of the brain. It is relatively nontoxic and can be given for prolonged periods.[60] More recently, urea and mannitol solutions have been used, particularly during or after surgical procedures on the central nervous system.[16]

The theory of action was that substances of higher osmotic effect, such as hypertonic solutions, would draw intracellular water out into the extracellular spaces. As the extracellular osmotic tension is lessened by dilution, the active ingredient in the former hypertonic solution penetrates the cell, increasing its osmotic concentration to the point that it draws water back into the cell. This effect is known as the "rebound effect." Since mannitol has the least cell penetration of the common hypertonic solutions, it has the least rebound.

Javid proposed that a 30 per cent sterile urea solution be prepared by adding 10 ml of 10 per cent invert sugar in water for every 30 gm of urea crystals. The invert sugar is necessary to prevent hemolysis of red blood cells. This solution is given intravenously at a rate of 60 drops/min and at a dose of 1 gm urea/kg body weight. Maximum shrinking of brain is seen within 1 hour and persists for 3 to 10 hours;[39] however, sucrose and urea solutions are somewhat nephrotoxic and are contraindicated in renal disorders.[96]

Both urea and dextrose, as explained previously, tend to cause a secondary or rebound rise in cerebrospinal fluid pressure after the initial dehydration. In man, the most marked effect of dehydration in the brain is usually seen in 20 to 30 minutes, whereas rebound overhydration of the brain reaches a peak between 12 and 18 hours. The pressure in the brain returns to normal at the end of 24 hours.[83] Frequent or continuous cisternal drainage to relieve increased pressure would not be practical in canine therapeutics.

Leonard and Redding[49] established the effects of urea and mannitol on the CSF pressure in the lateral ventricle of dogs for 9 consecutive hours. Both urea and mannitol at a dose of 1.5 gm/kg body weight proved to be highly effective in reducing CSF pressure. The effect was practically immediate and lasted an average of 1.5 hours. The second dose given 4 hours after the first produced a more prolonged effect (average 2¼ hours). When a 4.5 gm/kg dose was given the duration of effect was 3 hours. However, when this larger dose was repeated, two of the three dogs died. It was felt that repeated high doses of mannitol could be lethal, but that 1 gm/kg doses can be repeated if necessary. Intravenously administered lactate Ringer's solution and isotonic saline solution in a dose of 15 ml/kg body weight did not alter CSF pressure[49] (Table 12–3).

Further experimental work by Parker has established that mannitol is effective in reducing the edema seen in traumatized

TABLE 12–3 DURATION OF ACTION OF HYPERTONIC SOLUTIONS ADMINISTERED TO DOGS DURING A 15-MINUTE PERIOD*

Group II (1.5 gm. of mannitol/kg.)		**Group III (4.5 gm. of mannitol/kg.)**		**Group IV (1.5 gm. of urea/kg.)**		**Group V (1.5 gm. of mannitol/kg.)**			**Group VI (4.5 gm. of mannitol/kg.)**		
							Duration of Action (hr.)			*Duration of Action (hr.)*	
Dog No.	*Duration of Action (hr.)*	*Dog No.*	*Duration of Action (hr.)*	*Dog No.*	*Duration of Action (hr.)*	*Dog No.*	*First Injection*	*Second Injection*	*Dog No.*	*First Injection*	*Second Injection*
1	1¼	1	5½	1	1¼	1	2	3	1	2¼	4½
2	1¼	2	3½	2	1½	2	1¼	2½	2	4¼	.....
3	1¼	3	2	3	1½	3	1	1¼	3	3¾	.....
4	3	4	1½	4	1½	...	.....	.....	...	.....	.....
5	1¼	5	3¼	5	1	...	.....	.....	...	.....	.....
6	1¼	6	2	6	1¾	...	.....	.....	...	.....	.....
Range	1¾		4		¾		1	1¾		2	.....
Mean	1½		3		1½		1½	2¼		3½	.....

*From Leonard, J. L., and Redding, R. W.: Effects of hypertonic solutions on cerebrospinal fluid pressure in the lateral ventricle of the dog. Am. J. Vet. Res. *34*, 213, 1973.

spinal cords. When mannitol was given intravenously at a rate of 3 gm/kg of body weight, myelograms secured 2 hours later showed a significant reduction in diameter compared to pretreatment myelograms.[71] However, when 15 dogs with experimentally produced severe blood loss were treated with 3 gm/kg mannitol, 9 died. Death seemed to be associated with rapid large increases in central venous pressure. It was concluded that the hemodynamic changes that occur after mannitol administration could be dangerous in a dog suffering from severe vascular hypovolemia. Saline, plasma, or blood should be administered to restore blood volume before mannitol is given.[71]

The effect of mannitol in clinical practice is well established. Mannitol reduces intracranial pressure from 20 to 34 per cent in clinical patients as well as in experimental studies.[41, 57] There is a dramatic reduction in volume pressure response even though intracranial pressure response may be modest. Miller found that intravenous mannitol 0.5 gm/kg and intramusuclar betamethasone (26 mg) both reduce the volume pressure response more than they reduce intracranial pressure. Mannitol reduces the water content of the brain, and steroids inhibit CSF formation and improve local tissue perfusion as well as the bulk of areas affected by edema.[57] Pizzi recommends a continuous intravenous drip of 10 per cent mannitol to "titrate" intracranial pressure or neurological status. The maximal daily dose in man is 5 gm/kg for not more than 10 days.[80]

Although urea is highly effective, more surgeons are currently recommending the use of a solution of 20 to 25 per cent mannitol (Osmitrol or Mannitol) given intravenously at a dose of 1–2 gm/kg body weight. In appropriate clinical use, mannitol is nontoxic to the kidneys; in fact, it can be given to patients with nephritis.[32, 34, 36, 37] It causes little or no secondary rise of CSF pressure, or "rebound" effect, such as that characteristically seen with urea or dextrose solutions.[86, 90, 100]

In addition to its use for reducing CNS fluid and volume, mannitol has been used effectively in oliguria from renal shut-down in shock and postoperative procedures. The principal mechanism of mannitol diuresis in these patients is acute expansion of blood volume, with a subsequent increase in glomerular filtration rate.

In our hands, mannitol has been both safe and effective and is nearly always combined with dexamethasone. It is felt that mannitol will provide immediate improvement in CNS edema, while steroids will provide a response of longer duration. Hypertonic solutions should not be given in cases of intracranial hemorrhage, which can be determined by visual examination of CSF or by cranial bur holes. Shrinking the brain would promote greater accumulation of hemorrhage in such cases.[37] However, mannitol has been used in cases of hematomyelia (less danger of aggravating hemorrhage), in decompressive spinal surgery where marked damage to the cord was observed, and in craniotomies. General severe dehydration should be avoided or uremia will result.[37] Since severe distension of the bladder results from the diuresis, recumbent cases will require frequent catheterizations or an indwelling catheter. Replacement of body fluids should be initiated as promptly as deemed advisable.[27]

SURGICAL THERAPY

INDICATIONS FOR SURGERY

Cranial

The emergency surgery that is most valuable in determining the existence of *extracerebral hemorrhage* is the placement of bur holes. This procedure is safer and more diagnostic in the dog at the present time than such special diagnostic procedures as the cerebral angiogram. This procedure is the only one that will distinguish extracerebral hemorrhage from acute cerebral edema and brain swelling. Since the treatment for edema and swelling is contraindicated for space-occupying hemorrhages, bur placement becomes an absolute necessity in some instances.[32, 63, 64]

The placement of bur holes and possible craniotomy should be considered if the patient shows deterioration of vital signs (e.g., decreasing pulse rate, increasing blood pressure, ataxic respiration), decreasing level of consciousness, progressive hemiparesis, and unilateral pupillary dilation (or progression from unilateral to bilateral dilation). If surgery is performed during progressive loss of consciousness and

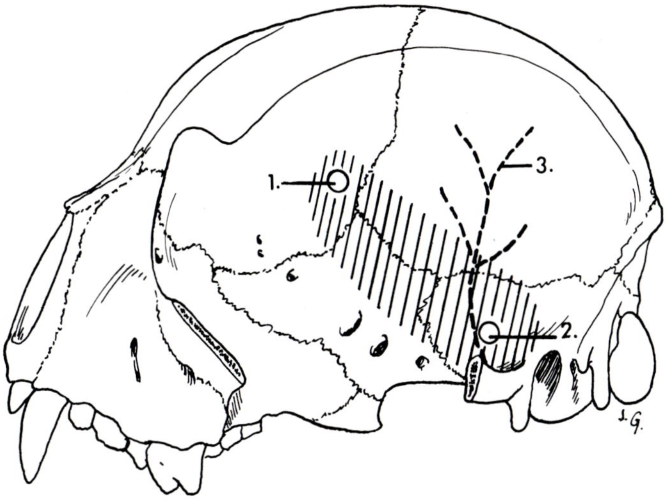

FIGURE 12-9 Bur holes (1 and 2) in the lower portion of the cranial vault and near the origin of the middle meningeal artery (3) will help determine the presence of probable extracerebral hemorrhage (hatched area). The middle meningeal artery is frequently lacerated in trauma to the head.

pupillary changes, the dog will have a much better chance of recovery than if surgery is performed when the vital signs are impaired. Prompt craniotomy will be the most effective[37, 40, 47, 48, 91, 93] (Figs. 12–9 and 12–10). Unilateral tentorial herniation and progressive brain swelling must be treated early and vigorously. Animals that have progressed to late midbrain signs (decerebrate rigidity) almost never recover[61] (Tables 12–4 and 12–5).

Craniotomy performed 24 to 48 hours after the accident would be acceptable when the aforementioned signs have *not* intervened in cases of various types of depressed skull fractures not causing rapidly progressive hemorrhage and of persistent CSF leaks (e.g., nose, ear, subcutaneous).[64]

Severe *cerebral edema* refractory to medical management may at least partially be relieved by bilateral subtentorial decompression, as discussed in Chapter 20.[32, 63, 64]

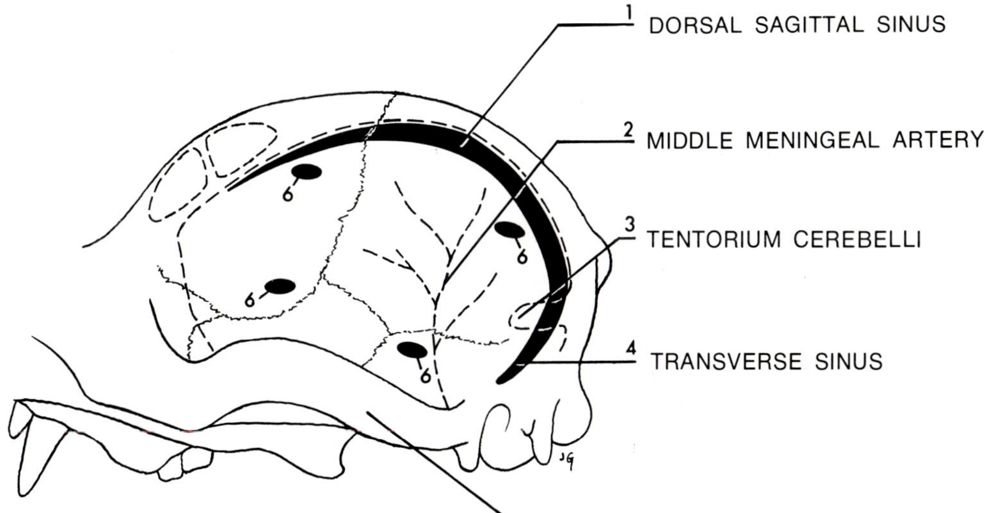

FIGURE 12-10 These bur holes are properly positioned in order to employ bone flaps to facilitate the relief of intracranial hemorrhage, or for decompression of generalized cerebral edema. In generalized cerebral edema, a bilateral bone flap should be made.

TABLE 12–4 UNILATERAL TENTORIAL HERNIATION*

Level	Consciousness	Pupils	Eye Movements	Motor	Autonomic
III N.	Normal to stupor	Ipsilateral dilatation	Normal to slight lateral strabismus	Normal to hemiparesis	Normal
Early midbrain	Stupor	Ipsilateral to bilateral dilatation	Ipsilateral ventrolateral strabismus	Hemiparesis ipsi or contralateral	Normal
Late midbrain to pons	Coma	Dilated, bilateral, to fixed midposition	Ventrolateral strabismus to fixed mid position	Decerebrate rigidity	Hyperventilation
Pons,	Same as Central Syndrome				
medulla	Same as Central Syndrome				

*From Oliver, J. E., Jr.: Neurologic emergencies in small animals. Vet. Clin. N. Amer. *2*(2):341, 1972.

Spinal Surgery

At the present time, the experimental and clinical forms of medical therapy for acute CNS injury discussed previously in this chapter are generally not employed with surgery in cases of spinal trauma. This differs from acute brain injury in that surgery is not mandatory nearly so often. The very confined spinal canal area occupied by the spinal cord in the dog probably makes compressive lesions much more damaging to normal neurological function. The major procedures considered in spinal cord injures are (1) decompression and (2) immobilization of the vertebrae. The decision for decompression is based on clinical signs, whereas the decision for immobilization may be based on clinical and radiographic signs and on abnormalities seen during surgery.

Acute compression of the spinal cord is a surgical emergency. An animal with complete paralysis must have decompressive surgery and vigorous medical treatment within minutes or hours in order to pre-

TABLE 12–5 CENTRAL SYNDROME*

Level	Consciousness	Pupils	Eye Movements	Motor	Autonomic
Early diencephalic	Apathy	Small but reactive	Normal	Hemiparesis	Normal to irregular respiration
Late diencephalic	Stupor	Same	Same	Hemiparesis to tetraparesis	Cheyne-Stokes
Midbrain	Coma	Dilated bilaterally	Poor oculocephalic response	Decerebrate rigidity	Hyperventilation
Pons	Coma	Midposition unresponsive	Oculocephalic response absent	Flaccid paralysis	Rapid, shallow respiration
Medulla	Coma	Midposition, dilated terminally	Absent	Flaccid paralysis	Irregular to apnea;, pulse slowing

*From Oliver, J. E., Jr.: Neurologic emergencies in small animals. Vet. Clin. N. Amer. *2*(2):341, 1972.

vent permanent cord damage. Assuming that immobilization is possible, the prognosis based on clinical signs can be summarized as follows:[61]

Paralysis with	Prognosis
1. Good conscious pain response, less than 24 hours duration	fair to good
2. No conscious pain response, less than 6 hours duration	poor to guarded
3. No conscious pain response, greater than 6 hours duration	unfavorable

The author feels strongly that in patients with acute spinal fractures or severe cord compression, medical and surgical therapy must proceed immediately. Frequently, immediate surgery with possible concomitant systemic shock can result in loss of the patient. The owner must know the possible results of such surgery and agree to the surgeon's recommendations. There will be little or no time for "thinking it over." If the owner wants a chance for normal recovery, decompressive surgery should be performed as soon as possible in spite of possible loss of the patient from shock.

Mendenhall *et al.*[56] have reported recently on aggressive pharmacological therapy (based on experimental work as previously discussed) combined with extensive decompressive surgery as employed on injured spinal cords in 22 dogs and three cats. The vertebral lesions varied from simple subluxations to comminuted fractures and were located in spinal segments C3 to L7. All animals were treated by the following procedures: administration of intravenous Ringer's solution containing sodium bicarbonate, epsilon-aminocaproic acid (EACA), dexamethasone, and chloramphenicol; reserpine (0.33 mg/kg) administered intracisternally; a three-segment, deep dorsal laminectomy (two vertebrae rostral and one caudal to the injured site); durotomy and catheterization of the subarachnoid space for perfusion with hypertonic solution (25 per cent dextrose or 15 per cent mannitol) containing 2 per cent lidocaine (200 ml/L) for 3 hours; vertebral stabilization effected by use of spinal and/or vertebral body plates; and a two-segment dorsal myelotomy immediately rostral to the lesion, extended to the level of the central canal. The recovery rate was 44 per cent for all 25 animals; however, not counting five animals that were destroyed at the time of surgery and five that died during surgery due to secondary lesions, the recovery rate was 73 per cent. This group was compared to a similar group of cases treated by more conservative methods at the same institution during an earlier period which had a recovery rate of only 39 per cent. Seven of the radically treated animals who did not have spinal cord transection and were treated within 4 hours of injury recovered. This points to the merits of early surgical intervention.[56]

Since so many different agents were used in combination with surgery in these cases, one cannot judge the merit of individual drugs or procedures. It is impressive, however, that aggressive and prompt surgical treatment (within 4 hours after injury) can be effective. There is a good possibility that the experimental drugs used—EACA and reserpine in addition to clinically accepted drugs, steroids, hypertonic fluids, and other drugs—increased the effectiveness of surgery.[56]

CARE OF URINARY TRACT IN ACUTE CNS INJURY[32]

The common urinary disorder associated with acute CNS trauma and general body trauma and shock is renal shutdown. Even if renal shutdown is not present, urinary retention or incontinence may occur. When the treatment involves methods designed to reduce CNS edema and swelling, it is important to monitor the urinary system for the presence of renal function and the removal of large quantities of urine promoted by diuretic therapy. Catheterization is useful for both monitoring kidney function and inhibition of bladder distention and atrophy. Monitoring the kidneys by measuring urinary output through catheterization is very important in the patient with an acute injury and can be simply accomplished in the recumbent or tranquil animal. Furthermore, a distended bladder causes discomfort and restlessness which can be hazardous in the patient with an acute CNS disorder.

Retention catheters are difficult to apply in the dog. Catheters equipped with inflatable balloons often are not available for small male dogs, although the inflatable catheter used in the female infant can sometimes be used in the bitch. The constant dribbling of urine from a retention catheter can make skin cleanliness difficult to maintain, and urine-soaked skin and bedding promotes the formation of decubital sores on the animal.

In our clinic, the problem of urine retention in paraplegic dogs is routinely handled as follows:

1. Manual expression of urine is employed in the bitch to empty the bladder completely. If complete elimination is in doubt, one should catheterize and flush the bladder at least once daily.

2. Usually, manual expression of urine in the male is not possible, but if it is, the prognosis is unfavorable. Frequently, however, a male will urinate spontaneously when gentle pressure is applied to the bladder area. If urination is incomplete, one should catheterize and flush the bladder once daily; if the dog cannot urinate at all, catheterization should be performed at least twice daily.

3. All catheters and specula should be sterile. The prepuce and vulva must be cleansed thoroughly before introduction of any instrument. All equipment must be well-lubricated with a sterile lubricant. Nupercaine ointment serves as a good lubricant, and its anesthetic qualities are of value in controlling urethral irritations.

4. A warm sterile saline solution can be used to flush the bladder until the return flow of fluid is clear. If blood is encountered, hemostatic agents such as Thrombin are instilled in the bladder. Frquently, broad spectrum antibiotics, such as penicillin and streptomycin, or chemotherapeutic agents, such as furacin solutions, are also instilled into the bladder after flushing.

5. Oral administration of urinary antiseptic preparations, sulfisoxazole, or nitrofurazone should be used routinely in all cases of incomplete urination or urinary retention.

It is emphasized that all instruments and equipment must be sterile, and must be inserted as atraumatically as possible. More details on the basic disorders of micturition are found in Chapter 13, Section 2.

CARE OF THE SKIN IN ACUTE CNS TRAUMA

The care of the integument in an acute neurological patient does not directly affect the outcome of the CNS disorder. However, acute neurological disease, whether primarily of the brain or cord, necessitates a recumbent position. If pressure spots are not anticipated or observed promptly, severe decubital lesions will occur. Although these lesions are rarely critical for the patient's recovery, they are painful and difficult to treat. Such lesions are a reflection of the general competence of nursing care.

In veterinary clinics, the recumbent animal must be kept clean and free of excretions, placed on foam rubber beds or even water mattresses, and frequently changed in position. Pressure spots should be protected by "donut"-shaped pads. When medically possible, animals should be placed in a frame or cart periodically to simulate a standing position. Whirlpool baths will stimulate circulation and help prevent decubital lesions.[90]

CONCLUSION

This section has emphasized the urgency and proper team management of the patient with an acute CNS injury from the immediate handling and transport of the patient through emergency and first aid care, diagnostic procedures, and medical and surgical care. Much of the management of acute CNS injury is the sole responsibility of the first veterinarian to see the patient. Frequently it is entirely inappropriate to send the patient elsewhere since the time and the additional hazards of transport endanger the patient's welfare. Recent methods of therapy such as oxygen, steroids, hypertonic solutions, hypothermia, anticatecholamine drugs and DMSO can greatly improve clinical management. Careful and persistent monitoring of vital and neurological signs is necessary. Occasional brain surgery is necessary in cranial trauma, whereas spinal cord decompression and immobilization surgery is frequently needed in the spinal injury. Proper management of a patient with an acute CNS injury will frequently be time-consuming and therefore expensive for the client;

however, when care is feasible it will be rewarding to patient, client, and clinician.

REFERENCES

1. Albin, M. S., White, R. J., Yashon, D., and Harris, L. S.: Effects of localized cooling on spinal cord trauma. J. Trauma *9,* 1000, 1969.
2. Allen, A. R.: Remarks in histopathological changes in spinal cord due to impact: An experimental study. J. Nerv. Ment. Dis. *41,* 141, 1914.
3. Allen, A. R.: Surgery of experimental lesion of spinal cord equivalent to crush injury of fracture dislocation of spinal column. Preliminary report. J.A.M.A. *57,* 878, 1911.
4. Allen, A. R.: Injuries of the spinal cord, with the study of nine cases with necropsy. J.A.M.A. *50,* 941, 1908.
5. Allen, G. S., Henderson, L. M., Chou, S. N., and French, L. A.: Cerebral arterial spasm. Part 1. In vitro contractile activity of vasoactive agents on canine basilar and middle cerebral arteries. J. Neurosurg. *40,* 433, 1974.
6. Allen, G. S., Henderson, L. M., Chou, S. N., and French, L. A.: Cerebral arterial spasm. Part 2. In vitro contractile activity of serotonin in human serum and CSF on the canine basilar artery, and its blockage by methylsergide and phenoxybenzamine. J. Neurosurg. *40,* 443, 1974.
7. Allen, G. S., Gold, L. H. A., Chou, S. N., and French, L. A.: Cerebral arterial spasm. Part 3. In vivo intracisternal production of spasm by serotonin and blood and its reversal by phenoxybenzamine. J. Neurosurg. *40,* 451, 1974.
8. Balentine, J. D.: Central necrosis of the spinal cord induced by hyperbaric oxygen exposure. J. Neurosurg. *43,* 150, 1975.
9. Belcher, W. R.: Evaluation of the lumbar myelotomy and durotomy in the dog. Senior Seminar Report, School of Veterinary Medicine, Auburn University *1,* 217, 1974.
10. Bingham, W. G., Ruffola, R., and Friedman, S. J.: Catecholamine levels in the injured spinal cord of monkeys. J. Neurosurg. *42,* 174, 1975.
11. Black, P., and Markowitz, R. S.: Experimental spinal cord injury in monkeys: comparison of steroids and hypothermia. Surg. Forum *22,* 409, 1971.
12. Brasmer, T. H., and Lumb, W. V.: Lumbar vertebral prosthesis in the dog. Am. J. Vet. Res. *33,* 493, 1972.
13. Brugghen, A. ver: *Neurosurgery in General Practice.* Charles C Thomas, Publishers, Springfield, Ill., 1962.
14. Campbell, J. B., De Cressito, V., Tomasula, J. J., Demopoulas, H. B., Flamm, E. S., and Ortego, B. D.: Effects of antifibrinolytic and steroid therapy on the contused spinal cord of cats. J. Neurosurg. *40,* 726, 1974.
15. Campbell, J. B., De Cressito, V., and Tomasula, J.: Experimental treatment of acute spinal cord contusion. Presented to the 40th Annual Meeting of the American Association of Neurological Surgeons, Boston. April, 1972.
16. Clasen, R. A., Cooke, P. M., Pandolfi, S., Boyd, D., and Raimondi, A. J.: Experimental cerebral edema produced by focal freezing. 1. An anatomical study utilizing vital dye technique. J. Neuropathol. Exp. Neurol. *21,* 579, 1962.
17. Clasen, R. A., Cooke, P. M., Pandolfi, S., Cornecki, G., and Bryar, G.: Hypertonic urea in experimental cerebral edema. Arch. Neurol. *12,* 424, 1965.
18. Clasen, R. A., Cooke, P. M., Pandolfi, S., Cornecki, G., and Hass, G. M.: Steroid–antihistamine therapy in experimental cerebral edema. Arch. Neurol. *13,* 584, 1965.
19. De la Torre, J. C., Johnson, C. M., Goode, D., and Mullan, S.: Chemotherapeutic reversal of experimental paraplegia. Neurology *24,* 387, 1974.
20. De la Torre, J. C., Kajihara, K., and Rowed, D. W.: Modification of experimental head and spinal cord injuries using dimethyl sulfoxide. Trans. Am. Neurol. Assoc. *97,* 230, 1972.
21. De la Torre, J. C., Rowed, D. W., Kawanago, H. M., and Mullan, S.: Dimethyl sulfoxide in the treatment of experimental brain concussion. J. Neurosurg. *38,* 345, 1973.
22. Denny-Brown, D., and Russell, W. R.: Experimental cerebral concussion. Brain *64,* 93, 1941.
23. Ducker, T. B., and Hamit, H. F.: Experimental treatment of acute spinal cord injury. J. Neurosurg. *30,* 693, 1969.
24. Eidelberg, E., Sullivan, J., and Brigham, A.: Immediate consequences of spinal cord injury, possible role of potassium in axonal conduction block. Surg. Neurol. *3,* 317, 1975.
25. Fox, M. W.: Gross structure and development of the canine brain. Am. J. Vet. Res. *24,* 1240, 1963.
26. Freeman, L. W., and Wright, T. W.: Experimental observations of concussion and contusion of spinal cord. Ann. Surg. *137,* 433, 1953.
27. Goldstein, S. L., Himwich, W. A., Knapp, F. M., and Rovine, B. W.: Effects of urea and other dehydrating agents upon dog brain. J. Neurosurg. *21,* 672, 1964.
28. Greene, C. E.: An experimental model for spinal cord compression simulating intervertebral disc disease in the dog. Thesis (M.S.), Auburn University, Auburn, Ala., 1976.
29. Griffiths, I. R., Rowan, J. O., and Crawford, R. A.: Spinal cord blood flow measured by a hydrogen clearance technique. J. Neurol. Sci. *26,* 529, 1975.
30. Guyton, A. C.: *Textbook of Medical Physiology,* 4th ed. W. B. Saunders Co., Philadelphia, 1971.
31. Hartzog, T. T., Fisher, R., and Snow, C.: Spinal cord trauma: Effect of hyperbaric oxygen therapy. Proc. 17th Veterans Administration Spinal Cord Injury Conference, Sept. 29–Oct. 1, 1969, p. 70.
32. Hoerlein, B. F.: *Canine Neurology,* 2nd ed. W. B. Saunders Co., Philadelphia, 1971.
33. Hoerlein, B. F., and Spano, J. S.: Nonneurological complications following decompressive spinal cord surgery. Arch. Am. Coll. Vet. Surg. *4,* 11, 1975.
34. Hoerlein, B. F., and Few, A. B.: Brain surgery in the dog—preliminary studies. J.A.V.M.A. *143,* 21, 1963.

35. Homburger, E., Himwich, W. A., Etstein, B., York, G., Maresca, R., and Himwich, H. E.: Effect of pentothal anesthesia on canine cerebral cortex. Am. J. Phys. *147,* 343, 1946.
36. Jackson, F. E.: The pathophysiology of head injuries. Clin. Symp. *18,* 67, 1966.
37. Jackson, F. E.: The treatment of head injuries. Clin. Symp. *19,* 4, March 1967.
38. Jamieson, K. G., and Yelland, J. D. N.: Extradural hematoma, report of 167 cases. J. Neurosurg. *29,* 13, 1968.
39. Javid, M., Gilboe, D., and Cesario, T.: The rebound phenomenon and hypertonic solutions. J. Neurosurg. *21,* 1059, 1964.
40. Jennett, W. B., and Stern, W. E.: Tentorial herniation, the midbrain and the pupil. J. Neurosurg. *17,* 598, 1960.
41. Johnston, I. H., Paterson, A., and Harper, A. M.: The effect of mannitol on intracranial pressure and cerebral blood flow. *In* Brock, M., and Dietz, H. (eds.): *Intracranial Pressure: Experimental and Clinical Aspects.* Springer Verlag, New York, 1972, p. 176.
42. Kajihara, K., Kawanaga, H., de la Torre, J. C., and Mullan, S.: Dimethyl sulfoxide in the treatment of experimental acute spinal cord injury. Surg. Neurol. *1,* 16, 1973.
43. Kelly, D. L., Lassiter, K. R. L., Vongsvivut, A., and Smith, J. M.: Effects of hyperbaric oxygenation and tissue oxygen studies in experimental paraplegia. J. Neurosurg. *36,* 425, 1972.
44. King, L. R., McLaurin, R. L., and Knowles, H. C.: Acid-base balance and arterial and CSF lactate levels following human head injury. J. Neurosurg. *40,* 617, 1974.
45. Kirk, R. W., and Bistner, S. I.: *Handbook of Veterinary Procedures and Emergency Treatment,* 2d ed. W. B. Saunders Co., Philadelphia, 1975, p. 96.
46. Kobrine, A. I., Doyle, T. F., and Martins, A. N.: Local spinal cord blood flow in experimental traumatic meylopathy. J. Neurosurg. *42,* 144, 1975.
47. Langfitt, T. W., Tannanbaum, H. M., and Kassell, N. F.: The etiology of acute brain swelling following experimental head injury. J. Neurosurg. *24,* 47, 1966.
48. Langfitt, T. W., Tannanbaum, H. M., Kassell, N. F., and Zaren, H.: Acute hypertension, cerebral blood flow, and the EEG. Electroencephalogr. Clin. Neurophysiol. *20,* 139, 1966.
49. Leonard, J. L., and Redding, R. W.: Effects of hypertonic solutions on cerebrospinal fluid pressure in the lateral ventricle of the dog. Am. J. Vet. Res. *34,* 213, 1973.
50. Lewin, M. G., Gausebaut, R. R., and Pappius, H. M.: Chemical characteristics of traumatic spinal cord edema in cats. Effect of steroids on potassium depletion. J. Neurosurg. *40,* 65, 1974.
51. Locke, G. E., Yasbon, D., Feldman, R. A., and Hunt, W. E.: Ischemia in primate spinal cord injury. J. Neurosurg. *34,* 614, 1971.
52. Luhan, J. A.: *Neurology, a Concise Clinical Textbook.* The Williams and Wilkins Co., Baltimore, 1968.
53. Lumb, W. V., and Brasmer, T. H.: Improved spinal plates and hypothermia as adjuncts to spinal surgery. J.AV.M.A. *157,* 338, 1970.
54. Matson, D. D.: Treatment of cerebral swelling. N. Engl. J. Med. *272,* 626, 1965.
55. McVeigh, J. F.: Experimental cord crushes with especial reference to the mechanical factors involved and subsequent changes in the areas of the cord affected. Arch. Surg. *7,* 573, 1923.
56. Mendenhall, H. V., Litwak, P., Yturraspe, D. J., Ingram, J. T., and Lumb, W. V.: Aggressive pharmacologic and surgical treatment of spinal cord injuries in dogs and cats. J.A.V.M.A. *168,* 1026, 1976.
57. Miller, J. D., and Leeck, P.: Effects of mannitol and steroid therapy on intracranial volume-pressure relationships in patients. J. Neurosurg. *42,* 274, 1975.
58. Naftchi, N. E., Demeny, M., De Crescito, V., Tomasula, J. J., Flamm, E. S., and Campbell, J. B.: Biogenic amine concentrations in traumatized spinal cords of cats; effect of drug therapy. J. Neurosurg. *40,* 52, 1974.
59. Nagai, H., Noda, S., and Mabe, H.: Experimental cerebral vasospasm. Part 2: Effects of vasoactive drugs and sympathectomy on early and late spasm. J. Neurosurg. *42,* 420, 1975.
60. Newkirk, T. A., Tourtellotte, W. W., and Reinglass, J. L.: Prolonged control of increased intracranial pressure with glycerin. Arch. Neurol. *27,* 95, 1972.
61. Oliver, J. E., Jr.: Neurologic emergencies in small animals. Vet. Clin. N. Am., *2*(2), 341, 1972.
62. Oliver, J. E., Jr.: Management of the patient with acute head injury. The newer knowledge about dogs. Gaines Dog Research Center, Ocotber 1969.
63. Oliver, J. E., Jr.: Surgical approaches to the canine brain. Am. J. Vet. Res. *29,* 353, 1968.
64. Oliver, J. E., Jr.: Canine brain surgery. Vet. Scope *13,* 13, 1968.
65. Osterholm, J. L.: The pathophysiological response to spinal cord injury: the current status of related research. J. Neurosurg. *40,* 5, 1974.
66. Osterholm, J. L., and Mathews, G. J.: Altered norepinephrine metabolism following experimental spinal cord injury. Part 1. Relationship to hemorrhagic necrosis and post-wounding neurological deficits. J. Neurosurg. *36,* 386, 1972.
67. Osterholm, J. L., and Mathews, G. J.: Altered norepinephrine metabolism following experimental spinal cord injury. Part 2. Protection against traumatic spinal cord hemorrhagic necrosis by norepinephrine synthesis blocked with alpha methyl tyrosine. J. Neurosurg. *36,* 395, 1972.
68. Osterholm, J. L., and Mathews, G. J.: Spinal pathways mediating traumatic hemorrhagic necrosis. Trans. Am. Neurol. Assoc. *97,* 187, 1972.
69. Pappius, H. M., and Gulati, D. R.: Water and electrolyte content of cerebral tissues in experimentally induced cerebral edema. Acta. Neuropathol. *2,* 451, 1963.
70. Palmer, A. G., and Walker, R. G.: Neuropathological effects of cardiac arrest in animals, a

study of five cases. J. Small Anim. Pract. *11,* 779, 1970.
71. Parker, A. J.: Blood pressure changes and lethality of mannitol infusions in dogs. Am. J. Vet. Res. *34,* 1523, 1973.
72. Parker, A. J.: Clinical significance of traumatic occlusion of segmental spinal arteries. J.A.V.M.A. *162,* 1041, 1973.
73. Parker, A. J.: Distribution of spinal branches of the thoracolumbar segmental arteries in dogs. Am. J. Vet. Res. *34,* 1351, 1973.
74. Parker, A. J.: Durotomy and saline perfusion in spinal cord trauma. J. Am. Anim. Hosp. Assoc. *4,* 412, 1975.
75. Parker, A. J., Park, R. D., and Stowater, J. L.: Reduction of trauma-induced edema of spinal cord in dogs given mannitol. Am. J. Vet. Res. *34,* 1355, 1973.
76. Parker, A. J., Park, R. D., and Stowater, J. L.: Traumatic occlusion of segmental spinal veins. Am. J. Vet. Res. *35,* 857, 1974.
77. Parker, A. J., and Smith, C. W.: Functional recovery from spinal cord trauma following delayed incision of spinal meninges in dogs. Res. Vet. Sci. *18,* 110, 1975.
78. Parker, A. J., and Smith, C. W.: Functional recovery from spinal cord trauma following incision of spinal meninges in dogs. Res. Vet. Sci. *16,* 276, 1974.
79. Parker, A. J., and Smith C. W.: Functional recovery following incision of spinal meninges in dogs. Res. Vet. Sci. *13,* 418, 1972.
80. Pizzi, F. J., James, H., Bruce, D., and Langfitt, T. W.: A protocol for the management of head trauma. Am. Family Pract. *10,* 163, 1974.
81. Preston, F. W., and Beal, J. M.: *Basic Surgical Physiology.* Year Book Medical Publishers, Inc., Chicago, 1969.
82. Rasmussen, T., and Gulati, D. R.: Cortisone in the treatment of postoperative cerebral edema. J. Neurosurg. *19,* 535, 1962.
83. Rosonoff, H. L.: Distribution of intracranial contents after hypertonic urea. J. Neurosurg. *19,* 859, 1962.
84. Sato, O., Hara, M., Asai, T., Tsugane, R., and Kageyama, N.: The effect of dexamethasone phosphate on the production rate of cerebrospinal fluid in the spinal subarachnoid space of dogs. J. Neurosurg. *39,* 480, 1973.
85. Shenkin, H. A., and Bouzarth, W. F.: Clinical methods of reducing intracranial pressure. N. Engl. J. Med. *282,* 1465, 1970.
86. Shenkin, H. A., Goluboff, B., and Hoft, H.: The use of mannitol for the reduction of intracranial pressure in intracranial surgery. J. Neurosurg. *19,* 897, 1962.
87. Sims, M. H., and Redding, R. W.: The use of dexamethasone in the prevention of cerebral edema in dogs. J. Am. Anim. Hosp. Assoc. *11,* 439, 1975.
88. Smith, C. W., and Parker, A. J.: Functional recovery from spinal cord trauma following normothermic irrigation in dogs. Res. Vet. Sci. *19,* 224, 1975.
89. Smith, R. R., and Upchurch, J. J.: Monitoring antifibrinolytic therapy in subarachnoid hemorrhage. J. Neurosurg. *38,* 339, 1973.
90. Swaim, S. F.: Unpublished data.
91. Tarlov, I. M., Grancotti, A., and Rapisarda, A.: Acute intracranial hypertension. Arch. Neurol. *1,* 3, 1959.
92. Tator, C. H., and Deeke, L.: Value of normothermic perfusion, hypothermic perfusion, and durotomy in the treatment of experimental acute spinal trauma. J. Neurosurg. *39,* 52, 1973.
93. Thompson, R. K., and Malina, S.: Dynamic axial brain-stem distortion as a mechanism explaining the cardio-respiratory changes in increased intracranial pressure. J. Neurosurg. *16,* 664, 1959.
94. Trotter, E. J.: Modified dorsal laminectomy and selective regional spinal cord hypothermia in the treatment of thoracolumbar disk disease. *In* Bojrab, M. J. (ed.): *Current Techniques in Small Animal Surgery* I. Lea & Febiger, Philadelphia, 1975, p. 406.
95. Trotter, E. J., Brasmer, T. H., and deLahunta, A.: Modified deep dorsal laminectomy in the dog. Cornell Vet *65,* 402, 1975.
96. Valls, M. B.: Effects of the administration of urea in neurosurgery. Rev. Esp. Otoneurol. *20,* 1, 1961. (Abstr. J.A.M.A. *176,* 179, 1961.)
97. Vise, W. M., Yashon, D., and Hunt, W. E.: Mechanisms of norepinephrine accumulation within sites of spinal cord injury. J. Neurosurg. *40,* 76, 1974.
98. White, R. J., Yashon, D., and Albin, M. S.: The acute management of cervical cord trauma with quadriplegia. Presented to the 40th Annual Meeting of the American Association of Neurological Surgeons. Boston, April 1972.
99. Wise, B. L., and Chater, N.: Use of hypertonic mannitol solutions to lower cerebrospinal fluid pressure and decrease brain bulk in man. Surg. Forum *12,* 398, 1961.
100. Wise, B. L., and Chater, N.: The value of hypertonic mannitol solution in decreasing brain mass and lowering cerebrospinal fluid pressure. J. Neurosurg. *19,* 1038, 1962.
101. Wurtman, R. J., and Moskowitz, M. A.: Brain catecholamines and neurological diseases. Trans. Am. Neurol. Assoc. *99,* 148, 1974.
102. Yashon, D., Bingham, W. G., Friedman, S. J., and Faddoul, E. M.: Intracellular enzyme liberation in private spinal cord injury. Surg. Neurol. *4,* 43, 1975.
103. Yturraspe, D. J., Lumb, W. V., Young, S., and Gorman, H. A.: Neurological and pathological effects of second lumbar spondylectomy and spinal column shortening in the dog. J. Neurosurg. *42,* 47, 1975.
104. Yturraspe, D. J., and Lumb, W. V.: Second lumbar spondylectomy and shortening of the spinal column of the dog. Am. J. Vet. Res. *34,* 521, 1973.

PART FIVE

THE SPINE

CHAPTER 13

GENERAL SPINAL DISORDERS

SECTION 1
CLINICAL SPINAL DISORDERS

To avoid repetition and present a more logical discussion of the etiology of spinal disorders, much of the material contained in this chapter in the last edition has been included in other chapters. Disorders affecting primarily the spinal cord are discussed in Chapter 11, and the muscle disorders are included in Chapter 9. This chapter has been divided into two sections: Section 1 describes the basic anatomy and physiology of the spine and cord and the clinical disorders attributed to poor nutrition, spinal malformations, and compressions, and Section 2 discusses the disorders of micturition. A better understanding of the problems of urination associated with spinal disorders may make possible a more intelligent prognosis and therapeutic regimen.

ANATOMY

The development of the spine can be classified into three stages: (1) mesenchymatous stage; (2) stage of chondrification; and (3) stage of ossification. The mesenchymatous stage begins with the early fetal differentiation of vertebral structures and continues to the stage of cartilage formation. The entodermal structure, the notochord, is surrounded by mesenchyma to form a cord between the brain and the tail. Segmentation of the mesenchymal sheath occurs, forming the sclerotomes that eventually make the vertebral body.

Chondrification of the mesenchymal sheath that surrounds the notochord proceeds rapidly. The cells of the notochord are forced into the portion of the dense area of the sclerotome, which forms the nucleus pulposus of the intervertebral disk.

The third stage of development is the ossification of the cartilaginous structure formed by the mesenchymal sheath. Centers of ossification appear in the dorsal and ventral portions of each half of the vertebral body. These centers soon fuse to form one center for each half of the vertebral body, then proceed to form a single center. Ossification centers later appear in the neural arches and include the spinous and transverse processes. The process of bone formation continues until maturity, when fusion of the different centers is complete. Abnormalities develop if the normal pattern of development becomes disturbed.[2]

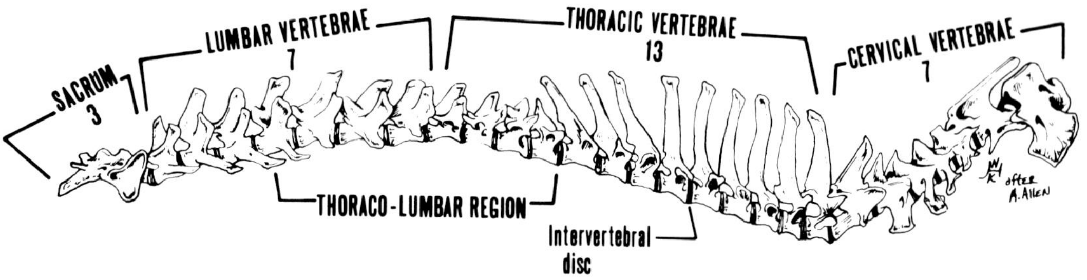

FIGURE 13–1 A schematic representation of the spinal column.

In the dog, the spinal formula is C7T13-L7S3Cy20, or approximately 50 irregular bones.[71] The spinal column from the cervical through the sacral vertebrae is most important neurologically. It consists of 30 vertebrae. According to Miller, the typical vertebra consists of a body, a vertebral arch with right and left pedicles and lamina, and processes for muscle or articular connections—the transverse, spinous, and articular processes. Together with the body, the arch forms a short tube called the vertebral foramen, which in combination with other vertebrae forms the vertebral (or spinal) canal. Caudal and cranial notches occur at the root of the vertebra. When the vertebral column is articulated in the natural state, the notches on each side of adjacent vertebrae, with the intervening fibrocartilage, form the right and left intervertebral foramina. Through these pass the spinal nerves, arteries, and veins[71] (Fig. 13–1).

The dorsal part of the vertebral arch is composed of right and left laminae, which unite at the midline to form the spine or spinous process. Each typical vertebra has irregularly shaped projections, extending laterally from the region where the pedicle joins the vertebral body, called transverse processes. Paired articular processes are present at both the cranial and the caudal surfaces of a vertebra, at the junction of the root and lamina (Fig. 13–2).[71]

The synovial joints of the vertebral column caudal to the axis appear in pairs between the articular processes of contiguous vertebrae and the joints between the ribs and the vertebrae. In the lumbar region, the articular surfaces are in a sagittal plane, whereas those cranial to the tenth thoracic

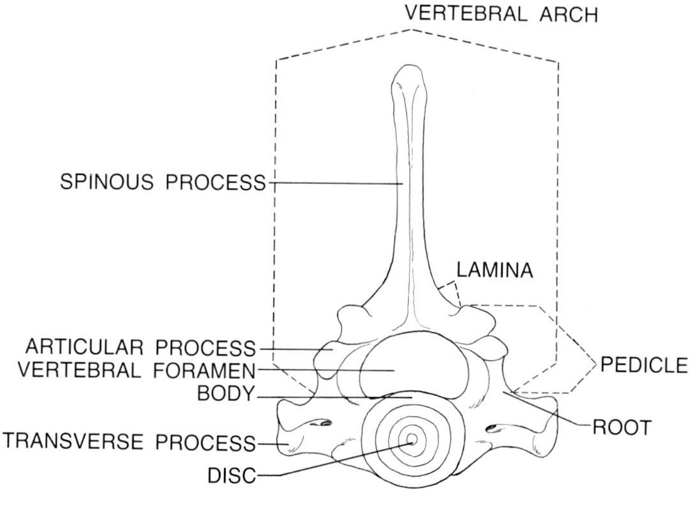

FIGURE 13–2 The anatomical features of a vertebra. (Adapted from Miller, M. E., Christensen, G. C., and Evans, H. E.: *Anatomy of the Dog.* W. B. Saunders Co., Philadelphia, 1964.)

vertebrae are in a frontal plane. In the latter case, the cranial articular processes face dorsally and the caudal articular processes face ventrally. Because of movement afforded by the intervertebral disks, one might consider these as fibrocartilaginous or secondary joints.[71]

The vertebral column is supported by various ligaments.

The supraspinous ligament unites the crests of vertebral spines. The interspinous ligaments attach the spines to each other. The yellow ligament attaches the adjacent vertebral arches. The dorsal longitudinal ligament attaches the vertebral bodies together on the floor of the spinal canal. The ventral longitudinal ligament attaches the vertebral bodies together at the ventral surfaces of the vertebrae. The ligament intercapitalis lies between the sternal pairs of ribs and forms the dorsal part of the intervertebral disk. The disks hold each pair of vertebrae together.[69] These structures are discussed in detail in Chapter 14 (Fig. 13–3).

The spinal cord lies in the spinal canal and is covered by three membranes called meninges. The pia mater lies adjacent to the cord, the arachnoidea next, and the dura mater lies outermost. The pia and arachnoidea are called leptomeninges, and the dura is termed a pachymeninge. The spinal fluid is contained between the pia and arachnoid membranes in what is termed the subarachnoid space. The spinal cord extends from the foramen magnum to the sixth lumbar vertebra, where it divides into terminal branches. It has two enlargements. One goes from sixth cervical to the second thoracic segment, which is the origin of the brachial plexus; the other enlargement occurs from the fourth lumbar to the second sacral segment, which constitutes the origin of the lumbosacral plexus.

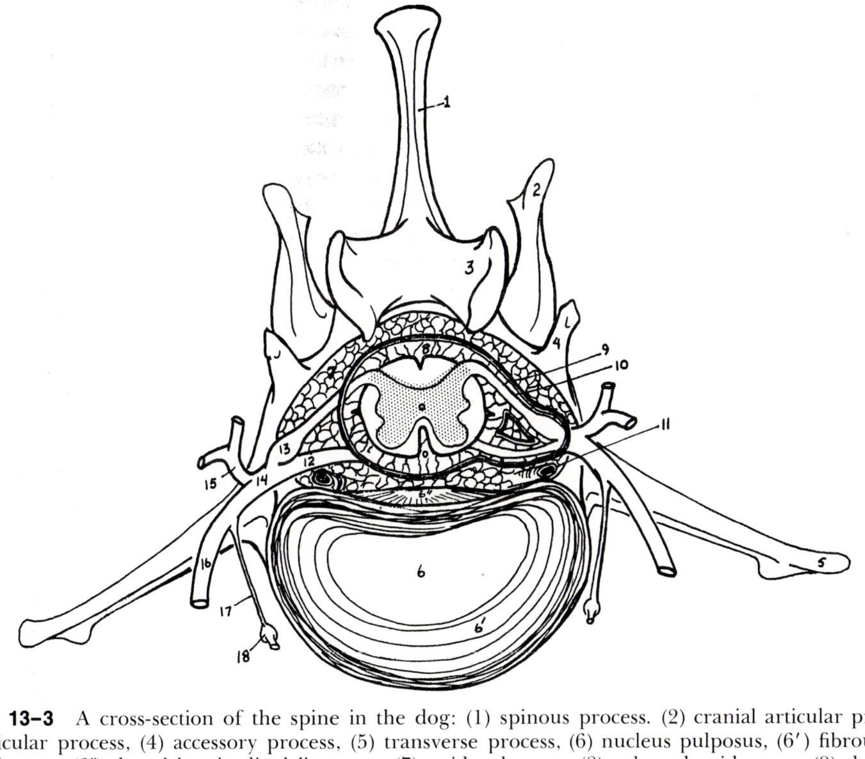

FIGURE 13–3 A cross-section of the spine in the dog: (1) spinous process. (2) cranial articular process, (3) caudal articular process, (4) accessory process, (5) transverse process, (6) nucleus pulposus, (6′) fibrous ring or annulus fibrosus, (6″) dorsal longitudinal ligament, (7) epidural space, (8) subarachnoid space, (9) dura mater, (10) arachnoid, (11) longitudinal venous sinus, (12) ventral nerve root, (13) dorsal root ganglion, (14) spinal nerve, (15) dorsal branch of spinal nerve, (16) ventral branch of spinal nerve, (17) ramus communicans, (18) sympathetic trunk ganglion. (From Worthman, R.: *The Nerve of That Dog*. Washington State University Press, Pullman, Wash., 1960.)

Each segment of the cord gives rise to a pair of spinal nerves that exit from the canal via the intervertebral foramina. There are 35 to 36 pairs of spinal nerves. Just outside the foramen, each spinal nerve divides into three parts; the dorsal branch supplies the dorsal muscles and the skin; the ventral branch supplies the lateral, ventral, and extremity musculature; and the visceral branch supplies the thoracic and abdominal viscera.

Fletcher has described the relationship of the spinal cord segments and the vertebrae. In general, the only spinal cord segments found to be entirely within their numerically corresponding vertebrae were the first cervical segment, the last two thoracic segments, and the first two or three lumbar segments. The remaining cord segments were positioned cranial to their corresponding vertebrae. The cord segment–vertebral relationship varies with the size of the dog. In small dogs (less than 7 kg), the lumbosacral cord segments tend to be positioned about half a vertebra caudal to those in larger dogs.[32]

Two regions of the spinal cord, the caudal cervical through the cranial thoracic region and the caudal lumbar through the coccygeal region, had shorter segments than the remainder of the cord. These segments had shorter lengths of spinal root attachment, shorter intervals between adjacent roots, and longer spinal nerve roots than did segments in other regions of the cord. As a consequence of their shorter lengths, these segments were shifted cranial with respect to their numerically corresponding vertebrae, and the longer roots were necessary to reach the appropriate intervertebral foramina (Figs. 13–4 to 13–6).[32]

The spinal cord is the main pathway of communication between the brain and the extremities. The gray and white matter concerned in neurological function has been described in detail in Chapter 2 (Fig. 13–7).

The longitudinal vertebral venous sinuses are situated within the spinal canal, and have been described by Worthman.[122] These sinuses are paired, thin-walled, flattened, valveless vessels that extend from the skull to the coccygeal vertebrae. They lie on the floor of the vertebral canal in the epidural fat. As paired trunks coursing through the canal, they diverge from each other at the intervertebral foramen and approach each other over the vertebral bodies. They are largest in the cervical area. Within the arch of the atlas, they originate as continuations of the ventral occipital sinuses and may appear to be ampullated. Within the atlas and axis, the large sinuses lie against the sides of the vertebral arches instead of on the floor of the canal. This fact is important in surgical procedures in the area and may account for the ease with which blood can be obtained in tapping the cisterna magna if the needle is not situated in the dorsal midline.[71]

Along the course of the sinuses, there are frequent anastomoses between the right and left channels, some superficial and others deep within the vertebrae or beneath the dorsal longitudinal ligament. Within the vertebral canal, the sinuses receive the spinal veins that follow along the nerve roots. Other anastomosing veins are the basivertebral, intervertebral, and arcuate. Since no valves are located in these sinuses and veins, these structures are the most accessible of all collateral routes of venous return in cases of vena caval occlusion. This accounts for the basis of venography discussed in Chapter 4 (Figs. 13–8 and 13–9).[71]

The arterial supply to the spinal cord and meninges arises from the spinal arteries that branch off from other main arteries in the various vertebral segments. These enter the canal through the intervertebral foramina shared by the spinal nerves and veins. These arteries divide into ventral and dorsal branches. The ventral arteries are united through the medium of the ventral spinal artery lying at the ventral median fissure. Branches or twigs go into the ventral medial fissure to supply the gray matter, and other twigs encircle the cord in the pia matter to supply the ventral and lateral white matter. The smaller dorsal branch follows the dorsal nerve root into the spinal cord, where it terminates (Fig. 13–10).[71, 121]

Contrast radiography, gross dissection, and vinyl resin injection techniques were evaluated as methods of counting the spinal branches of thoracolumbar segmental arteries in dogs. The study aimed to deter-

Text continued on page 420

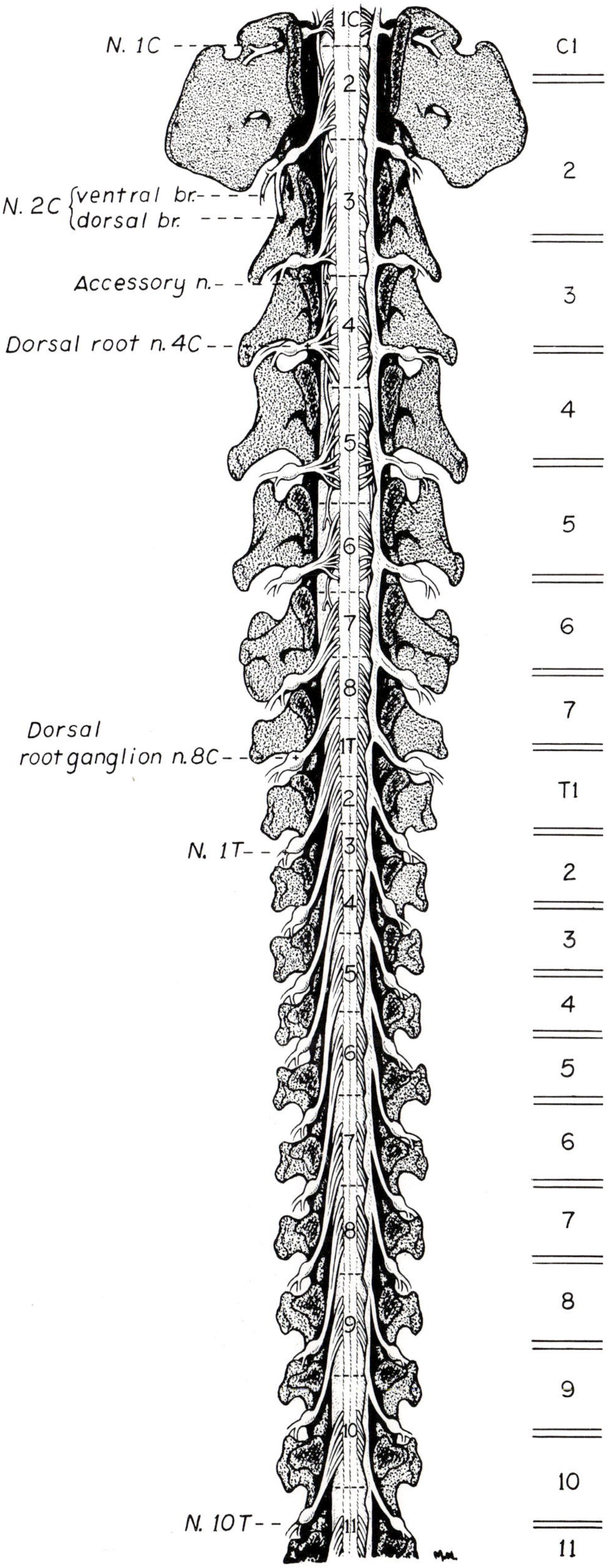

FIGURE 13–4 Dorsal roots of spinal nerves and spinal cord segments, cervical 1 to thoracic 11. Dorsal aspect. The dura mater has been removed except on the extreme right side. (The figures on the right represent levels of the vertebral bodies.) (From Fletcher, 1964. Thesis, University of Minnesota.)

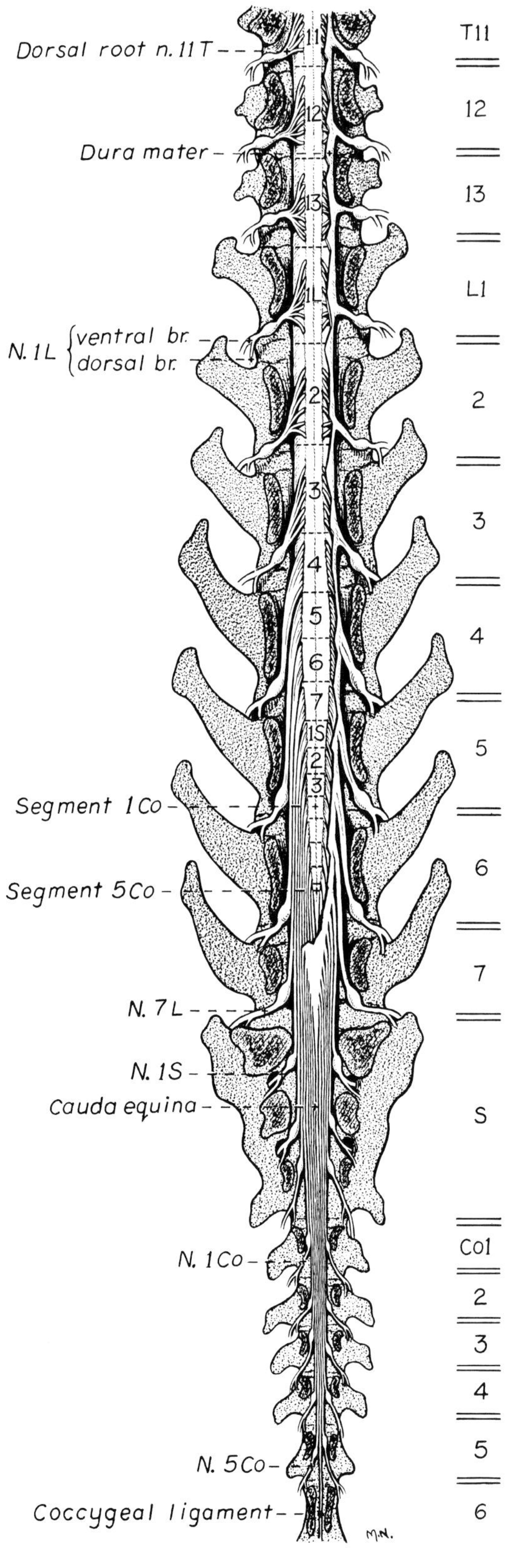

FIGURE 13–5 Dorsal roots of spinal nerves and spinal cord segments, thoracic 11 to coccygeal 5. Dorsal aspect. The dura mater has been removed except on the extreme right side. (The figures on the right represent levels of the vertebral bodies.) (From Fletcher, 1964. Thesis, University of Minnesota.)

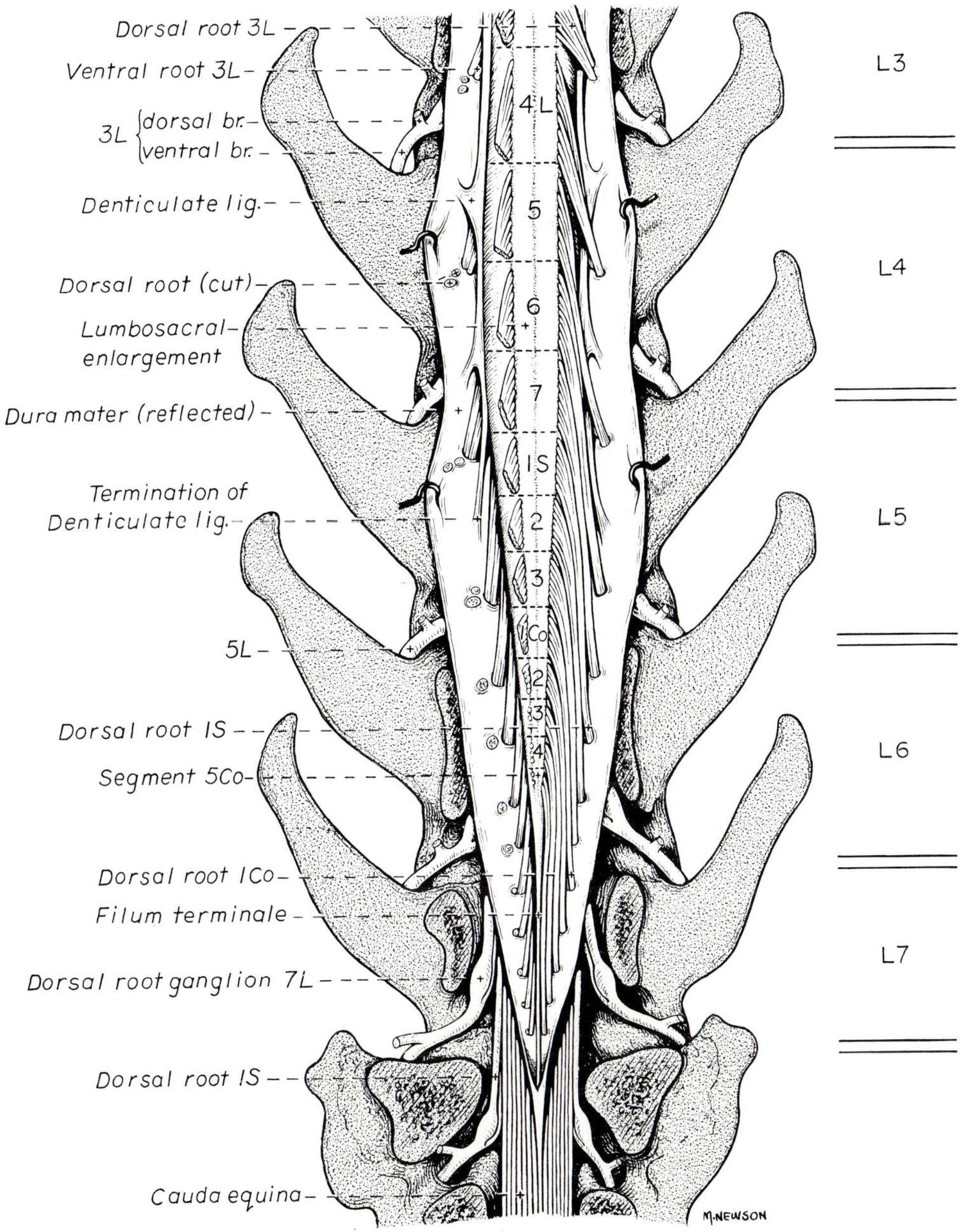

FIGURE 13–6 Distal end of spinal cord showing spinal cord segments. Dorsal aspect. (The dura mater has been cut mid-dorsally and reflected. The dorsal roots have been cut on the left side to expose the ventral roots and the denticulate ligament.) (From Fletcher, 1964. Thesis, University of Minnesota.)

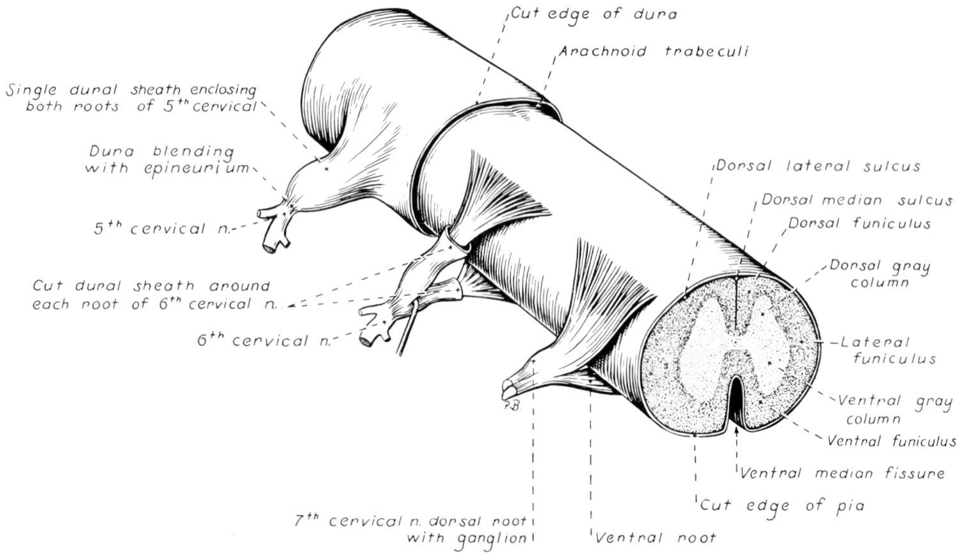

FIGURE 13–7 Cross section of spinal cord and meninges. (From Miller, M. E.: *Guide to the Dissection of the Dog.* Edwards Bros., Ann Arbor, Mich. 1952 © Dr. Malcom E. Miller.)

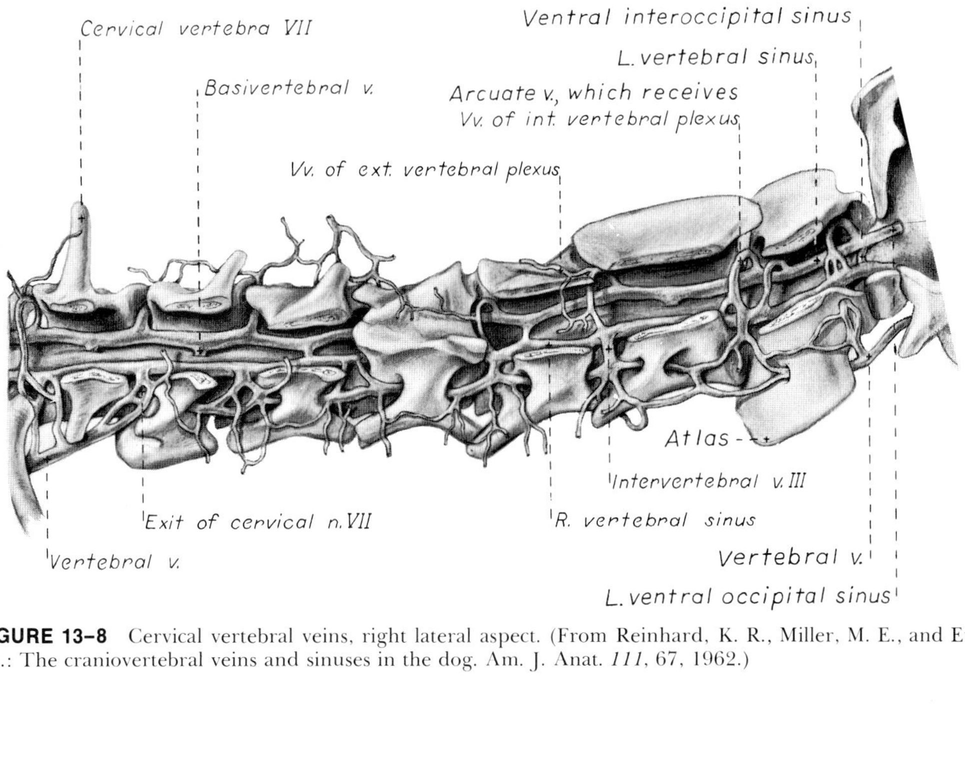

FIGURE 13–8 Cervical vertebral veins, right lateral aspect. (From Reinhard, K. R., Miller, M. E., and Evans, H. E.: The craniovertebral veins and sinuses in the dog. Am. J. Anat. *111*, 67, 1962.)

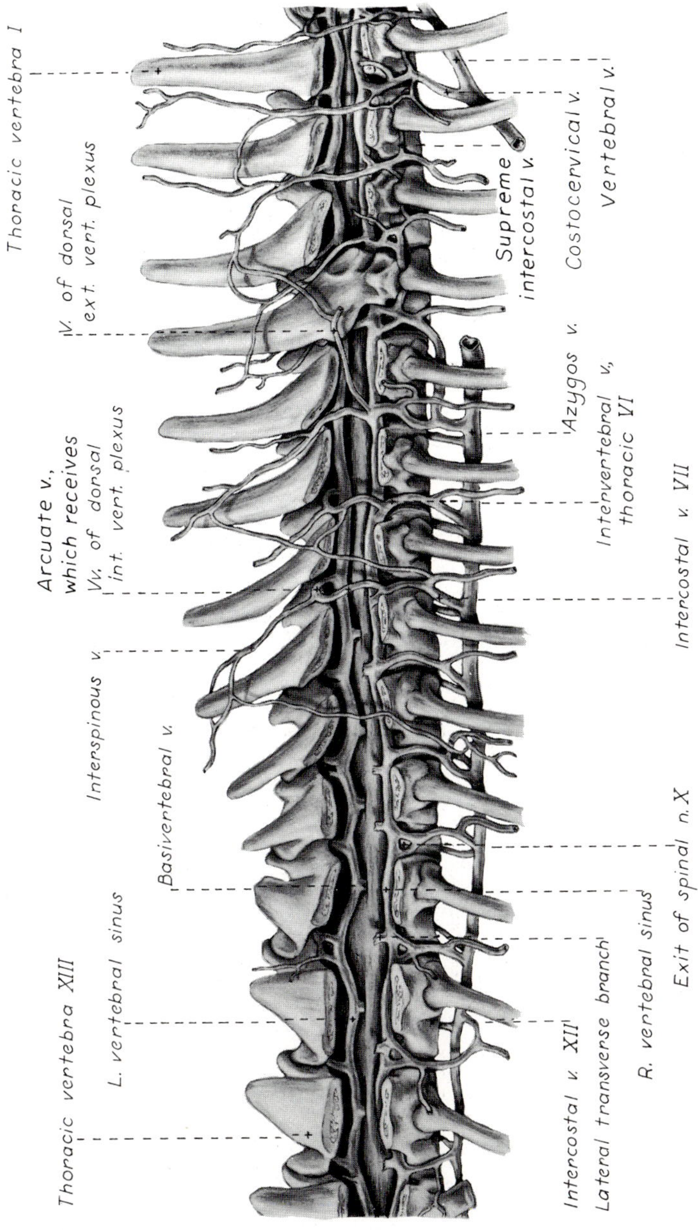

FIGURE 13–9 Thoracic vertebral veins, right lateral aspect. (From Reinhard, K. R., Miller, M. E., and Evans, H. E.: The craniovertebral veins and sinuses in the dog. Am. J. Anat. *111*, 67, 1962.)

mine why the spinal cord of the dog is so subject to ischemic changes, necrosis, and malacia.[88] Injection of the aorta with vinyl resin followed by dissection was the most feasible and accurate method and was used to count the spinal branches on each of the last four pairs of thoracic and the first five pairs of lumbar segmental arteries in 20 dogs.[88]

Parker found only five dogs with bilateral spinal branch arteries entering the canal at every intervertebral foramen from T10–11 through L5–6. In four dogs, the segmental arterial supply for up to seven cord segments was apparently precarious, as it depended on two to four spinal branch arteries. It has been shown that trauma can cause occlusion of these arteries, and if they are sparse in the normal dog, serious deficiency in arterial supply to the spinal cord can result.[86, 88]

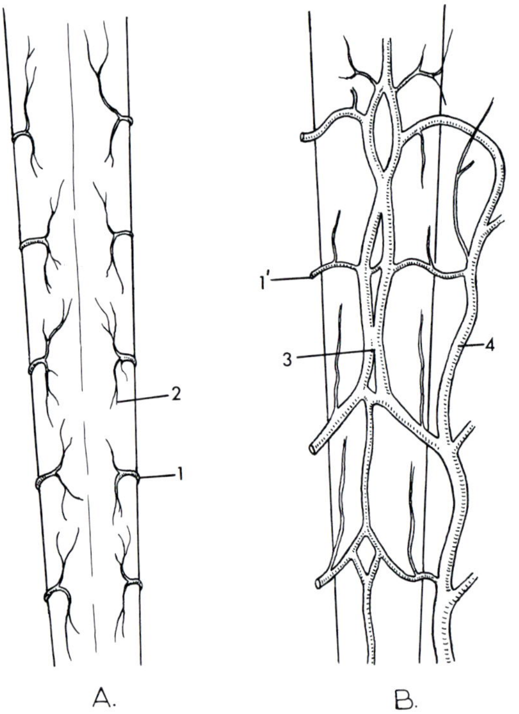

FIGURE 13–10 Blood supply to the cervical cord. *A*, Dorsal aspect. *B*, Ventral aspect. (1) dorsal branch; (1′) ventral branch; (2) dorsal spinal arteries; (3) ventral spinal artery; (4) vertebral artery. (Adapted from Miller, M. E., Christenson, G. C., and Evans, H. E.: *Anatomy of the Dog.* [W. B. Saunders Co., Philadelphia, 1964] and from Wilson, C. B., and Landry, R. M.: Experimental cervical myelopathy. I. Blood supply of the canine cervical spinal cord. Neurology, *14*, 809, 1964.)

Similar irregularities in arterial supply in the human cervical spinal cord have been noted. The anterior radicular arteries supplying the cervical cord vary in number from one to six, while the posterior radicular arteries vary from zero to eight. No arterial anastomoses could be found within the cord when it was examined under a dissecting microscope and by microangiography.[116, 117]

Various methods have been developed to outline the microvasculature of the spinal cord. The regional intrinsic functional integrity of the spinal cord is maintained by extensive anastomotic arterial networks on its surface called the pial-meningeal plexus. The closer experimental arterial obstruction is to the aorta and the further it is from the spinal cord, the greater are the possibilities for anastomotic substitution.[62] Terminal arterioles within the spinal cord do not interconnect but give rise to interlocking capillary networks which are more numerous in the gray matter than in the white matter. However, it has been confirmed that the white matter of the spinal cord, in contrast to the cerebral cortex, has a higher proportional blood flow than the gray matter. The spinal cord has autoregulation similar to that of the cerebral cortex. Regional blood flow is probably independent of the cerebrocortical circulation but depends on metabolic changes of hematologic and systemic origin.[45] Ventral-dorsal flattening of the spinal cord will elongate and occlude the intrinsic vessels, especially in the lateral columns. Dramatic alterations in blood flow occur on both local and systemic levels, and these may explain the resultant pathologic lesions.[116]

DIAGNOSTIC PROCEDURES FOR SPINAL DISORDERS[50–52]

As discussed in Chapter 3, the main procedures used in the diagnosis of spinal lesions involve a knowledge of neurological physiology as well as evaluation of the reflexes. These reflexes help the clinician to evaluate the dog's entire nervous system, the lower motor neuron (LMN), which is the cell body in the ventral gray column, and its processes, which terminate in the muscle, and the upper motor neuron (UMN), with the cell body in the brain stem, basal nuclei and cerebral cortex; its processes descend in the cord and control the lower motor neuron activity. The LMN carries out the motor component of the reflex. When the UMN is destroyed or damaged, the LMN is released, and the reflexes generally become spastic or hyperresponsive.

Lower motor neuron disease is characterized by hypotonia or atonia, hypoflexia or areflexia, and rapid atrophy of musculature. Typical cord lesions that cause LMN disease in the hind limbs involve the L4–6 area and affect the knee jerk, toe-pinch, and perineal reflexes. Typical cord lesions that produce LMN disease in the front legs involve the C6–T1 area and affect local tendon and toe-pinch reflexes. Signs of upper motor neuron disease are loss or decrease of voluntary motor contractions below the lesion, spasticity, presence of a crossed extensor thrust reflex, hyperreflexia, and loss of pain perception.

Typical UMN lesions would involve the cord above L4 in the hind legs. Lesions in C6–T1 would produce LMN signs in the forelegs and UMN signs in the hind limbs. Lesions cranial to C6 may produce UMN signs in all four limbs. Therefore, the segmented or spinal reflexes proposed by McGrath, such as the knee jerk and toe-pinch reflexes, other tendon reflexes, perineal or anal reflexes, and superficial skin prick, are all of value. The postural or attitudinal reflexes, such as tonic neck, placing, hopping, righting, extensor thrust, and crossed extensor thrust, determine the status of the whole nervous system and generally of the centers higher than the spinal cord.[98]

In Chapter 4, the diagnostic examination of the spine was emphasized as a most valuable aid in the determination of lesion location. The plain film screen and nonscreen Bucky techniques and the contrast techniques of myelography, discography, epiduralography, and venography were discussed. Radiography must be stressed as a most valuable diagnostic aid when combined with the physical neurological examination.

A diagnostic procedure that aids in the evaluation of the lower motor neuron and muscle receptors is electromyography (EMG). Botelho and workers used this technique in studying Weimaraner dogs affected with congenital spinal dysraphism or syringomyelia.[11] Since difficulty was experienced in the evaluation of the motor neuron by standard clinical responses to sensory stimulation and estimation of degree of muscle atrophy, EMG studies were initiated. Electromyographic evidence of denervation and reinnervation was found by spontaneous electrical potentials resembling denervation potentials in man or by reflex-induced motor unit potentials that were larger than those recorded from muscles of control dogs, or by both. Cummings reported abnormal EMG findings in the studies of polyradiculoneuritis. All dogs showed considerable fibrillation potentials and positive sharp waves.[18, 19] Breazile and workers used the EMG to study the cause of distemper myoclonus.[12, 13, 15] It is hoped that EMG procedures will become routine in clinical neurological centers in the future. Their usefulness is beyond question.

CLINICAL SPINAL DISORDERS

It has been said that in man a backache is one of the most common of all ailments—nearly as common as the headache. A physician once listed 57 causes of backache, some of which had no direct relation to spinal disease. Perhaps backache is just as frequent in the dog, and might have just as varied an etiology. The object of this chapter is to discuss diseases of the spine and spinal cord and their individual neurological signs.

An effort has been made to classify spinal disorders according to etiology and basic pathology. Infections, neoplasia, degenerative, congenital, and hereditary disorders, and toxic manifestations, all of which may affect both spinal cord and brain, are discussed in Chapter 11. The disorders that involve primarily the spinal column that will be discussed in this chapter are:

- Degenerative disorders
  - Nutritional
    - Avitaminosis

Hypervitaminosis
Mineral deficiencies
Dural ossification
Spondylosis deformans
Spinal osteoarthritis
Spondylolisthesis
Spondylolysis
Spinal osteochondrosis
Congenital and hereditary disorders
Hereditary spondylosis
Atlantoaxial subluxation
Abnormal odontoid process angulation
Canine wobbler syndrome
Malformations
Spina bifida
Hemivertebra
Scoliosis, kyphosis, lordosis
Block (nonsegmented) and fused vertebrae
Cervical vertebral deformity in basset hounds
Short spine deformity
Transitional vertebrae
Sacrococcygeal dysgenesis of Manx cats
Congenital deformity of the foramen magnum (occipital dysplasia)
Traumatic injury in the spinal cord
Concussion
Contusion
Hematorachis
Hematomyelia
Laceration
Compression of the spinal cord
Extravertebral
Vertebral

DEGENERATIVE DISORDERS

NUTRITIONAL DISORDERS

Avitaminosis

Vitamin deficiencies have been incriminated in neurological disturbances. Since these deficiencies are considered to be metabolic, multiple areas of degeneration occur that are not confined to the spine. In the growing dog, it has been shown that diets deficient in vitamin A may result in the formation of abnormally thick cranial and spinal bones. Nerve tissue in general grows normally while such bones have decreased growth, thereby causing a compression of nerves.[27, 68, 69, 70] It has been found that in growing animals diets deficient in vitamin A may also cause an increase in cerebrospinal fluid pressure, and therefore contribute to formation of hydrocephalus.

Niacin deficiency can cause widespread degeneration of nervous tissue, especially in the dorsal spinal horns, the dorsal and ventral spinal nerve roots, the ganglionic cells in the ventral spinal horns, and in the sympathetic ganglia. In blacktongue, or canine pellagra, weakness in the limbs from impaired nerve function can occur. Hysteria, coma, and convulsions have been seen.

Thiamine deficiency is said to cause negligible changes in the central nervous system, but lesions have been seen in the spinal ganglionic cells. The peripheral nerves show extensive changes and loss of function.[26] Thiamine deficiency can cause Chastek's paralysis in the fox, the mink, and the ferret.[33] Flaccid paralysis similar to Chastek's paralysis was seen in 14 dogs. All dogs had been fed a diet deficient in thiamine, such as boiled lungs, larynx, intestines, corn, and sugar. Recovery occurred in 2 to 3 weeks when B complex vitamins and additional vitamin B_1 were given.[105] Encephalopathy with clinical signs and lesions typical of Chastek's paralysis has been reported in four cats fed a diet of cooked or raw meat and/or canned pet food.[77] It has been shown that a cerebrocortical necrosis in cattle and sheep is a disease associated with some aberration in thiamine metabolism. Affected animals frequently respond to massive doses of thiamine. Thiaminases have been incriminated as the probable cause.[28, 31, 67, 96]

Riboflavin deficiency has been shown to cause substantial degeneration in brain and cord neurons in dogs. Muscle cramps, ataxia, and convulsions have been noted.[26]

The work of Newberne and O'Dell indicates that vitamin B_{12} deficiency promotes the development of hydrocephalus in rat pups.[80] Feeding a purified diet low in cobalt and vitamin B_{12} resulted in a high incidence of hydrocephalus. Future work may bear out this finding in dogs.

Although vitamin E deficiency is apparently not neurogenic, its effect on muscle tissue produces signs of weakness suggestive of a neurological disorder. Such deficiency has been reported in a litter of beagles and has been called "Scottie cramp." "Scottie cramp" has also been considered a hereditary disease, but the administration of vitamin E seemed to be efficacious; the beagle puppies responded well to vitamin E administration over a period of 10 days.[59] Vitamin E deficiency has been discussed in more detail under nutritional myopathy in Chapter 9.

Hypervitaminosis

Hypervitaminosis A has been seen in 2- to 4-year-old cats fed with diets rich in liver, causing primarily a cervical spondylosis. Clinical signs include anorexia, dullness, postural changes such as sitting like a kangaroo, inability to move head and neck, and lameness in the front limbs. As the spondylitic hypertrophic bone deposits encircle the spinal nerves and compress the cord, more severe neurological deficiencies can occur. English and Seawright, who studied 38 cases from 1953 to 1964, noted some cases of more generalized spondylosis.[29] These workers produced the condition experimentally by feeding excessive vitamin A to kittens.[16] A natural case of cervical spondylosis has been reported in England where the cat was fed a diet of raw liver and heart.[34]

Radiographic changes show confluent bone proliferation extending from the atlas to the thoracic vertebrae, and in some cases to the lumbar vertebrae, where the masses of bone envelop the dorsal spines and articular processes. As the disease progresses, the lateral and ventral surfaces become more involved, causing nerve compressions. Vertebral bodies are generally fairly normal. Exostoses of multifocal origin (ribs, hip, sternum, etc.) develop as subperiosteal new bone, characterized by peripheral development of trabecular bone. Often this undergoes resorption and is replaced with new cancellous bone. Experimental work has demonstrated that kittens fed a balanced commercial pet food but given additional high daily doses of vitamin A developed hyperemia, edema, and proliferation of the gums by 10 weeks of age, resulting in loss of teeth. Vitamin A fed in doses present in primarily liver diets also promoted tooth mobility and eventual loss of teeth owing to inadequate anchorage of the teeth in the alveoli.[103] Osteoporosis of the long bones, probably from disuse, has been seen in clinical cases of hypervitaminosis A, while experimental work with kittens also shows absence of epiphyseal plates and shorter malformed long bones.[16] Osteoporosis of long bones is seen in the front limbs.

The diagnosis is made from the characteristic dietary history, from typical clinical signs, and from radiographic changes.

The treatment includes a change of diet, which must be initiated in the early stages of the disease. Phenylbutazone and steroids may relieve the clinical signs, but remissions occur when the drugs are discontinued.[5, 29, 34, 65, 78]

Mineral Deficiency

Mineral deficiency probably has little direct effect on the nervous tissue, but since the central nervous system is encased in bone, abnormal growth or development of bone is bound to affect the system secondarily. Any metabolic mineral derangement, such as osteoporosis, frequently leads to pathologic fractures of the spine and a subsequent compression of the cord. It has been shown that copper deficiency in sheep causes spinal cord degeneration.[57] A report of selenium deficiency in dogs stated that symptoms resembled those of white muscle disease of sheep.[66] In the author's opinion, magnesium deficiency which is prevalent in the cow has not been reported in dogs.

Treatment

Nutritional deficiencies are treated by supplying the proper nutritive agent through therapeutic administration and diet. Since these deficiencies occur frequently in a secondary form, administration of vitamins and minerals is a routine part of any therapeutic regimen for a neurological disorder.

OTHER DEGENERATIVE DISORDERS

Spinal Dural Ossification

Dural ossification, ossifying pachymeningitis, or osseous metaplasia of the spinal dura mater is characterized by deposition of bone plaques on the inner surface of the dura. This bone is characteristic in that peripheral white cortical areas surround the central red marrow portions. These areas are found chiefly in the highly movable parts of the spine, namely the neck and lumbar segments.

Sandersleben and Sergony studied a group of 209 dogs. Ossifying spinal meningitis was found in over 50 per cent of the larger breeds and less than 30 per cent of smaller dogs.[99] The incidence in the various breeds was Alsatian—74 per cent; boxer—88 per cent; dachshund—24 per cent; and spaniels—23 per cent. The most frequently affected dural segments in this study were C2–4, C7, and L1–L7. The ossifying foci first appear in spaniels and dachshunds at 5 to 6 years of age and in boxers and Alsatians at 1 to 2 years of age. Spondylosis often accompanies dural ossification, but the two conditions are independent in both frequency and intensity.[99]

Morgan has more recently surveyed 114 dogs whose spines were carefully examined radiographically when the vertebral columns were dissected free of all soft tissue. The spinal cord was removed from the spinal canal, and the entire dura mater was incised and carefully examined for dural plaques of bone. The mean age was 8.06 years, and there were 55 males and 59 females. At least one bone plaque was seen in 74 of 114 dogs (65 per cent) representing 23 different breeds. Dogs as young as 2 years had a 40 per cent incidence and dogs weighing as little as 5 kg were affected. Little dogs were affected as frequently as larger dogs, a finding which varies somewhat from that of other workers. The highest incidence was seen in the cervical area and the next highest was seen in the lumbar area. Case histories on 78 dogs revealed that abnormal gait and hind leg weakness were noted in 23 per cent of affected dogs and 12 per cent of unaffected dogs. However, no positive clinical or pathological relationship could be established between the lesion and the clinical signs.[74, 76]

The cause of the condition, as described by Dexler in 1893,[21] was thought to be a low-grade inflammatory process, since the site of highest incidence was the most movable portion of the spinal column. This theory also seems logical when one considers the wear and tear on these segments over the period of years that elapses before the disorder becomes clinically evident. In America, this disorder seems to be more prevalent in the German shepherd and other large breeds, but it can occur in all breeds in middle to old age. Scherer in 1944 proposed the course to be that of osseous metaplasia.[100] This cause is confirmed by Sandersleben,[99] Morgan,[74] and other workers today. Spinal dural ossification is peculiar to the dog; however, calcification of the spinal arachnoidea has been reported in man.[81]

Most investigators consider dural ossification of little clinical importance primarily because of the demonstration of diffuse thoracic spinal cord degeneration in the German shepherd which was not associated with compressions such as disk protrusions, spondylosis, or dural ossification.[3] These spinal signs in German shepherds of middle to old age were formerly thought to be due to dural ossification. However, one must not discount the possibility that extensive dural ossification causes characteristic signs of pain, weakness, and other neurological deficits. These are seen more frequently in the giant breeds such as the Great Dane.[119, 120] The microscopic cord lesions associated with dural plaques include edema, necrosis, malacia, gliosis, and fibrosis of the adjacent nerve roots and spinal cord. No other reason for the clinical signs can be seen.

Positive antemortem diagnosis may be difficult. Typically, the dog is of an appropriate age and breed, and the disorder has progressed slowly. Radiographic interpretation sometimes reveals the lesion if it is dense and particularly if it is superimposed on an intervertebral foramen. If the history and symptoms are characteristic, and radiography reveals no other forms of chronic compression such as disk protrusion, spondylosis, spinal arthritis, or neoplasia, a tentative diagnosis of dural ossification can be made (Figs. 13–11 to 13–15).

Treatment

Treatment is not specific. On theoretical grounds, thyroid extract or iodine has been used to inhibit the ossification. Counterirritants, heat, and diathermy have been applied to the affected areas. Symptomatic treatment with enteric-coated aspirin, phenylbutazone (Butazolidin), adreno-

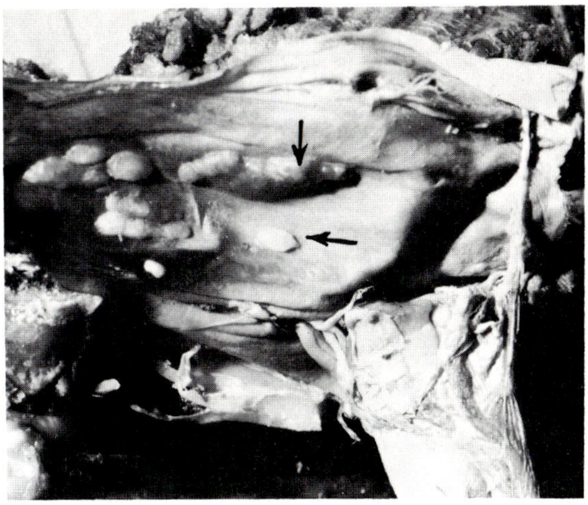

FIGURE 13–11 Dorsal ossification. Notice the circular and oblong areas of bone on the leptomeningeal surface of the dura mater.

corticoids, indomethacin (Indocin), and B complex vitamins is most commonly used.

Spondylosis Deformans

Disagreement as to a specific pathogenesis of this noninfectious, nonseptic spinal disorder has permitted a varied nomenclature. Earlier workers described the condition as a low-grade inflammatory disorder and used variations of the word spondylitis. Previous terms have included hypertrophic spondylitis, spondylitis deformans ossificans, bamboo back, rheumatoid spondylitis, ankylosing spondylitis, and Marie-Strümpell's disease. Hansen in 1952[46] introduced the term spondylosis into the veterinary literature, and recent extensive study by Morgan[73] has supported such nomenclature. Even though spondylitis deformans is a common term, it is felt that in order to promote academic accuracy and to lessen further confusion and controversy, spondylosis deformans should be the term for future usage. Forms of vertebral inflammations resulting from sepsis or combinations of factors have been discussed previously under osteomyelitis, septic spondylitis, and discospondylitis (see pages 329–332). Nutritional spondylosis was also discussed earlier.

Morgan's work has clarified many aspects of spondylosis deformans. It is defined as a disorder of the vertebral column characterized by the presence of vertebral osteophytes at the intervertebral spaces, resulting in the formation of spurs or complete bony bridges. These may be single or multiple in distribution and are frequently asymptomatic. The incidence is higher with

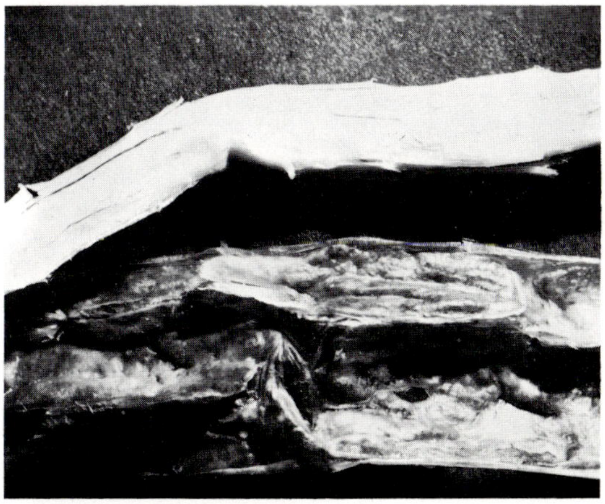

FIGURE 13–12 Dural ossification. Notice that practically the entire dura has ossified into a tube around the spinal cord.

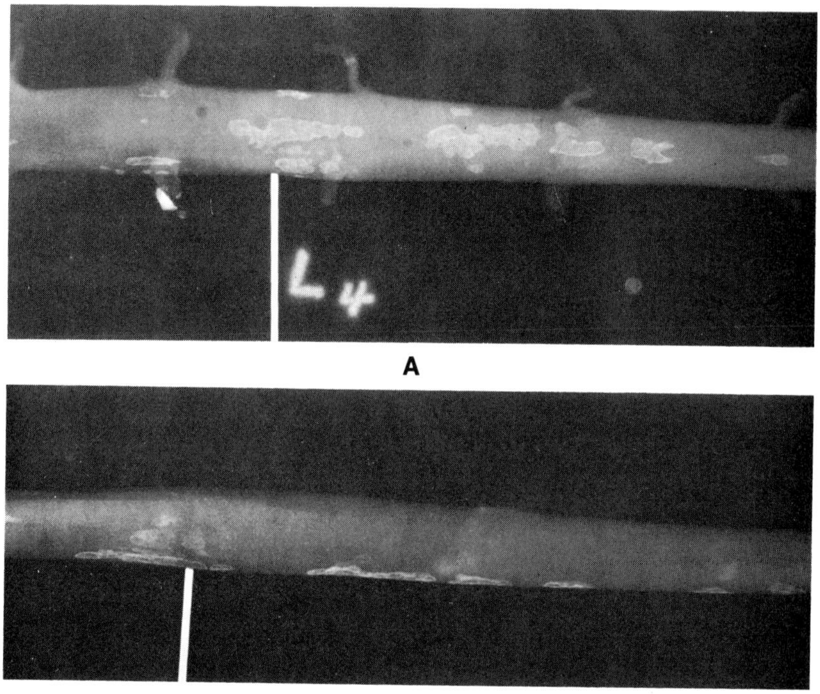

FIGURE 13–13 *A*, Radiograph of the spinal cord and meninges—dorsal view. Notice the plaques of bone in the dura mater. (Courtesy of Dr. J. E. Bartels.) *B*, Lateral view of the spinal cord and meninges seen in *S*.

increasing age, and size and number of osteophytes were greater in certain breeds. Species other than the dog, such as man, the cat, and the male bovine, are similarly affected.[73]

It was formerly felt that the disorder originated primarily from tears in the ventral longitudinal ligaments, but Morgan concluded that changes in the annulus fibrosus of the intervertebral disk led to fissures within the disk that predisposed to formation of osteophytes. The ventral longitudinal ligament influenced the direction of growth but played no role in its initiation. Osteophytes usually occurred at disk spaces of normal width. When they occurred at narrow disk spaces, they had a different shape. Osteophytes were located on the ventral, lateral, and dorsolateral aspects of vertebral margins. Osteophytic projections into the vertebral canal were rare,[73] and the radiographic appearance of a formation causing compression of the cord is usually an artifact. These artifacts are created by large dorsolateral spurs on the vertebral arch and laminae that when

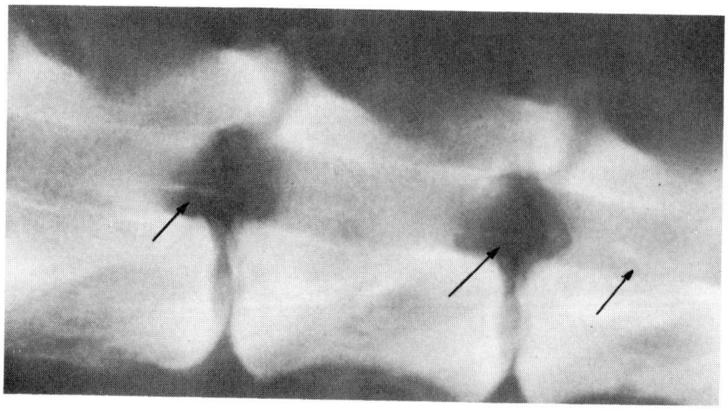

FIGURE 13–14 The appearance of dural ossification in a spinogram. The linear calcification is quite variable in appearance and is easily overlooked. (Courtesy of Dr. Jack Geary.)

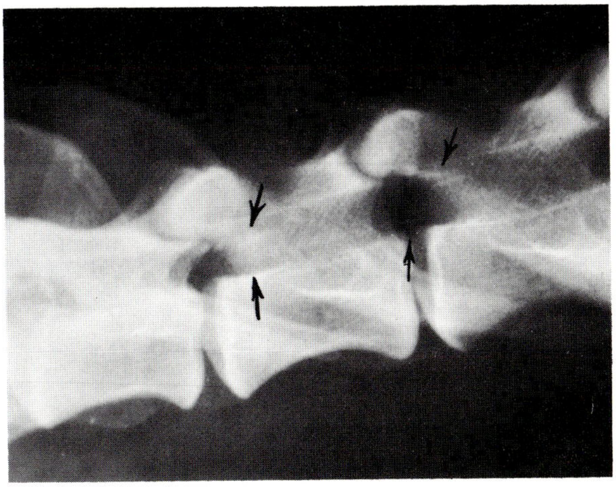

FIGURE 13–15 Dural ossification in a lateral radiograph. Notice the "streaks" of bone material as seen after careful examination of a radiograph made with good equipment, careful exposure, and proper processing technique.

projected on a lateral radiograph appear to extend dorsally, placing pressure on the cord.[73]

Morgan classified the size and shape of vertebral osteophytes in five stages (Fig. 13–16). He concluded that growth could cease at any age and at any stage. The number of stage 3 osteophytes was most frequent in all age groups of the 100 dogs studied, whereas stage 2 was the most frequent type in nine German shepherds. Stage 3 was seen most often in dachshunds (18) and boxers (18). Stage 5, the complete bony bridge, did not occur in the 9 German shepherds studied. The lesion sites most often affected were the T9–10 and L7–S1 areas (Fig. 13–17). The osteophytes were seen to be situated most frequently on the lateral surfaces of the body in the midthoracic areas, especially at T9–10, and were more ventral from T12–13 through L3–4. The distribution patterns suggested that dynamic and mechanical factors causing disk changes primarily in the annulus are of importance in the pathogenesis of spondylosis deformans.[73]

Morgan endeavored to note the probable cause of spondylosis deformans. A sharp line has not always been recognized in differentiating ankylosing spondylitis from spondylosis deformans. Ankylosing spondylitis in man is characterized by bony ankylosis across true synovial joints, ossification of ligamentous structures, or ankylosis across the vertebral space. Morgan states that none of the changes in the vertebral column that are typical of ankylosing spondylitis were found in the dog. The

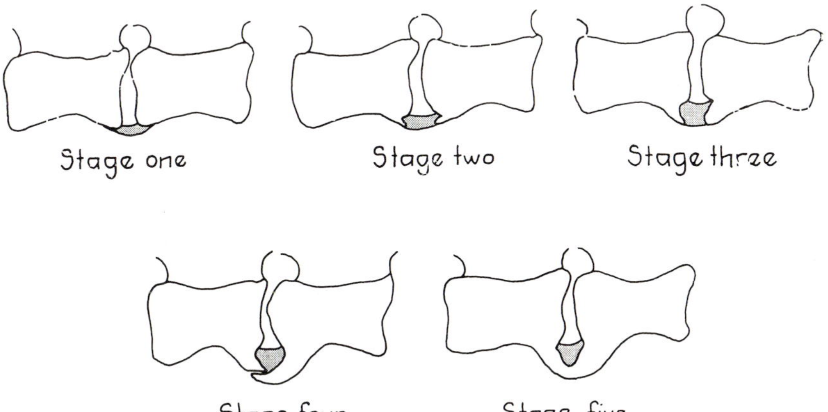

FIGURE 13–16 Five stages used in recording size and shape of vertebral osteophytes as determined grossly and macroradiographically. Stage one could only be identified grossly since it contained soft tissues. (The shading indicates soft tissue.) (From Morgan, H. P.: Spondylosis deformans in the dog. Acta Orthoped. Scand. *96*, 1967.)

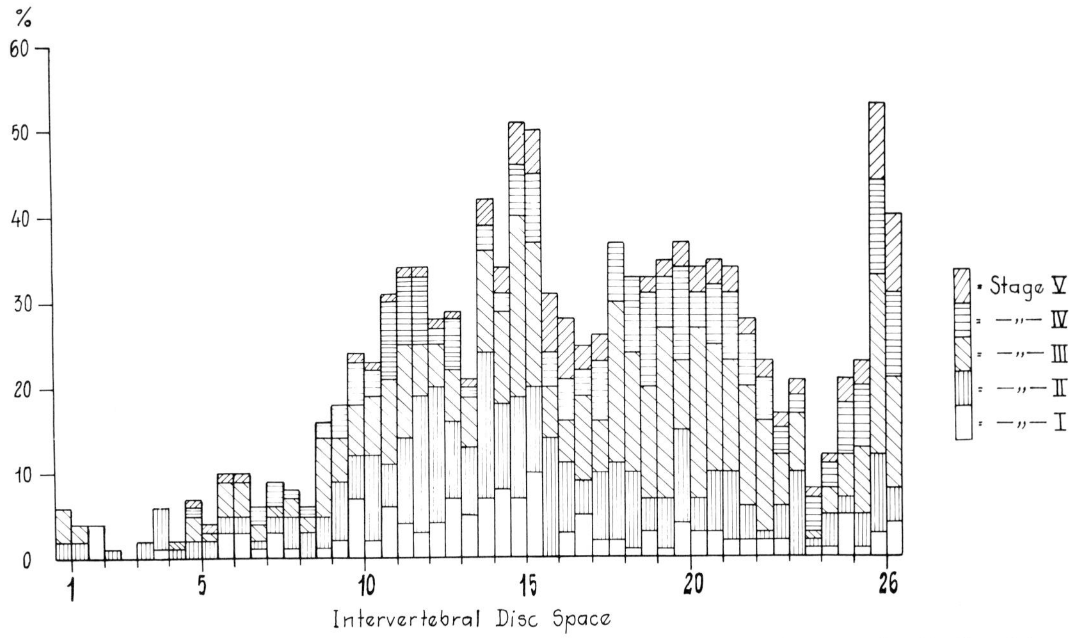

FIGURE 13–17 Frequency distribution of each of the five stages of spondylosis deformans in 100 affected dogs as it is related to both cranial and caudal aspects of each intervertebral disc space. (From Morgan, J. P.: Spondylosis deformans in the dog. Acta Orthoped. Scand. *96*, 1967.)

cause of spondylosis deformans will not be known until the etiology of disk degeneration is determined.[75]

Clinically, *localized* vertebral osteophytes can occur in middle-aged to old dogs of any breed, may bridge the vertebrae completely, and may or may not produce observable clinical signs. Although spondylosis occurred frequently in dachshunds in Morgan's survey, he readily admits that large osteophyte formations are rarely seen in chondrodystrophoid breeds frequently affected with disk disease. We have seen only one breeding line of dachshunds in which spondylosis was frequently seen. *Generalized* or diffuse osteophytes occur most frequently in working or sporting breeds and in large breeds. In 1974–75, the Auburn clinic saw 53 dogs (no cats) in which it was felt that the spondylitic changes were at least partially responsible for the clinical signs seen.

These dogs show *signs* of pain from pressure on or encirclement of spinal nerves. In cases of stage 5 vertebral osteophyte formation, trauma may fracture not only the bony bridge but the laminae and arch of the vertebrae, causing severe spinal cord compression.

Cervical spondylotic myelopathy has been the most important cause of progressive spinal cord and nerve root deterioration in man. It has been estimated that 75 per cent of persons over 50 years of age have narrowing of the spinal canal or intervertebral foramina and 50 per cent of these persons are symptomatic.[97] In a study by Crandall of 199 cases, cervical spondylosis was seen in a total of 581 spinal cord disorders for an incidence rate of 34.3 per cent. Seventy-eight of the 199 were severe enough to be referred for surgical treatment.[17] In a study by Stoops, cervical laminectomy and foraminotomy gave 83.3 per cent improvement to these patients.[107] Anterior cervical diskectomy and fusion is another procedure that is said to afford relief to this kind of patient.[55, 97]

Several studies of vertebral osteophyte formations have been performed in cats. These confirm many of Morgan's findings for the dog.[9, 79, 95]

The *diagnosis* depends on radiographic examination and characteristic local neurological signs involving lower motor neurons. Radiographic determination will aid in the differential diagnosis of bone or cord neoplasia, disk disease, and dural ossification (Figs. 13–18 to 13–22). Morgan emphasizes the radiographic differences

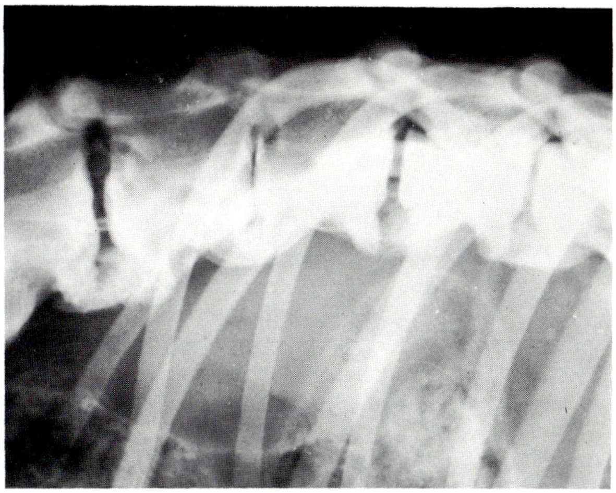

FIGURE 13–18 An advanced case of generalized spondylosis. Notice the collapsed disk space and the lack of articular involvement. (From Hoerlein, B. F.: Clinical spinal conditions of the dog. Vet. Med. *51*, 577, 1956.)

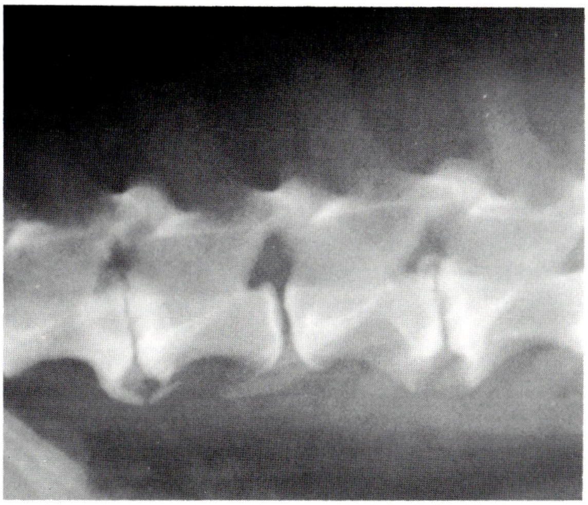

FIGURE 13–19 A case of localized spondylitis of two separate areas of the lumbar vertebrae probably due to sepsis. Notice the unusual dorsal ossification into the spinal canal and the very dense lateral bony proliferation. This type of spondylitis appears to fulfill the requirements of the term diskospondylitis.

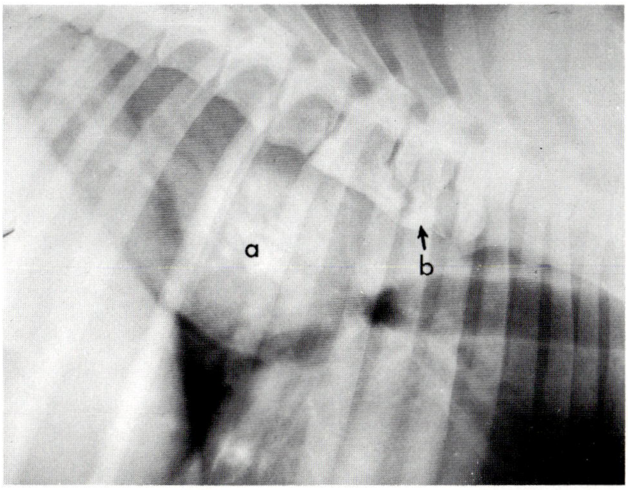

FIGURE 13–20 Spondylosis adjacent to a *Spirocerca lupi* tumor in the terminal esophagus: (a) tumor; (b) spondylosis. It is felt that this type of spondylosis is due to a larval migration.

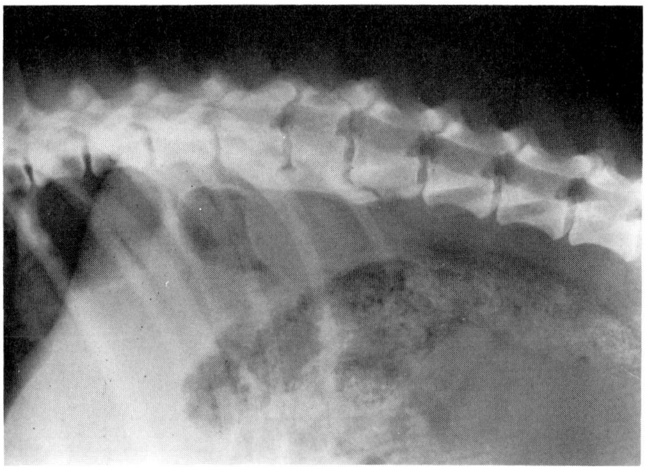

FIGURE 13–21 A complete and massive ventral spondylotic bridging of L1–3. L3 has fractured; the fracture line extends into the vertebral arch. This type of fracture generally causes extreme cord trauma, and immediate decompression may be indicated.

between spondylitis or neoplasia and typical spondylosis. Spurs of spondylosis are smooth, sharply outlined, bony growths originating from the circumference of the vertebral end-plate. The new bone growth of spondylitis or of tumors is irregular and usually involves the entire cortical surface of the vertebral body equally, or even the arch of the vertebra. The disk in spondylosis may be narrowed but the end-plates remain intact and actually become sclerotic. Spondylitis or tumors can invade the disk space and destroy the end-plates.[72]

Treatment

The treatment of spondylosis deformans in the dog has been nonspecific. In many cases there is little pain in dry, warm weather, but exacerbations occur on cold, damp days. Relief of periodic pain and inflammation has been enhanced by use of salicylates, phenylbutazone, indomethacin, thyroid extract, and adenocorticosteroids. Glenny has proposed the use of spinal fusion.[43] Our clinic has on occasion performed decompression and fusions or

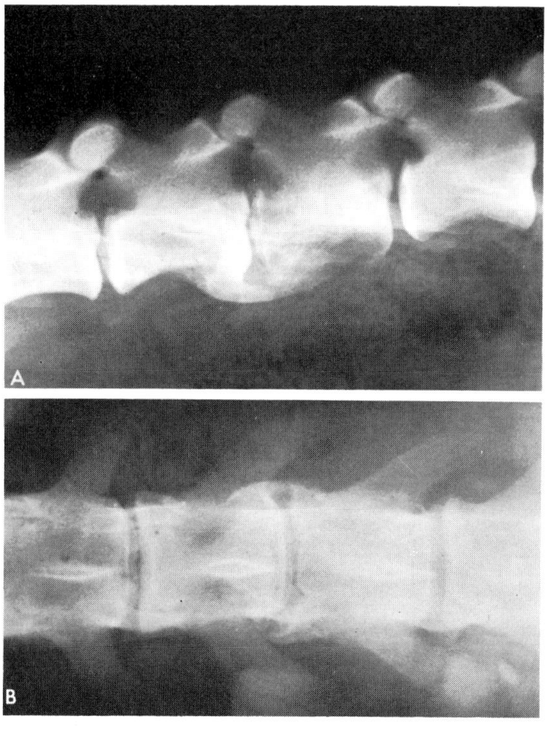

FIGURE 13–22 An apparent complete spondylotic bridge at L3–4 with considerable lateral osseous deposition, which is probably causing the uneven osseous density in the caudal third of L3. This could be mistaken for a septic process with destruction of bone. *A*, Lateral view. *B*, Ventrodorsal view.

skeletal plating in localized spondylotic compressions. Some cases of fracturing of the bony bridge and resultant trauma to the cord have been decompressed with satisfactory results. It is this author's opinion that more surgical decompressions and fusions probably should be done in localized lesions.

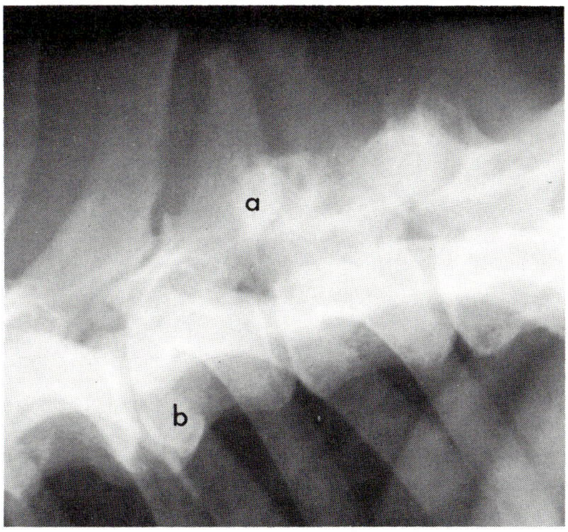

FIGURE 13–23 Degenerative spinal osteoarthritis of the terminal thoracic vertebrae. Notice (a) joint degeration and periarticular proliferation of bone and (b) local spondylitic lesion.

Spinal Osteoarthritis

Spinal osteoarthritis has in the past been considered one of the clinically significant painful spinal disorders seen in large dog breeds in middle to old age. Besides excessive pain on movement, occasionally posterior ataxia and weakness can also be observed. Radiography reveals no abnormalities such as disk compressions, luxations, mild fractures, spondylosis, or spondylitis. However, many of these animals show what appears to be periarticular hypertrophic osseous changes charactcristic of degenerative joint disease. Antiarthritic medications such as phenylbutazone, indomethacin, glucocorticosteroids, and salicylates generally give clinical relief[72] (Fig. 13–23).

However, Morgan's studies reveal that degenerative spinal arthritis in the dog is not commonly seen on necropsy examination. He felt that the radiographic signs are due to bony proliferations between the dorsal spinous processes on the dorsal midline of the arch of the vertebra. These pseudofacets are superimposed on the articular processes of the lateral radiographic projection. In man this entity is known as Baastrup's disease[72] (Fig. 13–24).

At this time, the clinical importance of spinal osteoarthritis in the dog may be questionable, and further work is necessary before a final conclusion can be drawn.[72]

Spondylolisthesis (L7–S1)

Spondylolisthesis in man is defined as a forward displacement of one vertebra over another.[22] In domestic animals a ventral displacement of the cranial vertebra compared to the caudal vertebra is probably infrequent. In the dog, the ventral spondylolytic bridge between L7 and S1 is frequently seen in routine radiography and is felt to be spondylolisthesis according to the above definition. Such slippage at this location results in a "dropping" of the sacrum relative to the lumbar segments. Secondary

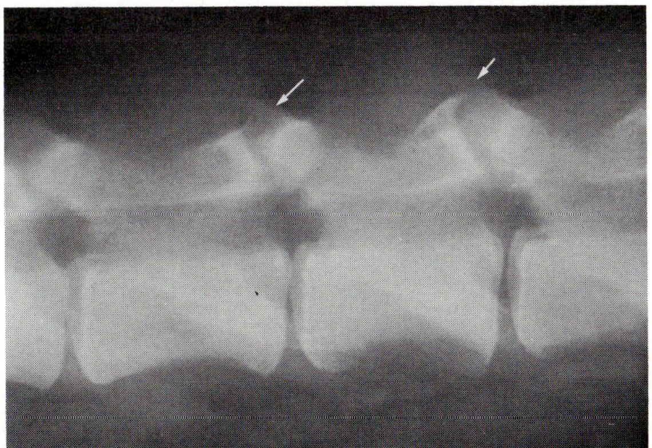

FIGURE 13–24 The typical "button-hook" proliferations of bone that Morgan refers to as Bastrup's disease in man. (Morgan, J. P.: *Radiology in Veterinary Orthopedics.* Lea & Febiger, Phildadelphia, 1972). These bony growths form at the base of the adjacent spinous processes on the dorsal midline of the vertebral arch. These pseudofacets are not necessarily indicative of degenerative spinal arthritis. Notice that the articular surfaces appear smooth and unaffected.

osteophytes develop to re-establish stability in the vertebral column[72] (Fig. 13–25).

It has been suggested that the cause in the dog is the result of a congenital anomaly, but probably more accurately it is the result of biomechanical stress or trauma. Most of the observed patients are not suffering clinical signs, but some affected dogs show some pain on movement and, if the dog is lean, possibly a change in conformation of the pelvic area. Treatment consists of rest and antiarthritic or anti-inflammatory therapy until stability has returned.

The term spondylolisthesis was used initially to refer to cervical vertebral instability, spinal anomaly syndrome, also called canine wobbler disease. This disorder will be discussed later in this chapter.

Spondylolysis

Spondylolysis is defined as a dissolution of a vertebra.[22] It is a cleft formation between the superior and inferior articular processes of a vertebra. When the vertebral bodies are displaced it is known as spondylolisthesis.[72] In man it occurs in about 5 per cent of the adult population. The average age of a human patient seeking treatment is 35 years. Pain and deformity are the chief signs.[124]

The disorder as seen in man is not well defined in dogs except as possibly associated with spondylolisthesis. Dissolution or destruction of a vertebra not associated with septic infections could result from vascular disturbances, as in possible trauma.

Spinal Osteochondrosis

Spinal osteochondrosis, as described by Alexander and Pettit,[1] refers to a bone disease in which one or more growth centers undergo a characteristic degenerative phase, followed by a regenerative stage. Theories of cause include embolism, acute or chronic trauma, congenital and hereditary factors, infection, and endocrine disturbances. One common denominator is resultant ischemia.[1]

Stages of the disease are necrotic, regenerative, and healing. The predominant clinical sign may be pain.[1] Hime[49] reports six cases in a pack of 75 foxhounds in which the puppies were poorly developed and walked abnormally by the age of 7 months. By 10 to 13 months of age, examination revealed a stilted gait, poor paraspinal muscle development, kyphosis, rigidity, and inability to extend the limbs properly at gallop.

Radiographic examination by Alexander of a similar case showed a shortened vertebral body with a deformity in the cranial articular surface with a distinct notch on its ventral half. Sclerosis of joint surfaces was visible.[1] Hime's cases seemed much more advanced, with similar but more pronounced osteolysis of bone at T5–6 and T7–9. In addition, there was a reduction in affected disk spaces, and advanced osteophytosis was present on the ventral aspects of vertebral bodies. Generalized spondylosis was noted in films in the report.[49]

Bartels and co-workers report a case in an 8-month-old male pointer who ap-

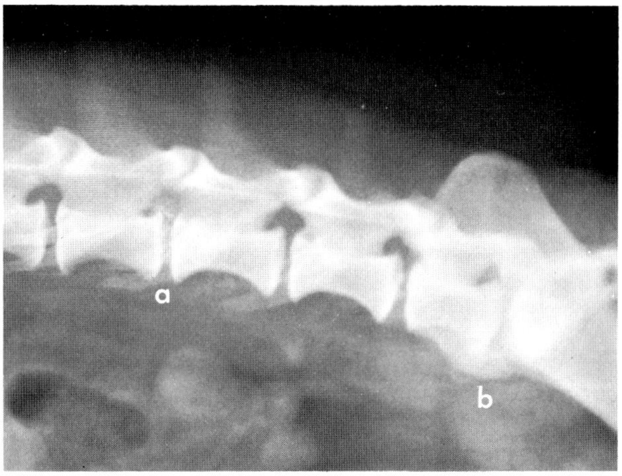

FIGURE 13–25 Lateral radiograph showing (a) calcific disk protrusion at L4–5 space and (b) spondylitic exostosis at L7–S1. The spondylosis at this area may have resulted from spondylolisthesis or unstable joint.

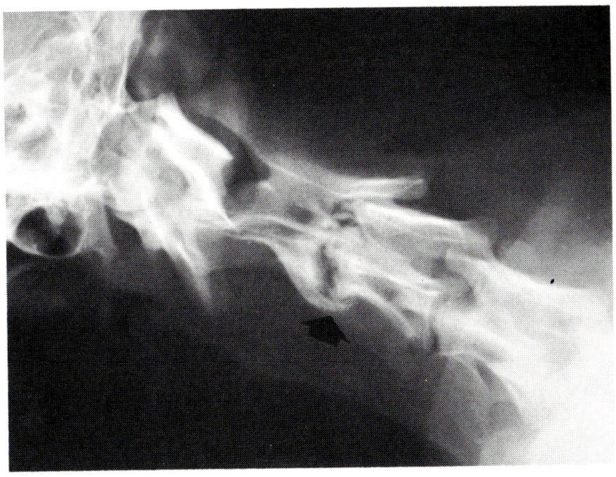

FIGURE 13–26 Osteochondritis dissecans (a form of osteochondrosis at C2–3 in a 7-month-old pointer. Note the ankylosis and sclerosis and vascular necrosis of the vertebral epiphysis. (From Bartels, J. E., Dorn, A. S., and Britt, A. L.: Osteochondrosis of the vertebrae in a dog. Canad. Vet. J. *11*, 47, 1970.)

peared sore and stiff when arising or moving quickly. The dog showed pain in the cervical area upon manipulation of the head and neck. A ventral spondylosis was seen at C2–3 and T4–5 interspaces on the 42nd day after initial examination, and osteolysis of the involved vertebral end-plates was seen on the 73rd day. Clinical improvement was noted after the 89th day, and marked radiographic improvement of the lesion was noted on the 104th day, at which time the dog was normal.[8]

In the two cases seen at this clinic, the clinical signs were relatively mild, consisted largely of pain, and were similar to Alexander's description. No treatment was attempted and recovery occurred spontaneously (Fig. 13–26).

Treatment in Alexander's report was radical surgical curettage, and slow, complete recovery took place.[1] Apparently no treatment was attempted in Hime's cases.[49]

CONGENITAL AND HEREDITARY SPINAL DISORDERS

HEREDITARY "SPONDYLITIS" (SPONDYLOSIS)

The occurrence of hereditary spondylitis (or spondylosis) in man is quite well established. Stephens noted its occurrence in identical twins at approximately the same time.[106] They were stationed at different military posts, and had been reared apart from infancy. O'Connell studied 70 families in which a member had ankylosing spondylitis;[82] in 16 families there were positive cases of familial ankylosing spondylitis, and in seven there were cases of rheumatoid arthritis. O'Connell felt that there was strong evidence for transmission through a simple dominant characteristic with variable sex penetrance.

In one family study, a 44-year-old man, his three brothers, and his eight children had ankylosing spondylitis, hyperuricemia, and anomalies of the lumbosacral junction.[115] No doubt work in the dog would substantiate a similar finding in our cases of spondylitis, since hereditary patterns have been seen in the occurrence of cataracts, glaucoma, and other disorders in dogs. We have noted a breeding line of dachshunds that appears to be frequently afflicted with a marked degree of spondylosis deformans, an unusual disorder in a chondrodystrophoid breed of dog.

CONGENITAL VERTEBRAL SUBLUXATION

Atlantoaxial Subluxation

Atlantoaxial subluxation in small dog breeds have been shown to be largely due to congenital absence, lack of fusion, or other anomalies of the odontoid process.[41, 42, 61, 90] The evidence has suggested an inherited problem in some breeding lines. Other breeds can have similar subluxations of the C1–2 area in fractures or ligamentous ruptures from trauma where the congenital weakness or heritable characteristics are probably lacking.

The anatomical development of the axis helps explain the pathogenesis of the disorder. The axis may arise from as many as seven centers of ossification. Four of these are present at birth: the main body, the dens, and one center for the arch and processes on each side. The centers for the cranial and caudal epiphyses of the axial body appear during the third week after birth. The cranial epiphysis develops between the body of the axis and the dens and unites during the fourth month. An accessory center for the apex of the dens is present in many dogs, and this center does not unite until the seventh to ninth month.[56, 83] This latter ununited ossification center may account for many subluxations of C1–2 in smaller breeds (Fig. 13–27).

The ligamentous support of the dens is unique in that it involves two other bones. The dens is attached to the *occipital* bone by three ligaments—the apical, which extends straight forward to the floor of the foramen magnum, and the two lateral or alar ligaments, which attach medially to the caudal part of the occipital condyles. The dens is additionally attached to the floor of the spinal canal of the *atlas* by the heavy transverse ligament and the smaller and less important deeper ligaments. Rupture of these ligaments is an important part of the pathogenesis in either the congenital or the strictly traumatic form of the condition[83] (Figs. 13–28 and 13–29).

As mentioned earlier, the disorder occurs most frequently in the smaller breeds in dogs that are 6 to 18 months of age, and usually under 1 year. Occasionally an older dog about 3 to 4 years of age is affected; in such a case the congenital weakness was clinically dormant until the right stress was applied. The clinical signs are similar to those of a severely protruding cervical disk in that there is extreme pain in the head and neck, and the head is rigidly held in a lowered position. The dog resists any type of manipulation of the head and neck, and due to the severity of the compression, he frequently develops motor deficits which may result in tetraplegia. The pain appears to be one of the most intense seen in canine practice. Careful palpation of the area may reveal a dorsal displacement of the C2 dorsal arch.

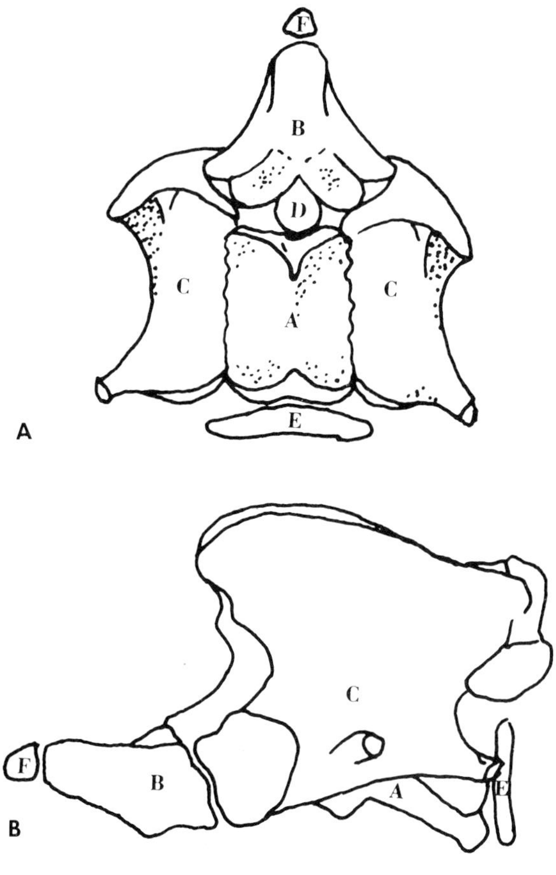

A

B

FIGURE 13–27 Ventral (*A*) and lateral (*B*) views of the axis illustrating centers of ossification: body (A), dens (B), arch (C), cranial epiphysis (D), caudal epiphysis (E), accessory center for apex of dens (F). (From Oliver, J. E., Jr., and Lewis, R. E.: Lesions of the atlas and axis in dogs. J. Am. Anim. Hosp. Assoc. *9*, 305, 1973.)

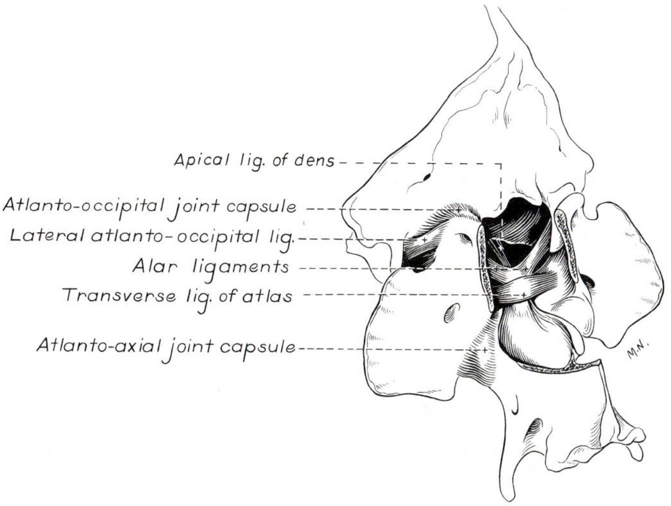

FIGURE 13–28 Ligaments of occiput, atlas, and axis. (From Miller, M. E., Christensen, G. C., and Evans, H. E.: *Anatomy of the Dog.* W. B. Saunders Co., Philadelphia, 1964.)

The causes can be classified as (1) absence or malformation of the dens, (2) fracture of the dens, or (3) insufficient ligamentous support of the dens. Any of these usually cause a rupture or severe stretching of the dorsal atlantoaxial ligament. The congenital absence of the odontoid process or dens leaves no internal support between the dens and the occipital or atlas bones, thereby causing a dorsal deviation or tilting of the anterior aspect of C2, which in turn ruptures the dorsal atlantoaxial ligament and compresses the cord. Odontoid fractures also cause a ruptured dorsal atlantoaxial ligament and, due to dramatic forces, a very severe compression of the cord which results in devastating clinical signs. Insufficient ligamentous support of the dens within the canal and the dorsal atlantoaxial ligament causes a C1–2 instability, possible rupture of the ligaments that are present, and a subluxating compression of the cord. Traumatic rupture of the ligaments that leaves the dens intact causes extremely severe compression of the cord and acute neurological signs[38] (Figs. 13–30 to 13–33).

The diagnosis in small breeds is aided by the history, breed predilection, and characteristic clinical signs. In traumatic subluxations of C1–2, the signs are so similar to fractures and luxations of the cranial por-

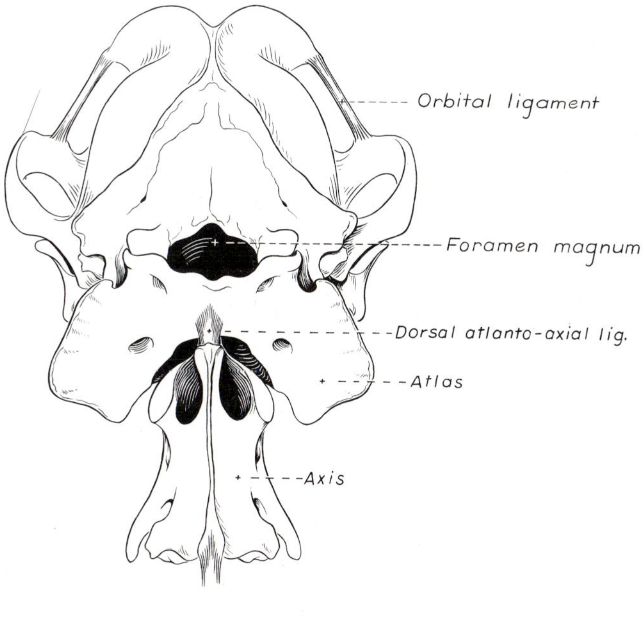

FIGURE 13–29 Atlanto-occipital space, head flexed, caudal aspect. (From Miller, M. E., Christensen, G. C., and Evans, H. E.: *Anatomy of the Dog.* W. B. Saunders Co., Philadelphia, 1964.)

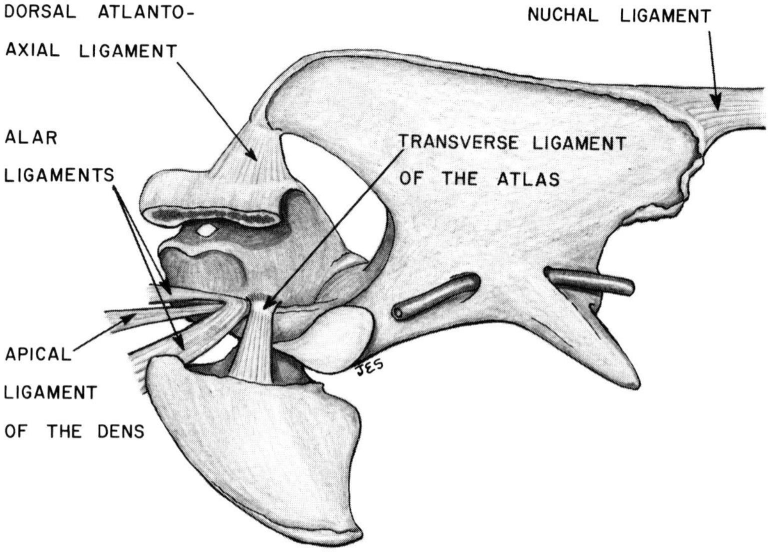

FIGURE 13–30 The normal relationship of the atlas and axis and the major anatomical structures. (From Gage, E. D., and Smallwood, J. E.: Surgical repair of atlantoaxial subluxation in a dog. Vet. Med. Small Anim. Clin. *65*, 583, 1970.)

tion of the cervical vertebrae that radiography is essential for even a tentative diagnosis. Radiographic examination should consist of extended and flexed lateral and ventrodorsal positions, and an occasional open mouth AP or basal view of the skull to demonstrate abnormal development of the dens. Other than initial scant films that can be made if the patient is cooperative, radiography should be performed under profound sedation or general anesthesia in order to minimize further injury to the cord and maximize interpretative detail of the lesion. The lateral projection characteristically shows the dorsal displacement of the atlas, particularly in a moderately flexed position of the head (Figs. 13–34 to 13–37).

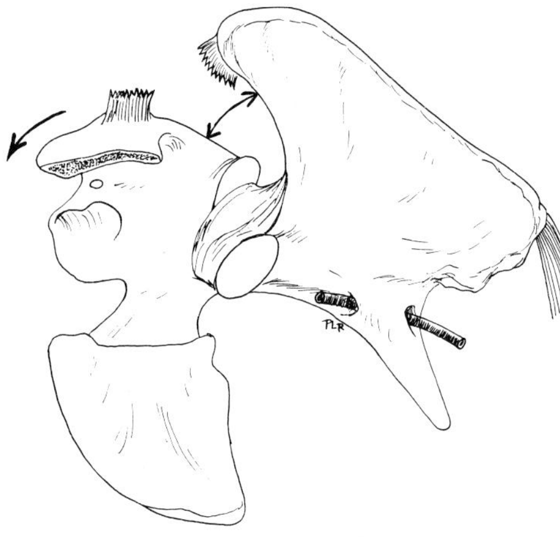

FIGURE 13–31 One cause of atlantoaxial subluxation is the congenital absence of the dens. The resulting lack of support of the ligaments of the dens leads to the rupture of the dorsal atlantoaxial ligament and a subluxation. (From Gage, E. D.: Atlantoaxial subluxation. *In* Bojrab, M. J. (ed.): *Current Techniques in Small Animal Surgery I.* Lea & Febiger, Philadelphia, 1975.)

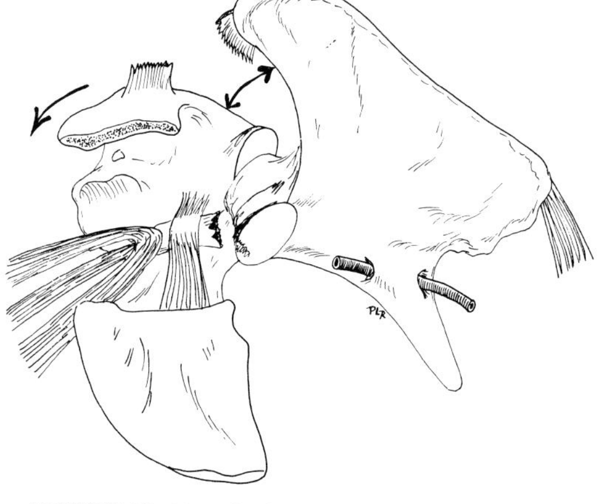

FIGURE 13–32 If a fractured dens occurs, the dorsal atlantoaxial ligament may rupture; a subluxation then occurs. (From Gage, E. D.: Atlantoaxial subluxation. *In* Bojrab, M. J. (ed.): *Current Techniques in Small Animal Surgery I.* Lea & Febiger, Philadelphia, 1975.)

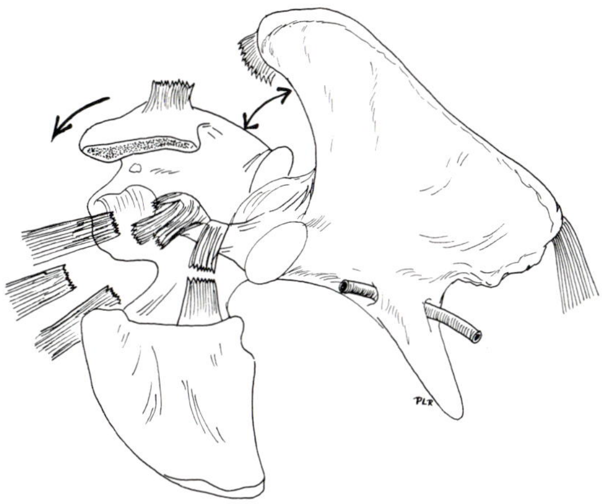

FIGURE 13-33 If a rupture of the dens ligament (alar and transverse ligament of atlas) occurs, undue stress on the dorsal atlantoaxial ligament may create a rupture that results in a subluxation. (From Gage, E. D.: Atlantoaxial subluxation. *In* Bojrab, M. J. (ed.): *Current Techniques in Small Animal Surgery I.* Lea & Febiger, Philadelphia, 1975.)

The prognosis for treatment is based on the extent and duration of the injury. If pain pathways are intact and motor deficits have not been present long enough to cause severe muscular spasticity, contractures, and atrophy, the prognosis is reasonably good.[83] The treatment generally consist of surgical reduction and immobilization of the C1–2 vertebrae with a decompression of the cord when needed. Occasionally a chronic, mild subluxation can be immobilized by coaptation splinting without surgery for 3 to 4 weeks, but usually even such cases do not heal without surgery.

The surgical approach is performed with the dog in a ventral recumbent position and the head in a padded and moderately flexed position or in a head stand used for cranial surgery. Care should be taken to minimize further compressions of the cord by manipulation or improper positioning. A dorsal midline incision is made over the caudal occipital bone to the caudal portion of the cervical spinal segment. The musculature is removed from the spine of the axis and from the arches of C1 and C2 by sharp or carefully blunt dissection. The periosteum is reflected from the arch of the atlas, and the spinal canal is carefully invaded on the cranial and caudal margins of the arch. Vascular damage should be avoided.

A hemilaminectomy is performed when decompression of the cord is needed in the acute case. In less severe cases, decompression takes place when the displacement of the atlas is reduced and C1–2 vertebrae are stabilized. Hemilaminectomy is performed

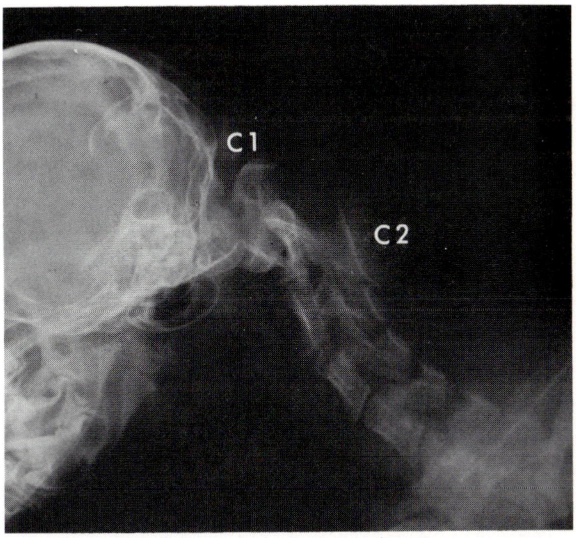

FIGURE 13-34 An atlanto-axial subluxation caused by an absence of the odontoid process and corresponding lack of ligamentous support and stabilization of C1–C2.

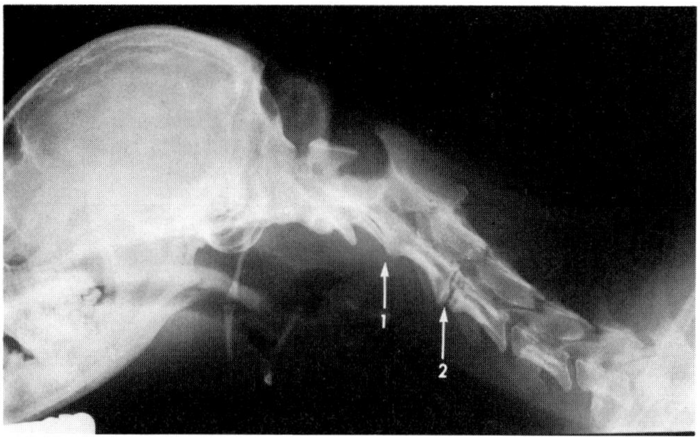

FIGURE 13–35 A less severe case of atlantoaxial dislocation. (1) A fusion of C2–3 vertebrae resulting from possible trauma. (2) Fragmentation at C3–4 that appears to have resulted from fracture. Because of lack of vertebral displacement, callous formation and fusion may result in C2–3.

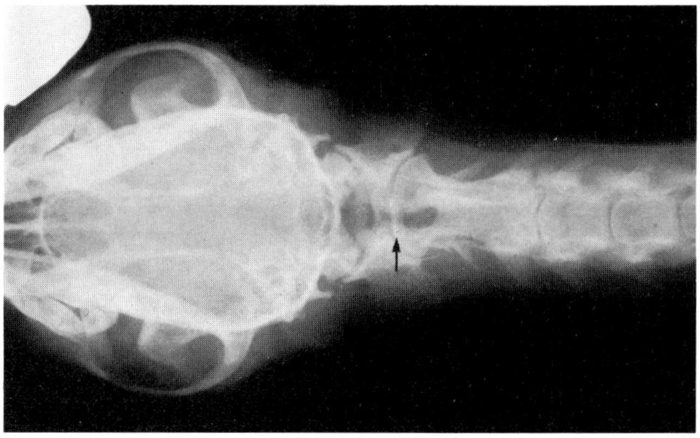

FIGURE 13–36 Ventrodorsal view of the case shown in Figure 13–35. Note the absence of the dens.

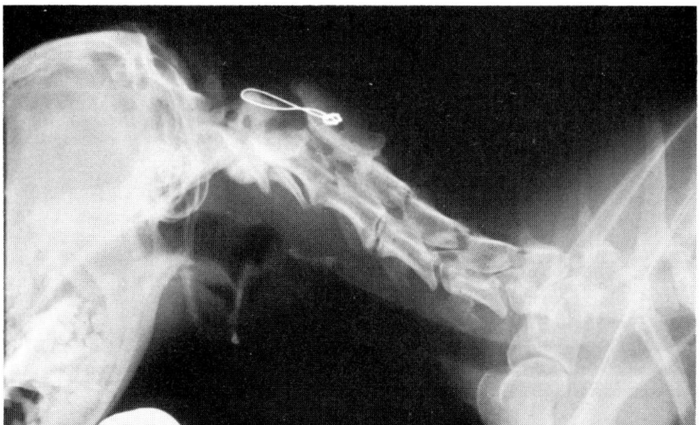

FIGURE 13–37 Same case as shown in Figure 13–35 after decompression and skeletal fixation.

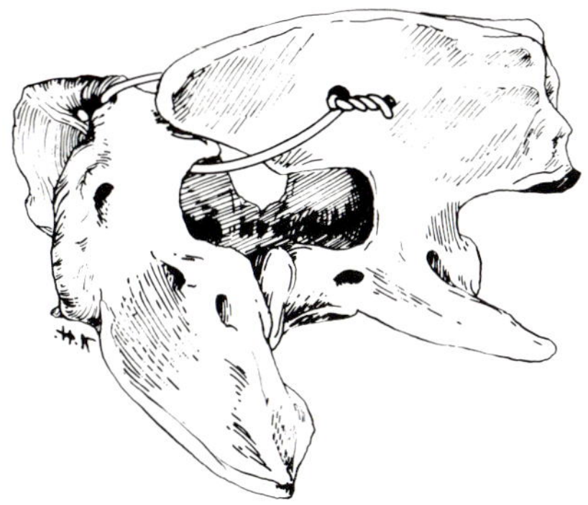

FIGURE 13–38 The single strand of orthopedic wire can be used as illustrated; however, the double strand affords better stabilization. (From Swaim, S. F.: Surgical approaches to spinal cord disease of small animals. Proc. Am. Anim. Hosp. Assoc. Vol. 1, 1975.)

by carefully removing the lateral lamina of the cranial aspect of C2 and the caudal aspect of C1. Care should be used to avoid the vertebral artery and anastomotic veins on the dorsolateral aspects of the cord.

The most suitable means of vertebral immobilization is use of single or double strand wiring of the involved C1–2 vertebrae. One method is to pass a looped 20 or 22 gauge malleable orthopedic stainless steel strand of wire longitudinally under the dorsal arch of the atlas from the caudal to the cranial aspect. This must be done carefully so as not to traumatize the cord. Flexion of the head or caudal traction of C2 by placing a small dural or ovarohysterectomy hook in the cranial brim of the C1 arch will facilitate the passage of wire. The soft tissue must have been dissected from the cranial and caudal rims of the C1 arch in order to expose the canal (Figs. 13–38 to 13–40). An alternate method used by the author is to drill small holes on each of the dorsolateral aspects of the arch of C1 and pass the looped wire transversely under the arch of C1 and dorsal to the cord. One or two holes are drilled in the spine of the axis at an appropriate distance from the atlas for maximal tension and reduction of the displacement. The wires are passed from the arch of C1 through the axial holes and are twisted together tightly after reduction has been accomplished. The looped wire can be cut so that each of the double strands are tied individually in a "saddle type" arrangement. This method affords maximum stability and strength[40, 83] (Fig. 13–41).

The tissues are approximated in individual layers for closure. A metal splint is sometimes applied from the dorsal aspect of the skull to the caudal cervical area in order to promote immobility during the postoperative healing period. Postoperative treatment may consist of drugs such as broad spectrum antibiotics, steroids, hypertonic mannitol solutions, and anticatecholamines. Good nursing care is essential in severe cases.

Abnormal Odontoid Process Angulation

An unusual disorder of the odontoid process angulation and cord compression has been seen by Parker[89] and Swaim.[110] The former case was a 6-month-old miniature poodle in whom the process projected upward into the spinal canal at a 45 degree angle, causing primarily ataxia and moderate spinal cord compression. At necropsy there was no evidence of a fracture, nonfusion of the dens, or abnormalities of the dens ligaments. Swaim's case was a male Pekingese, aged 6 months, who had profound neurological deficits over a period of 6 days after a fall. Surgical removal of the dens (also angled upward at 45 degrees) was performed by a ventral "slot" type of decompression. Clinical recovery was prompt and complete[110] (Fig. 13–42). It is felt that both cases are further evidence of odontoid abnormality but without the usual subluxation of C1–2.

Canine Wobbler Syndrome

This disorder is a progressive cervical spinal cord compression usually seen in Great Danes and Doberman pinscher dogs, but when appropriate trauma has occurred, it can be seen in any breed. In early reports[20, 25, 39, 42, 52] excessive mobility of the spine or spondylolisthesis was thought to be solely responsible for the spinal compression. Further studies have demonstrated that probably one of the basic defects is a malformation of one or more of the caudal cervical vertebrae that results in a smaller dorsoventral diameter in the spinal canal in the cranial part of the vertebra. Lateral stenosis of the spinal canal can exist from hyperostosis of the articular facets. Malfor-

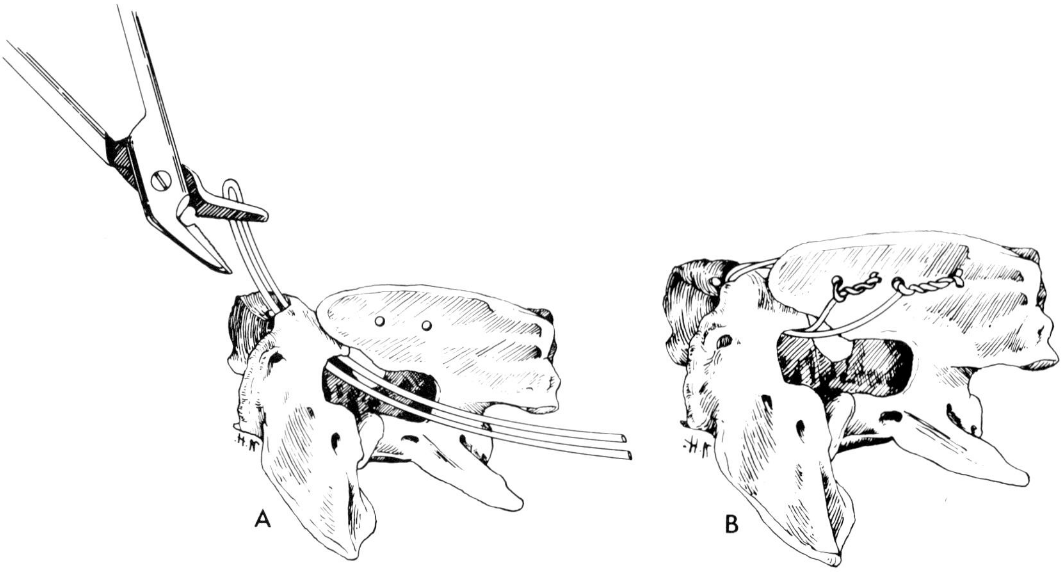

FIGURE 13–39 A double strand is placed on one side of the axis. *A*, After cutting the loop, both of these strands are tied on the other side of the axis to the original strands, which have been treated through the drilled holes (*B*). (From Swaim, S. F.: Proc. Am. Anim. Hosp. Assoc. Vol. 1, 1975.)

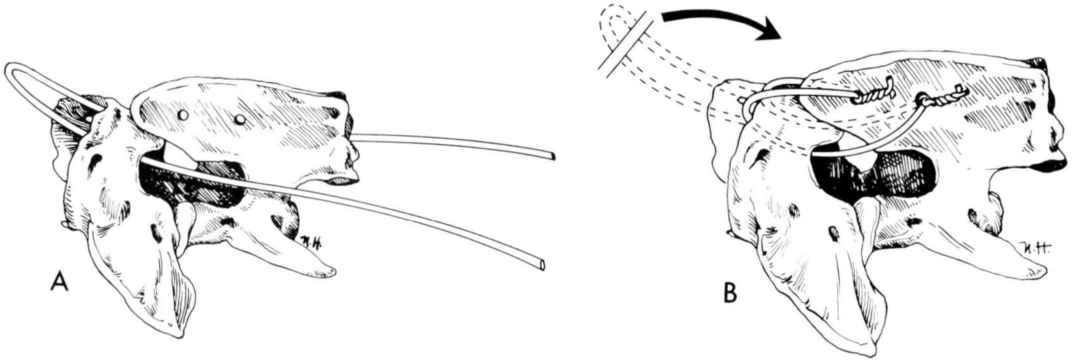

FIGURE 13–40 *A*, In this method, the caudal strands lie on opposite sides of the axis. *B*, The cranial and caudal pairs of strands are tied together in their respective drill holes, forming a true bilaterally symmetrical sling. (From Swaim, S. F.: Proc. Am. Anim. Hosp. Assoc. Vol. 1, 1975.)

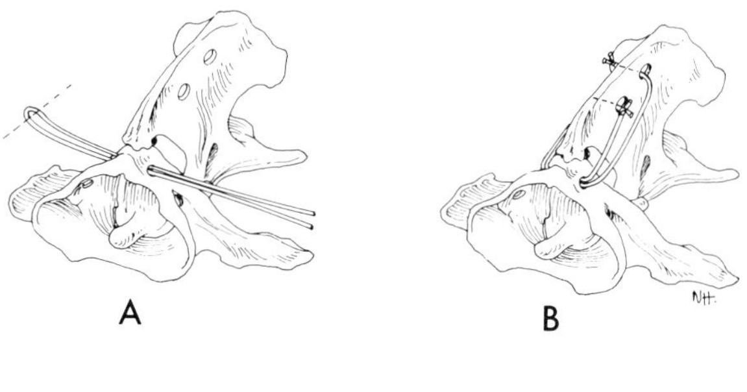

FIGURE 13–41 Another method used occasionally eliminates the tedious threading of the wire under the arch of the atlas (which may traumatize the cord). In this method, the wire is placed transversely through suitably placed drill holes. Trauma to the cord is minimized in this procedure; however, the bony support of the atlas may not be as great as in the longitudinal placement.

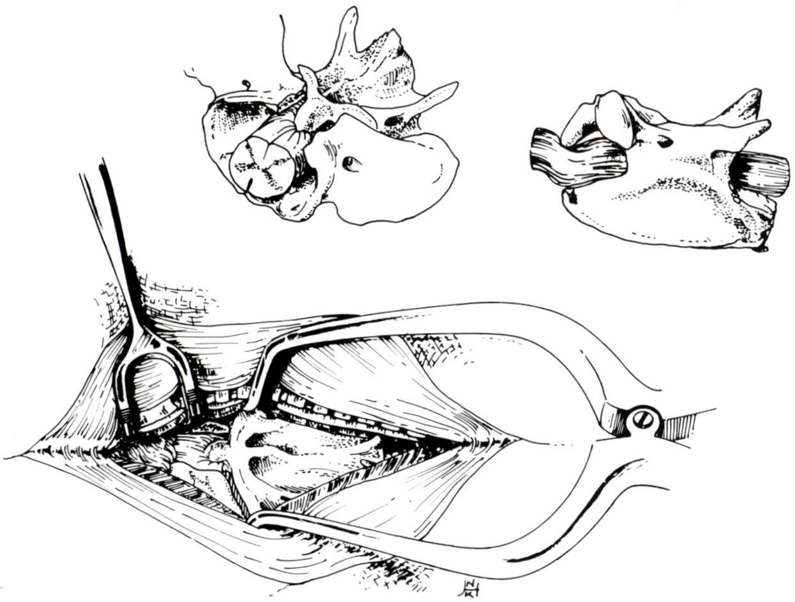

FIGURE 13–42 Angulation of the dens. The dog is in the dorsal recumbent position. The upper right view shows the dens or odontoid process angulated against the cord. In the ventral approach, the ventral arch of the atlas is burred off by means of a high speed drill, and the dens is removed from the cord. Recovery results. (From Swaim, S. F.: Odontoidectomy in the dog. J. Am. Anim. Hosp. Assoc. *11*, 663, 1975.)

mation of the vertebral body or its articulations can result in vertebral instability which may contribute to a hypertrophy of the ligamentum flavum, dorsal longitudinal ligament, or dorsal annulus. Frequently the surgeon observes what appears to be an annular constriction of fibrous tissue around the cord at the vertebral junction. Occasionally the syndrome is initiated by a "keel"-shaped vertebra or even a hemivertebra. One or all of these factors may be involved in the syndrome in Great Danes, Dobermans, and other large breeds of dog.[20, 104, 123] Wright feels that there are many similarities between the vertebral anomaly in Great Danes and Dobermans and that in young male basset hounds, ridgebacks, and thoroughbred horses in that it is a result of abnormal forces exerted on growing vertebrae[123] (Figs. 13–43 to 13–46).

The precise cause of the disorder is un-

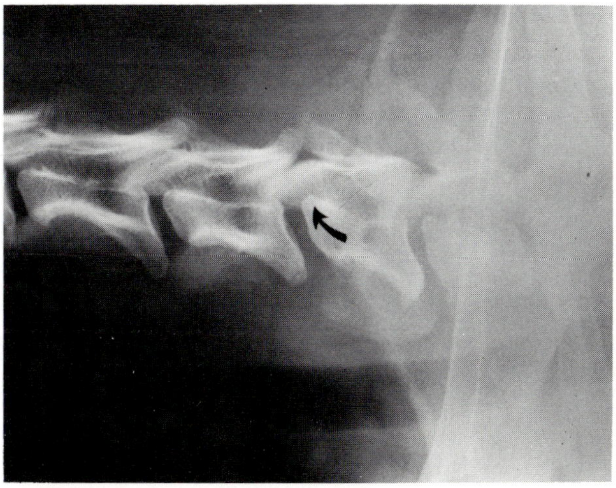

FIGURE 13–43 Canine wobbler syndrome in a 7-year-old Doberman pinscher manifested by a cervical vertebral instability and upward displacement of C6 (arrow), which resulted in a cord compression. Notice that this is the extended lateral projection.

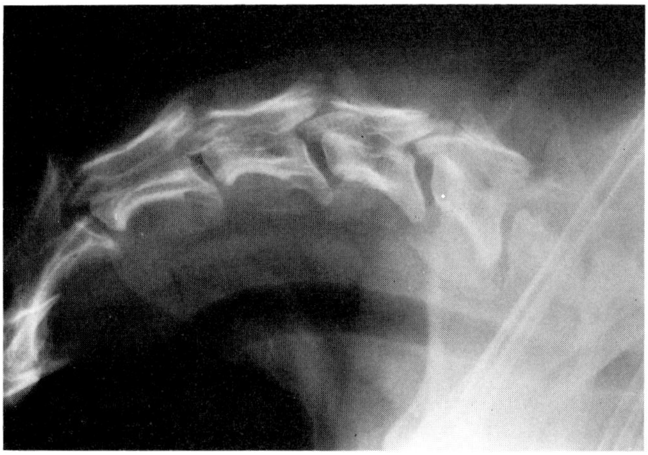

FIGURE 13–44 Same case as Figure 13–43. The flexed lateral projection still shows upward displacement of C6 but not as dramatically as in the extended position.

certain. The predilection for certain breeds and the tendency to occur in a certain breeding line and in littermates suggest a hereditary factor. The very large head of the Great Dane may exert an unusual force on the caudal cervical vertebrae in the growing puppy. A nutritional study in Great Danes has established the relationship between overnutrition (protein, calcium, phosphorus) and skeletal changes, including the cervical vertebrae.[49]

The clinical signs of the wobbler syndrome usually begin between 3 and 18 months of age; however, dogs up to 8 years old have been seen, especially Dobermans. Traumatic vertebral instabilities, luxations, and spondylolisthesis can occur in any breed, large or small, at any age. The typical signs are generally those of the UMN with varying degrees of bilaterally symmetrical paraparesis, tetraparesis, ataxia, wide-based stance, limbs crossing on turning, and knuckling of pelvic limbs. A spastic gait, hypermetria, hyperreflexia of the patellar reflex, poor postural reactions in the pelvic limbs especially, and a general clumsiness are also present. There generally is little cervical pain or rigidity. The onset is gradual and the course is progressive. The traumatic cases show more acute signs resulting from caudal cervical compression. The differential diagnosis excludes the possibility of disk protrusion, fractures, luxations, tumors, distemper myelitis, and the various musculoskeletal disorders of young, growing dogs of giant breeds.

The diagnosis in wobblers is suspected from the clinical history, breed, and characteristic signs. Since laboratory examinations are usually negative, radiographic examinations are necessary. Plain films may reveal the vertebral displacement in an extended lateral and occasionally in a flexed position. However, the flexion studies may be dif-

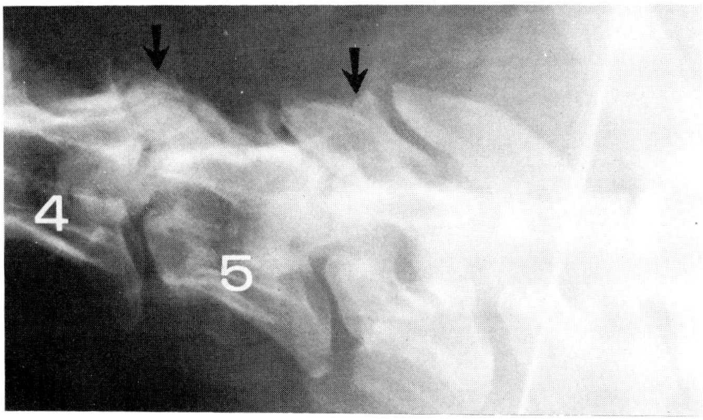

FIGURE 13–45 Cervical spondylopathy. Lateral view of the caudal cervical vertebrae. The dorsal spinous processes have an unusual shape, and there is new bone production on the dorsal aspects of the vertebrae (arrows). No site of cord compression can be identified. (From Bailey, C. S., and Holliday, T. A.: Diseases of the spinal cord. *In* Ettinger, S. J.: *Textbook of Veterinary Internal Medicine.* W. B. Saunders Co., Philadelphia, 1975.)

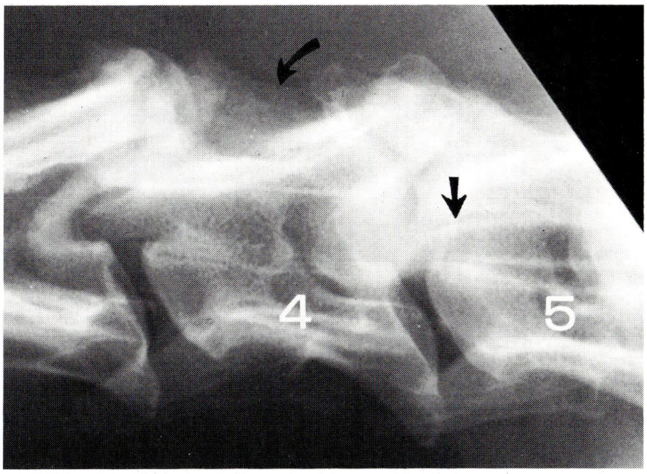

FIGURE 13–46 Water soluble myelography in same case as shown in Figure 13–45. The dorsal contrast column is depressed at C4–5 (straight arrow). Both the dorsal and ventral contrast columns terminate at this point, and the spinal cord is narrowed, suggesting compression by hypertrophic ligamentous structures. Note the new bone formation on the dorsal arches in this radiograph (curved arrow) as well as in Figure 13–45. This was a 3-year-old Great Dane that had a sudden onset of quadriplegia. (From Bailey, C. S. and Holliday, T. A.: Diseases of the spinal cord. *In* Ettinger, S. J.: *Textbook of Veterinary Internal Medicine.* W. B. Saunders Co., Philadelphia, 1975.)

ficult to interpret because the normal range of motion in these vertebrae is considerable. Plain films may demonstrate vertebral canal malformations, sclerosis and exostosis around vertebral joints, and sclerosis or ventral bridging of the vertebral body junctions. Subtle changes in spinal canal confirmation, fibrotic tissue proliferations, and concomitant disk protrusions may demand myelographic studies.

The histological changes in the affected cord are characteristic of cord compression and trauma. Swollen axons are prevalent throughout the white matter but are most prominent in the dorsal columns and dorsal spinocerebellar tracts. Demyelination and gliosis were prevalent in the traumatized area.[94]

The treatment generally involves surgical stabilization or decompression. Coaptation

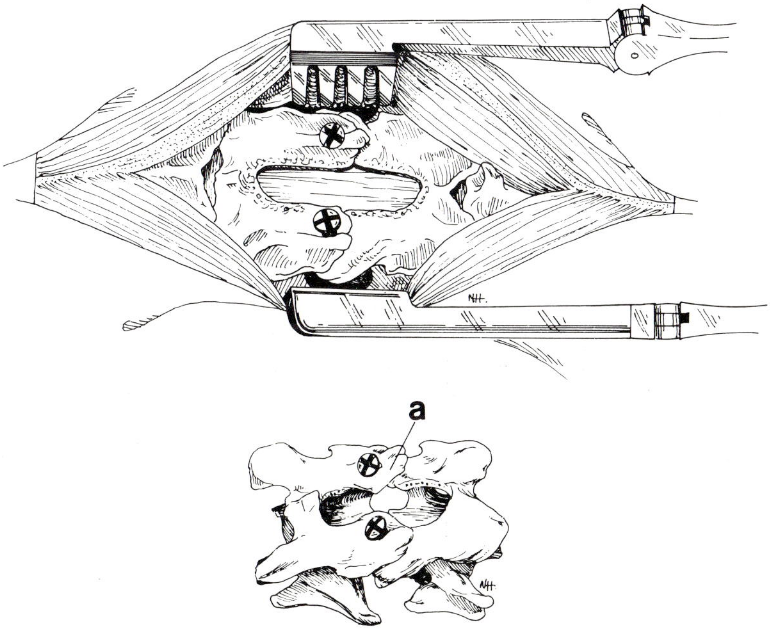

FIGURE 13–47 In the canine wobbler syndrome, a dorsal laminectomy is performed to relieve the fibrous and osseous constriction of the cord. Immobilization is obtained by bilateral placement of Bechtol radial-fluted point buttress-threaded screws in the heaviest portion of the overlapping articular processes (a) of the involved vertebrae. Notice the angulation of the screws in the insert drawing. (Courtesy of Dr. S. F. Swain.)

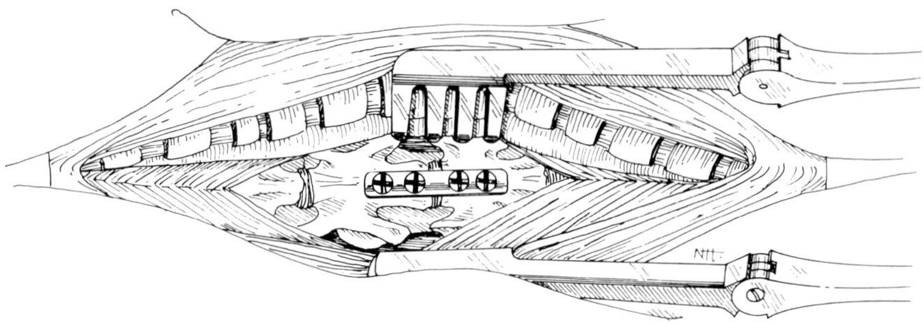

FIGURE 13–48 Bone screws and plates can be placed on the smooth ventral surfaces of the involved vertebrae for stabilization of unstable vertebrae (wobbler syndrome). This procedure may involve a separate surgical dorsal laminectomy for decompression of the cord. (Courtesy of Dr. S. F. Swaim.)

splinting or casting alone is usually difficult to maintain on the animal and is generally ineffective. Surgical dorsal decompressive laminectomy without further stabilization has been reported to be effective in alleviating progress of the signs.[20] Dorsal laminectomy with plating or stapling of the adjacent dorsal spines has been reported. Swaim[109] has proposed a midline dorsal laminectomy and careful bilateral placement of Bechtol radial, fluted-point, buttress-threaded bone screws through the heaviest portion of the overlapping articular processes of the affected vertebrae. He preferred this method to several other cervical fixation procedures investigated, including wiring articular processes, inserting bone screws in the bodies of involved vertebrae, and applying bone plates on the ventral surfaces of involved bodies with bone screws into the bodies.[109] Knecht and Oliver have proposed a peg bone graft placed in a trephine hole at the ventral intervertebral space of the vertebral bodies involved, reinforcing it with a long bone plate and screws affixed to the ventral involved and adjacent vertebral bodies.[60] Dueland proposed a dorsal decompressive laminectomy and stabilization by dorsal bone graft and wire fixation in the articular facet areas.[25] Gage and Hoerlein reported eight cases of vertebral instability in which bone screws were angled in the bodies of the affected vertebral junction from a ventral approach. This procedure may or may not be combined with a dorsal decompressive laminectomy, depending on the severity of the cord impingement[39] (Figs. 13–47 to 13–49).

The surgical approaches used in these methods are described in the chapters dealing with disks and fractures (Chapters 14

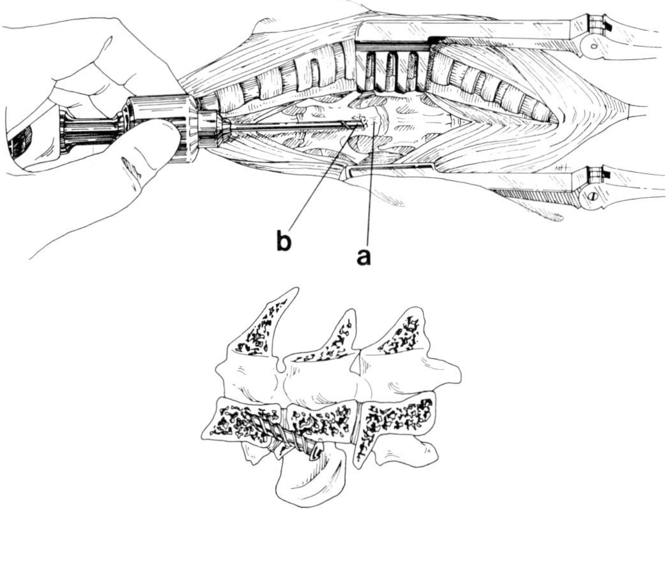

FIGURE 13–49 In cervical vertebral instability, the involved area can be stabilized by placing bone screws in the vertebral bodies. A drill (b) is directed from the body of the cranial vertebra downward and caudally into the body of the caudal vertebra in the ventral prominence cranial to the disk (a). Insert shows the placement of the screw.

and 15). At present the surgeon decides what method to use depending on what the patient needs and which method he can best perform. Surgical results will be most satisfactory if treatment is begun early, before permanent cord damage has occurred.

MALFORMATIONS

Morgan studied the incidence of congenital anomalies of the vertebral column in a total of 145 dogs 2 years of age and older who had been submitted for necropsy. An additional 26 dogs had been presented for destruction. A total of 84 congenital changes were found in 68 of the 145 dissected specimens (47 per cent). Changes were most common at the junctions between the major divisions of the spinal column. These included the cervical ribs, lumbarization of T13, sacralization of L7, lumbarization of S1, and fusion of S3 and Cy1. Hemivertebrae and block vertebrae were also seen. Change in position of anticlinal vertebrae was common. Almost all of the dogs had numerous minor changes of the articular facets of the true synovial joints of the vertebral column. No changes produced clinical signs.[75]

Vertebral and spinal cord anomalies can be classified into two major groups based on a common embryological origin: the vertebral body and intervertebral disk abnormalities, which are mesodermal in origin (e.g., block vertebra, butterfly vertebra, hemivertebra), and the vertebral arch and spinal cord anomalies, which are ectodermal in origin (e.g., spina bifida, syringomyelia, spinal dysraphism). Vertebral body–intervertebral disk abnormalities are usually traumatic or compressive due to instability or malalignment of the spinal canal. Clinical myelopathies associated with abnormalities of ectodermal origin are generally the result of spinal cord malformation and are usually not treatable.[4]

SPINA BIFIDA

Spina bifida may be defined as a defect in the closure of the arch formed by the dorsal laminae of the spinal vertebrae. As the term is commonly used, it also implies hernial involvement of the cord or meninges. The absence of dorsal laminae in spina bifida produces a sac-like protrusion that is called, if it involves the meninges, a meningocele, and a meningomyelocele if it includes the cord and nerve roots. Spina bifida occulta is a localized defect of one or more arches *without* protrusion of the meninges or cord.[10, 53, 69] The pathogenesis of the spina bifida complex is not known, but the theories include rupture of an already closed neural tube; hyperplasia and overgrowth of neural tube cells, preventing neural tube fusion; teratogenic drugs; and vascular defects.[93]

Frye has reported spina bifida with sacrococcygeal agenesis in a cat[35] and a spina

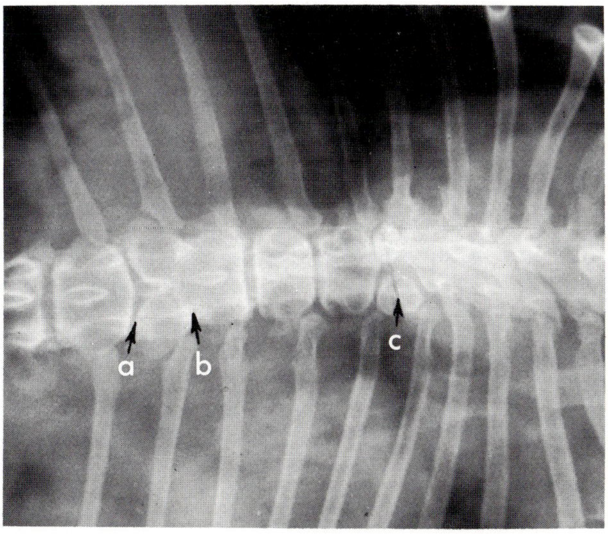

FIGURE 13–50 VD radiograph shows various spinal anomalies: (a) butterfly vertebra characteristic of hemivertebra, (b) block vertebra, (c) more extensive hemivertebrae with a probable slight spina bifida.

bifida with rachischisis.[37] The first case was a normally proportioned, bright and alert 8-week-old kitten who was studied for 18 months before euthanasia was performed. She walked on her hocks in the back legs and had urinary and bowel dysfunction (Fig. 13–50).

Case reports of spina bifida in dogs include Boston terriers, Dalmation puppies, a mixed breed, a Chihuahua, and an 8-month-old bulldog.[2, 14, 69, 102] The bulldog was diagnosed by normal and contrast radiography and necropsy as having a spinal bifida meningomyelocele; fecal and urinary incontinence and paralysis of the penis were the primary neurological signs.[93] The Chihuahua was a puppy a few days old with flaccid paraplegia and edematous hind legs. The dorsal arches of L5–Cy1 were absent, and a cleft in this area through all layers of skin, subcutaneous tissues, and meninges exposed the cauda equina.[14] Although published case reports of spina bifida in dogs and cats are few, the existence of the disorder is probably not too rare.

HEMIVERTEBRA

Hemivertebra results from the failure of the centers of ossification of the right and left halves of the vertebral bodies to fuse. This is due to the persistence of the dorsoventral septum, which arose from the remnant of the perichondral sheath surrounding the notochord. The various forms of hemivertebra result from the location of the remaining functional ossification center. If the defect extends throughout the length of the vertebral body, it is divided into nearly equal parts. The cranial and caudal vertebral end-plates have a funnel shape and in a dorsoventral radiograph the vertebral body looks like a butterfly, hence the term "butterfly" vertebra.[4] Another form of hemivertebra appears when a portion of hemivertebra is absent (unilateral ossification), making it appear to be cuneiform with the base lateral and apex extending across the midline. Scoliosis can result from this type of hemivertebra. If the dorsal or ventral halves of the vertebral ossification centers fail to develop, a cuneiform-shaped vertebra (as viewed laterally) results.[72] In lateral radiographs, the triangular shape is usually positioned with the apex ventrally and base dorsally; however, the reverse position may occur. If dorsal displacement from adjacent vertebrae occurs, compression of the cord may account for clinical signs. Trauma will either initiate or aggravate a clinical syndrome.[75, 101]

Since hemivertebra tends to accompany scoliosis or kinked tail, the condition is most frequently seen in the English bulldog and Boston terrier. Frequently, the animals are asymptomatic, although intermittent pain and posterior paresis or paraplegia have been seen.

The veterinary literature has in recent years dealt more with the clinical manifestations associated with hemivertebrae. One report cites three cases of hemivertebra diagnosed on plain film radiography; these had demonstrable spinal cord compression with myelography. A 3-month-old West Highland terrier, a 4-year-old beagle, and a 3-month-old Doberman were affected with varying degrees of neurological deficits.[91] A 7-month-old German shepherd puppy showed pelvic limb motor deficits due to a wedge vertebra at T13–L1.[64] Hemivertebrae from T5–11 caused severe kyphoscoliosis of the thoracic spine with pain and minor motor deficits in a 15-month-old pug.[44] Necropsies on ten bulldog puppies up to 12 weeks of age revealed a possible association of abnormal vertebral development and neonatal death. A 10-week-old puppy developed pelvic limb paresis because of a spinal cord compression at T10 from a hemivertebra.[23]

Hemivertebra generally necessitates little or no treatment. If symptoms are pronounced from malalignment and pressure on the cord, in dogs other than young puppies, a decompression and appropriate fusion or stabilization should be considered (Figs. 13–51 to 13–55).

SCOLIOSIS, KYPHOSIS, LORDOSIS

Scoliosis, kyphosis, and lordosis are disorders of the spine causing an abnormal curvature. A common cause of scoliosis or lateral curvature is the presence of hemivertebrae. Kyphosis, or dorsal arching, is frequently seen in cases of cord compression, arthritic spinal disorders, and spondy-

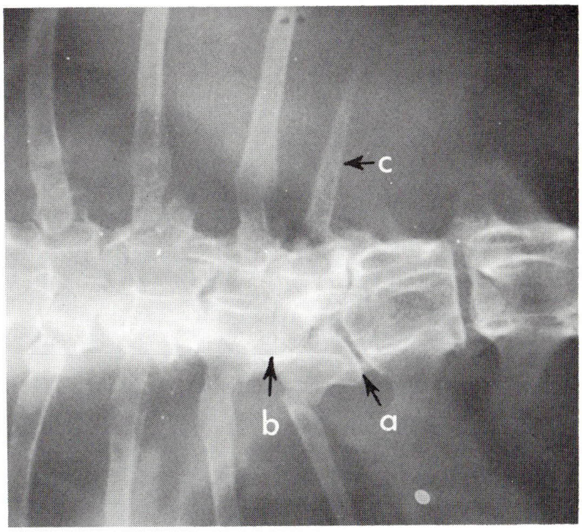

FIGURE 13–51 Hemivertebra at (a) T13; (b) nonsegmentation of T12–13; and (c) vestigial last rib.

losis. In disk protrusions, the protrusion can be flattened somewhat by extreme dorsal arching of the back, by which the dog apparently attempts to alleviate pain. Lordosis, or sway back (ventral arching), may result from hemivertebra in the thoracic region with a kyphosis caudal to this area. Lordosis in cats may result from hypomineralized bones, as in secondary hyperparathyroidism.[72] Extremely old and heavy dogs may show this defect, probably because of relaxation of the dorsal spinal musculature and fibrotic vertebral support (Fig. 13–54). A cervical kyphosis occurred in a 5-month-old Afghan hound with marked physical contour deformity and deficits in proprioception. Aplasia of the left articular facets in C2 and C3, reduction of length of the vertebral body of C3, and other defects were noted on radiographic and necropsy examination.[85]

BLOCK AND FUSED VERTEBRAE

Block or incompletely segmented vertebrae occur congenitally in areas of the spine in which two or more vertebrae appear as one. Bony structures are normal in appearance with no evidence of bone destruction or periosteal proliferation. If the spinal canal is of normal size and contour, no clinical signs will be noticed, but frequently the canal is not normal. Because of this consolidation, the movement of adjacent vertebrae may be so abnormal that periodic pain and motor dysfunction from compression of the cord result. This disorder may be caused by chondrification and ossification taking place in the portion of the sclerotome intended to become the intervertebral disk. Occasionally a remnant of the disk will be evident by a thin radiolucent line. Fusion of the vertebrae occurs

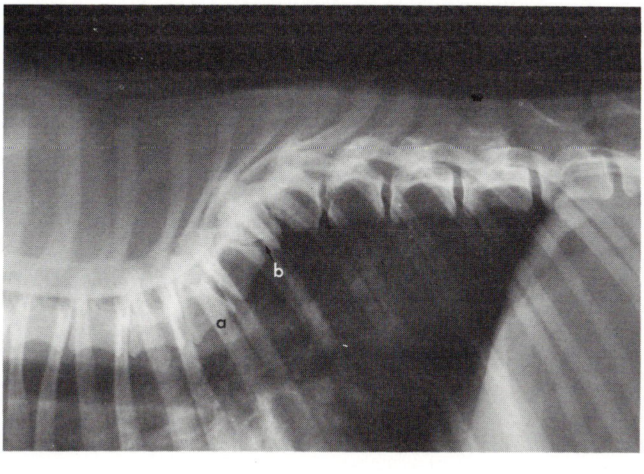

FIGURE 13–52 This lateral myelogram demonstrates (a) a severe spinal curvature and (b) a hemivertebra. Notice the dorsal displacement and spinal compression.

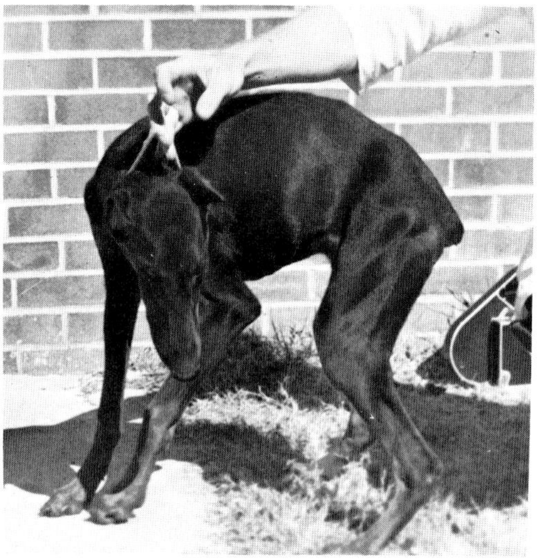

FIGURE 13–53 A 10-month-old Doberman pinscher. Notice the lateral and dorsal spinal curvatures.

following injuries and sepsis. Discospondylitis or other types of vertebral osteomyelitis may result in fused vertebrae,[73] and radiographs show evidence of inflammation, destruction, and proliferative changes.

If compression of the spinal cord has resulted from either type of vertebral consolidation, decompressive surgery should be performed. The results from hemilaminectomy or dorsal laminectomy have been gratifying (Figs. 13–56 and 13–57).

DEFORMATION OF CERVICAL VERTEBRAE IN BASSET HOUNDS

Palmer described six highly inbred basset puppies that showed ataxia initially from birth to 6 months of age.[84] The incoordination started in hind legs and later involved the front limbs. The dogs became totally recumbent. Necropsy showed a gross deformity of the third cervical vertebra that compressed the cord. The joints of C2–3 or C3–4 were the primary compressive sites. Severe degeneration of both white and gray matter resulted in the compressed area. The evidence shows it to be a heritable disorder. No treatment has been attempted; however, decompressive surgery could possibly be of value in mild or slight cases.[84]

SHORT SPINE DEFORMITY

Hansen[47] and Ueshima[118] have reported individually on short spine deformations. This disorder may be termed perocormus or perosomus. This condition was portrayed graphically in dogs as early as 1668, and there have been scattered reports of similar conditions in calves, goats, turkeys, and pigs. These monstrosities exhibit severe shortening of the vertebral column but the head and extremities are of normal length. There is a dextro rotation of the

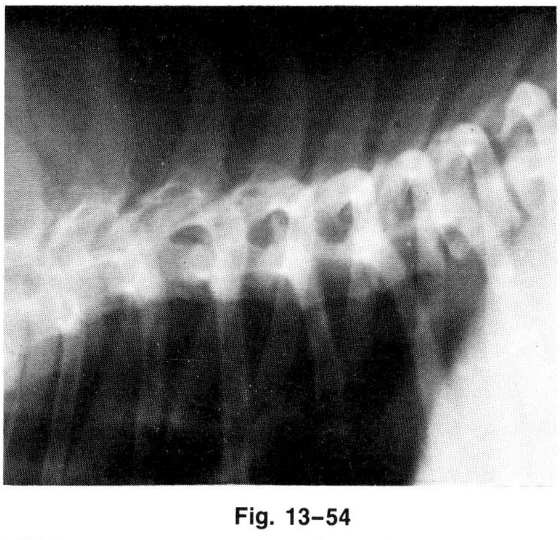

Fig. 13–54

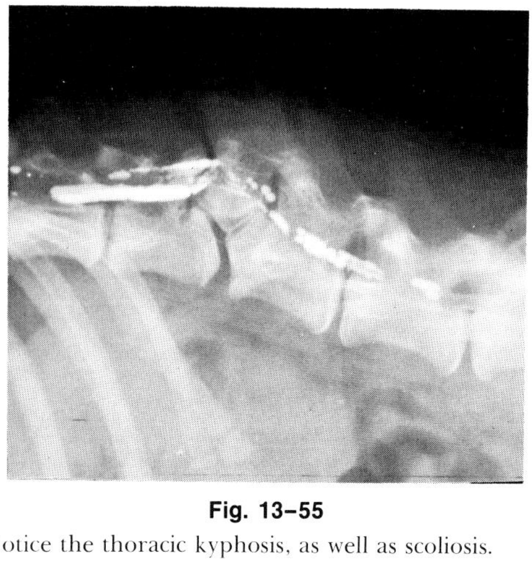

Fig. 13–55

FIGURE 13–54 Same case as shown in Figure 13–53. Notice the thoracic kyphosis, as well as scoliosis.

FIGURE 13–55 Same case as shown in Figures 13–53 and 13–54. Notice the dorsally displaced hemivertebra and subarachnoid blockage of Pantopaque. If the hemivertebra were counted, two other lumbar vertebra would be absent in this case of spinal deformity.

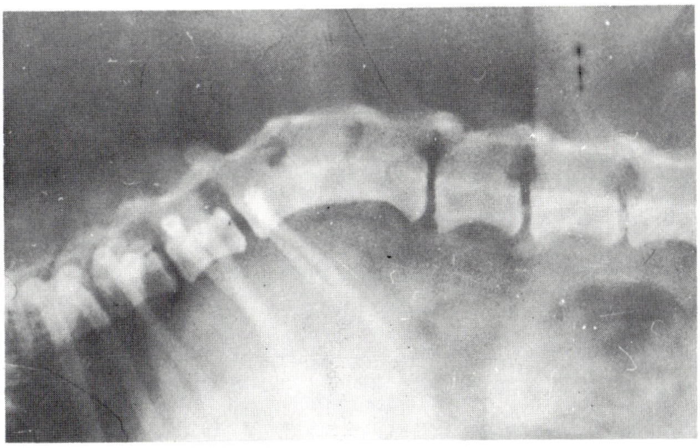

FIGURE 13–56 Fused T13, L1, and L2 vertebrae. Many authorities believe that this disorder is a case of nonsegmentation of vertebrae. This was a 3-year-old Manchester terrier who suffered from occasional atacks of spinal pain and weakness. (From Hoerlein, B. F.: Pathological conditions of the spinal cord in domestic animals. Auburn Vet. 9, 97, Winter, 1953.)

head, absence of cervical vertebrae, kyphosis in the shoulder and lumbar region, and shortening of the tail. The condition is similar to chondrodystrophy, and it results from a highly disordered vertebral ossification.[47, 118] Corresponding anomalies of the spinal cord develop from vertebral ossification disorders. The shortening of the cord is most conspicuous from the caudal cervical to the thoracic part, where two to eight spinal ganglia might have a common sheath.[108]

TRANSITIONAL VERTEBRAE

Morgan has described transitional vertebrae located at junctions of major divisions of the column, where a segment may assume the characteristics of either division. At the cervicothoracic junction, the change consists of a cervical rib on C7, unilateral or bilateral. At the thoracolumbar junction, changes are more common and may appear in either direction. The thirteenth thoracic segment may have a fused, thick, stubby, transverse process, unilateral or bilateral, instead of the normal thirteenth rib. Less commonly, the first lumbar vertebra may have a unilateral or bilateral rib that articulates with the vertebral body rather than the fused transverse process. At the lumbosacral junction, L7 may be fused with the sacrum either unilaterally or bilaterally. The large wing takes the place of the normally appearing lateral transverse process. The shift may be in the opposite caudal direction and S1 may possess transverse processes rather than normal alae that fuse with the ilium. These changes may be called *sacralization* of the last lumbar segment or *lumbarization* of the first sacral segment.[72]

SACROCOCCYGEAL DYSGENESIS OF MANX CATS

Manx cats are bred for absence of a tail, but numbers of these cats also have sacral deformities and spinal cord abnormalities.

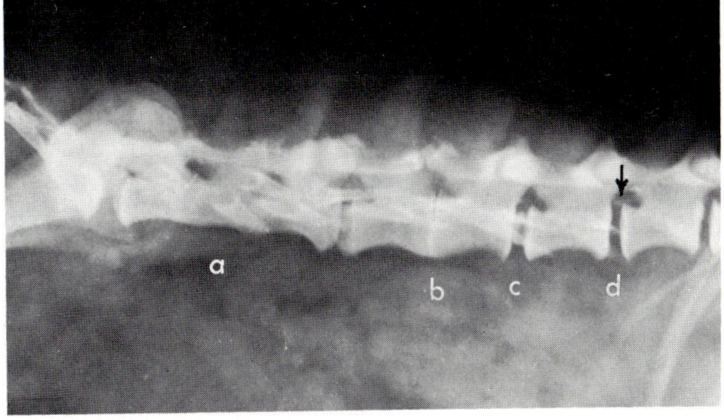

FIGURE 13–57 A case showing (a) fusion or nonsegmentation of L5–7 vertebrae. Notice the (b) partial fusion at L4–5, (c) calcified nucleus pulposus at L2–3, and (d) an osteophyte or calcification of the dorsal longitudinal ligament at L1–2. (From Hoerlein, B. F.: Clinical spinal radiography in the dog. J.A.V.M.A. *134*, 347, 1959.)

Osseous deformities are variable and range from spina bifida to complete sacrococcygeal agenesis. Spinal cord anomalies may include meningocele, meningomyelocele, syringomyelia, and spinal dysraphism. Pedigree analysis in five generations of Manx cats with these defects has indicated autosomal dominant inheritance for the Manx factor (taillessness), with incomplete penetrance of locomotor and fecal and urine incontinence abnormalities (Figs. 13–58 and 13–59).[4, 63]

CONGENITAL MALFORMATION OF THE FORAMEN MAGNUM (OCCIPITAL DYSPLASIA)

Bardens reports a disorder of toy breeds in which a malformation of the occipital bone results in an enlargement of the foramen magnum, which exposes the brain stem and the cerebellum.[7] Morgan has observed that congenital shortening of the atlas or C1 frequently accompanies the enlargement of the foramen magnum.[72] Some dogs remain asymptomatic, but others suffer sudden personality changes or pain. The time of appearance of the disorder has varied from birth to 4 years of age. Concomitant hydrocephalus has been seen in young dogs. Other dogs have demonstrated a caudal displacement of the brain stem into the spinal canal of the atlas and axis. There is evidence that this disorder is heritable.[7]

In dogs the changes in the base of the skull and first cervical vertebra resemble in part the so-called Arnold-Chiari malformation in man. In man, spina bifida with or without a myelomeningocele may be present. A similar disorder in man, Klippel-Feil syndrome, is characterized by several deformities in the cervical vertebrae, such as block vertebrae, defective segmentation, reduction in AP diameter of the individual segments, spina bifida, meningocele, the enlarged foramen magnum and malformed first cervical vertebra, and presence of a cervical rib.[72] Parker feels that since the disorder in the dog does not correspond exactly to either syndrome in man, the term occipital dysplasia would be descriptive[92] (Figs. 13–60 to 13–63).

Parker has graded the degree of severity of the foramen magnum enlargement as follows: grade 1 – a dorsal extension of less than one-half of the normal ventrodorsal (VD) dimension; grade 2 – dorsal extension of double the VD dimension; grade 3 – any dorsal extension that exceeds grade 2. The open-mouth AP radiographic position has been used to demonstrate the anomaly, but Parker feels that a modified AP position in which the dog's nose is flexed 25 to 40 degrees from the perpendicular is better. In the 29 cases reviewed approximately 25 per cent showed longitudinal shortening of

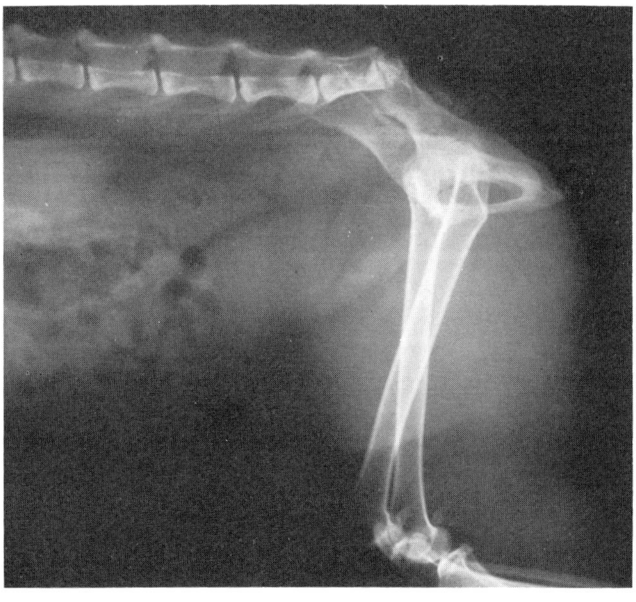

FIGURE 13–58 A Manx cat with a complete agenesis of the coccygeal vertebrae and segmental fusion defect with malformation of sacral vertebrae. A sacral iliac luxation is present on the right side.

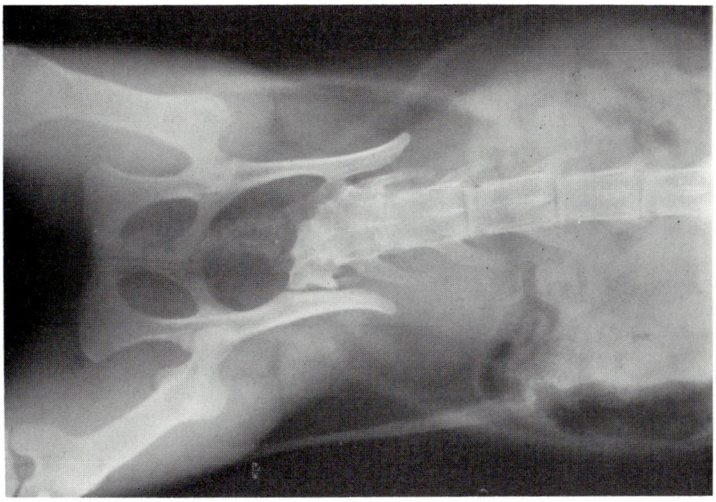

FIGURE 13-59 VD view of same case shown in Figure 13-58.

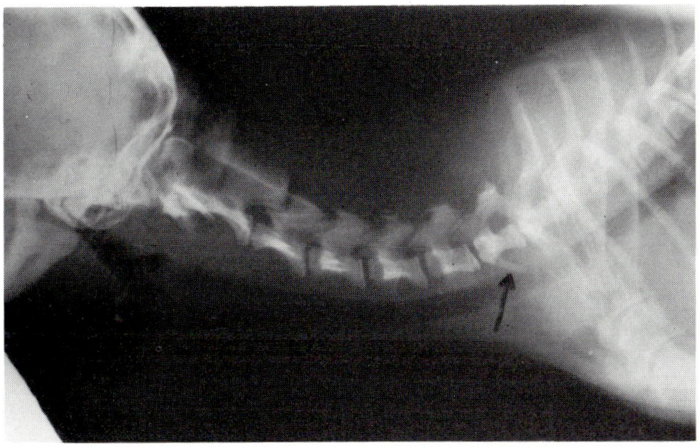

FIGURE 13-60 This case illustrates a cervical rib on C7 vertebra. This is frequently part of the Arnold-Chiari syndrome.

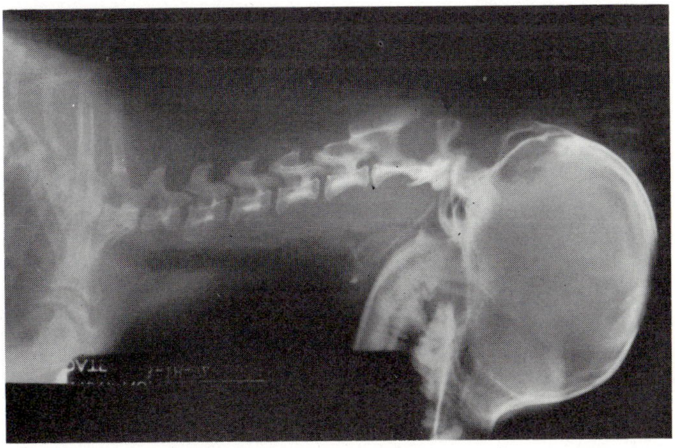

FIGURE 13-61 A 5-year-old Chihuahua has clinical hydrocephalus with the Arnold-Chiari syndrome and an enlarged foramen magnum. Notice the shortened arch of C1 and the stretched dorsal atlantoaxial ligament, the abnormal position of the osseous tentorium cerebelli, the lack of dural reflections (ground-glass appearance of cerebrum), and the forward displacement of the cribriform plate.

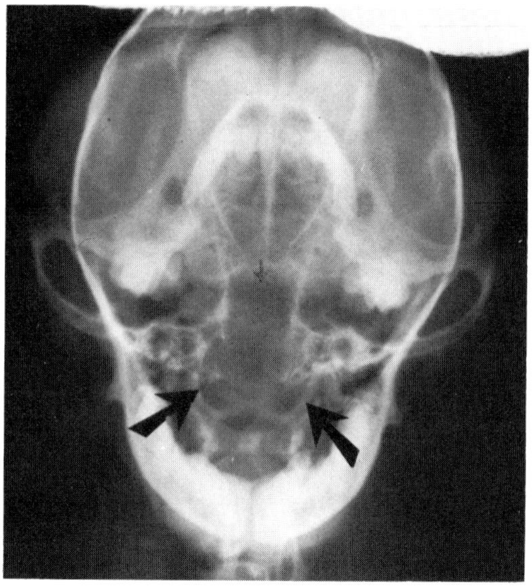

FIGURE 13–62 Open-mouth AP view of same case shown in Figure 13–61. Arrows indicate the ventral and dorsal limits of the enlarged foramen magnum. Immediately below the ventral arrows are the atlanto-occipital condylar articular surfaces.

C1 vertebra as the only cervical anomaly. The only sign attributable to a foramen magnum defect alone was ataxia and this was in grade 3 cases. In each of the three cases with grade 2 or grade 3 defects (graded by radiography) that were made available for necropsy, there was little evidence of cerebellar herniation or shift in position of the brain stem, but all had evidence of hydrocephalus.[92]

Diagnosis can be tentatively established by history, breed of dog, clinical signs, and palpation of a decrease in prominence of the external occipital protuberance, dorsal nuchal line, or even the outer borders of the enlarged foramen magnum. Radiographic examination is performed with the dog in the anteroposterior or frontal open-mouth position or in the AP position with the nose flexed 25 to 40 degrees from the vertical plane. A lateral position may show an enlarged intervertebral foramen between the atlas and axis and a shortened C1 vertebra. The EEG may demonstrate hydrocephalus. No treatment has been attempted other than treatment of the hydrocephalus when present.

TRAUMATIC INJURY OF THE SPINAL CORD

Injury to the spinal column and its contents is frequently received directly from automobile accidents, a blow or kick, a fall, or even a gunshot wound. However, an animal may *indirectly* injure his spine by running, jumping, or other movement, which may produce overextension, overflexion, or abnormal torsion. Injury can result in damage to the spinal column

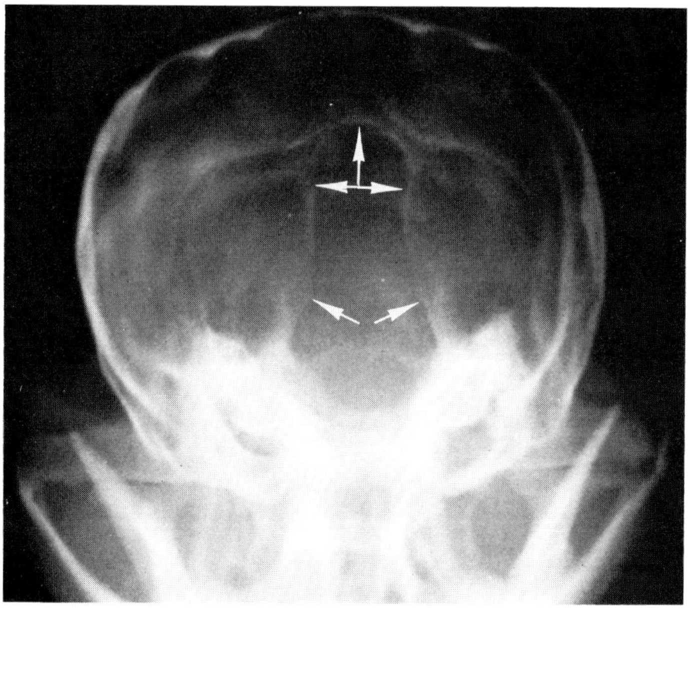

FIGURE 13–63 AP view of a grade III enlarged foramen magnum (occipital dysplasia) as classified by Parker. Notice the similarity to the disorder shown in Figure 13–61. (From Parker, A. J., and Park, R. D.: Occipital dysplasia in the dog. J. Am. Anim. Hosp. Assoc., *10*, 520, 1974.)

alone, to the cord alone, or to both the column and the cord. The discussion in this section is devoted to cord injury.

CONCUSSION

Spinal cord concussion results in a deficit of neurological function, usually temporary, following direct or indirect trauma. Some have called it a "shaking up" of neurological tissue. Although concussion is not a well-defined term, it usually implies a physiological dysfunction without gross pathologic change. There are no radiographic abnormalities, at least clinically. Paresis or paralysis may last from a few hours to several days to weeks.[69]

CONTUSION

Contusion of the spinal cord usually accompanies a severe trauma that is characterized by focal or diffuse lesions of ischemia, edema, hemorrhage, neuronal degeneration and necrosis, and malacia. The importance of edema of the cord has been and will be stressed frequently throughout the text (see Chapters 12, 14, and 15). When the cord swells so much that it fills the spinal canal, progressive counterpressure from the neutral arch may cause irreversible neural damage. See also Chapter 12 on CNS trauma for factors contributing to the cause of traumatic malacia of the spinal cord from hemorrhagic necrosis.

HEMATORACHIS

Hematorachis is hemorrhage into the subarachnoid, subdural, or epidural spaces from spinal injury. Neurological damage from compression is not frequently observed. A combination of hematorachis and intramedullary hemorrhage is frequently encountered.

A syndrome of pain and pyrexia characterized by remissions and recurrences in which the pathological finding was hemorrhage on or around the spinal cord has been described in dogs. Necropsy findings were given in six cases. The dogs were young, and neurological signs varied from pain to flaccid quadriplegia. Of the six dogs, one had extradural hemorrhage in the cervical spinal segment, two had generalized subdural hemorrhage, one had hematomyelia of C3–8, one had subdural hemorrhage at T10, and one had subdural hemorrhage and hematomyelia from T12 to the cauda equina. The confirmed cases were seen in a variety of nonchondrodystrophoid breeds: the suspect cases (nonconfirmed) were seen largely in beagles. A diagnosis can be tentatively made on clinical signs and the occurrence in a nonchondrodystrophoid breed, which helps to eliminate disk problems. No treatment has been effective.[58]

Two other case reports of idiopathic hemorrhage have been made. Eschenroeder observed areas of organized subdural hemorrhage in the lumbar spine and hemorrhages throughout the skeletal muscles and soft tissue of a miniature poodle.[30] Jackson reported widespread extradural hemorrhage in a dachshund that produced progressive quadriplegia and death.[54] In man, occasional spinal subarachnoid hemorrhage is due to coarctation or narrowing of the aorta. Rupture of large collateral vessels on the surface of the cord or meninges in times of stress can cause serious spinal subarachnoid hemorrhage.[6] This disorder could occur in domestic animals as well.

HEMATOMYELIA

Hematomyelia or hemorrhage into the cord substance is a frequent finding in acute ruptured disks and may result in progressive paralysis and death in 3 to 6 days. In our experience, hemorrhage usually progresses until hemorrhagic malacia or destruction of cord tissue results. This may be theoretically explained by the fact that arteriolar walls in the CNS have little contractile muscle tissue, which, when injured, promotes vasoconstriction. Future research may prove a tissue chemical (catecholamine) or immunological pathogenesis. When hemorrhage is localized, absorption of the blood clot begins on about the third day, and neurological function improves thereafter. A few dogs have regained normalcy when clinical signs of minor spinal hemorrhage appeared to be localized in the region of the ruptured disk.

LACERATION

Laceration or tearing of the spinal cord may occur in gunshot wounds and from penetrating fragments secondary to comminuted fractures. Since the dura mater is rather tough as well as elastic, penetration of fragments is rarely seen. We have seen several gunshot lacerations. Prognosis in spinal cord lacerations is generally unfavorable.

COMPRESSION OF THE SPINAL CORD

In the category of compression are discussed those conditions that cause compression of the spinal cord that gives rise to ischemia, edema, inflammation, and degeneration of the neural elements adjacent to the area of pressure. Compression can occur very easily in the dog, since the spinal cord occupies the spinal canal so completely. This is especially true in the thoracolumbar area; therefore, pressure on the cord may easily result in paralysis. In the cervical area, the canal-cord relations seem to be more comparable to those of man, and compression in this area more frequently causes pain rather than profound paralysis. When space-occupying masses develop in the canal, the cord is compressed since it is softer than bone. Compressions may be classified as extravertebral and vertebral.

EXTRAVERTEBRAL COMPRESSIONS

Extravertebral compression is caused by lesions that originate in structures adjacent to the vertebral column. Over an extended period of time, the resulting pressure causes a softening and necrosis of bone and subsequent compression of the cord (which may be due to neoplasm, abscess, cyst, aortic aneurysm, or hematoma).

VERTEBRAL COMPRESSION

Vertebral compression of the cord arises from the vertebrae themselves or within the spinal canal independently of the vertebrae. Vertebral compressions constitute a significant portion of the cases seen in small animal practice. At the Auburn University Small Animal Clinic during the year 1974–75, 513 clinical spinal compressions were seen out of a total of 15,012 individual cases (3.4 per cent). Due to traditional departmental research, this is a larger than normal accession rate, but we must emphasize the clinical importance of spinal compressions. We have previously considered many conditions that can conceivably cause crowding or compression of the spinal cord, such as osteomyelitis of the vertebrae, bone and meningeal cysts, meningitic and epidural abscesses, dural ossification, canine wobbler syndrome, multiple cartilaginous exostoses, vascular aneurysms, spondylosis deformans, spondylolisthesis, malformations of the spinal column, and vertebral and meningeal neoplasia. There are, however, other types of vertebral compression that arise from injuries. These include spinal fractures, spinal luxations, and disk protrusions. These conditions may cause not only violent and acute neuropathies but also systemic effects all of which require prompt treatment.

The systemic effects of spinal injuries include those generally seen in violent trauma. In Chapters 8, 12, 14, and 17, the consideration of shock, renal dysfunction, and other metabolic aspects are considered. Experimental work in cats has produced interesting data on the effect of acute compression of the cord and general cardiovascular physiology. Local cord compression evokes a transient, often marked rise in systemic arterial pressure that is proportionate to the degree of compression. The upper thoracic cord yields the most marked responses, and cardiac effects in the form of bradycardia and increased pulse-pressure amplitude are obtained exclusively from this region.

The pressor response is obtained also in the experimentally produced "spinal" animal in which the cord has been transected. The cardiac effects of bradycardia and increased pulse pressure are abolished by bilateral sinuaortic denervation and are absent also in the spinal animal. There is some evidence that baro-receptors are not involved. Most neurosurgeons have observed these cardiovascular changes in patients with acute cord compression, and perhaps this discussion will help to explain the physiological mechanisms.

It is interesting to consider the mechanism or effect of acute compression of the spine on the spinal cord. It has been said that the effects of compression producing complete sensorimotor paralysis are essentially the same as complete physiological transection. Tarlov and co-workers feel strongly that paralysis is caused by *mechanical deformation* of nerve tissue and not by ischemia or anoxia.[111-114] In the dog, about 35 minutes of spinal cord anoxia produced by thoracic aortic occlusion is usually the maximal period after which recovery will still occur, and after an hour of complete ischemia to the cord all nerve cells in the spinal cord are destroyed. On the other hand, dogs whose spinal cords had been compressed for 2 hours with forces producing instantaneous sensorimotor paralysis showed full functional recovery and little or no histological abnormality. In man, recovery from acute paralysis has occurred when the compressive force was removed within 24 hours; this could not have happened had paralysis been the result of ischemia or anoxia. Therefore, the pathological effect of compression in the cord is generally not due to reduction in the supply of blood or oxygen.

If Tarlov's theory of mechanical damage as the cause of cord trauma were entirely true, prompt decompression should be universally effective. However, every neurosurgeon knows that a portion of cases that should respond to appropriate decompression do not respond satisfactorily. Total segmental cord destruction and malacia follow injury in 24 or 48 hours. Recent research has indicated that a neurotransmitter vascular alteration of catecholamine metabolism is associated with these changes. Therefore, a new era of anticatecholamine and related therapy in conjunction with surgical decompression is rapidly developing.[111–114] (See Chapter 12).

The general signs of spinal compression are pain, paresis or weakness, and rigid or flaccid paralysis. As mentioned previously, violent trauma can cause cord contusion, laceration, and local or diffuse hemorrhage.

The signs of compression vary according to the site and are therefore called *segmental.* It must be emphasized at this time that spinal compressions generally do not cause unique clinical signs that other lesions at the same location would not cause. Clinical signs most frequently indicate the location and not the cause of the CNS lesion. The history and special examinations may indicate more clearly the cause of the lesion. Detailed discussions of clinical signs as related to spinal cord locations appear in Chapters 4 and 14.

If local damage is in the thoracic and lumbar areas, there may be pain, posterior paresis, paraplegia, urinary retention, fecal retention, exaggerated tendon reflexes (unless the specific area governing reflex is destroyed), diminished placing reflexes, and diminished to normal toe-pinch reflexes. If local damage is extensive, leaving few normal neural elements intact, the cerebral response to pain will be absent with the toe-pinch reflex. Widespread damage to a longer length of cord abolishes all leg, tail, anal, and urinary reflexes.

Compression in the posterior lumbar segment of the cord generally is not as serious as that occurring further forward. The spinal cord terminates at L6 into the cauda equina and filum terminale. Compression of L5–6, L6–7, and L7–S1 interspaces usually causes pain and may cause minor motor dysfunction. Inability to raise the tail has been seen. In fractures, urinary and fecal incontinence may be seen, as well as paralysis of the tail. Weakness and paralysis of the hind limbs may be seen if damage to the cord has beeen more extensive. Compressions of L3–4 to L6–7 spinal segments involve cord segments in the lumbosacral plexus, and LMN signs of individual motor nerves can be seen. Comparable compressions of C4–5 and T2–3 spinal segments can cause motor deficiencies of specific nerves in the brachial plexus.[87]

A compression in the cervical canal generally causes pain with little or no motor dysfunction. Extensive compression causes unilateral or bilateral motor dysfunction, depending upon the location. Tendon and toe-pinch reflexes are affected similarly in the hind legs. Extreme cervical pressure may cause a paralysis of all four legs, or tetraplegia. Cord compression rarely causes a unilateral paralysis (hemiplegia); this is most frequently seen with cerebral lesions. It should be mentioned here that anterior cervical trauma can occasionally cause a so-called Horner's syndrome, consisting of enophthalmos, upper eyelid ptosis, prolapse of the membrane nictitans, and miosis. In cervical trauma, the ascending cervical sympathetic chain is damaged, affecting innervation to the various cervical ganglia, trigeminal nerve, and eventually the globe.[36]

Besides the *location* of spinal compression, the *speed* of *occurrence* is extremely important. Minor compression occurring quickly and forcefully, as in a ruptured disk, can cause more neurological damage than a large lesion that has developed slowly. Obviously, a sudden and large compression will cause much neurological damage, and permanent dysfunction frequently develops.

Tarlov has compared experimentally the speed and duration of compression to the cord with the rate of recovery.[111-114] A small rubber balloon was introduced into the posterior portion of the thoracic epidural space and was filled, at varying speeds, with varying amounts of liquid. The animals so treated were studied over many months to determine the degree and speed of clinical recovery. The data are summarized in Table 13-1.

It is apparent that the speed of development and duration of the compression are crucial in the clinical recovery. Sudden and severe compression of the cord, as in fractures, causes spinal shock. Spinal shock manifests itself by a complete absence of muscle tonus and reflexes. In the dog, reflexes may begin to return after one to a few hours. The tendon reflexes are exaggerated, and respond in bizarre fashion to stimuli, while the front legs, head, and neck remain rigid and cannot be flexed (Schiff-Sherington sign, if the lesion is caudal to T3). This mechanism is controversial, but could perhaps be due to a release of the intersegmental inhibition of the tonic reflexes that maintain posture and supporting positions. Occasionally, in mild fractures, the pectoral limb extensor rigidity subsides, and this is a more favorable prognostic sign.

The establishment of a tentative diagnosis of the cause of compression can frequently be aided by a history of trauma (fracture), an insidious onset with slow progression (tumor), or recurrent attacks of pain or paresis (herniated disk). It is to be emphasized that the animal must be examined carefully; a complete neurological assessment should be made and recorded. Since many types of compression produce a similar pattern of symptoms, which vary only in degree and severity, radiographic examination is necessary for a more positive diagnosis. Radiographic standards discussed in Chapter 5 should be followed. Lesions commonly seen in spinal injuries are discussed in Chapters 12, 14, and 15.

TABLE 13-1 TEMPORAL RELATIONSHIP OF COMPRESSION AND RECOVERY*

Paralysis		**Recovery**		
Period of Development	*Maximum Duration Permitting Full Recovery*	*Period of Development of Paralysis*	*Duration of Compression*	*Interval Between Decompression and Initial Improvement*
(First sign of pain to complete paralysis)				
Sudden compression and paralysis	2 hours	Acute compression	10 minutes	2–3 days
			30 minutes	15–20 days
			50–120 minutes	20–30 days
Gradual compression to paralysis:		Gradual compression:		
75 minutes	9 hours	75 minutes	9 hours (max.)	1–3 days
20 hours	84 hours	20 hours	84 hours (max.)	4–32 days
18 hours	1 week	48 hours	1 week (max.)	4–10 days

*From Tarlov, I. M., Klinger, H., and Vitale, S.: Spinal cord compression studies. I. Experimental techniques to produce acute and gradual compression. Arch. Neurol. Psychiat. *70*, 813, 1953.

Treatment

The treatment of spinal compression resulting from trauma is centered upon prompt surgical relief, especially in cases of fracture and luxation. Immediate decompression is imperative. In more chronic compression resulting from disk protrusions, surgical correction may be delayed or may not be performed at all. However, many disk lesions also demand immediate surgical care (see Chapters 11 and 14).

The supportive therapy of hypothermia, hypertonic solutions, anticatecholamines, DMSO, and adrenocorticosteroids with or without surgical intervention is discussed in Chapters 8, 12, 14, and 15. When dogs were subjected to some standard procedures of experimental trauma known to produce paraplegia, a statistically significant rate of improvement and recovery of neurological function was seen. In well-established clinical practice, the supportive use of broad spectrum antibiotics, glucocorticosteroids, copious normothermic or hypothermic perfusion fluids in the surgical site, and timely mannitol dehydrants in conjunction with surgical decompression has proved to be valuable in cases of acute spinal cord compression.[24] Anticatecholamines, DMSO, and other experimental agents should be evaluated further before they are used extensively in clinical practice.

The supportive treatment of patients suffering from cord compression is extremely important. The care of the urinary system, the integument, and other aspects of supportive care are discussed in detail in Chapter 14.

REFERENCES

1. Alexander, J. E., and Pettit, G. D.: Spinal osteochondrosis in a dog. Can. Vet. J. *8,* 47, 1967.
2. Archibald, J., and Cawley, A. J.: The locomotor system. *In: Canine Medicine,* 2d ed. American Veterinary Publications, Santa Barbara, Cal., 1959.
3. Averill, D. R.: Degenerative myelopathy in the aging German shepherd dog: Clinical and pathological findings. J.A.V.M.A. *162,* 1045, 1973.
4. Bailey, C. L.: An embryological approach to the clinical significance of congenital vertebral and spinal cord abnormalities. J. Am. Anim. Hosp. Assoc. *11,* 426, 1975.
5. Baker, J. R., and Hughes, I. B.: A case of deforming cervical spondylosis in a cat associated with a diet rich in liver. Vet. Rec. *83,* 44, 1968.
6. Banna, M. M., Rose, P. G., and Pearce, G. W.: Coarctation of the aorta as a cause of spinal subarachnoid hemorrhage. J. Neurosurg. *39,* 761, 1973.
7. Bardens, J. W.: Congenital malformation of the foramen magnum in dogs. Southwest. Vet. *18,* 295, 1965.
8. Bartels, J. E., Dorn, A. S., and Britt, A. L.: Osteochondrosis of the vertebrae in a dog. Can. Vet. J. *11,* 47, 1970.
9. Beadman, R., Smith, R. N., and King, A. S.: Vertebral osteophytes in the cat. Vet. Rec. *76,* 1005, 1964.
10. Beeson, P. B., and McDermott, W.: *Cecil-Loeb Textbook of Medicine,* 14th ed. W. B. Saunders Co., Philadelphia, 1975.
11. Botelho, S. Y., Steinberg, S. A., McGrath, J. T., and Zislis, J.: Am. J. Vet. Res. *28,* 205, 1967.
12. Bowen, J. M.: Electromyography. *In* Klemm, W. R. (ed.): *Applied Electronics for Veterinary Medicine and Animal Physiology.* Charles C Thomas, Publishers, Springfield, Ill., 1976.
13. Breazile, J. E., Blaugh, B. S., and Nail, N.: Experimental study of canine distemper myoclonus. Am. J. Vet. Res. *27,* 1375, 1966.
14. Chesny, C. J.: A case of spina bifida in a Chihuahua. Vet. Rec. *93,* 120, 1973.
15. Chrisman, C. L., Wood, P. K., and Johnson, E. W.: Electromyography in small animal neurology. J.A.V.M.A. *160,* 311, 1972.
16. Clark, L., Seawright, A. A., and Gartner, R. J. W.: Long bone abnormalities in kittens following vitamin A administration. J. Comp. Pathol. *80,* 113, 1970.
17. Crandall, P. H., and Batzdorf, W.: Cervical spondylotic myelopathy. J. Neurosurg. *25,* 57, 1966.
18. Cummings, J. F.: Coonhound paralysis: A polyradiculoneuritis in dogs resembling the Landry-Guillain-Barré syndrome. Thesis, Cornell University, Ithaca, N.Y. 1966.
19. Cummings, J. F., and de Lahunta, A.: Acute polyneuritis (coonhound paralysis). *In* Kirk, R. W. (ed.): *Current Veterinary Therapy* VI. W. B. Saunders Co., Philadelphia, 1977, p. 825.
20. de Lahunta, A.: Progressive cervical spinal cord compression in Great Dane and Doberman pinscher dogs (wobbler syndrome). *In* Kirk, R. W. (ed.): *Current Veterinary Therapy V.* W. B. Saunders Co., Philadelphia, 1974.
21. Dexler, H.: Über Pachymeningitis spinalis ossificans chronica und compressions Myelitis beim Hunde. Wien. Med. Presse. *35,* 1998, 1893.
22. Dorland's Illustrated Medical Dictionary, 25th ed. W. B. Saunders Co., Philadelphia, 1974.
23. Drew, R. A.: Possible association between abnormal vertebral development and neonatal mortality in bulldogs. Vet. Rec. *94,* 480, 1974.
24. Ducher, T. B., and Hamit, H. F.: Experimental treatments of acute spinal cord injury. J. Neurosurg. *30,* 693, 1969.
25. Dueland, R., Furneaux, R. W., and Kaye, M. M.: Spinal fusion and dorsal laminectomy for midcervical spondylolisthesis in a dog. J.A.V.M.A. *162,* 366, 1973.
26. Eddy, D.: *The Avitaminoses,* 2d ed. The Williams and Wilkins Co., Baltimore, 1941.

27. Editorial: Bone overgrowth and nerve degeneration in vitamin A deficiency. Nutr. Rev. *1*, 419, 1943.
28. Edwin, E. E., Spence, J. B., and Woods, A. J.: Thiaminases and cerebrocortical necrosis. Net. Rec. *83*, 417, 1968.
29. English, P. B., and Seawright, A. A.: Deforming cervical spondylosis. Aust. Vet. J. *40*, 376, 1964.
30. Eschenroeder, H. C.: Lumbar pain syndrome due to subdural hemorrhage. Vet. Med. Small Anim. Clin. *59*, 1021, 1964.
31. Fenwick, D. C.: Polioencephalomalacia of sheep. Response to thiamine in a single case. Aust. Vet. J. *43*, 484, 1967.
32. Fletcher, T. F., and Kitchell, R. L.: Anatomical studies on the spinal cord segments of the dog. Am. J. Vet. Res. *27*, 1759, 1966.
33. Frauchiger, E., and Fankhauser, R.: *Die Nervenkrankheiten unserer Hunde.* Schmid et Cie., Bern, 1949.
34. Fry, P. D.: Cervical spondylosis in the cat. J. Small Anim. Pract. *9*, 59, 1968.
35. Frye, F. L.: Spina bifida occulta with sacrococcygeal agenesis in a cat. Anim. Hosp. *3*, 238, 1967.
36. Frye, F. L.: Horner's syndrome following cervical trauma. Vet. Med. Small Anim. Clin. *68*, 762, 1973.
37. Frye, F. L., and McFarland, L. Z.: Spina bifida with rachischisis in a kitten. J.A.V.M.A. *146*, 481, 1965.
38. Gage, E. D.: Atlantoaxial subluxation. *In* Bojrab, M. J. (ed.): *Current Techniques in Small Animal Surgery I.* Lea & Febiger, Philadelphia, 1975, p. 376.
39. Gage, E. D., and Hoerlein, B. F.: Surgical repair of cervical subluxation and spondylolisthesis in the dog. J. Am. Anim. Hosp. Assoc. *9*, 385, 1973.
40. Gage, E. D., and Smallwood, J. E.: Surgical repair of atlantoaxial subluxation in a dog. Vet. Med. Small Anim. Clin. *65*, 583, 1970.
41. Geary, J. C., Oliver, J. E., and Hoerlein, B. F.: Atlantoaxial subluxation in the canine. J. Small Anim. Pract. *8*, 577, 1967.
42. Geary, J. C.: Canine spinal lesions not involving disks. J.A.V.M.A. *155*, 2038, 1969.
43. Glenny, N. C.: Canine and feline spinal osteoarthritis (spondylitis deformans). J.A.V.M.A. *129*, 61, 1956.
44. Grenn, H. H., and Lindo, D. E.: Hemivertebrae with severe kyphoscoliosis and accompanying deformities in a dog. Can. Vet. J. *10*, 214, 1969.
45. Griffiths, I. R., Rowan, J. O., and Crawford, R. A.: Spinal cord blood flow measured by a hydrogen clearance technique. J. Neurol. Sci. *26*, 529, 1975.
46. Hansen, H. J.: A pathological anatomical study on disc degeneration in dog. Acta Orthop. Scand., Suppl. *11*, 1952.
47. Hansen, H. J.: Short spine deformity. J. Small Anim. Pract. *9*, 103, 1968.
48. Hartley, W. J.: Lower motor neuron disease in dogs. Acta Neuropath. *2*, 334, 1963.
49. Hedhammer, A., Wu, F., Krook, L., et al.: Overnutrition and skeletal disease. An experimental study in growing Great Dane dogs. Cornell Vet. *64* (Suppl. 5), 1974.
50. Hime, J. M., and Drake, J. C.: Osteochondrosis of the spine in the foxhound. Vet. Rec. *77*, 445, 1965.
51. Hoerlein, B. F.: Traumatic lesions of the canine spine. Mod. Vet. Pract. *39*, 31, 1958.
52. Hoerlein, B. F.: *Canine Neurology, Diagnosis and Treatment,* 2nd ed. W. B. Saunders Co., Philadelphia, 1971.
53. Innes, J. R. M., and Saunders, L. Z.: *Comparative Neuropathology.* Academic Press, New York, 1962.
54. Jackson, O. F.: Signs of cord compression caused by extradural hemorrhage in a dachshund. Vet. Rec. *75*, 964, 1963.
55. Jacobs, B., Krueger, E. G., and Leivy, D. M.: Cervical spondylosis with radiculopathy: Results of anterior diskectomy and interbody fusion. J.A.M.A. *211*, 2135, 1975.
56. Jenkins, F. A.: The evolution and development of the dens of the mammalian axis. Anat. Rec. *164*, 173, 1969.
57. Jensen, R., Maag, D. D., and Flint, J. C.: Enzootic ataxia from copper deficiency in sheep in Colorado. J.A.V.M.A. *133*, 336, 1958.
58. Joshua, J. O., and Ishmael, J.: Pain syndrome associated with spinal hemorrhage in the dog. Vet. Rec. *83*, 165, 1968.
59. Kaspar, L. V., and Lombard, L. S.: Nutritional myo-degeneration in a litter of beagles. J.A.V.M.A. *143*, 284, 1963.
60. Knecht, C. D., and Oliver, J. E.: Cervical vertebral fusion with rib graft and orthopedic plate. *In* Bojrab, M. J. (ed.): *Current Techniques in Small Animal Surgery I.* Lea & Febiger, Philadelphia, 1975, p. 387.
61. Ladds, P., Guffy, M., Blauch, B., and Splitter, G.: Congenital odontoid process separation in two dogs. J. Small Anim. Pract. *12*, 463, 1970.
62. Lazorthes, G., Gouaze, A., Zadeh, J. O., Santini, J. T., Lazorthes, V., and Burdin, P.: Arterial vascularization of the spinal cord, recent studies of anastomotic substitution pathways. J. Neurosurg. *35*, 253, 1971.
63. Leipold, H. W., Huston, K., Blauch, B., and Guffy, M. M.: Congenital defects of the caudal vertebral column and spinal cord in Manx cats. J.A.V.M.A. *164*, 520, 1974.
64. Loeffler, K., Volckart, W., and Homann, M.: Wedge vertebra formation: Case report. Kleintier Prax. *16*:107, 1971.
65. Lucke, V. M., Baskerville, A., Bardgett, P. L., Mann, P. G. H., and Thompson, S. Y.: Deforming cervical spondylosis in the cat associated with hypervitaminosis. A. Vet. Rec. *82*, 141, 1968.
66. Manktelow, B. W.: Myopathy of dogs resembling white muscle disease of sheep. N. Z. Vet. J. *11*, 52, 1963.
67. Markson, C. M., Terlecki, S., and Lewis, G.: Cerebrocortical necrosis in calves. Vet. Rec. *79*, 578, 1966.
68. McCay, C. M.: *Nutrition of the Dog,* 2d ed. Comstock Publishing Associates, Ithaca, N.Y., 1948.
69. McGrath, J. T.: *Neurologic Examination of the Dog with Clinicopathologic Observations,* 2d ed. Lea & Febiger, Philadelphia, 1960.
70. Mellanby, E.: *A Story of Nutritional Research.* The Williams and Wilkins Co., Baltimore, 1950.
71. Miller, M. E., Christensen, G. C., and Evans, H.

E.: *Anatomy of the Dog.* W. B. Saunders Co., Philadelphia, 1964.

72. Morgan, J. P.: *Radiology in Veterinary Orthopedics.* Lea & Febiger, Philadelphia, 1972.
73. Morgan, J. P.: Spondylosis deformans in the dog, a morphological study with some clinical and experimental observations. Acta Orthop. Scand., Suppl. *96,* 1967.
74. Morgan, J. P.: Spinal dural ossification in the dog: Incidence and distribution based on a radiographic study. J. Am. Vet. Rad. Soc. *9,* 21, 1969.
75. Morgan, J. P.: Congenital anomalies of the vertebral column of the dog: A study of the incidence and significance based on a radiographic and morphologic study. J. Am. Vet. Rad. Soc. *9,* 21, 1968.
76. Morgan, J. P.: Spinal dural ossification in the dog: Incidence and distribution based on a radiographic study. J. Am. Vet. Rad. Soc. *10,* 43, 1969.
77. Munday, B. L., and King, S. J.: A condition resembling Chastek paralysis in cats. N. Z. Vet. J. *20,* 80, 1972.
78. Myers, M., and Clerc, B.: Chronic hypervitaminosis A and cervical spondylosis. Rec. Med. Vet. *149,* 455, 1973.
79. Nathan, H.: Osteophytes of the vertebral column. J. Bone Jt. Surg. *44A,* 243, 1962.
80. Newberne, P. M., and O'Dell, B. L.: Histopathology of hydrocephalus resulting from a deficiency of vitamin B_{12}. Proc. Soc. Exp. Biol. Med. *97,* 62, 1958.
81. Nizzoli, V., and Testa, C.: A case of calcification in the spinal arachnoid giving rise to spinal cord compression. J. Neurol. Sci. *7,* 381, 1968.
82. O'Connell, D.: Heredity in ankylosing spondylitis. Ann. Int. Med. *50,* 1115, 1959.
83. Oliver, J. E., and Lewis, R. E.: Lesions of the atlas and axis in dogs. J. Am. Anim. Hosp. Assoc. *9,* 304, 1973.
84. Palmer, A. C., and Wallace, M. E.: Deformation of cervical vertebrae in basset hounds. Vet. Rec. *80,* 430, 1967.
85. Parker, A. J.: Cervical kyphosis in an Afghan hound. J.A.V.M.A. *162,* 953, 1973.
86. Parker, A. J.: Clinical significance of traumatic occlusion of segmental spinal arteries. J.A.V.M.A. *162,* 1041, 1973.
87. Parker, A. J.: Diagnosis and treatment of canine spinal cord disease. Scope, *18,* 1, 1974.
88. Parker, A. J.: Distribution of spinal branches of the thoracolumbar segmental arteries in dogs. Am. J. Vet. Res. *34,* 1351, 1973.
89. Parker, A. J., and Cusick, P. K.: Abnormal odontoid process angulation in a dog. Vet. Rec. *93,* 559, 1973.
90. Parker, A. J., and Park, R. D.: Atlanto-axial subluxation in small breeds of dogs. Diagnosis and pathogenesis. Vet. Med. Small Anim. Clin. *68,* 1133, 1973.
91. Parker, A. J., and Park, R. D.: Clinical signs associated with hemivertebra in 3 dogs. Canine Pract. *1,* 34, 1974.
92. Parker, A. J., and Park, R. D.: Occipital dysplagia in the dog. J. Am. Anim. Hosp. Assoc. *10,* 520, 1974.
93. Parker, A. J., Park, R. D., Byerly, C. S., and Stowater, J. L.: Spina bifida with protrusion of spinal cord tissue in a dog. J.A.V.M.A. *163,* 158, 1973.
94. Parker, A. J., Park, R. D., Cusick, P. K., Small, E., and Jeffers, C. B.: Cervical vertebral instability in the dog. J.A.V.M.A. *163,* 71, 1973.
95. Read, R. M., and Smith, R. N.: A comparison of spondylosis deformans in the English and Swedish cat and in the English dog. J. Small Anim. Pract. *9,* 159, 1968.
96. Reid, A. N. D., Clark, A., and Thomas, W. B.: Observations during an outbreak of suspected cerebrocortical necrosis in calves. Vet. Rec. *81,* 526, 1967.
97. Rosomoff, H. L., and Rossmann, F.: Treatment of cervical spondylosis by anterior cervical diskectomy and fusion. Arch. Neurol. *14,* 392, 1966.
98. Ross, G. E., Jr.: Surgical treatment of intervertebral disc disease. Proc. Am. Anim. Hosp. Assoc. 1969, p. 404.
99. Sandersleben, J., and Sergany, M. A. M.: Ein Beitrag zur sogenannte Pachymeningitis spinalis ossificans des Hundes unter berüchsichtigung pathogenetischer und ätiologischer Gesichtspunkte. Zentralbl. Vet. Med. *13A,* 526, 1966.
100. Scherer, H. J.: *Vergleichende Pathologie des Nervensystems der Saügetiere.* Georg Thieme, Leipzig, 1944.
101. Schiefer, B.: Über Keilwirbel beim Hund. Berl. Münch. Tierärztl. Wochenschr. *81,* 149, 1968.
102. Schlotthauer, E. S.: *In Canine Medicine,* 2d ed. American Veterinary Publications, Inc., Santa Barbara, Calif., 1959, p. 589.
103. Seawright, A. A., and Hrdlicka, J.: Pathogenic factors in tooth loss in young cats on a high daily oral intake of vitamin A. Aust. Vet. J. *50,* 133, 1974.
104. Selcer, R. R., and Oliver, J. E.: Cervical spondylopathy—wobbler syndrome in dogs. J. Am. Anim. Hosp. Assoc. *11,* 175, 1975.
105. Slesingr, L.: Flaccid paralysis due to nutritional deficiency. Berl. Münch. Tierärztl. Wochenschr. *82,* 91, 1969.
106. Stephens, F. E., and Nunemaker, J. C.: Spondylitis in identical twins reared apart. J. Hered. *41,* 283, 1950.
107. Stoops, W. L., and King, R. B.: Chronic myelopathy associated with cervical spondylosis. J.A.M.A. *192,* 281, 1965.
108. Suu, S., and Suzuki, Y.: Studies on the short-spine dogs, gross-anatomical observation on the spinal cord and spinal ganglia. Research Bulletin, Faculty of Argiculture, Gifu University, Gifu, Japan *33,* 152, 1972.
109. Swaim, S. F.: Evaluation of four techniques of cervical spinal fixation in dogs. J.A.V.M.A. *166,* 1080, 1975.
110. Swaim, S. F., and Greene, C. E.: Odontoidectomy in a dog. J. Am. Anim. Hosp. Assoc. *11,* 663, 1975.
111. Tarlov, I. M., Klinger, H., and Vitale, S.: Spinal cord compression studies. I. Experimental techniques to produce acute and gradual compression. Arch. Neurol. Psychiat. *70,* 813, 1953.
112. Tarlov, I. M., and Klinger, H.: Spinal cord com-

pression studies. II. Time limits for recovery after acute compression in dogs. Arch. Neurol. Psychiat. *71,* 271, 1954.

113. Tarlov, I. M.: Spinal cord compression studies. III. Time limits for recovery after gradual compression in dogs. Arch. Neurol. Psychiat. *71,* 588, 1954.
114. Tarlov, I. M.: *Spinal Cord Compression.* Charles C Thomas, Publisher, Springfield, Ill., 1957.
115. Thompson, G. R., Martel, W., Rakie, M. T., and Hayes, J. T.: Ankylosing spondylitis, hyperuricemia, and anomalies of the lumbosacral junction: A family study. Ann. Int. Med. *59,* 848, 1963.
116. Turnbull, I. M.: Microvasculature of the human spinal cord. J. Neurosurg. *35,* 141, 1971.
117. Turnbull, I. M., Brieg, A., and Hassler, O.: Blood supply of cervical spinal cord in man, a microangiographic cadaver study. J. Neurosurg. *24,* 951, 1966.
118. Ueshima, T.: Deformation of the vertebral column in the "short-spine dog." Jap. J. Vet. Res. *9,* 155, 1961.
119. Vandevelde, M.: In press
120. Wilson, J. W., Greene, H. J., and Leipold, H. W.: Osseous metaplasia of the spinal dura mater in a Great Dane. J.A.V.M.A. *167,* 75, 1975.
121. Wilson, C. B., and Landry, R. M.: Experimental cervical myelopathy. I. Blood supply of the canine cervical spinal cord. Neurology *14,* 809, 1964.
122. Worthman, R. P.: The longitudinal vertebral venous sinuses of the dog. I. Anatomy Am. J. Vet. Res. *17,* 341, 1956.
123. Wright, F., Rest, J. R, and Palmer, A. C.: Ataxia of the Great Dane caused by stenosis of the cervical vertebral canal: Comparison with similar conditions in the basset hound, Doberman pinscher, ridgeback, and the thoroughbred horse. Vet. Rec. *92,* 1, 1973.
124. Youmans, J. R.: *Neurological Surgery,* Vol. 2. W. B. Saunders Co., Philadelphia, 1973, p. 1179.

SECTION 2
DISORDERS OF MICTURITION

J. E. OLIVER, JR., D.V.M., M.S., PH.D.

Micturition, the physiologic process of storage and complete voiding of urine, has been described in detail in Chapter 2. Many areas of the nervous system influence the process of micturition, so it is reasonable that lesions in many areas can produce abnormalities of micturition.[16, 17] Abnormalities of micturition may include inappropriate voiding, inadequate storage of urine, incomplete voiding, or absence of voiding. Incontinence, the loss of voluntary control of micturition, may also be the result of non-neurogenic disorders such as congenital defects or calculi.[19] Only neurogenic disorders will be discussed here.

DIAGNOSIS

The primary complaint associated with disorders of micturition will usually include one of the following: inappropriate voiding; inadequate voiding with overflow or dribbling of urine; increased frequency, reduced capacity, or both; or incomplete voiding in which normal voiding reactions are interrupted by abrupt contraction of the sphincters (reflex dyssynergia).

The minimum data base recommended for an animal with a problem associated with micturition is listed in Table 13–2. The minimum data base is designed to reveal any additional problems as well as provide the information necessary to make a diagnosis and prognosis. Table 13–3 outlines the process of establishing a diagnosis. The specific items of information necessary to follow the algorithm will be discussed.[17]

HISTORY

In addition to the usual items in a history,[11] some specific information pertinent to micturition should be obtained. For instance, the pattern of micturition habits should be determined from as early an age as possible (see Chapter 19). Age at house training, frequency of micturition at various ages, and changes in habits may provide a clue to the onset of a problem prior to the owner's recognition of its significance.

Signs of abnormality in the nervous system or urinary tract or previous trauma may be important. Previous surgical procedures, especially neurological, abdominal, or pelvic (e.g., ovario-hysterectomy), should be analyzed in relation to the onset of the problem.

The onset and chronological course of the problem will allow construction of a sign-time graph which is useful for determining the etiology of the disease[13] (Chapter 4).

Voluntary control of micturition is often best established by the owner's observation. This can be supplemented and confirmed by direct observation of the animal in natural surroundings (e.g., outside on grass). If the animal can volitionally initiate voiding,

TABLE 13–2 MINIMUM DATA BASE FOR DIAGNOSIS OF URINARY INCONTINENCE*

History	
Physical examination	
Includes:	Observation of voiding and measurement of residual urine
Neurologic examination	
Includes:	Sphincter reflexes
Clinical pathology	
Includes:	CBC, urinalysis, BUN or creatinine
Radiology	
Includes:	Survey of abdomen and pelvis; contrast cystography and urethrography; intravenous pyelogram

*From Oliver, J. E., Jr. and Osborne, C. A.: Neurogenic urinary incontinence. *In* Kirk, R. W. (ed.): *Current Veterinary Therapy VI*. W. B. Saunders Co., Philadelphia, 1977.

TABLE 13–3 ALGORITHM FOR DIAGNOSIS OF DISORDERS OF MICTURITION*

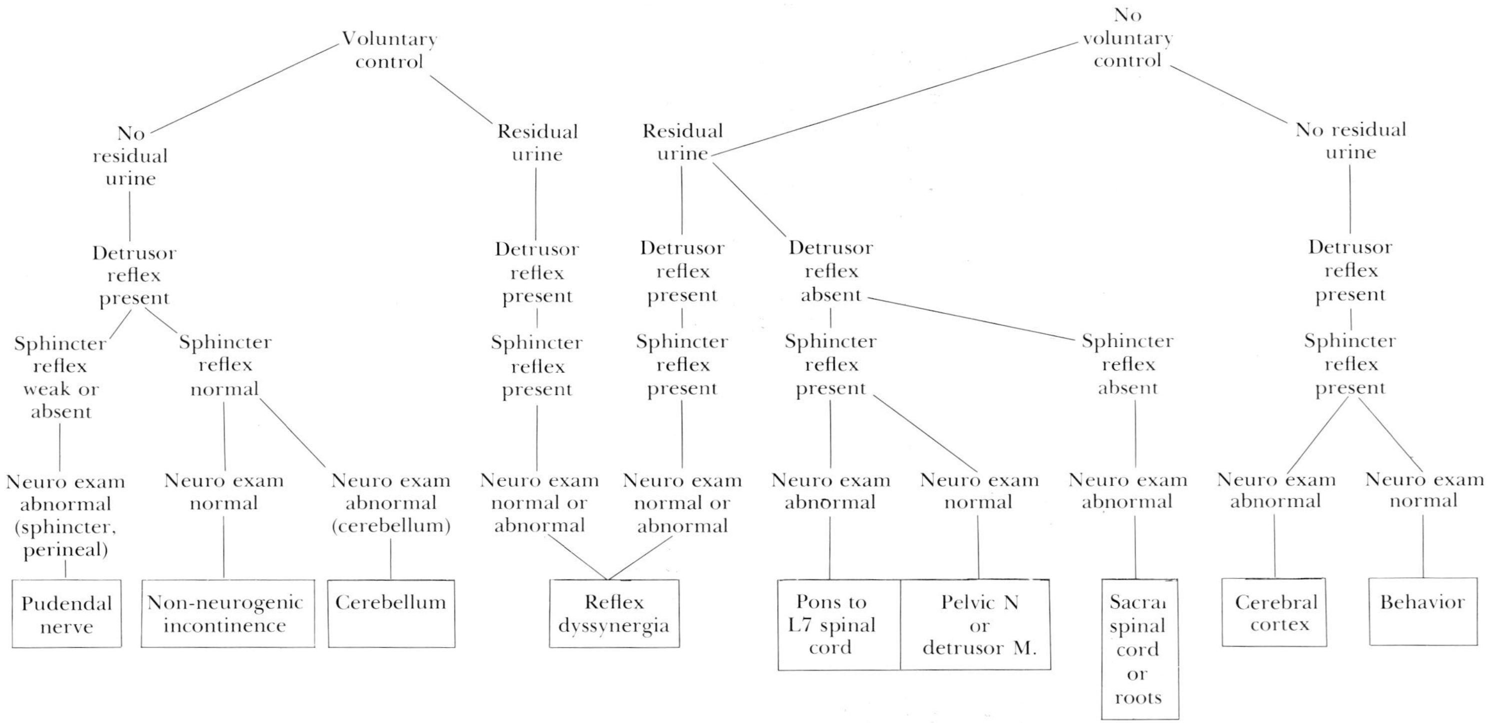

*From Oliver, J. E., Jr. and Osborne, C. A.: Neurogenic urinary incontinence. *In* Kirk, R. W. (ed.): *Current Veterinary Therapy VI.* W. B. Saunders Co., Philadelphia, 1977.

the *detrusor reflex* is probably present. Voluntary control also means that micturition can be withheld a reasonable length of time (house training) and can be interrupted if necessary. Interruption of micturition is more difficult to evaluate than voluntary initiation. A dog that is lead-trained can be interrupted by a pull on the lead and command to "come." Individual interpretation of interruption may be subjective.

Reflex dyssynergia will usually appear as normal initiation of voiding followed by narrowing of the stream and sudden interruption of flow. Straining will often continue and voiding may continue in brief spurts. Dyssynergia must be differentiated from partial obstruction (e.g., urethral calculi), which is usually recognized by catheterization and/or urethral contrast radiography.

Various types of incontinence may be described by the owner. Precipitate voiding, in which the animal voids suddenly in inappropriate places without apparent warning, is characteristic of cerebellar lesions and some partial spinal cord or brain stem lesions (Table 13–3). Differentiation of precipitate voiding from loss of normal voluntary control as in cortical lesions or behavioral changes may be difficult on the basis of the history alone.

Dribbling of urine may be the result of loss of urethral resistance or overflow from an areflexic bladder (Table 13–4).

PHYSICAL EXAMINATION

Observation of the animal may confirm the characteristics of micturition as described in the history. The difference between the various abnormalities of micturition may be very subtle, so it is critical that the problem described by the owner be verified by the examiner.

The presence of a *detrusor reflex* can be assumed if voiding is sustained (Table 13–3). However, bladder contractions with incomplete voiding are common in neurologic disorders. Such contractions are not the result of a true detrusor reflex. Therefore, every animal with a problem associated with micturition should have *residual urine* measured (Table 13–3). After the animal has voided, preferably outside in natural surroundings, the bladder should be catheterized and the residual urine measured. Residual urine should be less than 10 per cent of the normal volume, and most animals will have less than 10 ml remaining.

Except for urethral flaps (which are rare), obstructions in the urethra can be detected when the catheter is passed. A flap can be demonstrated only by excretory urethrography.[18]

Palpation of the bladder before and after voiding provides some information regarding bladder tone. The tone of the detrusor muscle is intrinsic and not directly related to innervation.[20] However, a normally functioning bladder will contract to accommodate the volume of urine present. An overdistended bladder with rupture of the tight junctions will not contract (Chapter 2). A chronically infected bladder will often be small and have thickened, fibrotic walls. A small contracted bladder with infection may not be the primary problem, as bladder infection is a common sequela to neurogenic disorders. Some of the nonneurogenic causes of incontinence such as tumors or calculi may also be identified by palpation.

Manual expression of the bladder provides some information on the tone of the urethral sphincters. Normally, expression of the bladder is more difficult in the male than in the female. Urethral sphincter tone will be decreased in lesions of the sacral spinal cord, sacral roots, or pudendal nerve (lower motor neuron) and increased in lesions between L7 spinal cord segment and the brain stem (Table 13–3). The sacral spinal cord segments lie within the body of the fifth lumbar vertebra, so lesions of the vertebrae from L5–6 caudally will affect the sacral roots (Fig. 13–64).

NEUROLOGIC EXAMINATION

The complete neurologic examination is described in Chapter 3. Reflexes related to the sacral spinal cord segments are especially important in neurogenic bladder dysfunction.

The anal and urethral sphincters are innervated by the pudendal nerve, primarily from sacral segments 1 and 2, but occasionally with fibers from S3.[12] It is easier to evaluate anal sphincter function because observation and palpation are more convenient.

TABLE 13–4 EFFECT OF LESIONS OF NEUROMUSCULAR SYSTEM*

Location of Lesion	Normal Function	Bladder					Sphincter			
		Voluntary Control	*Sustained Detrusor Reflex*	*Tone*	*Volume*	*Residual Urine*	*Voluntary Control*	*Reflexes (Perineal Bulbourethral)*	*Tone*	*Synergy with Detrusor*
Cerebral cortex to brain stem	Voluntary control to detrusor and sphincter	Absent	Normal	Normal	May be larger or smaller than normal	None	Absent	Normal to hyper-reflexic	Normal to increased	Normal
Cerebellum	Modulation (inhibition) of detrusor reflex	Normal, but increased frequency	Possibly hyper-reflexic	Normal	Small	None	Normal	Normal	Normal	Normal
Brain stem (pons) to sacral spinal cord	Sustained detrusor reflex	Absent	Lost early; small un-synchronized contractions late	Atonic early; possibly increased late	Large	Large	Absent	Normal to hyper-reflexic	Normal to increased	Absent
Partial lesions (reflex dyssynergia)	Sustained detrusor reflex	May be present	May be present	Normal to atonic	Large	Small to large	May be normal	Normal	Normal to increased	Absent
Sacral spinal cord or roots	LMN to detrusor and sphincter	Absent	Absent	Atonic	Large	Large	Absent	Absent	Flaccid	Absent
Disruption of tight junctions of detrusor	Spread of excitation in detrusor	Absent	Absent	Atonic	Large	Large	Normal	Normal	Normal	Normal (cannot evaluate, however)

*From Oliver, J. E., Jr. and Osborne, C. A.: Neurogenic urinary incontinence. *In* Kirk, R. W. (ed.): *Current Veterinary Therapy VI.* W. B. Saunders Co., Philadelphia, 1977.

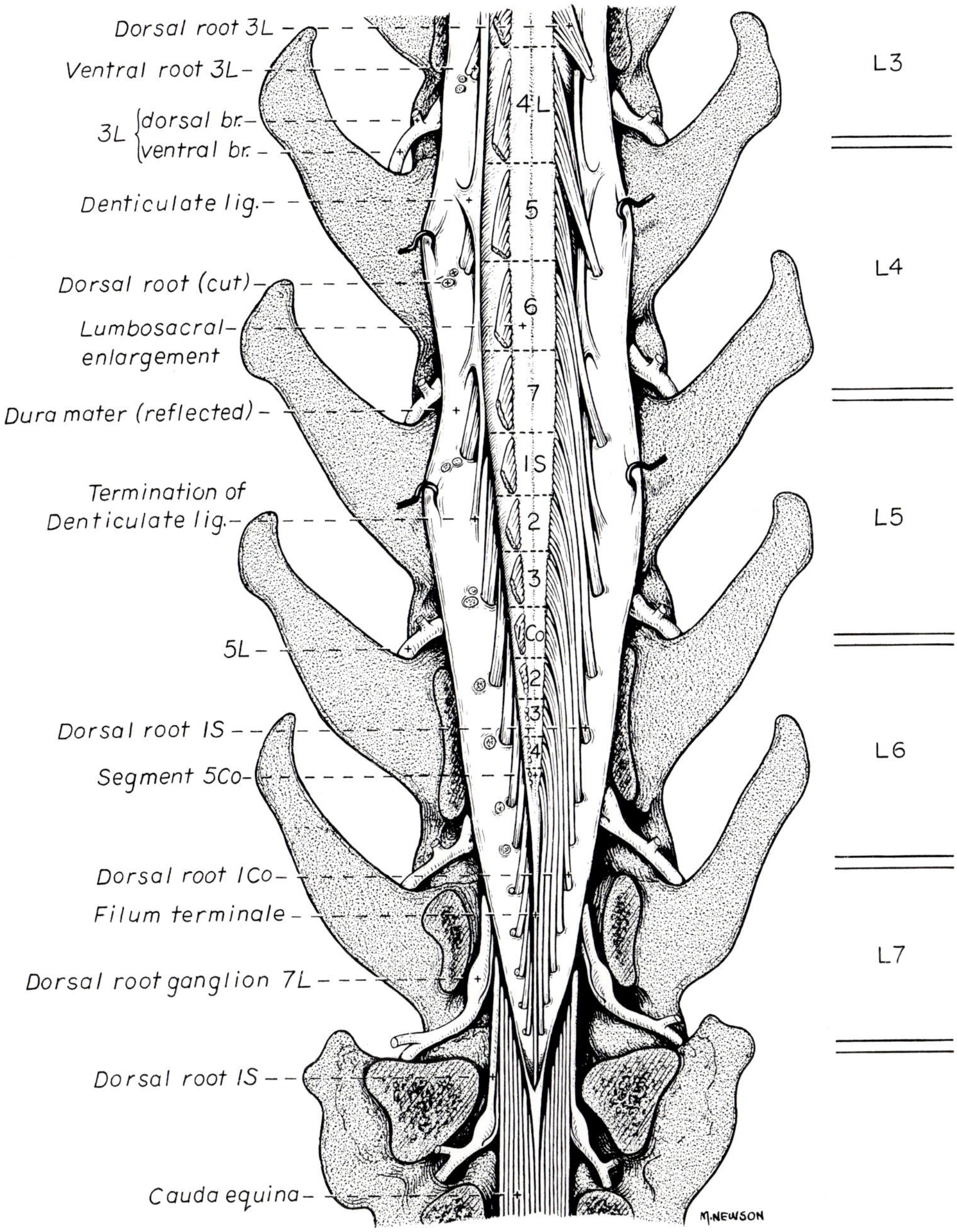

FIGURE 13–64 Distal end of spinal cord showing spinal cord segments. Dorsal aspect. (The dura mater has been cut mid-dorsally and reflected. The dorsal roots have been cut on the left side to expose the ventral roots and the denticulate ligament.) (From Fletcher, 1964. Thesis, University of Minnesota.)

The tone of the anal sphincter can be observed or it can be palpated with the gloved digit. Two sacral reflexes can also be evaluated. The *bulbocavernosus reflex* is a sharp contraction of the sphincter in response to a squeeze of the bulb of the penis or the clitoris. The *perineal reflex* is a contraction of the sphincter in response to a pinch or pin prick of the perineal region. The perineal reflex can also be used to test sensory distribution in the perineal region (see Fig. 9–25). Unilateral lesions can be detected in this manner.[2] Lesions of the sacral spinal cord, sacral roots, or pudendal nerves will diminish or destroy these reflexes, and the anal sphincter will be atonic.

The history, physical examination, and neurologic examination should provide sufficient data to differentiate neurogenic from non-neurogenic bladder disorders and to localize the lesion in the nervous system in neurogenic disorders (Tables 13–2 and 13–3, and Chapters 3 and 4). Additional data are necessary for an etiologic diagnosis and a prognosis.

CLINICAL PATHOLOGY

The minimum data base includes a complete blood count (CBC), urinalysis, and blood urea nitrogen (BUN) or creatinine values. Each of these is essential for prognosis of urinary tract dysfunction and may assist in diagnosis of non-neurogenic problems of micturition.[18, 19]

All animals with neurogenic bladder disorders are likely to have cystitis. Constant surveillance and appropriate treatment, when indicated, are imperative if a favorable outcome is to be expected. Ureteral reflux is also a frequent complication of neurogenic bladder dysfunction.[2, 6] Reflux when cystitis is present may lead to pyelonephritis, uremia, and death.[2]

RADIOLOGIC EXAMINATION

Radiography is important for differentiating non-neurogenic problems[19] and for evaluating the extent of urinary tract disease, which may be a complication of neurogenic disorders, and the primary neurologic problem (Chapter 5).

Contrast cystourethrography during voiding has not been adequately evaluated in animals but could provide considerable information about the functional morphology of the lower urinary tract.[1, 2]

ELECTROPHYSIOLOGY

Electrophysiologic tests have not been included in the minimum data base because they are not widely available at present. However, electrophysiologic tests may be necessary to make a definitive diagnosis in some cases. As more is learned about the pathophysiology of neurogenic bladder disorders, electrophysiology will be more important in the final diagnosis.

The cystometrogram (CMG) measures intravesical pressure during a detrusor reflex (Fig. 13–65). A sustained detrusor reflex may be difficult to document clinically in many cases. Additionally, the CMG provides data on threshold volume and pressure, capacity, the ability of the bladder to fill at a normal pressure (a measure of elasticity of the bladder wall), and presence of uninhibited bladder contractions (a sign of denervation). Normal data from the CMG of the dog are presented in Table 13–5.[15]

Electromyography (EMG) of the skeletal muscles of the anal and urethral sphincters

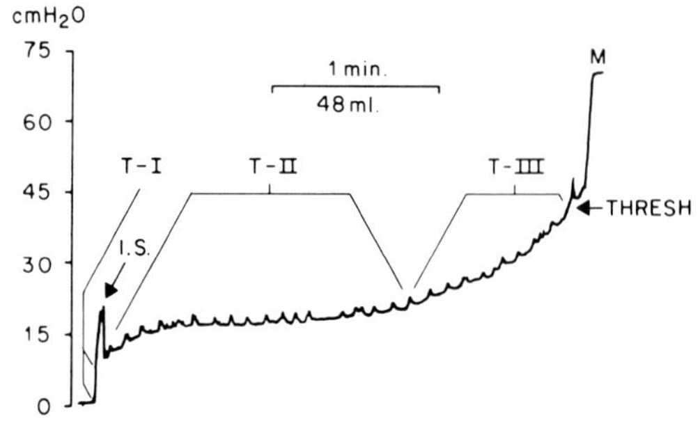

FIGURE 13–65 Cystometrogram of a dog showing segments of the tonus limb. T-I, resting pressure; T-II, bladder-filling pressure change (smooth muscle elasticity); T-III, bladder-filling pressure change after capacity is reached. Scale indicates time and volume. Thresh = threshold of detrusor reflex; M = maximal contraction; I.S. = initial spike, an artifact. (From Oliver, J. E., Jr., and Young, W. O.: Air cystometry in dogs under xylazine-induced restraint. Am. J. Vet. Res. *34*:1433–1435, 1973.)

TABLE 13–5 NORMAL VALUES FOR CYSTOMETROGRAMS (CMG) OF DOGS USING XYLAZINE FOR RESTRAINT*

Measurement	Mean ± SD Values of CMG (N = 41)[a] *(CM of Water)*
Tonus limb I	9.7 ± 4.3
Tonus limb II	12.6 ± 12.2
Threshold pressure	24.4 ± 10.0
Threshold pressure minus tonus limb I	14.4 ± 8.7
Threshold volume[b]	206.6 ± 184.4
Maximal contraction pressure	77.6 ± 33.8

*From Oliver, J. E., Jr. and Young, W. O.: Air cystometry in dogs under xylazine-induced restraint. Am. J. Vet. Res. *34*:1433–1435, 1973

[a]N = Number of CMG, other values defined in text and Figure 13–64.

[b]Value given in milliliters of air.

and other muscles in the pelvic diaphragm provides direct evidence of the status of innervation of these muscles. The perineal or bulbocavernosus reflexes can also be tested while recording directly from the muscles in animals in which clinical evaluation is equivocal (see Chapter 9).

EMG recording from the anal sphincter while stimulating the urethra or bladder with a catheter electrode has been termed electromyelography (EMyG).[3] Urethral stimulation evokes a response through the pudendal nerve, sacral segments, and pudendal nerve to the muscle, the same pathway as the bulbocavernosus reflex. Stimulation of the bladder wall evokes a similar response, but the afferent pathway is in the pelvic nerves. EMyG from bladder stimulation provides evidence of the integrity of the pelvic nerves. The other advantages of the electrical test are that the response is objective and can be measured, and latencies that provide information about partial denervation can be recorded.

Pressure measurements of the urethra offer the promise of more precise information about the functional integrity of the urethra.[5] A combination of CMG, urethral EMG, and urethral pressure recorded simultaneously would provide the best total functional evaluation of micturition and would show the synergistic relationship of detrusor and sphincter. These tests have not yet been developed to the point of application in clinical patients.

The final diagnosis should include (1) location of the lesion in the nervous system, (2) etiology of the lesion, (3) functional CNS deficit, and (4) functional deficit related to micturition.

TREATMENT

Management of a case depends on the final diagnosis. The treatment of primary CNS disease is described elsewhere in this text. Functional deficits of micturition secondary to CNS disease may be temporary or permanent, depending on the reversibility of the CNS lesion and the maintenance of integrity of the urinary system. If the bladder becomes severely infected with secondary sclerosis of the bladder wall, normal function will not be restored even if the CNS lesion is corrected. The management of the urinary tract will be discussed here in relation to the functional disorder of micturition that is present.

DETRUSOR AREFLEXIA, SPHINCTER HYPERTONUS

Lesions from the pons to L7 spinal cord segments may destroy the detrusor reflex while producing a UMN type sphincter characterized by hyperreflexia and increased tone (Table 13–3). The animal cannot void and it is difficult if not impossible to express the bladder manually.

The primary requirement in all neurogenic bladder disorders is complete evacuation of the bladder at least three times daily. Manual expression is not only ineffective but dangerous when tone in the urethra is exaggerated. Aseptic catheterization (three times daily) is required. Indwelling catheters should be avoided whenever possible because of the infection that accompanies their use. Detrusor areflexia from overdistention is an exception (see later discussion).

Urinalysis should be repeated weekly or at any time the urine does not look normal. At the first sign of infection quantitative urine culture and sensitivity tests should be obtained and appropriate antibiotic therapy begun.[18] Therapy should be continued until urinalysis verifies correction of the problem.

If catheterization is necessary for prolonged periods (over 1 week), prophylactic antibacterial agents such as methenamine may be indicated. These products should *not* take the place of an aseptic catheterization technique.

If the detrusor reflex returns with good voiding of urine, the bladder should be catheterized periodically to be certain there is no residual urine. Voiding is often incomplete in the early stages, and if 10 to 20 ml or more of residual urine is present, cystitis will probably result.

DETRUSOR AREFLEXIA, SPHINCTER TONE NORMAL

Some lesions of the spinal cord and brain stem may destroy the detrusor reflex without producing hypertonus of the urethral sphincter. The bladder can be manually expressed in many such cases. The urethra of the female dog is short enough that manual expression may be effective even if there is hypertonus of the sphincter. Manual expression, if adequate, is less likely to produce infection than repeated catheterization.

Other aspects of management are the same as those described for hypertonic sphincter above.

DETRUSOR AREFLEXIA, SPHINCTER AREFLEXIA

Lesions of the sacral spinal cord or roots will produce a lower motor neuron deficit of both the bladder and the sphincter. Management of the bladder is the same as that described for normal sphincter tone.

An additional management problem is created by the constant leakage of urine through the incompetent sphincter. More frequent evacuation of the bladder will reduce the problem but not entirely eliminate it. Continual soiling of the skin with urine will quickly lead to irritation and formation of decubital ulcers. Frequent hydrotherapy and protective emollients are useful adjuncts. Management of decubital ulcers is described in Chapter 14.

Long-term management of the patient with paralysis of the sphincter has not been completely successful. Surgical reconstruction of the bladder neck and urethra is sometimes successful in humans but has had no significant trial in animals.[9] Timm and others have developed prosthetic devices which offer promise of a solution;[21] however, the cost of these devices will probably limit their applicability in veterinary medicine.

DETRUSOR AREFLEXIA FROM OVERDISTENTION

Severe overdistention of the bladder can produce a separation of the tight junctions between detrusor muscle fibers, thus preventing excitation-contraction coupling.[10] The neural elements may be normal.

The bladder must be treated early if irreversible deficit is to be avoided after overdistention. Complete evacuation of the bladder must be accomplished and maintained for 1 to 2 weeks. Manual expression is not recommended because of the increased stress on the detrusor muscle. Intermittent aseptic catheterization can be performed at least three times daily but preferably four times a day. An indwelling catheter for the first 5 to 7 days followed by intermittent catheterization, if needed, is the procedure of choice. This is one of the few instances in which an indwelling catheter is recommended. Function should return in 1 to 2 weeks if treatment is successful.

Antibiotics or urinary antiseptics should be administered throughout the treatment period. Frequent urinalyses, with cultures when indicated, are mandatory. Infection in the overdistended bladder will lead to fibrosis, and adequate function will not be restored.

DETRUSOR HYPERREFLEXIA

Frequent voiding of small volumes of urine, often without much warning and with little or no residual urine, is characteristic of detrusor hyperreflexia. Partial long-tract lesions or abnormalities of the cerebellum may produce these signs. The condition is not usually detrimental to the patient, but it may be an early sign of a progressive disease of the nervous system. Additionally, it is socially unacceptable in the house pet. The condition must be differentiated from the small, contracted, irritable bladder associated with chronic cystitis.

If treatment is desired, anticholinergic medication may be of benefit. Propantheline (Pro-Banthine) has been used in doses of from 7.5 to 30 mg three or four times daily. The lowest dose should be tried first and increased in small increments until response is obtained. Overdosage may result in urinary retention in addition to the other side effects characteristic of this group of drugs.[4, 9]

REFLEX DYSSYNERGIA

Initiation of a detrusor reflex with voiding followed by uncontrolled reflex contraction of the urethral sphincter has been termed reflex dyssynergia. Partial lesions of the long tracts are presumed to be responsible, although the condition has been seen in a dog with a cauda equina lesion.

The problem may be related to uninhibited reflexes of the external urethral sphincter (skeletal muscle) or increased tonus in smooth muscle related to adrenergic innervation.[7,8] Because reports of therapeutic trials in humans are limited and only a few cases have been seen in dogs, definitive treatment is not available at this time. Skeletal muscle reflexes may be reduced with diazepam (Valium) or gamma aminobutyric acid (GABA). GABA is not currently available as a pharmaceutical. Sympathetic (adrenergic) activity can be reduced with an alpha-blocking agent such as phenoxybenzamine (Dibenzyline, 10 mg. capsules). Doses must be determined by trial, starting with 10 mg/day and increasing every fourth day if indicated. The major side effect of alpha-blockade is hypotension.

Management of neurogenic bladder disorders is critical for the ultimate prognosis of both reversible and irreversible CNS disorders. A study of chronically paralyzed people revealed that 75 per cent die of renal failure secondary to neurogenic bladder dysfunction.[22]

REFERENCES

1. Bates, C. P., Whiteside, C. G., and Turner-Warwick, R.: Synchronous cine/presence to stress and urge incontinence. Brit. J. Urol. *42*:714–723, 1970.
2. Bors, E., and Comarr, A. E.: *Neurological Urology.* University Park Press, Baltimore, 1971.
3. Bradley, W. E., Timm, G. W., Rockswold, G. L., and Scott, F. B.: Detrusor and urethral electromyelography. J. Urol. *114*:891–894, 1975.
4. Diokono, A. C., Hyndman, C. W., Hardy, D. A., and Lapides, J.: Comparison of action of imipramine (Tofranil) and propantheline (Probanthine) on detrusor contraction. J. Urol. *107*:42–43, 1972.
5. Jonas, U., and Tanagho, E. A.: Studies on vesicourethral reflexes. Invest. Urol. *12*:357–373, 1975.
6. Kelalis, P. P.: Proper perspective on vesicoureteral reflux. Mayo Clin. Proc. *46*:807–818, 1971.
7. Kiesswetter, H., and Schober, W.: Lioresal in the treatment of neurogenic bladder dysfunction. Urol. Int. *30*:63–71, 1975.
8. Krane, R. J., and Olsson, C. A.: Phenoxybenzamine in neurogenic bladder dysfunction. II. Clinical considerations. J. Urol. *110*:653–656, 1973.
9. Lapides, J.: Neuromuscular vesical and ureteral dysfunction. *In* Campbell, M. F., and Harrison, J. H. (eds.): *Urology,* 3rd ed. Vol. 2. W. B. Saunders Co., Philadelphia, 1970.
10. Lloyd-Davies, R. W., Clark, A. E., Prout, W. G., Shuttleworth, K. E. D., and Tighe, J. R.: The effects of stretching the rabbit bladder. Invest. Urol. *8*:145–152, 1970.
11. Low, D. G., Osborne, C. A., and Finco, D. R.: The pillars of diagnosis: history and physical examination. *In* Ettinger, S. J. (ed.): *Textbook of Veterinary Internal Medicine,* Vol 1. Philadelphia, W. B. Saunders Co., 1975.
12. Oliver, J. E., Jr., Bradley, W. E., and Fletcher, T. F.: Spinal cord distribution of the somatic innervation of the external urethral sphincter in the cat. J. Neurol. Sci. *10*:11–23, 1970.
13. Oliver, J. E., Jr.: Neurologic examination, taking the history. Vet. Med. Small Anim. Clin. *67*:433, 1972.
14. Oliver, J. E., Jr., and Young, W. O.: Evaluation of pharmacologic agents for restraint in cystometry in the dog and cat. Am. J. Vet. Res. *34*:665–668, 1973.
15. Oliver, J. E., Jr., and Young, W. O.: Air cystometry in dogs under xylazine-induced restraint. Am. J. Vet. Res. *34*:1433–1435, 1973.
16. Oliver, J. E., Jr., and Selcer, R. R.: Neurogenic causes of abnormal micturition in the dog and cat. Vet. Clin. N. Amer. *4*:517–524, 1974.
17. Oliver, J. E., Jr., and Osborne, C. A.: Neurogenic urinary incontinence. *In* Kirk, R. W. (ed.): *Current Veterinary Therapy VI.* W. B. Saunders Co., Philadelphia, 1977.
18. Osborne, C. A., Low, D. G., and Finco, D. R.: *Canine and Feline Urology.* W. B. Saunders Co., Philadelphia, 1972.
19. Osborne, C. A., and Oliver, J. E., Jr.: Non-neurogenic urinary incontinence. *In* Kirk, R. W. (ed.): *Current Veterinary Therapy VI.* W. B. Saunders Co., Philadelphia, 1977.
20. Tang, P. C., and Ruch, T. C.: Non-neurogenic basis of bladder tonus. Am. J. Physiol. *181*:249–257, 1955.
21. Timm, G. W.: Electromechanical restoration of voiding. Vet. Clin. N. Amer. *4*:525–533, 1974.
22. Tribe, C. R.: *Renal Failure in Paraplegia.* Pitman Medical Pub. Co., London, 1969.

CHAPTER 14

INTERVERTEBRAL DISKS

SECTION 1
DISK DISORDERS IN DOGS

HISTORY

In 130 A.D. Galen studied the spinal column in man and divided it into the cervical, dorsal, and lumbar areas. Galen's anatomical descriptions were used throughout the Dark Ages. In the early 1500's, Vesalius described the intervertebral disk and differentiated the annulus fibrosus and the nucleus pulposus. Further anatomical studies of the intervertebral disk were made in 1857 by Virchow and in 1858 by Von Luschka.[81] Charles Bell, in a book published in London in 1824, may have been the first to describe an intervertebral disk protrusion.[7] In 1896, Kocher described a case of spinal injury in which necropsy revealed a shattered first lumbar disk with the shattered parts protruding into the spinal canal.[81] Oppenheim and Krause in 1909 were the first to report the use of surgery in the treatment of intervertebral disk protrusion. This lesion was at the level of the third lumbar vertebra, and the patient was reported to have recovered.[81] In 1925, Schmorl, a pathologist in Germany, began to examine human spines, and over the five years that followed, he examined nearly 7000 spines at necropsy. Kyphotic deformities and the role of the disk in their formation were described. Schmorl also demonstrated a prolapse of the nucleus pulposus into the spongy part of the vertebral body. These lesions were then known as Schmorl's nodes.[181] In 1929, Dandy operated on two cases of intervertebral disk protrusion.[30] In 1932, Mixter and Barr started a series of publications concerning the true nature of disk protrusions and their pathologic importance in man; they demonstrated that so-called chondromata are actually intervertebral disk herniations and not neoplasias.[133]

A historical note should also be given on intervertebral disk protrusions in veterinary medicine. In 1881, Janson related a case of enchondroma in the vertebral canal of a young dachshund located at L4-5 interspace.[75] In 1883, Kitt and Stoss described a "circumscript pachymeningitis externa chronica" in a 3-year-old pinscher. The deposits outside the dura contained cartilage along with other material. In 1896, Dexler described two types of chronic spinal cord compression—one caused by a primary disease in one or several intervertebral joints that produced secondary ossifying pachymeningitis, and the other the consequence of a disseminated slowly progressive ossification in the dura. These cartilaginous masses, which sometimes became ossified, were situated in the epidural space, and therefore caused a compression myelitis.[34, 75]

In 1910, Jakob also made observations about disk protrusions and posterior paralysis or paraplegia.[98] Joest in 1921 and Wiedemann in 1922 contributed to the knowledge of disk protrusions in the dog, particularly the dachshund.[75] In 1937, Pommer did some original work on the radiographic nature of the intervertebral disk in the dog. He described primary degenerative changes but referred to them as cartilaginous tumors or proliferations originating from the intervertebral disk.[159] Tillmans in 1939 divided the intervertebral disk syndrome into two types, of which the first appeared in the dachshund and was manifested in solitary or unilateral protrusions, whereas the second appeared in various breeds and was manifested in multiple and symmetrical protrusions, especially in aged dogs.[75] In the 1940's, Schlotthauer,[180] Schnelle,[182] Riser,[169] and Fankhauser[38] published works which indicated the significance of intervertebral disk prolapse and disease in neurologic symptoms of paralysis or paraplegia.

In the 1950's, many papers were published regarding the various aspects of intervertebral disk disease in the dog. Hansen and Olsson described what seems to be the breed predisposition of the disease, particularly in the chondrodystrophoid group of dogs.[76] Olsson in 1951 proposed treatment with disk fenestration.[144] In 1951, McGrath described the pathologic and clinical symptomatology of disk protrusions.[126] Redding proposed treatment with hemilaminectomy,[168] and Greene proposed dorsal laminectomy.[66]

In 1952, Hoerlein reported a large number of cases in which hemilaminectomy and disk fenestration had been successful.[82] During the 1950's, Hoerlein and Olsson published numerous papers concerning the surgical treatment of disk protrusions.[83–88, 143, 145, 147–150] Smith in 1954 and Vaughan in 1958 described the general aspects of disk herniation,[187, 210] and in the early 1960's, Funkquist of Sweden published numerous articles on the use of water-soluble contrast media in canine myelography and also on the efficacy of decompressive laminectomy.[41–48]

Since 1970, there have been voluminous veterinary contributions to the literature on disk protrusions. Articles include discussions of the incidence, neurological signs, pathology, radiographic diagnosis, electrodiagnostics, and surgical therapy for disk disease. No special notations will be given here on leaders in the field because important contributors might inadvertently be omitted.

ANATOMICAL CONSIDERATION OF THE DISK

The function of the vertebral column is to provide a rigid structure for the attachment of muscles and bones and to protect delicate structures, especially parts of the nervous system, while being pliable enough to allow movement with maximal efficiency. These objectives are attained by the presence of a series of vertebrae connected by two types of intervertebral joints. The intervertebral disk is an important component in one of these types of articulations.[158]

A comparative study by King and Smith[103] has established that disk structures in man and the dog are very similar; hence, this discussion refers to the literature about both man and dog.

In the dog the intervertebral disks are spaced between some 50 irregular segments of bone in the vertebral column, starting cranially at the C2–3 interspace. As mentioned earlier in the section on anatomy of the spine (Chapter 13), the vertebrae articulate with each other at three points along each end, namely, the two articular processes and the body. The articular processes are supplied with joint capsules and are typically diarthrodial joints; the vertebral bodies have no such arrangement[129, 130] but are sometimes called amphiarthrodial joints.[189]

The intervertebral disk is composed of an outer fibrous structure called the annulus fibrosus, which invests the central homogeneous mass of fluid, gelatinouslike material called the nucleus pulposus. The annulus is composed of 25 to 30 concentrically placed lamellae which may divide and blend and often do not completely encircle the disk. The inner lamellae are derived from the cartilaginous plate and the outer ones are a continuation of Sharpey's fibers of the vertebral epiphyses. The lamellae pass from vertebra to vertebra, crossing each other at angles of 100 to 120 degrees as seen from the cranial or caudal side. The ventral part of the annulus is from one and half to three times as thick as the dorsal part, which means that the nucleus is always eccentrically placed.

The nucleus pulposus is a distinctly limited structure, originating from the notochord and composed in the young individual of a gelatinous or mucoid mass with a high water content. Between the uniform mesenchymal cells there is a three-dimensional lattice gel system consisting of poorly differentiated collagen fibrils and an amorphous mass and containing chondroitin sulfuric acid as well as keratan sulfate.[77, 129, 189]

The largest intervertebral disk is located at the lumbosacral junction (L7-S1), and the disks decrease in size progressively to the smallest, which is located at the junction of vertebrae C2–3. The thickness of the disk is directly proportional to the circumferential measurement; disk L7-S1 is the thickest (Fig. 14–1).[127, 129, 189]

The disk is bordered cranially and caudally by plates composed chiefly of hyaline cartilage, which adhere to the ends of the bony vertebrae by means of a thin layer of calcified cartilage. The annulus fibrosus binds itself not only to the cartilaginous plate, but also directly to the vertebral bodies. This arrangement enhances the elastic properties of the disk.[127, 129] The supportive area of disk is completed by the dorsal longitudinal ligament which is strongly attached to the median ridge of bone on the floor of the canal and spreads out to intermingle with the surface of the layers of the annulus between the consecutive vertebrae. A ventral longitudinal ligament runs in similar fashion on the ventral surface of many of the vertebral bodies.

The presence of a vascular system in the intervertebral disk has been questioned for many years. Keyes and Compere[102] have stated that avascularity exists in man from the embryonic stage throughout life, whereas Uebermuth[209] and Böhmung[8] agreed that vessels are present in the disk until after adolescence. Lee concluded from his studies in the cat that although vascularity in the disk declines from maturity to old age, blood vessels remain intact in the outermost layers of the annulus.[111] Since the disk performs a purely mechanical function, it is probably capable of maintaining itself on a very low rate of metabolism. Beadle proposed that the nourishment of the disk after adolesence (beginning in the third decade in man) is maintained by a cranial-caudal diffusion of blood elements from the bone marrow in the vertebral body to the intervertebral disks.[6] Brodin[14] has shown, by studying the penetration of fluorescent compounds in rabbits, that the nutrition of the disk is accomplished by diffusion currents from the vertebral bodies as well as from the periphery of the disk itself. Paulson[155] noted that within the nucleus the diffusion rate is dependent upon the size of the interfibrillary pores. These pores average 15 Å in the bovine nucleus.[14, 155]

It was believed formerly that the disk was devoid of nerves; however, Roofe has demonstrated copious nerve endings in the dorsal annulus and dorsal longitudinal ligament. Roofe also states that the type of terminal arborization in these nerves indicates that they are pain fibers.[170]

In man, Cloward postulated that the so-called sinovertebral nerve was responsible for carrying painful impulses from the annulus of the disk. This pain is often seen as

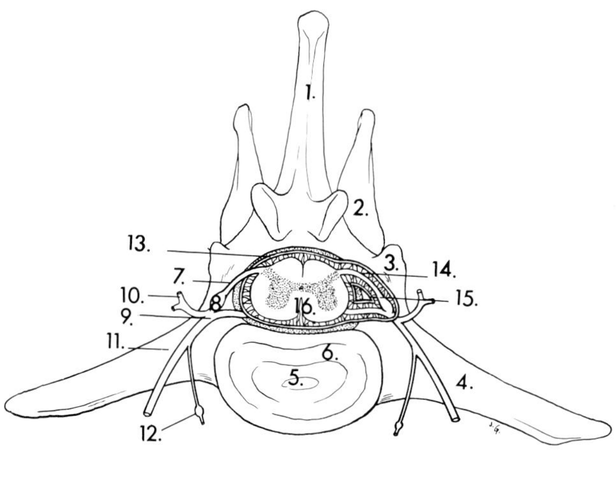

FIGURE 14–1 Intervertebral disk and associated structures. (1) Spinous process; (2) articular process; (3) accessory process; (4) transverse process; (5) nucleus pulposus; (6) annulus fibrosus; (7) dorsal root; (8) dorsal root ganglion; (9) ventral root; (10) dorsal branch; (11) ventral branch; (12) ramus communicans and sympathetic trunk ganglion; (13) epidural space; (14) dura mater and arachnoid; (15) subarachnoid space; (16) spinal cord.

referred pain to the scapular area.[23] Dohn feels that this nerve is largely responsible for the cervical syndrome consisting of pain in the head, neck, and shoulders from degenerated or unstable cervical disks that are not producing radicular or myelopathic involvement.[35] Many feel that there is clinical evidence that this syndrome also occurs in dogs.

The nucleus pulposus develops embryologically from the notochord and in turn is modified by the extension of tissue from the intervertebral disk anlage. In the 8-week-old human fetus, the nucleus pulposus is composed of notochord cells alone; however, it is being invaded by fibrocartilage cells from the fibrocartilage envelope. The annulus is better developed and already connects the bodies of the cartilaginous vertebrae. At the time of birth, the fibrocartilaginous cells are interspersed throughout the nucleus, and the notochord cells are inconspicuous. Differences in anatomical considerations in the various species will be elaborated upon in the section on the pathologic aspects of the disk.

Although the anatomy of the spinal canal was discussed in the preceding chapter, it should be emphasized at this point that the spinal canal of the dog is notably small, and therefore its contents are comparatively crowded. The vertebral canal is about 25 per cent longer and 20 per cent wider than the cord.

In the thoracic area, the intercapital ligament (formerly called the ligamentum conjugale costarum) covers the entire width of the disk dorsally and therefore largely replaces the dorsal annulus fibrosus.[88, 92] According to Miller, it is absent on the first, eleventh, twelfth, and thirteenth pairs of ribs,[129] which may be one factor that explains the lack of disk protrusions in the midthoracic area (Figs. 14–2 to 14–4).

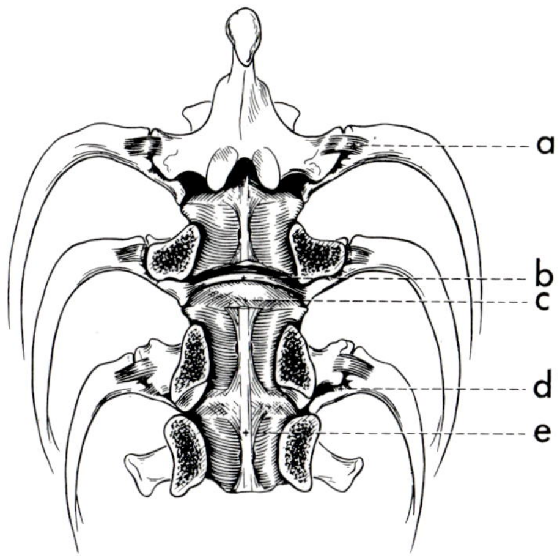

FIGURE 14–2 Ligaments of vertebral column and ribs, dorsal aspect: (a) costotransverse ligament; (b) intercapital ligament; (c) intervertebral disk; (d) ligament of neck; (e) dorsal longitudinal ligament. (From Miller, M. E., Christensen, G. C., and Evans, H. E.: *Anatomy of the Dog.* W. B. Saunders Co., Philadelphia, 1964.)

PHYSIOLOGY OF THE DISK

Physiologically, the intervertebral disk forms an elastic cushion between the bony vertebrae in order to allow movement, to

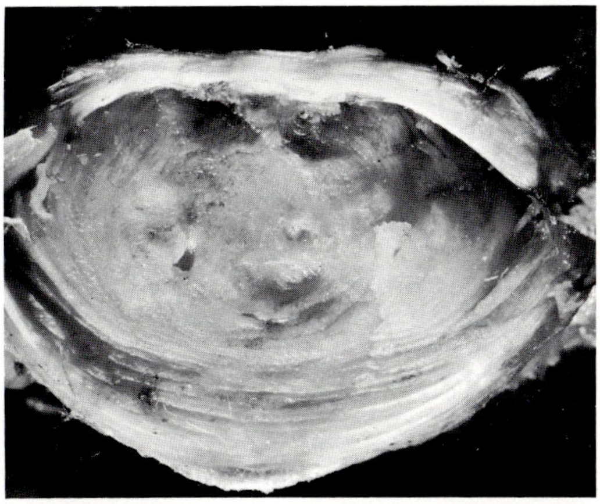

Fig. 14–3

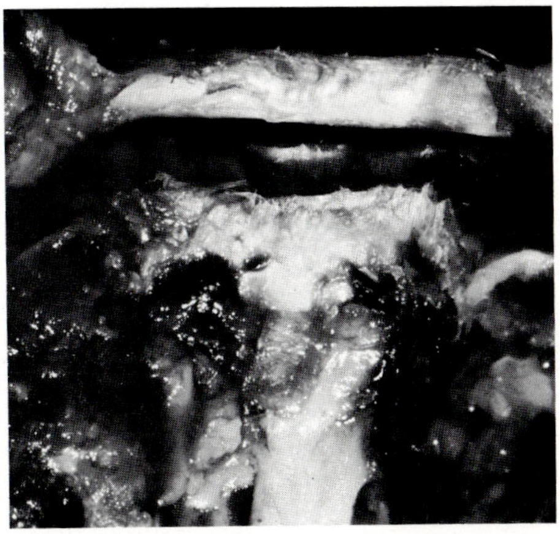

Fig. 14–4

FIGURE 14–3 Intercapital ligament (formerly the ligamentum conjugale costarum). Notice how it forms the dorsal annulus fibrosus.

FIGURE 14–4 Intercapital ligament. This ligament occupies the entire dorsal aspect of the disk between the adjacent vertebrae. (From Hoerlein, B. F.: Intervertebral disk protrusions in the dog. Am. J. Vet. Res. *14*, 264, 1953.)

minimize trauma and shock, and to unite the segments into a column.[1]

Armstrong has described the functions of the annulus as follows: (1) stability for the regional vertebrae, (2) allowance of movement between the vertebrae and prevention of excessive movement, (3) nuclear retention, and (4) shock absorption. The nucleus functions also to (1) absorb shock and facilitate movement between the vertebrae, (2) equilize stresses, and (3) facilitate fluid exchange between vertebrae and disks. The functions of the cartilaginous plates are (1) protection of vertebral bodies, and (2) facilitation of fluid exchange between disks and vertebral bodies.[1]

The vertebral column in four-footed animals is not a truss with its points of support at the two pairs of extremities, as it is in man. The mechanism that serves to bend or straighten the vertebral column should instead be compared to a bow and string, the bow being represented by the dorsal structures and the string by the sternum and rectus abdominus muscle. As far as the dog is concerned, the most important center of mobility is the region at and around the so-called anticlinal vertebra (T11), which marks the transition from the backward- to the forward-sloping spinous processes. It is interesting to note that the most frequent incidence of disk protrusions occurs immediately posterior to this area.[189]

Because of its design, the disk functions as a shock absorber as well as a distributor of pressure. When craniocaudal compression occurs, the shock is absorbed by the displacement of the incompressible nucleus in all directions and by distention of the annulus. All movements that cause compression of only part of the disk will, however, result in even distribution of pressure on the adjacent ends of the vertebral bodies because the pressure in a medium that contains a liquid is uniform. The fact that hydrostatic conditions prevail in the center of the disk has been shown by measuring intradiskal pressure.[96]

When the vertebral column is placed in the vertical position and thereafter loaded, the pressure on the annulus is three to five times greater in a tangential direction than in a vertical direction. Therefore, the normal annulus in an animal has to withstand a more severe stress through tension than through pressure. This ability to withstand severe stress is mechanically great, since violent physical strain more often results in fractures than in ruptured disks (at least in the nonchondrodystrophoid group of dogs).[77, 189]

The intradiskal pressure depends chiefly on two factors, the water-binding properties of the nucleus and the power of resistance and elasticity of the surrounding structures, particularly the annulus. The former is obviously closely connected with the content and proportions of the polysaccharides involved and also with collagen content. The water-binding ability of the nucleus, which some authors feel is the result of osmotic pressure and others feel is the result of imbibition pressure, decreases continuously with increasing age, paralleling the structural age changes.[77]

PATHOLOGIC ASPECTS OF THE DISK

After considering the anatomy and physiology of the disk, we should consider the pathologic changes that can develop. Most authorities agree that degeneration of the disk occurs constantly in the aging process. One of the significant features of degeneration is the loss of fluid not only from the annulus fibrosus but also from the nucleus pulposus. The water content of the disk in man has been calculated as follows:

Age *(Years)*	Annulus Fibrosus	Nucleus Pulposus
	(Per cent water)	
Newborn	78	88
18	72	80
30	70	
66		74
77	67	69

From these data, it can be seen that in the older person there is much less water in the disk than in the newborn infant. It has been stated that degeneration may be associated not only with dehydration but also with loss or reduction of hyaluronic acid and other mucopolysaccharides. Hyaluronic acid has only been isolated in immature human disks. The tissue is dull, gray, and less firm. The nuclear cells are reduced in number, and some of the fibers degenerate. The annulus also degenerates and may become brown. Usually, the outer rings of the annulus remain normal for a longer period than the inner ones, and at this stage the outer rings support the disk. Necrosis may cause yellowing of the disk;[217] when necrosis develops, the disk may undergo calcification.[20] In the dog, calcification frequently seems to start in the nucleus and perinuclear areas.

Hansen[74, 75] termed the process of disk degeneration in the dog systemic disk disease. He reports one form of systemic disk disease, which was related to pathologic forms of chondrodystrophy, to be prevalent in dachshunds, French bulldogs, and Pekingese. This was later confirmed by observation of achondroplasia (chondrodystrophy) as an occasional disease in miniature poodles. In these achondroplastic poodles, the histologic appearances of the costochondral junction, where endochondral ossification is best studied, and the intervertebral disk were in complete accord with the appearance of the same structures in normal puppies of chondrodystrophoid breeds. There was evidence that disk degeneration and disk prolapse in human chondrodystrophic dwarfs correspond to the conditions in chondrodystrophoid dogs.

The terms metamorphosis and degeneration are applied interchangeably to the disk process in veterinary literature. Hansen, as mentioned before, called the changes in the nucleus a systemic disease and used the word degeneration frequently.[74, 77, 95] However, the same author and others use the terms chondroid and fibroid metamorphosis for the changes occurring in disks. According to Dorland,[36] degeneration means a deterioration of tissue, usually from a higher to a lower functional form, while tissue metamorphosis refers to any change in tissue, either normal or pathologic. Therefore, degeneration could be considered a retrograde metamorphosis.[36] The author will continue to use the terms rather interchangeably but will emphasize degeneration as a more appropriate term.

The systemic disk disease in the dog appears in two morphologically distinct forms, one in dogs of the chondrodystrophoid breeds (dachshund, French bulldog, Pekingese) at a comparatively early age, and one in aged dogs of all other nonchondrodystrophoid breeds. The degeneration begins as a fibroid or chondroid metamorphosis or change at the periphery of the nucleus pulposus, and progresses centrally. In chondrodystrophoid animals this process takes the *chondroid* metaplastic form and occurs at 8 months to 2 years of age, whereas in nonchondrodystrophoid animals the change is *fibroid* and occurs at 8 to 10 years of age. Chondroid metamorphosis or changes at the center of the disk in chondrodystrophoid dogs might be interpreted as the result of deferral of the final embryologic stages because of the abnormally slow differentiation. Degeneration of the annulus fibrosus accompanies or possibly precedes the nuclear changes. As nuclear metamorphosis progresses, it loses its useful elasticity and thus the ability to act as an efficient shock absorber. A possible decrease in nuclear nutrition may result from an ineffective pumping mechanism potentiating further degeneration. As the nucleus continues to degenerate, a resulting diffuse disintegration occurs, leading to homogeneous calcification.[74, 75]

In chondrodystrophoid dogs at the age of 1 year, 75 to 100 per cent of all nuclei have been transformed into chondroid tissue and 30 to 60 per cent show macroscopic signs of degeneration, largely in the form of calcification. When dachshunds (at a mean age of 2 years) were surveyed radiographically, nearly 90 per cent of them showed disk calcification. When such dogs reach 6 or 7 years of age probably all of them will show macroscopically observable signs of disk degeneration, and about 75 per cent of them will have developed prolapse of some degree.[74, 75, 77]

Braund and associates[12, 58, 59, 205] recently reported the histochemical analysis and histologic examination of disks on greyhounds and beagles. The beagle was considered to be a chondrodystrophoid type of dog based on femoral epiphyseal growth plates and disk morphology. All beagle disks became chondroid (as defined by Hansen), and only the thoracic disks in the greyhound showed any sign of chondroid metaplasia. The disk annulus in the newborn beagle and greyhound contained hyaluronic acid, chondroitin sulfate, and keratin sulfate, while the nucleus and transitional zone contained no keratin sulfate but did contain the other two substances.[58, 59] Keratin sulfate was detected histochemically in the nucleus and transitional zone after 4 months. At 4 to 6 months of age in both breeds, hyaluronic acid disappeared from all regions of the disk, but the ratio of keratin sulfate and chondroitin sulfate steadily increased with age. The galactosamine/glucosamine ratio* of nearly 1.00 was present in all beagle disks and in the thoracic disk of the greyhound at 2 years of age.[12] In the greyhound thoracolumbar and lumbar disks this ratio of 1.00 was present at 4 to 5 years of age. Different functional responses to disk stresses were considered to account for the incongruity of the chemical parameters in the chondrystrophoid (beagle) and nonchondrodystrophoid (greyhound) dogs.[59]

Further work in two groups of 4-month-old beagles demonstrated that disk development is controlled at least in part by genetic determinants.[59] Group 1 was composed of half siblings and group 2 contained full siblings. Group 1 showed 10 to 15 times as much collagen in the nucleus as group 2, and there were significantly lower levels of hyaluronic acid (an index of hyaluronic acid and chondroitin sulfate) compared to group 2. Furthermore, acceleration in the glycosaminoglycan aging pattern was observed in immature disks which had been subjected to spinal arthrodesis.[12]

Further study of the histochemical changes in the aging disks of the chondrodystroid and nonchondrodystrophoid groups of dogs, as well as studies of the influence of stress and heredity on these changes will do much to clarify the pathogenesis of disk disease and will possibly aid in finding a means of prevention. The current practice is to treat only the clinical syndrome, and few suggestions have been offered for prevention.[12]

Hansen classified as type 1 chondroid degeneration those prolapses occurring frequently in the younger chondrodystrophoid dog that result from a total rupture of the annulus fibrosus and are therefore more or less massive. The senile or type 2 fibroid degeneration seen in nonchondrodystrophoid breeds is caused by a partial rupture of the annulus and causes a round domelike bulging of the dorsal surface of the disk. This type 2 disk degeneration has certain points in common with spondylosis deformans. Type 1 prolapses are caused by a more or less broad, linear rupture of the annulus and are large in a vertical or horizontal direction; their shape is irregular and their consistency brittle and grainy. Type 2 prolapses are usually smaller and smooth, and are cushion-shaped, hemispherical, or dome-shaped at or around the disk itself (Figs. 14–5 to 14–8).[74, 75, 77]

In the acute type 1 disk prolapse the rupture is accompanied by epidural hemorrhage, the volume of which may exceed that of the protruded material. The extruded nuclear material is gritty, cheese-like, hemorrhagic, or slate gray in appearance; it can be a somewhat circumscribed vertical mass or a widespread, horizontal,

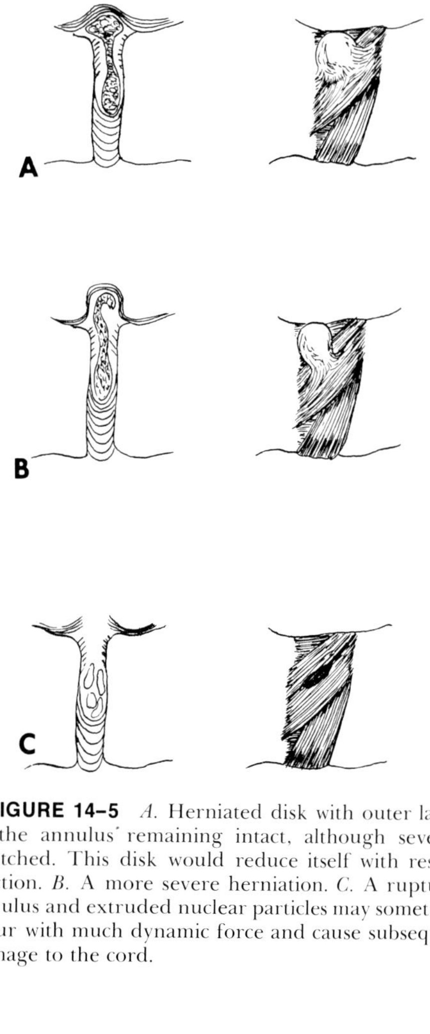

FIGURE 14–5 *A.* Herniated disk with outer layers of the annulus remaining intact, although severely stretched. This disk would reduce itself with rest or traction. *B.* A more severe herniation. *C.* A ruptured annulus and extruded nuclear particles may sometimes occur with much dynamic force and cause subsequent damage to the cord.

*An index of keratin sulfate/chondroitin sulfate in mature animals.

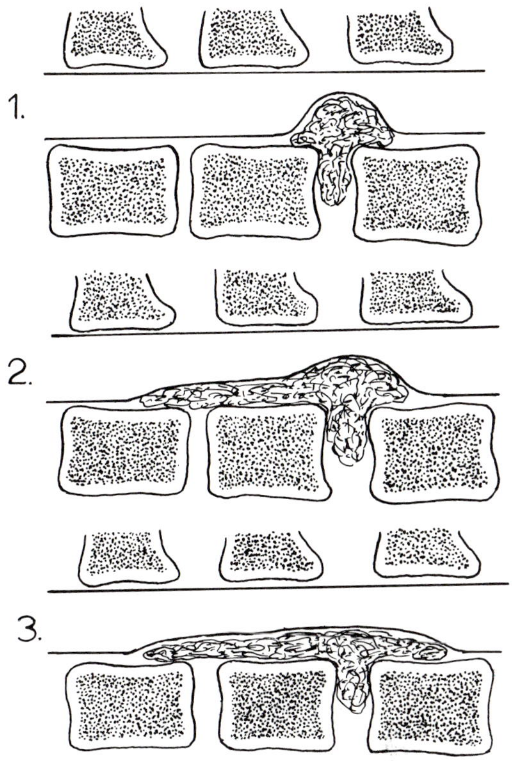

FIGURE 14–6 The stages of a ruptured disk, showing its distribution in the extradural space and subsequent spinal cord pressure. *1.* Initial stage of ruptured disk and protrusion. *2.* Migration of extruded nucleus pulposus. *3.* Note that nucleus may extend 1 to 3 vertebral lengths.

carpet-like mass extending around the sides of the dura. An inflammatory reaction occurs, causing a fibrinous adhesion between the protruding mass and the dura. The protrusion is composed of polymorphonuclear leukocytes, red cells, fibroblasts, large mononuclear cells, polynuclear giant cells, occasional chondrocytes, and much nondescript necrotic tissue debris. The inflammation is like that caused by a foreign body and is initiated by the irritating nucleus and the forceful ejection ("dynamic force" of Olsson) of the nucleus. The body tries to absorb the foreign material and frequently does so more or less completely. Incomplete absorption leaves a mass that organizes into a fibroid, cartilaginous, and frequently calcific protrusion. A subsequent rupture in the same disk creates a larger residual mass that is fairly characteristic of cervical or caudal lumbar disk disease. The thoracolumbar junction is frequently afflicted with a severe rupture of the annulus where the degenerated nucleus is driven against the cord with "dynamic force." Such a "blowout" causes severe neurological signs and occasionally a progressive hemorrhagic malacia of the cord which results in a progressive respiratory paralysis and death (Figs. 14–9 to 14–12).[82, 89]

An effort was made by the author to determine experimentally if the extradural reaction of a ruptured disk was due to the expulsion of the nucleus in the epidural space or whether the nucleus was an irritating substance. Nuclear material obtained from disk currettage was placed in the extradural space by means of a trephine opening into the spinal canal. The dogs were destroyed in 2 to 4 weeks. The most typical reproduction of the extradural deposit, as seen in clinical cases, was obtained when the nucleus from an aged cocker spaniel was placed in the extradural space of a mongrel puppy. The microscopic changes of the deposit were indistin-

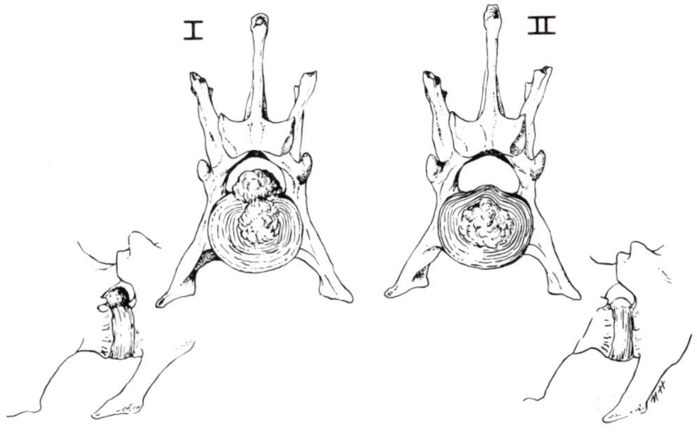

FIGURE 14–7 Hansen's classification of disk protrusions. Type I is the clinical ruptured disk with a massive extrusion of the nucleus and a compressive mass on the cord. This type is characteristic of the chondrodystrophoid group of dogs. Type II is typically a small round dome shaped protrusion seen in older dogs and generally produces very mild clinical signs or none. This type is characteristic of nonchondrodystrophoid groups of dogs.

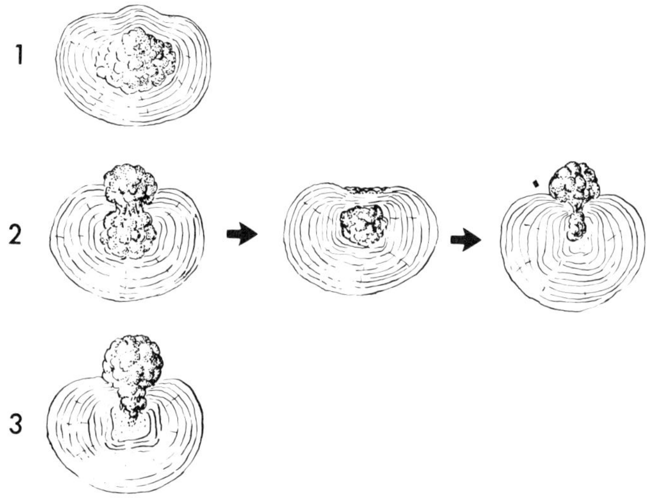

FIGURE 14–8 A sequence in a clinical disk (Hansen's type I). *1.* A partial rupture or stretching of the inner annular fibers, causing a small herniation of the nucleus. *2.* A complete rupture of the annulus which may be phagocytized by scavenger cells; the annulus heals with fibrous or scar tissue only to rupture again under clinical stress. *3.* A massive compression of the spinal cord results.

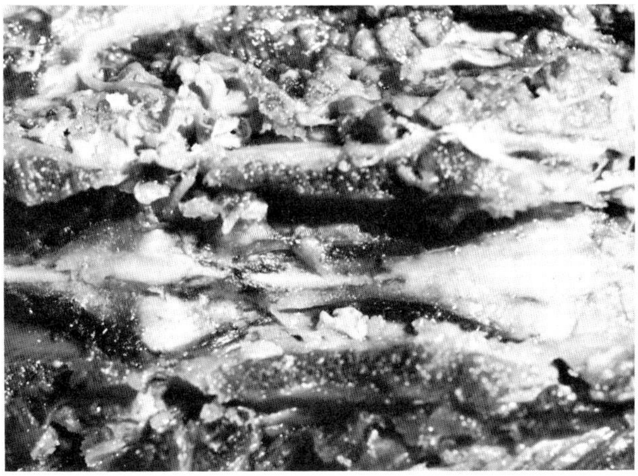

FIGURE 14–9 In disk protrusions of aged dogs without chondrodystrophy (Hansen's type II), small dome-like prominences are frequently seen. The disk in the center shows bilateral protrusions, while the one at the right shows a central protrusion in the dorsal longitudinal ligament. The roof of the canal and spinal cord have been removed.

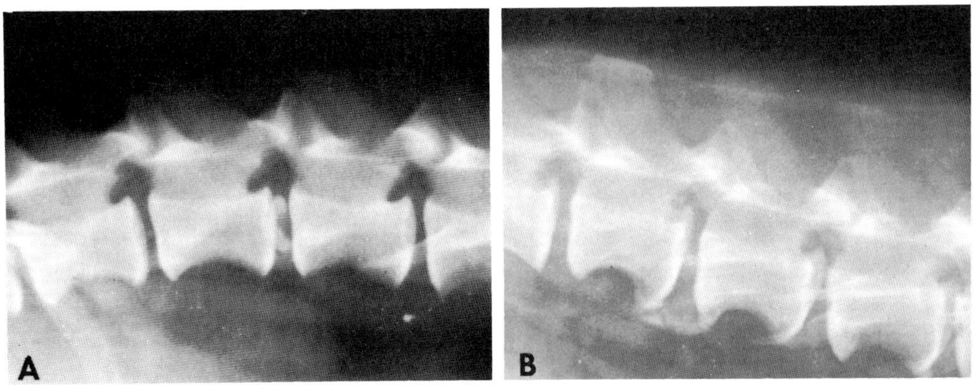

FIGURE 14–10 *A.* Calcified nucleus (L2–3) in a 2-year-old dachshund. *B.* The same disk, 9 years later, has lost nearly all its calcium, but the interspace is now stabilized by a ventral spondylitic "osseous bridge."

guishable from those of a deposit in a clinical case. This finding suggests that trauma is not an essential factor in the cause of this reaction, but that the nuclear substance, especially if it has undergone degeneration, initiates much of the extradural reaction.[82, 83, 89]

The terminology of the displaced mass has not been well defined by many clinicians. Most frequently the syndrome is called "disk protrusion," which might be an all-inclusive term for any mass originating from the disk and placing pressure on the cord, nerve root, or cord terminations. Figure 14–8 shows the stages of the pressure mass. An annulus that is partially ruptured while its outer layer is stretched but still contains the nucleus is shown as a *disk herniation;* a completely ruptured annulus from which the nuclear mass is forced out into the epidural space is called a *ruptured disk* or an *extruded* or *prolapsed disk;* an acute rupture or "blowout" refers to a sudden rupture that causes severe neurological signs; and finally, the protruding mass increases in size and density because of a series of small ruptures over a long period of time. Radiographically, these more chronic stages are accompanied by loss of disk spacing and fibrotic and calcific changes, not only in the protrusion but also in the residual part of the disk. The clinical signs and history are related to the type of disk disease present. The recurrences may be due to the same disk rupturing and consolidating or to the protrusion of another disk in the same general area.[89]

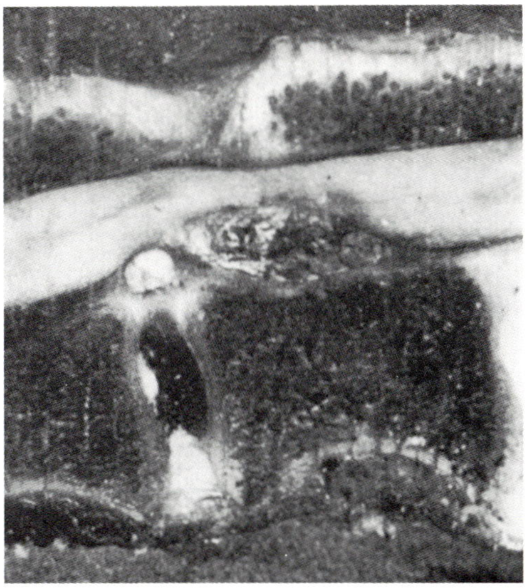

FIGURE 14–12 An epidural deposit of ruptured disk material and necrotic mass (2 mm lateral to the part of the spine shown in Figure 14–11). (From Gage, E. P., and Hoerlein, B. F.: The vertebral column. *In Canine Surgery,* 2nd Archibald ed. American Veterinary Publications, Inc., Santa Barbara, Calif., 1974.)

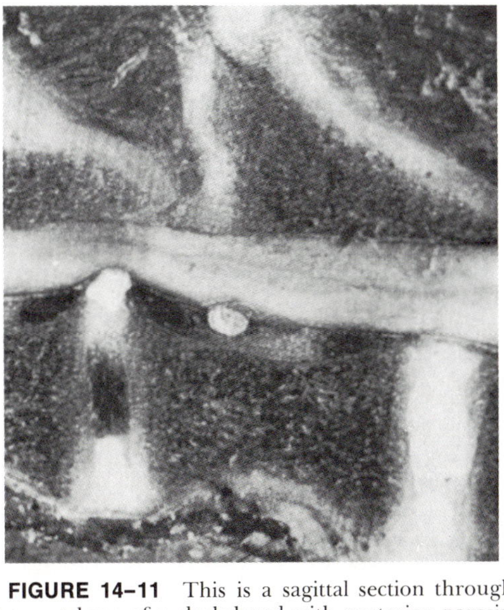

FIGURE 14–11 This is a sagittal section through the vertebrae of a dachshund with posterior paresis, showing a calcified disk protrusion. Notice the compression mass caudal to the protruding disk. (From Gage, E. P., and Hoerlein, B. F.: The vertebral column. *In Canine Surgery,* 2nd Archibald ed. American Veterinary Publications, Inc., Santa Barbara, Calif., 1974.)

These characteristics of the protruding mass and stages of prolapse in chondrodystrophoid breeds also apply in many ways to the protruded intervertebral disk in nonchondrodystrophoid breeds of dogs. Disk protrusion can occur in any breed, large or small, young or old, during certain types of stresses. The acute "blowout" may occur when the disk has not undergone chondroid or fibroid degeneration, but a ruptured disk has also resulted in an extruded nucleus, which causes an irritating, inflammatory reaction epidurally. The usual type of disk protrusion seen in a nonchondrodystrophoid dog is caused by a recurrent partial rupture in which the dome-shaped mass finally becomes large enough to cause clinical pain, paresis, and occasionally paralysis (Figs. 14–13 to 14–17).[89]

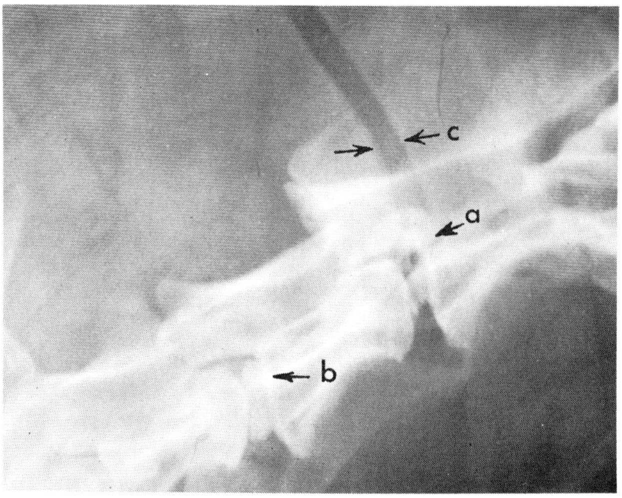

FIGURE 14–13 Radiograph of a disk protrusion (C2–3). (a) Notice the calcified disk at C3–4 (b) and the spastic musculature as evidenced by cross "streaking" (c).

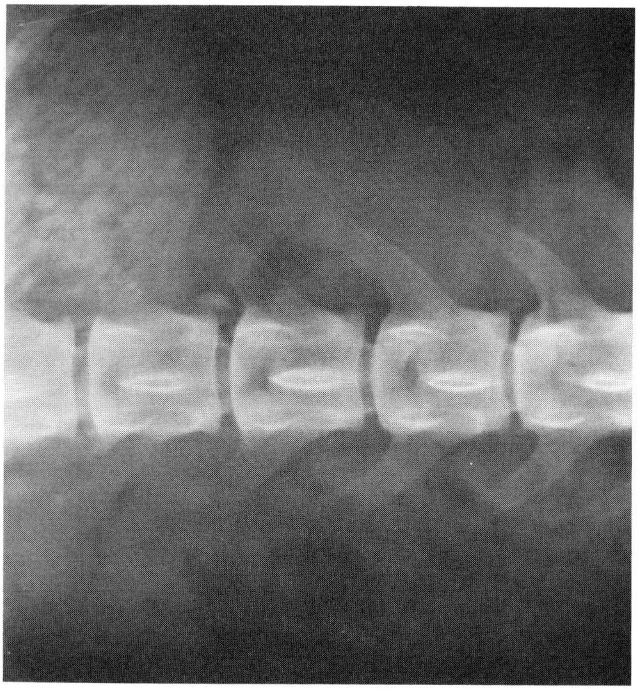

FIGURE 14–14 A ruptured disk in the *lateral* annulus has resulted in a calcific protrusion. This mass encircled the dorsal nerve root and produced considerable pain but no paralysis.

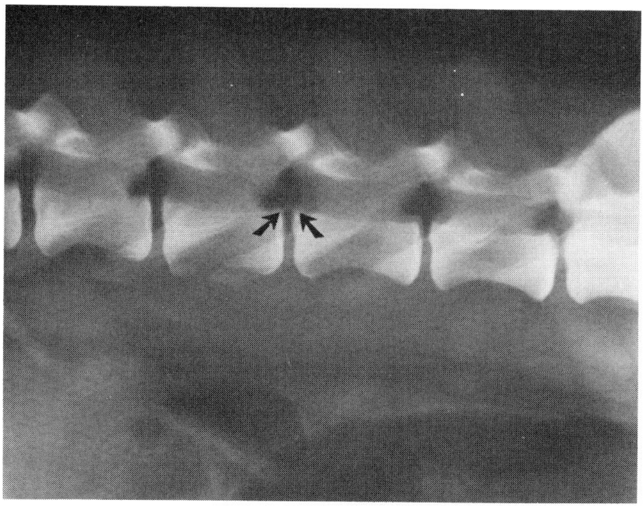

FIGURE 14–15 Calcified outermost layer of the annulus fibrosus, which could look grossly like a small disk protrusion seen in nonchondrodystrophoid dogs (Hansen type II).

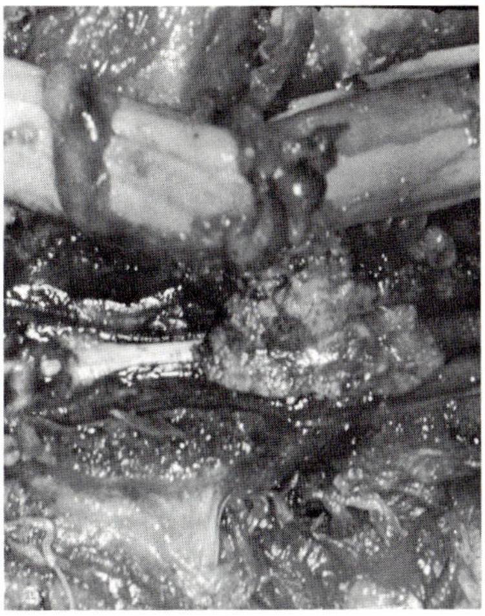

Fig. 14–16

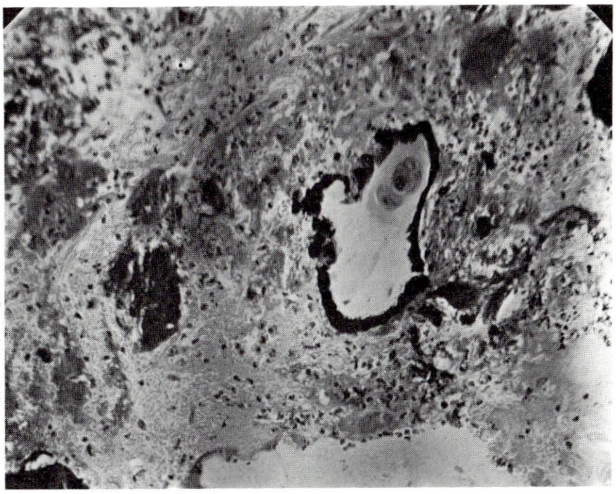

Fig. 14–17

FIGURE 14–16 Case of a large protrusion in a lumbar disk. The disk probably suffered from several partial ruptures and protrusions which organized into a mass, gradually increasing in size after each episode. Periodic attacks of pain occurred and paraplegia eventually resulted.

FIGURE 14–17 The compression mass presented in Figure 14–16 consisted of fibrotic, necrotic, hemorrhagic, calcific, and cartilaginous tissue. Notice the large cartilage cell slightly to the right of the center of the picture.

PATHOLOGIC CHANGES IN THE SPINAL CORD

Following consideration of the degeneration and changes that occur in the disk subsequent to localized disk protrusion, it is appropriate to consider the pathologic changes resulting in the spinal cord. As noted in Chapter 13, Tarlov has shown that compressions of the cord cause a mechanical derangement of nerve tissue that promotes the histologic changes noted. He felt that ischemia or local anoxia of the compression area therefore is not the chief cause of the changes. This is the reason why compressions lend themselves to surgical removal, which would not be the case if ischemia were the primary cause.[69, 201] However, there is a growing evidence that vascular factors can contribute significantly to the microscopic damage seen in the spinal cord with disk protrusion. When hemorrhage or edema from traumatic spinal cord insult causes a rise in intramedullary pressure, the intrinsic vessels become compromised and blood flow diminishes. An autodestructive process of ischemia causing further spinal cord damage occurs.[69, 89, 115, 149]

CHRONIC DISK PROTRUSIONS

Griffiths has classified pathological changes in the spinal cord caused by disk protrusions into three broad groups: (1) compressive changes, (2) malacia, and (3) diffuse demyelination. The compressive changes are distortions of shape of the cord by the "button-like" type 1 (Funkquist) protrusion masses. When the protrusion has spread out in the epidural space (Funkquist type 3), the compression is minimal. Occasionally it appears as if the denticulate ligaments anchoring the cord to the dural laterally prevent any gross displacement of the cord. White matter is usually more severely affected than gray. The lateral columns show the most damage, the ventral columns next, and the dorsal columns show the least. Patchy demyelination and phagocytic microglia, which eventually give a motheaten appearance, are seen. Usually a general astrocytic proliferation is seen. In a clinical syndrome that is gradually becoming more severe, there is an associated increase in vascularity, mainly of precapillary arterioles. Many arterioles and some veins have a thickened adventitia due to an increase in collagen.[69] Other pathologists have described a thickened dura and meningeal adhesion adjacent to the protrusion mass (Fig. 14–18).

Most cords with *malacia* have little evidence of compression. The malacia is not always present at the protrusion site but may be some distance from the lesion. It is present in the white matter, but only the periphery of the gray matter is affected.

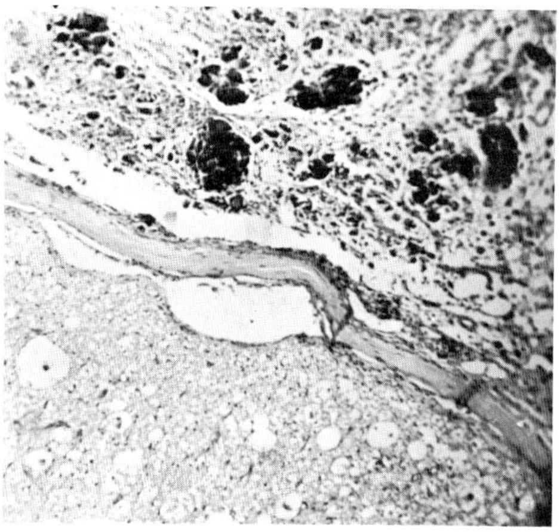

FIGURE 14–18 The changes in the spinal cord adjacent to the disk protrusion are characterized by demyelination, cavitation, gliosis, and dural thickening and adhesions. The pathologic changes are localized to the pressure area, and may be termed a *local* compression myelitis. (From Hoerlein, B. F.: Intervertebral disc protrusions in the dog. Vet. Scope *4*, Fall, 1959.)

Characteristic sites are the dorsolateral funiculus, lateral funiculus, the base and central area of the dorsal funiculus, and the ventral funiculus. The character of the malacia varies with the stage. In 8 days, the shortest duration studied, there was a well-established triangular area of malacia in one dorsolateral funiculus. The borders were ragged and ill-defined with capillary proliferation,whereas in older lesions the borders were clear-cut and well defined, and the vessels were surrounded by a thin sheath of collagen.[69]

Diffuse demyelination may be seen in cords with no evidence of compression and may be as severe as malacia. The demyelination appears in no obvious preferred site and may affect all columns of white matter or only small areas of one column. There is a moderate increase in small vessels, especially veins, in demyelinated areas.[69]

Changes in gray matter consisted of occasional malacia when the periphery of a dorsal horn was involved. Loss of neurons was common to all cords. Long-standing lesions showed fenestration of the gray matter due to loss of neurons and fibers. Microgliosis was never as marked as in the white matter, and lipid phagocytes were infrequent.[69]

Griffiths[71, 72] feels that there is a probable vascular factor in the pathogenesis of cord lesions in many disk protrusions. Many cords show no evidence of compression, and those with severe compression afterward have less severe lesions than those with compression. The site of maximal cord damage is not always opposite the protrusion, and many cords show lesser changes several segments away from the site of maximal damage. The appearance of many areas of malacia is wedge-shaped, and there may be an area of relatively normal white matter between the malacic area and the pia mater. It is suggested that these infarcts may be in areas supplied by the distal ramifications of the ventral spinal artery. The gray matter is usually spared infarcts. The reduced blood flow of the ventral spinal artery and intramedullary branches may be due to (1) compression by the disk material of branches of ventral spinal artery, (2) compression of ventral spinal artery itself, or (3) compression of a major artery in the intervertebral foramen before it can supply the ventral spinal artery. The fact that no marked pathological changes were found in these arteries by Griffiths indicates that the infarcts are due to compression and diminution of flow rather than to obstruction by thrombi.

It has been suggested that possibly nonmalacic lesions primarily involving the white matter are due to venous obstruction. Experimental obstruction of the sagittal vein in cats has shown that the major changes occurred in the white matter.[70–72]

Lindblad and associates, reporting on vascular disturbances resulting from disk protrusion in the dog, described their work with microangiography and phlebography. The disk protrusion caused a compression of veins which resulted in stasis and edema in the cord. In advanced cases, a disturbed arterial pattern was also seen. Retrograde contrast filling of longitudinal vertebral venous sinuses has not been observed in dogs with acute disk protrusions, even when there were no signs; however, retrograde filling was seen in chronic cases without symptoms.[115]

In cords with diffusely demyelinated white matter with minimal signs of compression, there is a reasonable possibility that venous obstruction may play an important part in the pathogenesis. If vascular changes contribute considerably to cord pathology from disk protrusions, then it is clear why some dogs make an incomplete clinical recovery even when prompt decompression of the cord and removal of the compressive mass is accomplished. On the other hand, the fact that most animals do recover when the mass is removed supports the theory that the most prominent cause and damage in these cases is the compression.

In recent years there have been several reports of spinal cord infarcts which appear to be caused by emboli originating from the intervertebral disk. Profound neurological signs may appear within a few hours after onset in these cases. Plain film radiography does not reveal major spinal compressions that would explain the existing clinical signs. Occasionally disk disease may be present, but generally it is not considered significant enough to account for the signs, since myelography does not demonstrate a significant extradural compression. The treatment is therefore generally medical, using corticosteroids, antibiotics, and good nursing care. (See Chapter 11 for a more complete discussion of spinal cord infarcts (Fig. 14–19).[33, 65, 71, 72, 101, 219, 221]

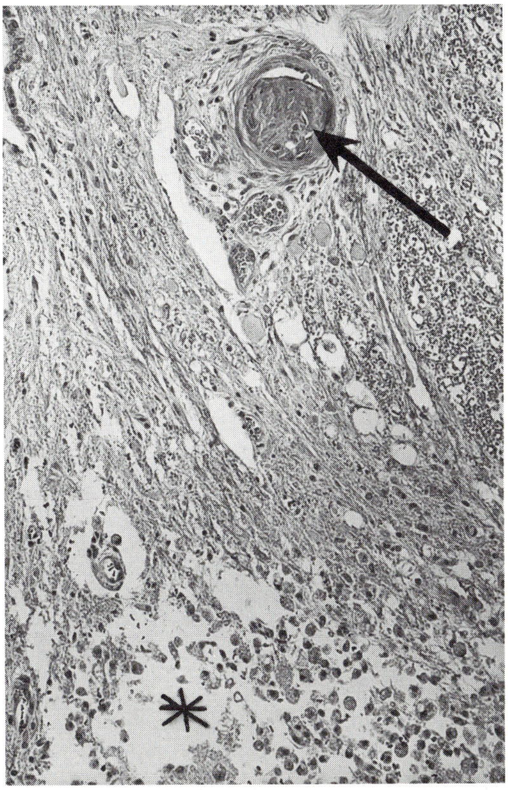

FIGURE 14–19 A spinal cord infarction is due to a fibrocartilaginous embolus which produces myelomalacia (asterisk). Note the small artery with embolus (arrow). Hematoxylin and eosin, medium power.

ACUTE RUPTURED DISKS CAUSING PROGRESSIVE HEMORRHAGIC MYELOMALACIA OR HEMATOMYELIA

Acute disk protrusion has been mentioned in veterinary literature by various workers, among whom are Fankhauser,[38] McGrath,[127] and Hutyra.[94] It appears that in man these pathologic changes do not result from disk protrusion. Grossly, there is a diffuse reddish-gray extradural necrosis, and there may be a subdural and medullary hemorrhage throughout the length of the cord. A ruptured disk on the floor of the canal can be demonstrated as a rent or tear in the dorsal annulus with widespread epidural necrosis extending along several vertebral lengths. Extradural hemorrhage may be marked, especially around the rupture (Figs. 14–20 and 14–21).

A section stained with hematoxylin and eosin shows a diffuse softening, hemorrhagic infiltration, extreme demyelinization, and large cavitations. Degenerated neurons and a marked polymorphonuclear infiltration can be seen in the cord substance.

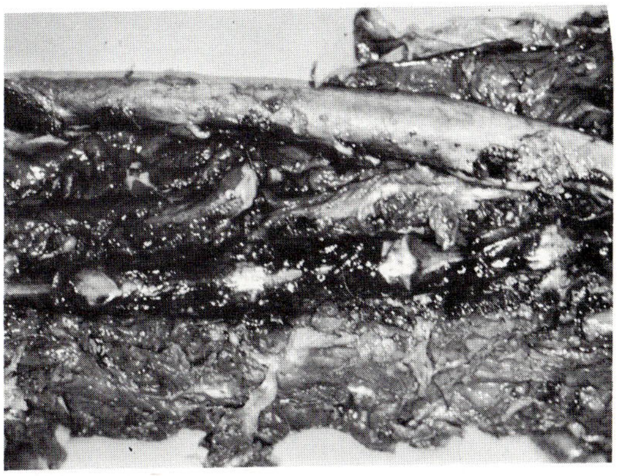

FIGURE 14–20 In contrast to what is seen in Figures 14–12 and 14–16, the patient suffered from an ascending paralysis which became generalized and caused death. Notice the diffuse subarachnoid hemorrhage evident in a "blue" spinal cord. Hematomyelia occurred from a sudden rupture of the dorsal annulus and an explosive blowout of the nucleus. A necrotic deposit is seen on the dura at the right of the picture. (From Hoerlein, B. F.: Intervertebral disc protrusions in the dog. Vet. Scope *4*, Fall, 1959.)

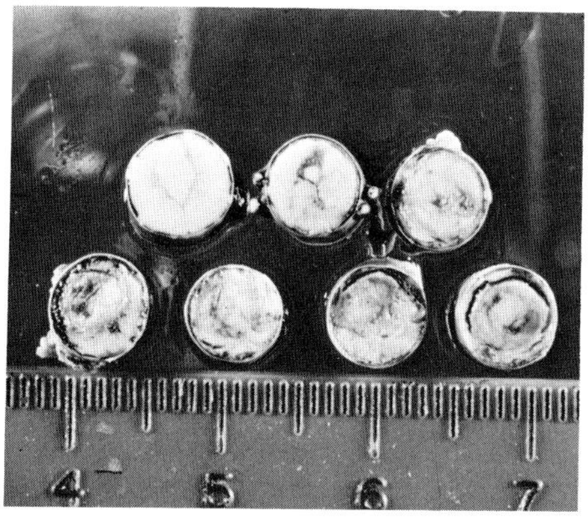

FIGURE 14–21 Cross sections of the spinal cord at various levels demonstrate medullary as well as subarachnoid hemorrhage. (Same dog as shown in Figure 14–20.) (From Hoerlein, B. F.: Intervertebral disc protrusions in the dog. Vet. Scope *4*, Fall, 1959.)

The disruption of normal architecture may be so marked that anatomical divisions of gray and white matter cannot be distinguished. The majority of intramedullary blood vessels may be necrotic, with hemorrhage more marked in the gray matter. The neurons show ischemic cell change varying from shrinkage and loss of Nissl granules to a more severe reaction in which the neurons stain homogeneously pink with a pyknotic nucleus. In less severely affected areas triangular infarcts with the apex toward the periphery may be found in the dorsal, lateral, and ventral funiculi. Patchy demyelination can be widespread in the white matter. Extramedullary vascular damage consisting of thrombosed arteries and veins is frequently seen. Many congested vessels may rupture, resulting in severe subdural and subarachnoid hemorrhage.[68, 70]

The pathogenesis of the sudden severe subdural, subarachnoid, and medullary hemorrhage is difficult to explain. In the concept of "dynamic force" expressed by Olsson the sudden powerful protrusion causes irreversible changes because the cord can endure only slowly increasing or large stable compression. However, it is not likely that the speed of occurrence is the sole causative factor. It is known that vasospasms result from subarachnoid hemorrhage and that vasoconstrictor substances are liberated during hemolysis.[68, 70] Previous discussions on the hemorrhagic necrosis syndrome seen in experimentally produced spinal cord compressions have centered around the release of norepinephrine and other catacholamine derivatives (see Chapter 12). Probably biogenic amine release, thrombosis of some vessels, and possibly vasospasms with a failure of the collateral circulation that has developed all contribute to the vicious hemorrhagic malacia seen. It has been stated that vascular hemorrhage progresses longitudinally because the vessel walls of arterioles in the CNS have little or no muscular tissue with which to promote vasconstriction and clotting. Therefore, a constant oozing of blood results in a progressive destruction of cord tissue.

Bacterial cultures have been prepared of the extradural deposits and of the cord substance itself; no organisms were found except some gram-positive anaerobic rods. The presence of these organisms may be due to agonal invasion, since the dogs are comatose and paralyzed for as long as 2 days before death. It is logical to assume that the inflammatory polymorphonuclear

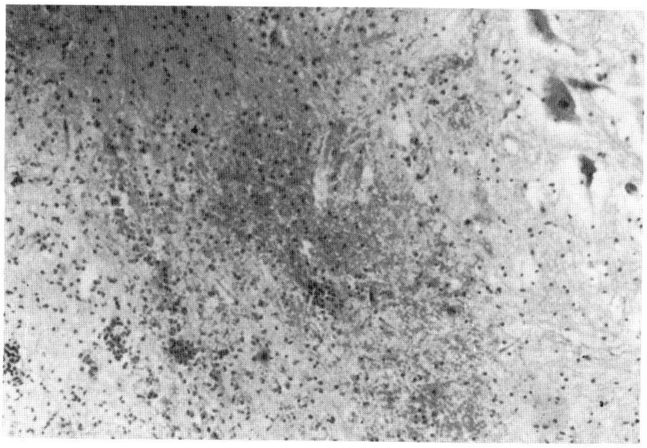

FIGURE 14–22 A histopathological section of the spinal cord shown in Figures 14–20 and 14–21 shows evidence of hemorrhage, aggregations of polymorphonuclear cells, demyelination, and necrosis. (From Hoerlein, B. F.: Intervertebral disc protrusions in the dog. Vet. Scope *4*, Fall, 1959.)

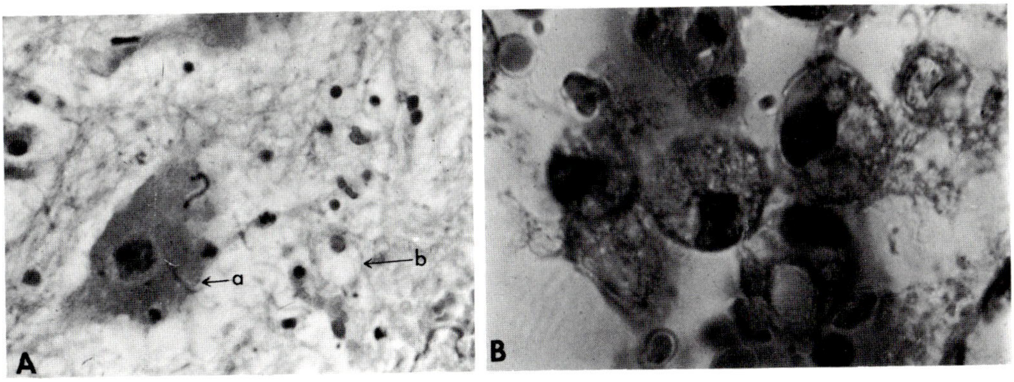

FIGURE 14–23 *A*. In a higher magnification of Figure 14–22, one can notice the degeneration of neurons (a) and the phagocytic Gitter cells (b). *B*. Gitter cells.

cell infiltration is a response to tissue necrosis or chemical change, or, at the least, that it is not due to an overwhelming bacterial invasion (Figs. 14–22 and 14–23).[81, 82]

INCIDENCE

The occurrence of disk disease in the dog is a significant clinical entity in small animal clinical practice. From the National Cancer Institute Veterinary Medical Data Program (VMDP), which has stored information collected for over 10 years from 13 colleges of veterinary medicine in the United States and Canada, 8117 cases of disk disease were reported in 356,954 dogs studied. These data indicated a crude hospital/clinic rate of 23 cases per 1000 dogs per year. For comparison, VMDP data from 1974–75 showed the following incidence of other entities (cases per 1000 dogs per year): posterior ectasia syndrome (collie eye), 9; otitis externa, 47; distemper, 10; perineal hernia, 2; allergic dermatitis, 24; and lymphoma, 4. Caution must be used in interpreting such institutional data, since they are likely to contain considerable bias because of selective referrals to veterinary schools for certain disorders.[163]

TABLE 14–1 INCIDENCE OF DISK DISEASE WITHIN BREED*

Breed	Number Affected	Population of Breed	Per Cent
Beagle	490	10,318	4.7
Dachshund	3898	16,315	23.8
Pekingese	389	4,282	9.1
Poodle (small)	753	32,082	2.3
Cocker spaniel	183	9,728	1.9
Mixed breed	1044	92,174	1.1
Doberman	69	5,278	1.3
Welsh corgi	20	230	9.0

*Raw data compiled by the author from computer data furnished by Dr. W. A. Priester, National Cancer Institute. These data have had no statistical treatment.

BREED

The clinical incidence of clinical disk protrusions in the dog has been reported by many workers.[46, 53, 61, 75, 82, 85, 89, 144, 159, 163, 169, 176, 187, 210, 215] It is generally agreed that the dachshund and members of the chondrodystrophoid group of dogs are more frequently affected with disk disease. However, the reports in the literature on clinical disk disease show that a great many breeds are affected and that there is a sizable incidence in nonchondrodystrophoid breeds and a low incidence in some chondrodys-

TABLE 14–2 BREED INCIDENCE OF DISK DISEASE (2395 Cases) (Auburn University 1952–1974)

Breed	Number	Per Cent
Dachshund	1557	65.0
Pekingese	201	8.4
Poodle (small)	150	6.3
Cocker spaniel	112	4.7
Beagle	85	3.5
Others	290	12.1

TABLE 14–3 PER CENT OF BREED INCIDENCE OF DISK DISEASE

Breed	Hoerlein	Wilcox[215] (thoraco-lumbar)	Russell[176] (neck)	Gage[53]	Goggins[61]	National Cancer Institute[162]
Beagle	3.5	1.9	28.2	3.6	6.2	6.0
Cocker spaniel	4.7	5.9	15.5	1.5	8.8	2.3
Dachshund	65.0	65.7	18.2	70.1	53.2	48.0
Pekingese	8.4	9.8	–	4.7	4.8	4.8
Poodle (small)	6.3	4.9	1.8	10.1	–	9.3
Mixed breeds	12.1	11.7	36.3	10.0	27.0	29.6
Total cases	2395	102	110	782	645	8117

trophoid breeds. In Priester's report from National Cancer Institute figures, there was at least one case of disk disease in 84 different breeds.[163] The reports of breed incidence from the literature are summarized in Tables 14–1 to 14–3.

In the 8117 disk cases reported by Priester, appropriate segments of the case series were related to the reference tabulation using estimated relative risk (R) techniques and chi-square tests of significance. The value R compares disease in a test group with that in a control group, so that R values greater than 1 indicate an increased relative risk. Breeds showing values significantly greater than R=1 (with $p<0.001$ in this compilation) are listed as follows:

Breed	Number with Disk Disease	R ($p < 0.001$)
Dachshund	3898	9.9
Shih tzu	9	3.9
Pekingese	389	3.5
Lhasa apso	24	3.0
Welsh corgi	38	2.3
Beagle	490	2.0

In comparison of case report data with statistical relative risk data, it is apparent that the cocker spaniel and small poodle are not statistically high risk breeds for disk disease. There were 753 cases in the miniature/toy poodle for an R of 0.8; in the cocker spaniel, 183 cases for an R of 0.7. The recent and past popularity of the poodle and cocker spaniel respectively is related to these case-related incidence figures.[163]

Goggins studied 645 cases of disk protrusion at the University of California teaching hospital and compared them to a group of cases by systemic sampling. It was determined that the risk of occurrence in dachshunds was 12.6 times greater than that for all other breeds combined. Excluding the dachshund, the risks of occurrence in the Pekingese, beagle, and cocker spaniel were, respectively, 10.3, 6.4, and 2.6 times greater than that of all other breeds combined.[61]

From these statistics, it is obvious that mixed or mongrel dogs are also affected with disk disease. One wonders, however, how many of these mixed breed animals reported in National Cancer Institute cases were predominantly of the chondrodystrophoid breed—for instance, predominantly dachshund. This author[83] surveyed 130 dogs in such a random group of necropsies and found disk lesions in 41.5 per cent. Twenty-two breeds were positive: cocker, 13; pointer, 4; beagle, 4; chow-chow, 3; and mixed collie, 5. These lesions were chiefly the domelike fibrotic protrusions of Hansen's type 2 classification that are characteristic of very small ruptures that have healed in nonchondrodystrophoid breeds. This work corresponds to that in surveys of human cadavers. Schmorl[181] found 38 per cent positive in 3000 cases; Haley and Perry[73] found 63 per cent in 99 cases; and Horwitz[92] found 66 per cent in 75 cases. The incidence of multiple changes was frequent in both dogs and man.

It is interesting to note not only the breed and body conformation but also the type of dog in which disk disease is prevalent. The cocker, dachshund, and Pekingese are kept as pets and are not used for extensive sporting activities. In America, beagles were formerly used primarily for sporting purposes but now are also pets. One might conclude that the relatively inactive dog, rather than the conditioned dog used for prolonged exercise, is affected primarily. The incidence in man is similar: Spurling and Grantham found that office workers, professional personnel, and executives accounted for 36 per cent of 378 cases of disk herniations.[191] The next largest incidence, 30 per cent, was among laborers, and no cases were recorded among athletes (Tables 14–1 to 14–3).

AGE

The numerous veterinary reports agree on the relative age incidence of disk disease in the dog. Among the various breeds, chondrodystrophoid and others affected with disk disease, the age incidence is similar. As Hansen mentioned, one frequently sees radiographic evidence of disk degeneration and calcification in dogs 1 to 2 years of age, especially in the susceptible breed groups. In the author's group of 2377 clinical cases, the group 3 to 6 years old accounts for 73.1 per cent of the total (Table 14–4).[176, 215]

Gage[53] determined that 81.3 per cent of 782 cases occurred between 3 and 7 years of age. Goggins[61] showed that, relative to distribution by age in the comparison group, Pekingese males with disk disease were the youngest, and males in cocker spaniels, dachshunds, beagles, and others were older in that order. A similar comparison among females showed that cocker spaniels were the youngest, followed by beagles, dachshunds, Pekingese, and other breeds. In dachshund females, age at admission was significantly greater in cases with cervical involvement than in those with thoracolumbar involvement. These differences in age and site of involvement were not seen in other breeds or in dachshund males.

TABLE 14–4 INCIDENCE OF DISK DISEASE ACCORDING TO AGE (2377 cases)*
(Auburn University, 1952–1975)

Age in Years	Number	Per Cent	
1 and under	26	1.1	
2	110	4.6	
3	338	14.2	73.1 (ages 3–6)
4	463	19.5	
5	571	24.0	
6	366	15.4	
7	239	10.1	
8	141	5.9	
9	61	2.6	
10 and over	62	2.6	

*The total number of cases varies from that in other tables because the age was not always known.

In the National Cancer Institute data of 8117 cases, the raw statistics of age–risk incidence within the various breeds is consistent with the clinical studies of age incidence just mentioned. Table 14–5 shows that 46.9 per cent of all 4- to 7-year-old dachshunds admitted to institutional teaching hospitals were admitted for disk disease. At 4 to 7 years of age the percentages for other breeds admitted for disk disease were: Pekingese, 16.2 per cent; small poodles, 4.4 per cent; beagles, 12.9 per cent; and mixed breeds, 4.2 per cent.[163]

Based on Hansen's work[74, 75, 77] on premature aging of disks in susceptible breeds, it would be logical to assume that clinical disk disease would also occur at an earlier age. However, the incidence curves are quite similar—a slightly later peak around 6 to 8 years of age occurs in low risk breeds, while a peak of 4 to 6 years occurs in high risk breeds. The Pekingese has the earliest peak (2 to 3 years), and the German shepherd (a low risk breed of $R = 0.3$) shows a slow rise to a peak at 7 to 9 years.[163]

Spurling and Grantham found that in man, 69.5 per cent of 378 cases were in the 30 to 50 year age group.[191]

In the survey of 130 random canine necropsies in nonclinical cases, the incidence of abnormalities increased with age. Twenty per cent of the 3-year-old dogs showed disease, while nearly 100 per cent of the 11-year-old dogs showed abnormalities (Fig. 14–24).[83]

SEX

The incidence is approximately equal in males and females. Riser concluded in 1946 that males were more frequently affected,[169] but most reports since that time have not confirmed this.[83, 85, 89, 131, 144, 192] Hoerlein through the years has analyzed 2395 cases (1952–1976) and has found that 1278 males (53.4 per cent) and 1117 females (46.6 per cent) were affected. Goggins (645 cases) found that 54.3 per cent of males and 45.7 per cent of females were affected.[61]

TABLE 14-5 INCIDENCE OF DISK DISEASE IN DACHSHUNDS BY AGE AND SEX*

	Age Groups							
	0–1 yr	*1–2 yr*	*2–4 yr*	*4–7 yr*	*7–10 yr*	*10–15 yr*	*Over 15 yr*	*Total*
Population – all sexes	2586	1353	2142	4860	2717	1690	118	16315
Number affected	25	48	530	2281	790	175	5	3898
Per cent	.97	3.5	18.6	46.9	29.0	10.3	4.2	24.0
Population – male	1258	615	1218	2151	1264	772	47	7399
Number affected	13	24	208	1059	438	100	3	1869
Per cent	1.0	3.9	17.1	49.2	34.7	13.0	6.4	25.3
Population – castrated male	–	–	36	70	56	38	2	221
Number affected	–	–	5	28	13	7	–	53
Per cent	–	–	13.9	40.0	23.2	18.4	–	24.0
Population – female	1247	575	1081	1624	727	389	30	5723
Number affected	12	24	203	736	177	26	3	1188
Per cent	.97	4.2	18.8	45.3	24.3	6.7	10.0	20.8
Population – spayed female	–	153	503	1009	668	491	39	2949
Number affected	–	4	113	457	162	22	1	785
Per cent	–	2.6	22.5	45.3	24.3	8.6	2.6	26.7

*Raw data compiled by the author from computer data furnished by Dr. W. A. Priester, National Cancer Institute. These data have had no statistical treatment.

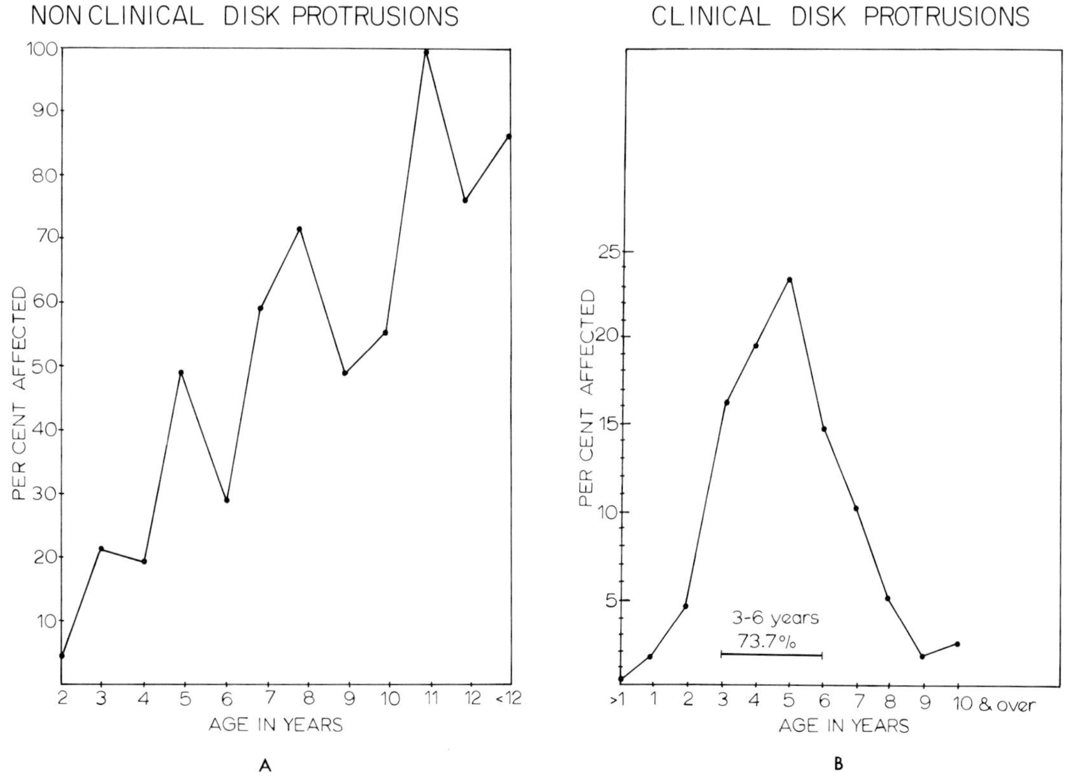

FIGURE 14-24 Age incidence in (*A*) nonclinical (Hansen type II) and (*B*) clinical disk protrusions (Hansen type I). *A*, Random necropsy survey on 130 dogs who showed no clinical signs of disk protrusion. *B*, Incidence of 1086 clinical cases of disk protrusion. Notice that this incidence is practically identical to the updated compilations on 2377 cases reported in Table 14-4.

In Gage's recent report of 782 cases, 50.8 per cent were males and 49.2 per cent were females. In cervical disk disease 51.6 per cent were males and 48.4 per cent were females.[53]

In 8117 National Cancer Institute disk case reports from institutional teaching hospitals, the R values by sex category can be summarized as follows*:

Sex Category	Number Cases Affected	R[a]
Female	2405	1
Female, spayed	1501	1.2[b]
Male	4063	1.2[b]
Male, castrated	141	1.1

[a]Each vs. "female" with adjustment made for age.
[b]R value significantly greater than R = 1 ($p < 0.001$)

The large number of cases in this study has suggested a subtle difference in R. One explanation is that female sex hormones may give some slight protection against the degenerative changes that predispose to disk disease[163] (Table 14-6).

In a compilation of 1400 cases in man, 63.7 per cent of those affected were males and 36.3 per cent were females.[81]

SITE OF LESION

The incidence according to site is generally agreed upon by workers in the veterinary literature. The presence of the intercapital ligament allows protrusion of the midthoracic disks to occur very rarely.[75, 76] Although cervical disk protrusions are seen frequently, protrusions of the terminal thoracic and cranial lumbar disks are most frequently observed.

In the various periodic surveys made by the author, there has been general agreement on site incidence. Cumulative data from 2395 cases, among which were 2620 clinically important individual disk protrusions seen on radiographs, surgery, or necropsy, showed that 22.8 per cent were seen at T12–13 disk space, 21.9 per cent at T13–L1, and 6.1 per cent at C2–3. The cervical area (C2–3 to C7–T1) accounted for 13.9 per cent, the thoracic segment T9–10 to T13–L1 for 55.5 per cent, the lumbar area (L1–2 to L7–S1) for 30.6 per cent, and the thoracolumbar junction (T11–12 to LI–2) for 65.6 per cent (see Tables 14–7 and 14–8).

Gage noted 16.4 per cent cervical disk lesions and 83.6 per cent thoracolumbar disk lesions in 782 cases. The T11–12 to L2–3 area accounted for 71.3 per cent of the lesions. The T11–12 to L1–2 area accounted for 63.5 per cent, a figure which is practically identical to that of Hoerlein.[53] Goggins noted lesions in 25.4 per cent in the cervical area, 66.0 per cent in the thoracolumbar area, 5.1 per cent in both areas, and 3.4 per cent nonspecified. Goggins noted a significant age difference in dachshund females suffering from cervical lesions.[61]

It is interesting to note the extreme similarity of site incidence in clinical disk disease and in the original necropsy survey of 130 cases of nonclinical disk cases in random breeds (Figure 14–24).[89]

Cervical disks occur infrequently in man. Raney and Raney analyzed 200 consecutive cases of disk disease and encountered no cervical ones[166]; however, Bradford and Spurling stated that cervical disks probably comprise 4 to 8 per cent of all disk lesions in man. Odom observed 70 per cent to occur at

*Table from Priester, W. A.: Canine intervertebral disk disease—occurrence by age, breed, and sex among 8117 cases. Theriogenology *6*, 293, 1976.

TABLE 14–6 PER CENT INCIDENCE OF DISK DISEASE WITHIN BREED BY SEX*

	Male	Castrated Male	Female	Spayed Female
Beagle	4.9	9.0	3.9	6.3
Dachshund	25.3	24.0	20.8	26.7
Pekingese	9.1	6.2	8.3	14.1
Poodle (small)	5.2	2.0	3.0	2.2
Cocker spaniel	1.9	2.0	1.5	2.7
Mixed breed	1.1	2.2	0.8	1.7
Average	7.9	7.6	6.4	8.9

*Raw data compiled by the author from computer data furnished by Dr. W. A. Priester, National Cancer Institute. These data have had no statistical treatment.

TABLE 14–7 SITES OF DISK LESIONS (2620 disks, 2395 cases) (Auburn University, 1952–1975)

Vertebral Space		Number of Cases	Per Cent
Cervical			
2–3		160	6.1
3–4		85	3.2
4–5		49	1.9
5–6		48	1.8
6–7		15	.6
C7–T1		6	.2
	Total	363	13.9
Thoracic			
9–10		2	.1
10–11		21	.8
11–12		259	9.9
12–13		598	22.8
T13–L1		574	21.9
	Total	1454	55.5
Lumbar			
1–2		287	11.0
2–3		183	7.0
3–4		165	6.3
4–5		124	4.7
5–6		33	1.3
6–7		10	.4
L7–S1		1	—
	Total	803	30.6
Thoraco-lumbar junction T11–12 to L1–2		1718	65.6

C6–7.[141] In Love's series, 0.25 per cent involved the thoracic area.[119, 120] Armstrong[1] listed the incidence of lumbar involvement in 1000 cases as follows:

L5–S1	–	46.8 per cent
L4–L5	–	40.4 per cent
L1– 2	–	2.1 per cent
Double lesions	–	10.7 per cent

CLINICAL SIGNS

For an understanding of clinical signs the reader is referred to the basic considerations of traumatic and compressive spinal disorders and the concept of upper (UMN) and lower (LMN) motor neuron disease (see Chapter 4). One of the major factors in consideration of clinical disk protrusions is the localization and evaluation of any other CNS disorder, particularly a spinal disorder. For instance, if an animal has a UMN and an LMN lesion in the same area of the spinal cord, only the LMN signs are observed. The neural pathways for expression of the UMN signs are destroyed by the LMN lesion. Therefore, if a dog has LMN signs in the hind limbs, examination of the spinal cord from T2 caudally for UMN lesions must be performed in addition to the terminal lumbar and sacral areas. If a dog shows LMN signs in the pectoral limbs, the cord from C1–T1 should be examined for possible additional UMN lesions. In addition, a dog with two or three UMN lesions may be indistinguishable clinically from a dog with one UMN lesion. These complex cases are particularly characteristic of degenerative disk disease, trauma, and systemic infections (Fig. 14–25).[4]

The clinical signs in clinical disk protrusions vary considerably. The owner frequently states that the dog was well the previous day and there is no known incidence of trauma. A sudden unaccustomed movement can precipitate the injury: jumping upon a bed, jumping over a fence, sitting, going up stairs, fighting with another dog, or mating. Love and Walsh found that in man 84 per cent of 500 subjects had inintermittent symptoms and remissions[120];

TABLE 14–8 INCIDENCE OF DISK LESIONS BY SITE (Per Cent)

	Hoerlein (2395 cases)	Gage[53] (782 cases)	Goggins[61] (645 cases)
Cervical	13.9	16.4	25.4
Thoracolumbar	86.1	83.6	66.0
Thoracolumbar junction T11–12, L1–2	65.6	63.5	
Both cervical and lumbar	–	–	5.1
Nonspecified	–	–	3.4

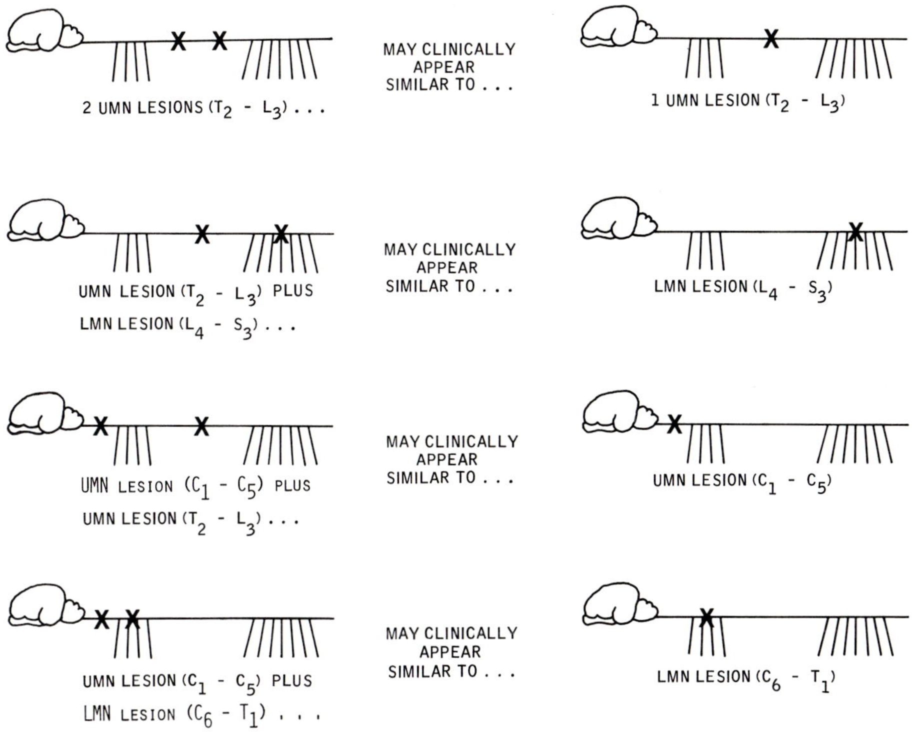

FIGURE 14–25 Multiple spinal cord lesions that can clinically resemble spinal cord lesions. UMN, upper motor neuron; LMN, lower motor neuron. (From Bailey, C. S., and Holliday, T. A.: Diseases of the spinal cord. *In* Ettinger, S. J. (ed.): *Textbook of Veterinary Internal Medicine.* W. B. Saunders Co., Philadelphia, 1975.)

similarly, the dog often recovers spontaneously only to suffer one or more relapses.

The stages of signs may be classified singly or in combinations as (1) pain; (2) paresis, incoordination, or both; (3) paralysis; and (4) progressive paralysis consequent to acute extensive rupture of the disk and generalized hemorrhage in the cord and myelomalacia. The pain, paresis, and paralysis are generally due to Hansen's type 1 disk protrusion, which causes a localized compressive or transverse myelopathy. The progressive paralysis (ascending and/or descending) is due to a more general myelopathy.

PAIN AND PARESIS

Pain arises from meningeal or nerve root irritation and is the most prominent sign in cervical disk protrusions. The head and neck are held low and rigid. Occasionally the dog is in such pain that he cries or whines continuously for no apparent reason. He may even refuse to drink or eat, or may do so with great difficulty. The owner may describe the dog as "standing on his head" and "bowing his neck." The dog may continuously or periodically resist any forceful movement of his head and neck (Fig. 14–26).

A cervical disk protrusion may compress the cord enough to cause UMN signs of paresis, ataxia, and proprioceptive deficits in the front and hind limbs. Frequently, clinical signs will be more pronounced in the hind limbs. Tetraparesis and paralysis can occur (Fig. 14–27). With caudal cervical lesions, LMN signs in one or both pectoral limbs can occur. Occasionally, disk protrusions in the cervical and cranial portion of the thoracic cord (C1 to T1–2) may cause Horner's syndrome (ptosis, miosis, and enophthalmus).[41] Intermittent pain from cervical disk protrusions is a characteristic clinical sign, whereas pain from thoracolumbar disks may be very transient before

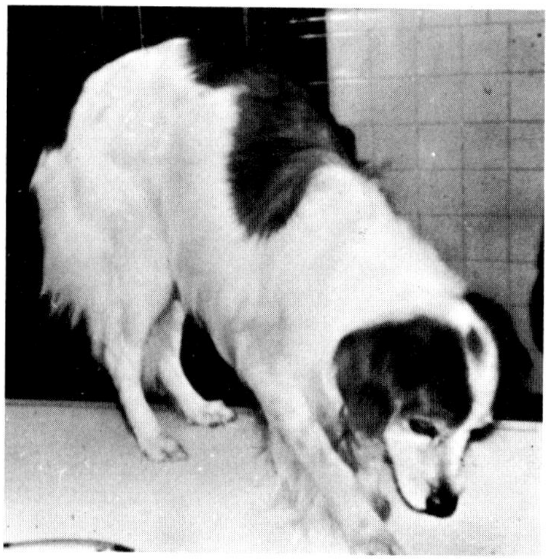

FIGURE 14–26 Dog suffering from a cervical disk protrusion. The head is held low and there are muscle spasms as well as acute pain on manipulation of the neck.

paralysis occurs. In more chronic cases pain may be a constant sign.

Terminal thoracic and lumbar disk lesions may cause generalized pain. Kyphosis or arching of the back may occur from the animal's effort to decrease the dorsal projection of the disk. Rarely, a scoliosis or lateral spinal curvature is seen with the convexity opposite the side of the lesion. When in pain, the dog will object to being forcibly moved or picked up, walking up stairs, or jumping into a car. He may awaken and cry frequently throughout the night. Tendon reflexes in this stage are usually exaggerated, and the limbs as well as the dorsal musculature may be rigid.

Pain may also be present with paresis or weakness. In thoracolumbar lesions, this condition may be manifested by posterior

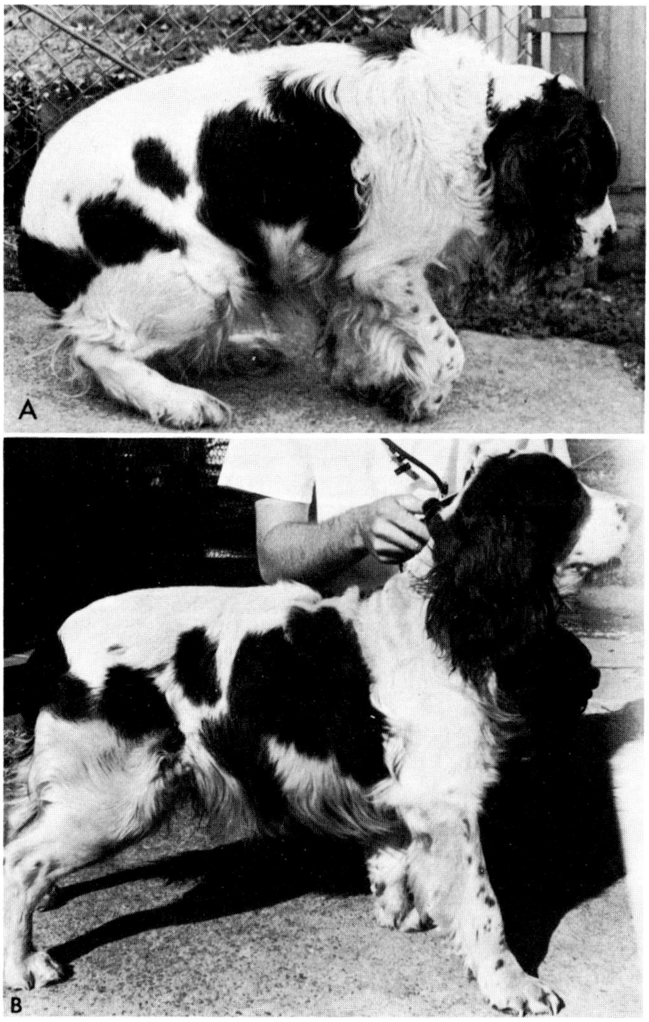

FIGURE 14–27 *A*. A cervical disk protrusion in a 6-year-old springer spaniel who is showing clinical signs of extreme head and neck pain and right front leg "knuckling." *B*. The same dog, completely devoid of pain and front limb weakness, 2 weeks after surgical correction.

incoordination if the lesion is bilateral or by dragging a toe or leg in extension if it is unilateral. As a result of the dog's effort to compensate for a unilateral paresis, the lumbar spine may show a scoliosis with the convexity opposite the affected side.

PARALYSIS

Paraplegia (hind leg or posterior extremity paralysis) may result concomitantly with or subsequent to the occurrence of pain. If the musculature of the posterior limbs is spastic, hypertonic, or rigid, the condition is termed a *spastic paraplegia.* Spastic paraplegia is generally present when some degree of pain is evident. The dog may "scoot," carry his hind legs under him, or drag them like stilts behind him.

Clinical signs will be due to UMN damage unless the lesion is at or distal to spinal segment L3–4. Upper motor neuron signs may include pain, paresis, and paraplegia (usually bilateral). Hind limb segmental reflexes are usually normal or hyperreflexic (usually hyperreflexic in rigid paraplegia). Muscle tone is normal or hypertonic in rigid paraplegia and a crossed extensor reflex may be present. Posture becomes worse as paralysis becomes more profound. The cutaneous sensation or reflex, when hyperesthetic, helps determine the site of the lesion. The usual animal with recent disk paraplegia shows a deep pain response to the toe pinch or flexor reflex; if this is not present the prognosis is guarded or unfavorable. In spastic paraplegia the urinary bladder generally retains urine at the onset, and then may become incontinent, or contract reflexively and partially empty as the disorder progresses (spinal bladder) (Figs. 14–28 to 14–31).

A *flaccid* paraplegia is seen in an advanced stage of paralysis (usually of several weeks' duration). It is one in which the musculature lacks tonus, the segmental reflexes and sensations are either normal, hyperreflexive, or diminished, and the urinary and defecatory sphincters do not function normally. There usually may still be urine retention, but there is usually incontinence, dribbling of urine, or a partial, "reflex" urination. The legs are carried flaccidly behind the body, rather than under it as in spastic paraplegia. Severe muscle atrophy takes place, decubital ulcers may appear, and the prognosis is generally unfavorable.

Frequently, LMN signs may be due to a disk lesion from L3–4 posteriorly. Protrusion at the L3–4 level may cause depression of the patellar or knee jerk reflex due to damage to the L4 cord segment that supplies some of the motor neurons to the quadriceps. Protrusions at L4–5 tend to damage the L7 cord segment, isolating sacral and coccygeal segments from the brain. If cord segments L4, L5, and L6 are spared, the dog is not paraplegic, but there may be weakness in the caudal thigh muscles and bladder dysfunction. Lesions at L5–6, L6–7, and the first sacral levels may carry some hind limb weakness, but incontinence, loss of anal reflexes, and loss of tail movement are frequent. The author feels that LMN signs from lesions in this area are variable clinically, depending on precise location and extent of the lesion.[68] These lesions that may cause arreflexia should be

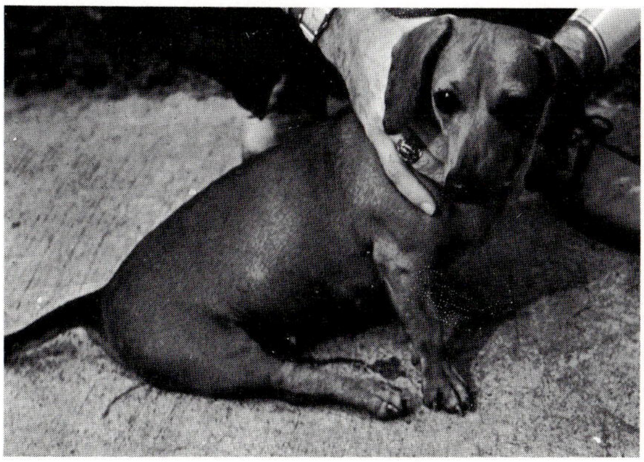

FIGURE 14–28 Characteristic case of a local compression myelitis resulting from a terminal thoracic or lumbar disk protrusion. The pelvic limbs are rigid or hyperflexic, and urinary and fecal retention is common. The front limbs, neck, and head of the animal are normal. If pain is not too severe, he may eat and may generally feel well.

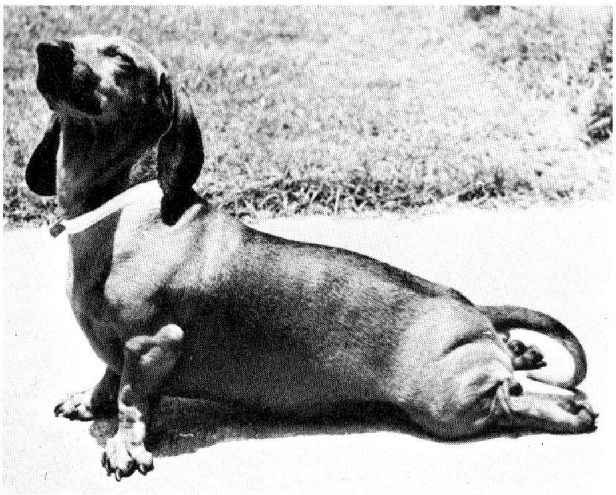

FIGURE 14–29 Dog suffering from a progressive hemorrhagic myelomalacia resulting from an acute rupture of the disk. The pelvic limbs are flaccid, the anal sphincter is relaxed, and the reflexes are either diminished or absent. The pectoral limbs are becoming rigid or spastic, the head and neck are rigid, the eyes are "glassy," and the animal does not feel well. (From Hoerlein, B. F.: Intervertebral disc protrusions in the dog. Vet. Scope *4*, Fall, 1959.)

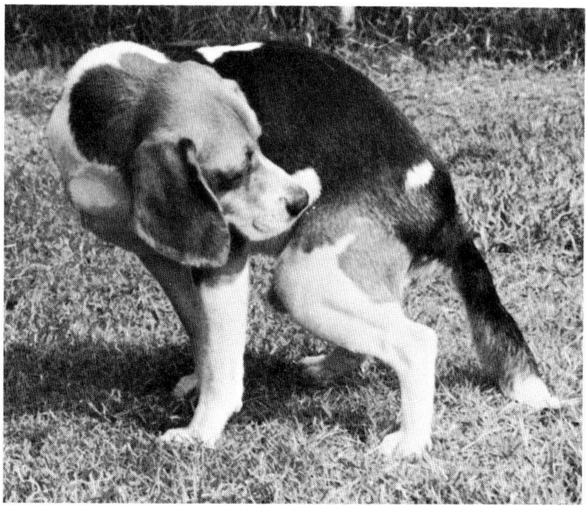

FIGURE 14–30 A paralysis of the tail may occur from a protrusion of L6–7 or L7–S1 disk. This dog could not raise his tail to defecate, a type of LMN manifestation.

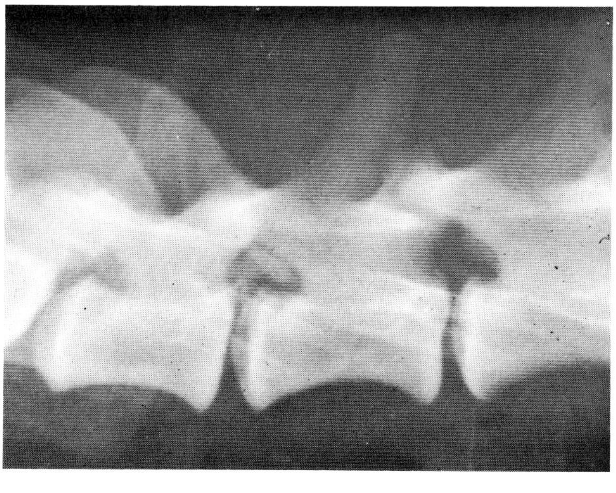

FIGURE 14–31 Radiograph of a calcific disk protrusion (L6–7), which produced the clinical signs seen in Figure 14–30.

differentiated from the initial stages of progressive myelomalacia caused by an acute blowout or ruptured disk.

PROGRESSIVE PARALYSIS

The ultimate clinical sign is acute progressive paralysis that usually results from an extensive, acute rupture of a thoracic or lumbar disk and causes a progressive, vicious myelomalacia. This is in contrast to the localized compressive or transverse myelopathy discussed previously. It has a poor prognosis. The onset is sudden and frequently follows an unusual movement or circumstance; the dog cries in pain and rapidly becomes paraplegic. The dog does not feel as well as he would in the usual case of disk protrusion and localized compression or transverse myelopathy. His eyes are glassy, his temperature may be elevated, and he does not eat. His head and neck are held rigidly upward, and he may not be able to fully control his front legs. Frequently, the dog is unable to properly support himself in the sitting position, and he falls over easily. He will not be able to "wheelbarrow" if one picks up his hind legs and forces him to walk on his front legs. Sensory and motor paralysis of the tail, hind legs, and anal and urinary sphincters rapidly develops. Progressive paralysis extends to the thorax, and intercostal paralysis causes respiration to become diaphragmatic. As myelomalacia progresses, the front limbs become more markedly rigid until they nearly simulate the Schiff-Sherrington reaction. When the cervical and thoracic cord segments are destroyed, the front limbs become flaccid, and finally death ensues from respiratory failure.

The cord pathology in progressive myelomalacia and paralysis from an acute blowout or ruptured disk has already been discussed (see p. 483). The pathogenesis, although not fully understood, probably involves not only vasospasm, thrombosis, rupture of vessels, hemorrhage, ischemia, and anoxia but also release of biogenic amines and catacholamines (see p. 389).[70]

INCIDENCE OF RECURRENT ATTACKS

It is well known that chronic disk disease tends to recur periodically when not treated with appropriate surgery. Wilcox[215] noted a 32.3 per cent incidence of more than one clinical attack in the history, Russell and Griffiths[176] noted 36.3 per cent, Jadeson 30.77 per cent,[97] and Funkquist 28.8 per cent.[43, 44] Recurrences frequently become acute and may cause irreversible pathological changes in the spinal cord.

FACTORS DETERMINING DEGREE OF PARALYSIS

The signs caused by disk lesion vary according to (1) the size of the lesion, (2) the rate of development, (3) the dynamic force behind the pressure mass, (4) the duration of pressure on the cord, and (5) the spinal level of the injury and area of pressure on the cord. Tarlov has demonstrated experimentally the factors in size, rate of development, and duration of pressure as they influence the speed of functional return to normalcy.[201] He has proved that a slowly increasing pressure is less deleterious than a sudden pressure, and that massive pressure needs to be relieved quickly.

The experience of Olsson,[148] Funkquist,[46] and Hoerlein[82-90] and others in clinical cases has substantiated Tarlov's experimental work. A gradual increase in a mass causing compression of the cord is better tolerated clinically than a sudden blowout or ruptured disk, which may cause death from generalized paralysis. During the past 25 years, Hoerlein has shown that prompt release of pressure on the cord from a disk protrusion or fracture helps effect rapid clinical recovery, whereas delayed relief usually fails to help the dog.

The level of injury is also important. Posterior lumbar protrusions generally do not cause the severe signs that result from protrusions of the anterior lumbar or terminal thoracic disks. In these instances, the major portion of motor innervation to the hind limbs lies anterior to the lesion and the spinal cord has terminated in smaller components that are better able to accommodate intraspinal canal pressures. The clinical signs of posterior lumbar lesions at L6–7 are rarely the paraplegias that are so characteristic of the thoracolumbar junction area. Since there seems to be more space extradurally in the cervical area, pressure here does not crowd the cord as severely as in the thoracolumbar junction. There is pain, but there is less motor dysfunction.

DIAGNOSIS

The diagnosis of disk protrusion is based on age, breed, history, clinical signs, presence or absence of infectious disease or other complicating disorders as evaluated by EEG and fundic examinations, laboratory diagnostics, radiographic examinations, and occasionally an EMG examination. The clinical disorders most frequently confused with disk protrusions are spinal cord tumors, mild luxations of fractures, infarcts caused by fibrocartilaginous emboli, and (in cats) malignant lymphomatous masses within the spinal canal. The differential examination must consider every other cause of meningeal and nerve root irritation, localized compressive myelopathy and transverse myelopathy. Therefore, spinal fluid analysis and cytology should be done in an atypical case of suspected disk protrusion to help differentiate infectious disease, inflammatory complications, or a spinal tumor. The age, breed, and history are all extremely important and will be most helpful diagnostically in the chondrodystrophoid dogs that suffer from premature disk degeneration. However, one must remember that a substantial number of cases occur in nonchondrodystrophoid dogs which may have a similar age, breed, and history, and the condition may be related entirely to trauma. In these traumatic cases, the clinical signs will of course be consistent with a compressive or transverse myelopathy.

The neurological examination proposed by McGrath[127] and outlined in Chapters 1 and 3 is helpful in providing more precise diagnostic information. It has been mentioned that compressions of the spinal cord, regardless of origin, may cause similar signs.

It is emphasized that reflexes are best elicited with the dog in a quiet place, away from the distractions of noise and movement. The clinician frequently needs a great deal of patience to obtain the animal's cooperation. A series of examinations may be needed to provide an accurate evaluation of reflex activity for either initial or progress examinations.

The segmental reflex patterns have been discussed under general clinical signs. Upper motor neuron signs of hyperreflexia, proprioceptive and motor deficits, and pain predominate unless nerve roots in the cervicothoracic and lumbosacral junction areas are involved. Total loss of segmental reflexes may reflect LMN deficits or the initial stages of progressive hemorrhagic myelomalacia. Dermal hyperesthesia helps to locate the approximate lesion site, and analgesic responses in a normally responsive area may indicate LMN sensory loss or progressive myelomalacic cord destruction. If the hind limbs are hyperthermic, it is possible that a central sympathetic deficit has occurred from a lesion rostral to L3, thus causing loss of vasomotor tone in the skin and increased dermal blood flow. The temperature difference may be as great as 10° C.[67, 68]

The reflex of most prognostic value is deep pain response to the toe pinch or pedal reflex. A favorable prognosis is indicated by the function of the ascending spinal sensory tracts as shown by the ensuing response in the eyes or voice, or by biting. Lack of such a normal response in several trials performed during a reasonably short period of time indicates a guarded or unfavorable prognosis. However, a stoic or frightened animal may not respond in a positive manner, so some doubt of neurologic deficit may exist. Hard sudden pressure on the base of the toenail will usually produce a response if there is sensation.

An electrical stimulus to the distal limb can be used to evaluate the presence of deep pain more critically.[68] Electrophysical measurement of afferent stimulation and recording of sensory impulses has provided a more sensitive prognostic assessment of spinal cord function with incomplete lesions. Unfortunately, implantation of electrodes on or near the dura or somatosensory cortex by means of craniotomy is usually necessary to detect impulses. The best results have been obtained by processing the information on an averaging computer or by superimposing tracings on a dual channel storage oscilloscope. More sophisticated methods of measuring evoked sensory responses include recording impulses from dorsal columns and spinal cord surfaces.[32, 64, 125, 203] Cortical evoked potentials as ascertained by EEG recordings and peripheral electrical stimulation are helpful but inaccurate and must be interpreted by a computer screening procedure.[168] In the future, cortical evoked potentials or surface cord recordings of neural transmission capabilities will greatly enhance evaluation of the sensorimotor reflexes in spinal cord injuries.

The use of EMG in the paraspinal musculature has been discussed in Chapter 9 as an aid in locating disk protrusions. EMG is most valuable when there are multiple radiographic lesions at various spinal levels and the use of myelography is contraindicated. The examination takes only a few minutes to perform and can be accomplished in the surgical case after anesthesia and initial patient preparation and before surgery.[21, 175]

DIFFERENCES IN CLINICAL MANIFESTATIONS IN DOG AND MAN

We have frequently mentioned the similarity of disk disease in man and the dog, which supports Riser's original report.[169] However, there is a marked difference in the way the clinical syndrome is manifested. Since many veterinarians gainfully seek advice from their physician colleagues, this difference must be emphasized or confusion will result. The chief differences are as follows:

The spinal cord terminates in man at L1, and in the dog at L6–7.[129]

In the dog, most disk protrusions occur at the thoracolumbar junction and exert full pressure on the cord, whereas in man most occur at L5–S1 or L4–5, and pressure is exerted on a terminal nerve root rather than on the cord.[1, 117]

In the dog, the spinal canal, especially in the thoracic and lumbar areas, seems to be relatively smaller in proportion to cord size than in man; therefore, the extradural space is smaller and extradural compressions cause more compression of the cord. The cervical epidural space seems larger and clinical signs are more similar to those of man.

Clinical signs differ dramatically. In the dog, thoracolumbar protrusions cause early paralysis, whereas in man lumbar protrusions cause pain predominantly. This is because in the dog pressure is exerted directly on the cord in an area in which the spinal cord is crowded into the spinal canal. In respect to clinical signs, disk injuries in the dog may be compared to cord tumors in man.

RADIOGRAPHIC LESIONS IN DISKS

STANDARD TECHNIQUE

The fundamental considerations in radiographic examinations of the spine were discussed in Chapter 5, which dealt with equipment, positioning, myelographic techniques and media, epiduralography, vertebral sinus venography, cerebral angiography, pneumoencephalography, ventriculography, and cranial sinus venography. It was emphasized that the nonscreen Bucky and newer high detail screen Bucky techniques are necessary for the maximal detail in spinal and disk cases. Both oil and aqueous contrast mediums are toxic and should be used sparingly in the diagnosis of disk lesions even though newer aqueous contrast media show promise to be less toxic.[56, 89] The interpretation of radiographic disk lesions will be stressed in this chapter.

It was emphasized in Chapter 13 that all spinal compressions may produce similar clinical signs. Therefore, one must employ careful radiographic examinations to differentiate them according to etiology and prognosis. Routine radiographic procedures should be concentrated in the hypersensitive cutaneous area as the most likely pathologic site. Routine films of the spine portray lateral and ventrodorsal views of the suspicious areas. The types of disk lesions that may be seen on radiography are as follows:

Calcified nucleus pulposus with little or no annular involvement.

Calcified nucleus with involvement of all or part of the annulus. The disk is completely calcified, but it rarely fuses with the vertebral bodies unless spondylitic changes are also present. A narrow disk space may also be present.

Narrowing of disk space.

Narrowing of the intervertebral foramina, abnormally spaced articular processes, or both.

Opacified mass in the canal above a normal, narrow, or calcified disk.

Osteophytes of the adjacent dorsal rims of the vertebral bodies or of the dorsal longitudinal ligament. This change is usually not accompanied by spondylitic changes.

Spondylitic exostoses are generally present on the ventral surfaces of the vertebral bodies, but there may also be arthritic changes or dorsal bridging. A collapsed disk space may be present (Fig. 14–32).[83, 144]

A *calcified nucleus* indicates previous dehydration and degeneration of the chondroid mass, as described by Hansen,[75] noncellular necrosis, and calcification. Calcification indicates degeneration and death of tissue but has no immediate significance in compression of the cord (Figs. 14–33 to 14–35).

When the *annulus* also becomes *calcified*, dysfunction of the disk becomes more marked. Infrequently, through stress and strain, it may become detached from the bony vertebrae and slip upward, causing a compression. A calcified nucleus and annulus can occur subsequent to a rupture and nuclear expulsion, causing a calcified protrusion, a narrow disk space, or both.

A *narrowing* of the disk space is highly significant radiographically, especially when combined with a local hyperesthesia of the dorsal skin. The structure of the disk is such that the dorsal annular layers are much thinner and weaker than the lateral and ventral layers. Since a narrow space usually indicates a rupture, it is most often a dorsal rupture against the cord. In a high percentage of cases, necropsy or surgery substantiates this observation. The relative width of disk spaces can best be visualized by radiographic examination, in which the tube portal is placed directly over the suspected lesion and the spine is kept parallel to the table surface. Adjacent spaces can be used for an accurate basis of comparison (Figs. 14–36 to 14–38).

The diameter of the intervertebral foramina and the position of the articular processes can also be used to estimate relative intervertebral spacing. A direct lateral superimposition of structures must be obtained in the film for accurate recording of these differences. In a narrow disk space, the involved intervertebral foramen or so-called "horse's head" is smaller than the adjacent foramen situated anteriorly or posteriorly. The articular processes also overlap in a markedly narrow space.

The finding of a *calcific mass* in the spinal canal is highly significant. Its presence must be confirmed in both lateral and ventrodorsal views; when it is seen in the radiograph and accompanied by an abnormal neurologic finding, it is positive proof of a spinal compression (Figs. 14–39 to 14–42).

Dorsal *osteophytic* formations may not represent significant spinal compression, as these often result from minor ruptures and tears in the dorsal longitudinal ligament, especially where it attaches to the vertebral bone. Periosteal exostosis develops. When these formations enlarge to produce significant pain, they are of neurological importance.

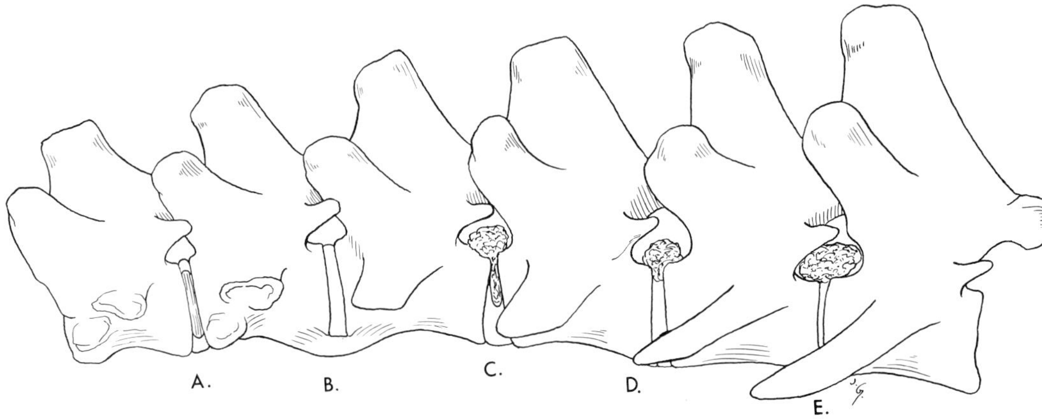

FIGURE 14–32 A drawing demonstrating various radiographic changes seen in intervertebral disks; (a) calcified nucleus; (b) spondylosis deformans; (c) calcified disk protrusion (nucleus has ruptured and organized into a calcific protrusion; (d) calcified dorsal annulus osteophyte formation, and partial ruptured disk; (e) narrow disk space resulting from a recent ruptured annulus causing a protruding disk and cord pressure.

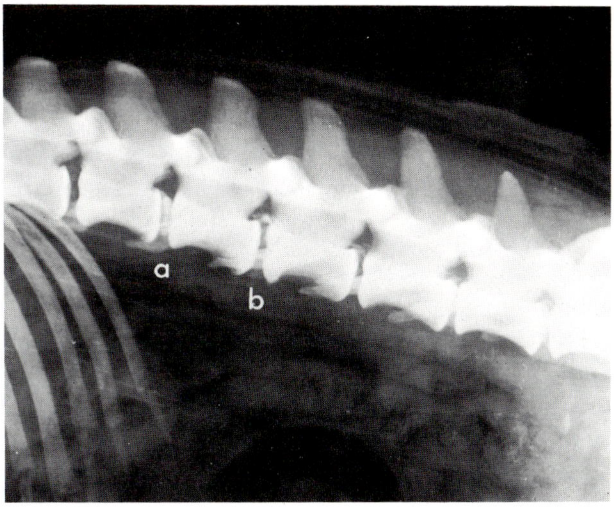

FIGURE 14–33 A radiograph showing some of the changes portrayed in Figure 14–32: (a) calcified nucleus and part of the annulus, (b) osteophyte formation. (From Hoerlein, B. F.: Clinical spinal radiography in the dog. J.A.V.M.A. *134*, 1959.)

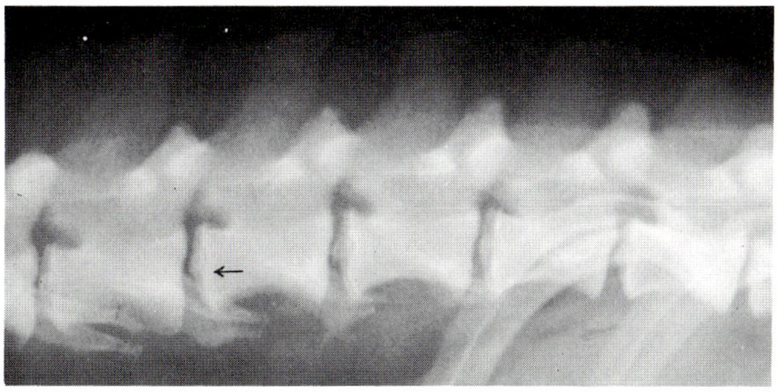

FIGURE 14–34 In this radiograph, one sees a systemic nuclear calcification, in a very early stage. Notice that all the disks show nearly identical changes.

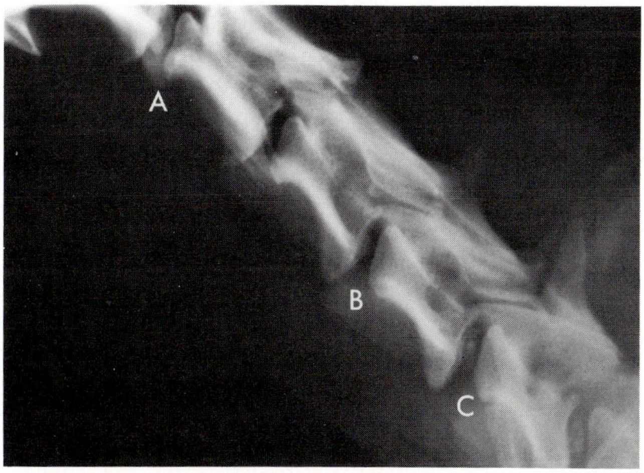

FIGURE 14–35 Cervical disks in various stages of calcification. (A) Calcified nucleus and annulus, (B) calcified nucleus and slightly narrower dorsal annular space; (c) larger calcified nucleus fragmented into two sections. (Courtesy of Dr. Jack Geary.)

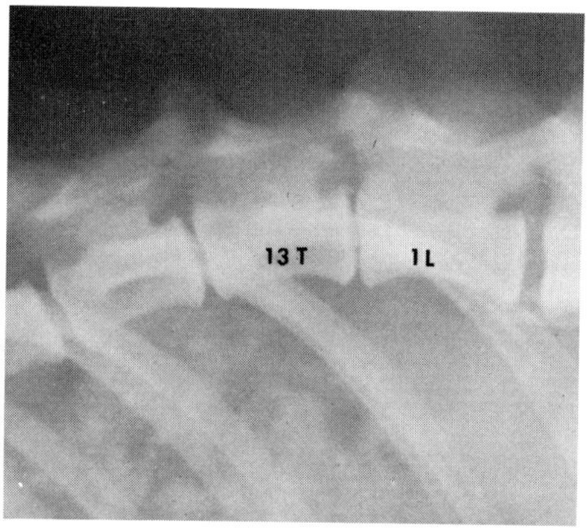

FIGURE 14–36 Two narrow disk spaces are seen in this radiograph. Notice that T13–L1 has collapsed and shows little or no protrusion mass.

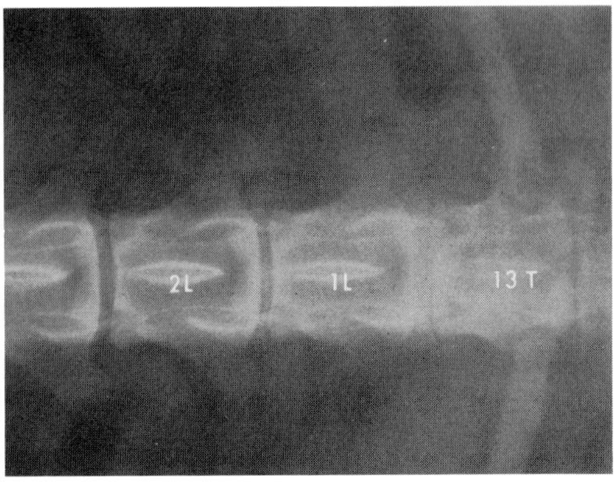

FIGURE 14–38 VD view of Figure 14–37. Notice the narrow space at L1–2.

Spondylitic exostosis causes minor neurological dysfunction in the dog. Only when exostoses narrow the spinal canal or surround or pinch spinal nerves are these changes clinically important. Generalized spondylosis may cause pain, a rigid spine, and possibly impaired movement of the limbs from compression of nerve tissue.

Routine radiographic examination should be employed in any clinical case of neural dysfunction, even if surgical procedures are not contemplated. Frequently, these films will establish the correct diagnosis, which may not have been considered on physical examination, and therefore may change the prognosis and course of therapy. In disk lesions, a series of films taken during recurrent attacks may be needed so that the correct therapy can be prescribed. This type of service is much appreciated by the owner (Fig. 14–43).

MYELOGRAPHIC TECHNIQUES

The cisternal and lumbar injection techniques and the use of contrast media for myelography were discussed in Chapter 5. Myelographic examinations for proposed surgical relief of disk protrusions need not be used routinely if proper procedures have been employed in the spinographic survey and if careful correlations of the

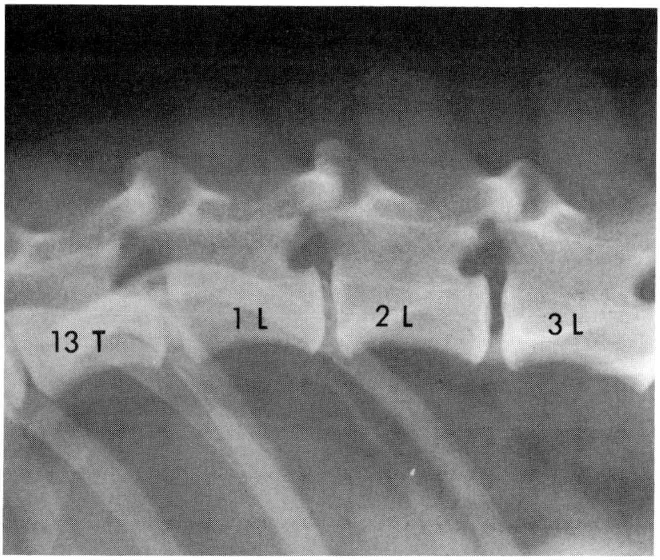

FIGURE 14–37 A narrow calcified disk is seen at L1–2 with some evidence of a protrusion into the canal. Careful study will also help visualize a smaller interverebral foramen. Notice the wide spaces at T13–L1 and L2–3; T13–L1 is calcified, while a small calcific deposit is seen in the dorsal longitudinal ligament of L1–2. Because the dorsal annulus is the weakest part of the annulus fibrosus, narrow disk spaces usually indicate a ruptured annulus and extruded nucleus against the spinal cord.

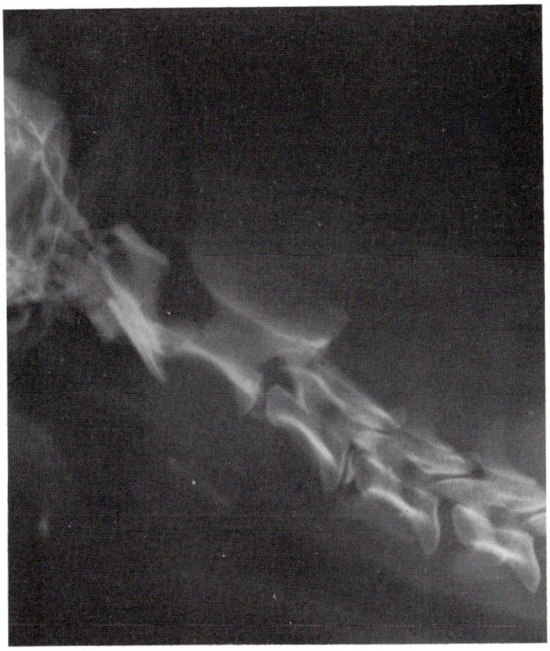

FIGURE 14–39 Radiograph shows a massive disk protrusion in C3–4 interspace. The protrusion has a pyramid shape with a narrow "stem" attachment to the narrowed calcified disk.

neurological examination and radiographic findings have been made. Even with development of a newer aqueous contrast medium, the media are still toxic and should not be used except when absolutely necessary.

Myelography, although potentially dangerous, can aid in the diagnosis of the nature and location of (1) extradural masses, (2) intradural–extramedullary masses, and (3) intramedullary cord lesions. These lesions all cause localized transverse myelopathies. Myelography is not indicated for diagnosis of disseminated myelopathies or meningopathies but only for reversible clinical lesions when decompressive surgery is need for therapy. The oil media such as Pantopaque are mainly useful for showing large extradural lesions such as disks or

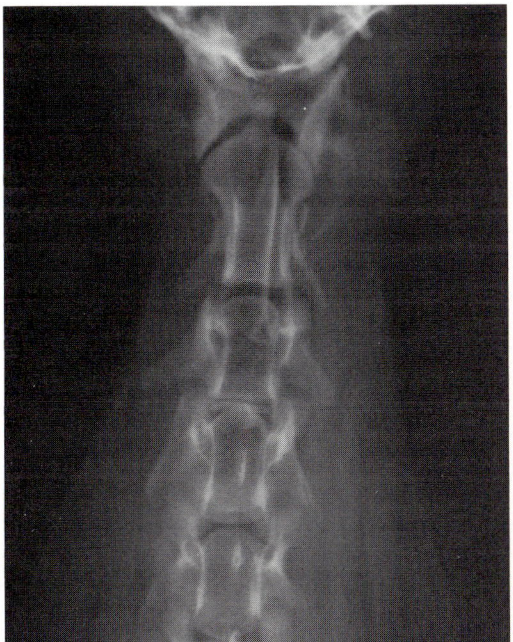

FIGURE 14–40 VD view of Figure 14–39.

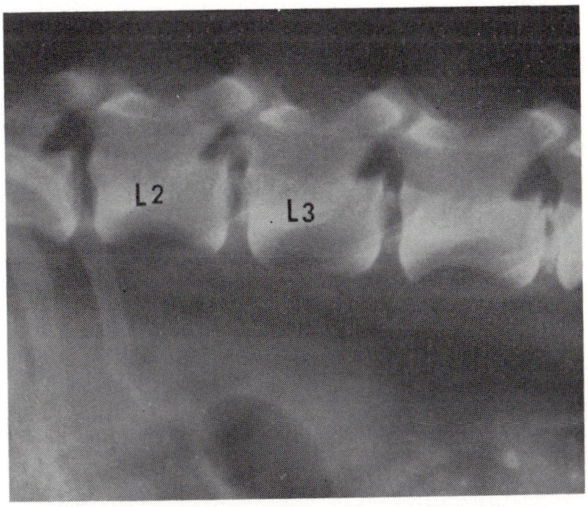

FIGURE 14–41 A mushroom calcified disk protrusion at L2–3. Notice that the protrusion has isolated itself from the parent calcified disk.

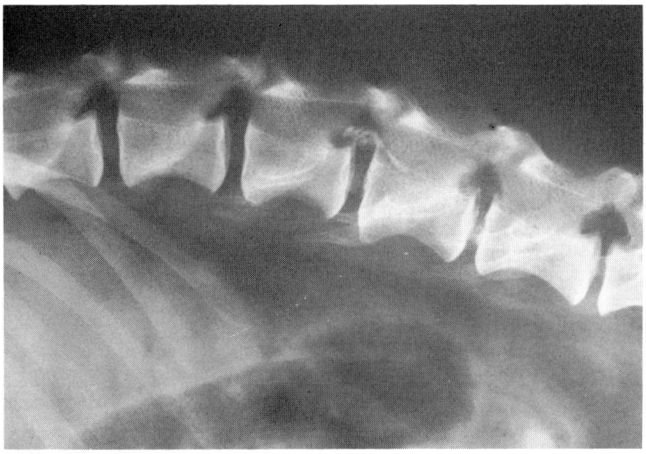

FIGURE 14–42 The protrusion mass has organized and calcified above the affected disk (L3–4). Also notice the residual fibrocalcific material in the nucleus and the relatively wide disk space. It is probable that this is an old lesion and that the disk space has assumed some of its original width by secondary fibrosis.

tumors, which cause a deviation of flow or a complete subarachnoid blockage. Generally, oil media will not flow in progressive hemorrhagic myelomalacia or hematomyelia, marked cord edema, and other disorders that tend to obliterate or diminish the subarachnoid space. However, because of their lack of viscosity, water contrast media (Skiodan or metrizamide) demonstrate small compressive lesions as well as other disorders of the cord such as edema, intramedullary lesions, and hematomyelia. In order to properly interpret aqueous contrast myelograms, one must have a

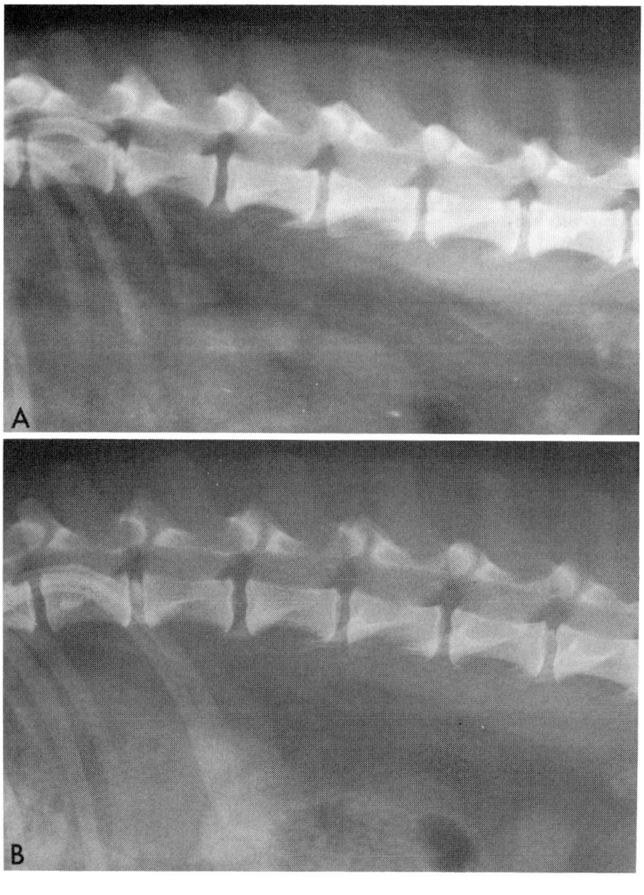

FIGURE 14–43 *A*. A radiograph of calcified disks at L1–2 and L3–4 taken with standard screen Bucky technique. *B*. This is the same dog, same view, but taken with a nonscreen Bucky technique. Notice the greater detail. The original film showed a protrusion of low density tissue at L3–4.

thorough knowledge of normal myelograms in normal, flexed, and extended spinal positions. Minor filling defects must be interpreted with caution since artifacts may be a factor. The most common change on the lateral view is narrowing and dorsal deviation of the ventral subarachnoid space at the level of the protrusion. The dorsal subarachnoid space is often narrowed or may be obliterated due to dorsal displacement and edema of the spinal cord. In cases of direct dorsal protrusion, the ventrodorsal view may show a narrowing of the lateral subarachnoid spaces with widening of the spinal cord. Lateral narrowing of the spinal cord may result if the disk protrusion extends to one side.[89, 193]

Myelography is extremely helpful as an aid in the location of cord tumors, cysts, vascular compressions, canine wobblers, and other lesions not readily discernible in plain films. The oil media, such as iophendylate (Pantopaque), tend to show filling defects from one-half to one vertebra away from the lesion, owing to a decreased subarachnoid space resulting from lesion pressure, hemorrhage, or edema. Water media such as sodium iodomethane-sulfonate (Skiodan) or metrizamide (Amipaque) give a more accurate location of the filling defect than oil media because of their aqueous densities. Occasionally, an atrophic myelomalacia will produce a localized smaller flow diameter of the entire contrast column around the lesion (Figs. 14–44 to 14–46).[89]

In conclusion, it is felt that the use of myelography in the diagnosis of disk disease is not routinely needed in the dog. At the present time, most radiologists are using Skiodan in some form or mixture as the aqueous contrast medium of choice in myelography. It is hoped that metrizamide may soon be available. The iodized oil, iophendylate (Pantopaque), is still probably the safest medium clinically (see page 107), but it has undesirable flow characteristics and causes histological arachnoiditis.

VERTEBRAL VENOGRAPHY

More recently, vertebral venography has been suggested as a radiographic aid in locating compressions of the spinal cord, swellings of the cord, or neoplasia of the cord or vertebrae. The technique is briefly described in Chapter 5 and in more detail in original reports and radiographic texts. More work should be done to evaluate the accuracy of this technique in diagnosis since it is probably safer than the existing contrast media used in myelography.[24]

EPIDURALOGRAPHY

This procedure was discussed in Chapter 5. It needs to be evaluated in clinical disk practice. It was used many years ago with oil contrast media and was considered inferior to myelography. This was no doubt

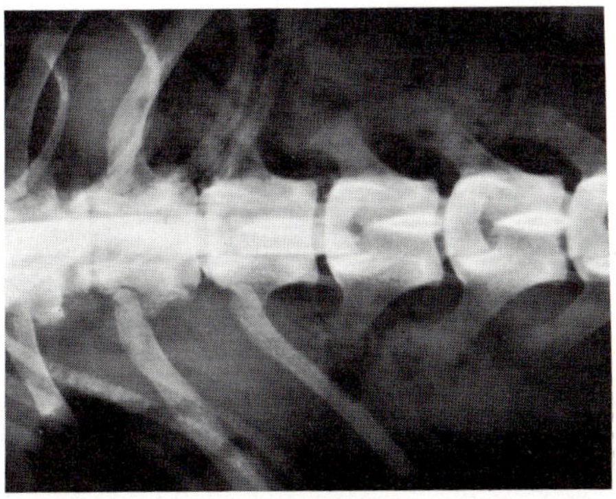

Fig. 14–44

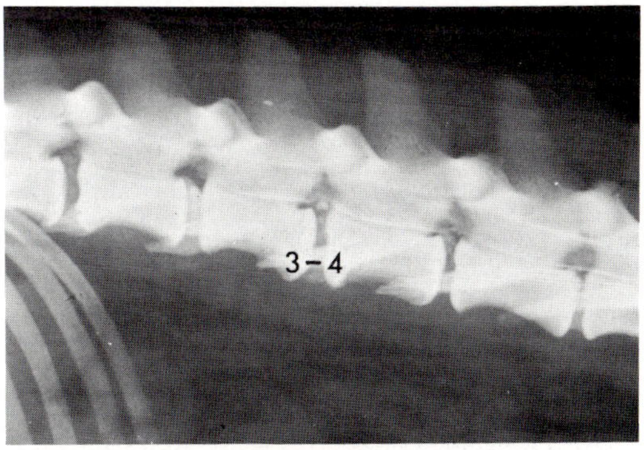

Fig. 14–45

FIGURE 14–44 A DV view of a Pantopaque myelogram demonstrates a complete subarachnoid blockage at T13–L1. Notice that the right thirteenth rib is absent. (Am. J. Vet. Res. *14*, 277, 1953.)

FIGURE 14–45 A lateral view of an aqueous contrast myelogram demonstrates a slight compression from an ossified protrusion of L3–4 annulus.

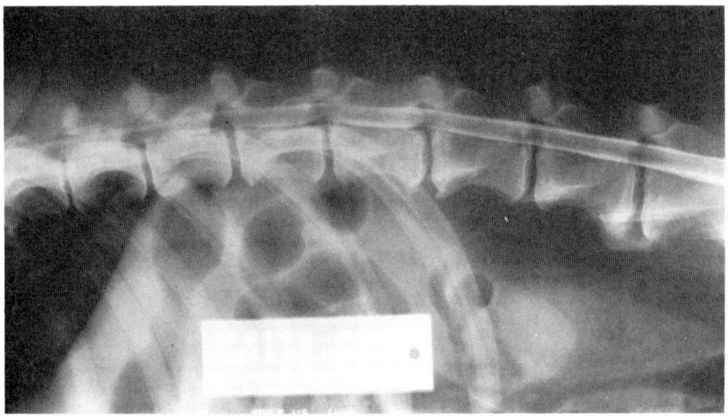

FIGURE 14–46 A myelogram on a 6-year-old German shepherd weighing 45 kg suffering from diffuse degenerative myelopathy. Notice the slight impaired flow of the ventral column of metrizamide at T13–L1 and L1–2, both of which have evidence of ventral spondylitic spurs.

due to the viscosity of the medium (Pantopaque) and the flow impairment caused by the extradural fat. The use of aqueous media should facilitate more accurate interpretation of compressions.[82, 89]

DISKOGRAPHY

Diskography has been discussed in detail in Chapter 5. This procedure has not gained widespread use in man and does not appear to have great promise in the dog.[55, 62, 79] The technical difficulties of proper injection, as experienced by Widdowson, seem to limit its clinical application.

NONSURGICAL TREATMENT

The sequence in the typical case of disk protrusion is degeneration, necrosis, and herniation or partial rupture, with subsequent resolution of the protrusion and repair of the remainder of the disk. Thus, neurological signs may diminish or disappear in the stage of resolution of minor protrusion, and the clinician may see spontaneous recovery from pain, paresis, and mild paraplegia, which accounts for the successful use of a variety of medications.

However, in a high percentage of cases exhibiting these signs, there are major relapses that cause much neurological damage. A significant number of patients also suffer a sudden complete paralysis from a major compression, for which surgical decompression is imperative. One must keep in mind that disk protrusions in the dog are characterized by *cord* pressure and are therefore more serious than those that routinely cause root pressure in man.

A careful neurological and radiographic examination should help the clinician to determine the course of therapy needed for each individual case. In the author's experience, the following types of cases should be considered for *nonsurgical* care:

Local compressive or transverse myelopathy
- Pain
- Paresis with pain
- Widespread or extensive spinal pathology. Presence of systemic disease or serious disorders of other organs.
- Complete paraplegia for more than 7 days with no sign of motor improvement.

Progressive paralysis produced by hemorrhagic myelomalacia.

In cases of *pain without* motor dysfunction, careful physical and radiographic examinations should be done, and the patient should be watched closely for progressive signs. The dog may recover without surgery, but recurrences are frequent.

In cases of *pain with* paresis, the dog generally has little loss of support, normal reflexes, and normal defecation and urination. If he has had no previous episodes, it would be well to keep him extremely quiet and hospitalized for complete observation. If he does not improve promptly or should suddenly become worse, surgical correction should be considered. Frequently, this type of case responds well to nonsurgical treatment, but recurrences may follow. Each recurrence tends to be more severe than the preceding one and causes more permanent cord changes.

Extensive disk lesions frequently occur in dogs, with evidence of cervical, thoracic, and lumbar disk degeneration with massive calcification of disks and protrusions. In some cases, spinal pathology in areas other than the disks occurs; examples are spondylosis, cervical wobbler syndrome, and bone degeneration. Nevertheless, disk disease in the cervical area and thoracolumbar junction has frequently been corrected by two surgical procedures.

Hemorrhagic myelomalacia from a sudden extensive and explosive rupture of the disk has been treated nonsurgically, since it was felt that surgery would merely aggravate the existing hemorrhagic process.

When biogenic amines and other neurochemical, endocrinological events seen in experimental cord trauma are fully understood, it is possible that immediate medical treatment to prevent spread of hemorrhagic necrosis, and concomitant surgical decompression may be advocated in clinical therapy. If there is some doubt that hemorrhagic myelomalacia exists, decompressive surgery and durotomy can be performed to determine the condition of the cord. In malacia, the medullary cord will flow out of the dural incision, confirming the diagnosis. The prognosis is grave.

OVERALL CARE OF LOCALIZED MYELITIS

Many features of the treatment of compression myelitis have been discussed in Chapter 13. The care of the urinary bladder was emphasized, and this of course applies equally to care of the disk protrusions. We believe that the bladder *must* be kept empty, and cystitis *must* be prevented if there is to be a successful recovery in a total paraplegic.

The therapy that the author has felt to be of most importance in the routine care of the paraplegic includes the following:

Maintain elimination of urine and feces.

Provide good nursing care and strict rest.

Maintain general nutrition.

Supervise exercise in an outdoor yard.

Give physical therapy, including hot water baths, ultrasound, and passive exercise of affected musculature.

Administer mild anodynes (salicylates, aspirin), sedatives, or tranquilizers to control *excessive* pain.

Administer anti-inflammatory drugs, such as phenylbutazone (Butazolidin), indomethacin (Indocin), and adrenocorticoids, only as needed.

Provide therapeutic levels of B complex vitamins (B_1, niacin, B_{12}).

We have discussed the use of catheters in care of the urinary tract. We must emphasize that the urinary bladder should be completely emptied twice daily, and it should be flushed after catheterization. Instillation of coagulants (topical thrombin) and antibiotics into the bladder after catheterization is accomplished when the urine appears bloody. The use of oral urinary antiseptics, sulfonamides (Manisul), or nitrofurazone is recommended to prevent urinary infection.

Every effort should be made to promote voluntary urination so that forceful manual expression of the bladder or catheterizations can be kept to a minimum. Placing the dog on the ground and applying mild pressure on the abdominal wall adjacent to the urinary bladder occasionally is all that is needed to initiate voluntary urination. Gentle pressure while the dog is in a hot "sitz" bath stimulates urination. Agents such as bethanechol chloride (Urecholine) may stimulate contraction of the bladder musculature and thereby promote voluntary urination.

When urinary retention exists, manual expression of the bladder is effective in the female. However, if the urine is concentrated, odorous, or bloody, the bladder must be flushed with warm saline and proper medication instilled via the catheter. Catheterization in the female must be done very carefully, with proper vaginal illumination, speculum, and a sterile, well-lubricated catheter. Traumatization of the external urethral orifice should be avoided. In the male, manual expression of the bladder is not easily accomplished unless total denervation exists. A sterile, well-lubricated, smooth (not cracked or rough) catheter should be inserted slowly and carefully, and the bladder should be flushed and medicated routinely.

Good nursing care and adequate rest are mandatory. The animal must be kept happy by careful handling and affectionate care, but still must be confined for the most part to a small cage or small pen such as a child's playpen. He must be kept clean and dry, as a severe dermatitis quickly results from urine and feces left on the skin. One must prevent the development of orchitis, vulvitis, or perineal dermatitis. A foam rubber cushion, a so-called "bean bag chair," or water mattress on the floor of the cage helps to prevent the development of decubital sores. Lambs' wool or synthetic fleece blankets used for human patients are also applicable for use in dogs. Animals in pens can be bedded in deep shavings. The use of ambulatory frames or carts periodically throughout the day affords relief from constant pressure on the tuber ischii.[15] The application of thick, tenacious medicaments such as zinc oxide ointment helps to protect the skin from excretory soiling.

Since many paraplegics have a negative nitrogen balance and a secondary anemia, good nutrition must be maintained. A heavy meat diet such as P/D,* supplemented with iron and liver, is desirable. All B complex vitamins should be supplied in therapeutic amounts. Injections of vitamin B_{12} and calcium have been used. If nephritis is present, K/D† is appropriate.

The author believes that personally supervised exercise is a very important part of care. This should be given twice daily, preferably early in the morning and late in the evening. The animal is taken outdoors to a grassy pen and is placed on his feet so that he will stand as long as possible. Gentle pressure on the posterior abdomen may stimulate urination. It is often best to leave the dog alone for several minutes to permit him to evacuate independently; however, one should observe his urinary action. The dog should be encouraged to walk following evacuation. He can be supported by the base of the tail or by placing a towel under his posterior abdomen to encourage his efforts. Since many of these patients normally relax by lying on their backs, "pumping" the legs (forced flexions and extensions) toward the abdomen is a relaxing type of passive exercise which the owner can effectively accomplish. The dog can be placed in an ambulatory device for a few minutes so that his feet touch the ground enough to encourage walking (Figs. 14–47 to 14–50).

Personal contact as described is most necessary for rapid rehabilitation of the paraplegic, in both nonsurgical and postsurgical care. In veterinary hospitals, one person who enjoys nursing care should be assigned so the patient can relate to that person as a friend. That person should feed the dog and assume total care if possible. The will to walk is essential to proper recovery of motor function.

*P/D, Prescription Protein Diet, Hill Dog Food, Topeka, Kansas.

†K/D, Prescription Kidney Diet, Hill Dog Food, Topeka, Kansas.

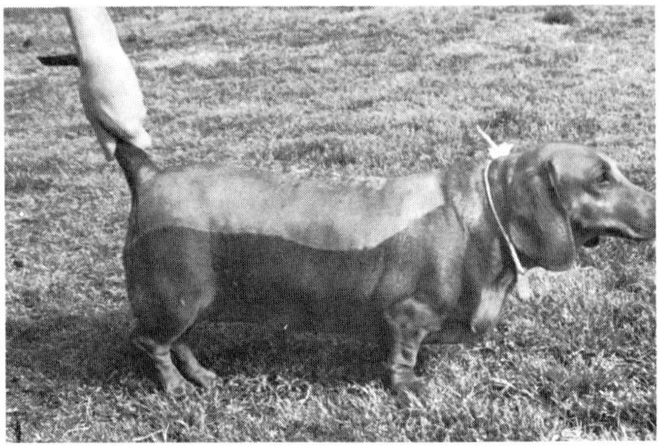

FIGURE 14–47 One should allow supervised exercise for a dog suffering from disk protrusion paraplegia. Supporting the animal by the base of the tail stimulates him to use his legs.

After exercising in the yard, the animal can be given some physiotherapy, either before breakfast or 2 to 3 hours later. Hot water baths are available in any veterinary clinic or home and require only a little time. The water is drawn in the tub until it covers the animal's back. It should be pleasantly warm to the touch, not uncomfortably hot. If the dog is in acute pain, a sitz bath is employed in which the dog sits in the water without being exercised. When pain has subsided, the feet are held down to the floor of the tub with one hand and the other hand is placed on the croup. The croup is forcibly moved toward the floor of the tub in order to flex and extend the limbs as in sitting and standing. Cranial-caudal movements of the legs are also beneficial. Such exercise done in warm water relieves muscle spasms and pain, helps to maintain cleanliness of the skin, increases circulation to the skin and hind parts, and helps to prevent muscle atrophy. Baths of 10 minutes' duration twice daily suffice. Many clinicians use whirlpool baths for the same amount of time for added passive exercise. Several patients can be exercised at once in the tub if constant supervision is available. Use of an antiseptic detergent in

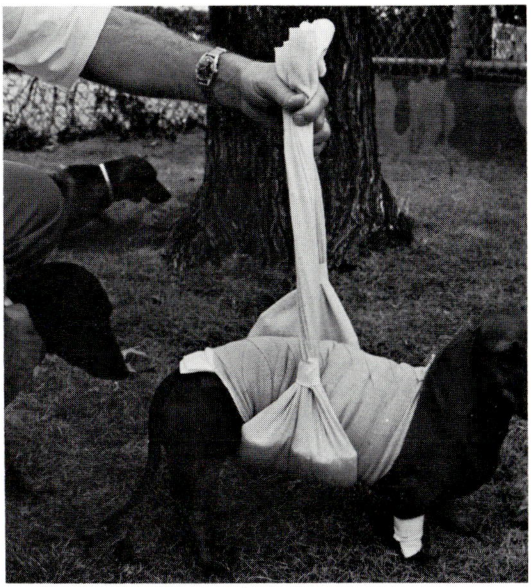

FIGURE 14–48 Some dogs object to the method of exercise portrayed in Figure 14–47 and prefer a "belly band" as a means of support.

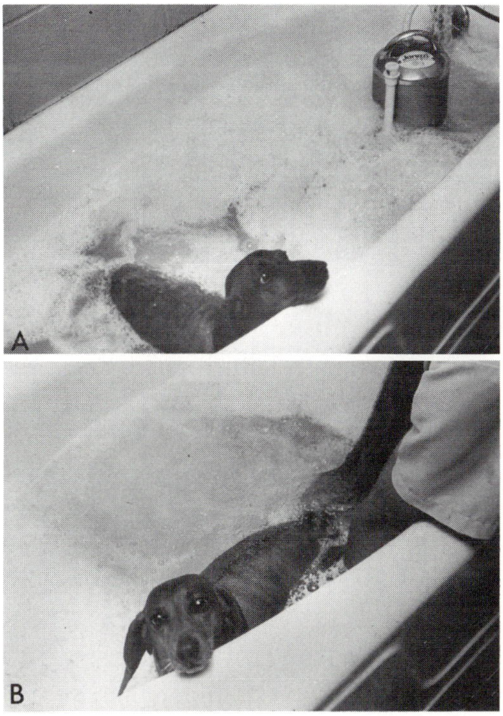

FIGURE 14–49 *A.* A whirlpool hot bath is an effective means of physical therapy. *B.* The feet are held on the floor of the tub and the other hand forces an extension and flexion action of the limbs by pushing the sacral area up and down.

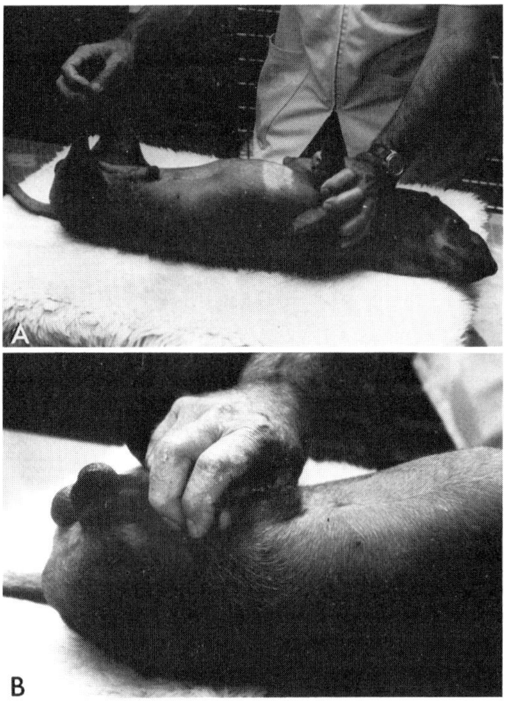

FIGURE 14–50 *A* and *B*. A means of exercise that the owner can do at home. Place the dog on a comfortable pad in the dorsal recumbent position and forcibly flex and extend the limbs continuously for 5 to 10 minutes, several times a day. Most dachshunds relax well in this position.

the water will promote dermal antisepsis and is good hospital practice.

Swimming is considered excellent exercise for paralytics and paretics. Many clients have encouraged the patient to swim in the family swimming pool or purchased a small child's pool for such exercise. Inflatable devices for the arms or limbs of humans learning to swim can be used around the body or neck of a dog to make such exercise safer.

MEDICINAL AGENTS

Among the most popular methods of treatment among American veterinarians is administration of the adrenocorticoid drugs,[123] phenylbutazone[142] and indomethacin. The corticoids and ACTH derivatives, such as hydrocortisone and dexamethasone, are anti-inflammatory, and are therefore anodyne in action. The anti-inflammatory dose of dexamethasone is believed to be 0.2 mg/kg, and this dose is fairly standard in routine cases of spinal compression. In severe cases of compression with deep pain deficit, antishock doses may be used (2 mg/kg or over) two to three times daily for 24 to 48 hours, with or without surgical decompression. Antacids or gastrointestinal protectives (e.g., Maalox) can be used to combat gastrointestinal inflammations and ulcerations that are prevalent in steroid therapy (see page 397).[91] These drugs create a sense of well-being. Phenylbutazone and indomethacin are very powerful antiarthritic and antirheumatic agents and are considered to be highly effective in relieving spinal pain. However, recent research in the use of phenylbutazone in experimental cord trauma found it to be ineffective in reducing the effects of trauma on the cord and promoting clinical improvement when 4.5 mg/kg were given intravenously twice daily.[64] The side effects of the corticoids have been well described, and these drugs should not be used in high dosages or for long periods of time. In addition, phenylbutazone is toxic, and can cause loss of weight, anemia, leukopenia, thrombocytopenia, and spontaneous hemorrhages.[130]

Indomethacin has not yet been used extensively in dogs. We have seen some dramatic clinical effects, particularly in cases of chronic spondylosis and spinal osteoarthritis. In man, indomethacin (especially in high doses) has caused CNS and gastrointestinal disorders. It is felt that it has ulcerogenic properties, at least in patients who have suffered with ulcers sometime previously. No blood dyscrasias have been noted. In the dog, we have seen few toxic effects with a dosage of one-half to three-fourths the amount recommended for man. In long-term or high-dose therapies, one should no doubt look for chronic gastrointestinal disorders such as those that may be seen in salicylate therapy.[172, 173] Vomiting and hemorrhagic gastritis have been our most common concerns.

The indiscriminate use of adrenocorticoids in outpatient practice is dangerous. The dog improves so quickly that he exercises beyond his capability, and more serious recurrences of neurological difficulties occur. In many such cases, there is permanent cord damage and paralysis. It is much safer to *reduce* the pain through drugs, rather than to *abolish* it, so that the dog will not be excessively active. He must rest until resolution and stabilization of the disk have occurred. *Rest* is the important aspect of treatment, not pain-killing drugs. The animal should usually be hospitalized when given corticoid drugs.

The local administration of hydrocortisone has been suggested for sciatica in man. Barbaso injected 25 mg of hydrocortisone acetate intraspinally with fairly good transient relief of pain.[5] The effects lasted from a few days to a few months.

Epidural administration of methyl prednisolone acetate (Depo Medrol) was reported in 91 dogs afflicted with paraplegia of varied etiology. Fifty-one dogs recovered. Dogs weighing less than 10 kg received 0.5 ml of a 40 mg/ml suspension initially; then 1 ml was given every 3 days thereafter. Larger dogs received twice this dose. The abstract article listed general diagnoses and made no mention of specific disk paraplegias. The injections varied from one to nine and were apparently given at the L7–S1 interspace.[114]

Another case report described the use of prednisolone acetate epidurally in 30 dogs with lumbar disk herniations. It was given at a dose of 1 mg per pound two to three times weekly. Very few failures noted were seen in the treatments administered. The failures noted were in cases of total flaccid paralysis, and in chronic cases characterized by recurrent episodes. There had been only one severe reaction, which appeared to be a violent anaphylactic shock. The dog recovered after intensive care. Pain was reduced or eliminated in about 12 hours, and ataxia and incoordination decreased in 2 days; paraplegia and paresis responded in 6 to 10 days. Injections were given epidurally at the lumbosacral junction.[212]

Nerve stimulants can be used, but of course they are difficult to evaluate. Certainly, the use of therapeutic amounts of thiamin, niacin, B_{12}, and the B complex vitamins is recommended, and may be helpful. Physostigmine has been proposed because of its cholinergic effect.[39] If the musculature and innervation of the bladder are functional but sluggish, bethanechol chloride will effectively stimulate urination. Thyroid extract is an effective stimulant to metabolism and is said to have an antirheumatic effect.[63]

In some practices, the use of vitamin E and selenium (Seletoc) has been popular for various arthromyopathies, including the disk syndrome. These agents are supposed to be anti-inflammatory, anodynic, catalytic for calcium and protein metabolism, and able to correct muscle deterioration by restoring normal protein metabolism. The usual dose of the preparation is 1 ml/10 kg of body weight daily for 3 to 5 days, and then 1 ml/10 kg every third day.[110, 154]

Muscle relaxants are occasionally useful in controlling muscle spasms. Methocarbamol (Robaxin) administered intravenously or intramuscularly at the rate of 0.34–3.00 mg/kg (or, in one report, 0.5 ml/kg[174]) has been used successfully.[37, 140] Mephenesin has been used with good results. A more recent product, chlorphenesin carbamate (Maolate), is an effective muscle relaxant. As muscle spasms can aggravate neurological pain and initiate an afferent-effector cycle, muscle relaxants should be used while the animal is forced to *rest.*

In 1964, Smith[188] and Saunders[177] reported on the use of chymopapain enzyme injections into the nucleus pulposus. The enzyme dissolved the nucleus and was thought to be of value in treatment of clinical disk protrusions. Smith reported the relief of back pain in seven of ten patients within 6 to 18 hours after injection. Radiography showed narrowing of the injected disks 4 to 8 days later. The injection consisted of 50 per cent sodium diatrizoate, to locate the disk via diskogram, and 4 to 16 mg of enzyme dissolved in saline. The posterolateral puncture technique was used. Saunders reported on its use in 75 dogs with suspected disk syndrome: 39 dogs walked, 14 improved, 16 did not improve, and 6 died within the 20 days postinjection observation period.

In 1967, Widdowson[213, 214] evaluated the enzyme in normal dogs and in dogs with clinical disk protrusions. This investigator experienced difficulty in proper administration in the nucleus even with a surgical exposure, and found the results somewhat inconclusive. He also found that the enzyme was toxic if given in the subarachnoid space, in the spinal cord, or even extradurally. This method of treatment has not seemed to gain much favor in the treatment of disk protrusion in veterinary medicine. However, there are increasing reports of its use in humans by orthopedists and adverse reports, mainly by neurosurgeons. Controversy concerning its impending release by the Federal Drug Administration is also increasing. It is possible that it will be fully approved in the near future.[183, 194, 211]

PHYSICAL THERAPY

The method of therapy just outlined has been used routinely by the author and has been satisfactory, while many other procedures of merit have been described in the literature. Jadeson has explored various methods of physical therapy, such as thermal therapy, massage, exercises and stretching, electrical stimulation, and ultrasonic therapy.[97] He concluded that when these modalities were used, the rate of recovery was faster, the incidence of relapse was decisively lower, and there was less pain and, consequently, reduced need for sedatives and analgesics. Jadeson feels that even though several forms of physical therapy have similar physical and physiological effects, more than one may be needed for improvement of dysfunction. For instance, preparatory application of heat facilitates manipulation and permits more intensive massage and exercise. Electrical stimulation enhances the effect of heat in stimulating muscle tone and deep circulation.

Ultrasonic applications have been used as a means of physical therapy. Jadeson feels that ultrasound is effective in reducing muscle hypertonia in the lumbar area and restoring muscle function, so that the protruding disk tends to return to its normal position.[97] The effects are as follows: high-frequency sound waves produce a pulsating action in tissue and cells; thermomechanical heat is induced; there is a biochemical effect; and neurotrophic action is produced by sonation of roots of autonomic nerves.

Schirmer has suggested that a series of ultrasonic treatments will permanently relieve pain from cervical disk protrusions.[178] Changes have been seen in the disk and the protrusions from ultrasound. The dog's hair is clipped and mineral oil is applied to the skin over the affected area. The applicator is moved gently over the area while a dose of 0.1 to 1 watt/cm^2 is used for 5 minutes. This treatment is repeated daily for 5 days and then every other day for a total of five treatments. In 102 cases, 90 per cent showed marked improvement in 30 days, and 4 per cent required a second course as outlined.

In a later publication, Schirmer reported that the use of ultrasound produced 100 per cent favorable results in 67 cases of chronic cervical disk disorders. Four cases were subjected to a second course of therapy following incomplete response from the first course. The dose in this series was 0.2 to 0.5 watt per sq cm applied to the dorsum of the neck, which had been clipped and liberally lubricated with mineral oil. Duration of application in this series was 3 to 5 minutes. Recovery time is usually 2 to 3 weeks, although a small percentage of cases requires 4 to 6 weeks. Schirmer used ultrasound in the healing stage of lumbar disk disease and felt that it hastened the rate of healing. Results in this area were not as dramatic. No statistics were given for recurrences.[179]

Swarts and Jefferies devised a truss or corset for use in canine paraplegics[200]; however, it is unavailable at the present time. A truss limits spinal movement during the stabilization period and may serve as an additional support to fix the skeleton in spinal fractures and spinal fusions. Casts, braces, corsets, and other devices have been used in man over a long period to bring about immobility in various spinal disorders (Fig. 14–51).

The use of ambulatory appliances has already been mentioned. Brooks,[15] Leighton,[112] Short,[186] Leonard,[113] and others have devised such carts. They are of definite benefit in helping the paraplegic to assume a relatively normal walking position so that he is not constantly sitting. If the feet touch the ground, walking movements are encouraged; however, one should not allow the dog to run about in a cart unless this helps him in walking movements. We use carts as a means of encouragement and to provide a change in position that discourages the formation of decubital lesions. We do not feel that using the cart as a "crutch" is helpful in total rehabilitation (Fig. 14–52).

Traction and manipulation have been used for years in man. Hansen reported on the use of traction and manipulation in 41 patients having lumbar disk lesions.[78] Surgical correction was thereby avoided in seven patients, and he concluded that traction was helpful only when the protrusion was not extensive enough to be positive on myelography. Spurling and Segerberg used

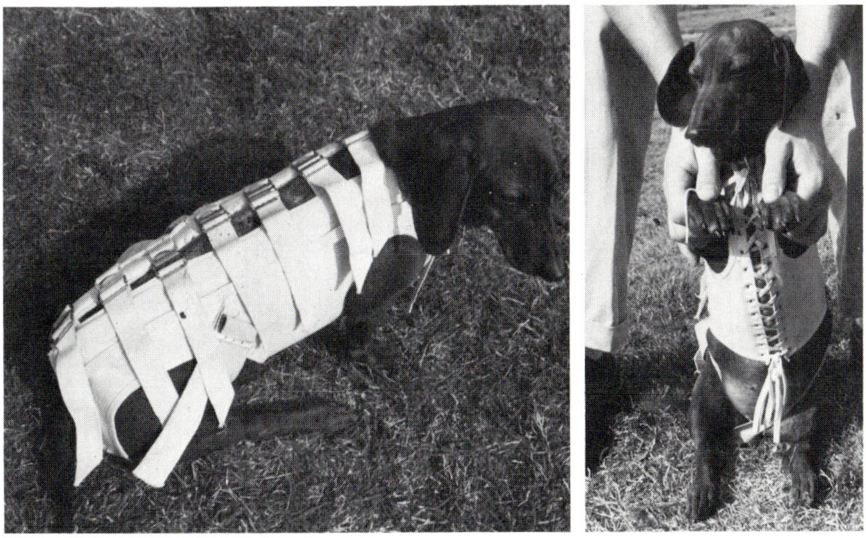

A B

FIGURE 14–51 *A*. A corset designed for the dog may help to enforce rest and partial immobilization of the spine. *B*. Another view of a canine corset.

traction in 110 patients, of whom 70 per cent responded and 30 per cent needed surgical treatment.[192]

Armstrong feels that traction and manipulation are becoming less popular as the dangers and limitations are becoming more widely appreciated.[1] He states that traction can relieve a patient only when separation of the vertebral bodies occurs, allowing an impacted sequestrum to slip forward (ventrally in the dog) into the central concavity between the bodies. Subsequent displacement will probably occur again unless the patient is then treated with rest and immobilization of the lumbar spine. It is also true that compressive forces on the disk are reduced during traction, and any tendency to nuclear retropulsion is temporarily di-

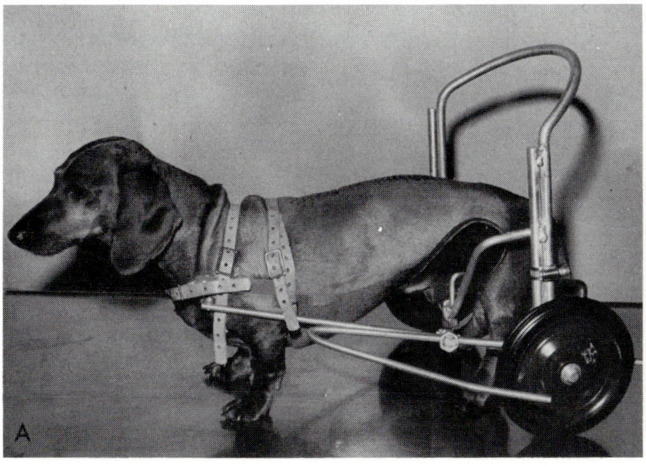

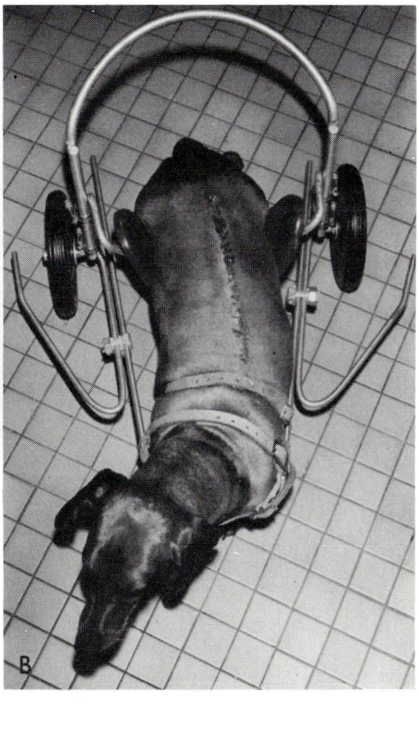

FIGURE 14–52 Ambulatory "carts" can be custom-made for each paraplegic with Thomas splint rods, or an adjustable commercial cart (*A* and *B*) can be purchased. This one is manufactured by Mustang Aviation Inc., 1874 Wooddale Court, Baton Rouge, La. 70806.)

minished. All other possible effects of traction are harmful to a greater or lesser degree, depending on the force used.

Cottle,[25-27] Moltzen,[134, 135] and Moody[136] have reported on the use of traction in canine protrusions. Moody placed a tie caudal to the shoulder and secured it to the table. He placed another tie cranial to the hips and secured it to a 14-lb weight suspended over a pulley. The dog was given a narcotic and a tranquilizer the first day and held in traction for 8 hours. Twenty-minute periods of traction were used on two consecutive days thereafter. The dog made a nearly complete recovery within 1 month. Apparently this was not a radiographically confirmed case of disk protrusion. More recently, Moltzen reported on manipulation therapy for disk protrusions in dogs and cats. Eighty-seven of 98 cases of moderate to severe enchondrosis with calcifications and protrusions (including several cases of spondyloarthrosis) were restored to normal, painless mobility. Thirty-four of these patients were manipulated only once, and others two to six times. Sixteen dogs suffered relapses several months to years later but again improved with renewed manipulation. Fourteen animals with total paralytic paraplegia were considered incurable and were destroyed.[135]

Cottle reports the use of a 5- to 10-kg weight traction under general anesthesia for a 30 to 60 minute period. Corticosteroids, antibiotics, and supportive care are used, and if needed, the traction may be repeated at a later time. Recovery has been complete in seven of eight dogs; one dog had a partial recovery.[25-27]

OVERALL CARE OF PROGRESSIVE OR HEMORRHAGIC MYELOMALACIA (HEMATOMYELIA)

The treatments mentioned previously apply chiefly to cases of local compression myelitis caused by protruding disks, with signs of pain, paresis, or paralysis. The treatment of a case of progressive hemorrhagic myelomalacia resulting from a severe rupture and blowout of the disk was given in Chapter 13, and may be summarized as follows:

1. Antibiotics (broad spectrum).
2. Adrenocorticoids for anti-inflammatory response (e.g., dexamethasone 1–4 mg/kg initially, repeated at lesser doses at 6- to 8-hour intervals for not more than 24 hours. Decrease gradually if the response is good. Watch for toxic signs (see p. 397).
3. Intravenously administered hypertonic solutions such as 20 to 25 per cent mannitol solutions[89, 185, 216] to combat edema of the cord, for not more than 24 to 36 hours.
4. Maintain urine elimination; flush bladder; instill hemostatics and antibiotics.
5. Maintain good nutrition, intravenously if necessary.
6. Keep animal as quiet as possible and handle very gently.

It may be possible with this regimen to stop the progressive hemorrhage and to limit cord destruction; however, most subjects die within 3 to 6 days. In the future, agents designed to combat production of catecholamines and their derivatives plus immediate decompressive surgery may be suggested for this syndrome.

SUMMARY

A routine course of conservative treatment has been outlined for disk protrusions in the dog. It is adapted particularly to cases showing pain and paresis. Some paraplegics respond to this treatment because resolution and repair in recent ruptures may take place before irreversible damage to the cord results. It is applicable to paraplegics chosen for *nonsurgical* therapy, but also can be used in the *postoperative care* of paraplegics. Supervised exercise, hot water therapy, and the use of ambulatory carts are important in patient rehabilitation. The veterinary literature has reflected little or no expanded use of manipulation, traction, ultrasound, or chymopapain injections since 1971.

The author concludes that nonsurgical treatment is centered around *rest* and the maintenance of body metabolism and excretion while the protrusion resolves or repairs itself and the cord regains its function.

SURGICAL TREATMENT

The surgery proposed for relief of disk protrusions in man has included hemiliaminectomy, dorsal laminectomy, removal of disk material with little or no removal of bone, and disk fenestration.[11, 28, 29, 119, 133] Various methods of fusion have been proposed, but this is not currently recommended in the routine case.[1, 22]

In dogs, surgical procedures advocated for cervical disk protrusion include ventral fenestrations,[84, 145] ventral decompression by means of a partial spondylectomy and diskectomy (ventral slot or trephination) with or without a graft,[60, 160, 161, 195, 196] dorsal laminectomy,[42, 89] and hemilaminectomy.[88, 157] Surgical operations proposed for thoracolumbar disk protrusions in the dog include ventral or ventrolateral fenestration,[113, 171] dorsolateral fenestration with or without a hemilaminectomy,[66, 84, 89, 145, 167] dorsolateral and lateral muscle separation approaches for disk fenestration,[40, 138, 184, 218] hemilaminectomy with or without fenestration of adjacent disks,[13, 84, 89, 167] doral laminectomy,[43, 66, 89] and modified dorsal laminectomy.[208] Other decompressive procedures which are not advocated for disk protrusions are the modified deep or total dorsal laminectomy in which the entire dorsal arch is removed,[267] and a bilateral hemilaminectomy extending over two vertebral lengths.[197]

Because the veterinary clientele is demanding more and better service, many practitioners have become interested and, in a few instances, enthusiastic about surgical therapy for severe protrusions. The growing popularity of the dachshund, Pekingese, and beagle breeds has also stimulated this interest. Every sizable urban community has or will have in the near future a trained clinician available for neurological consultations and surgery now that specialized training is available in this field.

Those cases recommended for nonsurgical treatment have been listed. In the author's opinion, *surgical* intervention is indicated with the following:

1. Recurrent attacks of neurological dysfunction due to disk protrusion, each attack being more severe than the previous one.
2. Pain and paresis that are unresponsive to nonsurgical care.
3. Profound paralysis with fecal and urinary dysfunction produced by a local compression. Conscious perception of pain on the pedal reflex should be present.

All surgical candidates should have a protrusion demonstrable on the plain or contrast roentgenogram. According to Olsson,[143-145] the rationale for disk fenestration is that removal of a large portion of the disk by currettage produces an acute inflammatory reaction which stimulates phagocytosis, resorption of necrosis, and the formation of a stable fibrosis in the disk. Through removal of the "foundation" of the disk, the herniation will recede.

The author agrees with some of the principles mentioned, but doubts that fenestration is sufficient for large calcific lesions, or for the acute blowout and massive soft protrusion that is accompanied by pronounced edema and swelling of the cord. In these, a more aggressive approach is necessary; one must decompress the edematous, swollen cord, and remove not only the protrusion but also the remainder of the disk. The paraplegic dog that is suffering from severe cord pressure can be helped by this method, and a high percentage of patients recover completely. However, surgical intervention must be accomplished promptly before irreversible damage to the cord has resulted. The outcome of surgery depends in part on the period of delay before surgery, the size of lesion, its rate of development, and the dynamic force behind it. Even some of the European workers[100, 210] that were reluctant to join American surgeons in recommending decompressive surgery for disk protrusions have been encouraged by Funkquist's work in Sweden on dorsal laminectomies. This technique will be described later.

THORACOLUMBAR DISK SURGERY

Dorsolateral Fenestration

The technique of fenestration as described by Olsson[144] involved a dorsolateral approach to the disks from T12–13 posteriorly. A pad was placed under the animal, which was then placed in the ventral recumbent position so as to produce a kyphosis suitable to the surgical approach. The skin and dorsal lumbar fascia were incised just lateral to the dorsal spines. In dachshunds the length of the incision was usually 5 to 6 inches. Dorsal musculature was removed from the vertebrae by a raspatory to expose three to four lateral pro-

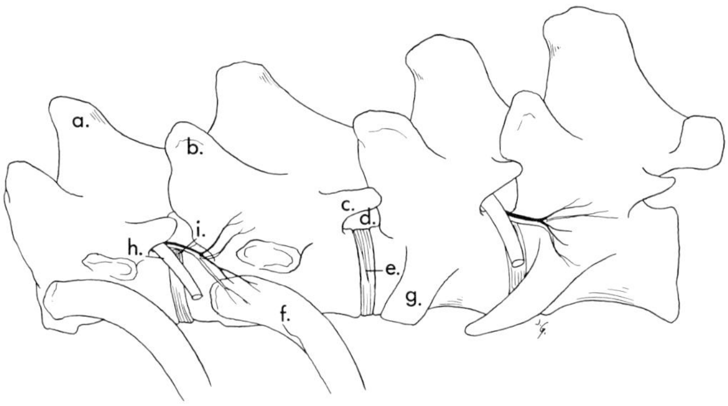

FIGURE 14–53 Anatomical structures involved in spinal surgery. (a) Dorsal spine; (b) articular process; (c) accessory process; (d) intervertebral foramen; (e) intervertebral disk; (f) ribs; (g) lateral process; (h) spinal nerve; (i) spinal artery and vein. Notice that the disk is located slightly cranial to the place at which the lateral process or rib joins the body of the vertebra.

cesses or ribs. Care was exercised to prevent injury to the intervertebral vessels and nerves. The disk was fenestrated dorsolaterally with a small knife or lancet to obtain a vertical incision 2 to 4 mm long. As much of the nucleus as possible was removed with a scoop or curette. The fascia was sutured with catgut, and the skin was closed with stainless steel wire. The sutures were removed in 8 to 10 days (Figs. 14–53 to 14–57).

In disks situated cranial to disk T12–13, fenestration was accomplished by a transthoracic approach. The animal was placed in the right lateral recumbent position, and the left thorax was entered. Trichloroethylene was administered with a positive pressure apparatus for anesthesia. A resection of 9 to 11 cm was performed on the rib just cranial to the protrusion, starting above the costochondral junction. A longitudinal incision was made through the remaining periosteum following the rib resection, and the cavity was entered. The pleura was separated from the disks with a blunt instrument, and the vessels and nerves were retracted. Fenestration was done as described previously. The pleura, rib periosteum, and muscles were sutured individually with catgut, and the skin was closed with stainless steel wire.[144]

Ventral Disk Fenestration

Leonard has modified Olsson's thoracolumbar disk fenestration to a ventral abdominal approach.[113] The animal is placed in the right lateral recumbent position, and a suitable lung ventilation apparatus is applied if the chest is to be entered. The skin incision is made over the thirteenth rib from the dorsal to the ventral midline. The subcutaneous tissues are dissected, and a paracostal incision is made into the abdomen. The left kidney is located and is reflected ventrally with the peritoneum. Frazier or other retractors are applied to

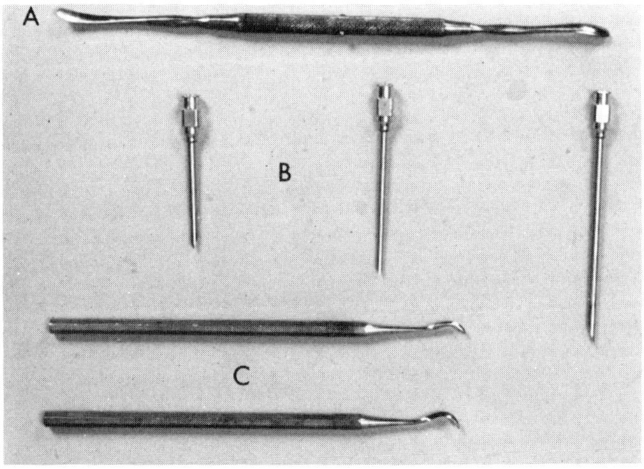

FIGURE 14–54 Instruments that are useful in disk fenestration procedures. (A) Periosteal elevator; (B) various lengths of 12 to 14 gauge intravenous needles; (C) various widths and curvatures of dental claw-type tartar scrapers. The needles and tartar scrapers are useful in removing extradural deposits of the protruding disk in decompressive surgery as well as in removing the disk in fenestration or curettage procedures.

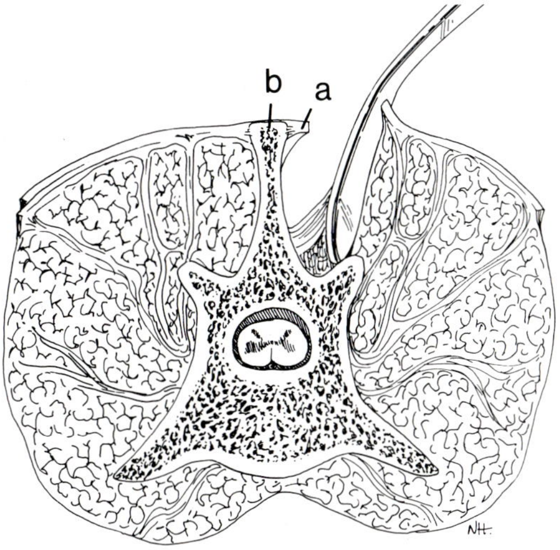

FIGURE 14–55 For the dorsolateral approach to the thoracolumbar spine for disk fenestration or hemilaminectomy, the incision is made on or 1 cm off the dorsal midline. The dorsal lumbar fascia (a) is incised lateral to the spine (b), and blunt dissection is employed to remove the musculature from the vertebrae.

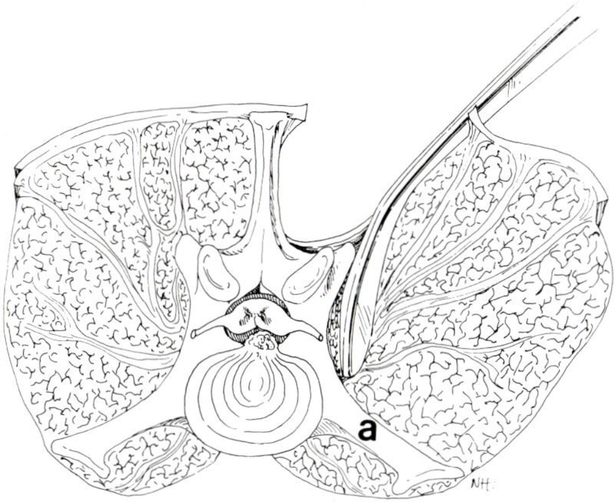

FIGURE 14–56 The musculature is reflected down to the lateral processes (a) or ribs.

spread the incision, and abdominal viscera are packed with a laparotomy pad. This retroperitoneal approach affords access to L1–2 through L5–6 intervertebral spaces.

When T9–10 through T13–L1 are to be fenestrated, the skin incision is "slid" forward so that an intercostal incision can be made between the tenth and eleventh ribs. The last rib is used as the key landmark in fenestrations. The disk is uncovered by blunt dissection, and the peritoneum, sympathetic nerve trunks, and aorta and its branches are carefully retracted from the area using the fingers or appropriate instruments. The whitish band of annular tissue (about 1 to 2 mm wide) is incised with the point of a scalpel. The nucleus is removed by a hooking motion (upward and outward) with a claw type tartar scraper.[9, 113, 171]

The pleura or peritoneum is closed with interrupted surgical gut sutures. Chest closure is facilitated by punching or boring three equally spaced holes in the two ribs adjacent to the incision, which are approximated by lacing with monofilament wire. Muscle, fascia, and skin are closed in the usual fashion. (It is assumed that any diaphragmatic incision is sutured, although Leonard does not mention this in his description).

Dorsal Laminectomy

After Greene's report on laminectomy in 1952,[66] Funkquist wrote extensively on dorsal decompression laminectomy in 1962.[42, 46, 50] Her procedure was developed in normal dogs and in those that had ex-

FIGURE 14–57 A disk can be curetted or fenestrated with a 12 or 14 gauge intravenous needle. The bevel of the needle is used as a scoop. The dental claw-type tartar scraper or a very small bone curet can be used to remove the disk.

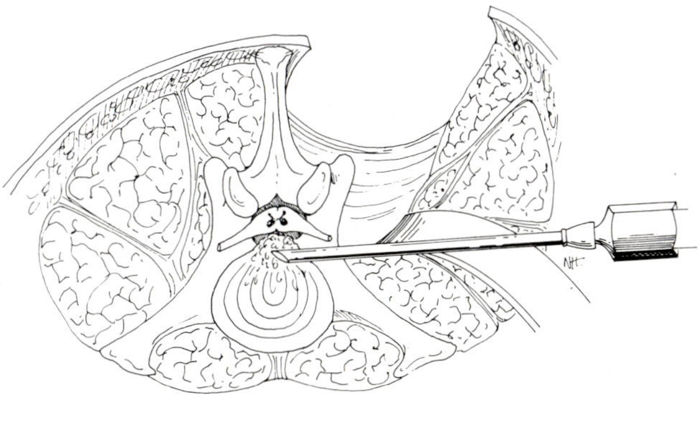

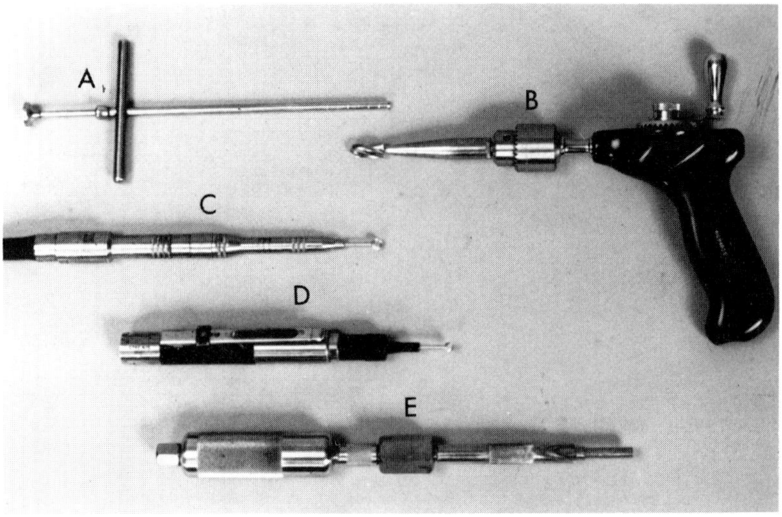

FIGURE 14–58 Instruments useful in laminectomies. (A) Michelle laminectomy trephine, 7/32-inch diameter; (B) orthopedic hand drill and bone bur (burring in spinal surgery can be utilized in lieu of trephination); (C) Stryker high-speed air drill; (D) Hall high-speed air drill; (E) Micrometer trephine with a preset depth guard.

perimentally produced compressions. The extensive thoracolumbar dorsal laminectomy (method A surgery), in which the dorsal arches were removed down to a horizontal line bisecting the spinal cord, resulted in a secondary compression of the cord because of the formation of scar tissue. However, when the compact bone of the dorsolateral portion of the dorsal arch (pedicle), including the articular process, was left intact (method B surgery), dorsoventral cord compression from fibrotic healing was prevented in experimental and clinical cases of disk protrusion.[42, 46, 50]

The technique for this procedure as described by Funkquist used a dorsal ap-

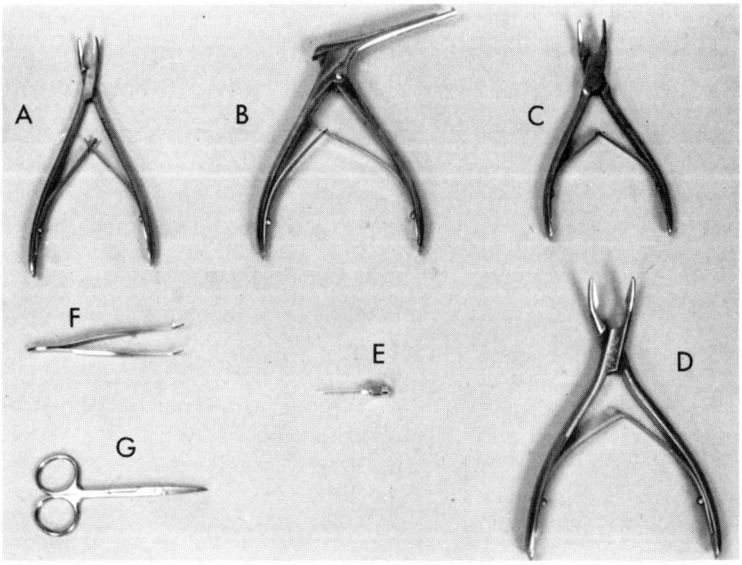

FIGURE 14–59 Instruments used in laminectomies. (A) Lampert rongeur; (B) Kerrison laminectomy rongeur; (C) Reiner rongeur; (D) mastoid rongeur; (E) 23-gauge intravenous needle that can be used to initiate a dural incision or to elevate the dura while using iris scissors in a durotomy; (F) an iris or dural forceps that can be used to grasp the dura to initiate a durotomy; (G) iris scissors. The cutting edge of the bevel of the injection needle (E) can be used to make a dural incision.

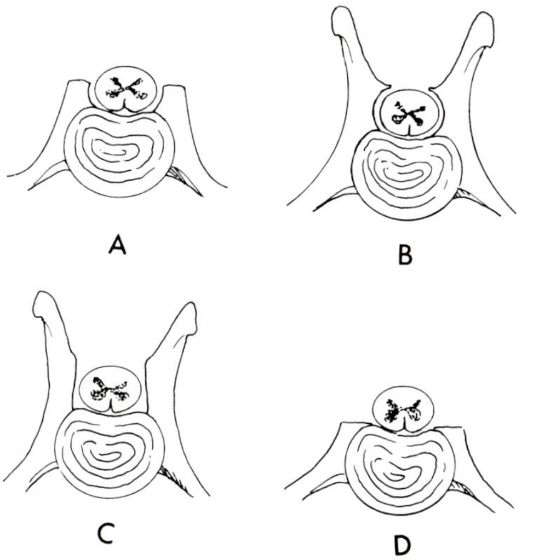

FIGURE 14–60 The different types of dorsal laminectomies. (A) Funkquist A, which is subject to secondary cicatricial compression. (B) Funkquist B, which is the standard dorsal laminectomy procedure. The dorsolateral arches remain above the cord, so that cicatricial compression is not a problem. (C) Modified dorsal laminectomy (Trotter), which provides a more spacious decompression. (D) Modified deep dorsal laminectomy (total dorsal laminectomy), which is recommended for severe cord trauma in spinal fractures.

proach. The dog was placed in the ventral recumbent position, and the incision was made in the dorsal midline. The musculature was bluntly dissected from each side of the spine and articular processes. The dorsal arches were freed of musculature. After the dorsal spines of two to six vertebrae were removed, a 50,000 rpm pneumatic dental drill was used to make a median groove in the dorsal arches. Round burs of 1.1 to 2.9 mm in diameter were used. The dorsolateral portions of the arches were excavated by removal of the cancellous bone and inner compact bone, while the outer compact bone was left intact. The outer articular processes were virtually undisturbed. The bone remnants were removed with a small-gauge forceps, the objective being to maintain the outer cortical areas of bone above the level of the cord, as far as possible. The protrusion was not removed unless it was above or lateral to the cord. The bone defect extended over a cranial-caudal dimension until normal cord and epidural fat relationships were observed on each end. This defect varied in extent from two to six vertebrae. No attempts were made to reconstruct the roof of the spinal canal. The dorsal lumbar fascia was not sutured. The skin was closed in a routine fashion.[42, 46, 50]

Funkquist referred to the procedure just described as method B, and believed that it was preferable to the more extensive laminectomy, called method A, in which fibrotic compression was seen in postoperative healing. Method A was used in 36 clinical cases and method B in 33 cases. In 14 dogs that had method A surgery, in which the laminectomy included the articular processes, attempts were made to reconstruct the dorsal arches by transplanting autogenous bone chips. The lumbodorsal fascia was sutured in 29 of the 36 cases (in ten of which bone chips were used), and in seven cases the fascia was not sutured. In the latter cases, fibrin foam was used on the dura. The results of the surgery are presented in a later section (Figs. 14–58 to 14–62).[42, 46, 50]

Modified Dorsal Laminectomy

The modified dorsal laminectomy as proposed by Trotter[206, 208] allows more spacious decompression and more adequate removal of disk protrusion material than the Funkquist type B method. The dog is placed in the sternal recumbent position, and a dorsal incision slightly off the midline is made to expose at least two vertebrae cranial and caudal to the involved disk. The thoracolumbar fascia is incised immediately lateral to the spines, and careful periosteal elevations are employed to dissect the epaxial musculature away from the arch of the vertebrae, ventral to the accessory processes. The spinous processes of the vertebrae involved in the decompression are removed by rongeurs. The outer cortical bones of the dorsal laminae are removed by a painting motion with a high-speed drill, utilizing a 4-mm, egg-shaped bur with notched flutes.* The drilling is continued laterally to the joint spaces between the lateral aspects of the caudal articular processes, leaving the cranial articular processes intact. The drilling of at least two vertebral lengths is continued until only the inner cortical layers are left intact. A 2.3- or 1.6-mm round carbide tip bur is

*Hall II Air Drill, Zimmer Manufacturing Co., Warsaw, Indiana.

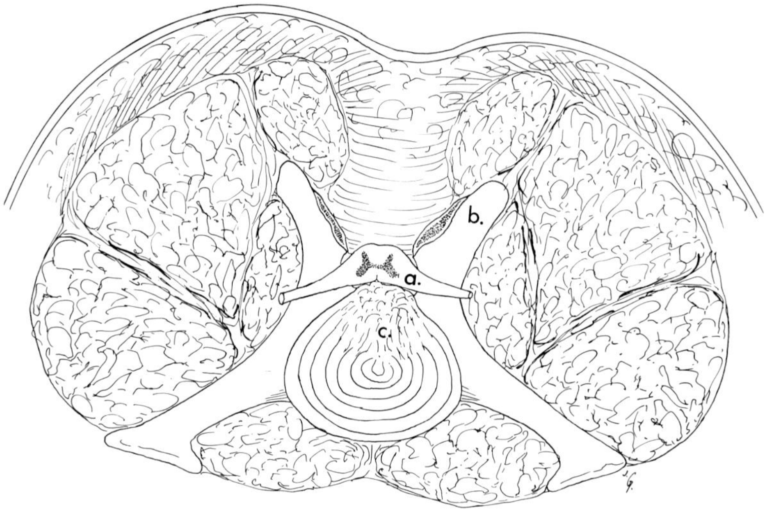

FIGURE 14–61 A cross section laminectomy decompression. (a) Spinal cord; (b) dorsolateral arch; (c) protruding disk.

substituted, and the last inner thin cortical bone is removed by drilling around the periphery of the laminectomy site with the bur held at a 45-degree angle from the spinal cord. Great care should be used not to penetrate the spinal canal at the interarcual spaces, which are devoid of a vertebral arch. "Sling" sutures of 5–0 cardiovascular silk may be placed transversely in the dura to allow the cord to be rolled laterally to facilitate removal of the protrusion mass. Lactate Ringer's slush is applied to the exposed cord routinely for at least 20 minutes. A pair of Potts Smith, 60-degree angled, cardiovascular scissors or a bent, disposable, 20-gauge injection needle is used to incise the dura on the dorsal midline the full length of the laminectomy site. The durotomy affords greater decompression of the cord when intradural hemorrhage or edema is present. It also is used to form a more accurate prognosis (Fig. 14–63).

Although Trotter does not describe the closure, his report of the modified deep dorsal laminectomy included use of absorbable gelatine sponge on the cord and the routine closure of the thoracolumbar fascia, subcutis, and skin. In addition, 20 per cent mannitol solution is administered in doses of 2 gm/kg body weight, repeated in 3 to 4 hours if necessary. Other postopera-

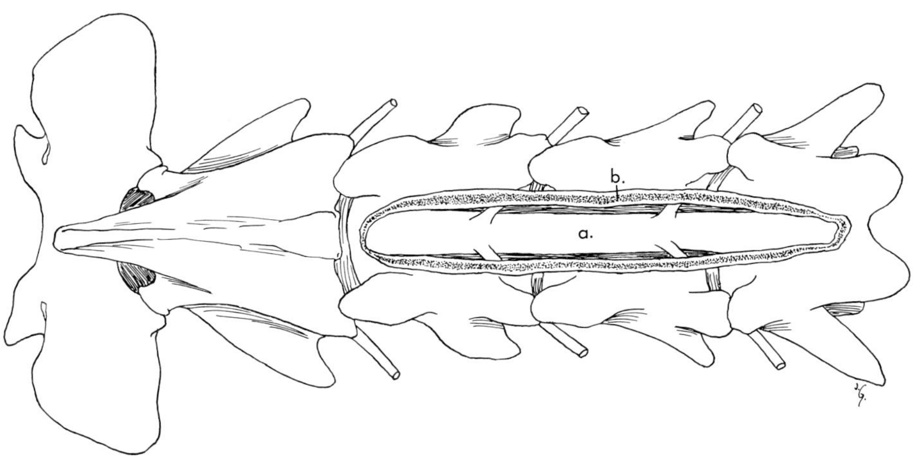

FIGURE 14–62 Dorsoventral view of a dorsal laminectomy decompression. The laminal defect must extend anteroposteriorly from the disk protrusion until normal spinal cord is seen in each direction.

tive care is similar to that previously described.[206-208]

There is a growing tendency among veterinary surgeons who employ extensive dorsal laminectomies and hemilaminectomies in the treatment of disk protrusions to use additional aggressive drug therapy to combat cord edema and catecholamine CNS changes.[57] The use of steroids, hypothermic or normothermic tissue irrigations, anticatecholamines, DMSO, and similar agents is becoming more prevalent. It is the opinion of this author that prompt decompression, steroids, and tissue irrigations during surgery are indicated, but more careful clinical evaluation of other agents is needed before widespread usage is recommended. See Chapter 12 for details of treatment of acute cord trauma.

The modified deep dorsal laminectomy has been discussed here as a radical decompression technique which may be applicable in severe spinal cord injury as in spinal fractures, especially of the vertebral arch[207] (see Chapter 15). When Mendenhall and associates[128] used the technique in spinal cord injuries, they used a very aggressive pharmacological approach as well as prompt, extensive decompression of an area that included at least three vertebral segments. They performed subarachnoid perfusions with hypertonic solutions for 3 hours, used myelotomies and durotomies, and administered steroids and anticatecholamines. It was concluded that the recovery rate was significantly higher in cases treated in this manner than in those handled in a more conservative fashion. Intervertebral disk cases were not included in this study.[128] It is generally agreed that modified deep dorsal laminectomies are not indicated for disk protrusions.

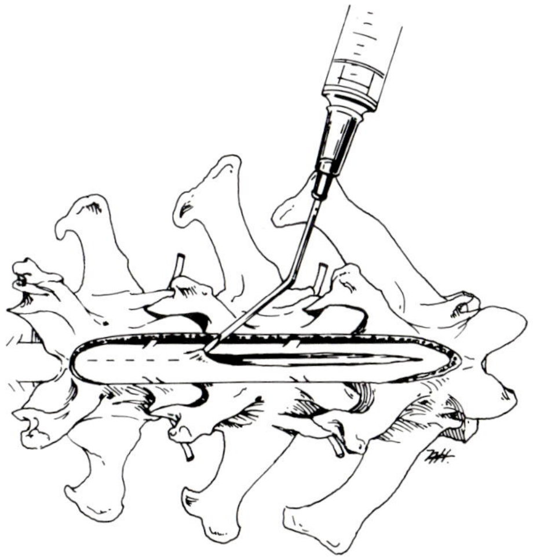

FIGURE 14–63 A durotomy can be performed using a dorsal or a hemilaminectomy approach for maximal cord decompression. In questionable cases of malacia, the durotomy is of prognostic value. The dural incision can easily be made with minimal cord trauma by bending a 23-gauge injection needle and using the cutting edge of the bevel for incising the dura.

Dorsolateral Fenestration and Hemilaminectomy

Hoerlein has suggested the dorsolateral approach to thoracolumbar disk lesions in order to fenestrate the disk, decompress the cord, and remove the compression.[82, 84-89] This surgical procedure involves fenestration and a hemilaminectomy. The dog is carefully prepared for extensive surgery in the usual manner, then placed in the ventral recumbent position with a sandbag of appropriate size, loosely filled, under the abdomen opposite the lesion. If a very large sandbag is used and considerable force is applied in the animal's position, compression of the vena cava and visceral veins will contribute to venous congestion of the venous sinuses and spinal cord. It sometimes helps the surgeon to have the animal's back rolled slightly away from him, thus rotating the lateral aspect of the spine more dorsally. The trachea is intubated and an intravenous infusion of an appropriate fluid is administered by means of a vascular indwelling catheter. The infusion also serves as a means by which to administer additional medication if needed.

The choice of anesthesia is important. Many paraplegics show signs of toxicity because of improper urine and fecal elimination. Nephritis frequently accompanies the disk syndrome, and laboratory tests for its presence should always be performed prior to surgery. Although pentobarbital sodium and oxygen were used for years, gaseous anesthesia has become and should be considered the standard method.[89, 121] In the critical patient especially, prudent monitoring of vital functions and rectal temperature during and after surgery is suggested. Postsurgical monitoring of kidney function by measuring the amount and rate of urine formation, as well as laboratory determination of nonprotein nitrogen and electrolyte imbalance, is recommended in nephritic patients. Blood gas and blood pH determinations and appropriate therapy are helpful in the critical patient when such laboratory service is available (see Chapter 8).

A dorsal midline or slightly paramedian skin incision, usually 9 to 11 cm long, is made, and the dorsolumbar fascia is incised just lateral to the spinous processes. Careful periosteal elevation is utilized to remove the musculature from the lateral surfaces of the spines to the articular processes. The muscle attachments to the articular processes are carefully severed, and the thin tendonous insertions of the muscle attachments to the accessory processes are identified and teased loose about 2 mm from the process. Care should be taken here not to injure the spinal vessels and nerves ventral to the accessory process. Blunt instrument and finger dissection is carried down to the lateral processes or the ribs of the vertebrae to be involved in the surgery. The causative disk should be in the most accessible portion of the surgical field. The author frequently performs the muscle-separating steps consecutively over the T13–L1 area for proper identification of landmarks (last rib and first lateral process). Gage suggests that the dissection of the field can be accomplished effectively in phases, e.g., the preparation of the spines, articular processes, accessory processes, and lateral process or rib on all the vertebrae to be involved in the surgery.[54]

Care is used in maintaining the spinal nerves and vessels emerging from the intervertebral foramina. The bone immediately surrounding the disk must be entirely free of flesh if proper curettage is to be done. The last rib is used as a landmark. The ventrodorsal radiograph should be properly marked (L or R) in case agenesis of a rib or an extra rib is found on either side.

It is optional whether the surgeon performs the decompression and removal of pressure mass or does the disk curettage first. The author prefers to locate the causative disk by hemilaminectomy and to decompress the cord before performing adjacent fenestrations. In this case, the surgeon can accomplish the fenestrations intermittently while the decompression is being carefully performed between saline tissue perfusions. This sequence may save operating time.

The disk that is actually pressing on the cord is explored with a hemilaminectomy. A rongeur or bone cutting forceps is used to remove the articular process over the disk, thus providing a flat surface for hand* or power† trephination or high speed drilling‡ *of the lateral lamina.* A laminectomy trephine or bur can be used to enter the dorsal lateral area of the canal. David has recently advocated a 12-mm skull trephine equipped with an automatic clutch and depth gauge and powered by an air-driven orthopedic drill.[31] The thin blade, claw-type tartar scraper is useful in removing bone dust and checking the depth of trephination. Frequent rocking of the trephine will determine the looseness of the plug so that it can be lifted out when it is ready. This procedure exposes the epidural fat or necrotic material of a recently ruptured disk. Trephination is a positive means of determining the site of the lesion, and does not create a serious bony defect in the lamina (Figs. 14–64 to 14–67).

Small rongeur forceps§ of varying sizes are efficient instruments for enlarging the trephine hole in order to facilitate exposure of the lesion and the dorsal aspect of the disk. Pressure is never exerted toward the cord, but always *away* from the cord (Fig. 14–68). In most small and "thin"-boned dogs, a small-nosed rongeur (Lampert) can be used to create the hemilaminectomy opening. This is especially useful when a high speed drill is not available. When the surgeon retracts the rostral dorsal spine forward and upward, the arches of the two vertebrae which have been pre-

---

*Hand trephines: Michele laminectomy trephine, available through various distributors; Micrometer trephine, California Surgical Design Corp., Gardena, California.

†Power trephine: Aesculap skull trephine, model DBP 105145, Aesculap-Werke AG, West Germany.

‡Power drills: Hall air drill, Hall International Inc., Santa Barbara, California; Stryker air drill, Zimmer Manufacturing Co., Warsaw, Indiana; Small air drill 511.10, Synthes Ltd., P.O. Box 529, Wayne, Pennsylvania.

§Rongeurs: Dean mastoid rongeur forceps, Reiner rongeurs, Lampert rongeurs, all available through various orthopedic instrument distributors.

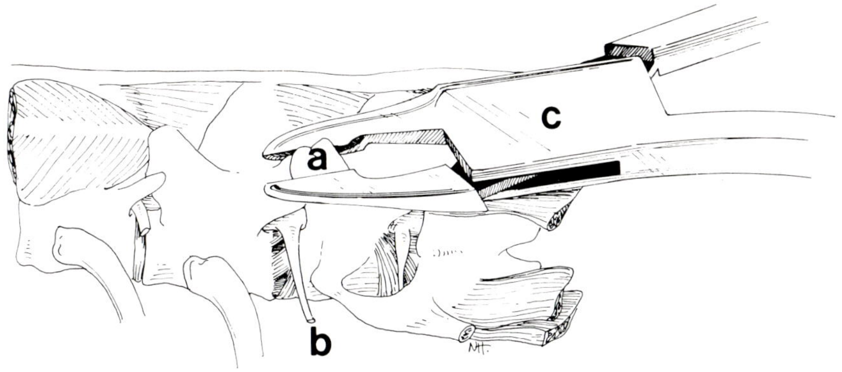

FIGURE 14–64 In the dorsolateral hemilaminectomy the articular process (a) is being removed to produce a flat surface for trephination or burring; (b) the intervertebral nerves and vessels; (c) rongeur.

FIGURE 14–65 A Michelle laminectomy trephine is used to expose the epidural space and spinal cord.

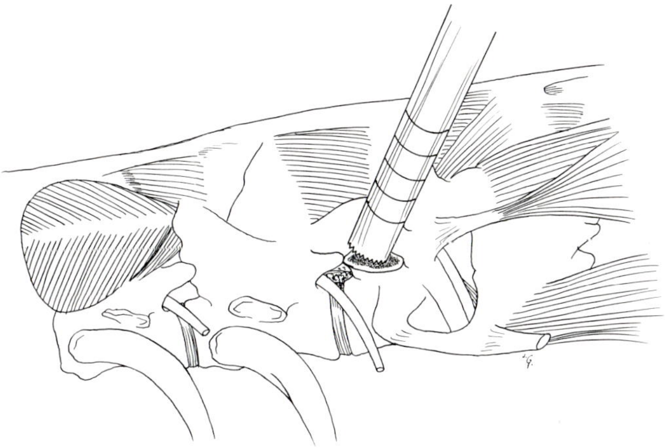

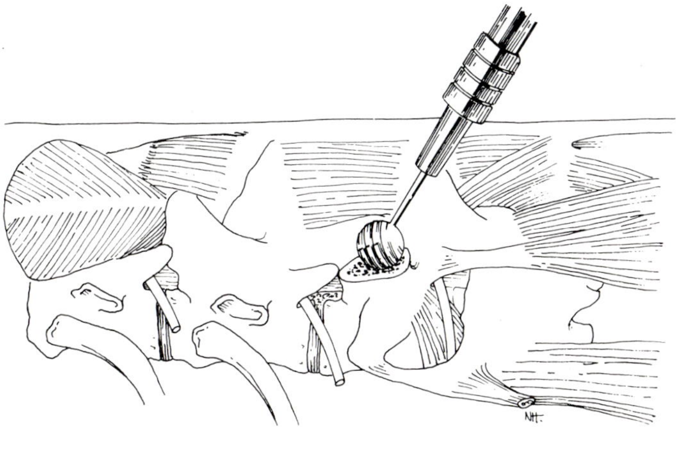

FIGURE 14–66 The air drill and spherical bur can be used instead of a trephine and rongeurs to create the bone defect. It is advisable to finish the decompression with the rongeurs in order to diminish the chance of cord trauma.

FIGURE 14–67 After a trephination, the epidural necrosis produced by a ruptured disk or the calcific protrusion mass is observed in the spinal canal.

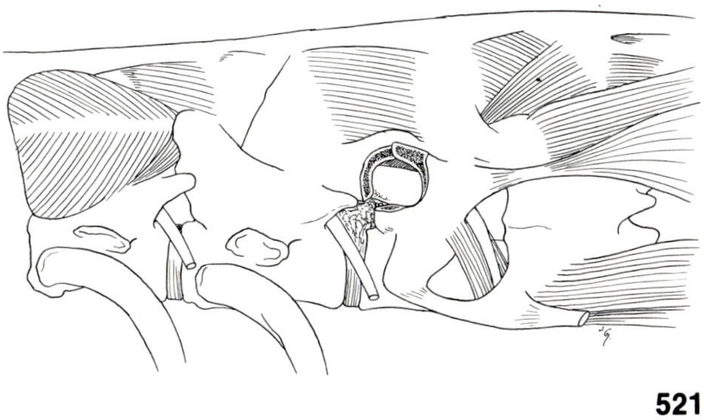

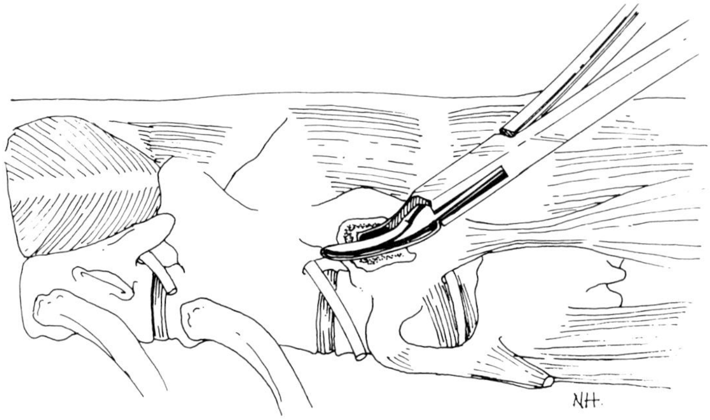

FIGURE 14–68 The trephine or bone defect created by high speed drilling is enlarged by use of a fine-nosed rongeur forceps (e.g., Lampert rongeur). The hemilaminectomy should extend well beyond the limits of the swollen cord for maximal decompression and removal of the protrusion mass.

pared separate sufficiently at the uppermost level of the articular facets so that a "toehold" can be obtained with the rongeur and the hemilaminectomy can be performed by using only the rongeurs (Fig. 14–69).[198]

The high speed surgical drill produces minimal heat. A variety of burs are available for removing the lamina. When the periosteal lining of the canal is exposed, it would be safer to complete the laminectomy with the rongeurs. The routine use of this instrument in spinal surgery requires that all soft tissue must be carefully removed from the area of lamina and pedicle, or the drill will be easily deflected. Therefore, the trephine and/or rongeurs may actually be faster in the smaller dog. The air drill is most effective, however, in large dogs who characteristically have heavy vertebral bones.

After the cord is exposed, the standard practice is frequent bathing of the tissues in the area with warm saline and subsequent aspiration. The protrusion and necrotic tissue are gently removed with the tartar scraper, tiny curette, or a similar instrument. The disk is then curetted from within the canal. The hook of the scraper is placed under the cord in a horizontal position, and the point is carefully rotated downward until it is directed into the annulus. The disk is removed in a downward and outward direction. At this point, considerable hemorrhage may occur from the venous sinus, which lies on the floor of the canal. Aspiration will speed the procedure from this point if the aspirator tip is placed carefully in the deeper recesses of the surgical area. Much damage to nerve tissue will occur if the sucker tip contacts the cord. Usually, pressure packing the area

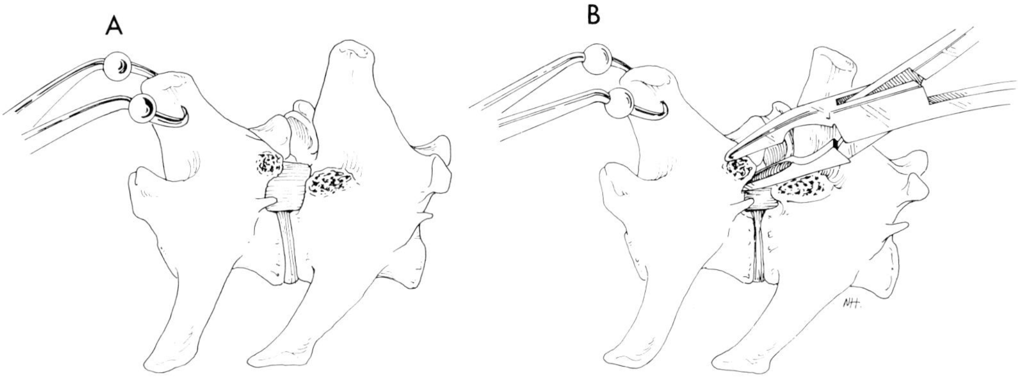

FIGURE 14–69 *A*. In small and "thin"-boned dogs, the articular facets can be opened far enough by traction on the rostral (or if necessary, the rostral and caudal) vertebra(e) to get a "toe hold" with a small rongeur (Lampert) to initiate a hemilaminectomy. *B*, The hemilaminectomy in progress. (From Swaim, S. F.: A rongeuring technique for performing thoracolumbar hemilaminectomies. Vet. Med. Small Animal. Clin. *71*, 172, 1976.)

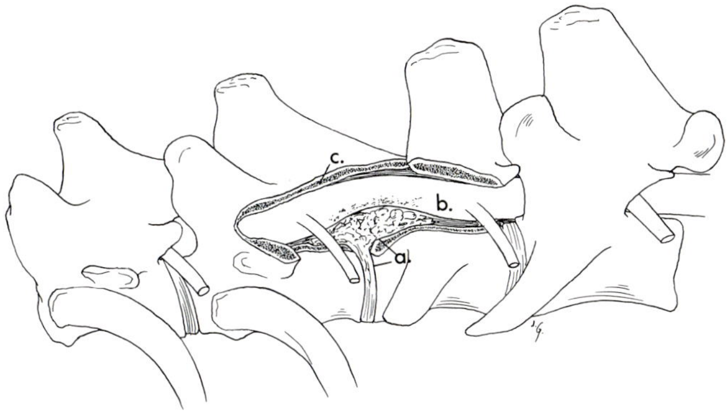

FIGURE 14–70 The hemilaminectomy has been completed. The compressive mass and its disk must now be removed to complete the decompression. (a) Disk and protrusion; (b) spinal cord; (c) edge of hemilaminectomy.

with surgical sponges will promote clotting, and absorbable gelatin pads are placed on the area before closure. Frequently, no blood from the sinus will be seen, since the sinus is thrombotic (Figs. 14–70 to 14–76).

In dorsal laminectomies, Funkquist was concerned with secondary cicatrix or fibrosis causing cord compression over the bony defect. However, since the cord is well below the cortical laminal level in a hemilaminectomy, secondary cicatricial cord compression has been no problem in this technique. Nevertheless, this phenomenon should be considered in extensive dorsal or dorsolateral decompressions that are sometimes necessary in neoplasia or fractures.[42, 46, 50, 51, 89, 90] In Figure 14–77, one can see that a decompression opening made by a hemilaminectomy is comparable to that made by a dorsal laminectomy.

After or during the hemilaminectomy procedure, the disk fenestrations or curettages are performed. The spinal vessels and nerves should be identified and retracted cranially when one is fenestrating a disk. A small-gauge spinal needle is used to locate the disk, which in the lumbar area is just cranial to the junction of the lateral process to the body of the vertebra; in the thoracic area, the disk is situated slightly more cranial to the junction of the rib with the vertebral body, usually about 1 to 2 mm. In this area, one should direct the instrument transversely, not downward, or the aorta may be encountered.

After the disk has been located, a 12- to 14-gauge intravenous needle (2 to $2^1/_2$ inches long) can be used to curette it, the needle being directed transversely into the disk over to the opposite annulus. By this "boring" action, several plugs of nuclear material are removed, and the disk material is scraped out with the bevel of the needle in a down and outward motion. A needle with a slight bend facilitates scraping toward the dorsal longitudinal ligament; a thin blade, claw-type tartar scraper, a very small bone curette, or a dental probe is helpful in this curettage.

When the affected disk is in the area of

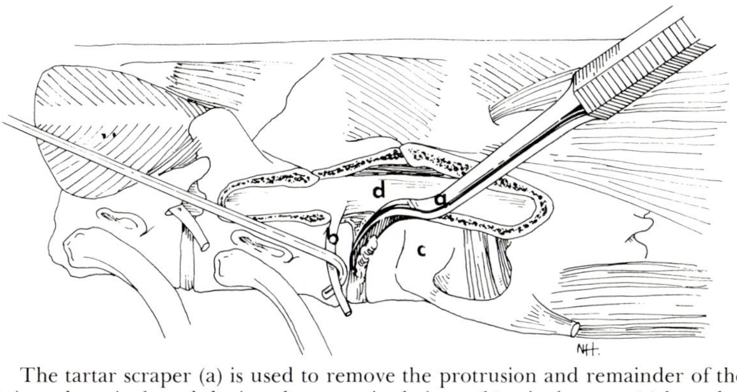

FIGURE 14–71 The tartar scraper (a) is used to remove the protrusion and remainder of the disk, care being employed not to injure the spinal cord during these manipulations; (b) spinal nerve; (c) lateral process; (d) spinal cord.

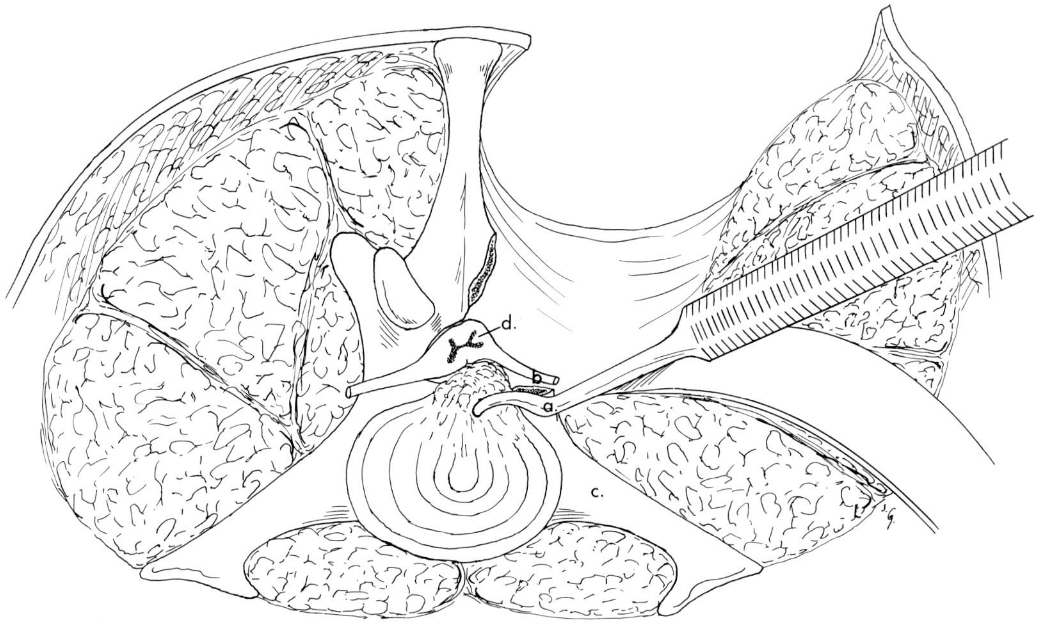

FIGURE 14–72 Cross section of a decompression through the hemilaminectomy. (a) Claw-type tartar scraper; (b) spinal nerve; (c) lateral process; (d) spinal cord.

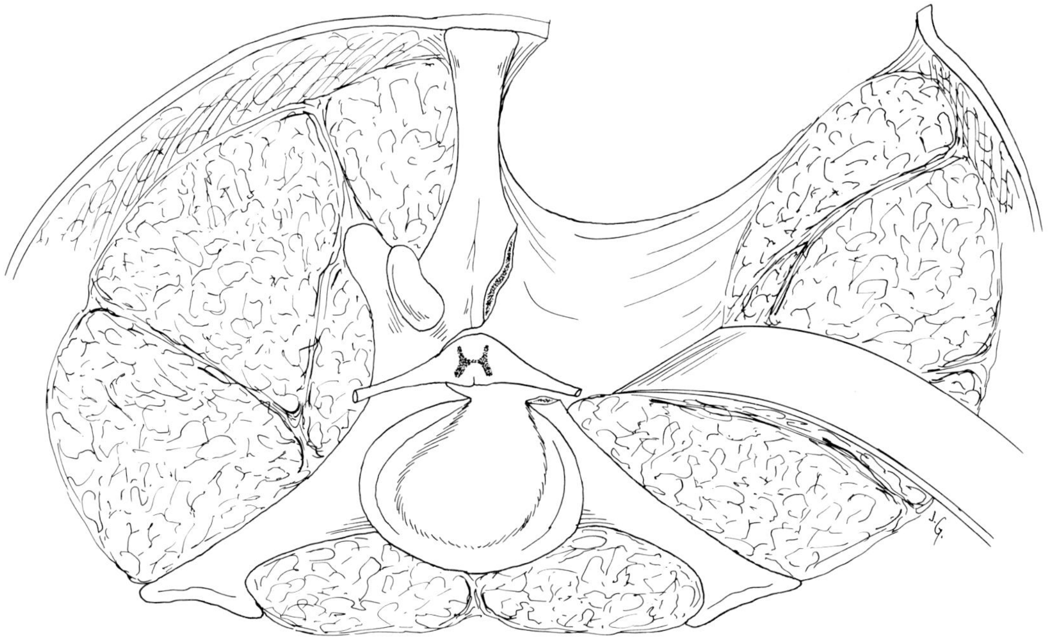

FIGURE 14–73 Sagittal view of completed hemilaminectomy, decompression, and disk curettage.

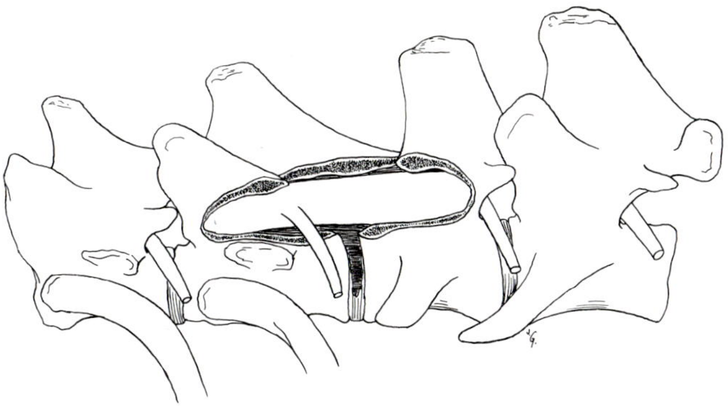

FIGURE 14–74 Lateral view of completed hemilaminectomy and disk fenestration. In the thoracolumbar region, T11–12 through L2–3 are fenestrated to avoid future disk protrusions in this region of high protrusion incidence.

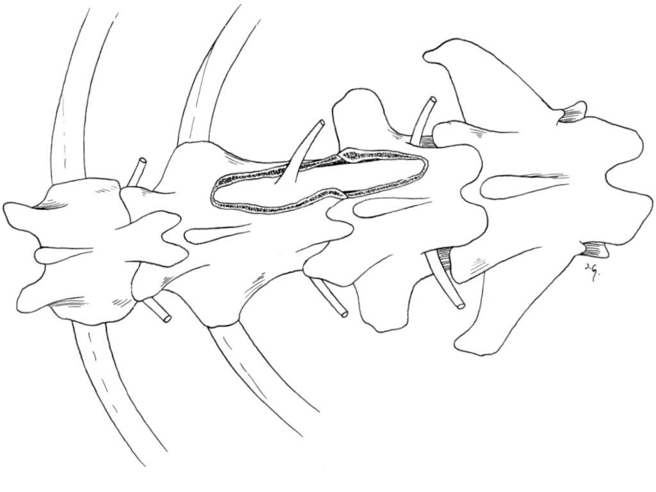

FIGURE 14–75 A dorsoventral view of a completed hemilaminectomy. Since the cord lies considerably medial to the edge of the hemilaminectomy, cicatricial contracture of cord tissue does not exist.

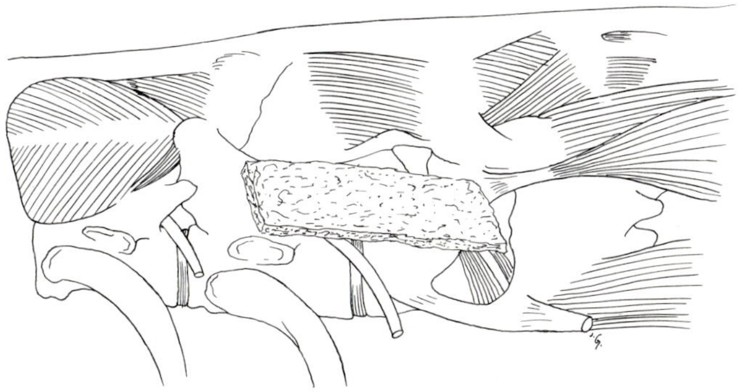

FIGURE 14–76 Absorbable gelatin sponge material is placed over the bone defect to promote local hemostasis.

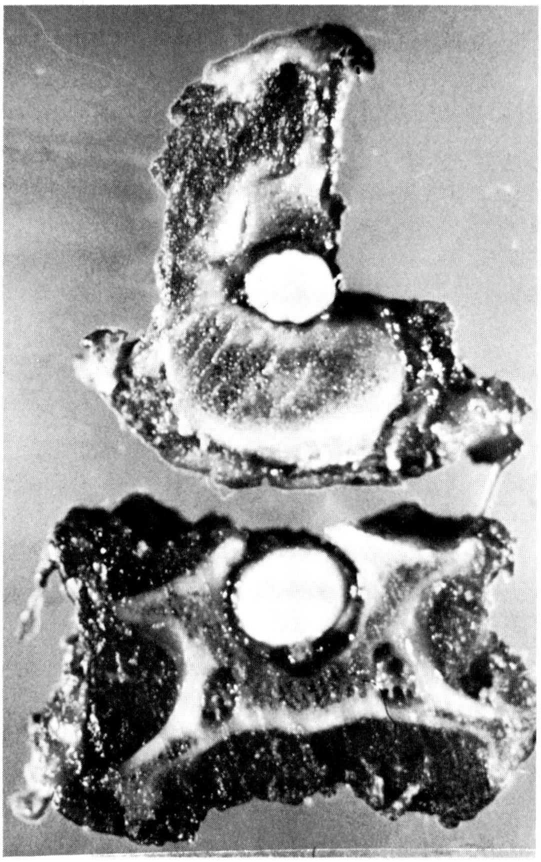

FIGURE 14–77 Cross section views of vertebrae on which a hemilaminectomy and a dorsal laminectomy had been performed. Their decompressive capabilities are comparatively equal. (From Hoerlein, B. F.: Various surgical methods for repair of intervertebral disc protrusions. Anim. Hosp. *4*, 12, 1968.)

the thoracolumbar junction, i.e., T12–13 or T13–L1, the adjacent disks frequently show radiographic evidence of degeneration, particularly in the dachshund and other susceptible breeds. It has also been shown that this is the area most frequently affected in disk paraplegia. Therefore, it has been standard practice in our clinic to fenestrate three to five (or even six) disks to prevent future lesions. Routinely, we curette T11–12 through L3–4 if the causative disk included one of these. We have rarely seen a protrusion recur when such a disk has been properly curetted (Fig. 14–78).

The curettage or fenstration procedure not only removes a large portion of the disk physically but, with its accompanying inflammatory tissue response, transforms the progressive degeneration into a stabilized fibrosis of disk tissue. Subsequent radiography reveals normal radiotranslucent tissue in the disk space.

Since little or no nucleus remains, the disk is then less susceptible to protrusion. One frequently sees slight localized spurs or lips of exostosis on the ventral borders of the vertebral bodies subsequent to disk curettage, but this has not been important clinically.

With closure, the area must be made completely hemostatic. Pressure packing the operative site with surgical sponges accomplishes this nicely in a few moments, after any arteries or arterioles have been ligated. A section of gelatin sponge (Gelfoam) is placed on the bone defect in the lateral lamina prior to closure (Figs. 14–79 and 14–80).

Although some of the first clinical trials of absorbable gelatin sponge material in veterinary medicine were performed in this clinic, its value for covering a laminectomy defect was not fully appreciated until a recent paper by La Rocca was published. La Rocca[109] performed a standard lumbar laminectomy at multiple levels in 30 dogs. The canal was scarified, packed with absorbable gelatin sponge (Gelfoam), or treated with three varieties of dimethyl siloxane

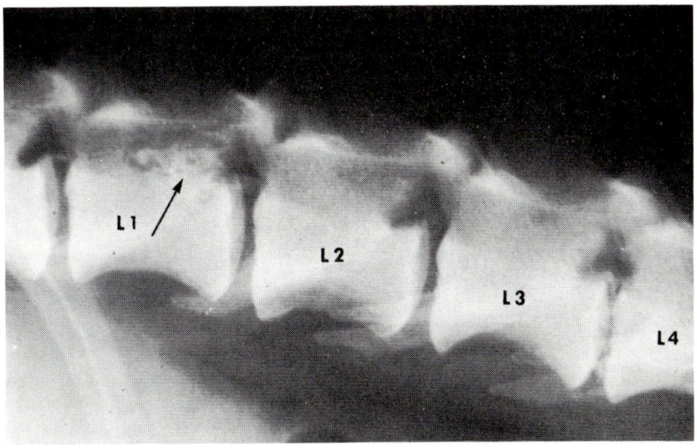

FIGURE 14–78 It is good practice to fenestrate all disks in the high incidence area when performing disk surgery. In this radiograph, a massive organized epidural mass has finally caused severe clinical signs. A hemilaminectomy was performed to decompress the cord and remove the mass (arrow), while disk fenestrations were performed on vertebrae from T11–12 through L3–4. Notice the calcified dorsal annulus at T13–L1 and L1–2 and the calcific narrow disk (some protrusion noted) at L3–4.

polymer sheeting (Silastic). The results were evaluated in 3 days to 12 weeks by a variety of observations and tests. It was seen that the scar, the laminectomy membrane, originates from the fibrous tissue elements of the dorsal erector spinal muscle mass. The scar covered the laminectomy defect and extended bilaterally to adhere to the dura and nerve roots. The gelatin sponge acted as an effective interposing membrane and did not contribute to the scar formation. The Silastic sheeting acted similarly. The advantage of gelatin is that it is completely resorbed by the fifth week. The author made the following general suggestions based on his observations:

1. The laminectomy should be only large enough to decompress the involved cord.
2. A dry field should be obtained and maintained.
3. At the conclusion of the decompression, the exposed nerve roots and the dura should be protected from the dorsal musculature by a barrier of impervious material.[109]

This clinic has persisted in the use of absorbable gelatin sponge material for nearly 30 years largely because of its hemostatic qualities. In that time there has been no clinical evidence of postoperative compressive dural adhesions.

The dorsolumbar fascia is sutured securely with the material of choice in a simple interrupted pattern. Subcutaneous tissues are approximated where necessary. Interrupted 3–0 braided or monofilament stainless steel wire is used routinely in the skin. Since the incision may be long, approximation will be improved if one or two perpendicular epidermal incisions have been made prior to the longitudinal skin incision. These points can be easily approximated and no gapping will occur in the incision.

A snug dovetail bandage is placed around the body. This keeps the incision clean, provides support, and helps prevent subcutaneous blood from accumulating into a hematoma or seroma. Hematomas and seromas are sequelae of spinal surgery, and every precaution must be taken to prevent their development.

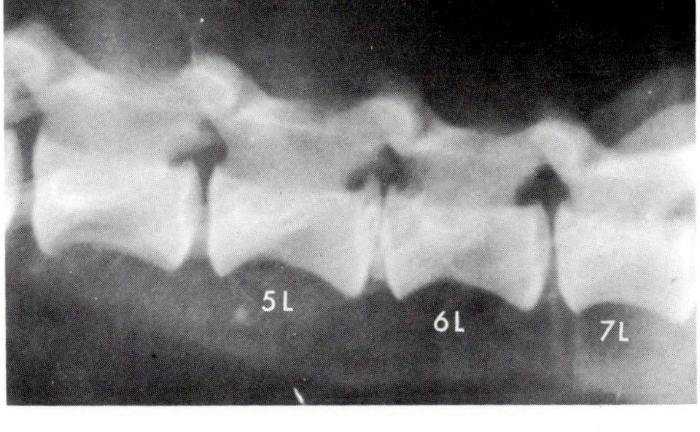

FIGURE 14–79 A calcific disk protrusion at L5–6 caused periodic pain and paraplegia.

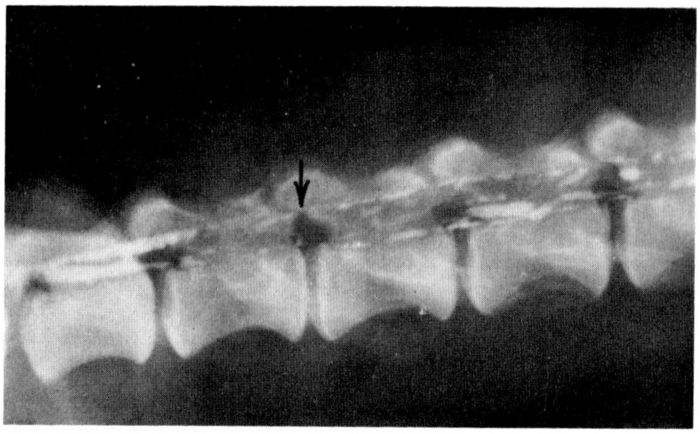

FIGURE 14–80 Same case as that shown in Figure 14–79. A hemilaminectomy was performed after a Pantopaque myelogram confirmed the compression at L5–6. The myelogram was performed as a teaching demonstration and was not indicated clinically. This film was taken 6 months after surgery. Notice that there are still sizeable amounts of contrast medium left in the subarachnoid space. Traces were still visible 1 year after surgery. No clinical meningeal signs were noted, but oil contrast media characteristically produce microscopic fibrotic leptomeningitis.

The bandage is removed on the third day, and flexible collodion may be placed on the incision. Hot water therapy is initiated at this point. The sutures are removed in 14 days, and the incision and operative site are usually cosmetically acceptable.

Swaim has recently explored the effectiveness of a bilateral hemilaminectomy for maximal decompression of the spinal cord. The procedure is basically the same as that used in the hemilaminectomy except that both lateral laminae are involved. The technique was found to be effective when no more than two vertebral lengths were involved and the adjacent articular processes remained intact. If longer decompressions are necessary, application of dorsal spinal plates is necessary, and frequently they are unsatisfactory. Indications for the two-vertebral length bilateral hemilaminectomy, which affords greater decompression than a single hemilaminectomy or a dorsal laminectomy, are (1) massive intervertebral disk protrusions, (2) spinal tumors or cysts, (3) fractures or luxations. This technique also provides dorsal cord protection and a better cosmetic appearance, the lack of which are deficiencies of dorsal laminectomies (Fig. 14–81).[197, 199]

Other Modified Thoracolumbar Approaches

During the last 10 years there have been modifications of the ventral and dorsal thoracolumbar disk fenestration approaches. Seemann[184] in 1968 proposed a hemilaminectomy of the causative disk by the approach described and adjacent disk fenestrations from a lateral muscle-separating approach. This involves retracting the longissimus dorsi muscle dorsomedially.[184] Flo has proposed making multiple disk fenestrations the sole objective of the surgery and has described the lateral approach in more detail.[40]

Flo places the dog in the right lateral recumbent position and makes a paramedial skin incision below the palpable level of the lateral processes of the lumbar spine and extending from T7 to L5. The subcutaneous tissue and fat are separated, and a curved Kelly forceps is forced through the

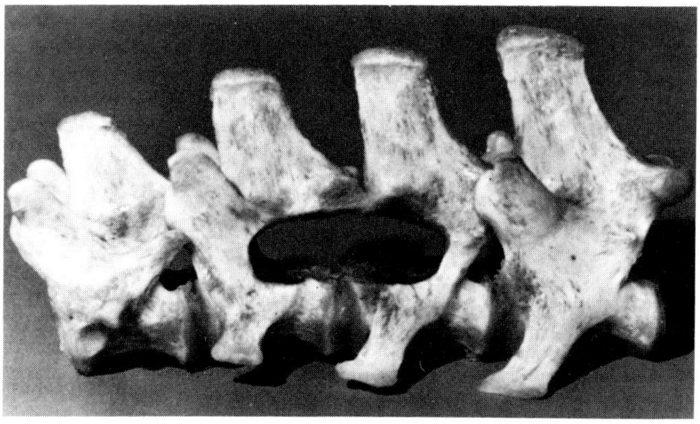

FIGURE 14–81 Bilateral hemilaminectomy. Note that the lateral lamina has been removed from both sides of the vertebral arch, leaving the dorsal lamina intact. No dorsal fixation is necessary unless more than one articular process is removed on each side. (From Swaim, S. F.: Bilateral hemilaminectomy: A technique for extensive spinal decompression. Auburn Vet. *32,* 67, 1976.)

slanting fibers of the iliocostalis lumborum muscle just dorsal to the lateral process. The musculature is bluntly separated by using the index finger and is then retracted toward the midline by a blunt retractor. A rectangular window is cut in each disk from the 2 to 4 o'clock position, and the nucleus is removed by an alligator or probe instrument. The thoracic disks are exposed similarly, but the levator costal muscle is detached from the anterior surface of the rib neck and is retracted ventrally. After all disks from T10 through L4 have been fenestrated, a chiropractic bending maneuver is used to loosen up and expose more disk nucleus. After recurettage of all disks, the wound is sutured routinely (Fig. 14–82).[40]

A dorsolateral muscle-separating approach for thoracolumbar disk fenestration has been described by Yturraspe.[218] The dog is positioned in a ventral recumbent position and a dorsal midline incision is made from T9 to S1. The skin, subcutaneous tissues, and fascia on one side of the incision are reflected laterally for a distance of 2 to 4 cm. The deep external fascia of the trunk and the aponeurosis of the longissimus lumborum muscle is incised 5 to 10 mm lateral and parallel to the dorsal midline. The lateral aspects of the intervertebral disks are exposed by separating the multifidus muscles medially and the longissimus thoracis et lumborum muscle laterally. The disks are exposed and incised with a scalpel, and the nucleus is removed with a tartar scraper. The fenestrations can be combined with a decompression if desired by using the approach already described for a dorsal or hemilaminectomy. The tissues are sutured in layers routinely after this type of disk fenestration.[218]

A ventrolateral approach to the T13–L1 to L6–7 disks has been developed by Northway[138] from work done on 11 normal dogs. The skin incision is made ½ to ¼ inch (½ to 1 cm) ventral and parallel to the transverse processes. The external abdominal oblique and transverse abdominal muscles are separated from the dorsal lumbar fascia, the lumbar nerves are severed, and the sublumbar muscles, ventral portions of the vertebral bodies, and disks are exposed. To reach the T13–L1 and L1–2 disks, part of the latissimus dorsi is severed and the diaphragm is dissected free. To reach the L6–7 disk, the sartorius, part of the tensor fascia lata, and the external abdominal muscles are severed. The disk is removed as in other ventral procedures.[113, 144, 145] During the 3 months of aftercare, no complications were noted and normal sensory and motor sensations were observed in the flank, abdomen, and genitals.[138]

Braund[13] has recently reported upon a muscle-separating approach similar to

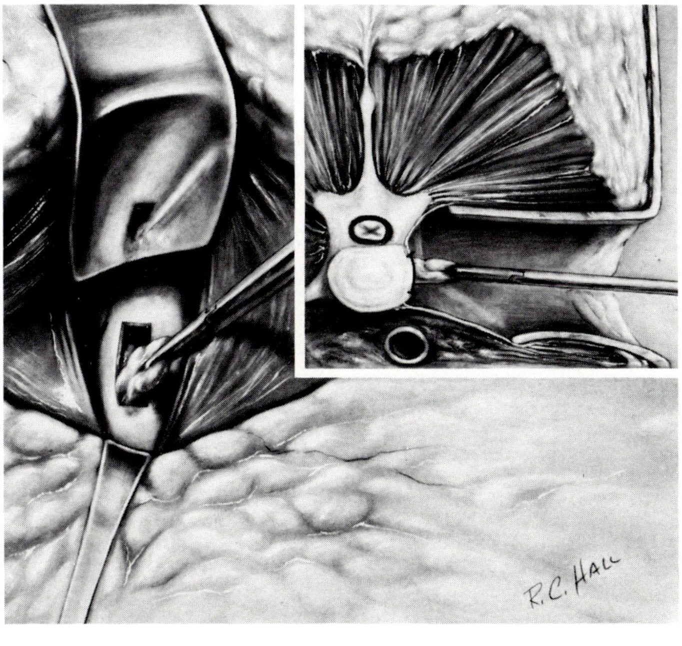

FIGURE 14–82 The muscle separation approach. The muscles are reflected as shown, and a rectangular window has been cut in the lateral annulus by a scalpel and is being removed by an alligator forceps. The nucleus is removed with a blunt probe. (From Flo, G. L., and Brinker, W. O.: Lateral fenestration of thoracolumbar discs. J. Am. Anim. Hosp. Assoc. *11*, 619, 1975.)

those previously described from which a lateral (hemilaminectomy) decompression and a concomitant prophylactic disk fenestration are performed. A skin incision is made 5 cm from the midline which can be extended if necessary from T9–10 through L5–6 vertebral levels. The incision is extended through the subcutaneous, deep lumbodorsal fascia and the subfascial adipose layers to expose the laterally lying iliocostalis muscle. The tips of the lumbar transverse processes are readily palpable and are exposed by blunt dissection. The thin fibrous periosteum on the dorsal surfaces of the transverse processes is elevated to the junction of the vertebral body. In cases of lumbar disk protrusion, the iliocostalis and medially lying longissimus muscles between the exposed transverse processes are separated from the intertransverse ligament and retracted dorsally, completely exposing the transverse processes and lateral aspect of the vertebral bodies adjacent to the involved disk. The periosteum is elevated to the dorsal border of the diarthrodial vertebral articulations, and the exposed muscle mass is retracted dorsally to expose the intervertebral foramen, segmented nerve, and vessels. After incising the membrane covering the intervertebral foramen, a fine-tipped ronguer or high speed drill is used to remove the lateral lamina from the adjacent vertebral segments, ventrally to the floor of the canal and dorsally to the diarthrodial joint.

If there is a caudal thoracic disk, the iliocostalis muscular system joining the ribs is exposed by extending the incision of the

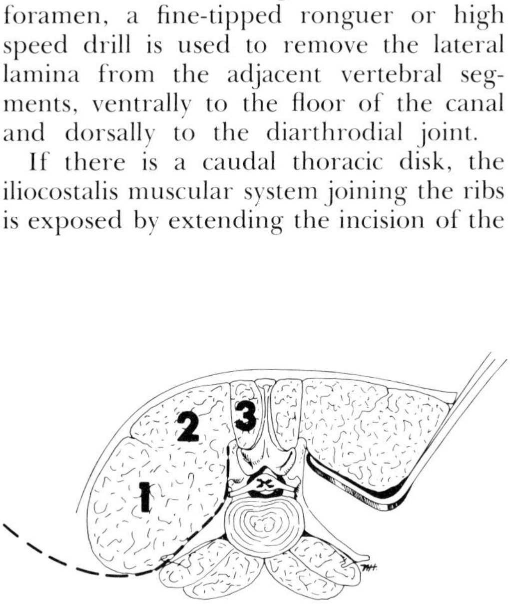

FIGURE 14–83 Lateral hemilaminectomy. The route of the proposed periosteal elevation and the dorsal retraction of the epaxial muscles (1, 2, 3) is shown on the left, and excised pedicular bone is shown on the right. (From Braund, K. G., Taylor, T. K., Ghosh, P., and Sherwood, A. A.: Lateral spinal decompression in the dog. J. Small Anim. Pract. *17*, 583, 1976.)

deep lumbodorsal fascia cephalad. After appropriate decompression of the offending disk, fenestration of this and adjacent disks can be accomplished in the highly susceptible area by using the lateral approach described by Flo. Decompression in larger areas can be performed by more extensive dissection and durotomy, and cord irrigations can be performed as in other decompressive procedures.[13] In addition to its muscle-separating advantage, Braund's procedure approaches the cord from a lateral ventral aspect instead of from the dorsal lateral aspect as in the standard hemilaminectomy, and this may have some advantages in removing the extruded compressive mass (Fig. 14–83).

CERVICAL DISK SURGERY

Ventral Fenestration

The usual disk surgery in the neck is ventral fenestration. Olsson reported this method in 1951,[144] and Hoerlein reported it in 1952.[84, 89] Fenestration is usually adequate, since pain is generally the predominant clinical sign; however, if a large protrusion mass is present in the canal causing prominent motor deficits, a decompression may be necessary. This is discussed in a later section.

The ventral fenestration[84, 144] is performed in the ventral midline with the dog in the dorsal recumbent position. Regardless of whether gas or intravenous anesthesia is used, an endotracheal tube is employed, and oxygen ventilation is given, since much tracheal manipulation is necessary. Since positioning is important for effective surgery, a loosely filled positioning bag is placed under the animal's neck, and the head is secured firmly to the table top. The front legs are restrained in a caudal position so as to leave the operative area entirely accessible. This position allows the neck vertebrae to be more easily explored (Fig. 14–84).

The incision is made in the ventral midline and is usually about 12 to 15 cm in length. The superficial muscle fibers are bluntly separated. The trachea, esophagus, vagus nerves, and carotid arteries are retracted laterally by means of a Frazier laminectomy retractor. It will be noticed that

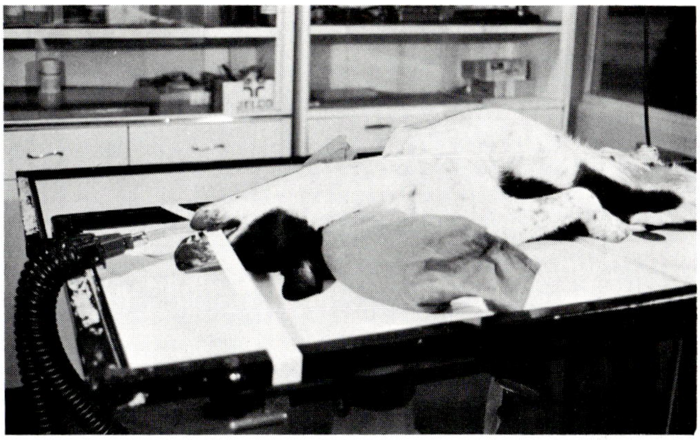

FIGURE 14–84 The proper positioning for ventral disk fenestration or curettage.

the ventral vertebral muscle fibers join the midline in a diagonal manner. The muscle fibers are then bluntly separated from the disk, which is located immediately behind the prominent ventral spinous process on the cranially situated vertebra. This process can be easily palpated.

The cranial landmark for cervical fenestrations is the wing of the atlas. If one follows the posterior border of the wing of the atlas to the midline, a very sharp ventral prominence is felt; this is counted as C1–2 interspace, and each successive caudal process is palpated and enumerated. The landmarks for more caudally located cervical disks are the expanded plate-like caudal portions of the transverse processes of the C6 vertebra. These plates extend prominently downward and outward from the vertebra. If there is any doubt, a radiograph can be taken during the surgical procedure to verify the position. Care must be taken not to mistake the transverse processes for the midline process, because such an error will lead to confusion and may cause excessive hemorrhage.

After the involved disk is located and exposed, a small-gauge needle is inserted into it in order to determine its direction and dorsoventral diameter. When the ventral surface of the dura is struck by the needle, a muscular flinch is generally seen. The usual distance is slightly greater than 1 cm, and the direction is downward and slightly forward from the surgical site. The ventral annulus is incised liberally with a scalpel, and the thin blade, claw tartar scraper as well as the conventional claw tartar scraper is used to tear out the disk. The entire disk should be "scooped out" as far dorsally as necessary to remove the protrusion (Figs. 14–85 to 14–88).

Since C2–3 and C3–4 are the cervical disks most frequently involved in protrusions, routine fenestrations should involve these two disks. In other words, it is felt that if C2–3 is protruding, fenestrating C2–3 through C5–6 is not necessary or especially desirable. Much loss of vertebral support could result. We would fenestrate C2–3 and C3–4 if no other disks showed degeneration. If others showed degeneration, we would perform curettage on those involved.

Little or no hemorrhage results from this approach. The vessels, trachea, and esophagus resume their customary positions when the retractor is removed. The superficial musculature is sutured with small interrupted sutures, and the subcutaneous fascia is handled in the same manner. The skin is closed routinely, and a loose bandage encircling the neck is applied. No special aftercare is needed in this type of cervical lesion.

Ventral Decompressive Surgery for Cervical Disks

In cases of motor deficits with cervical disk protrusions, the ventral fenestration procedure affords either little improvement or very slow improvement over a period of several weeks. Dorsal laminectomies have become the prescribed method of decompression for these cases; however, postoperative care is generally critical for 2 to 4 days, after which the dog shows good results. The ventral decompression proce-

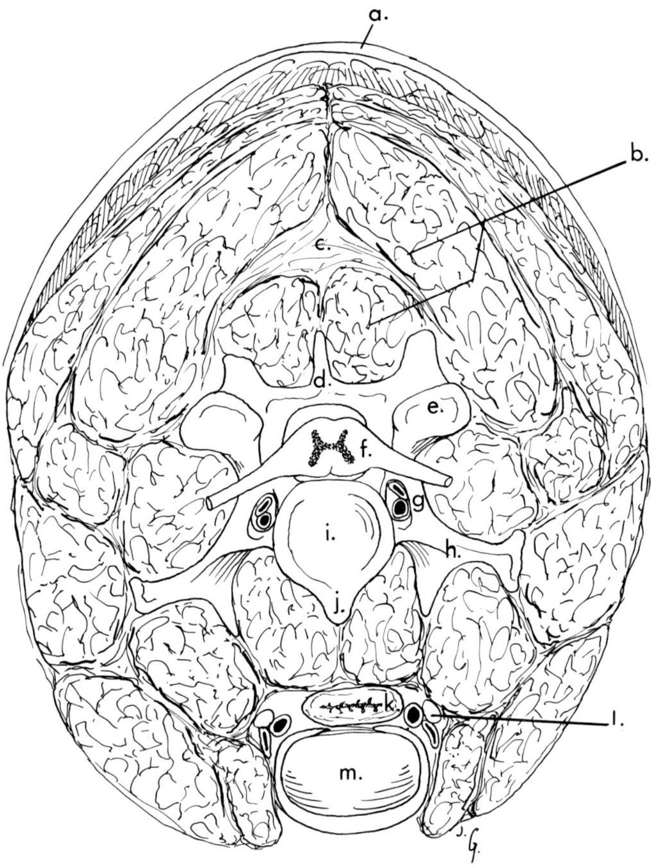

FIGURE 14–85 Cross section of the neck at about C2 or C3 level. (a) Skin; (b) dorsal cervical musculature; (c) ligamentum nuchae; (d) dorsal spine; (e) articular surface; (f) spinal cord; (g) vertebral artery and vein; (h) lateral process; (i) body of vertebra; (j) ventral protuberance; (k) esophagus; (l) carotid artery and vagosympathetic nerves; (m) trachea.

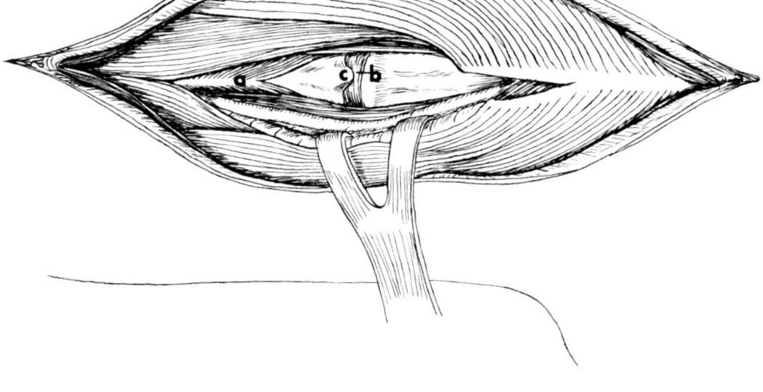

FIGURE 14–86 The fibers of the deep subvertebral musculature join in the midline (a) which should be identified so as to locate the midline vertebral prominences. The disk (b) is located immediately caudal to the prominent ventral protuberance (c) after blunt dissection is employed to remove muscle tissue.

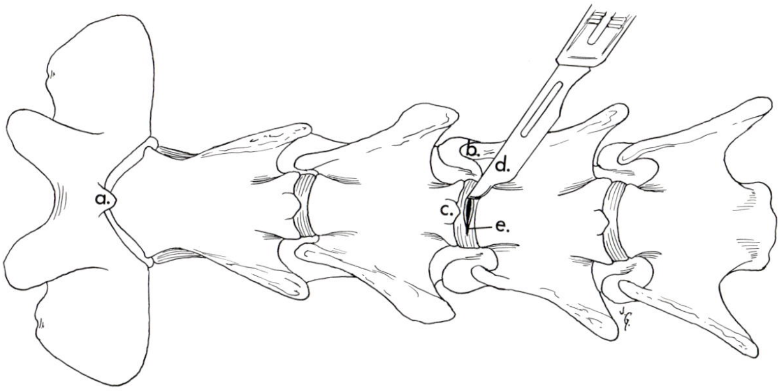

FIGURE 14–87 The ventral annulus is incised with a scalpel to facilitate curettage. The lesion site as seen on the radiograph can be located for surgery by counting caudally from the sharp C1–2 midline ventral prominence (a) or by counting cranially from the distinctly peculiar shape of the expanded plate-like caudal portions of the transverse processes of C6. (b) Lateral prominences; (c) ventral midline protuberance just cranial to the disk; (d) scalpel; (e) ventral annulus.

dure offers a direct approach in removing the protrusion mass and has a less traumatic effect on the patient.

Popvich described a ventral trephination over the disk space and adjacent vertebral bodies. After the entire disk was removed, a cylindrical bone graft was placed in the trephination hole to promote subsequent fusion. This technique was performed on clinically normal dogs and was not tried in animals with clinical disk disease (Fig. 14–89).[160]

Swaim[195, 196] developed a ventral midline spondylectomy and diskectomy without a bone graft for clinical disk disease. The dog is placed in the dorsal recumbent position, and the approach is the same as that described for ventral cervical fenestrations. The ventral spinous process is removed with a rongeur, and an oblong bur on a pneumatic drill is used to cut a slot in the adjacent ventral vertebrae across the disk space. The slot occupies about one-half of the width of each vertebra and extends longitudinally about one-third of the length of each vertebra. The point of a tartar scraper or a small bone curette is used to remove the disk mass from under the spinal cord through the bony slot. No graft is placed in the hole, and in 80 per cent of cases the defect fills up with osseous tissue in a few months (Figs. 14–90 and 14–91). An alternate technique which does not require a pneumatic drill makes use of a micrometer trephine set at a prerecorded depth determined from measuring the dorsoventral diameter of the vertebra from a radiograph. A trephine hole is made cranial and caudal to the disk, and a rongeur is used to remove the disk and intervening

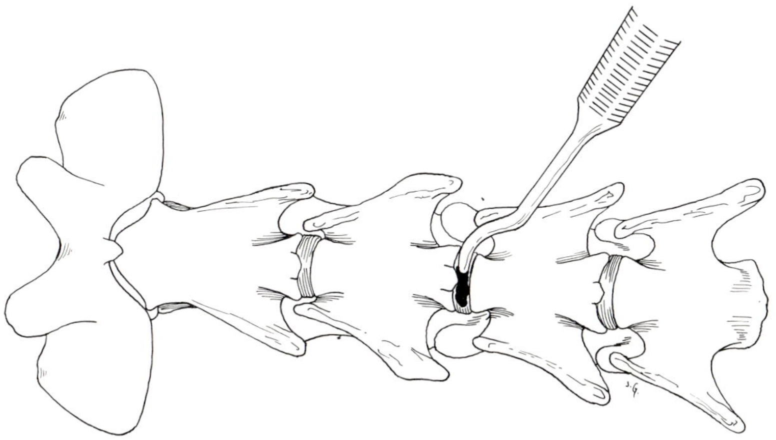

FIGURE 14–88 Curetting the disk with the claw-type tartar scraper.

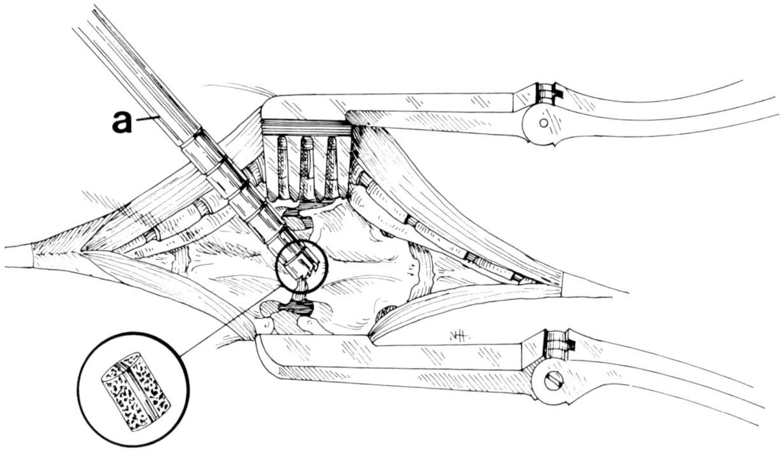

FIGURE 14–89 The approach used in the various ventral decompressive surgeries for cervical disk protrusions is essentially the same as that used for fenestration. A laminectomy trephine is used to expose the disk protrusion and spinal cord. After the protrusion is removed, some surgeons place a slightly oversized "dowel" bone graft in the trephination hole to aid in stabilization of the area. (From Popovic, N. A., Vander Ark, G., and Kempe, L.: Ventral approach for surgical treatment of cervical disk disease in the dog. Am. J. Vet. Res. *32*, 1155, 1971.)

bone down to the spinal canal and protrusion mass (Figs. 14–92 and 14–93). A laminectomy trephine (5/6 inch diameter) has also been used over the disk space, as described by Popovich.[160] Clinical results of the slot technique have been uniformly good, and the only concern is an occasional hemorrhage from laceration of a venous sinus or one of the anastomosing branches during manipulation of the tartar scraper while removing the protrusion mass. The hemorrhage can be terminated by packing the slot with a surgical sponge, relieving any pressure on the jugular veins, and raising the head a few minutes.[195, 196]

Prata and Stoll[161] employ ventral decompression similar to that of Swaim but place an iliac bone graft in the slot. The slot defect seems wider and shorter than the one described by Swaim. It is not more than three-fourths the width of the vertebral bodies and one-fourth the length of

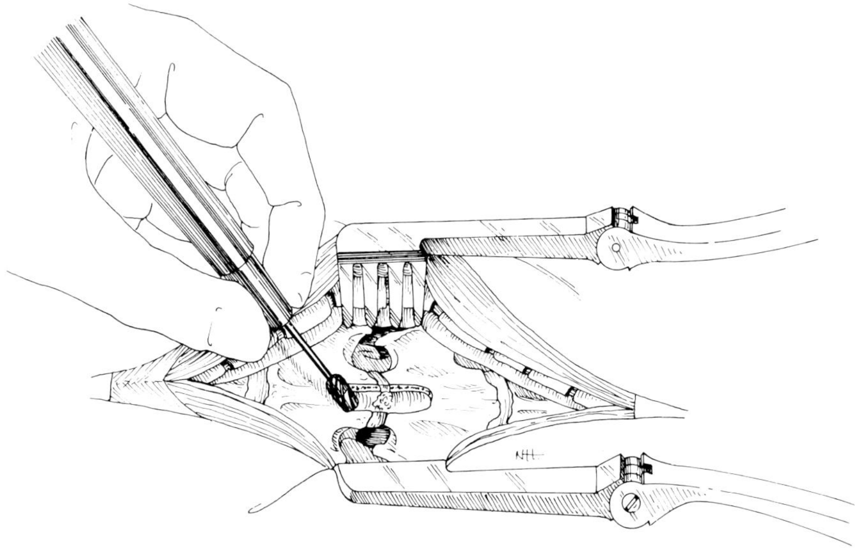

FIGURE 14–90 A more spacious ventral cervical decompression can be made by creating a slot by high-speed burring (one-half the width and one-third the length) in each vertebra bordering the disks. (Courtesy of Swaim, S. F.: Ventral decompression of the cervical spinal cord in the dog. J.A.V.M.A. *164*, 491, 1974.)

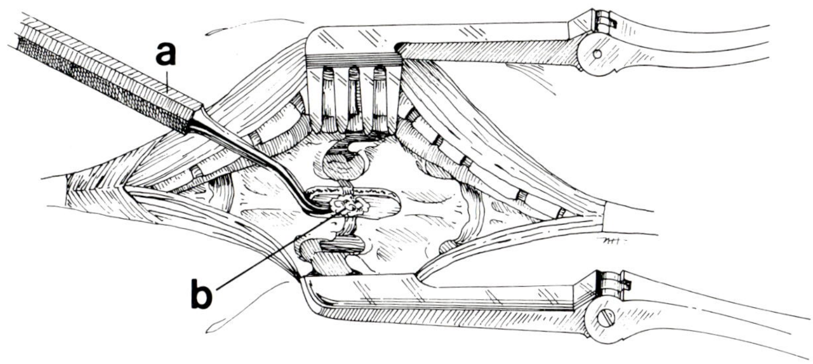

FIGURE 14–91 The protrusion mass (b) is removed by a small tartar scraper (a) or a small bone curette. No bone graft is necessary for stabilization. (From Swaim, S. F.: Ventral decompression of the cervical spinal cord in the dog. J.A.V.M.A. *164,* 491, 1974.)

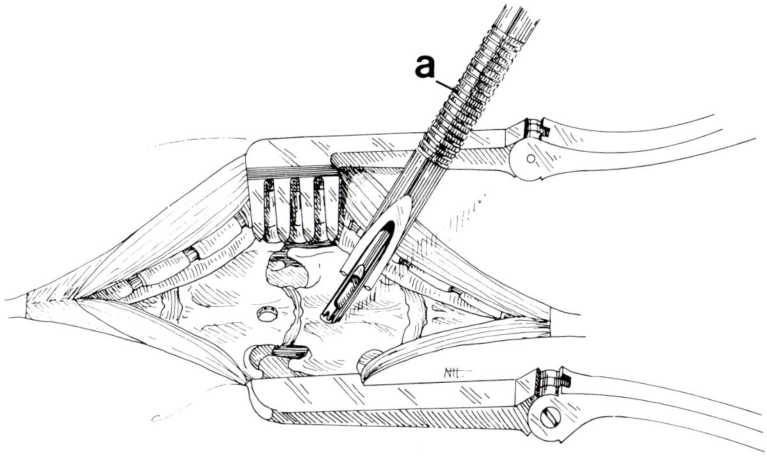

FIGURE 14–92 A micrometer trephine (a) with a preset depth guard can be used to create a slot-type ventral decompression if high-speed drill equipment is not available. Holes are drilled a small distance cranial and caudal to the disk. Caution must be used to avoid the cord. (From Swaim, S. F.: Ventral decompression of the cervical spinal cord in the dog. J.A.V.M.A. *164,* 491, 1974.)

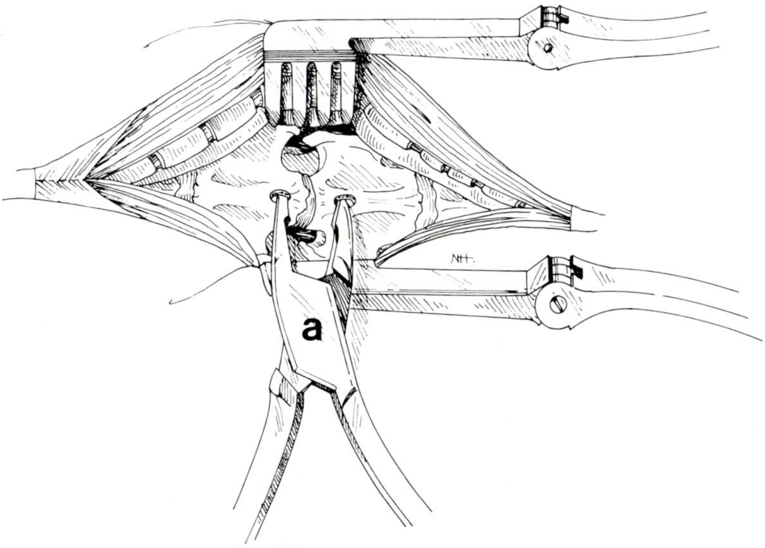

FIGURE 14–93 A rongeur (a) is used to remove the bone between the drill holes down to the protrusion mass and the canal. (From Swaim, S. F.: Ventral decompression of the cervical spinal cord in the dog. J.A.V.M.A. *164,* 491, 1974.)

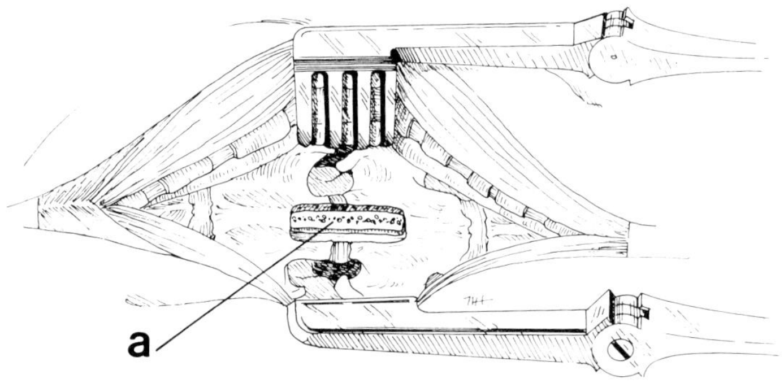

FIGURE 14–94 A bone graft (a) can be taken from the ilium or rib; the vertebrae are pulled apart, and the graft is placed into the bony defect to add stabilization if needed. (After Prata, R. G., and Stoll, S. G.: Ventral decompression and fusion for the treatment of cervical disc disease in the dog. J. Am. Anim. Hosp. Assoc. *9*, 462, 1973.)

each of the adjacent vertebrae. The graft is made 1 to 2 mm longer than the defect in full traction and is 2 to 5 mm thinner than the slot.[161] This method may leave the surgical area more stable; however, the surgical time is considerably longer, and danger of surgical infection if an autogenous graft is used is considerably greater (Fig. 14–94).

Gilpin[60] investigated more extensive ventral slotting of the cervical vertebrae in clinically normal dogs. Three dogs in group A had slots extending from the midpoint of C2 to C4 vertebrae and covering one-third of the width of the vertebral body on the midline (two vertebral lengths over two disk spaces) (Fig. 14–95). These dogs showed no adverse clinical signs, and normal healing of the defect occurred in 2 to 3 months in four dogs. Three dogs in group B had a slot which extended the total width of the vertebral body and one vertebral length over one disk. These dogs had no clinical signs and healed normally (Fig. 14–96). However, when the length of the total width slot covered two vertebral lengths and two intervening disks (three dogs, group C), two of the dogs showed mild clinical signs of pain. It was felt that the long wide slot destroyed much of the support of the vertebrae involved and resulted in instability (Fig. 14–97).[60]

The author feels that the development of ventral decompressive surgery in cases of cervical disk protrusion has been a very significant advancement in the past few years.

Dorsal Laminectomy or Dorsal Hemilaminectomy in Cervical Disks[42, 88, 158]

The dorsal hemilaminectomy for cervical disk protrusion is somewhat similar to that in the thoracolumbar area. This approach is more difficult in the neck, however, since the vertebrae are more deeply embedded in the surrounding tissue so that exposure is more difficult. Also, the presence of the vertebral vessels in the alar foramina limits the lateroventral exposure.

The dog is placed in sternal recumbency in a head-holder, as described for calvarial surgery, or with the neck padded upward as much as possible. In this position, pressure is exerted on the trachea; therefore tracheal intubation and oxygen administration are essential. The incision is made on the dorsal midline from occipital bone to the first thoracic vertebra. The supraspinous ligament is retracted by means of

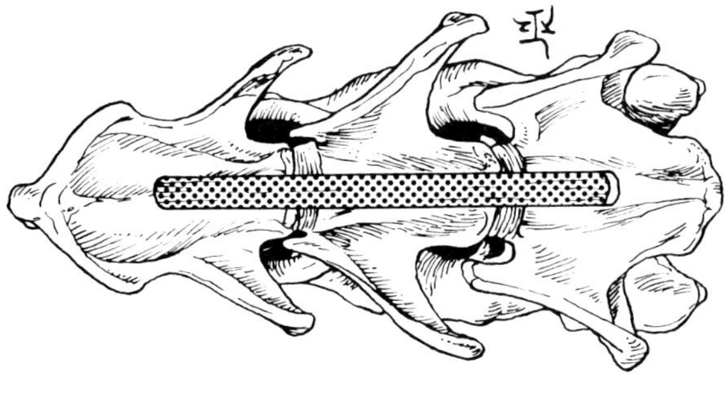

FIGURE 14–95 A long narrow ventral slot (one-third of a vertebral width and two vertebral lengths over two intervertebral spaces) produces no instability in experimental dogs. (From Gilpin, G. N.: Evaluation of three techniques of ventral decompression of the cervical spinal cord in the dog. J.A.V.M.A. *168*, 325, 1976.)

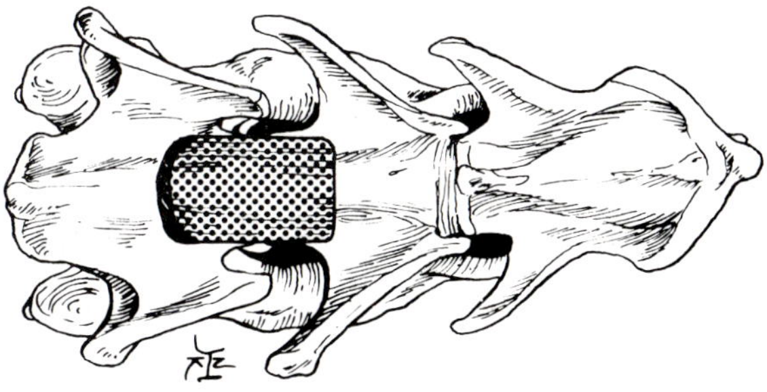

FIGURE 14-96 A full-width ventral decompression over one intervertebral space provides excellent exposure and produces no instability in experimental dogs. (From Gilpin, G. N.: Evaluation of three techniques of ventral decompression of the cervical spinal cord in the dog. J.A.V.M.A. *168*, 325, 1976.)

Frazier retractors, and the musculature adherent to the dorsolateral arches of the involved vertebrae is removed by blunt dissection on one side for a hemilaminectomy and on both sides for a dorsal laminectomy (Figs. 14-98 to 14-100).

The ligamentous attachments of the lateral laminae are carefully dissected free. The part of the lamina situated immediately above the lesion is removed carefully from each vertebra by means of the rongeur forceps or the air drill.

The hemilaminectomy is continued in the anteroposterior aspect until adequate decompression is effected—usually one to two vertebral lengths. The dorsal limit of the bony defect is nearly to the midline and as far ventrally toward the floor of the canal as possible. Care is exercised not to involve the vertebral vessels lateroventrally and to maintain some bone above the level of the cord. The protrusion mass is removed very carefully so as not to involve the cord by extensive manipulation or to lacerate the more laterally situated venous sinuses and their dorsal anastomotic branches. Removing the remainder of the disk by curettage is difficult with this approach and is rarely attempted (Fig. 14-101).

If the protrusion is massive and is situated entirely on the midline, the dorsal decompression described by Funkquist may be employed. The dorsal lamina is removed by means of the air drill or rongeurs, or both, for at least three vertebral lengths, or until normal cord exists at each end of the defect. Removal of the lesion is very difficult and is generally not attempted.

If the venous sinus ruptures upon removal of the lesion, aspiration will keep the field visible until the situation is corrected. Pressure against the sinus then must be maintained for a few minutes until clotting takes place. The defect is covered with an absorbable gelatin sponge and the dorsal musculature, fascia, and skin are routinely closed. The bandage is loosely applied around the neck. If curettage of the disk has resulted in an imperfect union between the two vertebrae, a ventral support should be applied to the head, neck, and body for 1 or 2 weeks. This splint is infrequently needed, however.

It should also be emphasized that considerable manipulation of the spinal cord in the anterior cervical area may lead to persistent respiratory arrest. This is undoubtedly due to a depression of the respiratory center in the medulla resulting from surgical edema. Respiratory stimulants seem to

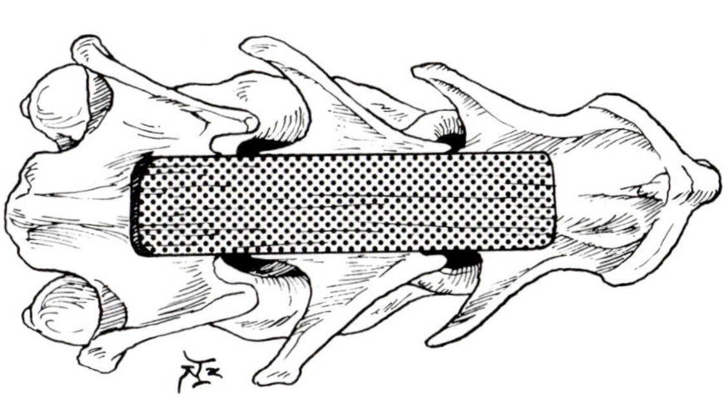

FIGURE 14-97 A full-width, two-vertebral-length ventral decompression is not advisable because of the risk of instability. (From Gilpin, G. N.: Evaluation of three techniques of ventral decompression of the cervical spinal cord in the dog. J.A.V.M.A. *168*, 325, 1976.)

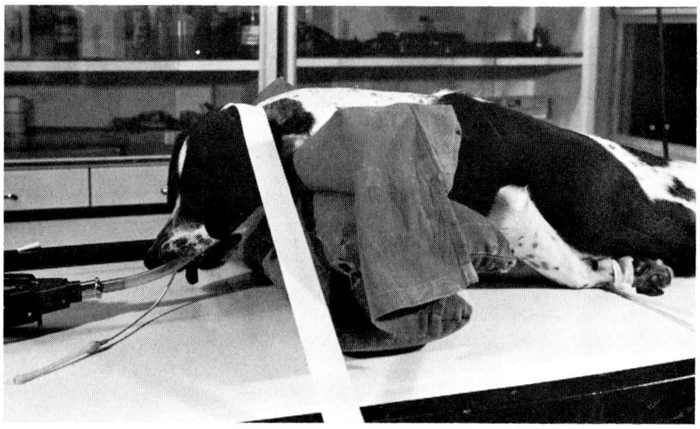

FIGURE 14–98 The position of the patient prepared for a dorsal cervical approach to the spine.

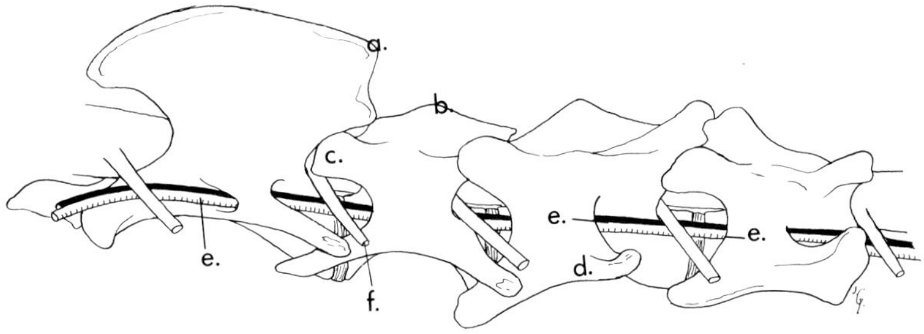

FIGURE 14–99 Structures involved in the dorsal or dorsolateral approach to the cervical vertebrae. (a) Insertion of ligamentum nuchae; (b) dorsal spine of cervical vertebra; (c) articular process; (d) lateral process; (e) alar foramina containing the vertebral vessels; (f) spinal nerve.

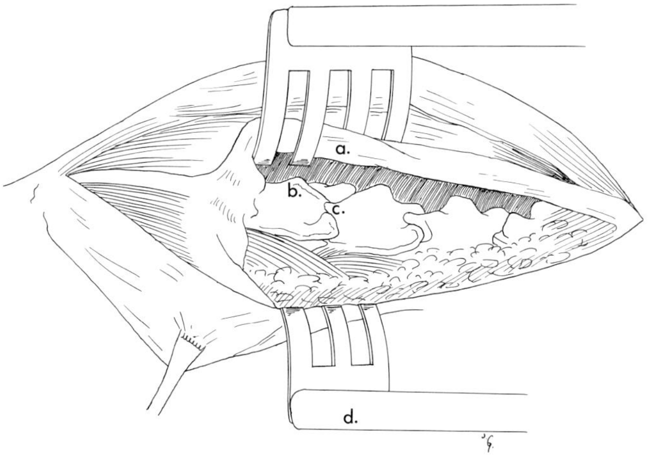

FIGURE 14–100 The nuchal ligament (ligamentum nuchae) is retracted laterally to help expose the vertebrae. (a) Nuchal ligament; (b) dorsal spine; (c) articular process; (d) Frazier laminectomy retractor.

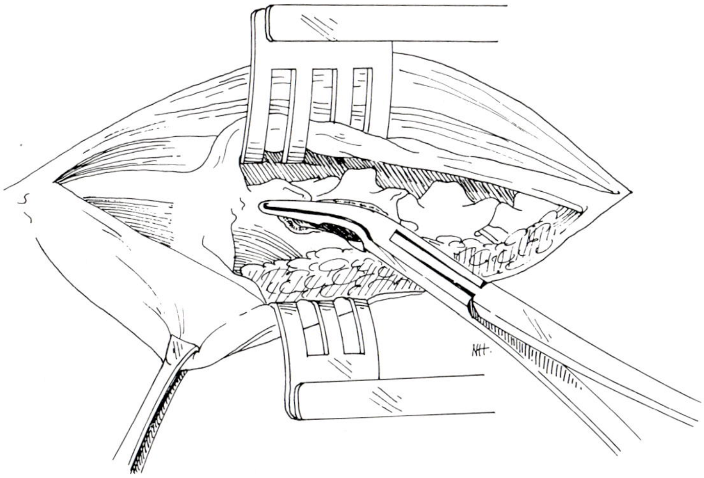

FIGURE 14–101 After the initial hemilaminectomy opening has been started with a trephine, bur, or air drill and bur, the rongeur is used to enlarge the opening to afford a more complete decompression.

have little or only transient effect. At the present time, we prefer to perform the dorsal laminectomy when expansive decompression of the cord is necessary, when the cord should be visualized for diagnostic reasons, or when a durotomy or possible myelotomy may be necessary. A ventral decompression is a direct means of removing a disk protrusion mass which generally cannot be removed by means of a dorsal laminectomy (Figs. 14–102 to 14–105).

Parker[152] has described an approach to the cervicothoracic junction for the dorsal laminectomy. The dog is placed in the sternal recumbent position with its forelimbs crossed under the sternum and tied in position laterally. Sandbags are placed on each side of the chest for stabilization. This position adducts the shoulder joints and pulls the wing of each scapula away from the dorsal midline. The incision is made on the dorsal midline from C4 to T4, and the trapezius and rhomboideus muscles are incised on the midline and reflected for the entire length of the incision. The splenius and serratus dorsalis muscles are incised close to the midline and are reflected. The longissimus cervicis, longissimus capitis, and semispinalis capitis are separated from the midline by blunt dissection. One should avoid the branch of the deep cervical artery that lies just lateral to the transverse process of C7 vertebra. The short intervertebral muscles can now be excised, completely exposing the dorsal spines and vertebral arches of the last three cervical and first three thoracic vertebrae. Since the nuchal ligament in effect originates caudal to the T3 dorsal spine by means of a fibrous midline raphe, the spines of T1, T2, and T3 can be severed if necessary for proper exposure. Brachial paralysis from

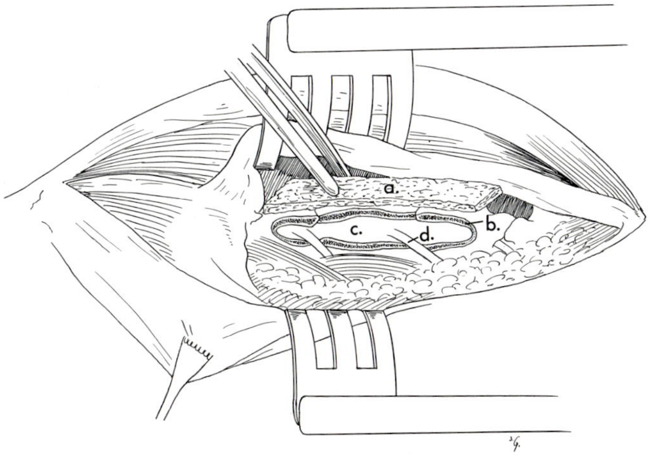

FIGURE 14–102 The completed hemilaminectomy decompression. Absorbable gelatin sponge or slightly crushed muscle is laid over the bone defect. (a) Gelatin sponge; (b) edge of hemilaminectomy defect; (c) spinal cord; (d) spinal nerve.

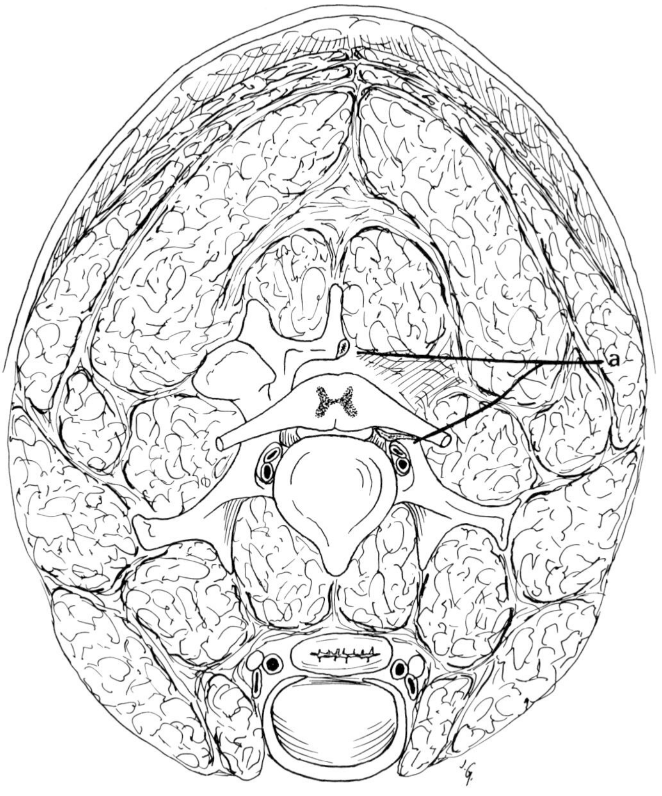

FIGURE 14–103 Cross section of neck after a hemilaminectomy. Notice the decompressive hemilaminectomy area (a).

FIGURE 14–104 *A.* The back of a dog operated upon 6 weeks previously. The surgical procedure involved disk curettage of disks T11–12 through L3–4 because of widespread pathologic changes. Hemilaminectomy was performed at T13–L1, a prominent disk protrusion. Even though the surgical area was extensive, minimal scar and conformation defect can be routinely obtained.

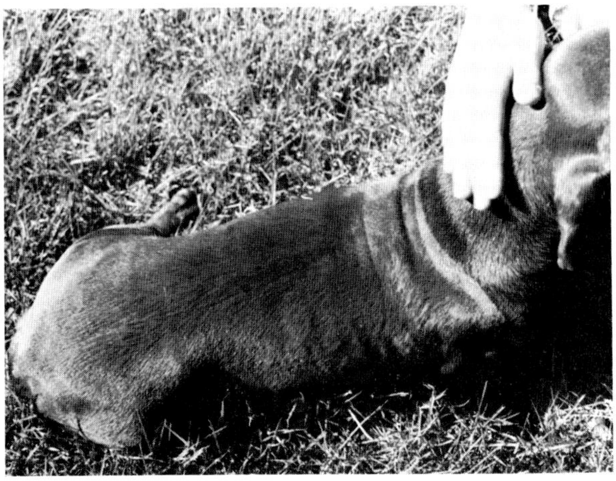

FIGURE 14–104 *B.* The same dog 6 years later.

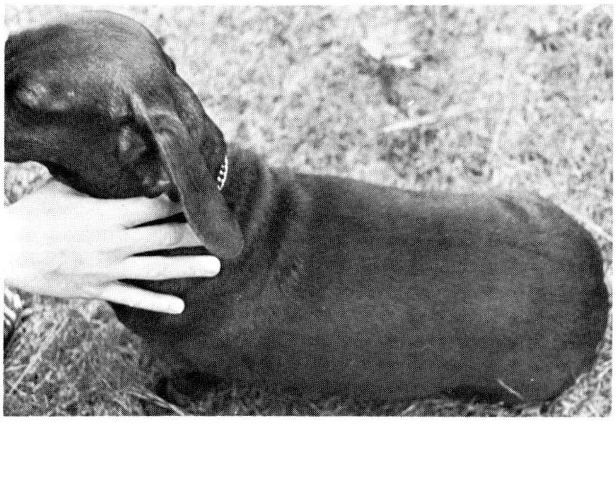

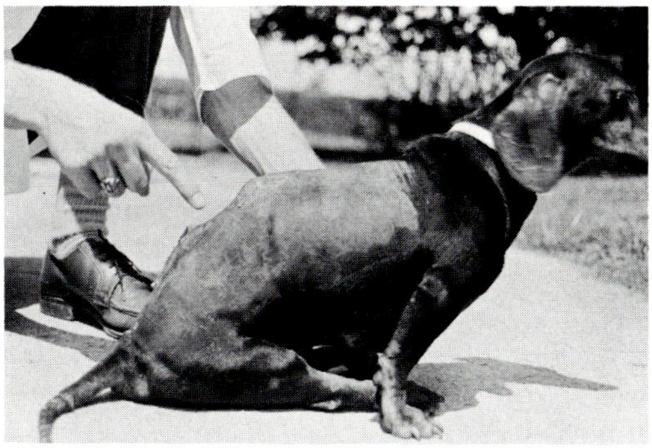

A

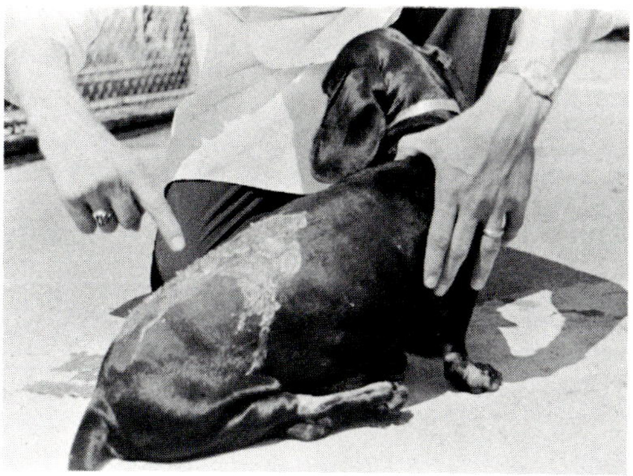

B

FIGURE 14–105 *A.* A dog who has had a dorsal decompressive laminectomy. Notice the cosmetic defect where the spine has been removed. *B.* A dog who has had a hemilaminectomy. Notice the relatively good cosmetic result. The skin has had flexible collodion placed on it to protect the incision during hot water soaks and exercise.

surgical positioning should not occur unless the wing of the scapula is retracted beyond a right angle to the ribs. The dorsal laminectomy is performed as already described. Closure is effected routinely by suturing muscle layers and obliterating any dead space resulting from surgery.[152]

SURGICAL SUMMARY

When a considerable percentage of cases respond at least temporarily to good nursing care and natural body healing, many modes of therapy will be utilized by those engaged in the different branches of medicine. As in many other recognized clinical entities, disk protrusions were not considered important in clinical practice until veterinarians became aware of the clinical signs and their pathological significance. In those early years, surgical relief was ridiculed as totally irrational.

Some 25 years later, we are still in the process of deciding which type of surgical relief should be used. It has been generally agreed recently that the chief value of disk fenestration is to correct pain and mild paresis and to prevent future acute attacks. Fortunately, this operation has never been taken as seriously as the appendectomy many years ago when high school athletes had preseason appendectomies to prevent acute attacks of appendicitis during the season. The appropriate removal of the disk from the lateral or ventral aspects of the cord prevents future protrusions and cord compressions.

It has also been established that an animal with sudden paralysis with a radiographically well-defined protrusion mass or evidence of a disk blowout should have appropriate decompressive surgery to relieve vascular embarrassments and medullary edema or hemorrhagic swellings. There is strong evidence that such decompression should be performed within hours after occurrence of paralysis—at most within 24 to 48 hours. Delayed decompression performed days or even a few weeks later can be effective when voluntary motor function and conscious pain responses are present. Formerly, extradural decompressions were generally considered adequate and appropriate clinically and probably are still effective in a high percentage of cases.

Recently, owing to the upsurge of research on the biogenic amines and biochemical—endocrinologic responses in experimentally produced spinal trauma, there have been suggestions that selective regional hypothermia, total deep laminectomies for severe injuries, durotomies, and myelotomies are appropriate for the most effective *intradural* decompression.[128] However, the experimental data and the subsequent conclusions are confusing because of differences in experimental procedures and species variations in experimental animal models.

It is felt that the conservative modern neurosurgeon will rely heavily on prompt *extradural* decompression in profound paraplegics, using plenty of normothermic saline perfusions during the surgical procedure, and using durotomies selectively only

TABLE 14–9 SUMMARY OF DISK SURGERY

Procedure and Reference	Indications	Advantages	Disadvantages
I. Thoracolumbar surgery			
A. Fenestration			
1. Dorsolateral (Olsson[145])	Pain Slight paresis Prophylaxis	Less cord trauma, as surgery does not involve cord Easily combined with hemilaminectomy	No means of observing lesion Probably more surgically traumatic than muscle separation procedures
2. Dorsolateral muscle separation (Yturraspe[218])	Same as A(1)	No cord trauma Probably less traumatic to spinal musculature	No observation of lesion Not easily combined with decompressive surgery
3. Lateral muscle separation (Seeman,[184] Flo[40])	Same as A(1) Flo also advocates this for paraplegia	Same as A(2)	Same as A(2)
4. Ventrolateral fenestration (Northway[138])	Lumbar disk problems Pain, paresis	Same as A(2)	No observation of lesion No data on clinical cases Traumatic to spinal nerves
5. Ventral–paracostal or intercostal (Leonard,[113] Ross[171])	Same as A(1)	No cord trauma Least traumatic to spinal musculature	No observation of lesion Decompressive surgery requires separate approach Need two body wall incisions for most thoracolumbar fenestrations
B. Decompressive surgery			
1. Dorsal laminectomy (Funkquist[43])	Resistant pain Paresis Paraplegia	Provides good vision for other pathological lesions Good for durotomy and myelotomy	Cannot remove protruding mass Prophylactic fenestrations not described—recurrences frequent Leaves cosmetic and structural defects
2. Modified dorsal laminectomy (Trotter[206])	Same as B(1)	Provides good observation of lesion Good for durotomy Can remove compressive mass but not the disk	Prophylactic fenestrations not described Leaves cosmetic and structural defects
3. Hemilaminectomy and disk fenestration (Hoerlein[85,89])	Same as B(1)	Provides good observation of lesion Good for durotomy Good decompression Effective prophylactic fenestration Cosmetically and structurally sound	Not good for myelotomy Venous sinus hemorrhage is possible
4. Hemilaminectomy–lateral muscle separation approach (Braund[13])	Same as B(1)	Less traumatic to spinal musculature Decompressive area to disk and floor of canal Same advantages as other hemilaminectomies	Same as other hemilaminectomies

TABLE 14–9 SUMMARY OF DISK SURGERY (*Continued*)

Procedures and Reference	Indications	Advantages	Disadvantages
II. Cervical disk surgery			
A. Fenestration			
1. Ventral (Olsson,[145] Hoerlein[84])	Pain Paresis	Easily performed with little postoperative reaction	Adequate removal of massive calcific protrusion is not possible If protrusion is large, recovery may be very slow or may not occur
B. Decompressive surgery			
1. Partial spondylectomy and diskectomy without graft (ventral slot) (Swaim[195])	Resistant pain Paresis and paralysis	Affords good removal of protruding mass and usually adequate decompression Moderate to slight postoperative reaction	Venous sinus hemorrhage is possible in removing mass
2. Partial spondylectomy and diskectomy with graft (Prata,[161] Popovich[160])	Same as B(1)	Same as B(1) Moderate postoperative reaction Possibly provides greater stability from graft	Same as B(1), although author does not stress it Surgical time is longer owing to graft procedures, therefore there is more chance of sepsis or shock
3. Dorsal laminectomy (Funkquist B[42])	Same as B(1)	Good exposure of cord for pathology other than disk problems Good decompression	No provision for removing protruding mass and causative disk lesion Severe postoperative reaction frequently occurs
4. Hemilaminectomy (Hoerlein,[88,89] Pettit[157])	Same as B(1)	Good exposure of cord Good decompression Possible to remove protruding mass	Difficult to remove causative disk lesion by fenestration Approach is more difficult than that of dorsal laminectomy Moderate postoperative reactions

when there is a need for a more accurate prognosis. One experimental series questioned the decompressive efficacy of durotomies, and another showed that durotomy performed 2 hours after experimental cord trauma had little significant effect.[153] If malacia has occurred and the spinal cord flows out of the durotomy incision, the animal should not be allowed to awaken from anesthesia. In severe injuries, such as spinal fractures, durotomy and myelotomy might have a therapeutic as well as a prognostic value. By using these guidelines in neurosurgery, the surgeon is using legally sound therapeutic procedures while allowing time for the scientific community to establish more facts concerning the temperature of saline perfusions in the surgical area and the value of extensive intradural decompression in disk protrusions.

The various types of surgery used in disk protrusions are summarized in Table 14–9.

RESULTS OF NONSURGICAL AND SURGICAL THERAPY

In a disorder such as disk protrusion, which because of its pathologic characteristics carries a rather high incidence of spontaneous improvement, the analysis of data concerning the efficiency of various treatment methods is most difficult. In the discussion of nonsurgical treatment it was emphasized that *rest* and maintenance of normal body metabolism and elimination were most important—in other words, one should not interfere with the natural course of mild disk protrusions. Since a sizable number of protrusions are not mild, but produce severe neurological dysfunction, surgical intervention might be considered.

COMPARATIVE RESULTS IN MAN

Before we consider the results of the two modes of treatment in dogs, let us consider the results in man. Reports vary considerably regarding results obtained by radical surgery; however, Higley[81] has compiled the following figures on surgery:

Lumbar Cases (2003)	
Recovered	46.8 per cent
Improved	39.9 per cent
Not improved or worsened	13.3 per cent

The results of a comparable group of cases treated by conservative methods are as follows:

Lumbar Cases (1582)	
Recovered	39.2 per cent
Improved	37.2 per cent
Not improved or worsened	23.5 per cent

The use of ultrasound seemed to produce the highest percentage of recovery in the various conservative treatments evaluated.[81]

DORSOLATERAL FENESTRATION COMPARED TO NONSURGICAL TREATMENT

Olsson in 1951 compared fenestration and nonsurgical methods in the dog. These results are abstracted briefly as follows:[144]

Pain or pain and slight paresis

- Fenestration: 11 of 13 recovered completely (85 per cent).
- Rest and administration of vitamin B_1: 5 of 10 recovered completely (50 per cent).

Severe paresis or paraplegia

- Fenestration: 12 of 15 recovered (80 per cent).
- Rest and administration of vitamin B_1: 5 of 11 recovered (45 per cent).

In 1958, Vaughan[210] reported on fenestrations in 13 dogs as follows:

- Seven cervical: all recovered in 6 to 42 days.
- Four paraplegics: two destroyed 4 months postoperatively; one died 24 hours postoperatively; one died 7 days postoperatively.
- Two lumbar pain and paresis: one died 24 hours postoperatively; one recovered.

Funkquist has reported upon lateral fenestration in 88 thoracolumbar disk cases that showed signs of pain or varying grades of paresis but retained the ability to walk on their hind legs. In all cases, fenestration and evacuation of degenerated disk material were performed in the region of T9–L6. The surgical results were compared to 128 similarly affected cases on which nonsurgery treatment was performed. No significant difference in respect to recovery time was seen. The chief advantage seen in the surgically treated cases was that almost 100 per cent of the dogs had no recurrences for some years postsurgically.[44] This is the reason that Hoerlein has for years combined the decompression hemilaminectomy and the fenestration.[82–90] It must be emphasized again that Funkquist's report was not on paralytic dogs but on those still able to walk.

Flo reports that 95 per cent of 67 cases were successful during a 2-year postsurgical period when a lateral approach from T10 through L4 was used for disk fenestrations. The clinical signs were pain or paresis in 31 cases, paraplegia with deep pain in 11 cases, and paraplegia with no deep pain in 6 cases.[40]

PHYSICAL THERAPY COMPARED TO CONVENTIONAL NONSURGICAL TREATMENT

Jadeson reported on the results of conservative treatment in 1961.[97] Eighty-two cases were described, in 35 of which the standard medical and conservative therapy was given (group I); in the remaining 47 the standard treatment and various types of physical therapy were given (group II). See Tables 14–10 to 14–12 for results.

CONVENTIONAL TREATMENT RESULTS

Wilcox conducted a survey among 38 veterinarians who contributed a total of 102 case histories for analysis of breed and age incidence, number of cases having prior attacks, variety of clinical signs, and functional recovery with conservative (nonsurgical) treatment. Of the 102 cases, 19 died and three suffered from hematomyelia. Thirty-seven (36.3 per cent) of the 102 dogs suffered from paraplegia, of which 18 (47 per cent) recovered and 16 (43 per cent) were destroyed. Of the 16 that were destroyed, five had no recovery, four had poor prognosis, four had a guarded prognosis, and three had a guarded to good prognosis. Of the 102 cases, 32.3 per cent had a history of having had one or more previous attacks.[215]

RECURRENCES IN SURGICALLY AND NONSURGICALLY TREATED CERVICAL DISKS

Russell and Griffiths analyzed 110 cases of cervical disk protrusion for recurrences. The recurrence in nonsurgically treated dogs over a 3-year period was 36.3 per cent, whereas it was only 5.6 per cent in dogs on which ventral fenestrations were performed. The nonsurgical treatment consisted of administration of analgesics, phenylbutazone, and corticosteroids in addition to the usual supportive therapy.[176]

Jadeson observed a smaller group of dogs for a period of 1 year and found that the incidence of recurrence was much lower in the group that had physical therapy (Table 14–10).[97]

TABLE 14–10 INCIDENCE OF RECURRENCE IN DOGS RECEIVING PHYSICAL THERAPY*

	Group I			Group II		
	Total	(No.)	Relapses (Per Cent)	Total	(No.)	Relapses (Per Cent)
Paralysis	13	4	30.77	23	1	4.35
Paresis	14	2	14.29	19	0	0.00

*From Jadeson, W. J.: Rehabilitation of dogs with intervertebral disk lesions by physical therapy methods. J.A.V.M.A. *138*, 411, 1961.

In some respects, Jadeson's results appear to be very good. One must remember that Jadeson is a registered physical therapist, apparently of unusual ability. The work was done in partial fulfillment of requirements for the Master of Science degree, so that it is certain that the patients received unusually fine care. Jadeson's methods were highly developed, and such equipment as an ultrasonic appliance, a diathermy machine, muscle stimulators, and carriages was available. Few practitioners could hope to achieve this degree of success with physical therapy.[97]

The results summarized in Table 14–10 indicate that the use of physical therapy in addition to conventional modalities increased the excellent results from 13 to 19 per cent in the various categories, based on severity of clinical signs (Table 14–11). In another series, the difference in "excellent" recovery rates of paretic and paralytic animals in the two treatment groups was only 7 per cent (Table 14–12).

TABLE 14–11 RESULTS OF CONSERVATIVE TREATMENT*

		Paralysis (Per Cent)	Paresis (Per Cent)	Total (Per Cent)
Group I	Excellent	9 (50.0)	10 (58.8)	19 (54.3)
	Good	4 (22.2)	4 (23.5)	8 (22.9)
	None	5 (27.8)	3 (17.7)	8 (22.9)
Group II	Excellent	18 (69.2)	15 (71.4)	33 (70.2)
	Good	5 (19.2)	4 (19.1)	9 (19.2)
	None	3 (11.5)	2 (9.5)	5 (10.6)

*From Jadeson, W. J.: Rehabilitation of dogs with intervertebral disk lesions by physical therapy methods. J.A.V.M.A. *138*, 411, 1961.

TABLE 14–12 RESULTS OF CONSERVATIVE TREATMENT AUGMENTED WITH PHYSICAL THERAPY*

	Conventional (Per Cent)	Conventional and Physical Therapy (Per Cent)
Excellent	189 (50.5)	54 (57.5)
Good	95 (25.3)	22 (23.4)
None	91 (24.1)	18 (19.1)
	375	94

*From Jadeson, W. J.: Rehabilitation of dogs with intervertebral disk lesions by physical therapy methods. J.A.V.M.A. *138*, 411, 1961.

DORSAL DECOMPRESSIVE LAMINECTOMY COMPARED TO NONSURGICAL TREATMENT

Funkquist has provided a highly comprehensive analysis of the recovery of neural dysfunction caused by protruding disks.[46] Her study offers the results of conservative treatment in 141 cases from Stockholm of complete and partial paralysis and other cases from two additional clinics in Sweden. These results are illustrated in Table 14–13.

Funkquist compared results of dorsal decompression when performed at various intervals after onset of paralysis. The incidence of ascending paralysis was 25 per cent when motor dysfunction occurred within 12 hours, whereas it was 4.5 per cent when dysfunction developed more slowly. Other than progressive paralysis, rapid development had no other obvious prognostic significance. In the Funkquist B dorsal decompression, the disk was not removed and 22 per cent of the recovered cases showed recurrences, while 28.9 per cent of the nonsurgery cases had recurrences. The observation time for recurrences was 11 months.[46] Subsequent disk fenestration after dorsal decompression has since been adopted by some workers in order to decrease the incidence of recurrences.[43]

TABLE 14–13 RECOVERY FROM PARALYSIS IN SWEDISH CASES (NONSURGICAL)*

	No.	Recovered Ability to Walk (Per Cent)
Stockholm Veterinary College	141	36.9
Animal Hospital (Hälsingborg)	94	45.7
Animal Hospital (Skara)	36	47.2

*From Funkquist, B.: Thoraco-lumbar disk protrusion with severe cord compression in the dog. I. Clinical and patho-anatomic observations with special reference to the rate of development of the symptoms of motor loss. II. Clinical observations with special reference to the prognosis in conservative treatment. III. Treatment by decompressive laminectomy. Acta Vet. Scand. *3*, 1962.

A more recent report by Funkquist states that 26 of 27 (96 per cent) disk paraplegics that she personally operated upon regained ability to walk. Seventy-three out of 82 (89 per cent) paraplegics that were operated upon at the Royal Veterinary College Clinic in Stockholm (including Funkquist's personal cases) by specially trained surgeons regained ability to walk. In emergency cases operated upon by surgeons with general training, 31 of 49 dogs (63 per cent) regained walking ability. In a control group treated by nonsurgical methods, 21 of 41 (51 per cent) regained walking ability. Incidence of relapses in surgical cases was at least as high as in those with conservative treatment except for the dogs that were subjected to a second disk fenestration procedure.[43]

Henry compared the results of two series of dorsal laminectomies when identical surgical procedures were used. In one series of 33 dogs who were operated upon within 24 hours of the onset of paralysis (upper limit, 48 hours), the recovery rate was 94 per cent. In 36 dogs, when the average time of surgical intervention was 4.6 days after onset of signs, the recovery rate was 47 per cent. When total paraplegics were compared, the first group had a recovery rate of 89 per cent, while that in the second group was 7 per cent. Henry concluded that animals with a sudden onset of paraplegia need surgery within 24 hours, whereas if the paralysis is not complete, the time interval is not as critical.[80]

DORSOLATERAL FENESTRATION, HEMILAMINECTOMY COMPARED TO NONSURGICAL TREATMENT

In 1956, Hoerlein reported on 154 clinicial cases of disk protrusion[85] that were observed or reported from 6 months to 4½ years after surgery.

The number of dogs considered to have had good recovery was 66 per cent in the surgically treated group, as opposed to 23 per cent in the nonsurgical group. This critical analysis on follow-up cases was the first study so conducted in veterinary medicine.[85]

Surgery consisted of multiple disk fenestration and hemilaminectomy. Twelve cases were not treated by either method because the symptoms were so mild that therapy was not needed, or because the condition was considered hopeless from the onset. Actually, many of the surgical cases would have been considered hopeless by our present standards; that is, there was complete voluntary motor and sensory dysfunction. The surgical group included many cases that did not respond or were considered too severe for conservative treatment. This fact makes the figures for surgical recovery much more significant.

Since 1952, the author has recorded periodically the long-term results of surgical and nonsurgical therapy as determined by evaluation of detailed questionnaires answered by clients. These findings of surveys conducted in 1956, 1964, and 1969 were charted in the last edition of this text.

The results of surgery were consistent in that about 80 per cent of the paraplegics regained normal function. The number of nonsurgical patients was much smaller and recovery of paraplegics varied from 13 to 50 per cent. In long-term surveys of cases of disk disease treated at the Auburn clinic from 1969 to 1975, 1150 cases were selected from 1309 cases seen, and questionnaires were sent to the owners. From these 1150, 215 were returned because the client had moved. Of the 935 delivered, 460 (49.2 per cent) were returned and evaluated. The results were consistent with previous surveys. The findings from these long-term surveys (1952–1975) are recorded in Table 14–14. In this period of 23 years, a total of 1007 surgical and 177 nonsurgical cases were reviewed during a postoperative period ranging from 6 months to over 6 years. Although this may not seem like a large number of cases, considering the present high incidence of residential mobility and a 50 per cent lack of response to the questionnaires, the number reported represents less than 50 per cent of the total number of cases studied (2395 cases in Table 14–2). Only cases with complete data and responsible follow-up information are included in the evaluation study (Figs. 14–106 and 14–107).

Paralysis was determined by complete absence of all voluntary motor control of the

TABLE 14–14 RESULTS OF TREATMENT OBSERVED 6 MONTHS OR LONGER IN 1184 CASES (Hoerlein, 1950–1975)

	Surgical Therapy						Nonsurgical Therapy					
	6 mo–1 yr	*1–2 yr*	*3–5 yr*	*6 yr & over*	*Total*	*Per Cent*	*6 mo–1 yr*	*1–2 yr*	*3–5 yr*	*6 yr & over*	*Total*	*Per Cent*
Paralysis												
Good	56	141	214	58	479	87.0	1	5	4	1	11	22.4
Fair	17	12	8	6	43	8.0	6	0	2	1	9	18.4
Poor	22	1	3	1	27	5.0	25	2	2	0	29	59.2
Total	95	154	225	65	539	100.0	32	7	8	2	49	100.0
Paresis												
Good	60	84	115	18	277	90.5	6	5	7	1	19	29.7
Fair	8	4	9	0	21	6.9	4	13	6	1	24	37.5
Poor	6	1	1	0	8	2.6	19	0	2	0	21	32.8
Total	74	89	125	18	306	100.0	29	18	15	2	64	100.0
Pain												
Good	44	29	44	17	134	82.7	9	3	10	2	24	37.5
Fair	3	5	3	2	13	8.0	11	10	7	1	29	45.3
Poor	6	3	3	3	15	9.3	6	2	2	1	11	17.2
Total	53	37	50	22	162	100.0	26	15	19	4	64	100.0
Total	222	280	400	105	1007		87	40	42	8	177	

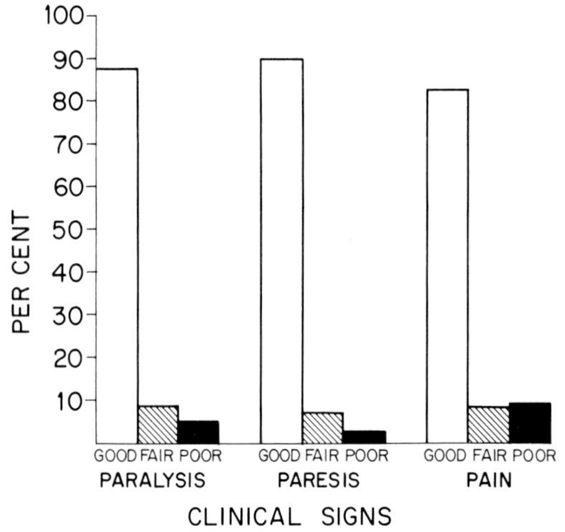

FIGURE 14–106 Surgical results in 1007 cases of disk protrusions (observed 6 months or longer) that had shown predominantly paralysis, paresis, or pain presurgically.

limbs. These animals had been affected with paralysis for 1 to 7 days. Nearly all had the usual urinary retention, hyperreflexia or exaggerated tendon reflexes, and some sensory function. Although animals showing no deep pain response on toe-pinch reflex were not recommended for surgery, many were operated upon at the owner's insistence. These were included in the statistics. Many animals already had or soon developed a hemorrhagic cystitis after admission to the clinic (comparable to Funkquist's Group II).

Paresis was termed a partial paralysis. These dogs had some degree of voluntary motor action but did not walk. Urinary retention was not as severe and cystitis did not develop as frequently as in the complete paralytic (comparable to Funkquist's Group I).

Pain was the dominant symptom, but weakness and incoordination were frequently observed in this group. Urinary function was frequently normal, and reflexes were nearly normal.

The categories of response to treatment were determined as follows:

Good—complete recovery of motor and urinary function.

Fair—some remaining dysfunction, either motor or urinary, but animal retained independent function and usefulness.

Poor—not enough improvement to be returned to owner as an independent pet or working animal. A case of recurrence was placed in this category.

To understand the data presented, additional information is given about the philosophy of the institution in which these cases were treated. It is a state-supported institution whose chief purpose is to train the professional student and postgraduate veterinarian. A random selection of treatment methods has been impractical, since the best possible care must be given each patient. This has been necessary not only because of the ethics involved, but also because the area is not highly urban and therefore potential teaching material (clinical accessions) is limited. The institution must therefore provide superior service, staff, and equipment. Comparable charges

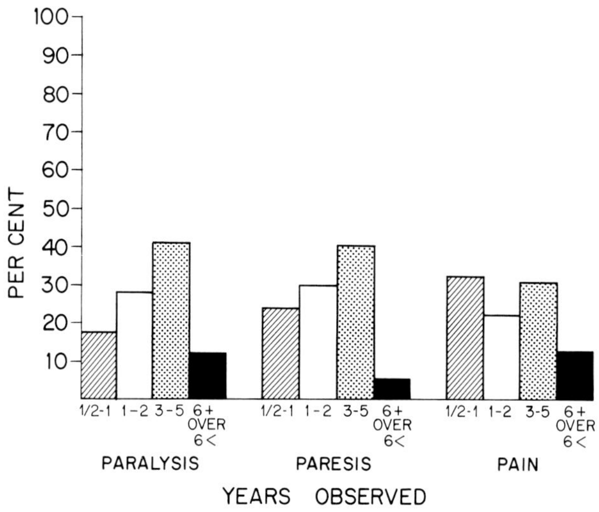

FIGURE 14–107 Postsurgical observation periods in 1007 cases of disk protrusion (observed 6 months or longer) that had shown predominantly paralysis, paresis, or pain presurgically.

must be made on all clinical services. In addition, the majority of spinal cases are referrals from practitioners, and considerable travel is sometimes involved. Such subjects are generally sent to the clinic specifically for surgical relief, since many have failed to respond to conservative care. Therefore, our results do not reflect a fair comparison between the two methods of therapy, but show only the effectiveness of the surgical relief.

Since the clinic staff numbers 19 professionals, and the annual accessions number approximately 27,000 cases, the surgical procedures over the years represent the work of not one surgeon but several. At the present time, six clinicians participate in spinal surgery, and in emergency hours, the surgery may be performed by a less experienced neurosurgeon. Therefore, the results reflect those that could be expected by the profession at large.

It is gratifying to note the lack of recurrence of neurological signs in the surgical cases. Occasionally, two separate operations were performed on one animal when the thoracolumbar and cervical areas were involved. It is also noted that approximately 72 per cent of the surgical cases and about 60 per cent of all cases were paralyzed. In Wilcox's study of 102 thoracolumbar cases, only 36 per cent were paralytic.[215] This figure excludes cases of cervical disks, which the Auburn data include. Dogs whose cervical disk is involved are generally not paralytic, but they suffer predominantly from pain (about 12 per cent of all disk cases involve the cervical disk). One must conclude that the pain and paresis cases are being treated by the private practitioner, while the paralytics are being referred. This adds further significance to the statistics presented. In the average cross-section of cases, much better surgical results could be expected.

According to the experience of Tarlov,[201, 202] Funkquist,[46] this author,[82-90] and others, the success of spinal decompressions depends largely upon the promptness of surgery. We have felt over the years that a persistent paralysis with no sign of motor improvement should not be considered for surgery after 7 days. We have observed a direct relationship between the duration of injury and duration of postsurgical rehabilitation. For example, a dog whose injury has lasted only 24 hours might take 3 to 4 days to walk; a dog who has been injured for 5 to 6 days might take 2 to 3 weeks to walk. However, Martin has statistics to show that in private practice situations, delayed surgery can be effective. In 53 paraplegics, 80 per cent (31 of 39) recovered with surgery when operated upon within 7 days, whereas 75 per cent (9 of 12) recovered when operated upon in 7 to 30 days.[124] Experiences of Henry,[80] Knecht,[107] and others differ from these unless the motor deficiencies are partial, in which case surgical intervention is not as urgent.

DISCUSSION OF TREATMENT METHODS

Although it is difficult to accurately compare the methods of treatment and their relative efficacy, the author feels that all have their merits and has presented them as objectively as possible. It appears that surgical treatment of selected cases is superior to nonsurgical care. It is felt that a specific treatment should be performed in a specific type of case. Since more cases of a surgical nature were referred to our clinic, more surgical interventions were performed. The average practitioner will generally not do as much surgical correction as he will nonsurgical treatment, unless he is also conducting a referral practice.

In the average small animal practice, both conservative and surgical treatments should be appropriately performed for maximal service to the client. The surgical service should be available to the client within a reasonably small geographic area.

It is not the intent of the author to promote controversy as to the merits of the various surgical methods. It is felt that each method—fenestration, hemilaminectomy, dorsal laminectomy, ventral cervical partial spondylectomy, diskectomy (slotting or trephination), and combination of hemilaminectomy and disk fenestration—has its specific indications, and the author and his associates have performed and do perform most of these basic procedures and combinations thereof on certain individual cases. Each surgeon must evaluate the purpose and surgical effects of each method and adapt these to his capabilities and the patient's needs.

Disk fenestration is a relatively simple,

safe, and effective procedure in dogs suffering from reversible cord damage manifested by pain and paresis. Some cases of paralysis, of course, will respond to fenestration. Fenestration is excellent for preventing future protrusions in the surgically involved disk and should be performed on disks showing degenerations that may lead to protrusion and on those located in the most susceptible protrusion area (T11–12 and L1–2). The more recent lateral muscle-separating techniques appear to have some advantages over the ventral or dorsolateral approaches.

Hemilaminectomy is effective for removing a massive protrusion and its causative disk, decompressing a swollen edematous cord, and providing a direct means of etiological diagnosis, prognosis, correction, and any additional procedure necessary for maximal effect, such as fusions and skeletal immobilizations. With modern surgical knowledge and equipment, it should be termed a conservative decompressive procedure. It is highly effective for the purposes outlined.

The Funkquist B and modified dorsal decompressive laminectomies provide spacious decompression with minimal manipulation of neurological tissue. The partial (nontotal) dorsal laminectomies are effective approaches for etiological diagnosis and prognosis of the compressive lesion. It is particularly indicated for massive disk lesions in the anterior cervical area, where any cord manipulation is especially hazardous. If aggressive anticatecholamine therapy, durotomies, and myelotomies are to be considered in massive cord trauma involving edema, swelling, and possible hemorrhagic malacia of the cord, the dorsal laminectomy provides the best approach. Its main disadvantages are that (1) it is difficult to remove the compressive lesions through the laminectomy opening, (2) the approach is not adaptable for conjunctive fenestrations, (3) a cosmetic defect results, particularly in the thoracolumbar area, and (4) great care must be exercised to prevent secondary cicatricial compression of the cord.

The modified deep or total dorsal laminectomy may be appropriate in spinal fractures and bone disease, but is rarely indicated for disk compressions. Future clinical trials will determine the more specific value of this procedure.

The combined hemilaminectomy–disk fenestration in thoracolumbar disks has been the routine method employed by the author for some 25 years. It satisfies the basic purposes of decompression—removal of the disk and its protrusion mass, and removal of disks that may cause future attacks—and it provides for a practical as well as a cosmetic approach. This method is indicated for motor paralysis. The results of some 1000 cases observed postsurgically were exceptionally good in view of their critical evaluation and documentation.

Nonsurgical care should be considered with the following:

1. Pain.
2. Paresis and pain.
3. Multiple disk protrusions and spinal disease disseminated throughout the spine.
4. Complete paraplegia (sensory and voluntary motor dysfunction) existing longer than 7 days.
5. Generalized myelitis and paralysis produced by hematomyelia unless diagnosis and prognosis are in question.

Surgical intervention should be considered in the following radiographically positive cases:

1. Recurrent cases.
2. Cases of pain and paresis unresponsive to nonsurgical care.
3. Cases of profound paralysis with urinary and fecal dysfunction caused by a local compression, and where conscious perception of pain is present on the pedal or toe pinch reflex.

Optimal routine conservative care and physical therapy should be given the nonsurgical patient and the surgical patient during the postoperative period. These factors are essential to recovery.

SECTION 2
DISK DISORDERS IN CATS

INCIDENCE

Disk disease in the cat has received very little attention, owing, no doubt, to its infrequent clinical incidence. Hoerlein has seen two cats with paraplegia due to a ruptured disk that resulted from trauma. A 4-year-old Siamese cat suffered a compression of the cord from a protrusion at T10–11 that was diagnosed by a myelographic examination; the animal had a sensorimotor paraplegia, and was destroyed. The other cat, a mixed breed tom also 4 years of age, was diagnosed at necropsy after being destroyed because of complete paraplegia. Both lesions were similar to ruptured disks in dogs, having a sizable amount of necrotic material present in the epidural space. The pathologic changes in the cord were characteristic of those discussed in Section I of this chapter.

There are other scattered reports of clinical disk protrusion in cats. Milnes cites three cases in cats 13, 15, and 8 years old. The 13-year-old demonstrated prominent protrusions at L4–5 and L5–6; L1–2 had a slight ridge. The 15-year-old cat, which had had otitis externa 6 weeks earlier, suddenly showed a posterior paresis and died within 24 hours. The spinal dura had adhered to the floor of the canal at C6–7, which showed a prominent protrusion, whereas L1–2 and L2–3 had minor protrusions. The 8-year-old cat had shown posterior weakness for several weeks. Necropsy showed only a small ridge at L1–2. Milnes had difficulty correlating the severity of clinical signs with the gross necropsy lesions seen. Apparently microscopic studies of cord sections were not performed.[132]

A Siamese cat that was a total and hopeless paraplegic was admitted to the Auburn clinic. The clinical signs, radiographic myelograms, and even physical appearance of the lesion at surgery were characteristic of a compressive myelitis caused by a disk protrusion. However, microscopic examination of the lesion demonstrated a lymphosarcoma. Since the occurrence of epidural lymphosarcomatous masses capable of causing signs characteristic of disk protrusions is fairly frequent in the cat, some reports of clinical disks in cats may have actually been due to lymphosarcoma. We have also seen lymphosarcomas cause occasional spinal signs in dogs in our clinic. This is a possible cause of paraplegia in the cat that resembles the disk syndrome (Figs. 14–109 to 14–111).

King and Smith have reported upon the incidence of protrusions in clinically normal cats.[104] One group of 100 cats was described in 1958 in which the ages were not known. Among these 100 random necropsies, there were 91 abnormal disks in 26 spines. King and Smith concluded that the dorsal protrusions were similar to those occurring in the nonchondrodystrophoid breeds of dogs. Protrusions in which the annulus was completely perforated appeared to be smaller in the cat than in the dog. Disks that showed only partial perforation of the annulus were about the same size as in the dog. It was noted that the disks that were supported dorsally by the conjugal ligament were seldom affected. Cervical protrusions were seen most frequently, protrusions at the thoracolumbar junction were seldom seen, and midlumbar lesions were often seen. Protrusions with a

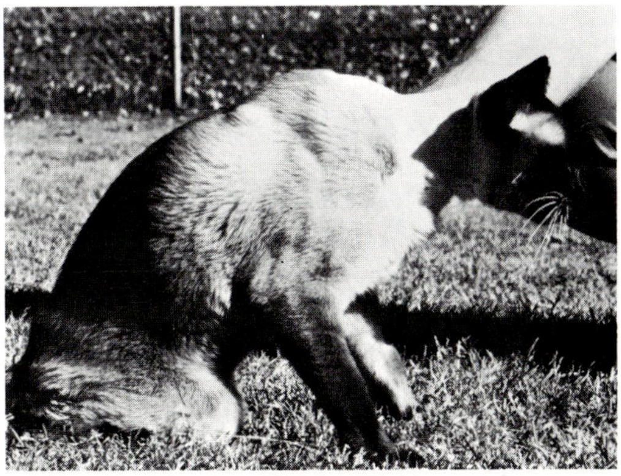

FIGURE 14–108 A 3½-year-old male Siamese cat showed a totally flaccid paraplegia. All segmental reflexes were absent. (Courtesy of Dr. S. F. Swaim, Auburn, Alabama.)

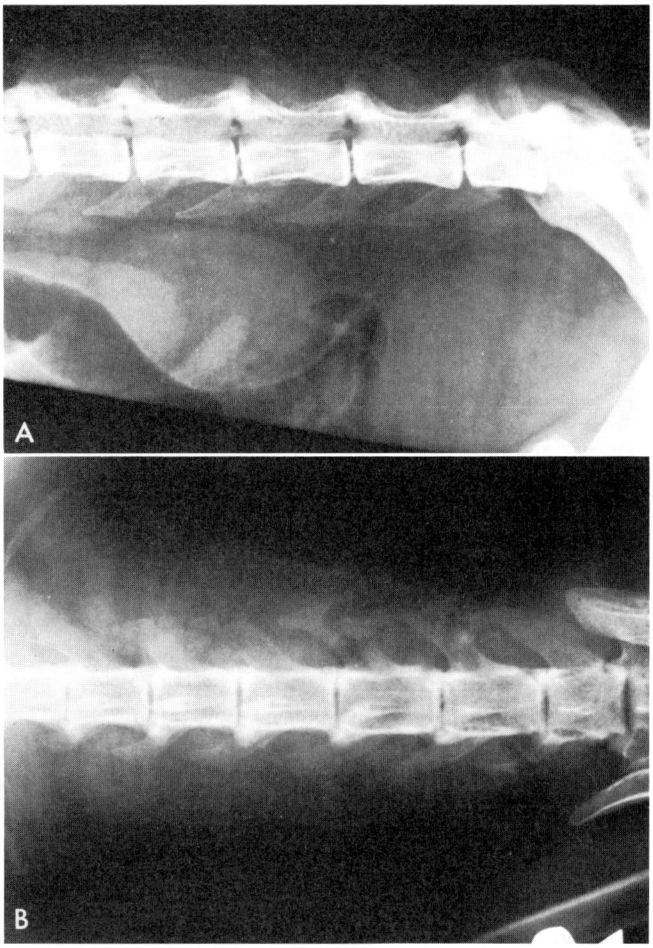

FIGURE 14–109 Normal contrast spinograms. Note the absence of disk or vertebral abnormalities that could result in a compressive myelitis. *A*. Lateral view. *B*. Ventrodorsal view. (Courtesy of Dr. S. F. Swaim, Auburn, Alabama.)

completely ruptured annulus accounted for only 16 of the 91 lesions.[104]

In 1960, King and Smith[105] reported another series of 100 cats, half of which had been included in the previous publication and half of which were new subjects. It was determined from the degree of epiphyseal fusion that the cats in this group were at least 2 years of age. The 135 dorsal protrusions among them were divided into three classes, and their percentage of incidence was recorded as follows:

1. Ruptured annulus, 20.7 per cent.
2. Large partially ruptured annulus, 34.1 per cent.
3. Small partially ruptured annulus, 45.2 per cent.

When all three types of protrusions were included, the cervical incidence was 51.1 per cent and the incidence of those occurring at T10–S1 was 41.5 per cent. When types 1 and 2 only were included, the cervical area accounted for 32; the area of T10–S1 had 36 lesions. When only type 1, or ruptured disks, were determined, the cervical frequency was nine and that of T10–S1 was 14. The incidence of protrusions was greatest at C2–3 and at L4–5. In this series of cats, the disks supported dorsally by the intercapital ligament also were virtually immune to dorsal protrusions.[105]

Later in the same year (1960), King and Smith reported on 60 cats of known age that had been examined for protrusions.[106] These cats were all destroyed for reasons other than the presence of spinal dysfunction. They were placed in four age groups of 1 to 5, 6 to 10, 11 to 14, and 15 to 20 years. The groups were designated young, early-middle-aged, late-middle-aged, and senile, respectively. There were 17 cats in the young category, 19 in the early-middle-aged group, 11 in the late-middle-aged group, and 13 in the senile group.

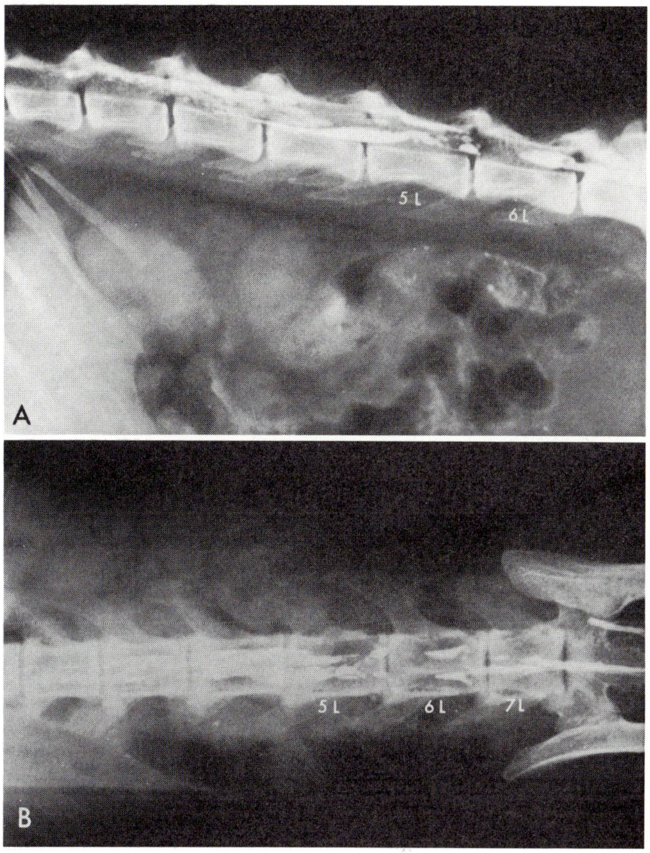

FIGURE 14–110 Myelograms with Pantopaque. Notice the partial obstruction of flow at L5–6 disk. *A,* Lateral view. *B,* Ventrodorsal view. (Courtesy of Dr. S. F. Swaim, Auburn, Alabama.)

It was found that 25 of the 60 cats had a total of 67 disk lesions. None were found in the young cats, but one-third of the early-middle-aged cats had lesions. Half the late-middle-aged and senile cats had them; in fact, 52 of the 67 lesions were found in the senile group. In the latter group, 11 of the 13 cats had multiple lesions, whereas fewer multiple lesions were seen in the younger cats.[106]

It is also interesting to note that the early-middle-aged cats and all but one of the late-middle-aged cats had protrusions in the cervical area. In the senile group there were 24 lesions in the cervical area and 23 in the area of T10–S1.[106]

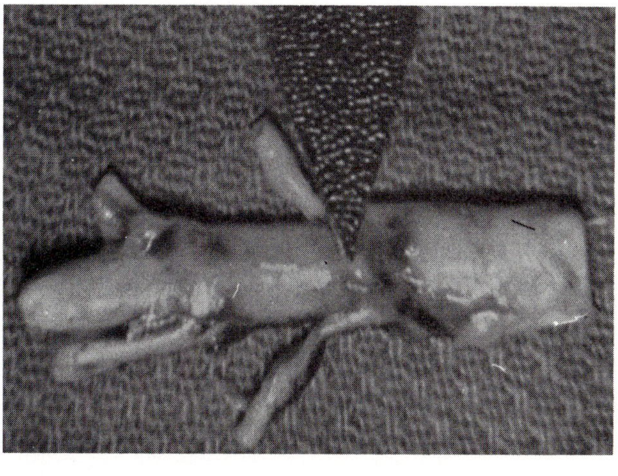

FIGURE 14–111 The cord was markedly compressed by an apparent disk protrusion, characteristic of those seen in the dog; however, microscopic examination demonstrated the lesion to be an extradural lymphosarcoma. The arrow designates the constricted and hemorrhagic spinal cord. (Courtesy of Dr. S. F. Swaim, Auburn, Alabama; diagnosis made by Dr. A. L. Britt, Auburn, Alabama.)

TABLE 14–15 TO SHOW THE RELATIVE INCIDENCE OF THE VARIOUS DEGENERATIONS IN THE THREE REGIONS OF THE VERTEBRAL COLUMN IN 100 ADULT CATS*

	Slight Degeneration No. of Disks	Advanced Degeneration No. of Disks	Very Advanced Degeneration No. of Disks	Partial Destruction No. of Disks	Total Destruction No. of Disks	Ankylosis No. of Disks	Grand Totals
Cervical region C2-T1 (6 disks)...	80	35	10	8	13	4	150
Region T1-T10 (9 disks)...........	110	88	51	33	20	0	302
Region T10-S1 (11 disks)..........	143	35	13	8	0	1	200
Totals..............................	333	158	74	49	33	5	652

*From King, A. S., and Smith, R. N.: Degeneration of the intervertebral disk in the cat. Acta Orthop. Scand. *34*, 139, 1964.

Seventeen ruptured disks occurred, one in each of the middle-aged categories and 15 in five of the senile group. Ten ruptured disks were in the area of T10–S1, two were in the cervical area, and three were in the region of the conjugal ligament.[106]

Butler and Smith[17-19] have continued to study the various aspects of the feline disk in recent years. They observed that maturation, which is a fibrous replacement of the nucleus, is found in 33 per cent of the disks, and degeneration is found in 25 per cent of the disks. These changes were uncommon in young cats, but sharply increased in the 11- to 14-year-old group and progressively increased with age. In Table 14–15, taken directly from King and Smith, the T1–T10 area was the most frequently affected and at an earlier age.

In further studies, these workers have noted that, generally, degeneration and ruptures start in the inner annulus of the disk, instead of in the nucleus, as described by Hansen for the dog. These ruptures progressed to involve the nucleus in cats aged 5 to 18 years, with the gelatinous nucleus pulposus gradually being lost between the lamellae.[17-19] Some of the distinctive features of disk degeneration with age in man, dog, and cat were discussed previously (p. 497).

Preliminary studies to determine the relative response in the dog and cat to experimental spinal compressions have been performed by Avadikian.[3] Based on work done in the dog by Botta,[10] stainless steel Steinmann pins were surgically placed transversely below the spinal cord in the canal. The pin was inserted and secured through the intervertebral foramen on each side of the spinal column. Results indicated that when 30 to 40 per cent of the ventrodorsal diameter of the canal was occupied by the pin, both the dog and cat suffered paraplegia. Study of the reflexes in the postsurgical period demonstrated similar duration of signs and recovery aspects in both species. He concluded that cats are not more tolerant or resistant to spinal compressions than dogs.[3, 10]

DISCUSSION

The work done in England should certainly stimulate further investigation of the intervertebral disk in the cat. It would be interesting to compare the relative size of the epidural spaces at various spinal levels in the dog and cat. Perhaps the cat has a proportionately larger extradural space, so that less spinal cord damage occurs with compressions. It would also be helpful to section the spinal cord adjacent to these protrusions. The large ones should produce evidence of histopathologic damage in the adjacent spinal cord.

Another basic concept that needs clarification is the relative sensitivity to pain of the cat. Is the cat less or more sensitive to pain originating from spinal compressions? Further work on the experimental production of well-controlled spinal compressions for the evaluation of pain and motor dysfunction needs to be done in the cat.

Radiographic examinations would be worthwhile in aged cats. Certainly, carefully executed radiographs would show evidence of spinal degeneration, calcification, calcified protrusions, and narrow disk spaces in the cat.

SUMMARY

The pertinent findings of the works by Butler, King, and Smith on disk protrusions in the cat might be summarized as follows:

1. Disk protrusions are seen frequently in clinically normal cats 6 years of age and older.
2. The incidence of clinical neural dysfunction resulting from disk protrusions in the cat is extremely low, and those cases that have been seen usually have been due to direct trauma. These are similar to the disk protrusion that occurs in nonchondrodystrophoid breeds of dogs.
3. The incidence of all types of protrusions increases with the age of the cat; however, partial ruptures are more frequent in the group 6 to 14 years of age, and complete ruptures are more frequent in the group 15 to 20 years of age.
4. The highest number of protrusions is in the cervical area, the next highest is in the midlumbar area, the next at the thoracolumbar junction, and the lowest in the conjugal ligament area, T2–T9. However, the highest incidence of degeneration in any form is in the T1–T10 area.

The interest in disk diseases in the cat seems to have diminished in the past 10 years. It is felt that the histochemical and histopathologic changes in the cat disk are comparable to similar changes in other species. The peculiar locomotor and behavioral characteristics of the cat may account for the lack of *clinical* disease. The likelihood of malignant lymphoma causing spinal compressions in the cat should be considered in such cases.

REFERENCES

1. Armstrong, J. R.: *Lumbar Disc Lesions,* 2d ed. E. and S. Livingstone Ltd., Edinburgh and London, 1958.
2. Austin, G.: *The Spinal Cord.* Charles C Thomas, Publishers, Springfield, Ill., 1961.
3. Avadikian, R. G.: A comparison of neurological signs seen in experimentally produced paraplegia in the dog and cat. Thesis. (M.S.) Auburn University, Auburn, Alabama, 1973.
4. Bailey, C. S., and Holliday, T. A.: Diseases of the spinal cord. *In* Ettinger, S. J. (ed.) *Textbook of Veterinary Internal Medicine.* W. B. Saunders Co., Philadelphia, 1975, p. 408.
5. Barbaso, E.: Observations on 100 patients with sciatica treated with intraspinal injections of hydrocortisone acetate. Minerva Med. *47,* 1152, 1956.
6. Beadle, O. A.: The intervertebral discs: Observations on their normal and morbid anatomy and relation to certain spinal deformities. Medical Research Council, Special Report Series No. 161. His Majesty's Stationery Office, London, 1931.
7. Bell, C.: *Observations on Injuries of the Spine and of the Thigh Bone.* Thomas Tegg, London, 1931.
8. Böhmung, R.: Die Blulgefassversorgung der Wirbelbandscheiben, das Verhalten des intervertebralen Chordasegments und die Bedeutung Heider für die Bandscheiben-degeneration. Arch. Klin. Chir. *158,* 374, 1930.
9. Bojrab, M. J.: Prophylactic thoracolumbar disk fenestration. *In Current Techniques in Small Animal Surgery.* Lea and Febiger, Philadelphia, 1975, p. 404.
10. Botta, J. A.: *An Evaluation of Experimentally Produced Paraplegia of the Dog.* Thesis, Purdue University, Lafayette, Indiana, 1965.
11. Bradford, F. K., and Spurling, R. C.: *The Intervertebral Disc,* 2d ed. Charles C Thomas, Publishers, Springfield, Ill., 1945.
12. Braund, K. G., Ghosh, P., Taylor, T. K., and Larsen, L. H.: Morphological studies of the canine intervertebral disc. The assignment of the beagle to the achondroplastic classification. Res. Vet. Sci. *19,* 167, 1975.
13. Braund, K. G., Taylor, T. K., Ghosh, P., and Sherwood, A. A.: Lateral spinal decompression in the dog. J. Small Anim. Pract. *17,* 583, 1976.
14. Brodin, H.: Paths of nutrition in articular cartilage and intervertebral discs. Acta Orthop. Scand. *24,* 177, 1955.
15. Brooks, E. L.: A preliminary report on the use of the Brooks paralysis carriage. Vet. Med. *46,* 241, 1951.
16. Butler, W. F.: Age changes in ruptured intervertebral discs. Res. Vet. Sci. *9,* 130, 1968.
17. Butler, W. F., and Smith, R. N.: Age changes in the intervertebral disc. Res. Vet. Sci. *6,* 280, 1965.
18. Butler, W. F., and Smith, R. N.: The nucleus pulposus of the intervertebral disc in newborn cats. Res. Vet. Sci. *5,* 71, 1964.
19. Butler, W. F.: Metachromasia and alcian blue staining of the intervertebral disc of the cat. J. Anat. *102,* 301, 1968.
20. Calve, J.: Le calcification du nucleus pulposus intervertébral. Rev. Orthop. *18,* 782, 1931.
21. Chrisman, C. L., Burt, J. K., Wood, P. K., and Johnson, E. W.: Electromyography in small animal clinical neurology. J.A.V.M.A *160,* 311, 1972.
22. Cloward, R. B.: The treatment of ruptured lumbar intervertebral discs; criteria for spinal fusion. Am. J. Surg. *86,* 145, 1953.
23. Cloward, R. B.: The clinical significance of the sinuvertebral nerve of the cervical spine in

relation to the cervical disc syndrome. J. Neurol. Neurosurg. Psychiatry *23,* 321, 1961.
24. Conrad, C. R.: Radiographic examination of the central nervous system. *In* Ettinger, S. J. (ed.): *Textbook of Veterinary Internal Medicine.* W. B. Saunders Co., Philadelphia, 1975, p. 333.
25. Cottle, L. W.: Traction for posterior paralysis in the dog. Mod. Vet. Pract. *43,* 74, 1962.
26. Cottle, L. W.: The use of traction for lumbosacral disorders of the dog. South Vet. *4,* 9, 1967.
27. Cottle, L. W.: Traction in the treatment of canine spinal disorders. J. Am. Anim. Hosp. Assoc. *8,* 332, 1972.
28. Crafoord, C., Hientoon, T., Lindblom, K., and Olsson, S. E.: Spinal cord compression caused by a protruded thoracic disc. Acta Orthop. Scand. *28,* 103, 1958.
29. Dandy, W. E.: Improved localization and treatment of ruptured intervertebral disks. J.A.M.A. *120,* 605, 1942.
30. Dandy, W. E.: Loose cartilage from intervertebral disk simulating tumor of the spinal cord. Arch. Surg. *19,* 660, 1929.
31. David, T.: Thoracolumbar hemilaminectomy in the dog using a power skull trephine. Vet. Med. Small Anim. Clin. *71,* 477, 1976.
32. Deecke, L., and Tator, C. H.: Neurophysiological assessment of afferent and efferent conduction in the injured spinal cord of monkeys. J. Neurosurg. *39,* 65, 1973.
33. de Lahunta, A., and Alexander, J. W.: Ischemic myelopathy secondary to presumed fibrocartilaginous embolism in nine dogs. J. Am. Anim. Hosp. Assoc. *12,* 37, 1976.
34. Dexler, H.: Beitrage zur Pathologie und pathologischen Anatomie der Compressionsmyelitis des Hundes-Osterreich. Z. Wissenschaftliche *7,* 1, 1896.
35. Dohn, D. F.: Anterior interbody fusion for treatment of cervical disk conditions. J.A.M.A. *197,* 897, 1966.
36. *Dorland's Medical Dictionary,* 25th ed., W. B. Saunders Co., Philadelphia, 1974.
37. Estrado, E.: Methocarbamol in the control of severe skeletal muscle spasms in small animals. J.A.V.M.A. *137,* 585, 1960.
38. Fankhauser, R.: Über die sogen. Dackellahmung. Schweiz. Arch. Tierheildk. *90,* 143, 1948.
39. Fittipaldi, S. A., and DeCamp, D.: Use of physostigmine and atropine in neuromuscular dysfunction in small animals. Vet. Med. *45,* 438, 1950.
40. Flo, G. L., and Brinker, W. O.: Lateral fenestration of thoracolumbar discs. J. Am. Anim. Hosp. Assoc. *11,* 619, 1975.
41. Funkquist, B.: Cervical myelography with a water-soluble contrast medium. An experimental study in dogs. Acta Radiol. *56,* 257, 1961.
42. Funkquist, B.: Decompressive laminectomy for cervical disk protrusion in the dog. Acta Vet. Scand. *3,* 88, 1962.
43. Funkquist, B.: Decompressive laminectomy in thoracolumbar disc protrusion with paraplegia in the dog. J. Small Anim. Pract. *11,* 445, 1970.
44. Funkquist, B.: Investigations of the therapeutic and prophylactic effects of disc removal in cases of thoracolumbar herniated discs in dogs. Unpublished data.
45. Funkquist, B.: Lumbar subarachnoid puncture and injection in the dog. Nord. Vet. Med. *12,* 805, 1960.
46. Funkquist, B.: Thoraco-lumbar disk protrusion with severe cord compression in the dog. I. Clinical and patho-anatomic observations with special reference to the rate of development of the symptoms of motor loss. II. Clinical observations with special reference to the prognosis in conservative treatment. III. Treatment by decompressive laminectomy. Acta Vet. Scand. *3,* 1962.
47. Funkquist, B.: Thoraco-lumbar myelography with water-soluble contrast mediums in dogs. I. Technique of myelography; side-effects and complications. II. Appearance of the myelogram in disk protrusion and its relation to functional disturbances and patho-anatomic changes in the epidural space. J. Small Anim. Pract. *3,* 53, 1962.
48. Funkquist, B., and Obel, N.: Effect on the spinal cord of subarachnoid injection of water soluble contrast medium. An experimental study in dogs. Acta Radiol. *56,* 449, 1961.
49. Funkquist, B., and Obel, N.: Tonic muscle spasms and blood pressure changes following the subarachnoid injection of contrast media. An experimental study in dogs with injection of Kontrast U and mixtures of Kontrast U and Xylocaine. Acta Radiol. *53,* 337, 1960.
50. Funkquist, B., and Schantz, B.: Influence of extensive laminectomy on the shape of the spinal canal. Acta Orthop. Scand. Suppl. *56,* 1962.
51. Gage, E. D., and Hoerlein, B. F.: Hemilaminectomy and dorsal laminectomy for relieving compressions of the spinal cord in the dog. J.A.V.M.A. *152,* 351, 1968.
52. Gage, E. D.: Disc syndrome in the large breed dog. Anim. Hosp. *5,* 93, 1969.
53. Gage, E. D.: Incidence of clinical disc disease in the dog. J. Am. Anim. Hosp. Assoc. *11,* 135, 1975.
54. Gage, E. D.: Modifications in dorsolateral hemilaminectomy and disc fenestrations in the dog. J. Am. Anim. Hosp. Assoc. *11,* 407, 1975.
55. Garrick, J. G., and Sullivan, C. R.: A technic of performing diskography in dogs. Proc. Mayo Clin. *39,* 270, 1964.
56. Geary, J.: Personal communication.
57. Gendreau, C., Stowater, J., and Menhusen, M.: Surgical treatment of thoracolumbar disc herniation. Vet. Med. Small Anim. Clin. *71,* 1051, 1976.
58. Ghosh, P., Taylor, T. K. F., Yarroll, J. M., Braund, K. G., and Larsen, L. H.: Genetic factors in the maturation of the canine intervertebral disc. Res. Vet. Sci. *19,* 304, 1975.
59. Ghosh, P., Taylor, T. K. F., Braund, K. G., and Larsen, L. H.: The collagenous and non-collagenous proteins of the canine intervertebral disc and their variation with age, spinal level, and breed. Gerontology *22,* 124, 1976.
60. Gilpin, G. N.: Evaluation of three techniques of ventral decompression of the cervical spinal cord in the dog. J.A.V.M.A. *168,* 325–328, 1976.
61. Goggins, J. E., Li, A. S., and Franti, C. E.: Ca-

nine intervertebral disk diseases; characterization by age, sex, breed, and anatomical site of involvement. Am. J. Vet. Res. *9,* 1687, 1970.
62. Goldie, I.: Intervertebral disc changes after discography. Acta Chir. Scand. *113,* 438, 1957.
63. Goodman, L., and Gilman, A.: *The Pharmacological Basis of Therapeutics.* The Macmillan Co., New York, 1941.
64. Greene, C. E.: An experimental model for spinal cord compression simulating intervertebral disc disease in the dog. Thesis (M.S.), Auburn University, Auburn, Alabama, 1976.
65. Greene, C. E., and Higgins, R. J.: Fibrocartilaginous emboli as the cause of ischemic myelopathy in a dog. Cornell Vet. *66,* 131, 1976.
66. Greene, J. E.: Surgical intervention for paraplegia due to herniation of the nucleus pulposus. No. Am. Vet. *32,* 411, 1951.
67. Griffiths, I. R.: A syndrome produced by dorsolateral "explosions" of the cervical intervertebral discs. Vet. Rec. *87,* 737, 1970.
68. Griffiths, I. R.: Some aspects of the pathogenesis and diagnosis of lumbar disk protrusion in the dog. J. Small Anim. Pract. *13,* 439, 1972.
69. Griffiths, I. R.: Some aspects of the pathology and pathogenesis of the myelopathy caused by disc protrusions in the dog. J. Neurol. Neurosurg. Psychiatry *35,* 403, 1972.
70. Griffiths, I. R.: The extensive myelopathy of intervertebral disc protrusions in dogs (ascending syndrome). J. Small Anim. Pract. *13,* 425, 1972.
71. Griffiths, I. R.: Spinal cord infarction due to emboli arising from the intervertebral discs in the dog. J. Comp. Pathol. *83,* 225, 1973.
72. Griffiths, I. R., Barker, J., and Palmer, A. C.: Cholesterol masses in association with spinal cord infarction due to intervertebral disc emboli. Acta Neuropathol. *33,* 85, 1975.
73. Haley, J. C., and Perry, J. H.: Protrusions of intervertebral discs. Am. J. Surg. *80,* 394, 1950.
74. Hansen, H. J.: A pathologic-anatomical interpretation of disc degeneration in dogs. Acta Orthop. Scand. *20,* 280, 1951.
75. Hansen, H. J.: A pathologic-anatomical study on disc degeneration in dogs. Acta Orthop. Scand. Suppl. *11,* 1952.
76. Hansen, H. J., and Olsson, S. E.: The indications for disc fenestration in dogs. Proc. 15th Int. Vet. Cong., Stockholm, Aug. 9–15, 1953.
77. Hansen, H. J.: Pathogenesis of disc degeneration and rupture. *In* Pettit, G. O. (ed.): *Intervertebral Disk Protrusions in the Dog.* Appleton-Century-Crofts, New York, 1966, p. 24.
78. Hansen, J. W.: Traction for lumbar disk herniation. J.A.M.A. *167,* 368, 1958 (Abstr.).
79. Harmon, P. H.: Saline injection test applied to lower lumbar disk degeneration: Comparison to Pantopaque myelography. Ann. Surg. *156,* 767, 1962.
80. Henry, W. B., Jr.: Dorsal decompressive laminectomy in the treatment of thoracolumbar disc disease. J. Am. Anim. Hosp. Assoc. *11,* 627, 1975.
81. Higley, H. G.: *The Intervertebral Disc.* National Chiropractic Assoc., Webster City, Iowa, 1960.
82. Hoerlein, B. F.: Intervertebral disc protrusions in the dog. A clinical and pathological study. Thesis, Cornell University, Ithaca, New York, 1952.
83. Hoerlein, B. F.: Intervertebral disc protrusions in the dog. I. Incidence and pathological lesions. II. Symptomatology and clinical diagnosis. III. Radiological diagnosis. Am. J. Vet. Res. *19,* 260, 1953.
84. Hoerlein, B. F.: The treatment of intervertebral disc protrusions in the dog. Proc. Am. Vet. Med. Assoc. *206,* June 23–26, 1952.
85. Hoerlein, B. F.: Further evaluation of the treatment of disc protrusion paraplegia in the dog. J.A.V.M.A. *129,* 495, 1956.
86. Hoerlein, B. F.: Traumatic lesions of the canine spine (Pt. 1 and 2). Mod. Vet. Pract. *39,* 24, 31, 1958.
87. Hoerlein, B. F.: The modern treatment of traumatic spinal compressions in the dog. Canad. Vet. J. *1,* 216, 1960.
88. Hoerlein, B. F.: Cervical spinal surgery—ventral and dorsal approach. Proc. Am. Vet. Med. Assoc. *103,* July 28–Aug. 1, 1962.
89. Hoerlein, B. F.: *Canine Neurology, Diagnosis and Treatment,* 2d ed. W. B. Saunders Co., Philadelphia, 1971.
90. Hoerlein, B. F.: Various surgical methods for repair of intervertebral disc protrusions. Anim. Hosp. *4,* 12, 1968.
91. Hoerlein, B. F., and Spano, J. S.: Nonneurological complications following decompressive spinal cord surgery. Arch. Am. Coll. Vet. Surg. *4,* 11, 75.
92. Horwitz, T.: Lesions of the intervertebral disc and ligamentum flavum of lumbar vertebrae; an anatomic study of 75 human cadavers. Surgery *6,* 410, 1939.
93. Hubert, J. D., Ectors, M., Ketelbant-Balasse, P., and Flament-Durand, J.: Fibrocartilaginous venous and arterial emboli from the nucleus pulposus in the anterior spinal system. Eur. Neurol. *11,* 164, 1974.
94. Hutyra, F., Marek, J., and Manninger, R.: *Special Pathology and Therapeutics of the Diseases of Domestic Animals,* 5th ed. Alexander Eger, Inc., Chicago, 1946.
95. Innes, J. R. M., and Saunders, L. Z.: *Comparative Neuropathology.* Academic Press, New York, 1962.
96. Inmann, V. T., and Saunders, J. B. de C. M.: Anatomico-physiological aspects of injuries to the intervertebral disc. J. Bone Joint Surg. *29,* 461, 1947.
97. Jadeson, W. J.: Rehabilitation of dogs with intervertebral disc lesions by physical therapy methods. J.A.V.M.A. *138,* 411, 1961.
98. Jakob, H.: Die Paraplegic resp. Paresis der Nochhand beim Dachshunde—eine Folge seiner ungunstigen Bauart. Munch. Tierartz. Wochenschr. *54,* 305, 1910.
99. Joest, E.: *Spezielle pathologische Anatomie der Haustiere.* Schoetz, Berlin, 1921.
100. Joshua, J. O.: The canine spine. J. Small Anim. Pract. *4,* 173, 1963.
101. Jurkovic, I., and Iben, E.: Fatal myelomalacia caused by massive fibrocartilaginous venous emboli from nucleus pulposus. Acta Neuropathol. *15,* 284, 1970.
102. Keyes, D. C., and Compere, E. L.: The normal

and pathological physiology of the nucleus pulposus of the intervertebral disk. J. Bone Joint Surg. *14,* 897, 1932.
103. King, A. S., and Smith, R. N.: A comparison of the anatomy of the intervertebral disc in dog and man with reference to herniation of the nucleus pulposus. Brit. Vet. J. *111,* 135, 1955.
104. King, A. S., and Smith, R. N.: Degeneration of the intervertebral disc in the cat. Acta Orthop. Scand. *34,* 139, 1964.
105. King, A. S., and Smith, R. N.: Disc protrusions in the cat: Distribution of dorsal protrusions along the vertebral column. Acta Orthop. Scand. *72,* 335, 1960.
106. King, A. S., and Smith, R. N.: Disc protrusions in the cat: Age incidence of dorsal protrusions. Acta Orthop. Scand. *72,* 381, 1960.
107. Knecht, C. D.: The effect of delayed hemilaminectomy in the treatment of intervertebral disc protrusion in dogs. J. Am. Anim. Hosp. Assoc. *6,* 71, 1970.
108. Knecht, C. D.: Results of surgical treatment for thoracolumbar disc protrusion. J. Small Anim. Pract. *13,* 449, 1972.
109. LaRocca, H., and MacNab, I.: The laminectomy membrane studies in its evolution, characteristics, effects, and prophylaxis in dogs. J. Bone Joint Surg. *56B,* 545, 1974.
110. Lecht, L., Bostic, J. B., and Stevenson, R.: Clinical use of selenium-tocopherol in treatment of orthopedic cases. Vet. Med. Small Anim. Clin. *63,* 493, 1968.
111. Lee, D. G.: The arterial supply of the intervertebral disk of the domestic cat (*Felix domestica*) from fetal life to old age. Am. J. Vet. Res. *23,* 1072, 1962.
112. Leighton, R. L.: A cart for small dogs with posterior paralysis. Vet. Med. Small Anim. Clin. *61,* 554, 1966.
113. Leonard, E. P.: *Orthopedic Surgery of the Dog and Cat,* 2d ed. W. B. Saunders Co., Philadelphia, 1971.
114. Lescure, F.: Treatment of paraplegia by epidural corticosteroids. Rev. Med. Vet. *120,* 519, 1969 (Abstr. Mod. Vet. Pract. Int. Vet. Ref. Service, 1970, F5-676).
115. Lindblad, G., Ljunggren, G., and Olsson, S. E.: On spinal cord compression in the dog; an angiographic study. Adv. Small Anim. Pract. *3,* 121, 1962.
116. Lindblom, K., and Hultquist, G.: Absorption of protruded disc material. J. Bone Joint Surg. *32A,* 557, 1950.
117. Lindgren, S.: Some problems concerning herniated intervertebral disc from the clinical point of view. J.A.M.A. *142,* 445, 1950.
118. Lippincott, C. L.: Use of the micrometer trephine in surgical treatment of the intervertebral disc syndrome. Vet. Med. Small Anim. Clin. *67,* 643, 1972.
119. Love, J. G.: Removal of protruded intervertebral disk without laminectomy. Proc. Mayo Clin. *14,* 800, 1939.
120. Love, J. G., and Walsh, M. N.: Intraspinal protrusions of intervertebral disks. Arch. Surg. *40,* 454, 1940.
121. Lumb, W. V.: Closed-circuit halothane anesthesia in the dog. J.A.V.M.A. *123,* 218, 1959.
122. Mantel, N., and Haenszel, W.: Statistical aspects of the analysis of data from retrospective studies of disease. J. Natl. Cancer Inst. *22*:719, 1959.
123. Martin, J. E., LeGrange, W. E., Fielder, F. G., Skelley, J. F., and Arnold, M. W.: The use of cortisone and hydrocortisone in veterinary medicine. Proc. Am. Vet. Med. Assoc. *115,* Aug. 23–26, 1954.
124. Martin, J. G.: The feasibility of delayed surgery in intervertebral disc protrusions causing paraplegia or paresis. 36th Annual Meeting, Am. Anim. Hosp. Assoc., 409, 1969.
125. Martin, S. H., and Bloedel, J. R.: Evaluation of experimental spinal cord injury using cortical evoked potentials. J. Neurosurg. *39,* 75, 1973.
126. McGrath, J. T.: Spinal paralysis of the dog. No. Am. Vet. *32,* 700, 1951.
127. McGrath, J. T.: *Neurologic Examination of the Dog,* 2d ed. Lea and Febiger, Philadelphia, 1960.
128. Mendenhall, H. V., Litwak, P., Yturraspe, D. J., Ingram, J. T., and Lumb, W. V.: Aggressive pharmacologic and surgical treatment of spinal cord injuries in dogs and cats. J.A.V.M.A. *168,* 1026, 1976.
129. Miller, M. E., Christensen, G. C., and Evans, H. E.: *Anatomy of the Dog.* W. B. Saunders Co., Philadelphia, 1964.
130. Miller, R. M., and Kind, R. E.: Phenylbutazone toxicity. Mod. Vet. Pract. *43,* 69, 1962.
131. Milnes, D. M.: Post-mortem findings in paraplegia and paraparesis in the dog. Vet. Rec. *72,* 511, 1960.
132. Milnes, D. M.: Nervous diseases of cats. Vet. Rec. *71,* 932, 1959.
133. Mixter, W. J., and Barr, J. S.: Rupture of the intervertebral disk with involvement of the spinal canal. New Engl. J. Med. *211,* 210, 1934.
134. Moltzen, H.: Treatment of spinal disorders by manipulation. J. Small Anim. Pract. *4,* 265, 1963.
135. Moltzen, H.: Manipulation as a method of therapy for spinal disorders in dogs and cats. J. Am. Anim. Hosp. Assoc. 7, 242, 1971.
136. Moody, P. W.: Suspected intervertebral disc protrusion in a dachshund. Vet. Rec. *74,* 420, 1962.
137. Munro, D.: Diagnosis of posterior herniation of lumbar intervertebral disc. New Engl. J. Med. *232,* 149, 1945.
138. Northway, R. B.: A ventrolateral approach to lumbar intervertebral disc fenestration. Vet. Med. Small Anim. Clin. *60,* 884, 1965.
139. O'Connel, F. B., Jr., and Gardner, W. J.: Metabolism in paraplegia. J.A.M.A. *153,* 706, 1953.
140. O'Doherty, D. S., and Shields, C. D.: Methocarbamol—new agent in treatment of neurological and neuromuscular diseases. J.A.M.A. *167,* 160, 1958.
141. Odom, G. L., Finney, W., and Woodhall, B.: Cervical disk lesions. J.A.M.A. *166,* 23, 1958.
142. Ogilvie, F. B., and Sutter, M. D.: Clinical uses of butazolidin. Vet. Med. *52,* 492, 1957.
143. Olsson, S. E.: Röntgenalogiska studier och operative Behandling av s. k. enchondrosis intervertebralis hos hund. Nord. Vet. Med. *2,* 1074, 1950.
144. Olsson, S.-E.: On disc protrusion in dogs. Acta Orthop. Scand. Suppl. *8,* 1951.
145. Olsson, S.-E.: Observations concerning disc fen-

estration in dogs. Acta Orthop. Scand. *20,* 349, 1951.
146. Olsson, S.-E., and Hansen, H.-J.: Cervical disc protrusion in the dog. J.A.V.M.A. *121,* 361, 1952.
147. Olsson, S.-E.: Studien über die Bandscheibenprotrusion beim Hund unter Spezieller Berücksichtigung der Chirurgishen Therapie. Wien. Tierärztl. Monatsschr. *44,* 329, 1957.
148. Olsson, S.-E.: The dynamic factor in spinal cord compression. A study on dogs with special reference to cervical disc protrusions. J. Neurosurg. *15,* 308, 1958.
149. Olsson, S.-E.: Diskbrack hos Hund. Medlemsbl. Sv. Vet. Förbund. *12,* 149, 1960.
150. Olsson, S.-E.: Disorders of the vertebral column and spinal cord. *In* Catcott, E. J. (ed.): *Canine Surgery.* American Veterinary Publications, Inc., Santa Barbara, Calif., 1965.
151. Paatsama, S., Rissanen, P., and Rokkanen, P.: Effect of estradiol, testosterone, cortisone acetate, somatotropin, thyrotropin, and parathyroid hormone on the lumbar intervertebral disc in growing dogs. J. Small Anim. Pract. *10,* 351, 1969.
152. Parker, A. J.: Surgical approach to the cervico thoracic junction. J. Am. Anim. Hosp. Assoc. *9,* 374, 1973.
153. Parker, A. J., and Smith, C. W.: Functional recovery from spinal cord trauma following delayed incision of spinal meninges in dogs. Res. Vet. Sci. *18,* 110, 1975.
154. Paul, E., and Wong, D.: Selenium-tocopherol therapy for lameness. Vet. Med. Small Anim. Clin. *61,* 726, 1966.
155. Paulson, S., Sylven, B., Hirsch, C., and Snellman, O.: Biophysical and physiological investigations on cartilage and other mesenchymal tissues. III. The diffusion rate of various substances in normal bovine nucleus pulposus. Biochem. Biophys. Acta *7,* 207, 1951.
156. Pettit, G. D.: The surgical treatment of cervical disc protrusions in the dog. Cornell Vet. *50,* 259, 1960.
157. Pettit, G. D., and Whitaker, R. P.: Hemilaminectomy for cervical disc protrusions in a dog. J.A.V.M.A. *143,* 379, 1963.
158. Pettit, G.: *Intervertebral Disc Protrusion in the Dog.* Appleton-Century-Crofts, New York, 1966.
159. Pommer, A.: Tierheilk und Tierzucht. Stang. Wirth. *11,* 134, 1937.
160. Popovic, N. A., Vander Ark, G., and Kempe, L.: Ventral approach for surgical treatment of cervical disk disease in the dog. Am. J. Vet. Res. *32,* 1155, 1971.
161. Prata, R. G., and Stoll, S. G.: Ventral decompression and fusion for the treatment of cervical disc disease in the dog. J. Am. Anim. Hosp. Assoc. *9,* 462, 1973.
162. Priester, W. A., and Mantel, N.: Occurrence of tumors in domestic animals. Data from 12 United States and Canadian colleges of veterinary medicine. J. Natl. Cancer Inst. *47,* 1333, 1971.
163. Priester, W. A.: Canine intervertebral disk disease—occurrence by age, breed, and sex among 8117 cases. Theriogenology *6,* 293, 1976.
164. Puschel, J.: Der Wassergehalt normaler und degeneriertez Zwischenwirbelscheiben. Beitr. Pathol. Anat. *84,* 123, 1930.
165. Ramsey, F. A.: Surgical correction of calcified lumbar intervertebral disk in a dachshund—a case report. J.A.V.M.A. *137,* 540, 1960.
166. Raney, A. A., and Raney, R.: A consideration of etiology in the development of the ruptured intervertebral disc. Calif. J. Med. *68,* 65, 1948.
167. Redding, R. S., and Braund, K.: Unpublished data.
168. Redding, R. W.: Laminectomy in the dog. Amer. J. Vet. Res. *12,* 123, 1951.
169. Riser, W. H.: Posterior paralysis associated with intervertebral disc protrusion in the dog. No. Am. Vet. *27,* 633, 1946.
170. Roofe, P. G.: Innervation of annulus fibrosus and posterior longitudinal ligament. Arch. Neurol. Psychol. *44,* 100, 1940.
171. Ross, G. E.: Surgical treatment of intervertebral disc disease. 36th Annual Meeting, Am. Anim. Hosp. Assoc., 409, 1969.
172. Rothermich, N. O.: An extended study of indomethacin. I. Clinical therapy. J.A.M.A. *195,* 531, 1966.
173. Rothermich, N. O.: An extended study of indomethacin. I. Clinical therapy. J.A.M.A. *195,* 1102, 1966.
174. Rowe, E. T., and Christian, C. W.: Clinical experiences with use of methocarbamol to control muscle spasms in the treatment of spinal lesions in dogs. Vet. Med. Small Anim. Clin. *65,* 1082, 1970.
175. Rowe, N. F.: Electromyographic study of the paraspinal muscles of the dog in clinical intervertebral disc disease. Thesis (M.S.), Auburn University, Auburn, Alabama, 1975.
176. Russell, W. W., and Griffiths, R. C.: Recurrence of cervical disc syndrome in surgically and conservatively treated dogs. J.A.V.M.A. *153,* 1412, 1968.
177. Saunders, E. C.: Treatment of the canine intervertebral disc syndrome with chymopapain. J.A.V.M.A. *145,* 893, 1964.
178. Schirmer, R. G.: Ultrasound therapy for intervertebral disc syndrome. *In* Kirk, R. W. (ed.): *Current Veterinary Therapy, II.* W. B. Saunders Co., Philadelphia, 1964.
179. Schirmer, R. C.: Ultrasound therapy. *In* Kirk, R. W. (ed.): *Current Veterinary Therapy III.* W. B. Saunders Co., Philadelphia, 1968.
180. Schlotthauer, C. F.: The incidence and pathology of various lesions of the nervous system. No. Am. Vet. *21,* 551, 1940.
181. Schmorl, G.: Zur pathologischen Anatomie der Virbelsaule. Klin. Wochenschr. *8,* 1243, 1929.
182. Schnelle, G. B.: *Radiology in Canine Practice.* North American Veterinarian, Inc., Evanston, Ill., 1950.
183. Scoville, W. B., and Silver, D.: Results of Scoville and Silver's questionnaire on chymopapain (Letter to the Editor). J. Neurosurg. *42,* 487, 1975.
184. Seemann, C. W.: Lateral approach for thoracolumbar disc fenestration. Mod. Vet. Pract. *49,* 73, July 1968.
185. Shenkin, H. A., Goluboff, B., and Haft, H.: The use of mannitol for the reduction of intracran-

ial pressure in intracranial surgery. J. Neurosurg. *19,* 897, 1962.

186. Short, T. R.: Experiences with a mobile support for paraplegic dogs. J.A.V.M.A. *152,* 973, 1968.
187. Smith, R. N., and King, A. S.: Protrusion of the intervertebral disk in the dog. Vet. Rec. *66,* 2, 1954.
188. Smith, L.: Enzyme dissolution of the nucleus pulposus in humans. J.A.M.A. *187,* 137, 1964.
189. Smith, R. N.: Anatomy and physiology. *In* Pettit, G. D. (ed.): *Intervertebral Disc Protrusion in the Dog.* Appleton-Century-Crofts, New York, 1966.
190. Smith, L., Garvin, P. J., Gesler, R. M., and Jennings, R. B.: Enzyme dissolution of the nucleus pulposus. Nature *198,* 1311, 1963.
191. Spurling, R. G., and Grantham, E. G.: Neurologic picture of herniation of the nucleus pulposus in the lower part of the lumbar region. Arch. Surg. *40,* 375, 1940.
192. Spurling, R. G., and Segerberg, L. H.: Lateral intervertebral disk lesions in the lower cervical region. J.A.M.A. *151,* 354, 1953.
193. Stowater, J. L., Menhusen, M. J., and Gendreau, C. L.: Canine myelography with Skiodan. Part 1: Indications and interpretations. Vet. Med. Small Anim. Clin. *71,* 1207, 1976.
194. Sussman, B. J.: Inadequacies and hazards of chymopapain injections as treatment for intervertebral disc disease. J. Neurosurg. *42,* 389, 1975.
195. Swaim, S. F.: Ventral decompression of the cervical spinal cord in the dog. J.A.V.M.A. *162,* 276, 1973.
196. Swaim, S. F.: Ventral decompression of the cervical spinal cord in the dog. J.A.V.M.A. *164,* 491, 1974.
197. Swaim, S. F.: Bilateral hemilaminectomy: A technique for extensive spinal decompression. Auburn Vet. *32,* 62, 1976.
198. Swaim, S. F.: A rongeuring technique for performing thoracolumbar hemilaminectomies. Vet. Med. Small Anim. Clin. *71,* 172, 1976.
199. Swaim, S. F., and Vandevelde, M.: Clinical and histopathologic evaluation of bilateral hemilaminectomy and deep dorsal laminectomy for extensive spinal cord decompression in the dog. J.A.V.M.A. (in press).
200. Swarts, R. J., and Jefferies, J. C.: The use of a truss in paraplegia of the dog. Vet. Med. *50,* 319, 1955.
201. Tarlov, I. M., Klinger, H., and Vitale, S.: Spinal cord compression studies. I. Experimental techniques to produce acute and gradual compression. II. Time limits for recovery after acute compression in dogs. III. Time limits for recovery after gradual compression in dogs. Arch. Neurol. Psych. *70,* 813, 1950; *71,* 271, 1954; *71,* 588, 1954.
202. Tarlov, I. M.: *Spinal Cord Compression, Mechanism of Paralysis and Treatment.* Charles C Thomas, Publishers, Springfield, Ill., 1957.
203. Tarlov, I. M.: Acute spinal cord compression paralysis. J. Neurosurg. *36,* 10, 1972.
204. Tator, C. H., and Deecke, L.: Value of normothermic perfusion, hypothermic perfusion, and durotomy in the treatment of experimental acute spinal cord trauma. J. Neurosurg. *39,* 52, 1973.
205. Taylor, T. K. F., Ghosh, P., Braund, K. G., Sutherland, J. M., and Sherwood, A. A.: The effect of spinal fusion on intervertebral disc composition: An experimental study. J. Surg. Res. *21,* 91, 1976.
206. Trotter, E. J.: Canine intervertebral disk disease. *In* Kirk, R. W. (ed.): *Current Veterinary Therapy V.* W. B. Saunders Co., Philadelphia, 1974, p. 666.
207. Trotter, E. J., Brasmer, T. H., and de Lahunta, A.: Modified deep dorsal laminectomy in the dog. Cornell Vet. *65,* 402, 1975.
208. Trotter, E. J.: Modified dorsal laminectomy and selective regional spinal cord hypothermia in the treatment of thoracolumbar disk disease. *In* Bojrab, M. J. (ed.): *Current Techniques in Small Animal Surgery I.* Lea and Febiger, Philadelphia, 1975, p. 406.
209. Uebermuth, H.: Die Bedeutung der Altersveranderungen der menschichen Bandscheiben für die Pathologie der Virbelsaule. Arch. Klin. Chir. *156,* 567, 1929.
210. Vaughan, L. C.: Studies on intervertebral disk protrusion in the dog. I. Etiology and pathogenesis. II. Diagnosis of the disease. III. Pathological features. IV. Treatment. Brit. Vet. J. *114,* 105, 1968.
211. Watts, C., Hutchinson, G., Stern, J., and Clark, K.: Comparison of intervertebral disc disease treatment by chymopapain injection and open surgery. J. Neurosurg. *42,* 397, 1975.
212. Whalen, R. F.: Lumbar disc hernia. Illinois Vet. *15,* 10, 1972.
213. Widdowson, W. L.: The effects of chymopapain on the normal and clinically protruded intervertebral disc and its related structures in the dog. Thesis, Auburn University, Auburn, Alabama, 1966.
214. Widdowson, W. L.: Effects of chymopapain in the intervertebral disc of the dog. J.A.V.M.A. *150,* 608, 1967.
215. Wilcox, K. R.: Conservative treatment of thoracolumbar intervertebral disc disease in the dog. J.A.V.M.A. *147,* 1458, 1965.
216. Wise, B. L., and Chater, N.: Value of hypertonic mannitol solution in decreasing brain mass and lowering cerebrospinal fluid pressure. J. Neurosurg. *19,* 1038, 1962.
217. Woodhall, B. J.: The study of ground substance in intervertebral disk degeneration. J. Bone Joint Surg. *36A,* 1112, 1954.
218. Yturraspe, D. J., and Lumb, W. V.: A dorsolateral muscle-separating approach for thoracolumbar intervertebral disk fenestration in the dog. J.A.V.M.A. *162,* 1037, 1973.
219. Zaki, F. A., Prata, R. G., and Kay, W. J.: Necrotizing myelopathy in five Great Danes. J.A.V.M.A. *165,* 1080, 1974.
220. Zaki, F. A., and Prata, R. C.: Necrotizing myelopathy secondary to embolization of herniated intervertebral disk material in the dog. J.A.V.M.A. *169,* 222, 1976.
221. Zaki, F. A., Prata, R. C., and Werner, L. L.: Necotizing myelopathy in a cat. J.A.V.M.A. *169,* 228, 1976.

CHAPTER 15

SPINAL FRACTURES, LUXATIONS, AND FUSIONS

SECTION 1
FRACTURES AND LUXATIONS

Spinal fractures and luxations in the dog are often seen in clinical practice. This can be explained by the aggressiveness or preoccupation of dogs in respect to autos. Many dogs like to chase autos and bite at the wheels, and finally they are struck down. Others are so preoccupied with other matters, such as hunting or crossing a street to greet the owner or another dog, that they do not even see the vehicle.

Generally, spinal fractures and luxations occur at the junctions of movable and stable spinal segments. Such areas are close to the skull or the thorax in the cervical portion, and to the pelvis or thorax in the lumbar portion. The thoracic vertebrae comprise the most immobile section of the spinal column, and probably the most frequent site of spinal fracture in the dog is the terminal thoracic vertebral area.

Hansen studied the clinical effect of a single violent traumatic accident on the spine of the dog.[25] This study consisted of 122 cases, examined roentgenologically or pathologico-anatomically, in which the dogs had been subjected to various kinds of violent trauma from accidents. They had been run over by cars, had fallen from heights, or had been injured in fights. They were divided into the chondrodystrophoid breeds, which are especially subject to disk disease, and the nonchondrodystrophoid breeds. A distinction was made between dogs under and over 1 year of age.

When the data were studied in respect to changes in the disks and the vertebral bodies, the most frequent finding was a fracture of the vertebral body. Of the 122 dogs, 79 had fractures, 35 had ruptured disks, and 8 had both. Age and breed have no significant bearing on these findings; therefore, the breeds predisposed to disk disease did not show a greater frequency of traumatically ruptured disks than of fractures. Hansen concluded that bone may have degenerated at a rate similar to that of disks and was therefore just as vulnerable to a single violent trauma.[25]

TYPES OF FRACTURES AND LUXATIONS

Fractions and luxations of the spine may be classified according to the degree of resulting neurological dysfunction. Fractures of vertebral bodies might also be classified as transverse or compression. Dislocations without concurrent fractures can be classed as subluxations with minor displacement or luxations with major displacement. Transverse fractures generally result from direct trauma and usually compress the cord. Compression fractures of the verte-

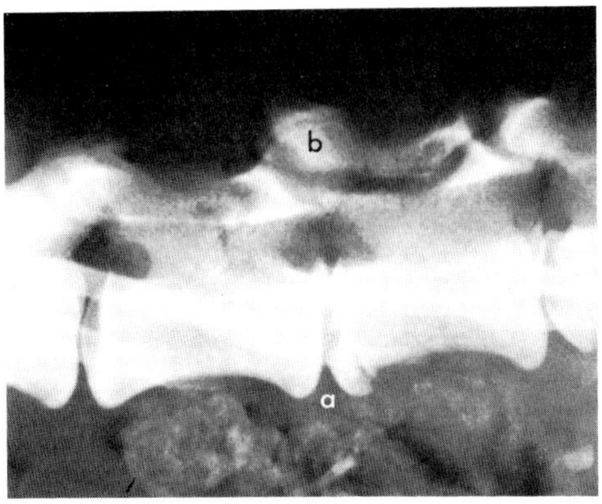

FIGURE 15–1 Radiograph demonstrates a spinal fracture with a fragment displaced ventrally (a) and a dorsal laminal defect (b). The dog was not paraplegic but suffered considerable pain.

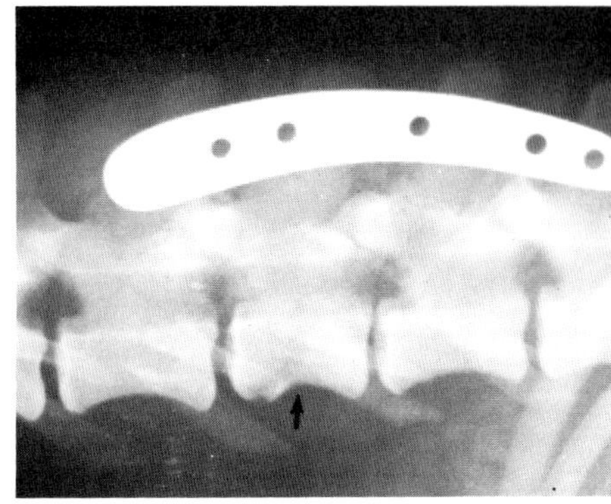

FIGURE 15–2 A case of compression fracture of the vertebral body. Decompression and skeletal fixation with Wilson laminectomy plates and bolts was accomplished. Notice the shortened length of the involved vertebra. (From Hoerlein, B. F.: Traumatic lesions of the canine spine. Mod. Vet. Pract. 39, Oct. 15, 1958.)

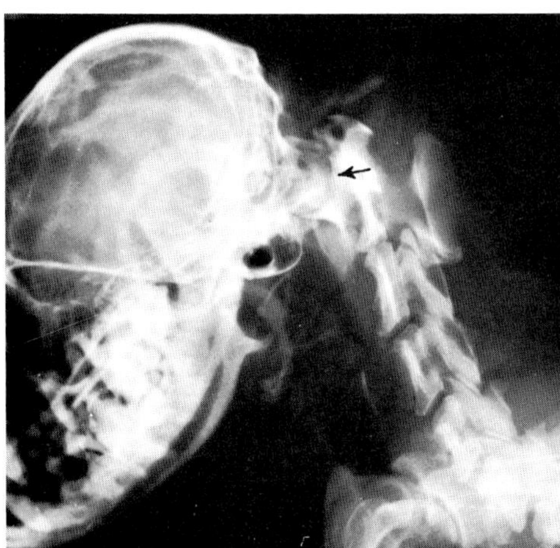

FIGURE 15–3 A combination atlantoaxial subluxation and fracture of the first cervical vertebra. Severe compression of the spinal cord resulted.

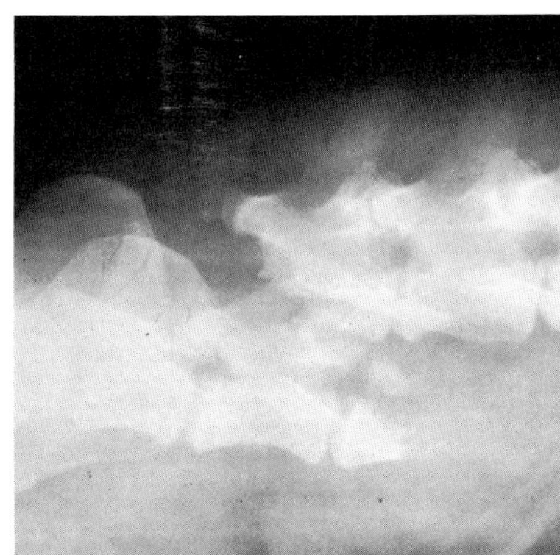

FIGURE 15–4 A transverse fracture has completely severed the spinal cord and cannot be corrected surgically.

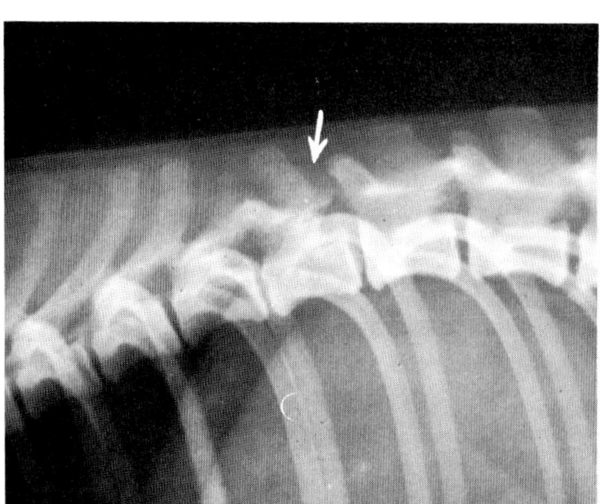

FIGURE 15–5 This radiograph shows an unusual case of a fractured articular process at T11-12, with little apparent spinal displacement.

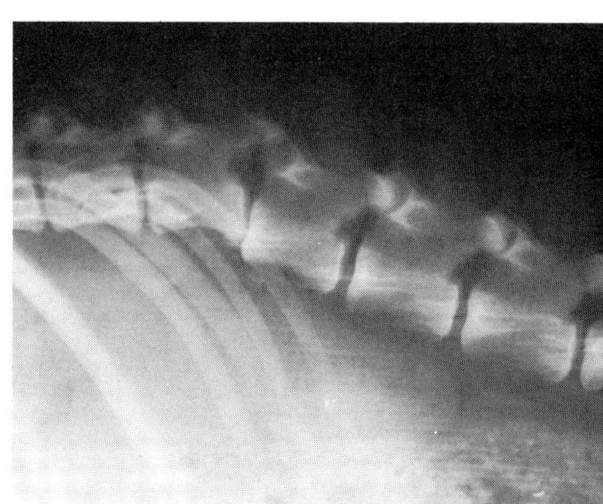

FIGURE 15–6 Spinal luxation with gross rupture of collateral ligaments and muscle support. Surgery was successful in this case because it was done shortly after luxation occurred.

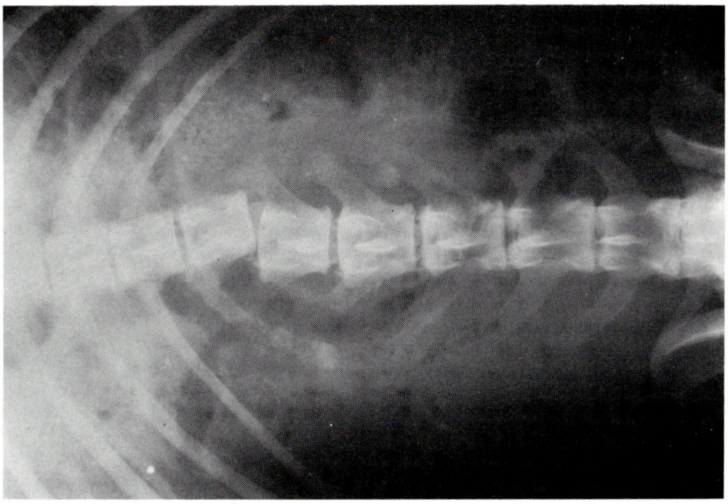

FIGURE 15–7 Same case as shown in Figure 15–6. A VD radiograph shows the lateral displacement and compression. Notice the agenesis of the thirteenth rib on one side.

bral bodies result from trauma to the head or rear parts of the animal's body and cause a longitudinal shortening of the vertebral body. These fractures also compress the cord to some degree. Fractures of the spinous and lateral processes may not involve the cord directly, and in such cases neural dysfunction may result from spinal concussion rather than from direct compression. A fractured articular process generally causes some displacement of the laminae (Figs. 15–1 to 15–5).

It is possible to have a complete interruption of ligamentous support without a fracture (Figs. 15–6 and 15–7). This may cause a luxation with severe neuronal disturbances or may result in recurrent subluxations or a so-called "loose joint," with pain being the dominant sign. Occasionally, a luxation will reduce spontaneously or will be reduced by movement made just before the radiograph is taken, and thus the appearance will be normal radiographically. If severe damage to the cord occurred prior to reduction, paralysis would be permanent.

ATLANTOAXIAL SUBLUXATIONS AND CANINE WOBBLER SYNDROME

Atlantoaxial subluxations and canine wobbler syndrome have been discussed in Chapter 13.

CLINICAL SIGNS AND INDICATIONS FOR SURGERY

The clinical signs noted for spinal fractures and luxations have been described in Chapter 13 in the discussion of compressions. They will of course vary according to degree of compression and the concomitant dynamic force (Figs. 15–8 to 15–10). The speed of compression in fractures or luxations is nearly always instantaneous because of the nature of the trauma. The location of the fracture also influences the clinical effect. The areas of the spinal cord

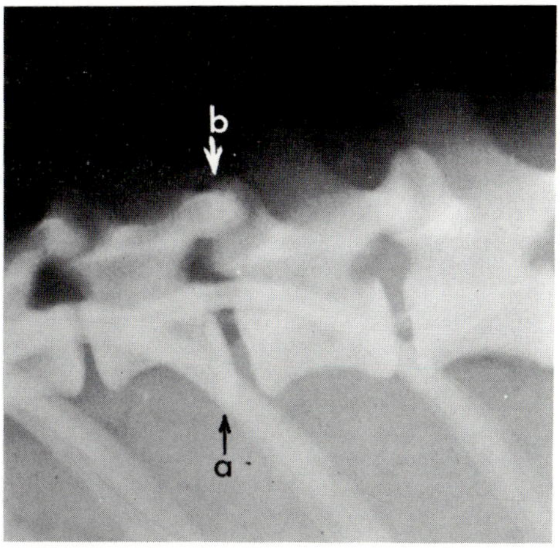

FIGURE 15–8 A fractured vertebral epiphyseal fragment has displaced itself ventrally (a). Notice the spinal canal displacement as seen at the articular process area (b).

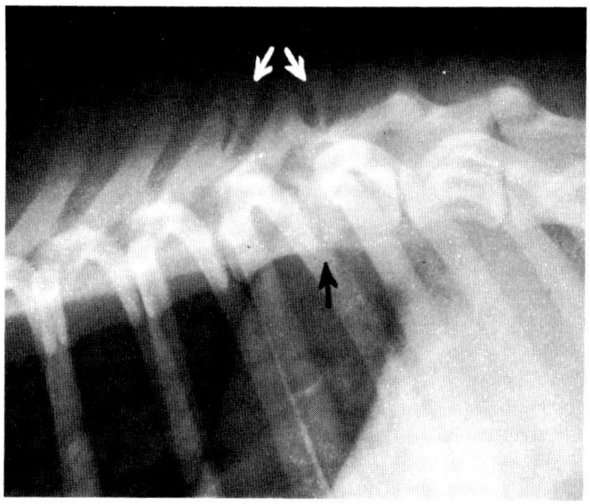

FIGURE 15–9 Vertebral fracture at T11. Notice the dorsal fragmentation compressing the cord.

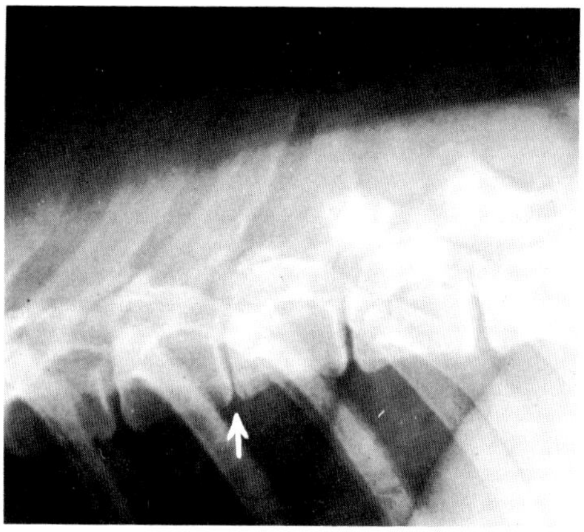

FIGURE 15–10 Careful observation reveals a linear fracture of T10 vertebral epiphysis.

that have more epidural space to accommodate the displaced fragments—such as the cervical and terminal lumbar areas—are less vulnerable to mild compressions.

The severe fracture produces evidence of spinal shock. The stages of spinal shock have been described as (1) an immediate and complete flaccid paralysis; (2) loss of sensibility; (3) suppression of reflex activity posterior to the lesion; and (4) retention of urine and feces.

When presented for treatment, the typical dog with a severely fractured thoracic or lumbar vertebra may show evidence of partial recovery from spinal shock. The hind limbs may still be atonic and flaccid, but the front limbs will have acquired extensor rigidity (Schiff-Sherrington phenomenon) (Fig. 15–11). In some cases, the front limbs may be so rigid that they resist forceful flexion. The head and neck may appear to be relatively normal. In one or more days, the hind limbs may regain reflex ability, but the reflexes will generally be exaggerated and uncontrollable. This is *hyperreflexia,* which is characteristic of upper motor neuron disorders. Extensor rigidity in the front limbs may persist indefinitely, but generally the intensity diminishes after several days. This type of case is usually hopeless, and radiographic examination may reveal gross displacement or fragmentation of the vertebrae involved, or even severance of the cord. Surgical correction should not be attempted.

If the severe fracture occurs in the cervical area, much systemic involvement may be seen. Fractures in the area are frequently fatal because of respiratory failure resulting from phrenic nerve paralysis or from depression of the respiratory center in the medulla. In such animals, hemor-

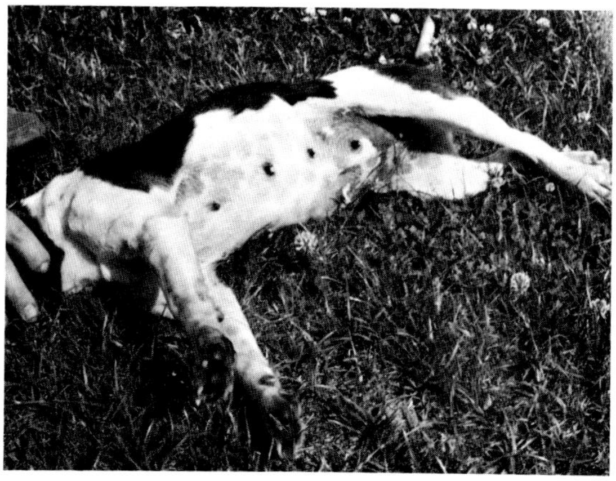

FIGURE 15–11 Spinal fracture demonstrating extensor rigidity in the pectoral limbs. This is seen in severe traumatism and compression of the spinal cord in the thoracic or lumbar spinal segment.

rhage and edema of the brain stem are frequently seen. Neurological signs may include flaccid tetraplegia. Surgical correction is generally not feasible in such cases unless the animal is seen immediately after the injury and before cord damage has become irreversible.

Surgical correction *should* be considered in cases of incomplete paralysis in which some voluntary muscle activity and tone remain. In addition to nonparalytic cases, surgical correction should be considered when some reflex ability is present caudal to the lesion and when extensor rigidity occurs only periodically or is stimulated by handling. When an animal so affected is seen promptly after the accident and the radiographic examination shows a moderate displacement of less than one-third the diameter of the canal, the case may be surgically correctible.

Occasionally, one can be optimistic about a case that is presented within minutes after the accident. Since spinal shock may have occurred, neurological damage may not be ascertained on examination. If the radiograph demonstrates a compression that has displaced not more than one-third the diameter of the canal or at least has not severed the cord, immediate surgical correction might be considered. However, the possibility of complete recovery in such cases may be remote and the prognosis should indicate this fact. The experimental work on spinal cord compression described in Chapter 12, as well as clinical experience, demonstrates that *immediate* surgical relief should be performed in such cases.

NONSURGICAL TREATMENT

The handling of spinal injuries in the early stages was described in Chapter 12. The emergency treatment of nonneurologic disorders such as shock, hemorrhage, collapse, and cyanosis must be performed with dispatch. Disorders of nerve tissue, such as hemorrhage, edema, and histochemical changes in the CNS from trauma, must also be treated appropriately.

Occasionally, the neurological damage from a fractured vertebra is mild enough to be handled conservatively. This happens most frequently in or caudal to the sixth lumbar vertebra. Pain, urinary and fecal dysfunction, and impairment of voluntary tail movement may be seen in such cases (Fig. 15–12). Confinement to a cage combined with general nursing care may suffice for this type of fracture. Occasionally, mild fractures of the cervical, thoracic, or lumbar vertebrae respond to immobilization with partial or full-body casts or splints; however, spinal cord compression may develop secondarily from the resulting abnormal callus formations when surgical decompressions are not performed also.[18, 27, 29, 30, 44]

SURGICAL PROCEDURES

Surgical procedures generally involve the dorsal or dorsolateral approach and are similar to those described for hemilaminectomy or dorsal laminectomy for protruding disks (Figs. 15–13 to 15–16).[1, 27, 29, 30] The animal is placed in a ventral recumbent position. The area is prepared for surgery. The skin and dorsal fascia are incised and both sides of the spines are exposed by blunt dissection. Removal of musculature by blunt dissection can usually be discontinued somewhat ventral to the articular processes (see Chapter 14).

DECOMPRESSION

The first stage of the surgery is a decompression of the cord. The depressive bone fragments must be removed, and their location should determine whether the decompression approach should be a hemilaminectomy or a dorsal laminectomy. The dorsal or the lateral lamina is removed, as necessary, to provide the cord with ample space for expansion, so that pressure from any abnormal contour of the canal can be relieved. Decompression is needed also because the cord is swollen from traumatic edema and, possibly, hemorrhage. The amount of lateral or dorsal lamina that should be removed varies. The usual approach is to decompress by a lateral laminectomy or hemilaminectomy, if possible. This allows the dorsal lamina and spine to remain intact, promoting stability and protection of the cord against future trauma, and affording possible use of the vertebral arch in subsequent immobilization proce-

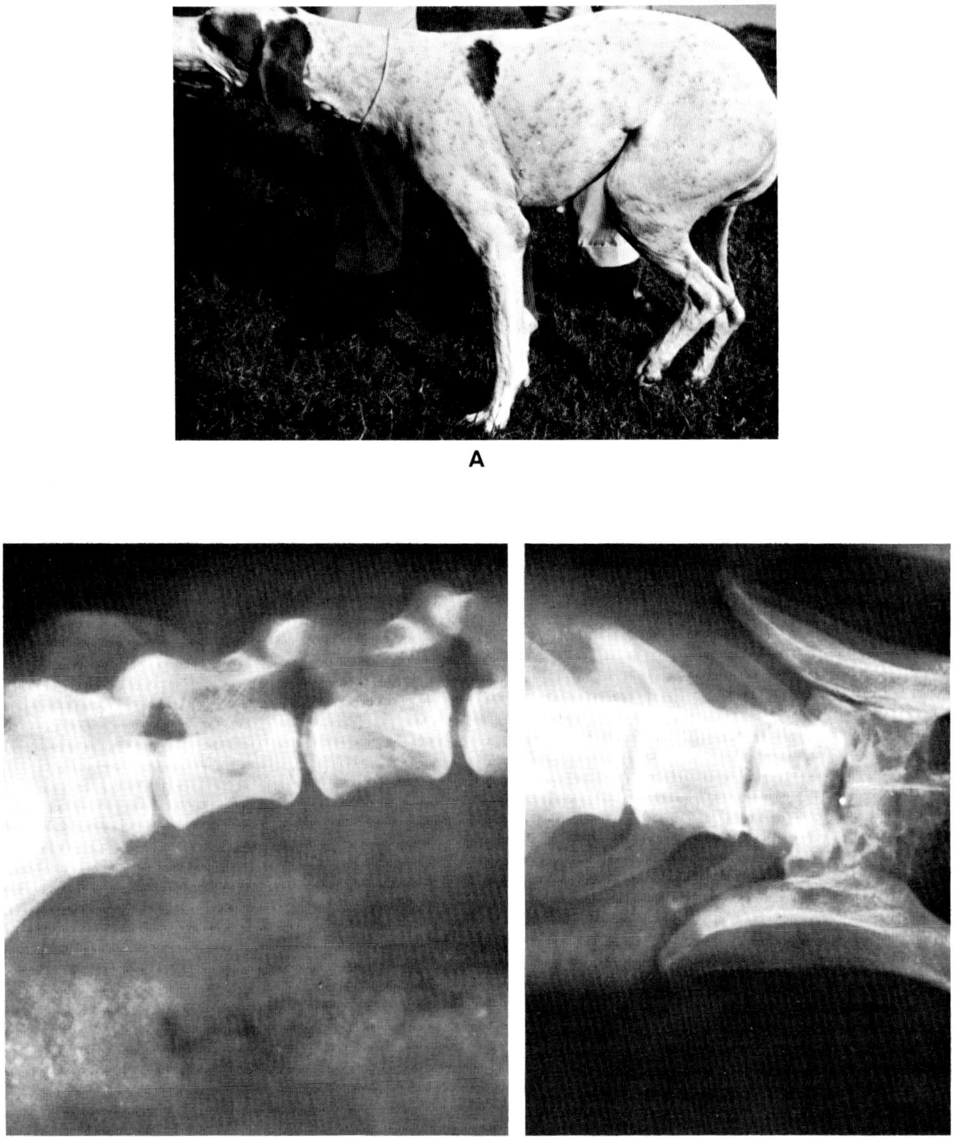

A

B C

FIGURE 15–12 *A,* A pointer showing pain and some locomotor weakness from a fractured L6 vertebra. A dorsal laminectomy relieved the pressure, and the dog recovered. *B,* Lateral view. *C,* Ventrodorsal view.

dures. If a hemilaminectomy suffices, the procedure is much the same as that described for disk surgery. The lateral defect should always be made at the point of greatest pressure, as determined by previous radiographic examination. The lateral laminal defect can extend the length of one or more of the vertebrae involved until all of the pathological area of the cord has been decompressed. In the dorsoventral dimension, the cord is exposed but not subject to additional trauma (Fig. 15–17).

If a unilateral decompression would not relieve the fragmentation, compression, and associated edema and pathology of the cord,[30] a bilateral hemilaminectomy[48] or a dorsal laminectomy of some type should be considered.[19, 50, 51] Dorsal laminectomy procedures include a Funkquist type B procedure,[19] Trotter's modified dorsal laminectomy,[50] and a total laminectomy which involves the removal of the entire arch of the spine and leaves the cord lying open on top of the body of the vertebra.[51] The level

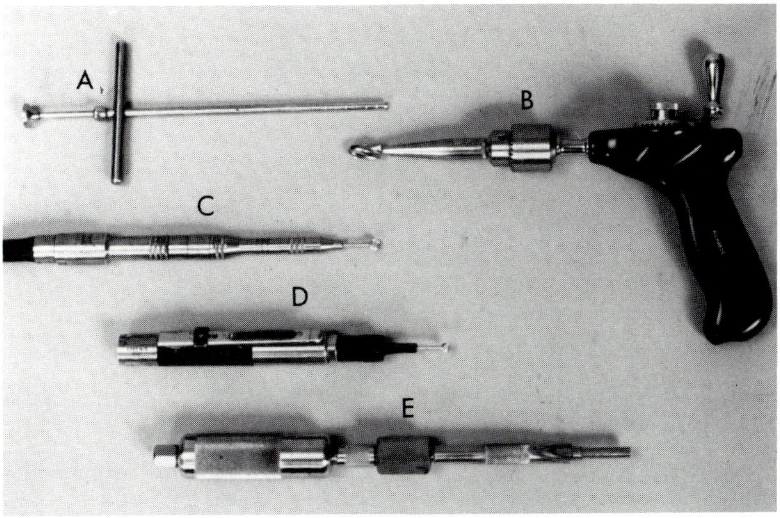

FIGURE 15–13 Instruments useful in laminectomies. (*A*) Michelle laminectomy trephine, 7/32-inch diameter; (*B*) orthopedic hand drill and bone burr (burring in spinal surgery can be utilized in lieu of trephination); (*C*) Stryker high-speed air drill; (*D*) Hall high-speed air drill; (*E*) Micrometer trephine with a preset depth guard.

of the bone around the cord in a dorsal laminectomy should extend above the cord (as in the Funkquist B and Trotter modified procedures), or else the lateral lamina should be removed completely to the level of the body of the vertebra. Any lamina left, as in the Funkquist A procedure, will promote secondary cicatricial compression of the cord. These laminectomy procedures have been discussed previously in Chapter 14.

In severe fractures, luxations, and compressions of the cord when edema, swelling, and hemorrhagic necrosis are possible, medical therapy (discussed in detail in Chapter 12) should be initiated as well as decompressive and skeletal fixation procedures. A durotomy and possibly myelotomy

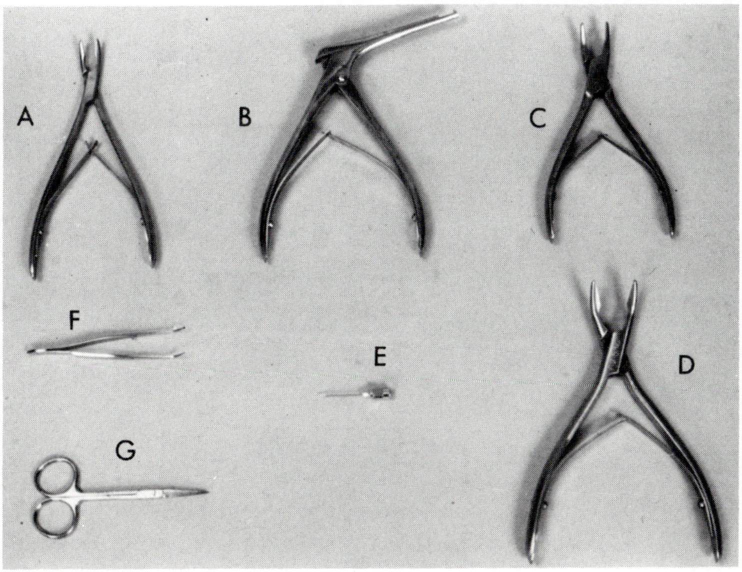

FIGURE 15–14 Instruments used in laminectomies. (*A*) Lampert rongeur; (*B*) Kerrison laminectomy rongeur; (*C*) Reiner rongeur; (*D*) mastoid rongeur; (*E*) 23-guage intravenous needle that can be used to initiate a dural incision, or to elevate the dura while using iris scissors (*G*) in a durotomy; (*F*) an iris or dural forceps.

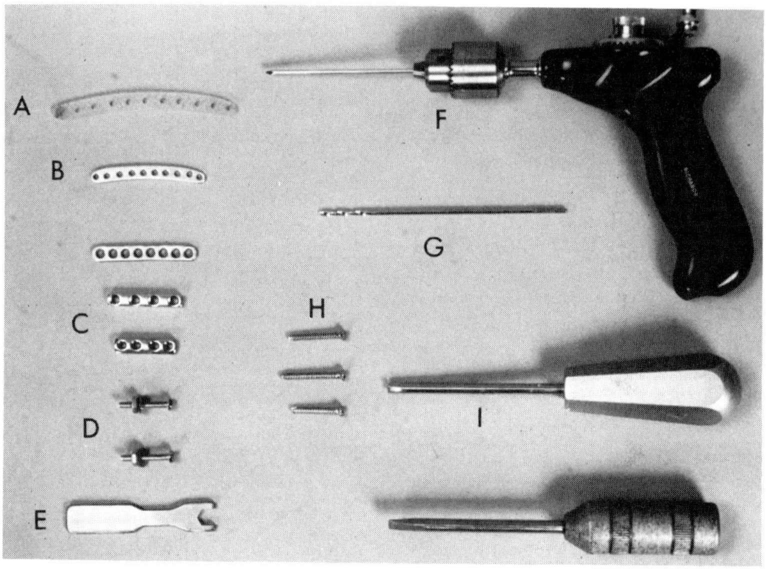

FIGURE 15–15 Additional instruments used in spinal fractures. (*A*) Plastic plates; (*B*) stainless steel (Richards) plates; (*C*) small stainless steel body plates, 1½ to 2 inches long (Richards); (*D*) stainless steel bolts, nuts, and washers; (*E*) wrench, open-end; (*F*) hand drill and Steinmann pin; (*G*) drill bit; (*H*) Bechtol screws (7/16-inch diameter); (*I*) screw drivers.

may also be appropriate in severe cases. Massive dorsal decompressions may need vertebral body fixation, or the defect may have to be spanned with long dorsal spinal plates for effective vertebral immobilization.

IMMOBILIZATION

The second phase in correction of spinal fractures or luxations is immobilization. Experimental work reported in 1956 was done in an effort to determine the best means for immobilization of spinal fractures.[28] The procedures included grafting of bone; placement of bone grafts and plates on the vertebrae; application of bone plates and screws to spines, lateral processes, and ventral vertebral surfaces; placement of bone plates with bolts and nuts applied to the spines; wiring the spines together; and finally, application of a body cast without skeletal fixation.

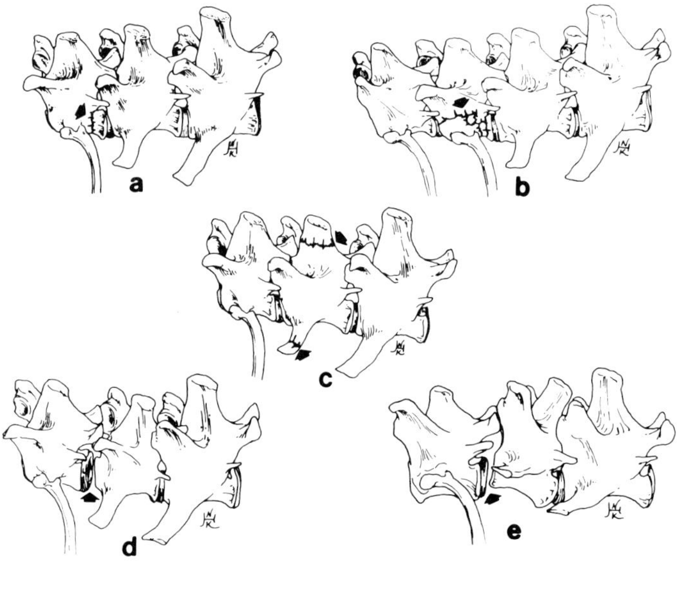

FIGURE 15–16 Five basic types of spinal fractures and luxations (arrows). (a) Transverse fracture; (b) compression fracture; (c) spinous and lateral process fractures; (d) subluxation; (e) luxation. (From Swaim, S. F.: Thoracolumbar and sacral spine trauma. *In* Bojrab, M. J. (ed.): *Current Techniques in Small Animal Surgery I.* Lea & Febiger, Philadelphia, 1975.)

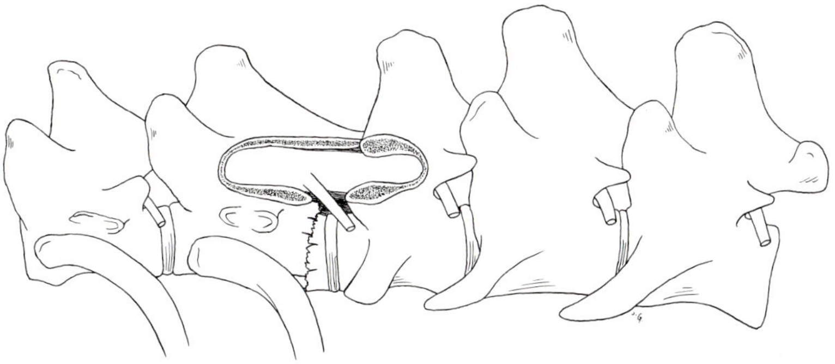

FIGURE 15–17 In the surgical relief of spinal fractures, the dorsal approach described in Chapter 14 is used. Here, the trephine opening has been made as part of extensive hemilaminectomy or partial dorsal laminectomy in order to adequately decompress the area.

Based on the results of this research in 1956,[28] fixation with stainless steel plates and bolts and nuts supplied with washers was considered the most satisfactory procedure. The plates and bolts were secured to the spinous processes. This apparatus should also be reinforced with an external cast or splint that is applied immediately following surgery and is allowed to remain in place for 10 to 14 days. The most suitable plates have been custom-made,* although standard bone plates of various types have been used on occasion (Fig. 15–18). More recently, plastic plates made of a vinylidine fluoride resin† have been developed. They have the advantage of some flexibility in thickness but sufficient dorsoventral stability to afford immobilization when applied to the dorsal spinous processes.[56]

Application of Steel Plates[28, 30]

The surgical procedure for applying steel plates is not difficult. The pair of plates best suited for the individual case is long enough to include at least one normal vertebra on each side of the fractured one. However, in larger dogs it is more effective to include at least two vertebrae on each side of the affected one. The musculature must be removed adequately from both sides of the spines to facilitate the application of the plate and bolt assemblies. Orginally, it was recommended that a bolt be placed in each dorsal spine; however, with plastic plates the bolts should be placed between the spines.[56] Occasionally, it is desirable to do this with steel plates also. For effective application, it is imperative that the bolts be placed in the heaviest and most central part of the spine, and that plates be placed as close to the dorsal lamina as practicable. This may necessitate the removal of articular processes and/or grooving slightly with a rongeur forceps in order to insure the proper position of plates, nuts, and bolts in the vertebrae. Proper positioning prevents friction or rubbing of plates against the dorsal fascia and skin, and affords more stability to the spine.[30]

Holes can be drilled in the spines with a drill bit or intramedullary pin whose diameter is slightly larger than the bolt. For greatest efficiency, these holes should be drilled with one plate in place. Bolts should be inserted as the holes are drilled to keep the spines and plate in position during the remaining drilling procedure. Correct positioning of the involved vertebrae must be maintained while one is drilling. The fractured fragments should be aligned in as nearly normal a position as possible.[30]

After the holes are drilled and the bolts are in place, the second plate is applied to the other side of the spine and the washers and nuts are secured. Excessive force should not be exerted or the spines will be crushed. With the usual equipment available, this crushing is not apt to occur. The excess bolt is cut with a side-cutting pin cutter as close to the nut as possible. Crimping of the bolt occurs, so that the nut must remain tight. The sharp edges of the bolt may be filed (Figs. 15–18 to 15–20).

Frequently, one must modify the proce-

---

*Richards Manufacturing Co., Memphis, Tennessee.

†Lubra Co., Fort Collins, Colorado.

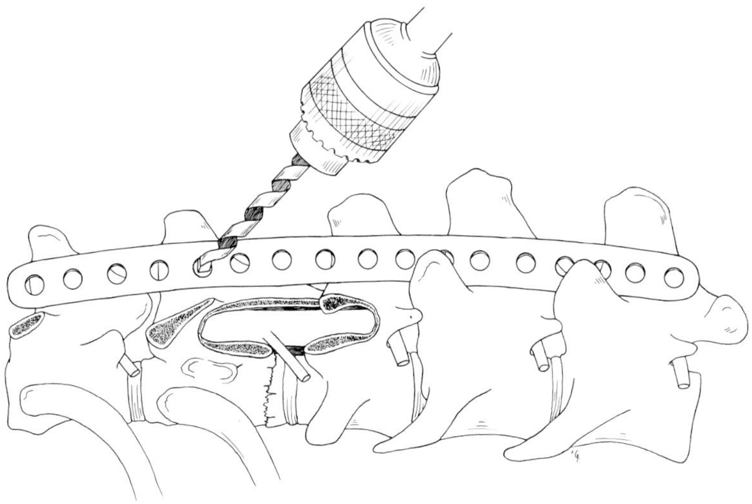

FIGURE 15–18 The drill holes are made in the spinous processes after the plates have been positioned, so that the bolts will afford the greatest stability and immobilization.

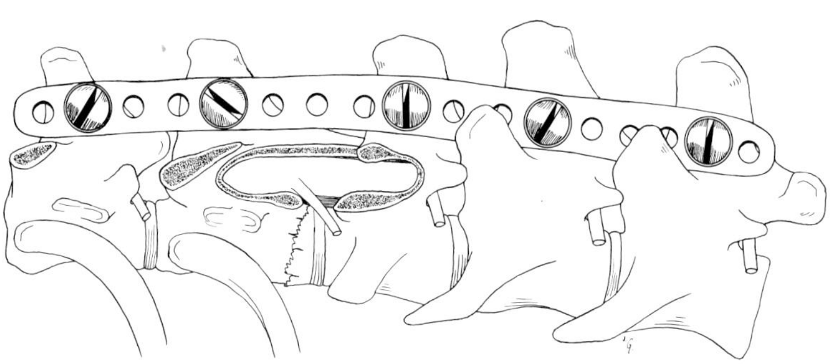

FIGURE 15–19 The plates and bolts have been secured to effect skeletal immobilization; at least three, and occasionally four or five, vertebrae should be incorporated in the plate application. Bolts should be placed in the thickest portion of the spine as close to the lamina as possible for most effective stabilization.

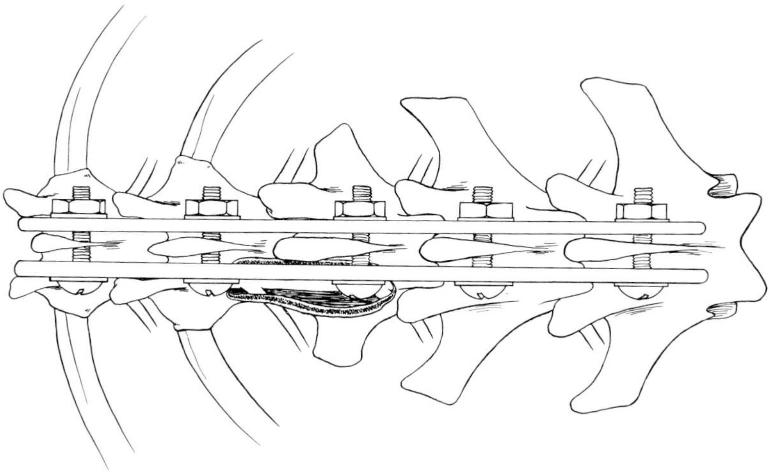

FIGURE 15–20 Dorsal view of illustration shown in Figure 15–19.

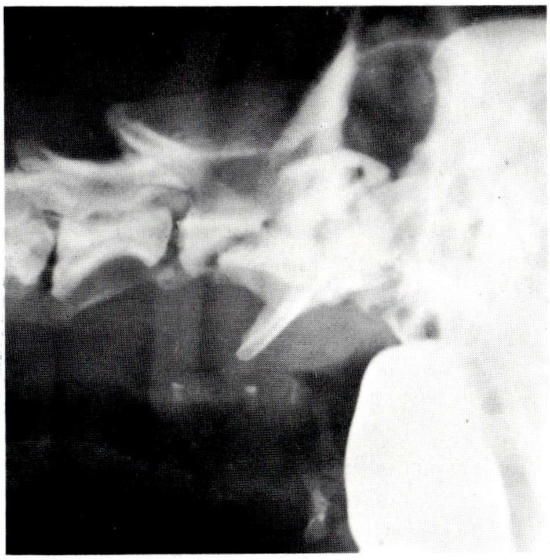

FIGURE 15–21 A transverse fracture involving the first and second cervical vertebrae and causing tetraplegia. (From Hoerlein, B. F.: Clinical spinal radiography in the dog. J.A.V.M.A. *134,* April 15, 1959.)

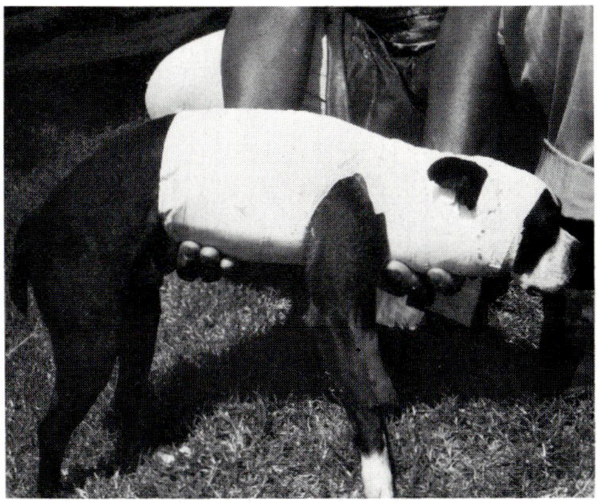

Figure 15–22 Same case as shown in Figure 15–21. After surgical decompression the dog was placed in a full-body, plaster of Paris cast. A length of yucca board was fitted on the padded ventral surface of the head, neck, and chest and was incorporated into the cast for support.

dure for maximum immobilization. This may involve wiring the spines to the plates. The stainless steel wire should be of orthopedic rather than of suture type. Orthopedic wire of sufficient diameter affords better support, and since it is malleable, it can be twisted upon itself for taut fixation. Occasionally, the adjacent spines should be wired together, as well as the spines and the plates. In fractured spines, it may be necessary to wire the dorsal arch to the plate (Figs. 15–21 to 15–28).[30]

Application of Plastic Plates

Plastic plates are similar in design to stainless steel ones, and the surgical preparation for application is the same as that previously described. With the gripping surface of the plates toward the exposed bone, one plate is placed on each side of the dorsal spines, and the bolts are directed between the spines instead of into them as prescribed for steel plates. Because of their flexibility, the plates then tend to wrap themselves around the spines when the nuts and bolts are tightened. If stainless steel nuts, bolts, and washers are used, the nuts and washers should be placed on both sides so they can be locked to prevent loosening. If vitallium nuts and bolts are used,[55] loosening is less likely to occur because of their design. Yturraspe and coworkers report that placing the nuts and bolts between the spines affords greater strength and decreases the chances of fractured spinous processes after surgery (Fig. 15–29).[56]

Occasionally, spinal fractures involve not

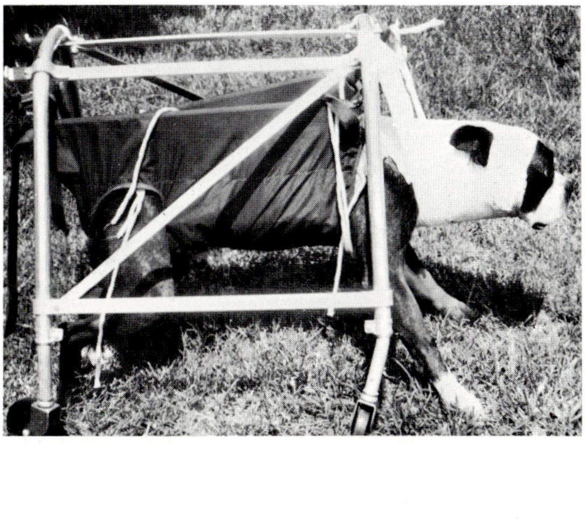

FIGURE 15–23 Same dog as shown in Figure 15–22. After a few days in the "walker" the dog walked by herself, and the cast was removed in 3 weeks. Full recovery occurred.

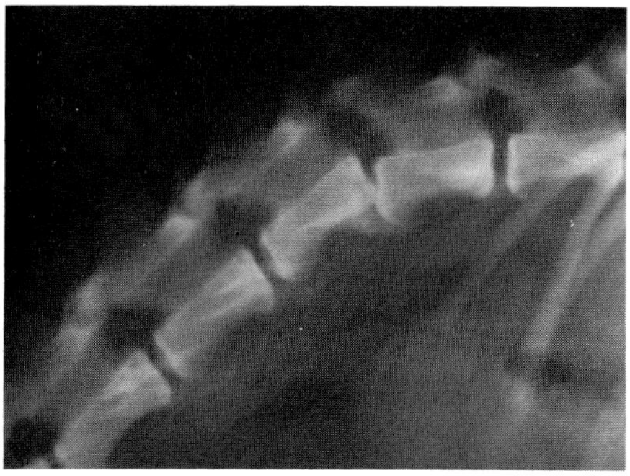

FIGURE 15–24 A spinal luxation and possibly a very slight fracture of the articular processes at L2–3.

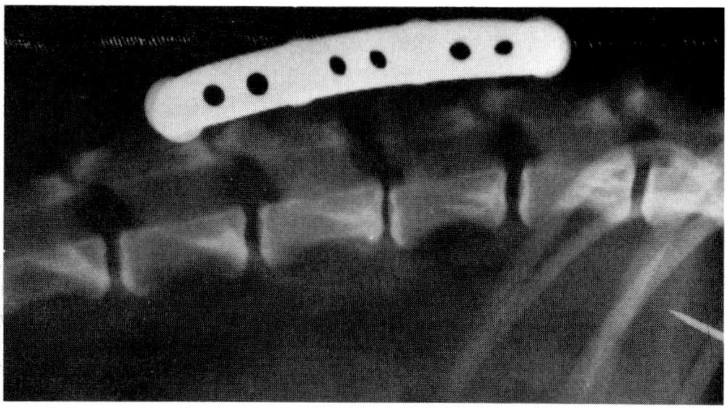

FIGURE 15–25 Same case as shown in Figure 15–24. Radiograph was taken after prompt decompression and immobilization with bone plates.

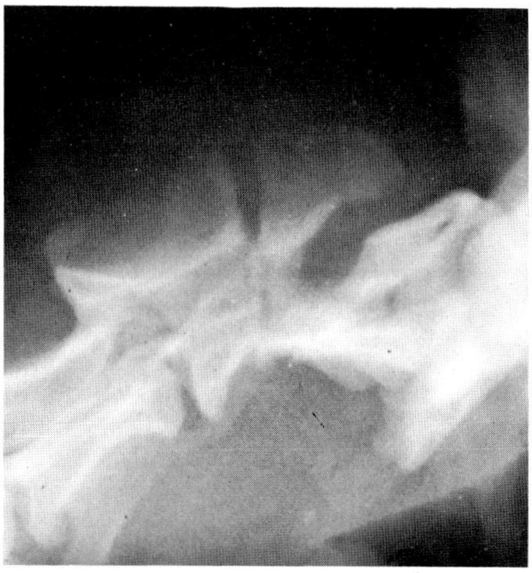

Fig. 15–26

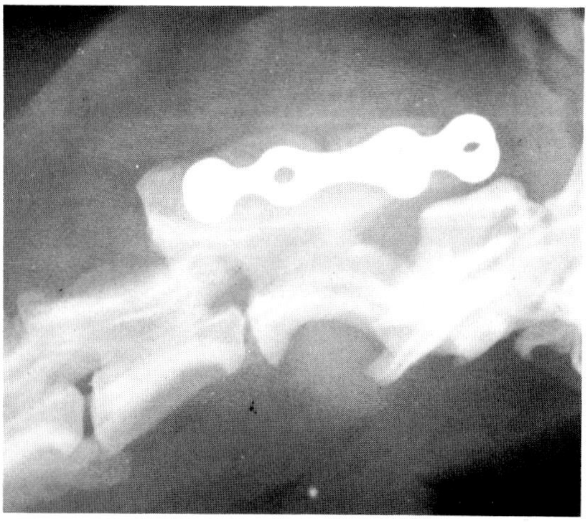

Fig. 15–27

FIGURE 15–26 A fractured axis was compressing the cord, producing marked clinical pain but no motor dysfunction. (From Hoerlein, B. F.: Traumatic lesions of the canine spine. Mod. Vet. Pract. *39*, Oct. 15, 1958.)

FIGURE 15–27 Same fracture as shown in Figure 15–26, 2 years later. (From Hoerlein, B. F.: Traumatic lesions of the canine spine. Mod. Vet. Pract. *39*, Oct. 15, 1958.)

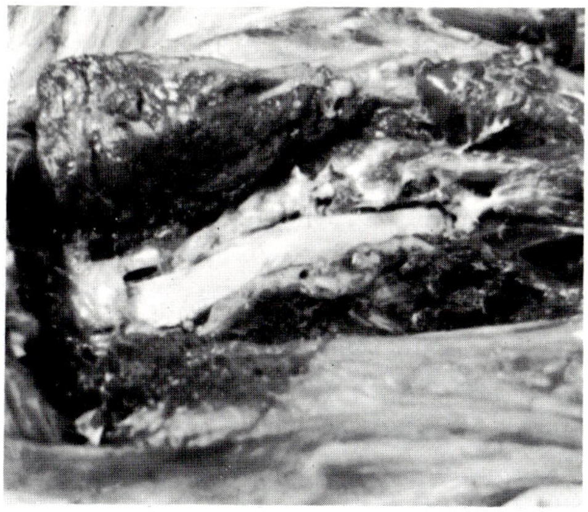

Figure 15–28 Same case as shown in Figure 15–27. The dog died from nephritis 5 years after fixation. The spine of the axis was removed at necrospy, and the spinal cord appeared to be entirely normal. Notice the slight curve of the spinal cord.

only the bodies of the vertebrae but also the arches. Bridging of one or two affected vertebrae with dorsal plates can be done in fractures of the arches and spines, but bridging alone may not be entirely satisfactory. Large dogs may fracture the dorsal spines to which the plates are attached or tear the plates loose from the spines, and vertebral displacement and compression of the cord may recur. Swaim[45] has developed an alternate method of applying plates to the vertebral bodies. If dorsal plates are used across a gap, conjunctive body fixation may be desirable.

Application of Vertebral Body Plates and Pins[45]

In the *body plating* method of immobilization, the approach to the vertebrae and the decompression procedure are the same as those already described. It is helpful if the dog has been placed in a ventral recumbent position with the operative side slightly elevated by means of positioning bags placed under the limbs of that side. Since the dorsal spines are not utilized in this procedure, the musculature need not be removed from both sides of the spines. The musculature is bluntly removed from the lateral aspects of the vertebrae as far as the rib heads or transverse processes of the vertebrae to be plated. Care is exercised not to injure the spinal nerves and vessels emerging from the various intervertebral foramina.[45]

The spinal vessels and nerves emerging from between the vertebrae to be plated are isolated, ligated, and severed near the foramina. This prevents them from being compressed or damaged during plating and causing pain following surgery. A stainless steel plate of the proper length (1½ to 2 inches) is secured and laid on the dorsolateral aspects of the vertebral bodies just ventral to the hemilaminectomy decompression. If the transverse processes or any part of the vertebrae prevent the plates from lying perfectly flat and in good contact with the entire surface, the offending part is removed or remodeled with a rongeur forceps. Two screw holes in the plate must involve each of the affected vertebrae. With the plate in place, a small hand drill with a 5/64-inch diameter drill bit is directed through the most caudal hole in the plate and vertebra, angling it slightly downward across the body of the vertebra. A bone depth gauge is used to facilitate selection of the proper length screw for each hole; the screw should protrude slightly through the hole in the opposite bony cortex of the vertebra. A 7/64-inch drill is used for a short distance in the same hole to facilitate the first turns of the screw. Radial, fluted-point bone screws (7/16-inch diameter) with cruciate heads and buttress threads (Bechtal screws) are used (Richards). All four screws are placed and tightened appropriately (Figs. 15–30 and 15–31).[45]

In the thoracic area, the method is modified to include the ribs. The tops of the ribs are exposed and a small intramedullary bone pin is used to drill dorsoventral holes in them just lateral to the site of articulation with the vertebrae. The ribs are sev-

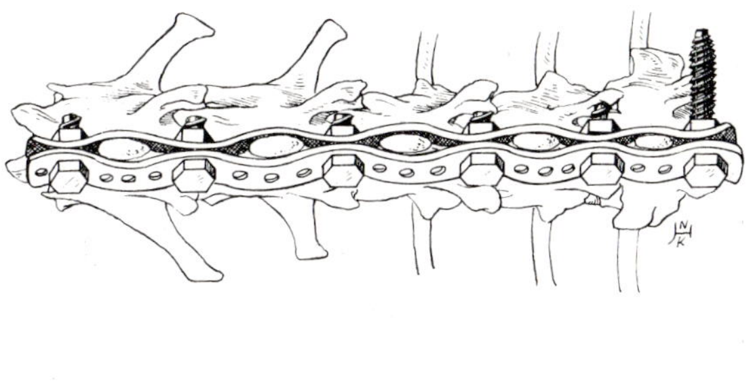

FIGURE 15–29 The spinous processes are sandwiched between the friction grip surfaces of the plastic plates. The bolts and nuts almost pull the plates into apposition between the spines, and this tends to wrap the plates around the spines. (From Swaim, S. F.: Thoracolumbar and sacral spine trauma. *In* Bojrab, M. J. (ed.): *Current Techniques in Small Animal Surgery I.* Lea & Febiger, Philadelphia, 1975.)

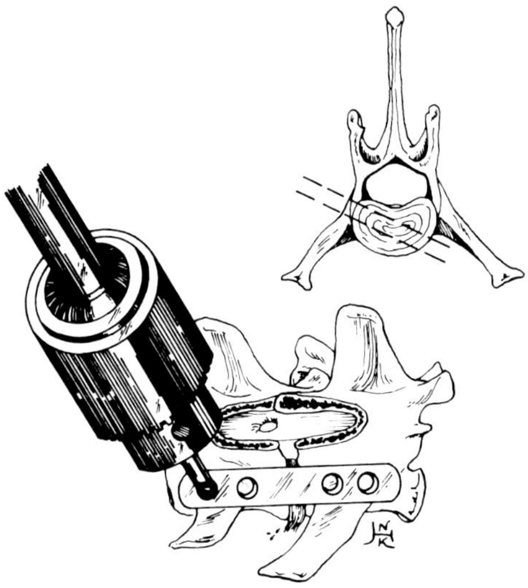

FIGURE 15–30 In Swaim's body plating, the cord is decompressed by a hemilaminectomy. With the plate in place, a drill bit is used to drill two holes in each vertebra involved. Notice the slightly ventral path of the drill holes across the body of the vertebra. (From Swaim, S. F.: Thoracolumbar and sacral spine trauma. *In* Bojrab, M. J. (ed.): *Current Techniques in Small Animal Surgery I.* Lea & Febiger, Philadelphia, 1975.)

ered as close to the vertebral bodies as possible, and the exposed vertebral surfaces are made flat with a rongeur to accommodate the plate. After plating, the severed ribs are elevated to their normal position, and a hole is drilled in the base of each corresponding dorsal spine. Orthopedic wire is passed through the predrilled

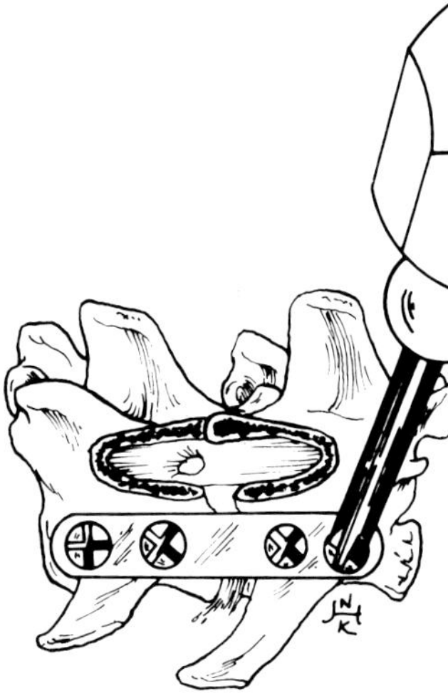

FIGURE 15–31 A depth gauge is used to select the correct length for the screws. The screws should have Bechtol radial-fluted points with buttress threads (Richards) and are applied firmly so that there will be no movement of the plate. (From Swaim, S. F.: Thoracolumbar and sacral spine trauma. *In* Bojrab, M. J. (ed.): *Current Techniques in Small Animal Surgery I.* Lea & Febiger, Philadelphia, 1975.)

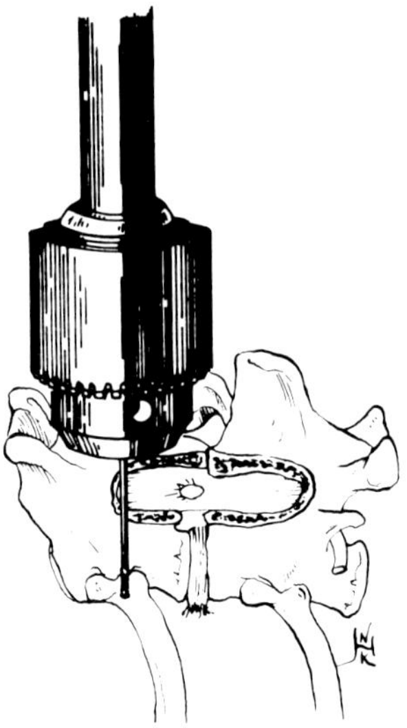

FIGURE 15–32 In the thoracic area, the ribs must be removed to place the plates. A dorsoventral hole is drilled in the ribs prior to the disarticulation of the rib from the vertebra. (From Swaim, S. F.: Thoracolumbar and sacral spine trauma. *In* Bojrab, M. J. (ed.): *Current Techniques in Small Animal Surgery I.* Lea & Febiger, Philadelphia, 1975.)

holes in the rib and the spine, and the ribs are secured in their normal position by twisting the wires at the appropriate length (Figs. 15–32 to 15–35).[45]

The advantage of body plating is that a small segment of spine is immobilized very securely because of the substantial amount of bone involved, and less prosthetic material is thereby necessary.[45, 47]

Gage has devised a method of spinal fixation by cross-pinning the involved vertebral bodies. The pins are inserted into the fractured vertebral body from the vertebral bodies anterior and posterior to the fracture. They can be used either in conjunction with dorsal bone plates in very large dogs or alone when pathological changes in the dorsal spines (degenerate or traumatic)

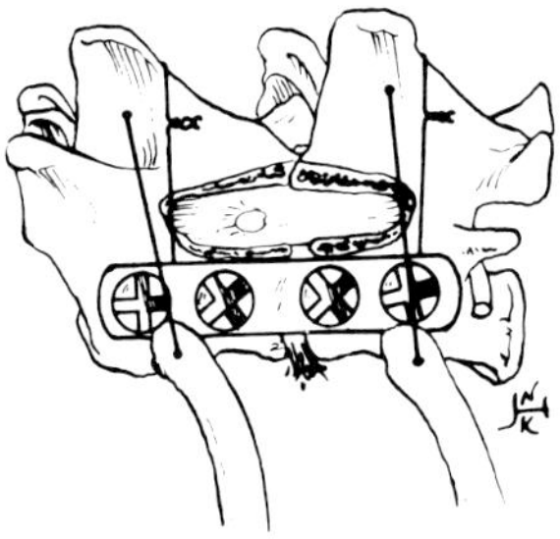

FIGURE 15–33 After the body plate is applied to the involved thoracic vertebrae, the ribs are wired in place as shown to hold them in their original position. (From Swaim, S. F.: Thoracolumbar and sacral spine trauma. *In* Bojrab, M. J. (ed.): *Current Techniques in Small Animal Surgery I.* Lea & Febiger, Philadelphia, 1975.)

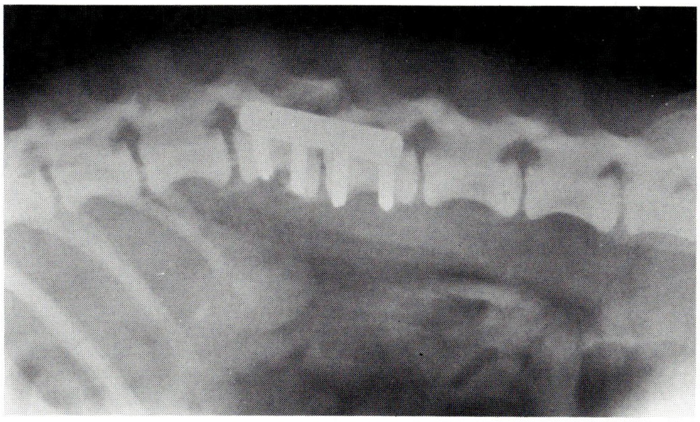

FIGURE 15-34 The plate placed on L3 and L4 vertebral bodies. The L3 body is fractured. This dog recovered completely and required no external cast for further stabilization. (From Swaim, S. F.: Vertebral body plating for spinal immobilization. J.A.V.M.A. *158*, 1683, 1971.)

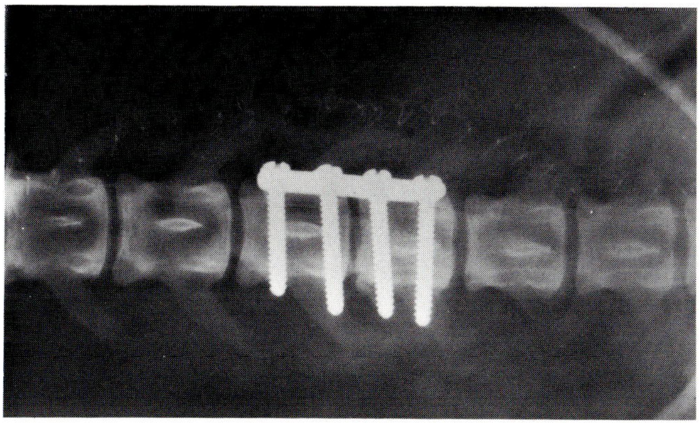

FIGURE 15-35 Ventrodorsal view of the dog shown in Figure 15-34. (From Swaim, S. F.: Vertebral body plating for spinal immobilization. J.A.V.M.A. *158*, 1683, 1971.)

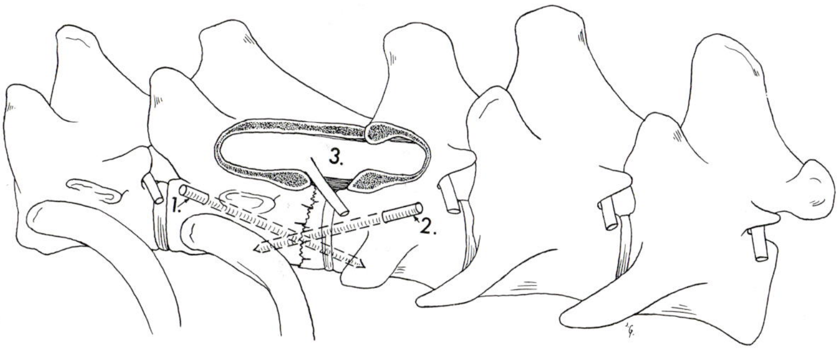

FIGURE 15-36 Stabilization across a single intervertebral space by means of cross-pinning the involved vertebral bodies. (1) Pin directed caudally; (2) pin directed cranially; (3) area of hemilaminectomy and decompression. (After Gage, E. D.: A new method of spinal fixation in the dog. Small Anim. Clin. *64*, 295, 1969.)

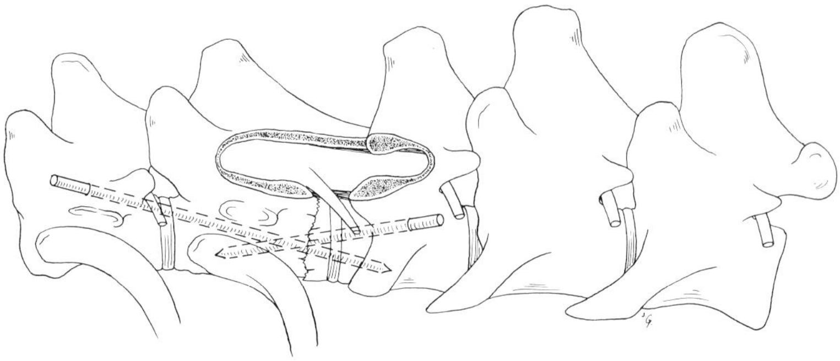

FIGURE 15–37 Stabilization across two intervertebral spaces with pins anchored from adjacent normal vertebral bodies into the fractured body. (After Gage, E. D.: A new method of spinal fixation in the dog. Small Anim. Clin. *64*, 295, 1969.)

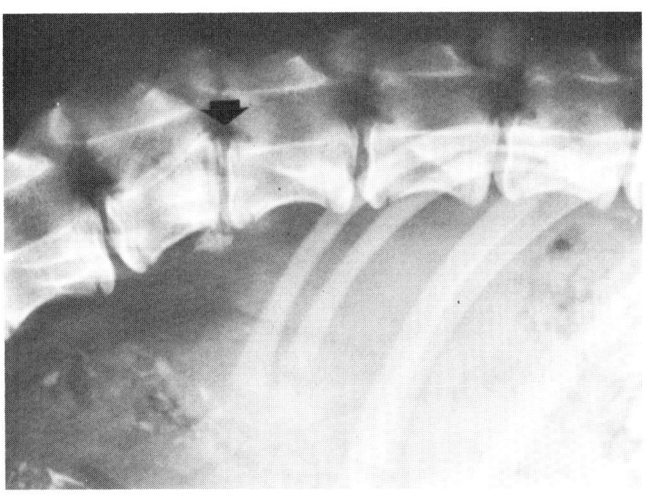

FIGURE 15–38 A lateral radiograph of a compression vertebral fracture. The compression of the cord resulted in clinical paraplegia. (After Gage, E. D.: A new method of spinal fixation in the dog. Small Anim. Clin. *64*, 295, 1969.)

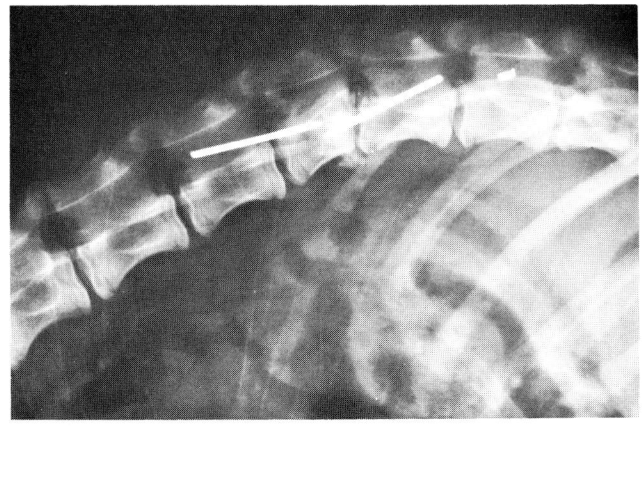

FIGURE 15–39 Same case as shown in Figure 15–38, after decompression and stabilization of vertebral bodies by pinning. (After Gage, E. D.: A new method of spinal fixation in the dog. Small Anim. Clin. *64*, 295, 1969.)

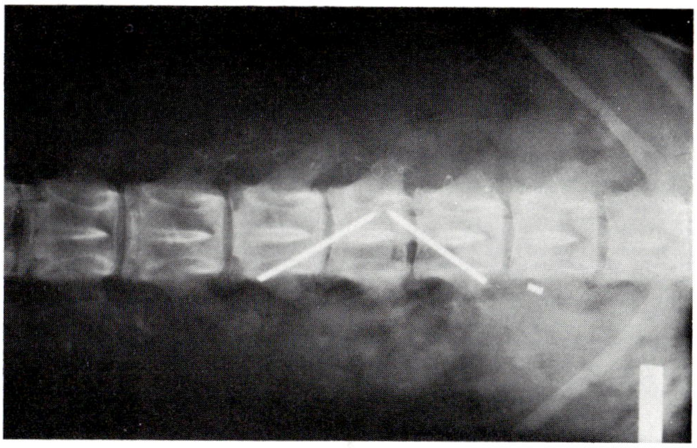

FIGURE 15-40 Ventrodorsal radiograph of the case shown in Figures 15-38 and 15-39. (After Gage, E. D.: A new method of spinal fixation in the dog. Small Anim. Clin. *64*, 295, 1969.)

would make the spines unstable for plating (Figs. 15-36 to 15-40).[21]

Other Methods of Internal Fixation

Gage[22] has proposed the "stapling" method of fixation for vertebral fractures in small breeds of dogs with intact dorsal spinous processes. The decompression should be done by means of a hemilaminectomy. Small holes are drilled in all the spines to be involved in the immobilization (usually five), as close to the base as possible. The holes in the most cranial and caudal spines should be large enough to accommodate a small, semiflexible, stainless steel intramedullary pin (0.045-0.062 cm in diameter). The pin is bent at right angles at each end of the appropriate length for the spinal segment to be immobilized, and the right angle arms, which are 2 to 3 cm long, are inserted through the holes in the end spines. The ends of the right angle arms are then "crimped" around the end spines, and the pin is wired at each intervening spine with 22-24 gauge orthopedic wire (Fig. 15-41).[22] Hoerlein's modification of this method allows one long right angle arm to be doubled back the entire length of the immobilized segment. All aspects of the pin are wired to the intervening spines to afford double strength immobilization. Swaim has modified the procedure by bending the pin in an exaggerated U shape, cutting the full-length, double-legged U pin to the desired length of the segment of spine to be immobilized. The pin is inserted in the most caudal hole so that the base of the U is firmly placed in this spine. Both arms of the U pin, which may be bent slightly dorsoventrally to fit the contour of the spine, are wired to each intervening dorsal spine (Fig. 15-42).[47]

Other methods or modifications of internal fixation of fractured vertebrae have been described in the literature. Dorsal spines have been wired to each other for

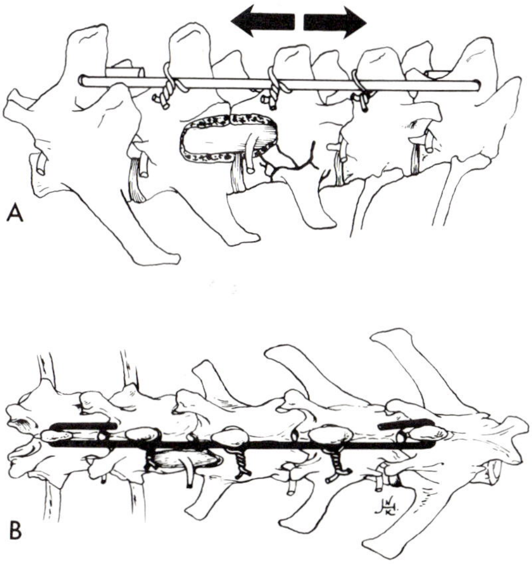

FIGURE 15-41 Gage's "stapling" method in small dog breeds. Holes are drilled in the cranial and caudal spines of the area to be immobilized. The small, semiflexible, stainless steel intramedullary pin is bent at right angles at the appropriate length, and the bent arms are inserted into the holes and crimped as shown. The intermediate spines are wired to the pin. *A*, Lateral view. *B*, Dorsoventral view. (From Swaim, S. F.: Thoracolumbar and sacral spine trauma. *In* Bojrab, M. J. (ed.): *Current Techniques in Small Animal Surgery I*, Lea & Febiger, Philadelphia, 1975.)

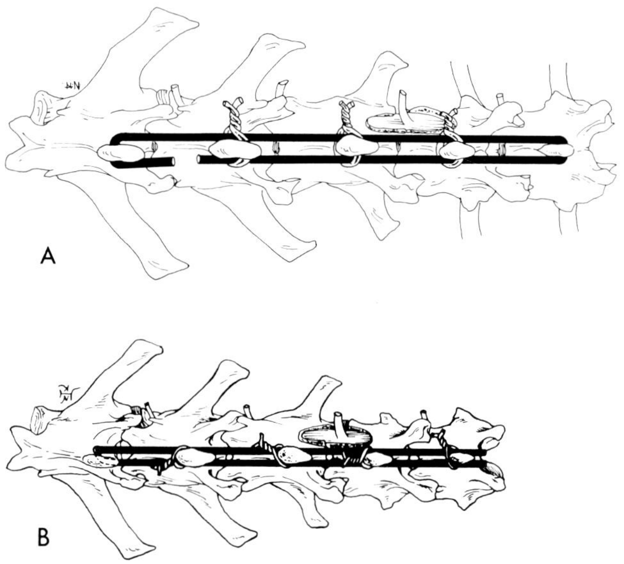

FIGURE 15–42 *A*, Hoerlein's modification of Gage's method, which provides double strength. *B*, Swaim's "U" modification, which allows the open end of the bent pin to rest at the cranial-most spine of the segment to be immobilized. (From Swaim, S. F.: Thoracolumbar and sacral spine trauma. *In* Bojrab, M. J. (ed.): *Current Techniques in Small Animal Surgery I.* Lea & Febiger, Philadelphia, 1975.)

stabilization[28] or to intramedullary pins that have been placed on each side of the spines in the involved area.[5] The latter method was a precursor of the "staple" pin method and has the disadvantage that the pins frequently migrate. Slotted bone plates have been used in place of plates with multiple holes on the dorsal spines. These plates are easier to apply but generally are not as strong and are not curved to the shape of the spine.[18, 32, 34]

CLOSURE

The defect in the laminae in all of the aforementioned methods should be covered with a gelatin sponge (Gelfoam) and the dorsal fascia sutured in a simple interrupted pattern. The skin is closed in a routine manner. A body splint can be applied immediately after surgery to reinforce the skeletal fixations if so desired. This is especially important in young and large breeds of dogs in which the bones are soft and the bodies or spines of the vertebrae can be broken when dorsal arching of the back occurs after surgical intervention. Casting or splinting tends to prevent this.[30]

OTHER SURGICAL PROCEDURES

Fractures of the L7, sacral, and coccygeal vertebrae generally do not cause major motor deficits to the limbs. However, micturition, defecation, and tail movement are frequently impaired. Usually decompression of L7 and sacral fractures is all that is needed, and immobilization may not be necessary. Wiring, small pins, or screws are occasionally used to align coccygeal displacements. Fixation of the L7 vertebra using a para-anal insertion of an intramedullary pin through the bodies of the sacrum and L4-L7 vertebrae has been reported.[38] Slocum and Rudy reported on 18 cases of fracture-luxation of the L7 vertebra, including 10 dogs who were treated by open reduction and transilial stabilization. A dorsal midline incision was made from L5-6 to the midsacral area and the musculature was separated. The dorsocaudal displacement of a luxated L7 was reduced by placing the tip of a heavy forceps between the L7-S1 dorsal arches and prying S1 upward until the L7 vertebra assumed its normal position. Dorsal decompression was performed as needed by removing the remains of the interarcuate ligament covering the dorsal lumbosacral space and as much of the arch of the sacrum and L7 as necessary to release pressure on cord terminations and nerves. Reduction of L7-S1 luxation was maintained by a transilial Steinmann pin placed between the wings of the ilia dorsocaudal to the base of the spine of the L7 vertebra.[43]

Recently a surgical technique for spinal fractures utilizing a dorsal laminectomy to decompress the cord was described. Two Steinmann pins were placed in the dorsolateral aspect of the midbodies of the vertebrae in front of and behind the fractured vertebra; these pins were cut at the height of the articular processes, and the involved spinal segment was then encased in *methylmethacrylate.* The spinal cord and exposed nerves were covered with an absorbable gelatin sponge soaked in cold lactate Ringer's solution to protect them from the acrylic mass. The vertebral displacement or malalignment was reduced and immobilized for approximately 5 minutes while the mass was polymerizing and hardening. The mass was molded around the pins, laminectomy defect, and adjacent dorsal spines, and irrigated with iced lactate Ringer's solution to dissipate the heat of hardening. Preliminary work with this method has resulted in a firm immobilization and good tissue tolerance of the acrylic mass.[41]

BODY CASTS

As mentioned earlier, body splints or casts are needed occasionally to promote immobilization of spinal fractures when internal fixation is not indicated or to provide additional support for internal fixation. In the latter instance, the need is usually most urgent in the immediate postoperative period when arching of the spine is most prevalent. Special requirements for accomplishing effective and comfortable casting include: (1) the cast should be applied under profound sedation or anesthesia (preferably after surgery); (2) appropriate support material of thin plywood, bass-board, aluminum splint, or other material should be selected and cut to the appropriate length; (3) the material should be over-padded at each end of the support so that there will be no pressure on the incision; (4) the skin must be protected from moisture irritation by the application of compound tincture of benzoin; (5) the area of body to be splinted should be wrapped with cast padding material* and gauze bandage; and (6) the support material and body area should then be covered with any choice of casting material such as plaster of Paris or plastic casting material[30, 44]

The casting material should be applied so that the cast will fit snugly; cranially it should be anchored slightly to the hair to prevent caudal slipping, and there should be special tension in the flank area so it does not fit too loosely. The cast material should be applied over the external genitalia if necessary, cutting out an aperture for the prepuce after the cast has hardened. All pressure spots must be observed and relieved appropriately before decubital lesions occur.[44]

The hind limbs can be incorporated in a body cast if necessary by applying a T-shaped splint to the dorsum of the area, taping or casting the padded abducted flexed limbs to this splint, and applying skids to the cast so that the legs and ventral area do not drag on the floor of the cage. Proper apertures for the genitals are necessary so that urine and feces do not accumulate between the cast and the skin. It is

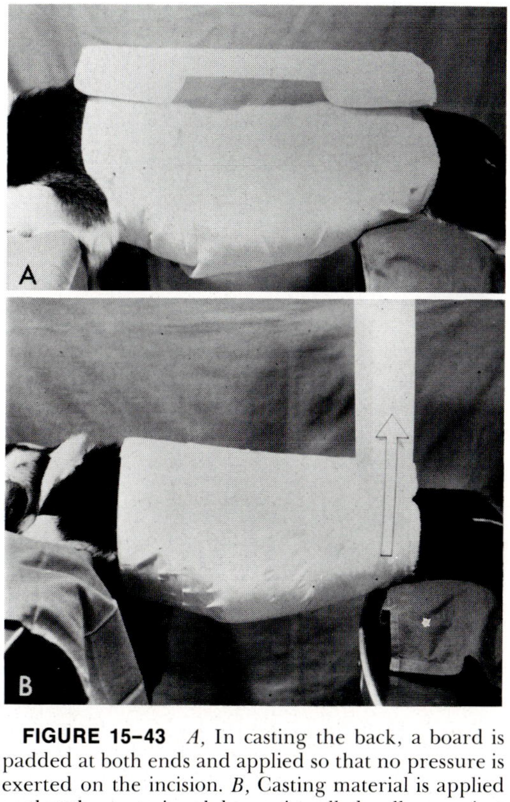

FIGURE 15–43 *A,* In casting the back, a board is padded at both ends and applied so that no pressure is exerted on the incision. *B,* Casting material is applied so that the posterior abdomen is pulled well up against the splint. (From Swaim, S. F.: Body casts. Vet. Med. Small Anim. Clin. *65,* 1179, 1970.)

*Composite Padding Roll, Parke, Davis & Co., Detroit, Michigan.

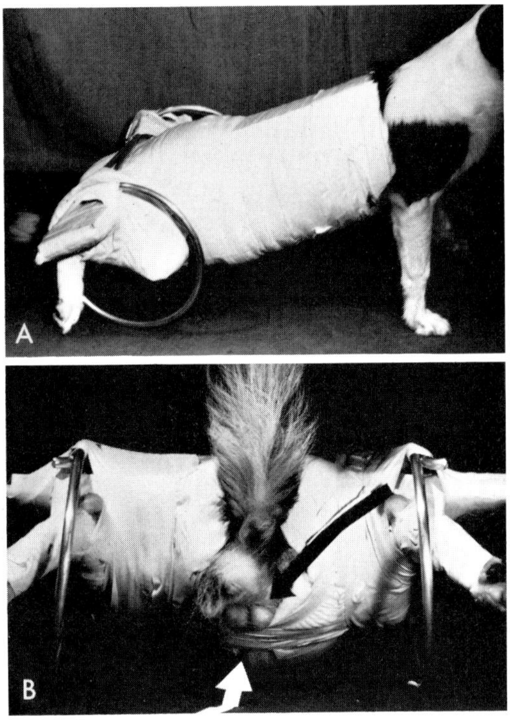

FIGURE 15–44 A full body cast with runners on the Ehmer sling. *A* Lateral view. *B*, Posterior view. Notice that apertures are cut in casts for the scrotum and prepuce of the male dog. (From Swaim, S. F.: Body casts. Vet. Med. Small Anim. Clin. *65*, 1179, 1970.)

emphasized again that great care should be taken to anticipate pressure sites when applying casts so that decubital infections and patient discomfort can be avoided (Figs. 15–43 and 15–44).[44]

ADVANTAGES OF IMMOBILIZATION METHODS

Each of these methods of spinal immobilization has its advantages and disadvantages. The stainless steel plates have been used with generally good results when the dorsal arches are intact. It is common practice to reinforce internal fixation with external casting or splints for 5 to 14 days, especially in large or young dogs in which there is danger that the bolts may be torn out of the spines or the spines may break. The metal plates are readily available, well designed, and polished, so that the danger of infection is minimized and general tissue acceptance is good.

The flexible plastic plates have the advantage of affording perhaps better holding power and allowing less chance of the spines breaking or the bolts tearing out. However, they are generally considerably more expensive and do not have highly polished, smooth surfaces. Therefore, the rough "gripping" surface especially may contain infectious organisms and surgical infections might be more prevalent.

The use of "staple pins" is limited to smaller dogs, generally less than 7 kilograms or 15 pounds in weight. Economy of application is a real advantage of staple pins. Body casts or splints in addition to staple pins should also be considered in some cases.

The use of vertebral body plating has several advantages when the dorsal arches are badly damaged. Generally, it requires a shorter length of spinal segment immobilization and therefore permits better postoperative function. Since body plating has not been used nearly as long as dorsal spine plating, unforeseen disadvantages may yet develop. But thus far, there seems to be a higher degree of stability in body plating because of the greater amount of osseous tissue in the vertebral bodies, and body casting is therefore less important postsurgically. The chief disadvantage is the greater difficulty of application in thoracic and terminal lumbar-sacral areas.

The cross-pinning of the vertebral bodies is advantageous because it is economical and requires a minimal amount of prosthetic material to be left in the area. Body pinning, however, is difficult, especially in thoracic areas. Pins may work loose and migrate to other areas, necessitating removal.

Other methods either are used infrequently or are too new to evaluate properly. The use of the acrylic mass may open a new field in spinal fixation. This author wonders about tissue acceptance and the consequences of sepsis, since the possibility of surgical "slips" in asepsis, or the existence of sepsis before surgery, is always present in traumatic injuries.

RESULTS

The clinical results depend on the severity of the fracture and the resulting neurological damage, the speed with which decompression was initiated, and the effectiveness of surgical correction and postsurgical care based on the aforementioned nursing practices.

Means of controlling edema, swelling, and hemorrhagic necrosis of the cord should be employed when appropriate. Such therapy as hypertonic solutions (25 per cent mannitol), corticosteroids, and perfusions of normothermic or hypothermic solutions of the surgically invaded tissues, and other means of limiting CNS deterioration from trauma should be considered. These matters were discussed in detail in Chapter 12. Elimination of feces must be maintained, and care of the urinary organs must be meticulous. Broad spectrum antibiotics and urinary antiseptic agents are routinely employed. Good nutrition must be maintained. Decubital sores resulting from wearing the cast or from recumbency must be avoided. Some spinal fracture cases can be extremely discouraging considering the expense, time, effort, and tender loving care that are necessary in the total patient program. However, if the cases are properly selected and if the client has been properly informed on all aspects of cost and prognosis, the surgical correction of spinal fractures or luxations can be a most rewarding experience for all concerned.

Spondylectomy and Vertebral Prosthesis

In cases of gross disease of a vertebra resulting from infection, neoplasia, or severe trauma, it would be highly desirable if the vertebra could be removed and replaced by a prosthesis. Brasmer and Lumb reported on a *vertebral prosthesis* successfully applied in 12 normal experimental dogs. Total body hypothermia was employed with gaseous anesthesia. A complete dorsal laminectomy was performed on the L2 vertebra, after which polyvinylidene fluoride spinal plates were applied to the dorsal spines of T13 to L5. The vertebral body was then removed and a specially designed prosthesis was applied in the area of the spondylectomy. All 12 dogs recovered from the surgery; 10 of them regained motor function within 48 hours after surgery, and two remained paraplegic. Four dogs were called long-term survivors after a 58- to 400-day observation period. The prosthesis and modified plating technique provided stability for the spine, and the prosthetic materials caused no observable local tissue reaction.[8]

Yturraspe and co-workers have reported on a spondylectomy of the L2 vertebra in 10 experimental dogs. The shortened vertebral column was stabilized by internal fixation with two types of plastic plates. The standard vinylidene fluoride spinal plates were attached to dorsal spines of the three vertebrae cranial and caudal to the removed vertebra. A specially designed single plate was attached dorsolaterally to the adjacent vertebral bodies with bone screws. Shortening of the spinal column was usually not associated with a marked clinical neurological deficit. However, there was histological evidence of widely disseminated areas of axonal degeneration, gliosis, and atrophy of spinal nerve roots in the surgical area. The spinal cord became intrinsically shorter rather than being displaced within the spinal canal.[57]

SUMMARY

The surgical correction of spinal fractures and luxations is effective in cases in which neurological and radiographic examinations have revealed favorable signs. Such correction also depends on how quickly the case is presented following the accident. Prompt lateral or dorsal decompression of the cord and effective immobilization of the involved vertebrae by fixation devices applied to the dorsal spines and/or vertebral bodies results in a gratifying recovery in most instances. Supportive body casts or braces are used occasionally to provide additional support.

Some cases in which slight compression of the cord has resulted from fracture displacement can be corrected by body casting without surgical decompression and skeletal fixation. However, secondary compressions of the cord can develop from improper healing processes with this method.

Spondylectomy with or without a vertebral prosthesis may become a more common clinical procedure in the future. Infections, tumors, or degeneration disorders of the vertebra constitute the primary indications for this procedure.

SECTION 2
SPINAL FUSIONS

Various methods of producing spinal fusions by means of bone grafts have been used in man for many years. Fusions are used occasionally in conjunction with disk surgery, and Compere has suggested that spinal fusions should be done in all cases in which disks have been removed.[13] Cloward advised vertebral body fusions by means of the intervertebral "plug" graft in disk surgery on patients whose occupations involved heavy labor.[12]

Most surgeons at the present time do not routinely perform a spinal fusion with standard disk surgery. The prolonged bed rest necessary and the need to use a jacket or cast for the ambulatory patient when extensive fusions are performed have discouraged many surgeons.[37] Armstrong[3] expressed the opinion that arthrodesis or fusion of the affected joint could not be justified as an immediate and routine measure in all patients undergoing disk surgery. Arthrodesis should be reserved for a later, second-stage procedure in selected patients, and should be carried out initially only in special circumstances.

INDICATIONS FOR SPINAL FUSION

Spinal fusion by means of bone grafts has been used frequently in arrested cases of spinal tuberculosis as well as in selected cases of disk disease in man.[9] Other diseases that might be treated by fusions are arrested septic osteomyelitis, spondylosis, degenerations and malformations resulting from trauma, metabolic bone conditions, and vertebral instabilities.

In our experience, we have used spinal bone grafts in disk disorders and in concomitant bone disease. When a lack of vertebral support results in a traumatic rupture of the disk, a bone graft should be used. This is especially true in a working or sporting dog, or in large pets. Disk disease and adjacent spondylosis or spondylarthritis in the same dog would be an indication for a spinal bone graft and fusion. A bone graft could be done in a dog with a large decompression which has left an unstable intervertebral joint or a large dorsal bone defect. The advent of ventral cervical decompressive surgery has stimulated the use of bone grafts to stabilize the vertebrae involved and to facilitate closure of the body defect. Surgical relief of the wobbler has promoted use of bone graft fusions for spinal immobilization.

BASIC CONCEPTS IN BONE GRAFTS

The types of bone graft generally recognized are (1) autogenous—bone taken from the host himself; (2) homogeneous—bone taken from the same species as the host, but a different individual; and (3) heterogeneous—bone from a different species. Homogeneous and heterogeneous grafts may be preserved and become part of a "bone bank."[34]

There are various opinions as to the most effective type of bone to use and how it should be placed or fixed. Campbell states that osteogenic cells and osteocytes survive only in fresh autogenous bone grafts.[10] Autogenous bone grafts are also better tolerated in tissue than preserved or fresh homogeneous grafts. Wilson, on the other hand, has suggested that the healing of "bone bank" grafts and fresh autogenous grafts takes place chiefly by a process of invasion, absorption, and replacement.[55] Both of these types are indistinguishable several months after implantation; however, fresh autogenous grafts become incorporated more rapidly. Austin[4] states that the ideal bone graft for vertebral body fusion is obtained from a bone bank; that frozen cadaver bone preserved in blood plasma is as good as or superior to bone obtained from the patient. Gurdjian[24] states that the incidence of infection is greatest when autopsy bone grafts are used. Gallie and Robertson state that such osteoblasts that stay alive do so because they have access to a surrounding supply of blood and lymph.[23] These cells proliferate and form new living bone along the framework of bone that has died from lack of fresh blood and lymph.

Armstrong has outlined the basic conditions of bone grafting in man as follows.[2]

1. There should be close and stable contact between large areas of raw bone on the graft and host.
2. Fixation of the graft and fracture must be mechanically stable.
3. Before grafting, the fractured surfaces should be cleared of fibrous tissue and sclerotic bone.
4. Normal apposition and alignment of the fragments of the host bone should be restored.
5. The architecture of the reconstructed bone should as far as possible approximate that of the normal bone at the conclusion of the operation.

If growth is to take place, the bone should be cut, prepared, and placed so as to utilize fully the revascularization process. The graft should be in contact with a vascular area.[2] The deeper layers of the cortex and medullary cavity are more vascular than the superficial cortex. The graft will be more easily vascularized if it contains, at least in part, soft cancellous endosteal bone that is in immediate contact with the host bone. Finally, the larger the areas of graft and host that are brought into contact, the more rapid will be the revascularization of the graft and its subsequent replacement by living bone. Since osteoblasts are found chiefly under the periosteum and the endosteum, osteogenesis will take place much more rapidly if one or both of these structures can be included in the graft.[36]

In general, it would seem from the literature that fresh autogenous grafts are accepted by the host more quickly than homogeneous or bank grafts, but that the end result is the same. A graft should be prepared so as to have an abundant supply of osteoblasts as well as of blood for nutrition.

TYPES OF SPINAL BONE GRAFTS

INTERVERTEBRAL BONE GRAFT

An intervertebral bone graft[12] is shaped like a disk, block, or dowel and is inserted between the bodies of the vertebrae in the disk space (Fig. 15–45).

CLOTHESPIN GRAFT

A clothespin graft[7] is an H-shaped graft wedged between the spinous processes with the spines notched to keep the graft fixed (Figs. 15–46 and 15–47).

HIBB'S METHOD

Hibb's method[42] was one of the first to be successful. It consists of splitting the spinous processes into small fragments, chipping the outer surfaces of the arches of the laminae, removing the cartilage from the articular facets, and placing the bone chips as bridges across the denuded bone of the vertebral arches. Additional bone chips from the ilium or tibia can be used to reinforce the area.

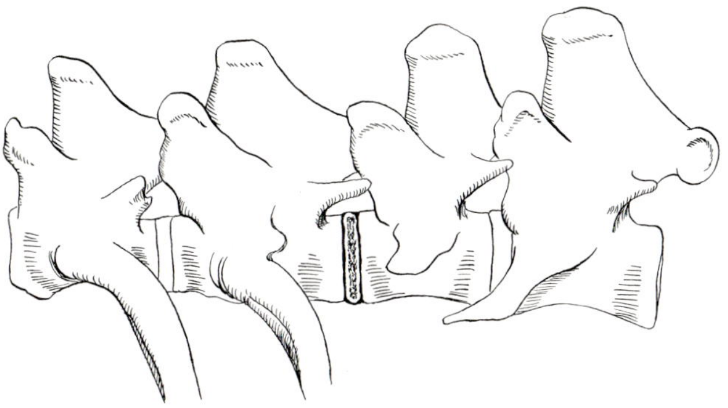

FIGURE 15–45 The intervertebral graft is a disk-like piece of bone forcibly placed between the vertebrae to replace the disk, which has been removed.

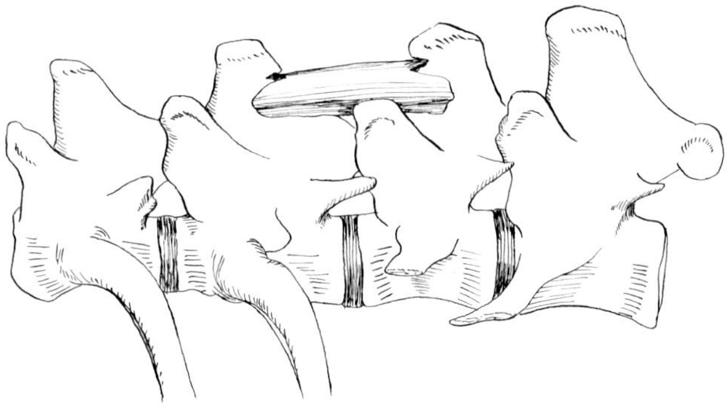

FIGURE 15–46 The clothespin or H graft is placed between the spines, which have been specially notched and pulled apart to promote stability when the graft is inserted.

FIGURE 15–47 A dorsal view of the graft shown in Figure 15–46. This graft maintains pressure against the spines, thereby promoting rigidity.

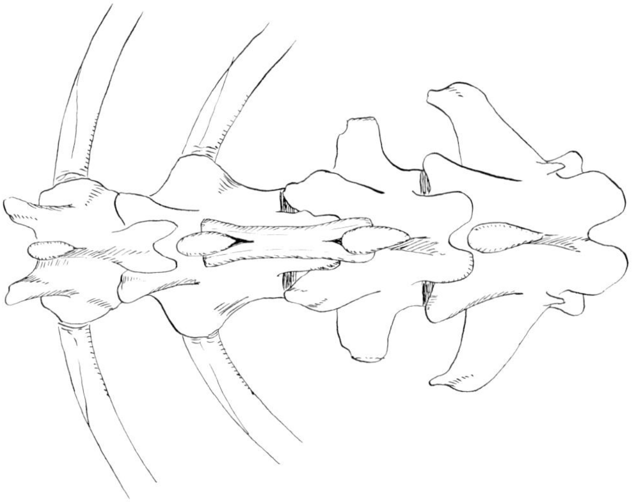

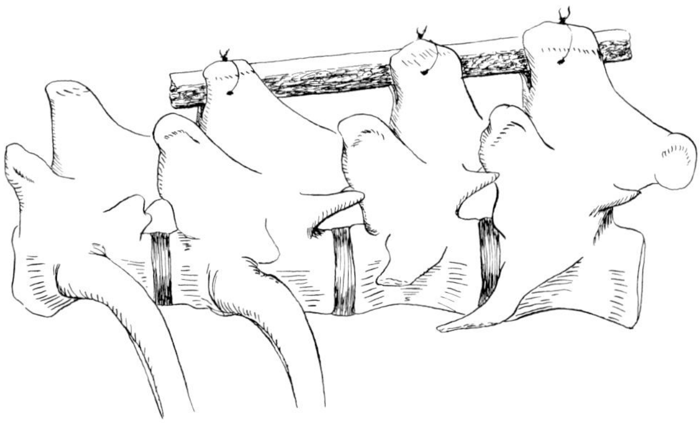

FIGURE 15–48 The wedge or inclusion graft is placed between the split sections of the spines.

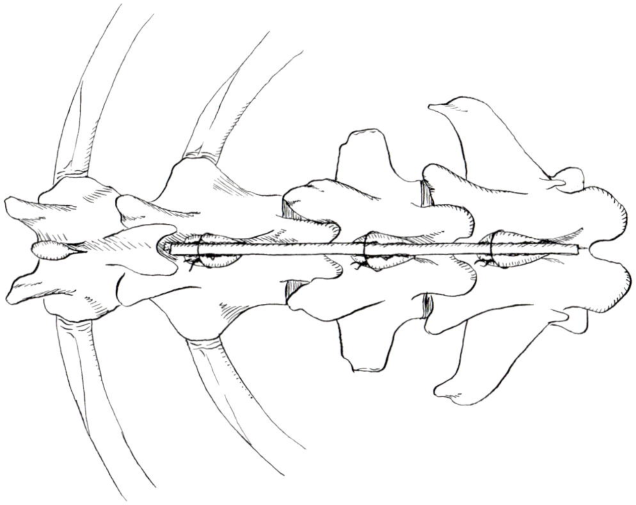

FIGURE 15–49 Holes are drilled through the split sections of the spines and the graft (Fig. 15–48). The graft is secured with stainless steel wire.

ALBEE'S METHOD

Albee's method[42] makes use of a "wedge" or an "inclusion" graft, and consists of placing a rigid graft between the split spinous processes and securing it by means of wire or other suture material (Figs. 15–48 to 15–50).

ONLAY GRAFT

An Onlay graft[2] is used frequently on long bones, and involves placing a rigid bone graft on a properly prepared area of host bone and securing it by means of screws or similar equipment (Fig. 15–51).

ANTERIOR (VENTRAL) FUSION

The anterior (ventral) approach to fusion consists of one or two grafts inlaid on the anterior (ventral) surfaces of the affected vertebrae. This method was designed primarily for fusion in cases of spondylolisthesis.[3, 37]

PROCEDURE IN DOGS

In 1956,[28] experimental methods of performing spinal bone grafts and vertebral immobilization, including those just mentioned, were reported. It was determined that an autogenous rib graft was possible. In surgical interventions of the spine, the spinal and terminal rib areas can be prepared as one surgical field. The subject experiences no discomfort from the removal of one or two terminal ribs, which provide cancellous bone from an autogenous source (which is said to be ideal for grafting).[34] The use of long bones as a source of graft material may be associated with rather persistent pain and disuse of the leg, and this is especially true of the tibia.[28] The one disadvantage in using a rib is that it is curved. However, it can be straightened by partial cortical sectioning and bending by means of a small rongeur or power-driven bur.[30]

The varieties of grafts tried included: (1) single and double onlay grafts second to

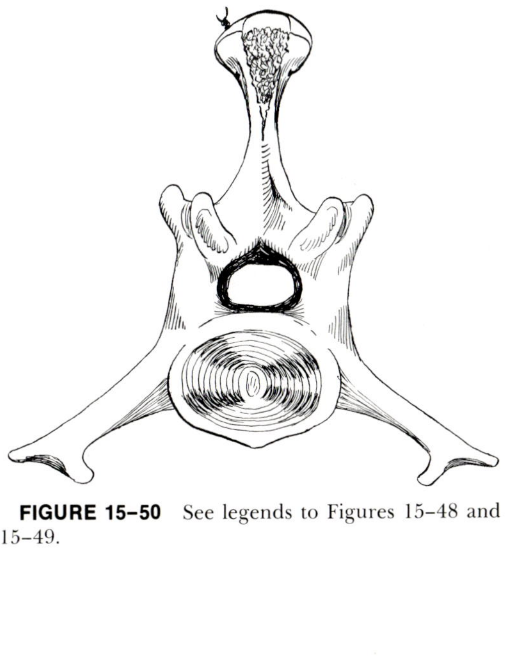

FIGURE 15–50 See legends to Figures 15–48 and 15–49.

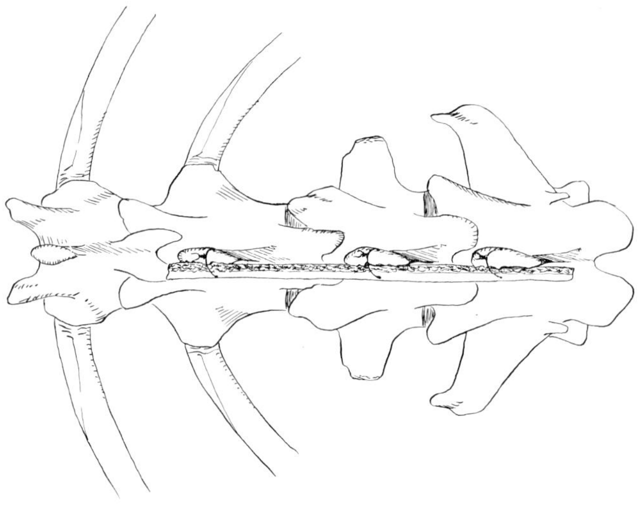

FIGURE 15–51 Onlay graft which is secured to the spines with stainless steel wire.

dorsal spines by means of screws, nylon suture, wire strands, and small pins; (2) clothespin or H grafts forcibly applied between the adjacent dorsal spines; and (3) wedge or inclusion grafts placed between split dorsal spines and secured by wire or small pins.[28]

The methods of immobilization for these experiments consisted primarily of external full body casts made from plaster of Paris and synthetic or plastic materials. The cast or support was allowed to remain in place for 3 months. Periodic radiographic examinations of each animal were made. Necropsies were performed from 3 to 7 months following the surgical application of bone grafts. In a few instances, the immobilization methods consisted of plates and bolts secured to the dorsal spines or to the lateral processes, or plates screwed into the ventral surfaces of the involved vertebrae.[28]

The study indicated that the wedge graft seemed to provide the most effective fusion (Figs. 15–54, 15–55, 15–57). The H graft provided the best initial support but might have resulted in a pseudoarthrosis instead of a fusion (Fig. 15–56). Onlay grafts pro-

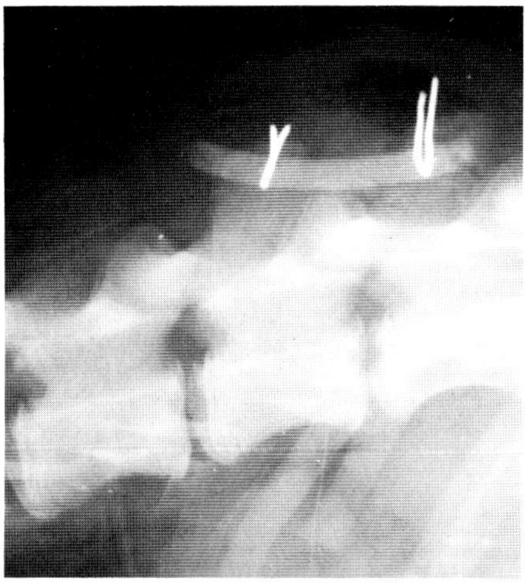

Fig. 15–52

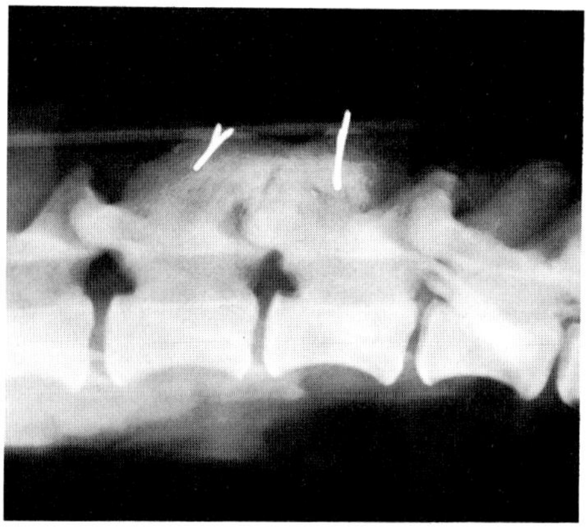

Fig. 15–53

FIGURE 15–52 A onlay graft which had been implanted 2 days previously.

FIGURE 15–53 Radiograph of a section of spine 4 months after the onlay graft had been performed on the dog in Figure 15–52. (From Hoerlein, B. F.: Method of spinal fusion and vertebral immobilization in the dog. Am. J. Vet. Res. *17*, Oct., 1956.)

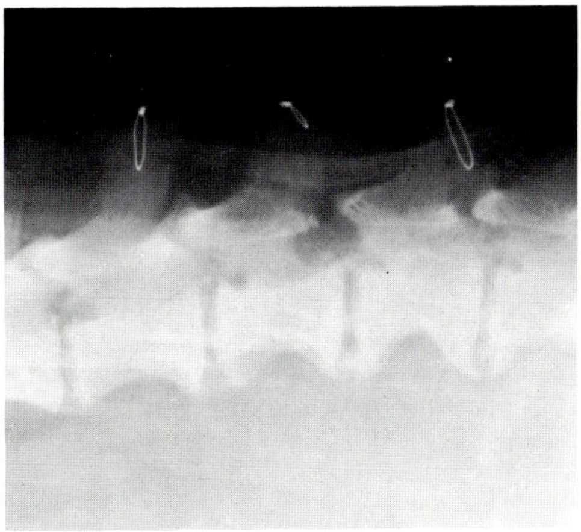

Fig. 15–54

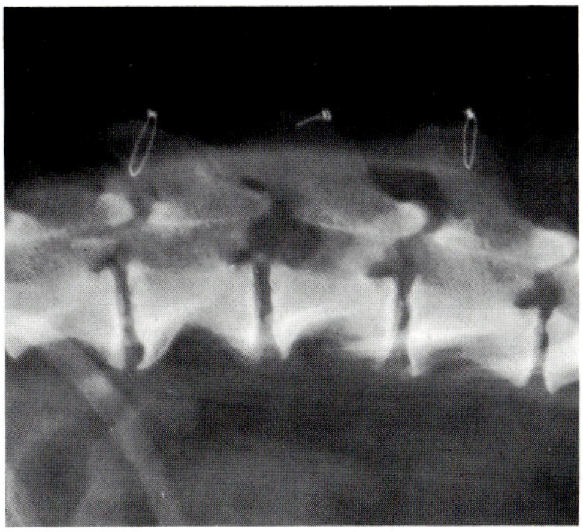

Fig. 15–55

FIGURE 15–54 Clinical disk paraplegia in a 5-year-old dachshund was fused with a wedge graft.
FIGURE 15–55 Fusion observed 1 year later in the case shown in Figure 15–54.

vided a satisfactory fusion when wired securely to the spines (Figs. 15–52 and 15–53).[28]

Skeletal fixation did not produce the best acceptance; it appears that a slight degree of movement is necessary to stimulate osteogenic activity. Therefore, the use of body casts seemed satisfactory and desirable for immobilization following grafting.[28] Clinical applications based upon these findings have substantiated the experimental results.

The literature on spinal fusion in humans in recent years deals largely with anterior (ventral) cervical fusions.[11] White reports a series of 65 patients in whom curettage of the disk interspace had been done and a horseshoe-shaped portion of iliac bone had been inserted. In two-thirds of the cases there were good or excellent results during a follow-up period averaging 3½ years.[53] Many other methods of spinal fusions are now being used in man.[14]

In the dog, Popovic[39] has proposed a dowel graft for a trephination type of ventral cervical disk decompression (Fig. 15–58). Prata and Stoll[40] have proposed a cortical graft to fill in the decompression defect and add stability to the area in a slot type of ventral cervical disk removal (Fig. 15–59). However, Swaim[46] feels that this is

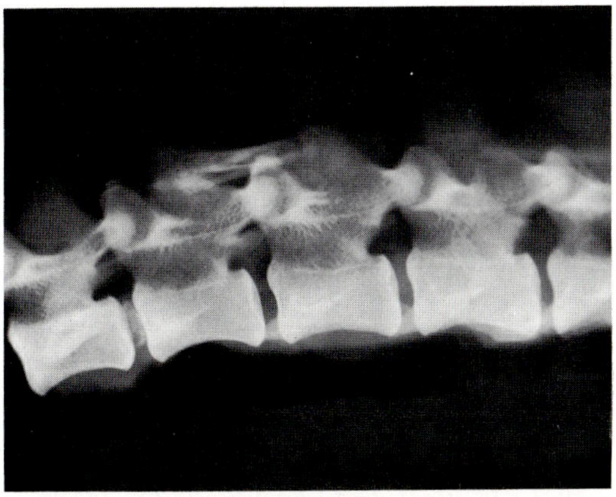

Fig. 15–56

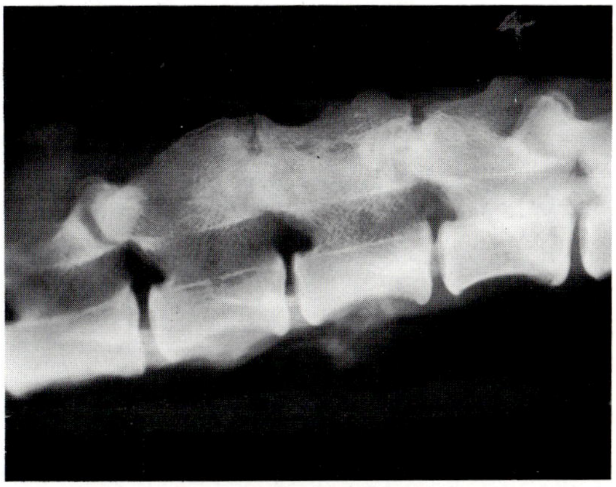

Fig. 15–57

FIGURE 15–56 Radiograph of a specimen 4 months after an H or clothespin graft had been performed. (From Hoerlein, B. F.: Method of spinal fusion and vertebral immobilization in the dog. Am. J. Vet. Res. *17*, Oct., 1956.)

FIGURE 15–57 Radiograph of a section of the spinal column 6 months after implantation of a wedge graft. Notice the heavy fusion of bone which has resulted. (From Hoerlein, B. F.: Method of spinal fusion and vertebral immobilization in the dog. Am. J. Vet. Res. *17*, Oct. 1956.)

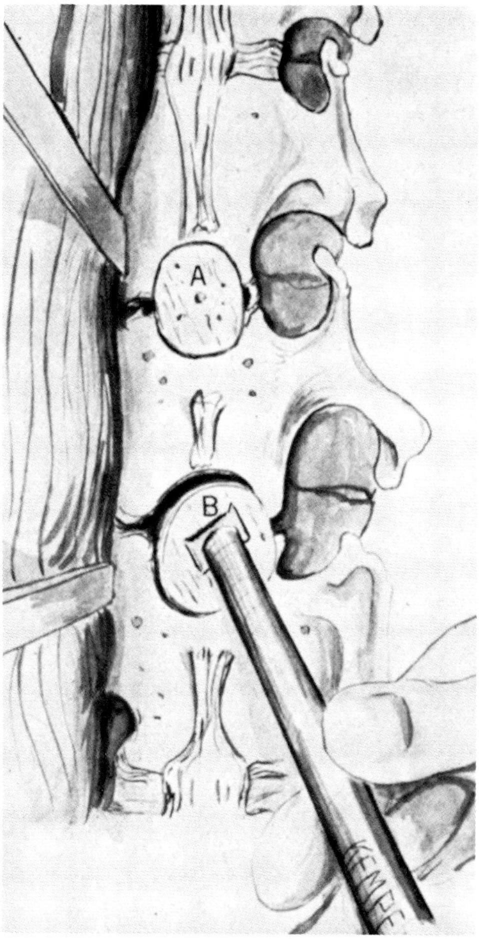

FIGURE 15–58 Ventral view of the cervical vertebrae of a dog, showing one bone graft in place (A) and a second bone graft (B) being gently tapped into place. (From Popovic, N. A., Vander Ark, G., and Kempe, L.: Ventral approach for surgical treatment of cervical disk disease in the dog. Am. J. Vet. Res. *32*, 1155, 1971.)

unnecessary since the defect will reossify and the area will remain stable unless the defect covers more than 1 vertebral length. Dueland[15] has described surgery on a dog with the wobbler syndrome (cervical instability) involving dorsal lay-on grafts wired in thc unstable area (Fig. 15–60). Flo[16] has reported the use of clothespin or H grafts forced between thoracic dorsal spines with conjunctive lay-on grafts wired in place to stabilize spines when hemivertebrae are present (Fig. 15–61). In dogs with cervical vertebral instabilities, Knecht and Oliver[33] have used ventrally placed dowel grafts in the affected intervertebral spaces, overlayed by steel plates fixed to the involved vertebrae by screws (Fig. 15–62).

It appears to this author that more vertebral bone grafts will be used in the future, probably combined with other means of at least partial internal immobilization or fixation. External casts in some spinal areas and in certain breeds of dogs are difficult to apply and are uncomfortable to the average patient. However, in original investigative work on spinal fusions (1956),[28] this author found that better "graft takes" resulted when rigid internal fixation was not used instead of external casts or corsets.

SURGICAL PROCEDURE[30]

The wedge graft has occasionally been used with satisfactory results in the circumstances outlined. The bone graft is obtained by making a longitudinal incision directly over the terminal rib. The lateral periosteum is incised over the full length of the rib, extending from the costochondral

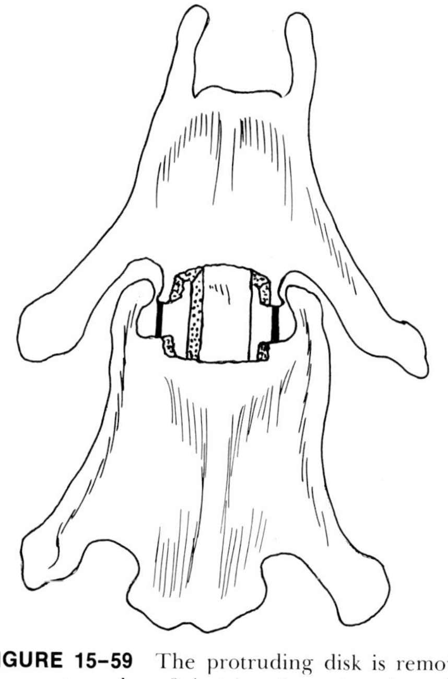

FIGURE 15–59 The protruding disk is removed, and a contoured graft is taken from the wing of the ilium and positioned after traction is placed on the cervical spine. The thickness of the graft is 2 to 5 mm less than the defect to prevent impingement of the graft on the cord. (From Prata, R. G., *In* Bojrab, M. J. (ed.): *Current Techniques in Small Animal Surgery I.* Lea & Febiger, Philadelphia, 1975.)

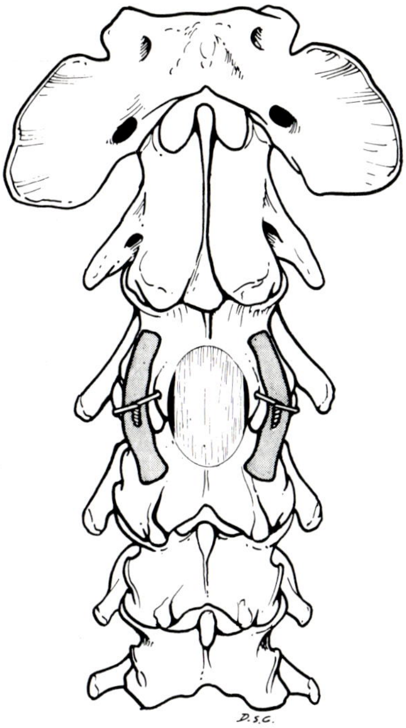

FIGURE 15–60 A dorsal laminectomy, partial fascetectomy, and wire fixation of lay-on bone grafts to stabilize a canine wobbler. (From Dueland, R., Furneaux, R. W., and Kaye, M. M.: Spinal fusion and dorsal laminectomy for midcervical spondylolisthesis in a dog. J.A.V.M.A. *162*, 366, 1973.)

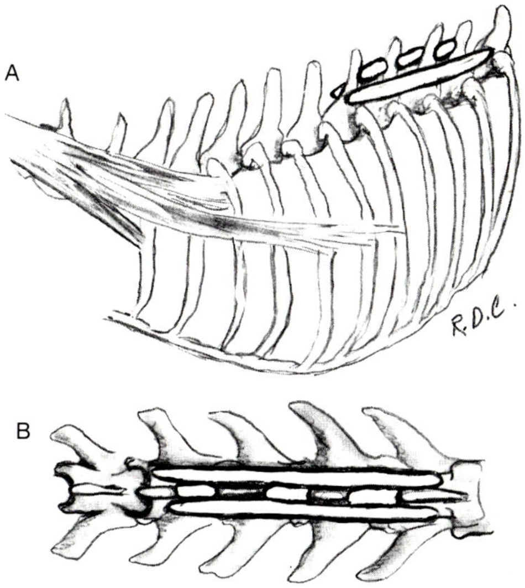

FIGURE 15–61 Rib grafts are wedged longitudinally (using the clothespin technique) between the dorsal spines, and lay-on grafts, which are split longitudinally, are packed tightly around the spine for stabilization of a hemivertebra. *A,* Lateral view. *B,* Dorsoventral view. (From Flo, G. L.: Serial fusion for the treatment of hemivertebra. *In* Bojrab, M. J. (ed.): *Current Techniques in Small Animal Surgery I.* Lea & Febiger, Philadelphia, 1975.)

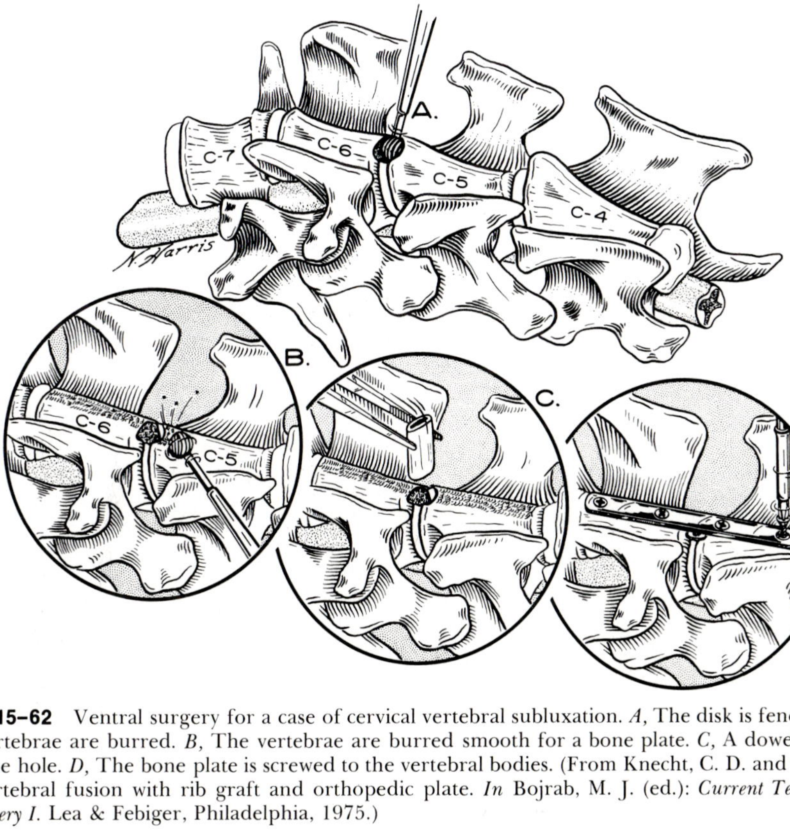

FIGURE 15–62 Ventral surgery for a case of cervical vertebral subluxation. *A,* The disk is fenestrated, and the adjacent vertebrae are burred. *B,* The vertebrae are burred smooth for a bone plate. *C,* A dowel-shaped graft is placed in the hole. *D,* The bone plate is screwed to the vertebral bodies. (From Knecht, C. D. and Oliver, J. E., Jr.: Cervical vertebral fusion with rib graft and orthopedic plate. *In* Bojrab, M. J. (ed.): *Current Techniques in Small Animal Surgery I.* Lea & Febiger, Philadelphia, 1975.)

junction to a point as close to the vertebra as possible. A periosteal elevator or the White thin blade tartar scraper can be used to lift the rib out of its periosteal envelope. The rib is severed at its ventral attachment to the cartilage and is lifted upward as it is dissected free of surrounding tissue. The bone cutting forceps is used to sever the rib as close to the vertebrae as possible. If the periosteum has been removed with the rib, the surrounding musculature is sutured carefully with interrupted sutures. If the periosteum has been resected from the rib, the periosteal envelope is sutured in like fashion, and the bone should replace itself within a few months. Since the terminal rib has little or no function, it appears to be unnecessary to preserve the periosteal sleeve.

The rib is kept moist in warm saline until the spinal correction has been made and the fusion is to be performed. The wedge graft method consists of carefully splitting the spinous processes by means of a scalpel or a thin chisel. A motor-driven appliance can be used. Since the spine is quite thin, splitting may be difficult and must be attempted carefully. After this, the graft is shaped for proper application.

The rib is somewhat curved, and part of the convex side usually must be resected in order to straighten it for use in a wedge graft. This can be done with the Dean mastoid rongeur, which has probably been used previously in some phase of the spinal surgery. With the graft shaped and placed in its proper location, holes are drilled into the split spines and graft. Generally, No. 0, 1, or 2 stainless steel wire is used to secure the graft in place by inserting it into the holes and tying a square knot or twisting it.

The closure of the fascia and skin is routinely performed. The cast is applied around the body as described for fracture fixations. It may be left in place for 8 to 12 weeks. During this period, the dog is allowed restricted and supervised exercise. A corset may be applied to a dog of a quiet and easily controllable disposition after the sixth week. An active dog should not be permitted unrestricted exercise for a 6-month period.

In the H or clothespin graft, the rib is shaped as illustrated in Figures 15–46 and 15–47. The spines are notched as indicated. With the spines pulled apart by means of forceps, the graft is placed between the spines. The forceps are released, and the graft holds the spines rigidly apart. Bone chips or "shingles" (Hibb's method) can be placed around the area for added osteogenic effect. A moistened piece of absorbable gelatin sponge placed as a blanket on the bone chips will help confine them to the area during closure.

Onlay grafts should be placed as close to the base of the spine as possible, with cancellous bone of the graft contacting cancellous bone of the host. Generally, best results will be obtained when substantial grafts are placed on each side of the spines and holes are drilled through grafts and spine and secured with orthopedic wire.

In ventral cervical decompressive disk surgery, the dowel graft placed in a trephine hole is obtained from either a rib or the ilium. In a slot type of decompression, the block graft most commonly used is obtained from the ilium. Air-driven burs can facilitate the shaping of both the donor site and the graft for maximal effect.

SUMMARY

Bone grafts may be applied to the dog's spine in pathologic disorders of the vertebral and articular joints or in extensive decompression procedures. It is felt that if rigid and immediate skeletal stabilization is needed in the area, direct skeletal appliances should be employed, as in a fracture. If osteogenic material is needed for eventual healing of a degenerative process, a bone graft is used. In recent years some surgeons prefer to use bone grafts (block or dowel) in ventral disk decompressions.

The rib or ilium may be used as a desirable source of an autogenous bone graft. A wedge graft has given the best results in the dog, although H or onlay grafts can be used for dorsal spinal grafts and fusion. Body casting for a 3-month period seems to provide satisfactory immobilization that promotes acceptance of the graft. Only restricted exercise should be allowed during this period.

REFERENCES

1. Archibald, J., Pennock, P. U., and Cawley, A. J.: Trauma of the vertebral column in dogs. Vet. Med., *54*:518, 1959.

2. Armstrong, J. R.: *Bone Grafting in the Treatment of Fractures.* The Williams and Wilkins Co., Baltimore, 1946.
3. Armstrong, J. R.: *Lumbar Disc Lesions.* E. and S. Livingstone, Ltd., London, 1958.
4. Austin, G.: *Basic and Surgical Considerations.* 2nd ed. Charles C Thomas, Publishers, Springfield, Ill., 1972, p. 416.
5. Bartels, M.: Observations on spinal injuries. Small Anim. Clin., *2,* 679, 1962.
6. Betts, C. W., Kneller, S. K., and Skelton, J. A.: An unusual case of traumatic spondylolisthesis in a red bone hound: diagnosis and therapy. J. Am. Anim. Hosp. Assoc. *12,* 470, 1976.
7. Bosworth, D. M.: Clothespin or inclusion graft for spondylolisthesis or laminal defects of the lumbar spine. Surg. Gynecol. Obst. *75,* 593, 1942.
8. Brasmer, T. H., and Lumb, W. V.: Lumbar vertebral prosthesis in the dog. Am. J. Vet. Res. *33,* 493, 1972.
9. Brugghen, A. V.: *Neurosurgery in General Practice.* Charles C Thomas, Publishers, Springfield, Ill., 1952.
10. Campbell, C. J., Brower, T., McFadden, O. G., Payne, E. B., and Doherty, J.: Experimental study of the fate of bone grafts. J. Bone Joint Surg. *35A,* 332, 1953.
11. Clark, K.: Anterior operative approach for benign extradural cervical lesions. *In* Youmans, J. R. (ed.): *Neurological Surgery.* W. B. Saunders Co., Philadelphia, 1973, p. 1213.
12. Cloward, B.: The treatment of ruptured lumbar intervertebral discs; criteria for spinal fusion. Am. J. Surg. *86,* 145, 1953.
13. Compere, E. L., Schmite, U., Compere, C. L., and Thompson, R. G.: Intervertebral disc removal and spine fusion. Am. J. Surg. *96,* 624, 1958.
14. De Palma, A. F.: *The Management of Fractures and Dislocations,* 2d ed. W. B. Saunders Co., Philadelphia, 1970, p. 419.
15. Dueland, R., Furneaux, R. W., and Kaye, M. M.: Spinal fusion and dorsal laminectomy for midcervical spondylolisthesis in a dog. J.A.V.M.A. *162,* 366, 1973.
16. Flo, G. L.: Spinal fusion for the treatment of hemivertebra. *In* Bojrab, M. J. (ed.): *Current Techniques in Small Animal Surgery I.* Lea and Febiger, Philadelphia, 1975, p. 392.
17. Frazier, C. H., and Northway, R. B.: Intramedullary immobilization of the lumbar spine of the dog. J.A.V.M.A. *148,* 676, 1966.
18. Frye, F. L., and Cucuel, J. E.: Fracture of the second cervical vertebra in a dog treated with an extension collar. Anim. Hosp. *4,* 193, 1968.
19. Funkquist, B., and Schantz, B.: Influence of extensive laminectomy on the shape of the spinal canal. Acta Orthop. Scand. Suppl. *56,* 1962.
20. Gage, E. D.: Surgical repair of a fractured cervical spine in the dog. J.A.V.M.A. *153,* 1407, 1968.
21. Gage, E. D.: A new method of spinal fixation in the dog (a preliminary report). Vet. Med. Small Anim. Clin. *64,* 295, 1969.
22. Gage, E. D.: Surgical repairs of spinal fractures in small breed dogs. Vet. Med. Small Anim. Clin. *66,* 1095, 1971.
23. Gallie, W. E., and Robertson, E. E.: The transplantation of bone. J.A.M.A. *70,* 1134, 1918.
24. Gurdjian, E. S., and Thomas, L. M.: *Operative Neurosurgery,* 3rd ed. The Williams and Wilkins Co., Baltimore, 1970, p. 418.
25. Hansen, H. J., and Olsson, S. E.: The effect of a single violent trauma on the spine of the dog. Acta Orthop. Scand. *24,* 1, 1954.
27. Hoerlein, B. F.: Successful correction of a vertebral fracture in a dog. Case report. Auburn Vet. *10,* 15, 1953.
28. Hoerlein, B. F.: Methods of spinal fusion and vertebral immobilization in the dog. Am. J. Vet. Res. *17,* 685, 1956.
29. Hoerlein, B. F.: Traumatic lesions of the canine spine. Mod. Vet. Prac. *39,* 24, Oct. 15, 1958; *39,* 31, Nov. 1, 1958.
30. Hoerlein, B. F.: *Canine Neurology, Diagnosis and Treatment,* 2d ed. W. B. Saunders Co., Philadelphia, 1971.
31. Hurov, L.: Spinal fracture plating. Small Anim. Clin. *2,* 441, 1962.
32. Kavit, A. Y.: Hemilaminectomy in a dog with bone graft and metal internal fixation. J.A.V.M.A. *132,* 16, 1958.
33. Knecht, C. D., and Oliver, J. E.: Cervical vertebral fusion with rib graft and orthopedic plate. *In* Bojrab, M. J. (ed.): *Current Techniques in Small Animal Surgery I.* Lea and Febiger, Philadelphia, 1975, p. 387.
34. Leonard, E. P.: *Orthopedic Surgery of the Dog and Cat.* W. B. Saunders Co., Philadelphia, 1960.
35. Lumb, W. V., and Brasmer, T. H.: Improved spinal plates and hyperthermia as adjuncts to spinal surgery. J.A.V.M.A. *157,* 338, 1970.
36. Markowitz, J.: *Experimental Surgery,* 3d ed. The Williams and Wilkins Co., Baltimore, 1954.
37. Mullen, S.: *Essentials of Neurosurgery.* Springer Publishing Co., Inc. New York, 1961.
38. Northway, R. B.: Fusion of the lumbar vertebrae in the dog. Vet. Med. Small Anim. Clin. *61,* 1190, 1966.
39. Popovic, N. A., Vander Ark, G., and Kempe, L.: Ventral approach for surgical treatment of cervical disk disease in the dog. Am. J. Vet. Res. *32,* 1155, 1971.
40. Prata, R. G., and Stoll, S. G.: Ventral decompression and fusion for the treatment of cervical disc disease in the dog. J. Am. Anim. Hosp. Assoc. *9,* 462, 1973.
41. Rouse, G. P., and Miller, J. I.: The use of methylmethacrylate for spinal stabilization. J. Am. Anim. Hosp. Assoc. *11,* 418, 1975.
42. Shands, A. R.: *Handbook of Orthopedic Surgery,* 3d ed. C. V. Mosby Co., St. Louis, 1948.
43. Slocum, B., and Rudy, R. L.: Fractures of the seventh lumbar vertebra in the dog. J. Am. Anim. Hosp. Assoc. *11,* 167, 1975.
44. Swaim, S. F.: Body casts: technics of application to the dog. Vet. Med. Small Anim. Clin. *65,* 1179, 1970.
45. Swaim, S. F.: Vertebral body plating for spinal immobilization. J.A.V.M.A. *158,* 1683, 1971.
46. Swaim, S. F.: Ventral decompression of the cervical spinal cord in the dog. J.A.V.M.A. *162,* 276, 1973.
47. Swaim, S. F.: Thoracolumbar and sacral spine trauma. *In* Bojrab, M. J. (ed.): *Current Techniques in Small Animal Surgery I.* Lea and Febiger, Philadelphia, 1975, p. 393.
48. Swaim, S. F.: Bilateral hemilaminectomy: a tech-

nique for extensive spinal decompression. Auburn Vet. *32*, 62, 1976.
49. Trotter, E. J.: Canine intervertebral disk disease. *In* Kirk, R. W. (ed.): *Current Veterinary Therapy V.* W. B. Saunders Co., Philadelphia, 1974, p. 666.
50. Trotter, E. J.: Modified dorsal laminectomy and selective regional spinal cord hypothermia in the treatment of thoracolumbar disk disease. *In* Bojrab, M. J. (ed.): *Current Techniques in Small Animal Surgery I.* Lea and Febiger, Philadelphia, 1975, p. 406.
51. Trotter, E. J., Brasmer, T. H., and de Lahunta, A.: Modified deep dorsal laninectomy in the dog. Cornell Vet. *65*, 402, 1975.
52. Trotter, E. J., de Lahunta, A., Geary, J. C., and Brasmer, T. H.: Caudal cervical vertebral malformation-malarticulation in Great Danes and Doberman Pinschers. J.A.V.M.A. *168*, 917, 1976.
53. White, A. A., Southwick, W. O., Deponte, R. J., Gainor, J. W., and Hardy, R.: Relief of pain by anterior spine fusion for spondylosis: report of 65 patients. J. Bone Joint Surg. *55A*, 525, 1973.
54. Whittick, W. G.: *Canine Orthopedics.* Lea and Febiger, Philadelphia, 1974, p. 407.
55. Wilson, P. D.: Experiences with the use of refrigerated homogeneous bone. J. Bone Joint Surg. *33B*, 301, 1951.
56. Yturraspe, D. J., and Lumb, W. V.: The use of plastic spinal plates for internal fixation of the canine spine. J.A.V.M.A. *161*, 1651, 1972.
57. Yturraspe, D. J., Lumb, W. V., Young, S., and Gorman, H. A.: Neurological and pathological effects of second lumbar spondylectomy and spinal column shortening in the dog. J. Neurosurg. *42*, 47, 1975.

PART SIX

THE BRAIN

CHAPTER 16

PARACRANIAL DISORDERS

There are four structures associated with the skull that may, if diseased, cause infections to extend into the cranial cavity: the eye, the ear, the sinuses, and the nasal passages.

The eye has a direct pathway to the brain by means of the optic nerves. These nerves are surrounded by sheaths that are formed by extensions of the meninges of the brain and include a minute quantity of cerebrospinal fluid. The sheaths therefore are extensions of the subdural and subarachnoid spaces,[36] and a massive infection of the eyeball can easily spread to the brain and meninges (Fig. 16–1).

The ear is also in close association with the brain, anatomically and functionally. An infection of the outer ear can easily spread to the middle and inner ear, and an inner ear infection can spread to the brain by extension through contact with the dura and endolymphatic sac and along the vessels and nerves that pass through the internal acoustic meatus.[36] Infections of the inner ear can affect position, balance, and movement (Fig. 16–2).

Infections of the sinuses and nasal passages in the dog are frequently seen. The frontal sinuses are situated dorsally to the anterior cerebrum and are separated from

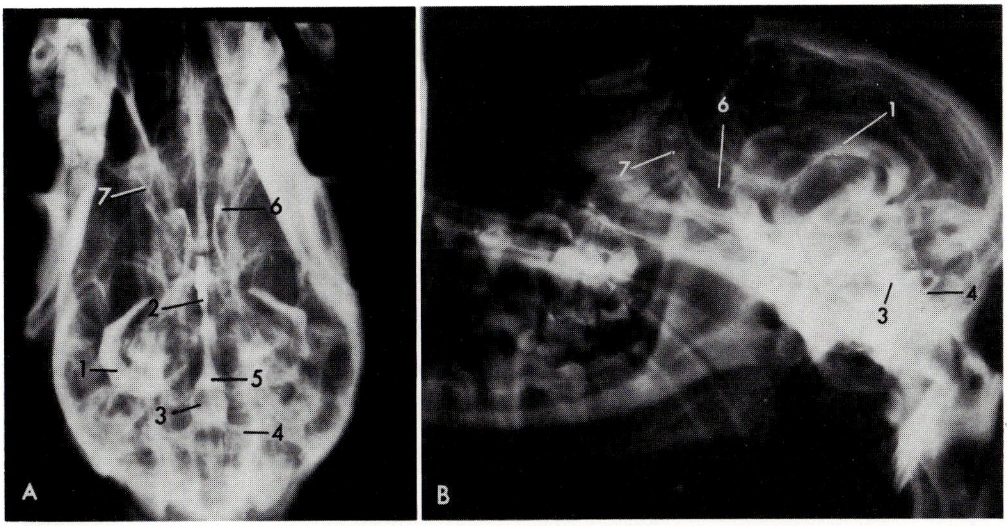

FIGURE 16–1 These radiographs were made following the administration of meglumine iothalamate (60 per cent) into the lateral ventricle. Notice the filling of the optic nerve tracts. Radiographs demonstrate the proximity of the eyes to the brain and the CSF system, and the importance of the eyes in possible metastatic infections to the brain. (1) lateral ventricle; (2) third ventricle; (3) rostral position of the fourth ventricle; (4) lateral recess of the fourth ventricle; (5) cerebral aqueduct; (6) olfactory recess; (7) optic tracts.

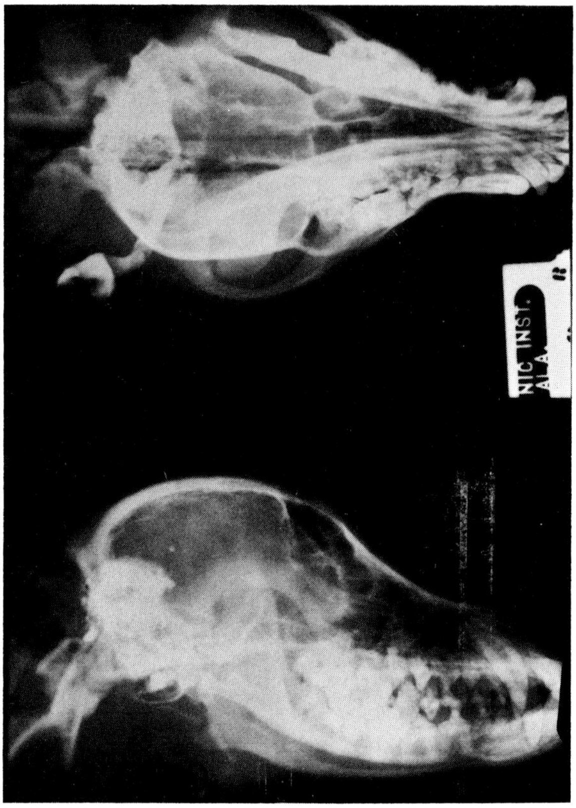

FIGURE 16–2 The cerebellum has been rendered radiopaque with barium sulfate. The ear canal has also been filled with barium sulfate solution. Notice the proximity of the ear to the cerebellum.

the cranial cavity by the internal table of the frontal bone. Infections characterized by large amounts of thick semisolid exudate may by pressure cause a necrosis of this very thin plate of bone and thereby create a communication with the cranium. The cribriform plate is extensively perforated by olfactory nerves that enter the large olfactory bulbs of the brain. The perineural sheaths of the olfactory nerves are in direct communication with the pia arachnoid spaces of the brain. Studies involving iodine isotopes injected into the cisterna magna of healthy dogs revealed a significant flow into the nasal submucosal space and hence into local lymphatics in the nasal cavity.[10] It is apparent that from this initimate contact of the two areas, infections and neoplasia can easily spread from the nose to the brain.[6] Since surgery in the sinuses and nasal passages can easily affect the cribriform barrier, antibiotics must be administered for 4 to 6 days after such surgical procedures (Figs. 16–3 and 16–4).

THE EYE

Panophthalmitis or neoplasia of the eyeball may spread to the brain as well as to the opposite eye. Every means of diagnosis should be used to determine the definitive lesion. Retrograde contrast radiography of the infraorbital artery is helpful in diagnosing orbital and nasolacrimal tumors that may invade the nervous system.[13] In case of infections, it should be routine practice to administer an appropriate parenteral antibiotic as well as a local one. If ablation of the eyeball is a necessity, antibiotics should be given as far in advance of surgery as practicable in order to establish a therapeutic level in the brain and blood.

In extensive infection or neoplasia of the eyeball, ablation should be of the radical type, and every precaution should be taken to prevent mechanical spread of the pathologic lesion. After the area is prepared, an incision is made peripheral to the lid margins, which have been sewn or clamped together. All tissue should be excised at a safe distance from the eyeball, and the optic vessels and nerves should be ligated as deep in the socket as possible. Handling of tissue must be gentle to inhibit the spread of the infection or tumor. The socket is packed with bacteriostatic or antibiotic surgical powder after the ablation, and drainage is instituted in case infection is present in the socket. The animal should be kept as quiet as possible during the postsurgical period in order to reduce the possibility of mechanical metastasis. In addition to administration of antibiotics before surgery when practicable, antibiotic therapy should be maintained at least 4 to 5 days after surgical removal of the eye. If an abscess forms in the anterior brain or meninges, drainage may be established through the socket or through the frontal sinus. Cosmetic defects can be corrected at a subsequent date if desirable.

THE EAR

Although the tympanic membrane is an effective barrier to the spread of infections from the outer to the middle ear, it is frequently perforated by infective processes. This penetration may be stimulated by the careless use of instruments in cleaning the ears, by parasitic migrations, or by sharp foreign bodies such as sticks or awns gaining access to the ear canal. Longstanding otorrhea in the dog has been observed to spread to a middle ear infection. No attempt will be made here to elaborate on the various accepted treatments for otitis externa. Proper treatment will in most instances prevent the progression of the disease. Surgical drainage or ablation of the ear canal may be effective (Fig. 16–5).

OTITIS MEDIA

Infection in the middle ear is called otitis media and may affect the inner ear and disturb the neurological functions of the animal. Denny describes 12 cases of otitis media and interna, of which 11 had perforated tympanic membranes and evidence of otitis externa.[9] However, Moltzen analyzed 210 cases and decided that the most common route of infection was the eustachian tube, not the external ear canal.[28] It is possible that very few clinicians consider the role of the eustachian tube as a possible source of infection in otitis media. Most clinicians feel that otitis media is generally caused by an extension of otitis externa.[22, 25, 26, 34, 37-39] A hematogenous origin of infection is possible in a systemic pyogenic infection, and in this instance would be termed a primary otitis media.

Incidence and Clinical Signs

The incidence of otitis externa in the dog is relatively high. Spreull analyzed 100 cases of otitis media. Sixteen of the early cases also had otitis externa, and over 50 of the chronic cases were affected in both areas.[39]

The clinical signs attributed to otitis media in veterinary literature are very confusing. This is probably because otitis media frequently extends into an otitis interna, which can disturb neurological function. Spreull and Denny feel that the clinical signs of otitis media are like those of otitis externa and include discharge from the external auditory meatus and inflammations of the ear canal. Clinical signs include hyperkeratosis, fibroplasia, ulceration, and cystic changes in the sweat glands. Such irritations cause the dog to paw and rub his ear and to shake his head.[39] In addition, the dog may be in extreme pain and hang his head with the affected ear downward. Pain may be due to an affection of the temporomandibular joint. Pyrexia may be seen. Signs involving neurologic and motor function are generally not attributable to otitis media but rather to otitis interna.[9, 30]

Otoscopic examination of the tympanic membrane usually requires the dog to be under sedation, tranquilization, or general anesthesia. Cleansing of the outer ear is frequently necessary before examination can be done. This should be accomplished by flushing with a syringe and special otoscopic cannula or a small flexible tube until the backwash fluid is clean. Gently drying with an aural probe and small pledgets of cotton should precede the otoscopic examination. Harsh dry swabbing should not be the sole means of cleaning the external ear canal in the vicinity of the tympanic membrane.

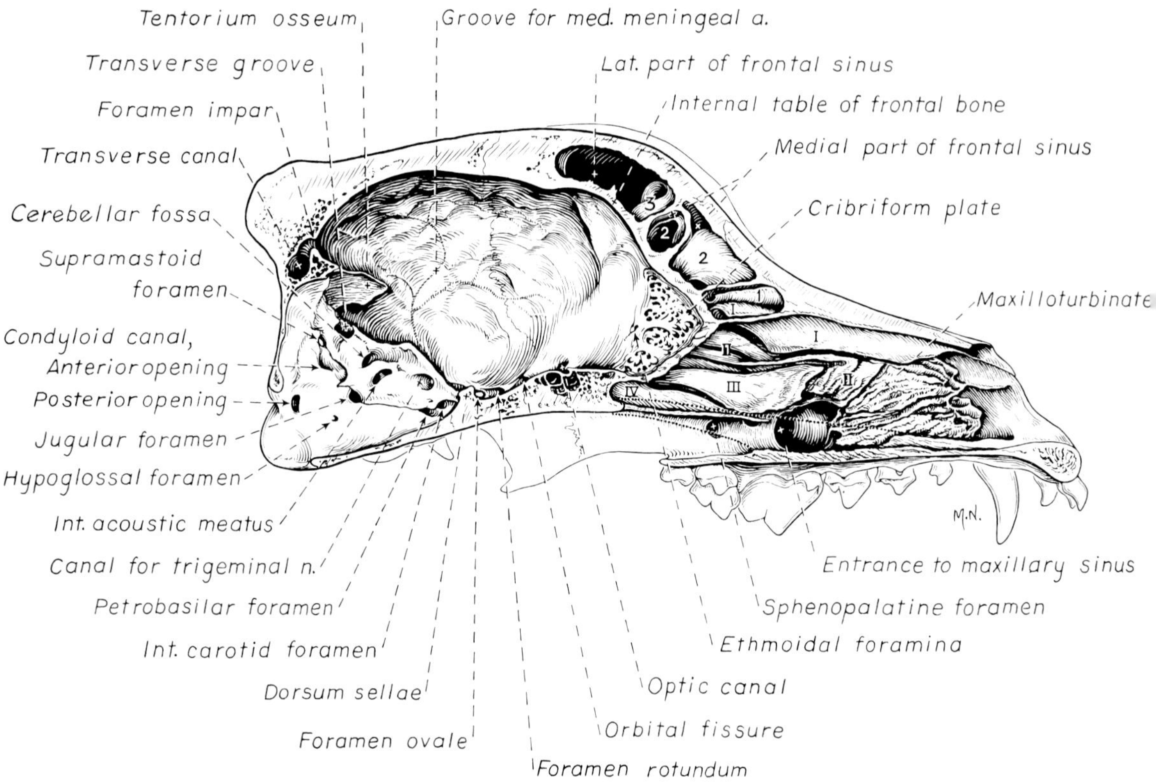

FIGURE 16–3 *A*, Sagittal section of skull. The position of the vomer is indicated by a dotted line. Roman numerals indicate endoturbinates. Arabic numerals indicate ectoturbinates. (From Miller, M. E., Christensen, G. C., and Evans, H. E.: *Anatomy of the Dog.* W. B. Saunders Co., Philadelphia, 1964.)

Illustration continued on the following page

The external ear may show signs of a longstanding, destructive infection. Parasites or foreign bodies may be present. If the tympanic membrane is destroyed, exudate, fibrous neoplasia, or raw bone in the area of the middle ear may be visible. If the membrane is intact, it may vary in color from a normal, glistening, semitransparent white to an abnormal gray or yellow (caused by the exudate). It may bulge toward the examiner. For further details, the reader is urged to study Spreull's notable work on examination of the ear.[39]

Diagnosis

The diagnosis is important, since otitis media may develop into otitis interna and cause neurological signs. The characteristic signs and history of chronic otitis externa support a tentative diagnosis of otitis media. Frequently, the appearance of the tympanic membrane confirms the diagnosis. Radiographs often reveal a sclerosis and dense exudate within the bulla and ear canal. Inflammatory or degenerative changes in osseous structures are noted in infections of long duration (Figs. 16–6 and 16–7). If chronic otitis externa makes examination of the tympanic membrane impossible, radiography using an oil-based radiographic contrast medium in the ear canal may demonstrate the medium in the bulla, indicating a perforated eardrum and otitis media.[9]

Medical Treatment

The medial treatment of otitis media involves the elimination of any secondary cause, such as parasites, foreign bodies, or infections of the external ear. Thorough flushing and cleaning not only of the ear canal but also of the tympanum itself is of prime importance. Normal saline and a cleansing antiseptic agent such as 0.5 per

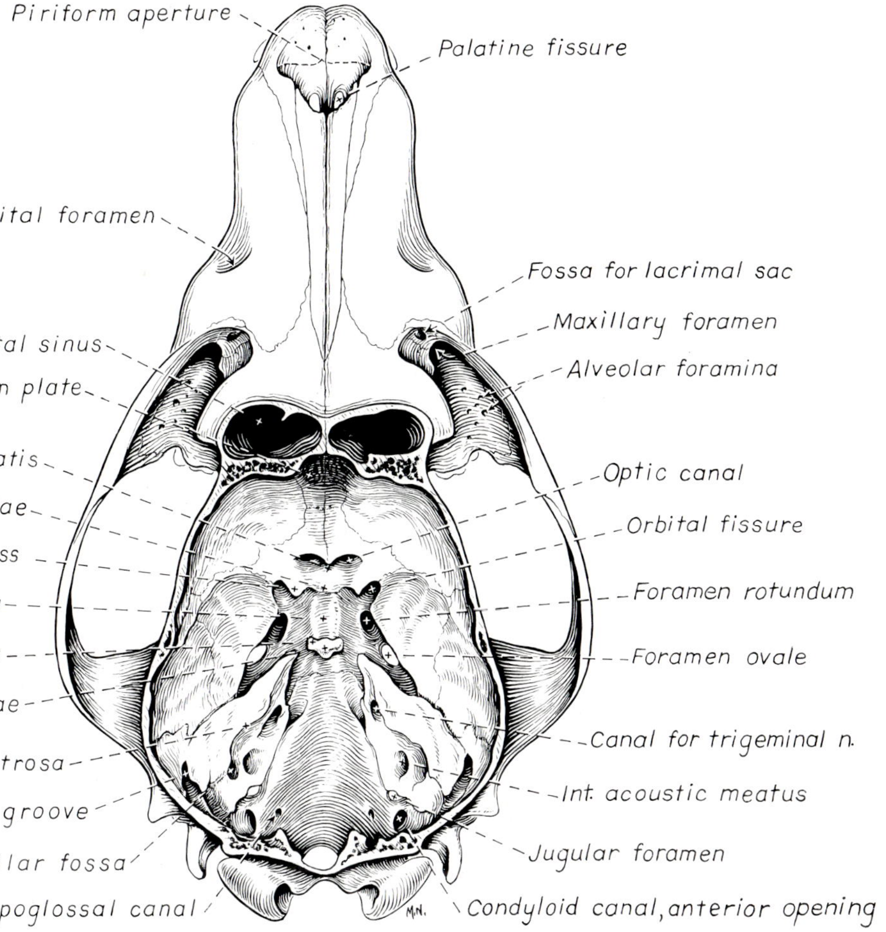

FIGURE 16–3 *Continued* *B*, Skull and calvarium removed, dorsal aspect.

cent cetrimide (Cetrimide B.P.) should be used.[37-39] In either primary or secondary otitis media, antibiotics should be used locally and systemically. A full strength or half strength organic iodide solution (Betadine solution) has been reported useful as a flushing antiseptic. The antibiotic of choice can be ascertained by sensitivity studies of the culture of a specimen of exudate. Gentamicin drops or ointment often gives good results in treating an outer ear infection but should be well diluted when instilled into the bulla in middle ear infection. If clinical improvement is not seen within a few days, surgical therapy should be considered.

Surgical Treatment

If one is unable to correct an otitis externa, external ear drainage may be considered. This surgical procedure facilitates drainage and medication of the external ear canal and affords aeration, which in turn improves the outlook in a secondary otitis media caused by otitis externa. In some instances, refractory cases of otitis externa and otitis media have apparently been cured by ablation of the infected ear canal.[31, 43]

Myringotomy

Occasionally, a myringotomy or incision into the tympanic membrane is used in treating a primary otitis media. This procedure is designed to relieve pressure and to provide drainage when the membrane is bulging and the pain is intractable. Drainage by this means is incomplete and may not be effective except to relieve symptoms. Myringotomy is carried out by incising the

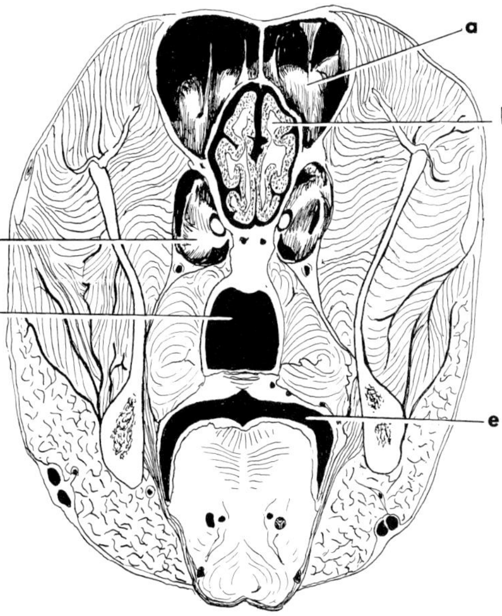

FIGURE 16–4 Cross section emphasizes the extent and proximity of the (a) frontal sinuses to the (b) prefrontal lobes of the brain; (c) orbits, (d) nasal passages, (e) oral cavity.

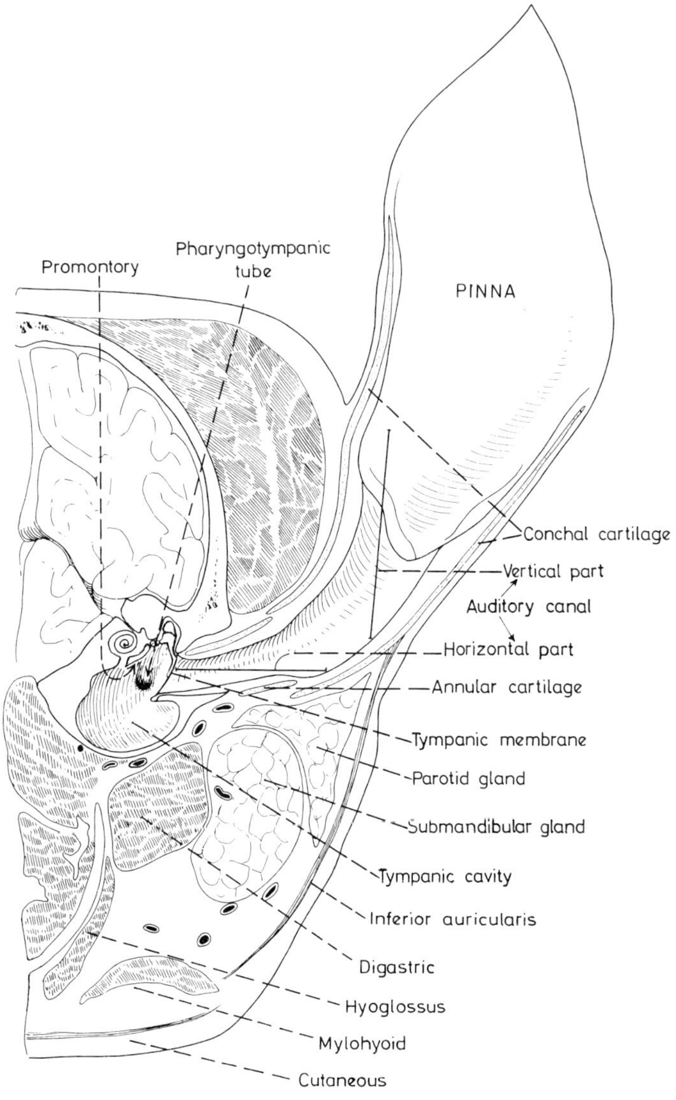

FIGURE 16–5 The anatomic structure of the outer, middle, and inner ear and their surrounding tissues. (From Spreull, J. S. A.: Ablation of ear canal. *In* Bojrab, M. J. (ed.): *Current Techniques in Small Animal Surgery I.* Lea & Febiger, Philadelphia, 1975.)

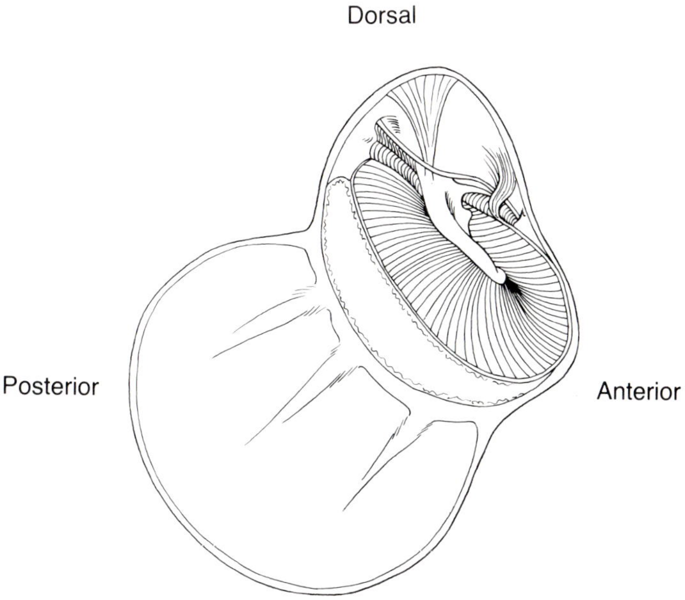

FIGURE 16–6 Medial face of the lateral wall of the tympanic cavity (right ear). (From Spruell, J. S. A.: Treatment of otitis media in the dog. J. Small Anim. Pract. 5, 107, 1964.)

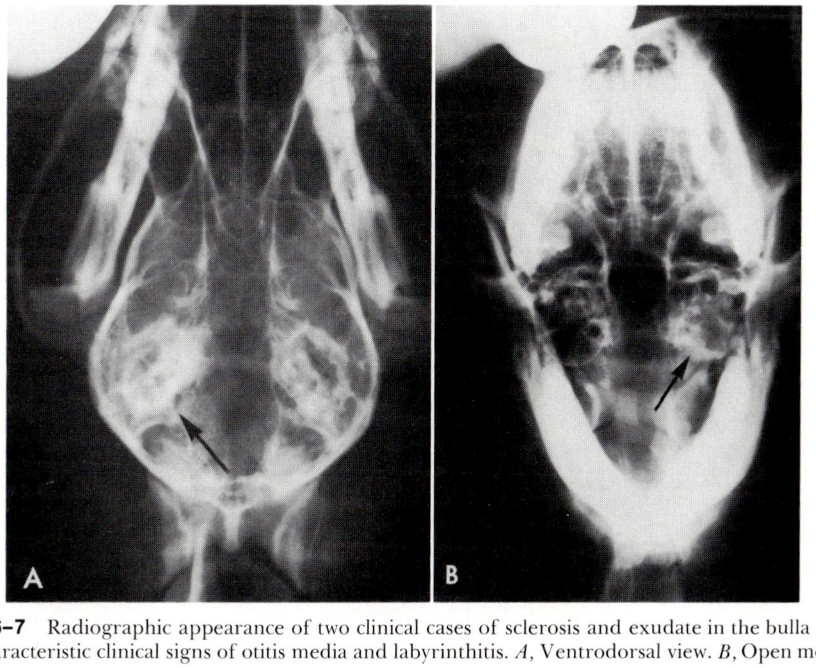

FIGURE 16–7 Radiographic appearance of two clinical cases of sclerosis and exudate in the bulla ossea, which produced characteristic clinical signs of otitis media and labyrinthitis. *A*, Ventrodorsal view. *B*, Open mouth antero-posterior view.

membrane with a von Graefe cataract knife passed through the speculum of the otoscope. General anesthesia is necessary. Antibiotics are administered locally and parenterally.[31]

Parker has reported a small series of chronic, nonresponsive cases of otitis media which he felt responded better to curettage of the bulla combined with lateral external ear resection than to myringotomy alone. A ventral cartilage flap was established in the external ear canal, and the bulla was curetted with a 1/8-inch bone curet pushed through the tympanic membrane. Ampicillin or chloramphenicol with dexamethasone was given for up to 1 month after surgery. In five of ten dogs, head carriage became normal 2 to 8 weeks after surgery and remained so for at least 18 months.[32]

Eustachian Tube Insufflation

In many cases of otitis media, direct drainage of the middle ear is essential. Drainage through the tympanic membrane generally is not effective. A method has been described by Moltzen in which the eustachian tube is insufflated through the opening in the tympanic membrane,[26] and an otoscopic speculum is passed deep into the middle ear cavity until the opening of the eustachian tube is seen. A small rubber catheter is inserted into the opening, and a bulb syringe is used to blow into the eustachian tube. Antibiotics are instilled into the canal. The procedure is repeated four to five times at 48-hour intervals. It is felt that this procedure is too delicate to be done by most clinicians, and the middle ear is usually drained by means of a bulla osteotomy.[26, 28]

Bulla Osteotomy

The bulla osteotomy, which is comparable to the classic surgery in man, was described by McNutt and McCoy using a ventral approach[25] in 1930 and has been developed further since then by Spreull.[39] The approach is readily performed in most brachycephalic breeds but can be difficult anatomically in some animals of dolichocephalic breeds. This method can be performed aseptically, and if continuous drainage is necessary, the tube can be conveniently placed exterior to the wound and dressed.[9, 12, 25, 39]

The ventral bulla osteotomy is performed in a dorsal recumbent position with the head extended. A longitudinal paramedian incision is made immediately over the bulla just medial to the digastric muscle. The incision extends 4 cm anteriorly and 4 cm posteriorly to the angle of the mandible. The skin and cutaneous muscles are incised, and blunt dissection between the digastric and mylohyoid and hyoglossus muscles is performed. The digastric muscle is retracted laterally, and the mylohyoid and hyoglossus muscles and the hypoglossus nerve are retracted medially. The bulla can occasionally be palpated medial and slightly posterior to the vertical ramus of the mandible and medial to and just anterior to the stylohyoid bone.[39, 40]

The tensor of the palate and connective tissue are bluntly removed from the bulla, taking care not to damage large vessels (e.g., the internal maxillary vessels). A bone gouge is used to open the cavity widely; the septic material, granulation tissue, or other pathologic tissue is gently but completely removed or flushed out. An antibiotic is applied, a sterile Silastic drain tube is secured tightly in the surrounding tissue, and the surgical closure is made. The tube may be left in place for 4 to 7 days while saline flushes and antibiotic instillations are applied through it daily. A Silastic or soft rubber tube may also be placed in the incised tympanic membrane via the external ear canal. Flushing this tube through the ventral bulla tube with Betadine solution (half or full strength) has been advocated by Bojrab.[3] Parenteral antibiotics of choice, appropriately selected from results of sensitivity tests should be used[39] (Fig. 16–8).

The methods of bulla osteotomy performed frequently are the pharyngeal approach, as described by Ehmer,[11] and the Rudy–McBride approach through the ear canal into the bulla in the pharynx.[22, 31] The pharyngeal approach is done through the mouth with the dog under general anesthesia. The mouth is held open with a speculum, and the bulla is located by passing a finger caudal to the last cheek tooth. The sharp ridge of the pterygoid bone is palpated caudally and slightly medially to this tooth. Caudal and some-

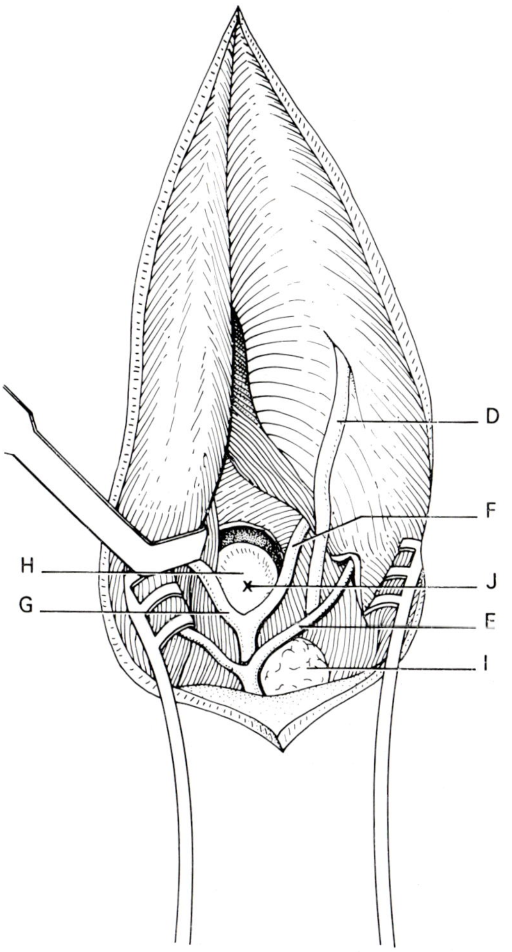

FIGURE 16–8 Ventral approach for bulla osteotomy—the dissection between the digastric muscle laterally and the styloglossus and hyoglossus muscles medially. (D) Hypoglossal nerve; (E) lingual vein; (F) lingual artery; (G) external carotid artery; (H) tympanic bulla; (I) submandibular salivary gland; and (J) the point through which a hole is drilled into the tympanum. (From Denny, H. R.: The results of surgical treatment of otitis media and interna in the dog. J. Small Anim. Pract. *14*, 585, 1973.)

what lateral to the pterygoid bone is a dome-like eminence called the bulla tympanica.[36]

A small incision is made in the mucosa on the anterolateral portion of the bulla. A large intramedullary pin or a small chisel is placed on the bone, and by tapping it gently with a mallet, an opening is created for drainage. The cavity is flushed very thoroughly and an antibiotic is instilled; however, unless a drain is secured in place, the mucosa will heal and seal the defect in a few hours. A short rubber tube or the end of a rubber urinary catheter can be inserted into the cavity and sutured securely to the surrounding mucosa. The sides of the catheter or tube should be fenestrated with a sharp pair of scissors.

The chief precaution necessary with this procedure is to avoid the external carotid or maxillary artery, which lies toward the rostrolateral aspect of the bulla. Injury to this vessel would be serious, and ligation would be difficult (Fig. 16–9).

The chief disadvantage of this method is the difficulty of maintaining drainage for an extended period. If no tube is inserted, surgery would need to be repeated several times. A drainage tube is difficult to keep in place, and even if the tube is secure, the animal must be sedated to permit flushing of the tube and instillation of antibiotics each day during the treatment period.

The drainage tube or seton inserted from the outer ear has definite advantages. It provides constant drainage and a means of flushing or instilling medicants. The method of McBride[22] and Rudy, as described by Ott,[31] consists of modifying an intramedullary pin so that there are no cutting edges, only a point remaining on the tip. A hole is drilled through the end of the pin. A piece of fenestrated rubber or Silastic tubing of slightly larger diameter than the pin is used. A rubber urinary catheter works well, since the tapered point facilitates insertion. The pin, Jacob's chuck, suture wire, tube, and other instruments are sterilized in the autoclave.

The animal is placed in the sternal recumbent position under general anesthesia, and the affected ear is prepared for surgery as aseptically as possible. Frequently, an external ear drainage operation (Zepp's method[46]) not only facilitates the bulla osteotomy from this approach, but also aids in treating the otitis externa that may be the cause of, or coexistent with, a middle ear infection.

The pin is fastened to the chuck and is inserted through the remnant of the tympanic membrane into the middle ear cavity. A finger of the opposite hand is placed on the pharyngeal bulla. Light tapping on the pin is palpated by this finger. When the tapping vibrations have located the pin in the proper position, it is driven through the floor of the bulla into the pharynx. A stainless steel wire suture is threaded

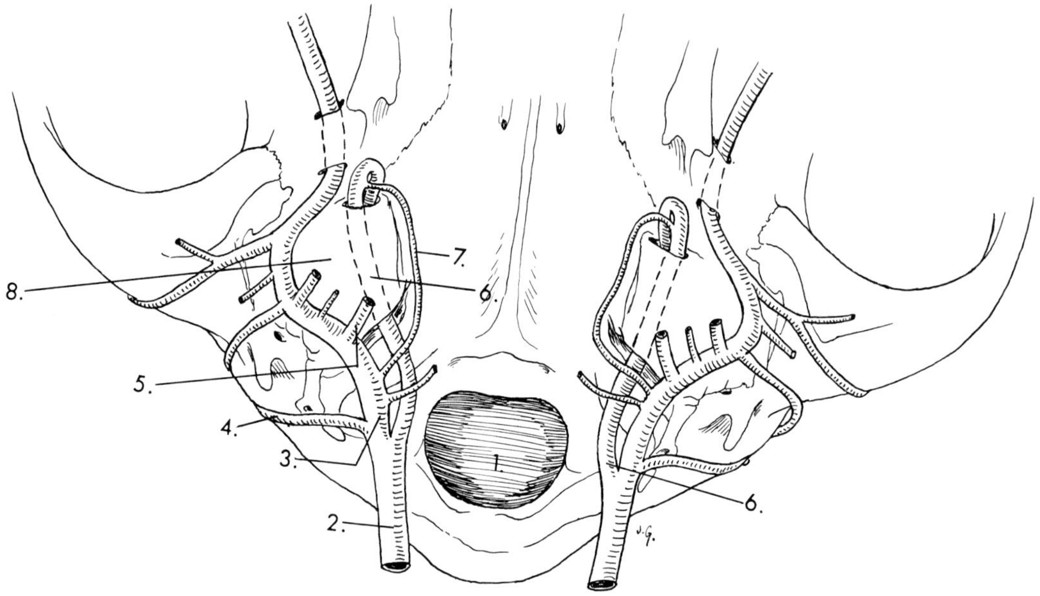

FIGURE 16–9 A diagram depicting anatomical considerations in a pharyngeal approach to a bulla osteotomy. (1) Foramen magnum; (2) common carotid artery; (3) external carotid artery; (4) occipital artery; (5) facial artery; (6) internal carotid, which also lies dorsal to the tympanic cavity; (7) ascending pharyngeal; (8) area of preferred pharyngeal drainage of the bulla ossea.

through the hole in the pin, and the pin and wire are withdrawn through the external ear canal. The tapered end of the rubber tube is securely fastened to the wire, and the tube is stretched so that it passes through the hole easily. The tube is pulled through the middle ear, trimmed flush with the pharyngeal mucosa, and secured to the mucosa with silk sutures. Since the tube is larger than the hole, it should fit tightly after the tension applied to it is relaxed. The other end of the tube should be sutured to the external ear flap.

A proteolytic enzyme and antibiotic solution is flushed through the tube three times daily for 3 to 4 days. The tube is then removed, after the dog has been anesthetized with a short-acting agent.

A grooved director can be substituted for a pin in cats and small dogs. The Rush intramedullary pin with the hook removed or a large fascia needle has been used successfully. A probe or seton needle can be used to pull through a tube or umbilical tape. Umbilical tape is tied on the outside of the mouth as it is drawn tightly behind the last cheek tooth.[31]

Our experience with this method has been fairly favorable; however, we are doing more ventral approaches than previously. Concomitant antibiotic therapy is always necessary. Recovery may be prompt, or it may take months for the head tilt and incoordination indicative of otitis interna to subside, depending on the amount of damage present (Figs. 16–10 to 16–15).

Recently, a lateral bulla osteotomy has been proposed. The same principle of exteriorizing one end of the tube draining the bulla into the caudal oropharynx is used; however, through an appropriate skin incision, the bulla is approached aseptically from the dorsolateral aspect immediately *below* the cartilaginous ear canal instead of *in* the usually highly contaminated ear canal. A Steinmann pin is used to penetrate the bulla, first on its caudal-lateral aspect and second on its cranial-medial wall into the pharynx. A fenestrated Silastic tube can be inserted by the same devices used in the Rudy–McBride approach.[31] Postoperative treatment can be given as previously described. This method may be difficult for the novice until he has mastered the anatomical relationships, but it has the advantage of providing a more aseptic area for the tube insertion than through the ear canal. The flushing and instillation of medication

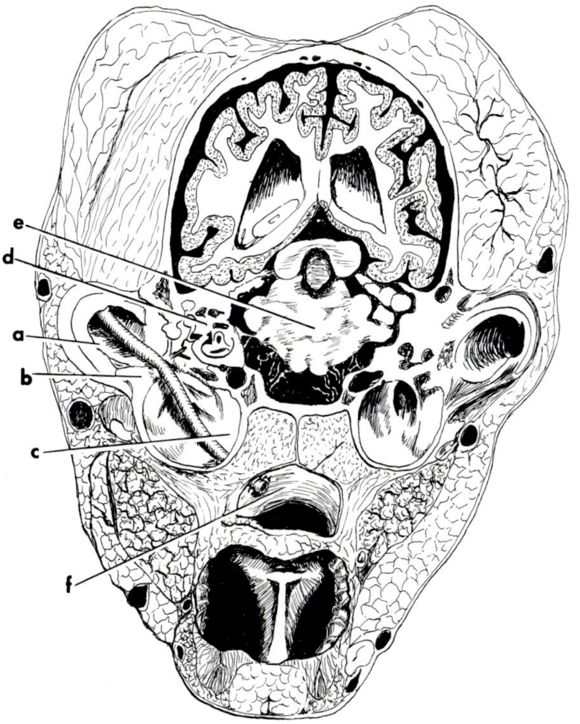

FIGURE 16–10 Placement of a drainage tube from the outer ear through the bulla into the pharynx for the surgical treatment of otitis media and interna. (a) External ear canal; (b) tympanic membrane; (c) bulla ossea; (d) internal ear; (e) cerebellum; (f) pharynx.

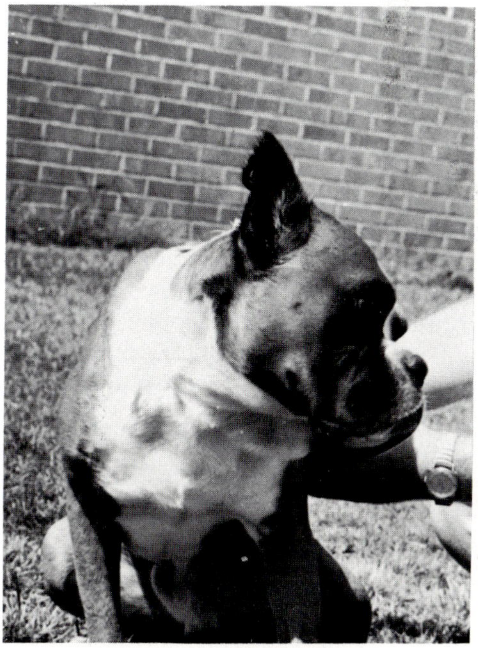

Fig. 16–11

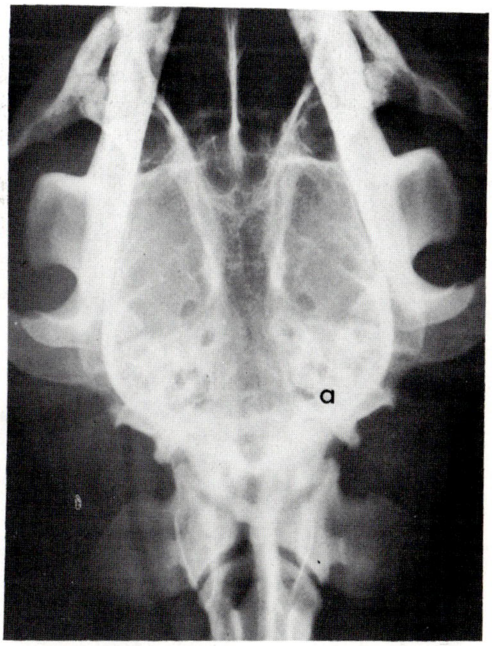

Fig. 16–12

FIGURE 16–11 A 4-year-old boxer shows signs of left labyrinthitis, such as tilting the head, falling to the left side, and nystagmus.

FIGURE 16–12 Radiograph shows a sclerosis and density (a) in the left bulla. Same case as shown in Figure 16–11.

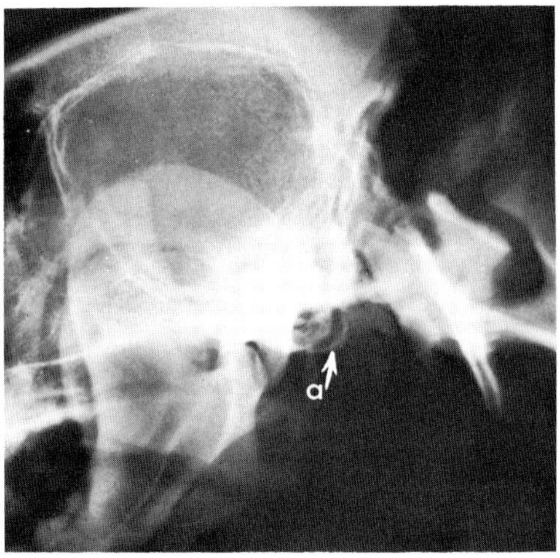

Fig. 16–13

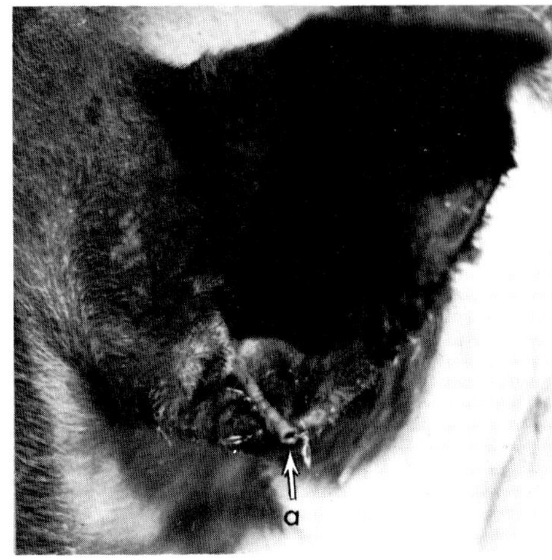

Fig. 16–14

FIGURE 16–13 Same case as shown in Figure 16–11; lateral view. The bulla ossea is at *a*.
FIGURE 16–14 Same case as shown in Figure 16–11. The drainage tube (a) is sutured to the external ear flap after a bulla osteotomy.

is facilitated by having both ends of the tube available for manipulation, as in this method, whereas in the ventral approach only one end is available.[1]

LABYRINTHITIS (Otitis interna)

An inner ear infection may be called labyrinthitis or otitis interna. In the discussion of the applied physiology of the central nervous system in Chapter 2, it was stated that the inner ear, or labyrinth, consists of two intercommunicating portions: (1) the anterior labyrinth, consisting of the cochlea, housing the 32,000 hair cells concerned with hearing, and (2) the posterior labyrinth, which contains the three semicircular canals, the utricle, and the saccule, all of which are concerned with equilibrium. All of the vestibular structures are encased within hollowed-out bony canals that are considerably larger than their membranous contents. Each canal is lined with a fibroserous membrane enclosing perilymph, which surrounds the vestibular apparatus. Perilymph acts as a hydraulic shock absorber for the membranous semicircular ducts, which normally occupy less than one-fourth of the diameter of the bony canals.[45] Disorders of the posterior labyrinth may be called vestibulitis.

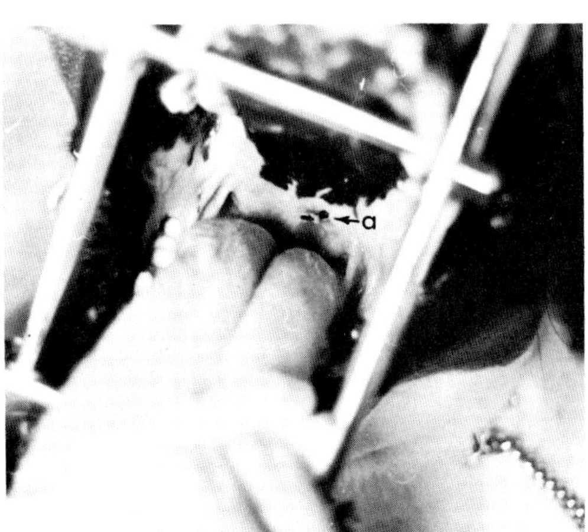

FIGURE 16–15 Same case as shown in Figure 16–13. Exit of the drainage tube (a) in the mouth.

The semicircular ducts contain a fluid called endolymph. Endolymph is high in potassium and low in sodium (like intracellular fluid), whereas perilymph is low in potassium and high in sodium. This disparity of chemical composition could help to explain some of the disorders of the vestibular system. The endolymph communicates with the auditory portion of the ear, the cochlear duct, via the ductus reuniens.[45] This fact helps to explain auditory signs and equilibrium disorders seen in human labyrinthitis (Meniere's disease) that could also be present in animal disorders.

The semicircular canals lie at right angles to each other, and each is stimulated in certain positions. Vestibular impulses are conducted by the eighth cranial nerve, which enters the brain stem just below the pons and anterior to the cerebellum. Impulses are further distributed to the four vestibular nuclei—the superior, medial, lateral, and spinal—and to the cerebellum. From the vestibular nuclei, axons enter the medial longitudinal bundle, which conveys impulses to the eye, head, and neck muscles. Also from the nuclei, axons enter the lateral vestibulospinal tract, which descends in the cord to the body and limb musculature. These pathways explain nystagmus, motor muscular efforts to compensate during attacks of vertigo, and autonomic reactions of nausea and vomition in man. The vestibular centers are inhibited and coordinated by higher centers, usually cerebral (Figs. 16–16 and 16–17).[24, 45]

The destruction of the labyrinth in the dog and cat affects the complex coordination of nerve functions of the inner ear, with consequent abnormalities of posture and movement. Head tilt and falling and rolling *toward* the side affected can be seen. Clinical signs are severe in proportion to the amount of damage. Nystagmus is frequently encountered; nystagmus and the caloric test as aids in differential diagnosis were discussed in Chapter 3. Auditory deficits can occur in extremely severe cases.

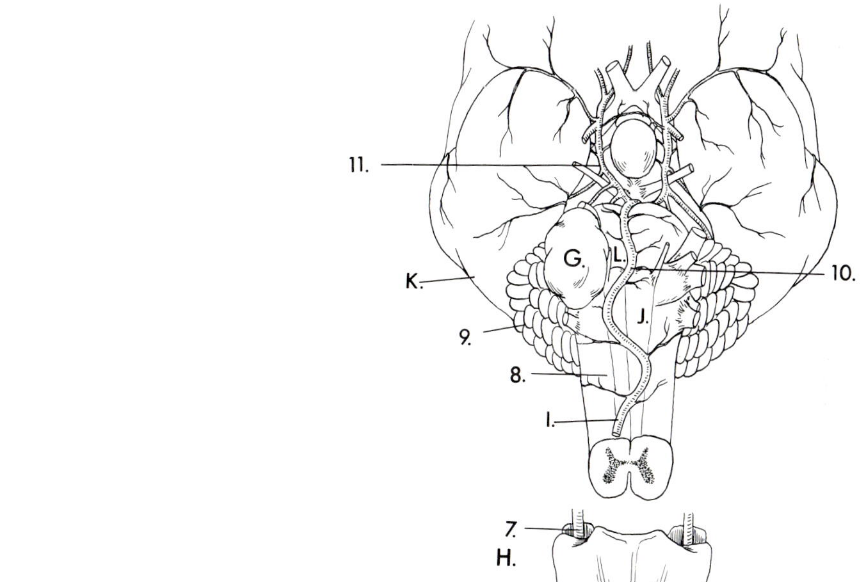

FIGURE 16–16 Some pathological causes of vertigo. (1) Tympanic membrane; (2) auditory ossicles; (3) bulla ossea or tympanic cavity; (4) labyrinth; (5) cochlea; (6) vestibular and cochlear nerves; (7) vertebral artery; (8) medulla; (9) cerebellum; (10) basilar artery; (11) circle of Willis. Disorders associated with these areas are: (A) acute otitis media; (B) chronic otitis media; (C) labyrinthitis, from drugs, toxins, edema, or secondary infection; (D) trauma in area of labyrinth (fracture); (E) vestibular neuritis; (F) neuroma; (G) cerebellopontine angle tumor; (H) spondylosis causing vascular disorder; (I) vascular disorders, e.g., hemorrhage, aneurysm, and thrombi; (J) CNS trauma; (K) vertiginous epilepsy; (L) CNS degenerative disease (distemper) (Adapted from Wolfson, R. J., Schlosser, W. D., and Winchester, R. A.: Vertigo. Ciba Symposium *17*, 99, 1965.)

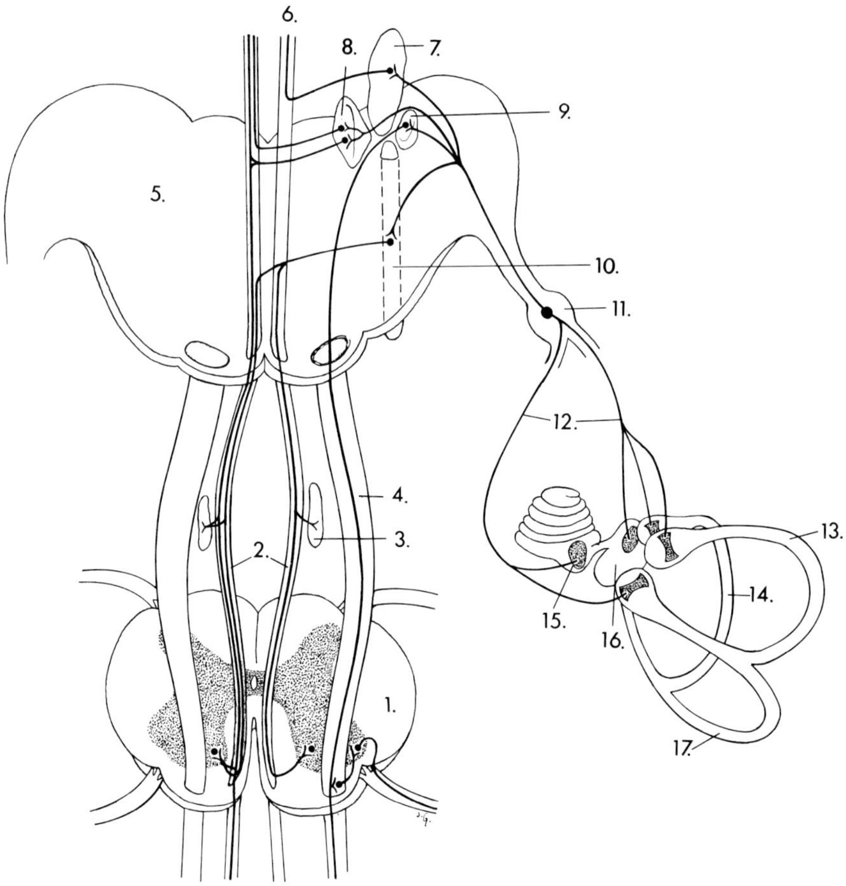

FIGURE 16–17 The vestibular system. (1) cervical cord; (2) medial longitudinal fasciculus; (3) spinal accessory nucleus; (4) lateral vestibulospinal tract; (5) upper medulla; (6) third, fourth, and sixth motor nuclei; (7) superior vestibular nucleus; (8) medial vestibular nucleus; (9) lateral vestibular nucleus; (10) inferior spinal vestibular nucleus; (11) vestibular ganglion; (12) vestibular nerve; (13) superior canal; (14) lateral canal; (15) sacculus; (16) utriculus; (17) posterior canal. (Adapted from Wolfson, R. J., Schlosser, W. D., and Winchester, R. A.: Vertigo. Ciba Symposium *17*, 99, 1965.)

However, the case reports of congenital deafness in various breeds have not involved vestibular dysfunction.[2]

Labyrinthitis can frequently be the result of an extension of external and middle ear infections. Parasitic infections and foreign bodies can stimulate such progression, or the infection can be hematogenic.

Treatment

Since both labyrinthitis and otitis media are frequently present, the treatments outlined for otitis media would apply. These include thorough cleansing of the ear canal and the tympanic cavity, administration of an antibiotic to which the microorganism is sensitive, and bulla osteotomy as a last resort. External ear canal surgery (drainage or ablation) may be appropriate if otitis externa is present.

Most neurologists feel that chloramphenicol is the most effective antibiotic for treating infections of the central nervous system (CNS). We have found this drug to be effective when administered in 50 to 60 mg/kg doses for 2 to 3 days and maintained on 25 to 50 mg/kg doses for an additional 10 to 20 days. One must watch for hematopoietic depression upon prolonged adminstrations; however, we have seen this occur infrequently when proper dosage is given. Antibiotics are always given in conjunction with bulla osteotomy. Some clinicians find that cephalosporin antibiotics (cephaloridine) are satisfactory in CNS diseases. Results of such therapy will depend on the amount of damage to the CNS.

It is possible that in dogs, infection and tumors might not be the only causes of the vestibular syndrome. In Chapter 3, lesions in the nervous tissue other than the labyrinth were discussed as causes of vestibular disorders. It is possible that dogs may have periodic vertigo, tinnitus, and related signs, which characterize Meniere's disease in man. Clinical signs included severe ataxia, nausea, vomition, and depression. In most instances, spontaneous recovery occurred in 3 weeks; however, some cases suffered remissions.[33]

The cause of Meniere's disease is in question, but it frequently is described as "labyrinthine hydrops" because excess endolymph is observed on necropsy examination. The disease may be associated with so-called "cluster headaches"—a type of vascular headache seen in patients who get migraine headaches.[14]

The treatments for Meniere's disease have included pilocarpine sweats and diuretics; vasodilating drugs such as histamine, niacin; anticholinergic drugs such as atropine, methantheline, and propantheline; citrus bioflavonoids and vitamin B complex; antimotion drugs such as dimenhydrinate (Dramamine), meclizine (Bonamine or Bonine), and trimethobenzamide (Tigan); and sedative and tranquilizing drugs.[35] Other therapies have included a vasoconstrictor agent instead of a vasodilator, such as ergotamine tartrate or methysergide maleate.[5]

It is not known whether these drugs would be of value in relieving the pronounced signs associated with labyrinthitis in the dog. In our experience, antimotion drugs, such as meclizine, have seemed to be beneficial. However, it is generally recognized that this type of medical therapy affords only symptomatic relief and may abort an attack if given during the very initial phase; it will not cure or alter the progress of the disease.

The classic surgical relief of Meniere's disease has been a labyrinthectomy. McCrady reports the clinical improvement of chronic labyrinthitis in a dog treated by this method.[23] A labyrinthectomy involves the total removal of the pathologic membranous inner ear. Total deafness occurs and therefore is indicated only in a unilateral disorder. Spreull has reported a vestibular osteotomy in cases in which a septic otitis media is not present. In the ventral bulla osteotomy the osseous promontory is chipped away so that the vestibule of the inner ear is extensively opened (Fig. 16–18).[40]

Cryosurgery of the labyrinth has led to encouraging results. Animal experiments suggest that vestibular function could be eliminated without deleteriously affecting the cochlea or facial nerve. Temperatures of −80° C to −120° C applied to the horizontal canal for 12 to 25 minutes in 15 human patients with Meniere's disease produced nine cures, two patients with recur-

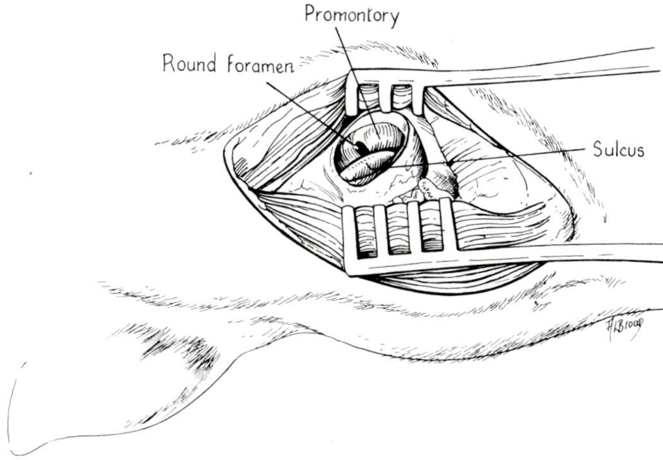

FIGURE 16–18 Landmarks for a vestibular osteotomy (Spruell). The medial wall of the promontory is chipped away to open the vestibule of the inner ear. (From Spruell, J. S. A.: Ablation of ear canal. *In* Bojrab, M. J. (ed.): *Current Techniques in Small Animal Surgery I.* Lea & Febiger, Philadelphia, 1975.)

rent attacks, and four failures.[44] It is possible that in further refinements of technique, cryosurgery will prove very effective in man and can be applied in the treatment of labyrinthitis in the dog.

IDIOPATHIC FELINE VESTIBULAR DISEASE

This disorder, the etiology of which is unknown, has puzzled many veterinarians. De Lahunta[8] found that it occurs primarily in late summer and fall, with peracute onset, and that it is characterized by loss of generalized head and body equilibrium. Ipsilateral head tilt and falling occur. Contralateral quick phase nystagmus is generally horizontal but occasionally rotatory. The head oscillates from side to side or in a rotary fashion. The postural reactions of placing, hopping, and extensor thrust and the tonic neck and eye reflexes are usually deficient on the side of the head tilt. The cat generally makes steady spontaneous improvement, and after 3 to 4 weeks the only signs are a slight head tilt and occasional ataxia.[8]

Since the pathogenesis of the disease is unknown, therapy, consisting of antibiotics, corticosteroids, calcium gluconate, vitamins, or antimotion drugs, is somewhat empirical. Vestibular disease caused by suppurative otitis media and interna can be diagnosed by physical, laboratory, and radiographic examinations and treated accordingly.[8]

THE NOSE

SINUSES AND NASAL PASSAGES

The anatomical proximity of the nasal passages and the cribriform plates to the olfactory bulbs and brain has been emphasized previously. Infections and tumors of the nasal passages can easily spread to the brain. The paranasal sinuses, by virtue of their anatomical locations, are also important as possible causes of CNS disorders. The maxillary sinus communicates directly with the nasal passages and is referred to actually as a recess of the nasal cavity. The maxillary sinus frequently becomes involved through suppurative infections of the carnaissal or upper fourth premolar tooth.[5]

The frontal sinus is more isolated from the nasal passage and communicates with it medially through the small nasofrontal opening.[27] The frontal sinus overlies a considerable portion of the brain and is separated from it by only the internal plate of the frontal bone. Infections of the frontal sinus, because of its natural poor drainage opening, are frequently characterized by extensive thick and heavy exudates. The accumulation of such material may create pressure necrosis and bulging in the facial contour bones or penetrate through its interior plate into the cranium. In the latter circumstance, meningitis and brain abscesses can result (see Fig. 16–3).

Acute rhinitis may result from trauma or it may occur in primary viral infections and subsequent secondary bacterial infections (canine distemper, feline viral rhinotracheitis). Chronic nasal and sinus diseases resulting from primary bacterial and viral infections and from fungal or yeast infections are common and cause granulomatous lesions. In addition, foreign bodies such as grass awns and sticks and parasites such as *Pneumonyssus caninum* or *Linguatula serrata* can cause nasal or sinus disease.

The Veterinary Medical Data Program has recorded 300 cases of primary neoplasms involving the nasal cavity or paranasal sinuses among 12,300 microscopically confirmed neoplasms of many animal species. Significant numbers of tumors were seen in dogs, horses, and cats. Intranasal tumors were more frequent than paranasal sinus tumors in dogs and cats. Only cats showed a sex difference in nasal tumors, with a male predilection. Incidence increased with age, but no relationship was established between incidence and nose length. Of the 300 tumors, 239 occurred in dogs and 35 in cats. The number of tumors and estimated neoplasms per 100,000 patient years was listed as follows:

Species	Number of Tumors		No. Tumors per 100,000 Patient Years
Dog	Nose	193	65
	Sinus	46	16
Cat	Nose	34	38
	Sinus	1	1

In the dog, 80 per cent of the tumors were malignant, whereas in the cat 91 per cent were malignant. Of 49 canine nasal tumors studied in detail, 27 were carcinomas and 22 were sarcomas. The estimated relative risk of intranasal tumors in dogs was highest in the miniature or toy poodle, German shepherd, collie, basset hound, airedale, Scotty, and keeshond breeds.[21] O'Brien observed that, among 116 nasal and sinus tumors of dogs, 19 occurred in spaniels.[30] In another study of 70 intranasal tumors in dogs, the majority of the dogs weighed over 20 kg, and only 4 were brachycephalic breeds.[29]

Diagnosis of Nasal and Sinus Disease

In some instances there may be bulging of the facial bones over the affected sinus, or pain may be exhibited on percussion of the area. Since the sinusitis is generally unilateral, a unilateral nasal discharge may occur. Clinical signs also include sneezing and dyspnea or mouth breathing. When the lesion invades bilateral structures, the discharge becomes bilateral and must be distinguished from such systemic diseases as distemper. Tumors generally affect middle-aged and old animals, whereas most systemic diseases such as distemper are seen in young dogs.

With a metastatic infection to the brain, dullness, stupor, periodic convulsions, papilledema, and locomotor dysfunction may be seen. Laboratory analysis of blood may demonstrate leukocytosis and neutrophilia, and the protein and total cell count of the spinal fluid may be elevated. Frequently, neurological signs are vague and diagnosis is difficult.

Direct examination of the nasal passages is difficult and in the paranasal sinuses it is virtually impossible. The use of a dilatable nasal speculum, head mirror, and reflected light provides a clear view of the anterior portion of the nasal chamber and nostrils.[6] Occasionally, foreign bodies can be seen and removed by such a procedure. An otoscope can in some cases be useful. However, the author strongly suggests the use of general anesthesia or heavy dose of tranquilizer and 8 per cent Pontocaine locally for this examination. Even so, if the discharge is copious, it is a most difficult examination and should only be used in conjunction with radiology. Nasal washings or smears of pathological tissue (although not really dependable) can be a diagnostic aid if examined by a competent cytologist. Positive findings are diagnostic, but negative results may require a surgical biopsy examination.[6]

A direct examination of the posterior nasal chamber can be made by administering general anesthesia, withdrawing the soft palate anteriorly, and visualizing the nasopharyngeal area by means of reflected light and mirrors. These procedures are best accomplished in conjunction with the radiographic examination, which generally is by far the most effective diagnostic procedure.[6, 7]

Radiographic examination is the most effective means of demonstrating a lesion and its extent. It must be emphasized that proper demonstration will require absolute immobilization, proper positioning, good exposure and processing techniques, and careful interpretation. To completely eliminate motion, heavy tranquilization or short acting anesthesia must be given. If the direct examinations discussed previously are also planned, anesthesia will be a necessity. Since advanced cases show marked dyspnea, endotracheal intubation and oxygen should always be provided in general anesthesia. In many cases, anesthesia will be safer than the air hunger and possible cardiac failure seen from the excitement associated with manual restraint.[16-19]

The x-ray positions should include the ventrodorsal, lateral, anteroposterior or frontal, and the open-mouth ventrodorsal. The last view is the most rewarding when one uses nonscreen film, opens the dog's mouth wide, and angles the central x-ray beam substantially. This view keeps the mandible from obliterating any portion of the lesion. The findings in disease processes are usually asymmetrical alterations in the appearance of the turbinates. They may be replaced or masked by extensive zones of homogeneous soft tissue density, representing granulomatous or neoplastic tissue. Opacities in one or both sets of paranasal sinuses may be observed. The nasal septum or facial bones or both may be incomplete or obviously eroded and the lesion will be seen protruding through the defect (Figs. 16–19 to 16–27). If tumor cells

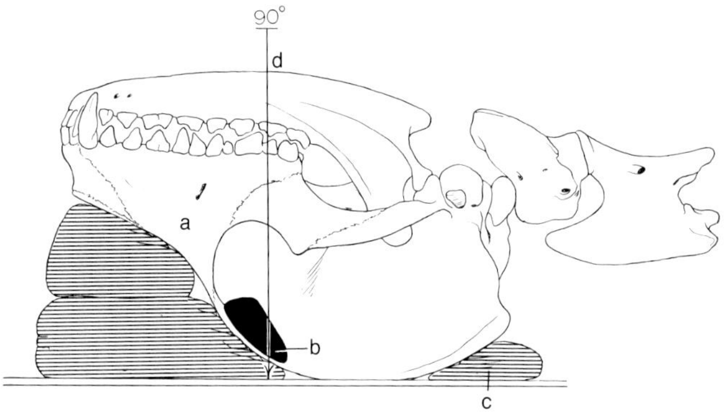

FIGURE 16–19 Ventrodorsal positioning for radiographic demonstration of the nasal passages (a) and sinus cavities (b); (c) cushions; (d) central x-ray beam.

have been identified and classified by direct smears or by biopsies taken by nostril or pharyngeal approaches, radiographic therapy in lieu of surgery could be used. However, if the etiology or the location of the lesion has not been established by radiographic and possibly direct examination, the surgical exploration not only will help to establish the positive diagnosis but will afford an effective means of treatment. Since the frontal sinuses have a meager blood supply, antibiotic therapy and other medications alone are usually ineffective. Drainage can be accomplished only by a surgical procedure. Chronic mycotic granulomatous lesions and tumors require surgical removal. Chronic bacterial infections usually accompany mycotic lesions or tumors and therefore also are best treated surgically. It is strongly felt that treating chronic lesions with drugs for prolonged periods of time is a gross injustice to the client. The best form of treatment may be radiographic demonstration of the lesion and prompt surgical intervention.[16-19]

In a recent study[4] of the therapy of intranasal neoplasms, 15 dogs were treated surgically; 13 of them were destroyed within 4 months of treatment, and 2 were lost to follow-up information. Four dogs were treated with radiation and survived for 6, 12, 26, and 52 months after the initial therapy. The radiation was administered from a 250 kvp orthovoltage therapy unit with a 1.1 cu mm half-value layer, and the total absorbed dose ranged from 2500 to 5000 rads. These workers stress that cytological examination does not provide a satisfactory method of early diagnosis because of the difficulty of interpreting cells from nasal washings. The difficulty then is to diagnose the tumor type early enough to

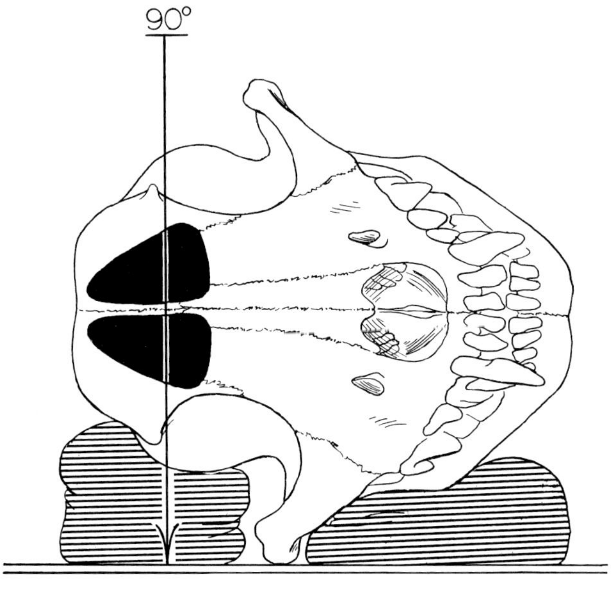

FIGURE 16–20 Lateral positioning for radiography. Note the use of cushions to promote superimposition of anatomical structures.

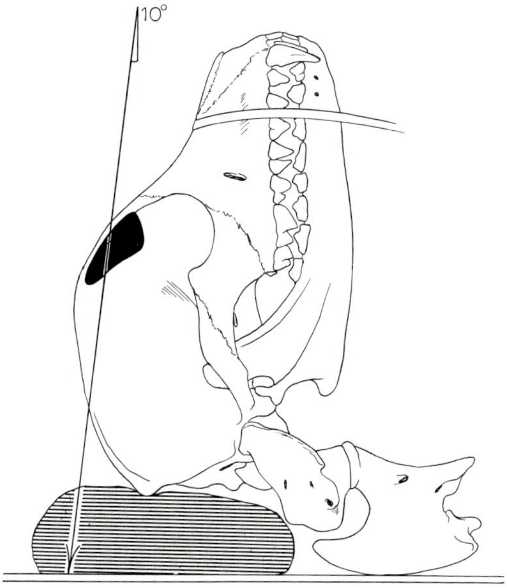

FIGURE 16–21 Anteroposterior positioning for radiographic examination of the sinuses.

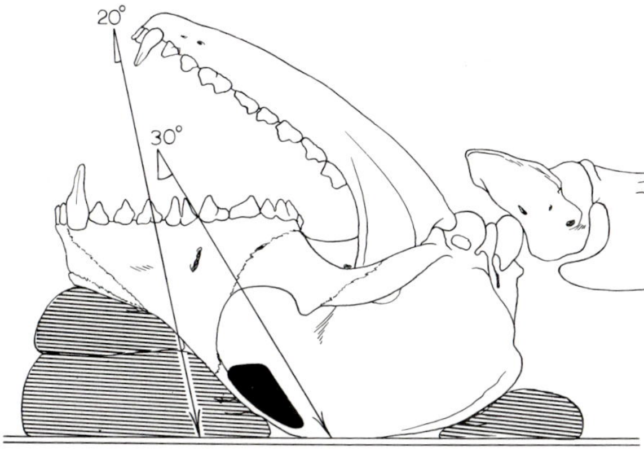

Figure 16–22 The open mouth ventrodorsal position, in which the central x-ray beam is directed between the jaws in order to prevent the mandibles' obscuring visualization of the nasal passages.

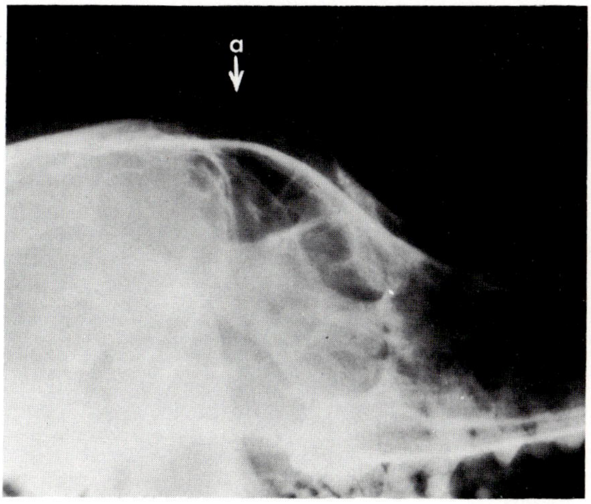

Fig. 16–23

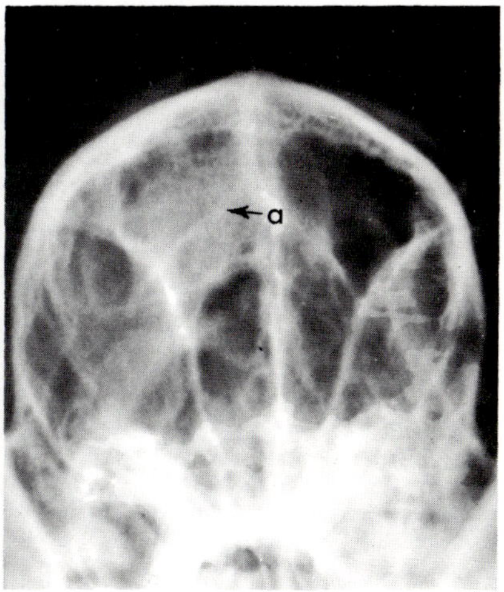

Fig. 16–24

FIGURE 16–23 A lateral radiograph of a sinus infection. Notice the fuzzy appearance of the exudate.
FIGURE 16–24 Same case as shown in Figure 16–23; frontal view. Notice the density (a) in one frontal sinus.

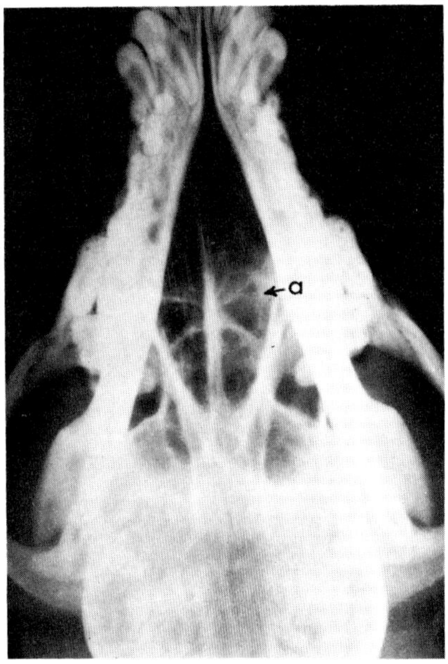

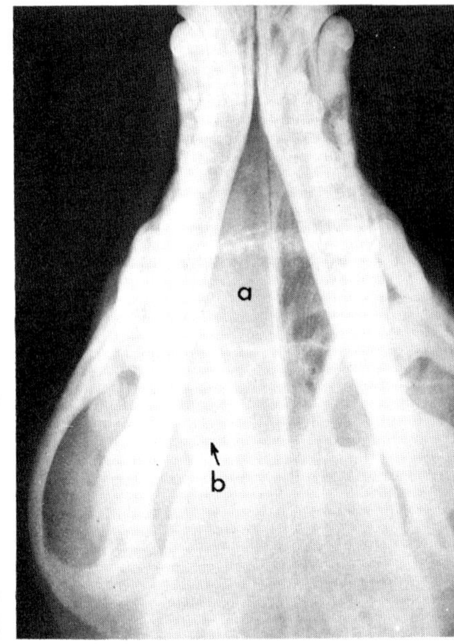

Fig. 16–25

Fig. 16–26

FIGURE 16–25 VD radiograph of nasal tumor (a). (From Hoerlein, B. F., and Evans, L. E.: Clinical diagnosis and surgical removal of nasal tumors in dogs. Small Animal Clin. *2*, 65, 1962.)

FIGURE 16–26 A unilateral nasal (a) and sinus (b) infection is seen in this VD radiograph. (From Hoerlein, B. F., and Evans, L. E.: Clinical diagnosis and surgical removal of nasal tumors in dogs. Small Animal Clin. *2*, 65, 1962.)

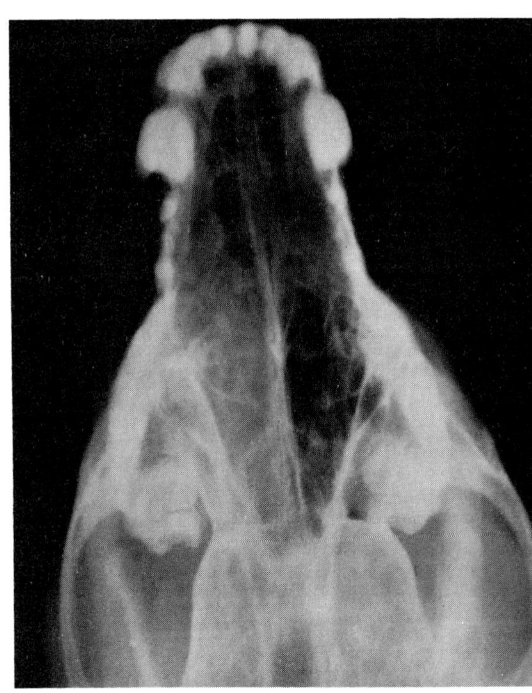

FIGURE 16–27 An open-mouth ventrodorsal radiograph (see Fig. 16–22) showing neoplastic opacities of the nasal passages and sinuses, predominantly on the right side.

permit effective use of surgical or radiation therapy. It is apparent that a patient with advanced neoplasia which has invaded the facial bones, the pharyngeal area, and possibly the sinus and cranial cavities is not a candidate for surgery, and radiation may be palliative for only a short period of time. Since most intranasal tumors are carcinomas, it might be appropriate to initiate radiation therapy promptly without waiting for a surgical biopsy. It has been our experience that the spacious dorsal flap approach is the most satisfactory method for diagnosis of the tumor type. A biopsy of the tumor may be difficult to obtain through a small trephine opening or through the nostril.[4]

Surgical Treatment

As mentioned, some cases of chronic infectious sinusitis and rhinitis in dogs and cats are virtually impossible to cure by local or parenteral antibiotic therapy or other drugs. Removal or drainage of infectious material is necessary not only for proper drug therapy but for a definitive diagnosis. Occasionally the disorder is caused by a combination of neoplasia and infection. Surgical procedures therefore vary from trephinations and insertion of drain tubes to expansive dorsal flap exposures of sinuses and nasal passages. In humans and cats, chronic sinusitis has been treated best by osteoplasty and obliteration of the sinus cavity. Tomlinson[42] describes this procedure in a cat—first, a dorsal bone flap over both frontal sinuses was made, and the mucosa of both sinuses was removed using a small periosteal elevator and electrically driven bone burr. The nasolacrimal duct was then enlarged to allow aspiration of exudate and to stimulate scar tissue closure, and finally, both cavities were filled with autogenous fat removed previously from the subcutaneous area of the ventral abdo-

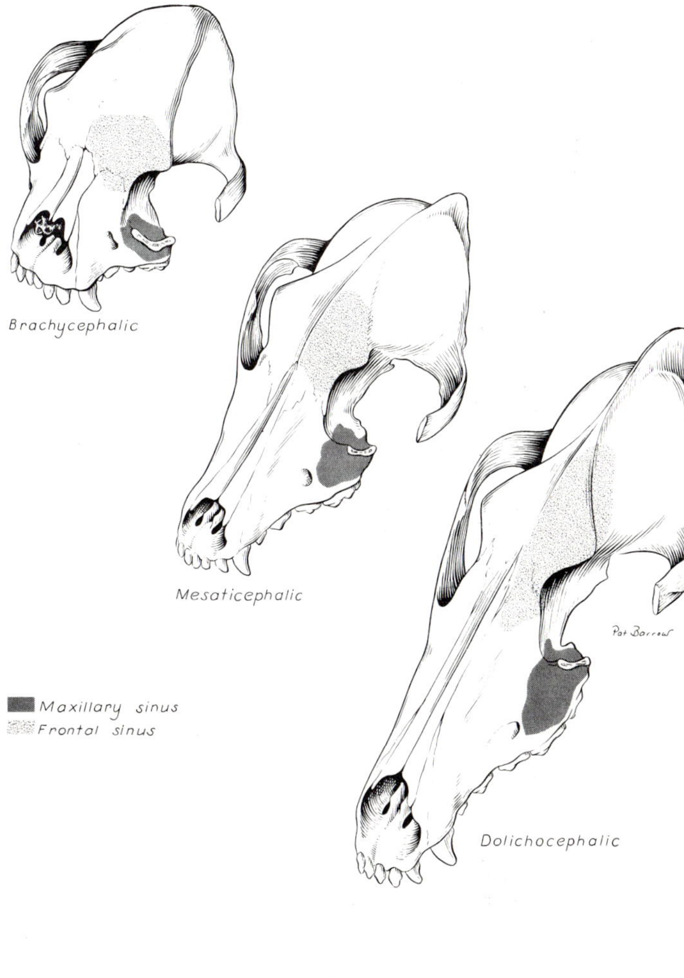

FIGURE 16–28 The extent of the frontal sinuses in three types of skulls. (From Miller, M. E., Christensen, G. C., and Evans, H. E.: *Anatomy of the Dog*. W. B. Saunders Co., Philadelphia, 1964.)

men. The bone flaps were replaced, the periosteum resutured, and the wound closure completed. Although this procedure has been used only in humans and cats, it could be considered in selected cases of sinusitis in the dog.[42]

In the dorsal bone flap exploration,[16-19] the animal is placed in a sternal recumbent position with the head on a cushion or sandbag. The trachea should be intubated with the cuff on the tube completely inflated so that no blood from the nasal passages can be aspirated into the lungs. Oxygen and a gaseous anesthesia should be administered in a semiclosed or closed system.

The skin is incised at the dorsal midline of the affected areas of the nasal passages, sinuses, and cranium (Fig. 16–28). The skin, fascia, and periosteum are dissected laterally from the bone on the affected side or sides. A power driven oscillating saw, a small curved handsaw, a narrow pneumatic surgical drill, or a suitable bone chisel can be used to cut a rectangular section of bone diagonally from the pathologic area.[19, 20, 41] The section of bone is removed by prying it out with a sharp chisel or elevator, thus exposing the sinus and nasal passages (Figs. 16–29 to 16–33).

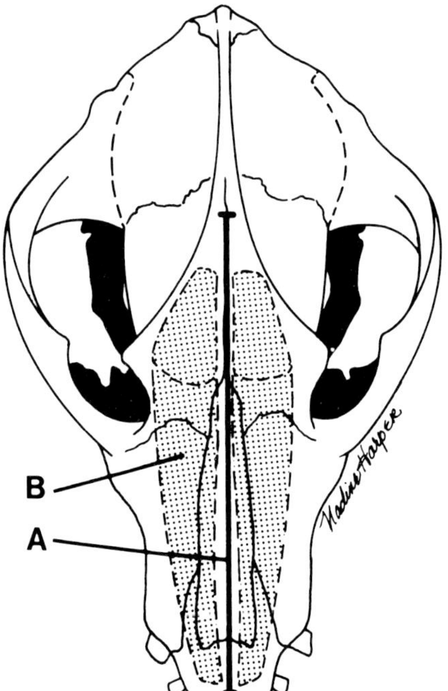

FIGURE 16–29 In the dorsal bone-flap nasal surgery, the incision (A) is made from the nostril caudal to the calvarium (B) nasal passages. (From Hoerlein, B. F.: Disorders of the nasal passages and sinus cavities. *In* Bojrab, M. J. (ed.): *Current Techniques in Small Animal Surgery I.* Lea & Febiger, Philadelphia, 1975.)

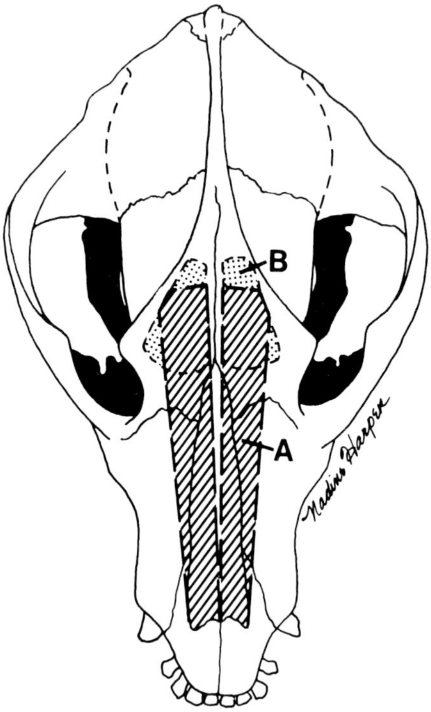

FIGURE 16–30 The proposed flaps. (A) Nasal passage area; (B) Frontal sinus area. (From Hoerlein, B. F.: Disorders of the nasal passages and sinus cavities. *In* Bojrab, M. J. (ed.): *Current Techniques in Small Animal Surgery I.* Lea & Febiger, Philadelphia, 1975.)

The exudate or neoplastic tissue is removed and the affected tissue in the nasal passages and/or sinuses, or both, is examined. The internal plate of the frontal bone can be removed with a mastoid rongeur forceps in order to properly expose or explore the olfactory and frontal poles of the brain. The frontal sinus resection must be very carefully accomplished, since the brain is immediately adjacent to the bone in this area. After the infection is drained and antibiotics are applied, a tube or seton can be placed in the flap area, draining through the bone flap and skin, or through the nasal passages and the nostril. In some instances, tubes or setons could be placed so that they drained in both directions; flushing could be through the upper end and drainage through the lower one. In order to control hemorrhage, the author generally packs the resected nasal passage and sinuses with a gauze bandage, leaving one end protruding through the nostril.[19] Other surgeons prefer not to pack the passage, and some do not even use tube drainage.[20] This packing is removed (Figs.

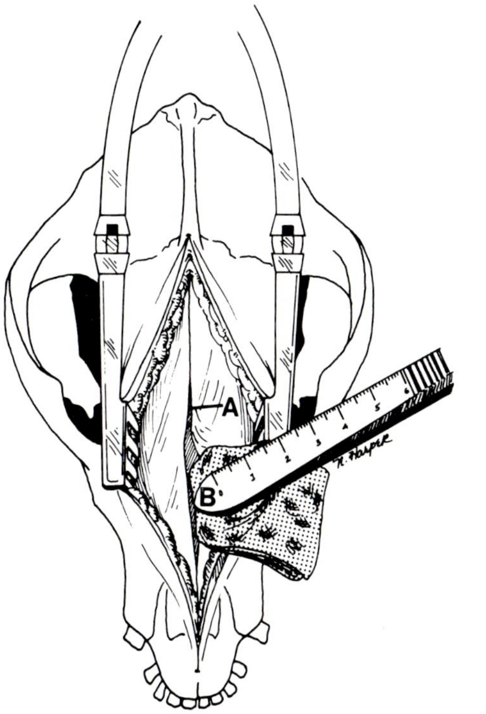

FIGURE 16–31 The periosteum and fascia are reflected from the nasal and facial bones by placing a dry surgical sponge upon the tissue with a lateral action of the scalpel handle. When the reflection is started the periosteum peels off readily. (A) Incision in fascia and periosteum; (B) Scalpel handle on the sponge. (From Hoerlein, B. F.: Disorders of the nasal passages and sinus cavities. *In* Bojrab, M. J. (ed.): *Current Techniques in Small Animal Surgery I.* Lea & Febiger, Philadelphia, 1975.)

16–34 and 16–35) in such a way that the possibility of subcutaneous emphysema is diminished. Sedation for 1 to 4 days after surgery may be necessary to diminish efforts to sneeze.

The bone flap is replaced, and if it was cut initially so that the sides beveled inward, no suturing need be done. If this was not done, holes can be drilled in two or more corners of the flap and nasal bones to facilitate suturing with malleable stainless steel wire. The periosteum, fascia, and skin are closed routinely, and a stint bandage is sutured to the incision. Head bandages can be applied if necessary. A tracheostomy is performed regularly as soon as the endotracheal tube is removed. This is especially important when extensive nasal surgery has been done in massive destructive or neoplastic lesions. Packing is used to control hemorrhage. The tube is necessary to maintain respiration and can usually be removed in 4 to 7 days (Figs. 16–36 to 16–38).

Parenteral and local antibiotics should be used. Again, the agent chosen depends upon the antibiotic sensitivity determinations previously made from culture of the specimen. If the lesion is neoplastic, postsurgical radiographic therapy should be considered. Frequently irradiation will prevent a recurrence of the tumor. In our experience, malignant tumors in this area are

FIGURE 16–32 The bone flaps are made with the edges beveled inward. (a) The oscillating power bone saw (Stryker); (b) Air-driven bone drill (Hall). (After Hoerlein, B. F.: Disorders of the nasal passages and sinus cavities. *In* Bojrab, M. J. (ed.): *Current Techniques in Small Animal Surgery I.* Lea & Febiger, Philadelphia, 1975.)

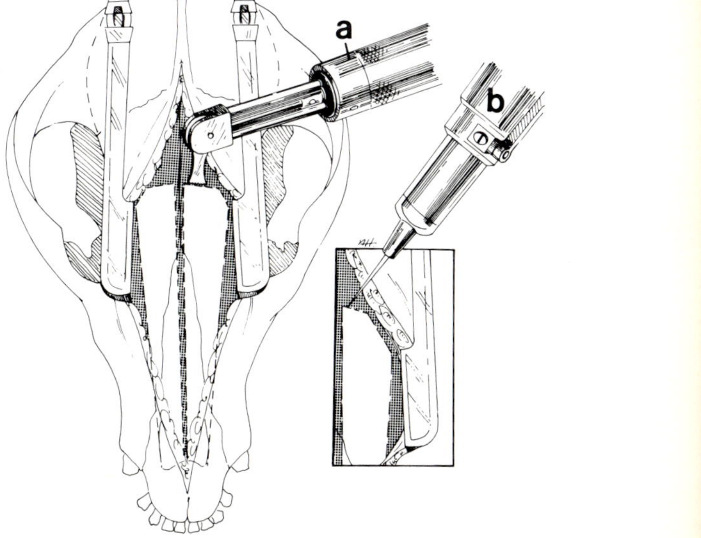

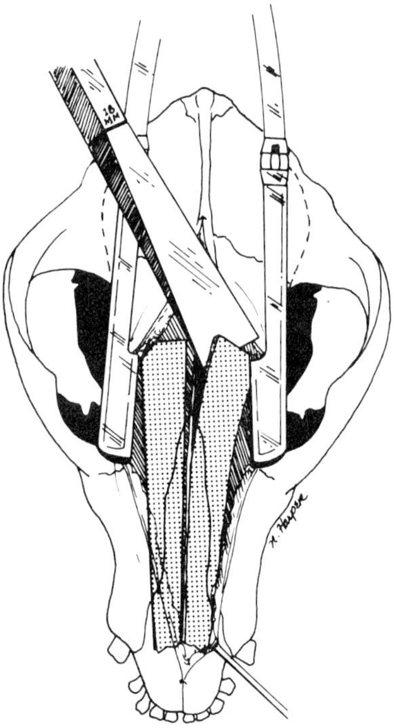

FIGURE 16–33 The flap or flaps may be pried loose from interior attachments by means of a small bone chisel. (Figures 16–33 to 16–37 from Hoerlein, B. F.: Disorders of the nasal passages and sinus cavities. *In* Bojrab, M. J. (ed.): *Current Techniques in Small Animal Surgery I.* Lea & Febiger, Philadelphia, 1975.)

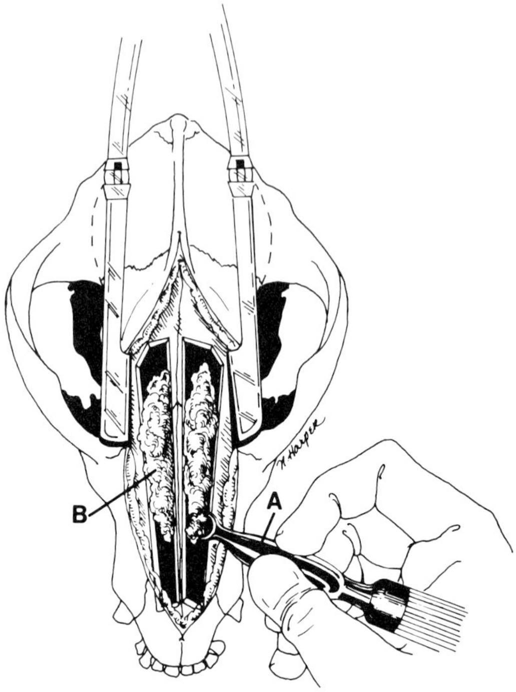

FIGURE 16–34 The lesions are removed by means of a bone curette. (A) Curette; (B) tumor.

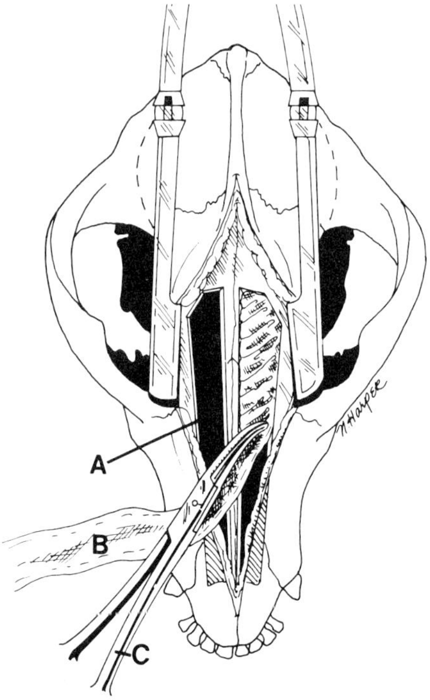

FIGURE 16–35 Gauze bandage may be used for packing and can be soaked in a medication if necessary. The packing is started at the caudal portion, and an end is left protruding through the nostril. (A) Nasal passage with tumor removed; (B) gauze packing; (C) hemostatic forceps.

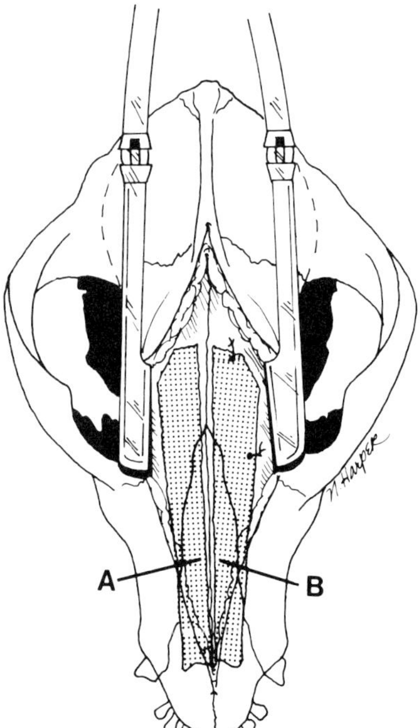

FIGURE 16–36 The inner surfaces of the bone flaps are made smooth with a rongeur and are secured in place. (A) This bone flap, which is in one piece and is beveled properly, doesn't need suturing. (B) This flap is sutured where necessary so that it can't fall into the passage.

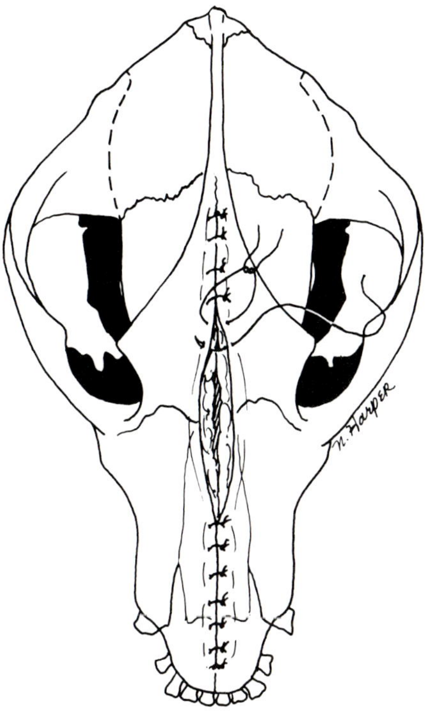

FIGURE 16–37 The periosteum and fascia are sutured with interrupted 00 or 0 absorbable material, in this case, 5–0 monofilament stainless steel suture material.

not highly metastatic but will recur if not irradiated properly. Amphotericin B can be administered in certain mycotic infections; however, the kidney function must be monitored periodically during its administration. Dermal sutures are generally removed in 10 to 14 days.[17, 18]

The flap method of exploration is superior cosmetically to trephination into the sinus, because trephination and removal of sufficient bone to permit exploration or drainage of the infection may create such a large defect that subcutaneous emphysema will result. A bone graft, wire mesh, metal plate, or plastic may be required to repair the bony defect. The bone flap fulfills the requirements of good exposure, ample opportunity for surgical correction, and complete obliteration of the defect. There is generally therefore no need for secondary surgical repair.[16–19]

REFERENCES

1. Barrett, R. E., and Rathfon, B. L.: Lateral approach to a bulla osteotomy. J. Am. Anim. Hosp. Assoc. *11*, 203, 1975.

FIGURE 16–38 A stent bandage is sutured to the skin over the incision area. Notice that the gauze bandage ends at the nostril and the tracheostomy tube. *A*, The one-piece stent bandage. *B*, The double stent bandage with an area sutured open in the center of the incision to discourage the chance of subcutaneous emphysema. (After Hoerlein, B. F.: Disorders of the nasal passages and sinus cavities. *In* Bojrab, M. J. (ed.): *Current Techniques in Small Animal Surgery I.* Lea & Febiger, Philadelphia, 1975.)

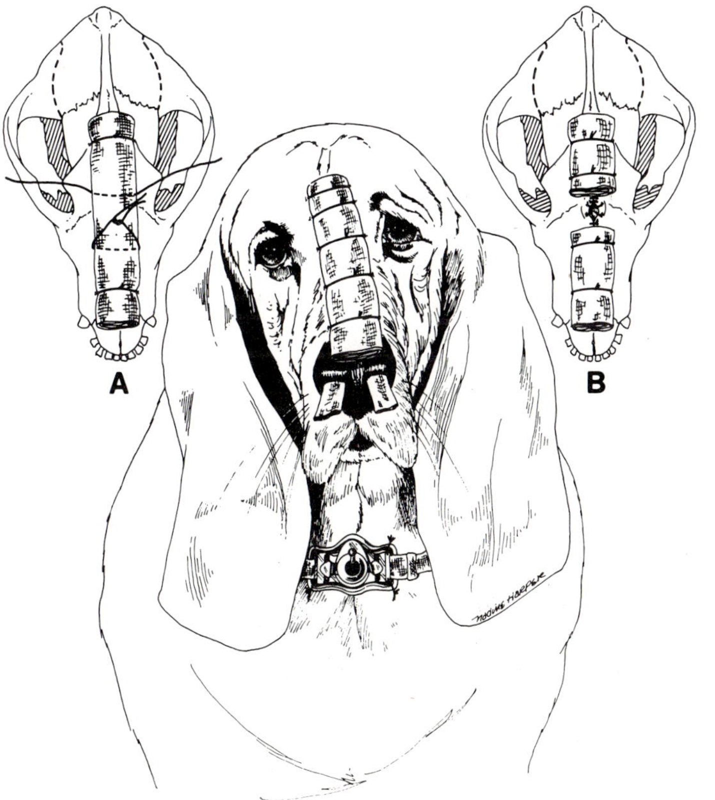

2. Blakemore, J. C.: Diseases of the ear. *In* Catcott, E. J. (ed.): *Canine Medicine.* American Veterinary Publications, Inc., Santa Barbara, Cal., 1968, p. 739.
3. Bojrab, M. J.: Personal communication.
4. Bradley, P. A., and Harvey, C. E.: Intranasal tumors in the dog: an evaluation of prognosis. J. Am. Anim. Pract. *14,* 459, 1973.
5. Carpenter, J. L.: Sinusitis. *In* Kirk, R. W. (ed.): *Current Veterinary Therapy III.* W. B. Saunders Co., Philadelphia, 1968, p. 151.
6. Cook, W. R.: Observations on the upper respiratory tract of the dog and cat. J. Small Anim. Pract. *5,* 309, 1964.
7. Cook, W. R.: A routine for the clinical examination of the nasal chambers and nasopharynx in the dog. Vet. Rec. *76,* 859, 1964.
8. de Lahunta, A.: Feline vestibular disease. *In* Kirk, R. W. (ed.): *Current Veterinary Therapy IV.* W. B. Saunders Co., Philadelphia, 1971, p. 484.
9. Denny, H. R.: The results of surgical treatment of otitis media and interna in the dog. J. Small Anim. Pract. *14,* 585, 1973.
10. Di Chiro, G., Stein, S. C., and Harrington, T.: Cerebrospinal fluid rhinorrhea in normal dogs. J. Neuropath. Exp. Neurol. *31*:447, 1972.
11. Ehmer, E. A.: Modified bulla ossea operation. N. Am. Vet. *15,* 44, 1934.
12. Fraser, G., Gregar, W. W., Mackenzie, C. P., Spreull, J. S. A., and Withers, A. R.: Canine ear disease. J. Small Anim. Pract. *10,* 725, 1970.
13. Gelatt, K. N., Guffy, M. M., and Boggess, T. S.: Radiographic contrast techniques for detecting orbital and nasolacrimal tumors in dogs. J.A.V.M.A. *156,* 741, 1970.
14. Gilbert, G. J.: Meniere's syndrome and cluster headaches. J.A.M.A. *191,* 691, 1965.
15. Goodger, W. J., and Carlson, L.: Surgical removal of a neoplasm from the nasal cavity of a dog. J.A.V.M.A. *160,* 726, 1972.
16. Hoerlein, B. F.: Nasal and sinus surgery. *In* Kirk, R. W. (ed.): *Current Veterinary Therapy III.* W. B. Saunders Co., Philadelphia, 1968.
17. Hoerlein, B. F.: *Canine Neurology, Diagnosis and Treatment,* 2d ed. W. B. Saunders Co., Philadelphia, 1971, p. 425.
18. Hoerlein, B. F., and Evans L. E.: Clinical diagnosis and surgical removal of nasal tumors in dogs. Small Anim. Clin. *2,* 65, 1962.
19. Hoerlein, B. F., and Geary, J. C.: The radiographic diagnosis and the cosmetic surgical removal of nasal and sinus lesions in the dog. Animal Hosp. *2,* 1975, 1966.
20. Hughes, C. D.: Surgery of the nasal cavity. Scientific presentation and seminar synopses to the Am. Anim. Hosp. Assoc., 1974, p. 21.
21. Madewell, B. R., Priester, W. A., Gillette, E. L., and Snyder, S. P.: Neoplasms of the nasal passage and paranasal sinuses in domestic animals as reported by 13 veterinary colleges. Am. J. Vet. Res. *37,* 851, 1976.
22. McBride, N. C.: Persistent otorrhea in the dog. Proceedings book, 90th annual meeting of the American Veterinary Medicine Association, 1953, p. 217.
23. McCrady, J. D., and Alford, R. R.: Surgical correction of labyrinthitis. S. West. Vet. *17,* 29, 1963.
24. McGrath, J. I.: *Neurologic Examination of the Dog with Clinicopathologic Observations,* 2d ed. Lea and Febiger, Philadelphia, 1960.
25. McNutt, G. W., and McCoy, J. E.: Bulla-osteotomy in the dog. J.A.V.M.A. *77,* 617, 1930.
26. Meynard, J. A.: Treatment of otitis media in the dog. Rev. Med. Vet. *111,* 119, 1960.
27. Miller, M. E., Christiansen, G. C., and Evans, H. E.: *Anatomy of the Dog.* W. B. Saunders Co., Philadelphia, 1964.
28. Moltzen, H.: Otitis media in the dog and cat. Adv. Small Anim. Pract. *3,* 56, 1961.
29. Morgan, J. P., Suter, P. F., O'Brien, T. R., and Park, R. D.: Tumors in the nasal cavity of the dog: a radiographic study. J. Am. Vet. Rad. Soc. *13,* 18, 1972.
30. O'Brien, J. A., and Harvey, C. E.: Diseases of the upper airway. *In* Ettinger, S. J. (ed.): *Textbook of Veterinary Internal Medicine.* W. B. Saunders Co., Philadelphia, 1975, p. 581.
31. Ott, R. L.: Ears. *In* Archibald, J. (ed.): *Canine Surgery,* 2d ed. American Veterinary Publications, Inc., Santa Barbara, Cal., 1974.
32. Parker, A. J., Schiller, A. G., and Cusick, P. K.: Bulla curettage for chronic otitis media and internal in dogs. J.A.V.M.A. *168,* 931, 1976.
33. Redding, R.: Personal communication.
34. Rocken, H.: Beitrag zur operativen Behandlung der Otitiden des Hundes. Berl. Munch. Tierärtzl. Wochenschr. *67*:357, 1954.
35. Simonton, D. M.: Meniere's disease and the medical treatment of vertigo. Mayo Clin. Proc. *44,* 81, 1969.
36. Sisson, S., and Grossman, J. D.: *The Anatomy of the Domestic Animals,* 5th ed. W. B. Saunders Co., Philadelphia, 1975.
37. Spreull, J. S. A.: Treatment of otitis media in the dog. J. Small Anim. Pract. *5,* 107, 1964.
38. Spreull, J. S. A.: Otitis media. Animal Hosp. *2,* 80, 1966.
39. Spreull, J. S. A.: Otitis media of the dog. *In* Kirk, R. W. (ed.): *Current Veterinary Therapy III.* W. B. Saunders Co., Philadelphia, 1968, p. 482.
40. Spreull, J. S. A.: Tympanotomy, bulla osteotomy, and vestibular osteotomy. *In* Bojrab, M. J., (ed.): *Current Techniques in Small Animal Surgery I.* Lea and Febiger, Philadelphia, 1975.
41. Swaim, S. F.: Use of pneumatic surgical instruments in neurosurgery: Part 2. Cranial and paracranial surgery. Vet. Med. Small Anim. Clin. *68,* 1404, 1973.
42. Tomlinson, M. J., and Schenck, N. L.: Autogenous fat implantation as a treatment for chronic frontal sinusitis in a cat. J.A.V.M.A. *167,* 927, 1975.
43. Tufvesson, G.: Operation for otitis externa in dogs according to Zepp's method. Am. J. Vet. Res. *16,* 565, 1955.
44. Wolfson, R. J., Cutt, R. A., Ishajama, E., and Myers, D.: Cryosurgery of the labyrinth – preliminary report of a new surgical procedure. Laryngoscope *76,* 733, 1966.
45. Wolfson, R. J., Schlosser, W. D., and Winchester, R. A.: Vertigo. Ciba Symposium *17,* 99, 1965.
46. Zepp, C. P.: Surgical technique to establish drainage of the external ear canal and corrections of hematomas of the dog and cat. J.A.V.M.A. *115,* 91, 1949.

CHAPTER 17

THE BRAIN AND RELATED DISORDERS

SEIZURES[49-51]

The word epilepsy in Greek means seizure, or "to be seized." The terms seizure, fit, convulsions, and epilepsy are used to identify and describe a group of acute or chronic disorders that are manifested by abnormal body movements, a loss or disturbance of consciousness, abnormal behavior, involuntary urination and defecation, or a combination of these. This disease, which we will refer to as seizure, is a common clinical sign of CNS disturbance.

Croft[12, 13] analyzed the records of 570 dogs with suspected CNS disorders and found that 260 had the presenting sign of seizures. Epilepsy was diagnosed in 167 dogs. The remainder of cases were due to: encephalitis (23 cases), cardiovascular disorders (17), internal hydrocephalus (10), space occupying lesions (9), encephalopathy (7), metabolic disorders (5), hysteria (5), head injury (3), poisoning (1), and miscellaneous causes (13).[12, 13] Cunningham has reported that seizure disorders constitute about 1 per cent of all canine diseases, whereas the prevalence of epilepsy in man is about 0.5 per cent.[15] Palmer studied neuropathological changes in 40 dogs suffering from fits. Idiopathic epilepsy was diagnosed in 12, cerebral neoplasia in 9, encephalitis in 7, and laminar necrosis of the cerebral cortex in 3; various neuropathies accounted for one each in the remainder.[46]

Seizures may be classified by their signs or characteristics. *Grand mal* is a general tonic-clonic convulsion with syncope that is associated with severe and spreading cerebral arrhythmia. This type of seizure is the usual one in the dog. *Petit mal*—like seizures are brief, frequent attacks accompanied by blinking, nodding, jerking of legs or loss of posture, and, often, impaired consciousness. However, the occurrence of EEG patterns (spike and dome) characteristic of petit mal in man have been observed infrequently in dogs.[49-51] *Psychomotor* or *behavioral* seizures are poorly coordinated, purposeful movements characterized by behavioral abnormalities. They can be manifested by what appears to be taste sensation—salivation, vomiting, and retching (visceral seizures); auditory sensation or hallucinating sensation (perhaps this accounts for the "fly catchers"); or by paroxysmal rage reactions (the dog attacks his owner). So-called "hysterical" seizures might be included as a form of behavioral or psychomotor seizures.[30] *Thalamic* and *hypothalamic* seizures are preceded by dizziness, nausea, fear, and pain in the abdomen, head, or thorax. *Focal* seizures (sometimes called partial seizures) are asymmetrical contractions of a limb or other muscle group referable to a small portion of the motor cortex. Common focal seizures include lifting the paw, unilateral facial twitching, and turning of the head. The contractions may "march" or spread to other areas and end in grand mal or jacksonian seizures (Fig. 17-1). A *myoclonic* seizure is a sudden jerk of the head, limbs, or trunk that usually lasts only a second or two. Sometimes groups of four or

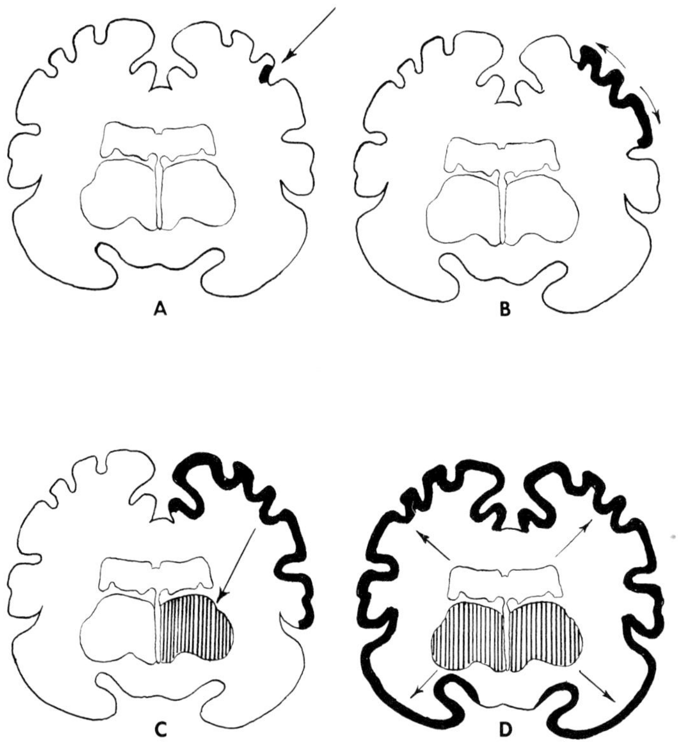

FIGURE 17–1 The "seizure" spread in a jacksonian attack of epilepsy. *A*, Histochemical short-circuiting causing a jerking of a part. *B*, Severe jerking in one or more parts as the reaction spreads. *C*, As reaction spreads to deeper centers of the brain the convulsion becomes generalized. *D*, Generalized tonic–clonic seizures and loss of consciousness. (Based on Mullan, S.: *Essentials of Neurosurgery for Students and Practitioners.* Springer Publishing Co., New York, 1961.)

five of these will occur at intervals of 3 to 6 seconds. Jerking in sleeping dogs has been considered possibly as myoclonic. *Status epilepticus* is a series of convulsions rapidly repeated without intervals of consciousness.[44, 49-51]

The essential disturbance in epilepsy could be described as a physicochemicoelectrical malfunction in a focal area that is usually located in the cerebral cortex. Any physical, electrical, or chemical alteration of the affected cell may lead to a spread of discharges, though no histological change may be detectable. When the barrier to such changes breaks down, a spread of the discharge results in a seizure that continues until oxygen and glucose are exhausted. If therapy isn't instigated, permanent neuronal damage ensues. The paroxysmal cerebral dysrhythmia produced will vary with the type of seizure, being fast in grand mal attacks, slow in psychomotor attacks, and alternately fast and slow in petit mal attacks.[66] There are a multitude of disorders that may stimulate or contribute to seizures, such as disturbed metabolism of amino acids, changes in sodium and potassium ion concentrations, cerebral ischemia, hypoxia, hypocapnia, hypoglycemia, hypocalcemia, congenital defects, cerebral trauma during parturition, infectious diseases, neoplasia, poisoning, cardiovascular disease, hepatosis, nephrosis, and head trauma.[44, 49-51]

The components of an epileptic attack should be understood by the clinician and the owner so that an accurate history can be secured. The preictal stage or aura is a series of events preceding the actual attack; these include restlessness, nervousness, whining, shaking, salivation, affection, wandering, and hiding. The duration of this phase may vary from a few seconds to several days and may be unnoticed by the owner. On the other hand, the aura may be so prominent that the owner can quickly give increased anticonvulsant medication to lessen the severity of the actual attack.[30]

The ictus or actual epileptic attack can last from a few seconds to several minutes unless status epilepticus develops. Most attacks last from 1 to 3 minutes. The nature of the ictus depends on the type of epileptic episode. Generalized or grand mal seizures are characterized by bilateral and symmetrical tonic, clonic, and running movements; loss of consciousness; and autonomic signs such as salivation, urination, and defecation; all of which occur usually in the lateral recumbent position.[30]

The postictal phase is characterized by confusion, disorientation, salivation, pacing, wandering, restlessness, unresponsiveness, and transient blindness. This period can vary in duration just as the preictal phase does. There seems to be no correlation between the severity of the ictus and the duration of the postictal stage. It must be emphasized that, to qualify as epileptic episodes these paroxysmal attacks must be repetitive and generally similar, and occur in the characteristic preictal, ictal, and postictal stages.[30]

There has been much controversy concerning the nomenclature and classification of the various etiological forms of so-called epilepsy. Redding has formulated an etiological classification of seizures that seems logical and accurate and probably won't promote controversy in academia.[49-51]

TYPES OF SEIZURES[49-51]

I. Acquired seizures. All acquired seizures are caused by damage to brain tissue, which acts as a focus for seizures.
   A. Viral. Distemper is the most common cause of acquired seizures in the dog. The history, clinical signs, and EEG are aids in clinical diagnosis. Serological and histological examinations are means of definitive diagnosis.
   B. Protozoan. Toxoplasmosis, a protozoan infection, may be responsible for seizures in dogs and cats. This disease clinically resembles distemper as a neuropathy. The EEG, serological, cultural, and histological examinations are useful aids in diagnosis.
   C. Metabolic. Seizures of metabolic origin are not focal in nature and are related to some alteration in blood chemistry, ionic constituents, or blood gas tension of the extracellular fluid.
      1. Hypoxia. A lowered oxygen tension of the blood and extracellular fluid usually causes syncope or fainting, but it can cause seizures. Cardiac and pulmonary disorders frequently are the basic cause. Carbon monoxide poisoning, seen in hunting dogs transported in the trunk of a car, is seen occasionally. Carboxyhemoglobin interferes with the formation of oxyhemoglobin, and seizures result from cerebral hypoxia after 5 to 15 minutes of hunting. Hypocapnia in absence of hypoxia has been found to cause coma by reflex vasoconstriction of the CNS vasculature.
      2. Hypoglycemia and hypocalcemia. Hypoglycemic seizures are associated with a reduced level of blood glucose and have been discussed previously. Functional hypoglycemia in working dogs, glycogen storage disorders in puppies, hyperinsulinism, and malabsorption seen in heavily parasitized puppies can all cause types of seizures. Hypocalcemia, which can also cause seizures, is seen most often in young puppies and nursing bitches.
      3. Chemical intoxication. There are many insecticides and herbicides responsible for abnormal motor activity that may mimic other causes of convulsions. These poisons include organic phosphates, chlorinated hydrocarbons, strychnine, and cyanide. Other chemicals and drugs have been mentioned elsewhere.
   D. Cerebral trauma. Cerebral trauma and resultant scar tissue may promote seizure activity up to 3 to 6 months after injury. History, EEG, radiographic, and neurological examinations are helpful aids in the diagnosis.
   E. Cerebral neoplasms. Cerebral neoplasms have been discussed in

Chapter 11 and frequently initiate seizures by encroaching upon and irritating surrounding normal tissue. A focal lesion will frequently cause abnormal reflexes. If the tumor is in the motor cortex, a jacksonian type of seizure will take place. If the lesion is deepseated, the seizures will be generalized, with several in a series. Each series is apt to become more frequent and severe. Diagnosis can be facilitated by careful physical, radiographic, laboratory, and EEG examinations.

F. Mycotic (e.g., cryptococcosis, blastomycosis, etc.). Cryptococcosis is one of many mycotic infections that can affect the CNS and cause neurological signs. Frequently, this disease localizes in the cerebral meninges and cortex, causing seizures. Diagnosis is best made clinically by isolation and culture of the organism from spinal fluid.

G. Hydrocephalus (acquired). This type of hydrocephalus is not necessarily hereditary and may be the result of paraventricular or ventricular infections, trauma, neoplasms, or disorders upsetting the balance of production, circulation, and absorption of CSF. In addition to clinical signs, diagnosis may be aided by the EEG or ventriculography (see pages 127 and 182).

II. Familial (congenital) seizures. The familial or congenital epilepsies are seizures in which there is an apparent associated genetic transmission. The genetic defect may be an inherited metabolic dysfunction in the CNS that is responsible for the initiation of seizures.

A. Idiopathic epilepsy. Idiopathic epilepsy is reported to occur most frequently in poodles and the spaniel breeds, although this may be debatable. It is believed that idiopathic epilepsy is an inherited defect in the metabolism of brain neurons. The usual age of onset is from 6 to 18 months, and there is nothing unusual in the history nor any sign of other disease. There is usually an aura, in which the animal apparently anticipates the seizure by perception of some sensory sensation. The observant owner recognizes the aura. The seizure period is usually quite short (one-half to 2 minutes), and may occur at regular intervals. Recovery is rapid, with few residual after effects. Neurological, radiographic, and EEG examinations are usually negative during the period between seizures. Occasional interseizural EEG recordings may be diagnostic (see Chapter 7).[49-51]

Heritable seizures have been reported in certain families and breeds of dogs such as the Alsatian, beagle, cocker spaniel, dachshund, keeshond, miniature poodle, and Tervuren shepherd dog.[5, 7, 20] Croft's studies of EEG interpretation in detecting preclinical manifestations of familial seizures, or heritable epilepsy, in the keeshond breed in England were initially very encouraging. She felt that the EEG could predict those puppies destined to be epileptic before clinical disease developed.[12-14] Wallace has recently critically analyzed data from 321 keeshond dogs and 108 close ancestors and concluded that there was little or no correlation between EEG readings and the incidence of epilepsy. There did seem to be a high incidence in families, which points to a hereditary component in its etiology.[63]

The various diseases of congenital, degenerative, and hereditary origin discussed in Chapter 11 frequently progress to the stage of seizures. Examples of these are gangliosidosis disorders, ceroid lipofuscinosis, leukodystrophy in cats, and lissencephaly.

B. Congenital or inheritable hydrocephalus. Hydrocephalus can be congenital (and probably heritable) or acquired. Probably many cases of hydrocephalus, regardless of the age at which clinical signs occur, have a heritable predisposition, and certain stresses promote the clinical drome. Congenital hydrocephalus is more common in the Chihuahua and brachycephalic breeds. As mentioned in Chapter 21, hydrocephalus can cause a wide variety of neurological signs, and seizures can be one of them. Obvious hydrocephalus with the enlarged cranium and open fontanels is no problem to diagnose. The latent, and sometimes acquired type, characterized by normal skull size and contour and showing seizures, may be a diagnostic problem. Evidence of retarded intelligence, incoordination, and depression; abnormal plain and contrast radiography; and characteristic EEG tracings can establish a definitive clinical diagnosis.[49-51]

DIFFERENTIAL DIAGNOSIS

The differential diagnosis is based upon the evaluation of a very detailed, carefully secured history, a thorough physical examination, selective laboratory examinations, plain and appropriate contrast radiography, and electroencephalography. The history is one of the most important aids in determining familial or idiopathic epilepsy and would be helpful in differentiating distemper, trauma, and other causes for seizures. The physical examination is essential in diagnosing the multitude of metabolic disorders that could be contributing to seizures. Radiography is most useful in confirming a traumatic, neoplastic, and hydrocephalic lesion. Laboratory examination is particularly helpful in confirming the presence of infections; abnormal levels of blood glucose, calcium, and electrolytes; and identification or culture of infectious protozoan, mycotic, and bacterial organisms. The EEG is a helpful aid in differentiating the various inflammatory infectious encephalitides, such as distemper, toxoplasmosis, or systemic mycoses, as well as neoplasia, trauma, and hydrocephalus. Positive EEG findings are generally not seen in the interseizural stage of idiopathic epilepsy (Table 17–1).

TREATMENT[49-51]

The treatment of all cases of seizures other than idiopathic epilepsy obviously involves eliminating the primary cause. Since hard or continuous seizures are devastating to the CNS, anticonvulsants may be used to control seizures while the primary disorder is being treated. For instance, Redding has established that when an EEG pattern is characteristic of distemper encephalitis, anticonvulsant therapy for 30 to 60 days may prevent seizures from occurring. In seizures due to trauma, anticonvulsants may be given during other medical therapy after surgery, or both.

The *objectives* of therapy in seizures are to save the patient's life in the acute emergency, such as status epilepticus, and to prevent recurrences or continued attacks. The emergency case should be hospitalized, while routine interseizural therapy would be given largely on an outpatient basis.

The drugs used are not curative but prophylactic. They act by preventing the spread of an abnormal discharge from a diseased area to the surrounding tissue, thereby preventing abnormal motor activity. In acute attacks, the drug must stop motor activity and allow the animal to recover. The anticonvulsant must insulate the abnormal focus by preventing spread to normal surrounding tissue.

The *principles* of anticonvulsant therapy must be known and understood by the owner of the animal if satisfactory results are to be obtained. The client must be fully aware of the facts and problems associated with therapy, such as the initial and maintenance dosage of the drug, the need for continuous medication, the possibility that other drugs or combinations may be necessary, and the importance of proper environmental management of the patient. Several days of the therapy are required for many anticonvulsants to reach maximal effectiveness. With average oral dosages of diphenylhydantoin (Dilantin), 5 to 15 days may be needed for maximal effect.[35] Primidone (Mysoline, Mylepsin) and phenobarbital may be effective within 1 to 3 days.[67] During this period, seizures may occur, and the owner is likely to feel that the drug is ineffective and to stop medication.

The dosage must be adapted to the individual by trial and error methods. The owner must be acquainted with the side-effects of sedation that may accompany anticonvulsants. Sedation should not always mean that the drug should be discontinued, since continued therapy may promote

TABLE 17–1 DIFFERENTIAL DIAGNOSIS OF SEIZURES (after Redding[51])

Acquired Seizures	
Viral encephalitis	History of previous symptoms suggestive of viral invasion (distemper complex). Hyperexcitability or depression. Electroencephalography is useful for diagnosis.
Toxoplasmosis	Previous chronic disease signs, i.e., anorexia, weakness, emaciation, pulmonary symptoms, ocular lesions, seizures progressively more frequent and occasionally of long duration. (Test: serum titer.) Electroencephalography is useful for diagnosis.
Cerebral neoplasia	Neurological examination usually suggestive of focal abnormality, abnormal reflexes, "Jacksonian" fit. Seizures progressively more frequent. Electroencephalography and radiography (plain and contrast) are useful for diagnosis.
Trauma	History of injury to skull, unconsciousness followed by incoordination. Seizures may start 3 to 6 months after injury. Electroencephalography and radiography are useful for diagnosis.
Cryptococcosis	Variable neurological signs, occasional seizures. Culture of cerebrospinal fluid.
Familial (Congenital) Seizures	
Idiopathic epilepsy	Neurological examination negative in young animal 6 to 18 months old with no previous illness. Aura, short seizure period (20 to 90 seconds), rapid recovery after seizure. Seizures may occur at regular intervals. Electroencephalographic findings usually negative.
Hydrocephalus	Retarded intelligence, incoordination, lethargy. May or may not have increased head size and open fontanelles. Seizures start at 3 to 9 months of age. Electroencephalography and radiography (plain and contrast) are useful for diagnosis.
Metabolic Seizures	
Carbon monoxide poisoning	History of riding in truck or trunk of automobile prior to seizure, which occurs 5 to 15 minutes after muscular activity. Pink mucous membranes.
Parasitism	Very young puppies affected. Low blood calcium, low blood sugar, anemia. Frequent seizures of short duration.
Hypoglycemia	Muscular twitching, hunger, low blood sugar. Seizures occur 30 to 60 minutes after exercise and are related only to the exercise. (Exception: islet cell tumor.) Interseizural electroencephalogram nondiagnostic.
Hypocalcemia	Muscular twitching, anxious attitude, low blood calcium associated with pregnancy, whelping, and parasitism in puppies. Seizures of the tonic type.
Drug-Induced Seizures	
Organophosphate poisoning	Gastrointestinal hypermotility, salivation, miosis, dyspnea. Muscular twitching followed by seizures of long duration.
Chlorinated hydrocarbon poisoning	Hyperexcitability, tremors followed by tonic-clonic seizures of long duration.
Cyanide poisoning	Weakness, tremors, rapid deep respirations, seizures tonic in nature. Bright red mucous membranes.
Other Causes of Seizures	
Hypothalamic syndrome	Hypothermia or hyperthermia, polyuria, polydipsia. Occasional seizures with postseizural confusion. Electroencephalography is useful for diagnosis.
Tetanus	Muscular stiffness, hypertonus of extensor musculature, ears pulled back, nictitating membranes protruding.

tolerance of this effect. Metabolic tolerances, absorption efficiency, and existing disorders such as liver disease may mean that the dose must be varied appreciably. Some animals may require medication for the balance of their lives; others may be "weaned off" anticonvulsants after a period of time. If one drug is not effective, other drugs or combinations must be tried. Occasionally, the effectiveness of one drug may diminish, and the dog will require a higher dose or another agent.[49-51]

In an idiopathic epileptic, the anticonvulsant of choice should be efficient at low doses, economical in cost, widely available in suitable dose ranges for various sizes of patients, easily administered, and lacking in undesirable side effects. It is obvious that the ideal drug has not yet been developed. The four most effective drugs in small animal practice are diphenylhydantoin (Dilantin), phenobarbital, primidone (Mysoline, Mylepsin), and diazepam (Valium).[30]

Diphenylhydantoin is thought to exert its anticonvulsant activity at the neuronal dendritic levels, thus preventing the spread of the spontaneous electrical discharge. It is effective in generalized major motor seizures, focal motor seizures, and psychomotor-behavioral-hysterical seizures. Diphenylhydantoin does not generally promote sedation and it is effective, low in cost, nontoxic in normal use, and widely available. Its disadvantages include the possibility of transient ataxia in high doses, slow action (maximal effectiveness is not obtained until 5 to 15 days after initiation of therapy), rapid metabolism in dogs (it must be given three to four times daily), and general ineffectiveness in parenteral injections. It is therefore not effective in status epilepticus. Polyphagia, polydypsia, and polyuria are frequent side effects. Diphenylhydantoin is not given in cats because it is so slowly metabolized that the dose is difficult to regulate. The usual dose is 2 to 50 mg/lb/day divided into three or four doses. In a normal size dog (30 to 40 pounds) most clinicians use 30 to 90 mg three times daily.[30]

Phenobarbital has been widely used in man for some 60 years and is an extremely effective anticonvulsant. It is thought to act at the nerve cell body and therefore prevent the initial ictal discharge. Phenobarbital is said to be effective in any type of seizure disorder in dogs and cats. It is highly effective with little time lag in efficacy, low in toxicity, low in cost, and widely available. It can be administered by several routes and is the ideal drug for either single or status attacks. Its disadvantages include its sedative effect and the fact that it is a control drug except when used in combination with diphenylhydantoin. Polyphagia, polydypsia, and polyuria are routine side effects, and sometimes phenobarbital promotes restlessness and irritability. Because its effect is prolonged, a neurological examination cannot be performed for several hours or even a day or so after its administration for a seizure. It is the drug of choice in the cat. The usual dose is 0.5 to 1 mg/lb given once or twice daily.[30]

Primidone is a good anticonvulsant in the dog but is not recommended for the cat. The action of primidone is similar to that of phenobarbital in that about 25 per cent of it is converted to phenobarbital by the liver. It is effective against all types of seizures, has a rapid action when given orally, is widely available, and is not a controlled drug. The disadvantages of primidone include sedation (sometimes transient), wide variation in dose ranges, lack of a parenteral form, and routine side effects of polyphagia, polydypsia, and polyuria. High doses over a long period of time may cause liver disorders. The usual dose is 4 to 25 mg/lb/day given in one or two doses.[30]

Diazepam is usually given parenterally in control of exacerbated or status seizures. It is the only tranquilizer that is not epileptigenic; its mode of action is believed to be at the presynaptic level, and it has anticonvulsant properties. The drug can be given as a preanesthetic in epileptics undergoing surgery. The advantages of diazepam are its effectiveness in controlling status epilepticus,[3] its rapid and brief action in preparation for a neurological examination, and its usefulness in parenteral or oral form in cats. Its disadvantages include its brief action when prolonged control is needed, high cost, and its tendency to become less effective in prolonged usage. The usual dose is 0.5 to 1 mg for toy breeds; in larger dogs 10 to 50 mg parenterally to effect (usually IV).[30]

It is confusing to have a large number of anticonvulsants in the pharmacy when a thorough knowledge of the big four and their effects singly and in combination is more useful. In brief, a dog with a routine case of grand mal epilepsy will generally do well on diphenylhydantoin alone or in combination with phenobarbital if a slight sedative effect or quick action is desired. Phenobarbital is best for an immediate effect but causes sedation which in some cases is undesirable. Primidone is also good for a quick effect but has some sedative effect. Diazepam is generally reserved for status epilepticus. For psychomotor efficacy, primidone is the drug of choice. Petit mal is not seen frequently; however, these four drugs are not thought to be particularly effective, with the possible exception of phenobarbital. Trimethadione (Tridione), paramethadione (Paradione), and phensuximide (Milotin) are said to be effective against petit mal. Some clinicians use mephobarbital (Mebrol) instead of phenobarbital, since it has a less sedative effect.[30]

Many clinicians treat routine cases of epilepsy with increasing doses of diphenylhydantoin until the seizures are controlled. Phenobarbital may be added when necessary for control of seizures or when some sedation is desired. Primidone may be added if the first two drugs have not controlled the seizures. Doses of each drug and combinations of drugs should be increased until they have proved to be ineffective. There should be several days or weeks overlap of medication when the intention is to eliminate one drug and start another. Combinations of anticonvulsants and antibiotics may alter therapeutic effects and dosages.

Treatment failures may result because (1) the client failed to give the drug as prescribed, (2) the doses were too low, (3) an inadequate overlap of anticonvulsants occurred when the drugs were changed, (4) the cause of the seizures was a progressive organic disease, or (5) diseases or stressful environment caused the seizures in a highly nervous dog.[30]

TREATMENT OF STATUS EPILEPTICUS

This continuous convulsive disorder is truly a neurologic emergency that can lead to irreversible coma and death. An animal that has had continuous seizures for 12 to 36 hours before therapy or effective control may suffer postictal signs of coma, semiconsciousness, nonresponsiveness to normal stimuli, general hyperreflexia, and hypertonicity. A general rigidity may be maintained in various positions for prolonged periods of time, and stages of cataplexia may occur. These signs are thought to be due to general hypoxia and subsequent neural toxicity from prolonged violent activity of the brain in long-term seizural activity. Status epilepticus must be considered an emergency and an intensive care situation by both veterinarian and owner. The therapeutic regimen should include the following steps:

1. Stop the seizure.
   (a) Diazepam, 10 to 35 mg IV, should be used to effect; if diazepam is ineffective, phenobarbital, 60 to 120 mg IV, to effect should be tried.
   (b) If diazepam or phenobarbital fails to stop the seizure, anesthetize the patient with the least amount of anesthetic possible. Sodium pentobarbital or a gaseous anesthetic can be used.
2. Since continuous medication and laboratory blood specimens may be needed, an indwelling catheter should be used in an appropriate vein.
3. Tests for blood glucose electrolytes, pH, and pCO_2 should be run. If hypoglycemia is present, 50 per cent dextrose should be given in a 2 to 50 ml dose, depending on the patient's size and need. Fluids should be administered appropriately as determined by laboratory results.
4. The animal must be in intensive care until the seizures have subsided and until a neurological examination and diagnosis can be established.[30]

In the quest for more effective methods of seizure control, new anticonvulsants and other supportive drugs are constantly being investigated. A recent study reports that paramethadione (Paradione), a drug designed for control of petit mal in man, is effective in problem cases of epilepsy. It is generally felt that this class of drugs may potentiate grand mal seizures. In preliminary work, Parker stated that 65 per cent of the problem cases showed improvement with this drug.[47] Bartels in Germany reported on the use of carbamazepine (Tegretol) in 148 dogs with various types of epileptiform fits. The drug was felt to be best adapted to controlling vegetative psychomotor seizures.[6]

Some of the newest experimental work in seizure control deals with the use of corticosteroids and ACTH. ACTH in doses of 5 mg/kg/day, intramuscularly, is used for a 4-week period. Then ACTH is replaced by corticosteroids such as dexamethasone 3 to 5 mg/kg/day for a full 4-week period, and the dose is decreased every 3 weeks. This regimen has proved to be effective in very resistant cases of psychomotor or behavioral epilepsy. The dog should be maintained on any prescribed anticonvulsant drug in addition to steroids. The use of progesterone has also been used for resistant psychomotor seizures.

POSSIBLE TOXIC EFFECTS WITH ANTICONVULSANT THERAPY

Since anticonvulsants have been used for years by epileptic persons, there are numerous scattered reports of toxic sequelae in the human literature. Diphenylhydantoin and primidone have been reported to cause hepatosis when used for long periods of time. Since the liver is involved in the metabolism and detoxification of most of these drugs, doses vary tremendously when there is a liver disorder. Diphenylhydantoin has been implicated in peripheral neuropathies and in cerebellar ataxia.[36, 56] Long-term treatment of epileptics with primidone has been associated with alterations in calcium metabolism that resemble vitamin D deficiency.[17] Anticonvulsant drugs, including primidone, seem to accelerate the degradation of vitamin D, resulting in a need for dietary supplements to maintain normal values.[18] Megaloblastic anemia with primidone therapy was attributed to a drug-induced disturbance in folic acid metabolism.[48]

These are only examples of some reports of toxic sequelae from anticonvulsant therapy in the human literature. Scattered reports of serious toxic effects are appearing in the veterinary literature. Jennings has reported ataxia, incoordination, anorexia, and tachycardia with primidone in a 3-month treatment period in a toy poodle. Upon cessation of the drug, the animal returned to normal, but reinstatement of the drug caused a recurrence of signs.[27]

One must be aware of the possible toxic effects of anticonvulsants in animal practice and also that anticonvulsants have pharmacologic actions on other organs; for example, diphenylhydantoin may increase the heart rate and coronary blood flow.[70] Diazepam may have a prophylactic effect on cardiac arrhythmias.[40] Phenothiazine tranquilizers other than diazepam lower the seizure threshold, and the same is true of some antibiotics, such as penicillin and chloramphenicol. Therefore, when giving medication to an epileptic animal the veterinarian must be sure that he is not using a drug that may promote seizures even when an anticonvulsant is used also.[16, 51]

NARCOLEPSY—CATAPLEXY SYNDROME

Narcolepsy was first reported in a dog and cat by Knecht and co-workers,[34] and since then it has been reported by others.[8, 39] Narcolepsy is a disorder of the central nervous system and is characterized by sudden recurring attacks of sleep. In man it may be accompanied by cataplexy, hallucinations, and sleep paralysis in 70, 30, and 25 per cent of the cases, respectively. Blauch has compared the tetrad of signs in human narcoleptics—daytime sleep, cataplexy, sleep paralysis, and hypnogogic hallucinations—to the syndrome as seen in the dog.[8]

Daytime sleeping in humans is characterized by rapid eye movement (REM) onset of sleep, as shown on the EEG. In normal nighttime sleep, REM sleep does not occur until about 90 minutes of ordinary sleep have passed. REM sleep may last for only 15 minutes, after which the person either wakes up or passes into ordinary sleep. The second part of the tetrad is cataplexy, which is seen in 50 to 75 per cent of human narcoleptics. In cataplexy, there is a sudden loss in muscle tone of part or all of the voluntary muscles, except for the extrinsic eye and respiratory muscles, but the person remains conscious. The EEG findings are similar to those in an alert person. These attacks may last for a few seconds or as long as 30 minutes. The third phase in the tetrad is sleep paralysis—the sensation of being unable to move while drifting into sleep or awakening from it. The final phase consists of hypnogogic hallucinations, which differ from dreams in their intensity, completeness of visual or auditory recollections, and time of onset. In veterinary medicine, only REM sleep and cataplexy are recognizable in animals with narcolepsy.[8]

The cause of narcolepsy is not known, but it is thought to be a pathophysiological disorder of the reticular activating system (RAS), perhaps related to a neurohumoral deficiency. There are two functional units of the RAS; one is located in the caudal pontine medullary area and governs motility, and the other is located in the rostral medullary area and governs consciousness, arousal, and wakefulness. It is possible that the inhibitory component of REM sleep may be involved in the sudden atonia and areflexia characteristic of cataplexy.[8]

In dogs and cats the disease is characterized by a sudden collapse to the ground when walking, sleep lasting for a few seconds, and then wakefulness. Eating frequently stimulates an attack of cataplexy and sleep even while food is in the mouth. In the Auburn Clinic, a young Irish setter was observed to take several hours to eat a pan of food because he continuously suffered loss of supporting muscle tone when the food dish was approached, and cataplexy and sleep continuously interrupted the prehension and swallowing of food. Most attacks of sleep or cataplexy can be avoided if the animal is stimulated by people or other dogs. One young giant schnauzer did not sleep but had recurrent "bouncing" attacks or cataplexy that involved all limbs simultaneously when he was involved in relaxed exercise. However, he was entirely normal when playing and romping with other dogs.

The diagnosis is based on clinical signs, EEG findings, a negative response to neostigmine to rule out myasthenia, and a positive response to imipramine or amphetamine. Generally, all laboratory tests and clinical examinations are negative. Electroencephalograms show characteristic sleep spindles preceding slow activity of 2 to 4 Hz, 75 mV. The patient can be alerted by auditory or tactile stimulus to 12 to 20 Hz, 5 to 10 mV activity but will return to a slow wave pattern within 5 to 10 seconds. The pattern is symmetrical.[8]

The treatment has consisted of use of CNS stimulants. Dextroamphetamine (Dexedrine) given orally in doses of 5 to 6 mg or 0.25 to 0.50 mg/lb two or three times daily has been effective. Imipramine (Tofranil) at 0.2 to 0.4 mg/lb orally up to three times daily can be used. Long-term treatment with methylphenidate (Ritalin) at 0.1 mg/lb may be better than dextroamphetamine. The best drug and optimum dose must be established for each individual.[8, 34]

METABOLIC DISEASES

PHYSICAL AGENTS

Cerebral Anoxia

The term cerebral anoxia is used to indicate oxygen deprivation of the brain severe and prolonged enough to result in permanent damage to the tissue. Courville classified anoxias as (a) stagnant anoxia as seen in cardiac failure, (b) anemic anoxias as in carbon monoxide poisoning, (c) anoxia proper from anesthesia, (d) histiotoxic anoxia as in cyanide poisoning, and (e) neonatal anoxia.[11] Most researchers feel that there are variations in the neurons regarding metabolic rate and oxygen need. The need is highest in the cerebral cortex and decreases progressively in other areas in the direction of the medulla; therefore, the signs and pathological sequences vary according to the degree of anoxia.

The signs of cerebral anoxia include dilated pupils, convulsions, collapse, and coma. Anoxic convulsions are clonic when blood oxygen is higher. EEG impulses gradually decrease with the development of anoxia.[38]

One of the chief signs of cerebral hypoxia (chronic lack of oxygen) is cerebral edema and swelling. If the brain is allowed to swell appreciably in its tight-fitting bony encasement, irreparable compressive damage will occur to nerve tissue. One of the chief causes of cerebral hypoxia is head trauma in which the air passages are partially occluded. Maintaining an open airway and a high concentration of oxygen in respiratory air is essential. Other common causes of cerebral hypoxia and syncope may stem from cardiovascular origins, as seen in heartworm disease and aortic stenosis.

Occasionally, carbon monoxide poisoning is seen in dogs being transported in the trunk of a car. Carbon monoxide combines with hemoglobin in a stable form so that oxyhemoglobin cannot be formed. The clinical signs are dilated pupils, rapid shallow respiration, stupor, convulsions, and unconsciousness. Necropsy reveals cherry red blood and mucosa. Treatment includes oxygen therapy and blood transfusions, and recovery depends upon the extent of the cerebral damage.[38]

Perhaps the most common cases of cerebral anoxia in dogs are those developing during anesthesia and surgical procedures. A patent airway must always be maintained or acute hypoxia will result. An inadequate oxygen supply often occurs with gaseous anesthesia when the mask or open method of administration is used. The practice of draping the head area heavily when performing surgery with intravenous anesthesia may lead to hypoxia unless oxygen is given via an endotracheal tube. Although death from anoxia does not always follow this sequence of events, hypoxia may explain the depressed attitude of the patient after awakening or his slow recovery from anesthesia. It has been determined that the dog's metabolism remains aerobic during asphyxia, and its cerebrum does not tolerate hypoxia. Reversible hypoxic EEG patterns appear when pO_2 reaches 14 mm Hg in arterial and 9 mm Hg in sagittal-sinus blood. Blood pH then ranges from 6.95 to 7.4, pCO_2 from 40 to 135 mm Hg, with no difference in arterial and venous lactate. Within 2 minutes after the start of asphyxia, the heart rate falls from 100 to 30, or to 60 if atropine has been given.[32]

Cases of cardiac arrest or fibrillation in which cardiac resuscitation is successful may leave the patient suffering from brain damage. In man, the total period of blood or oxygen privation of the brain before permanent damage occurs is 5 to 10 minutes,[23] according to the onset of oxygen loss. If the anoxia is sudden and profound, damage can occur in 3 minutes.[64] In dogs, this period may be greater. Neely and Youmans experimentally increased the intracranial pressure in dogs to retard cerebral circulation.[42] When an intracranial pressure of 100 mm of mercury was applied to the brain of 23 dogs that did not receive artificial respiration, death occurred in 9 to 12 minutes. In five dogs, artificial respiration was given while similar intracranial pressures were exerted for 5, 10, 15, 20, and 25 minutes, respectively. All could stand, see, and hear the next day, and all survived at least 48 hours. In six dogs in which elevations of pressure were exerted for longer than 25 minutes, the maximum survival period was 24 hours. Neely and Youmans concluded that the mechanisms of survival in cerebral anoxia were the following:

If blood pH falls below a certain point, minute thrombi form which cause tissue damage.

In the bloodless brain, lactic acid, which is a product of anaerobic metabolism, will not accumulate because no blood glucose is present to be converted by anaerobic glycolysis to lactate. Other tissues have stores of glycogen, whereas the brain does not; therefore, these tissues form lactic acid in the absence of blood.[42]

In a study of 100 human open-heart surgery patients, half showed neurological damage following recovery from anesthesia. Forty-three per cent (43 per cent) of survivors developed behavioral abnormalities preceded by focal neurological damage and decreased intellectual function. Although most patients were normal by the time of discharge from the hospital, 15 per cent of the survivors had signs of cerebral damage at discharge. Cerebral damage was closely related to increasing age and depression of arterial pressure. Neuropathological findings suggested cerebral ischemia.[62]

Palmer studied five animals who had suffered cardiac arrest during surgery. The clinical signs in two dogs and two cats (one sheep is not included) resulting from 7 to 45 minutes of cardiac arrest included decerebrate rigidity, paddling, seizures, and blindness with dysfunction of the pupil which later returned to normal. Extensor rigidity generally improved or disappeared within 1 to 3 days. The histopathological lesions were widely distributed, not only in the cortex but also in the basal nuclei, thalamus, and inferior colliculi. Hemorrhage occurred in the cortex, and ischemic necrosis involved certain individual cranial nerve nuclei. The white matter was not severely involved.[46]

Hoerlein studied two dogs in which cerebral anoxia resulted from cardiac arrest. In both dogs, the intervals between the arrest and the administration of cardiac massage and oxygen were over 10 minutes. The dogs, a 4-year-old Pekingese and a 4-month-old mongrel, both had signs of severe brain damage, remaining comatose for several days after resuscitation. Except for hearing, vision, and reasoning, the Pekingese became relatively normal within 2 months. Locomotion was normal. Sight was impaired severely, apparently from cortical, retinal, and corneal ulcerative damage.[24]

The mongrel suffered similar brain derangement for weeks. He made steady progress, however, for 6 months, at which time locomotion was fairly normal. He ate normally and had normal growth and other body functions. There was a noticeable sight and auditory dysfunction, although at times this was not recognizable.

These cases were interesting in that presumably extreme cerebral damage from anoxia is apparently not as incapacitating in the dog as in man. The dogs were vegetative specimens initially but improved remarkably.

Cerebral Hyperoxia

There has been little work on hyperoxia in animals, although it is common knowledge that prolonged hyperoxia in the human infant promotes retinal damage and blindness. In an experimental study, the blood flow of two day-old puppies decreased 20 to 30 per cent in nearly all areas of the brain they breathed 80 to 90 per cent oxygen for 1 hour; arterial pO_2 increased from 48 mm Hg to 349 mm Hg without affecting blood pressure, pH, or pCO_2. At 3 weeks of age, the pO_2 of controls was 74 mm Hg, but with hyperoxia it increased to 357 mm Hg, about 60 per cent of the level achieved by adults breathing 80 to 90 per cent oxygen. When newborn puppies breathed oxygen continuously for 1 week and then were removed to air for 2 to 3 days, there were no major changes in cerebral blood flow. The cerebral vessels of the young puppy, like those of the retina, have an exaggerated response to hyperoxia, but the cerebral blood flow response appears to be reversible, unlike that in the retina. The vasoconstrictive action of oxygen on cerebral vessels of the newborn may serve to limit oxygen concentration in the brain when the arterial pO_2 is elevated.[31]

Hyperthermia (Heat Stroke)

Heat stroke is characterized by acute cerebral hyperemia as well as congestion of all viscera. The vessels of the brain, spinal cord, and meninges are extremely congested. The Purkinje cells of the cerebellum are particularly susceptible.[65, 66] Armistead[1] classified disturbances of heat-regulating mechanisms into three types:

Heat prostration or heat exhaustion is characterized by fatigue and circulatory collapse but not necessarily a marked rise in body temperature. A failure of peripheral circulation causes weakness, muscle tremors, and cyanosis. This disorder is usually seen in heart diseases, following major surgery during the hot summer, or in an overheated environment. Sodium chloride deficiency is a predisposing cause.[1, 24]

Heat cramp is characterized by severe muscle spasms from extreme sweating while working in high environmental temperature. It is caused by considerable deficit in sodium chloride. The loss of salt in man occurs primarily through prolonged and profuse sweating. The loss of salt in the dog through sweating (because of his relative inability to sweat) would probably be insufficient to cause heat cramp unless the salt intake were inadequate or physiological abnormalities contributed to the syndrome. Failure to provide salt along with water would be an important contributing cause to heat cramps and heat exhaustion. Heat cramp is seen infrequently except in working or racing dogs (e.g., the greyhound) during extreme heat.

Heat stroke, sunstroke, or *insolation* has a sudden onset, characterized by high body temperature and collapse.[1] It has been said that an average man doing light work dissipates approximately 3000 calories daily in the following proportions: radiation, convection, and conduction—65 per cent; evaporation of water from the skin and lungs—30 per cent; warming of inspired air—3 per cent; and excretion of urine and feces—2 per cent. When the environmental temperature approaches body temperature, radiation, convection, and conduction losses cease. If environmental temperature exceeds that of the body, then the body absorbs heat via this route unless other mechanisms compensate. In man and some other mammals, sweating is the chief mechanism of heat loss.[22] Because the dog has a poorly developed sweat gland system, loss of body temperature must be largely accomplished by panting—that is, from the respiratory system. Respiratory loss of heat is more efficient in dogs than in other mammals.[22]

Heat stroke is probably caused by a failure of the heat-regulating mechanism of the hypothalamus, associated with lack of sweating or respiratory loss of heat, and subsequent anoxic damage to various organs of the body. The brain may be affected, with disturbances of mentality, consciousness, ataxia, seizures, and severe motor deficit. The heart may experience congestive failure, myocardial damage, and hypotension. Systemic shock is frequently seen. Abnormal function of the kidneys is shown by proteinuria and pyuria. Elevated blood urea nitrogen strongly indicates an unfavorable prognosis. Oliguria is often a fatal complication. Liver damage frequently accompanies cases of heat stroke. Hematological changes include hypoprothrombinemia, thrombocytopenia, generalized hemorrhage, and hyperkalemia.[22]

Several theories have been proposed to explain heat damage at the cellular level. Among these are the following: (1) Heat may inactivate enzymes to a denatured form. (2) Heat may cause some damage in the lipids of the cell membrane, resulting in an increase of its permeability. (3) Heat may produce alterations in intramolecular and intermolecular bindings.[22]

Factors other than temperature and humidity that predispose to heat stroke include various surgical procedures, drugs, and febrile disease. We have seen extreme postsurgical hyperthemia following operations on the cervical spine and brain. The use of atropine or related drugs, antihistamines, and tranquilizers predispose to heat stroke. The aged person, who may have diabetes or cardiovascular, cerebrovascular, or renal disorders, is predisposed to heat stroke. Any febrile disease or abnormality of the air passages especially predisposes dogs to heat stroke. One must bandage the head and neck with caution to avoid interference with respiratory exchange of air, which will promote hyperthermia. Obesity reduces dissipation of heat by radiation and conduction because of the subcutaneous insulating effect. Nervousness or anxiety in a hospitalized pet, when added to other metabolic disorders, may promote heat stroke.[1, 22]

Environmental factors that predispose dogs to heat stroke are: high atmospheric temperature, high humidity, poor ventilation, loss of sodium chloride, excessive exercise, high specific dynamic action of food, breed predisposition, and poor health. Certain factors must be present to produce heat stroke; others are less vital. In the dog, ventilation is essential; a dog kept outdoors in a shaded, breezy area can easily withstand temperatures of over 100°F, whereas heat stroke may occur at 80° F to 90°F in a poorly ventilated room if other conditions are favorable. The calorigenic action of food can be important, since the dog eats a high proportion of protein, which has the most specific dynamic effect. It is a good practice to feed a dog late in the evening in hot weather.[1]

In our experience, the breed predisposition and temperament are important factors. Brachycephalic breeds such as boxers, Bostons, pugs, bulldogs (especially the English bulldog), and Pekingese are most frequently affected. These breeds are anatomically abnormal because of inadequate development of the nose and throat and therefore are unable to dissipate much heat by panting like other dogs. Many cannot breathe easily under normal conditions, and with the added stress of heat they are severely handicapped. The glottis, soft palate, and pharyngeal tissues often become edematous. If, in addition to being brachycephalic, these dogs are of a nervous temperament, they are much more apt to suffer from heat stroke.

Lack of acclimatization to heat and lack of proper physical conditioning due to poor training practices in working, sporting, or racing dogs are other contributing factors to hyperthermia. Partial acclimatization can occur within 2 weeks, but full acclimatization may require up to 2 months. The process of acclimatization promotes greater efficiency of the cardiovascular system, changes in sweating or heat loss mechanism (respiratory loss through panting), and an increase of adrenocorticosteroid activity.[22]

CLINICAL SIGNS. Early signs of heat stroke are extreme panting, a staring or blank expression, and a high temperature. The dog is weak, falls easily, has a pounding fast pulse, and is very dyspneic. Cyanosis develops rapidly because of pulmonary congestion and edema. Hysteria and vomiting occur frequently, and finally, terminal coma develops, during which the heart action and respiration become weak and irregular. After recovery, slight stress may cause a recurrence.

Clinical signs of heat prostration are weakness, mild muscle tremors, and dyspnea and cyanosis. Body temperature is mildly elevated or normal. Cardiovascular disease, surgical procedures, or salt depletion are frequently associated with its occurrence.

Clinical signs of heat cramps are due to plasma sodium and chloride depletion after undue exercise in hot weather. Severe, painful cramps in the skeletal muscles used most during the exercise are characteristic signs. The diagnosis must be differentiated from disorders that the layman might mistake for seizures, such as epilepsy and heart attacks.

DIAGNOSIS. Establishment of a diagnosis of heat stroke is aided by recognition of temperatures above 106°F or 107° F, exceeding the recording capacity of the thermometer. A history of previous attacks, rapid onset, and characteristic signs aid in diagnosis. Signs of eclampsia in a nursing bitch may be similar to those of heat stroke. Heat prostration and heat cramps must be largely diagnosed from history and clinical signs.

TREATMENT. Heat stroke in advanced stages may be fatal in up to 50 per cent of cases in man. The dog must be cooled promptly, or permanent brain damage will occur. Placing the animal in the bath tub and soaking him with cold water is beneficial. Ice applied to the head and cold water enemas are helpful. If the animal is hysterical, tranquilizers are beneficial, but the use of morphine is contraindicated. When the dog's temperature has fallen to about 103° F, intravenous dextrose and saline fluids can be given slowly, but care must be exercised not to overhydrate the animal. Many clinicians feel that adrenocorticoid preparations are indicated to boost the stress mechanism. Most dogs experience panting, hyperventilation, and alkalosis. Calcium gluconate, 5 ml of a 10 per cent solution per 15 kg body weight, given intravenously may be indicated. The packed cell volume (PCV) may be as high as 75 per cent. Intravenous fluids must be given and kidney function must be monitored by continuous catheterization. If blood gas analysis is available, the actual acidic or alkalotic state of the animal should be determined before such therapy is initiated. Empirical treatment for heat stroke can be detrimental to the patient. If the animal is in shock, he should be treated with steroids, antibiotics, and other drugs according to the methods described in Chapter 8. The animal should be hospitalized in an air-conditioned room for at least 24 hours after return to normalcy. The owner should be advised concerning the probability of recurrences.

The treatment of heat exhaustion consists of correcting the causative condition and giving isotonic saline parenterally. Care must be exercised if extreme cardiovascular or pulmonary disorders (or both) exist; otherwise, overhydration will add to the patient's distress. Administration of oral saline in drinking water or by stomach tube is generally adequate in treating heat cramps; however, intravenous saline can be used if necessary. Good nursing care is essential in all three of the hyperthermic disorders that have been discussed.

PREVENTION. Prevention of heat stroke is based on the following provisions: (a) adequate ventilation, (b) protection from the direct rays of the sun, (c) free access to cool drinking water (0.2 per cent salt added in very hot weather), and (d) keeping the animal quiet and avoiding strenuous exercise. A nervous animal should be tranquilized or kept away from exciting influences. Susceptible breeds, when hospitalized, must be kept out of the sun, preferably in air conditioned quarters. Special care must be taken with hospital driers in hot weather.[1]

Hypothermia

Hypothermia or accidental exposure to extreme cold may cause convulsions, irreversible coma, cardiac arrest, and death. Frostbite is commonly seen on the tips of the ears in cats and small prick ear dogs. Occasionally frostbite affects the scrotum of dogs, resulting in erythema and scaliness of the skin. Dogs that have become conditioned to living outdoors develop very thick coats and survive cold temperatures very well, especially if some shelter from winds and moisture is provided. Accidental exposure of the unconditioned house pet can lead to disaster. It has been shown during experimental procedures that hypothermia of less than 12°C (53.5° F) will consistently cause brain damage.[19]

Hypothermia of 34.5°C to 36.1°C (94°F to 97°F) is normal in young puppies in the first 2 weeks of life. However, the temperature of young puppies can become much lower if the litter is neglected or if they are orphans. Shivering is not seen until after 1 week of age. Hypothermia routinely occurs in anesthesia and surgery. It is not unusual for a small lean dog to show a rectal temperature of 33.3° C to 35° C (92° F to 95° F) during or following surgery. Since all metabolic processes, including elimination of the anesthetic agent, are greatly reduced at such temperatures, clinical recovery will be slow and postoperative sequelae can easily develop. Surgical hypothermia is discussed in detail in Chapters 8 and 12.

The treatment of hypothermia consists of elevation of the body temperature by immersion in warm water, heating pads, or circulating water blankets. Care must be taken not to burn the skin. Frostbite is treated like an open wound. Surgical debridement of necrotic tissue, antibacterial dressings, and systemic antibiotics may be needed.

Neuropathies Caused by Toxic Agents

See Chapter 11.

ENDOCRINE DISORDERS

The glands of internal secretion and the organs of the nervous system are intimately related morphologically, anatomically, physiologically, pharmacologically, and clinically. Disorders resulting from endocrine dysfunction that may be involved in the diagnosis of neurological diseases include: (1) hypoglycemia from hyperinsulinism and other causes; (2) hyperadrenocorticalism and hypoadrenocorticalism; (3) hypothyroidism; (4) hyperthyroidism; (5) diabetes mellitus; (6) diabetes insipidus; and (7) hypoparathyroidism.

Hypoglycemia

Kirk has divided the causes of hypoglycemia into two categories. In one group blood glucose is removed at an accelerated rate because of excess exogenous insulin, excess insulin produced by beta cells, pancreatic insulinoma, or carcinoma, or feeding leucine or sulfonylurea. Phlorhizin toxicity and congenital renal tubular defects also cause excessive removal of glucose from the body. Severe muscular exercise causes increased utilization of glucose. In the other group of causes of hypoglycemia, glucose is introduced into the blood at an inadequate rate because of chronic starvation, malabsorption, severe liver damage due to poisons or disease, or deficient glycogen storage.[33]

Hyperinsulinism

Insulinomas—functional tumors of the beta cells of the islets of Langerhans which produce excessive quantities of insulin—result in severe neurologic abnormalities. The clinical signs are exactly like those of hypoglycemia. Unlike muscle cells, neurons cannot store significant quantities of glycogen. Neurons depend almost exclusively upon glucose for energy, and unless the blood contains sufficient glucose, an "energy crisis" will occur in the cerebral cortex. Causes of such crises include fasting, exercise, excitement, and eating. Hypoglycemia caused by eating is a potent stimulus for insulin production. L-leucine, an amino acid found in most proteins, also stimulates insulin production. Eating can therefore initiate hypoglycemia, especially in an insulinoma patient.[28]

Insulinomas occur most frequently in older dogs. In dogs 69 per cent are malignant, while in man 90 per cent are benign. Clinical signs can develop very gradually; they include general weakness, paraparesis, muscle twitching, disorientation, apparent blindness, and seizures in the final stages. Signs may be intermittent. The differential diagnosis includes epilepsy, brain tumor, lead poisoning, distemper, and cerebral hypoxia, as well as other causes of hypoglycemia such as hypoadrenocorticism, hypopituitarism, hepatic lipidosis, hepatic glycogen storage disease, hepatic cirrhosis, and massive mesodermal tumors that utilize huge quantities of glucose (e.g., metastatic mammary tumors or primary pulmonary carcinomas). Diagnoses in specific cases may be difficult, and fasting blood glucose determinations, plasma insulin levels, and the glucose tolerance test are recommended. Surgical laparotomy, biopsy, or ablation of the tumor and subsequent histopathological examination give the definitive diagnosis. However, many of these patients are difficult surgical candidates.[28]

The hypoglycemia-neurological crisis must be treated vigorously with massive infusions of dextrose, soluble glucocorticosteroids such as flumethasone (Flucort), prednisolone, diazepam, mannitol, and possibly hypothermia. If surgery is to be attempted, normal glycemic levels must be established by dextrose infusions. Steroids should be used at least 48 hours before surgery. Postoperative therapy may be as intensive as if pancreatitis were present, and may include use of broad spectrum antibiotics, steroids, dextrose infusions, and daily laboratory work. Chemical therapy can be attempted with diazoxide, which has a hyperglycemic effect. The effect of diazoxide (Hyperstat) might be increased by using hydrochlorothiazide (Oretic). Glucocorticoids, a high protein diet, and frequent feedings may help control hypoglycemia.[28]

Functional hypoglycemia is seen frequently in hunting dogs that collapse in the field after work and in puppies, especially of the toy breeds. At the onset, clinical signs include mild incoordination, confusion, bewilderment, and trembling. As the condition progresses, the dog's eyes are sunken, he is unable to stand, his extremities are cool, his body temperature falls, and he becomes comatose. Grand mal seizures prior to losing consciousness are frequent. The owner of a hunting dog frequently says that his dog "falls out" in a seizure. If a blood sample can be taken during the acute episode, frequently the blood sugar will be below 50 mg/100 ml.[33]

The differential diagnosis involves distinguishing organic from functional causes of hypoglycemia. Organic lesions such as insulinomas may cause fasting hypoglycemia, although it may be necessary to fast for as long as 72 hours. Functional hypoglycemia usually shows normal levels of blood sugar during fasting. Hypoglycemia caused by insulinomas has been demonstrated to be prolonged (90 to 180 minutes) after injection of 1 gm of tolbutamide, whereas in functional hypoglycemia the blood glucose level returns to 60 mg/100 ml blood or higher by 90 minutes.[33]

Bardens[4] has divided glycogen storage problems in puppies into three groups, based on their response to glucagon: (1) generalized glycogen storage disease, (2) von Gierke's disease, and (3) Cori's disease or limited dextrinosis. The generalized glycogen storage disease is seen in puppies of toy breeds at 6 to 12 weeks of age. Acute episodes are precipitated by stress, overactivity, exposure, and overmedication. There is said to be no deficiency of glucose-6-phosphate in such cases, and therefore intravenous administration of 0.5 mg of glucagon to fasted patients produces a rise in blood glucose.

In von Gierke's disease, there is said to be a deficiency of glucose-6-phosphate, and affected pups do not respond to glucagon either in a fasted state or after a meal.

Cori's disease, or limited dextrinosis, is a disorder in which there is said to be a deficiency of amylo-1,6-glucosidase, or debrancher enzyme. Affected dogs do not respond to glucagon administration in a fasted state, but if it is given after a meal there is a limited glucose response. Bardens feels that the disorder is the same as that seen in hunting dogs: The dogs are nervous and have an insatiable desire to hunt, and they are frequently used for hunting in a fasted state.[4]

TREATMENT. The objectives of treatment of functional hypoglycemia are quick restoration of blood glucose to normal in the acute attack, elimination of any positive underlying cause, and maintenance of a homeostatic glucose level by frequent feeding of food low in carbohydrates and high in protein and fat. Exercise should be restricted. Corticosteroids, sedatives, or both should be used as needed. Many dogs recover spontaneously after hypoglycemic attacks, but 1 ml of 10 per cent glucose per kg of body weight administered intravenously or intraperitoneally will act as a satisfactory emergency treatment. Subcutaneous 2.5 per cent glucose in half-strength saline may be given for prolonged effect.

Puppies with generalized glycogen storage disease may outgrow the disorder at six to eight months of age. High-protein feedings at 6-hour intervals and avoidance of stress will help in the interim period. Prednisolone in 1 to 2 mg doses every 12 hours for several days may be helpful. Corn syrup and water should be given to help treat minor relapses. Puppies with von Gierke's disease respond to glucose therapy but usually relapse.[33]

In dogs with limited dextrinosis (Cori's disease), the problem can best be controlled with careful management. Hunting dogs should be fed twice a day, and a small high-protein meal 1 hour before hunting is recommended. The main meal should be in the evening. Some owners will feed sugar to the dogs during hunting, or provide high-caloric foods used in human diets prior to hunting. Mild sedatives, tranquilizers, or parasympatholytic drugs (Darbazine) may be useful to counteract nervousness. The hyperglycemic effect of adrenal steroids such as prednisolone, may be useful in aborting an attack. The peak effect of prednisolone occurs 4 to 6 hours after oral administration (0.25 to 0.5 mg/kg). Steroids should be used as a last resort.[33]

Hyperadrenocorticalism (Cushing's Syndrome)[59]

Hyperadrenocorticalism in the dog is a progressive disease caused by adrenocorticoid hyperfunction. It is characterized by bilaterally symmetrical hair loss, polydipsia, polyuria, a pendulous abdomen, lymphopenia, eosinopenia, slight hyperglycemia, and occasional electrolyte disturbances. Signs associated with Horner's syndrome such as hypothalamic damage by pituitary tumor growth may be present. In the dog, the main abnormality is usually the increased secretion of the glucocorticoid, cortisol.

In spontaneous hyperadrenocorticism, the excessive hormones may result from secretory activity of: (1) hyperplastic adrenal cortices without another clinically evident endocrine lesion (this is the most frequent disorder); (2) adrenal cortical adenoma or carcinoma; (3) ectopically located adrenal-like tumor, such as an ovary; (4) ACTH-secreting tumor of the anterior pituitary associated with adrenal cortical hyperplasia; or (5) nonpituitary carcinoma, such as carcinoma of the lung or pancreas, which secretes an ACTH-like material. It should be noted that adrenocortical tissue can be normal both grossly and histologically and yet be hyperfunctional. Hyperfunction can result from a defect in the negative feedback mechanism in the hypothalamus whereby increasing levels of circulating cortisol do not result in physiological inhibition of ACTH production. The syndrome can also result from administration of therapeutic amounts of corticosteroids over a long period of time.[59]

The diagnostic features of hyperadrenocorticism include the characteristic clinical signs that have already been mentioned. Pituitary tumors will frequently produce additional neurological signs of change in disposition, pressure on optic nerves causing visual defects, and seizures. Electrolyte disturbances are not as frequent in the dog as in man, but when they do occur, hypokalemia is the most significant change. Severe hypokalemias cause marked EKG changes, such as prolongation of the Q-T interval and existence of U waves. The EMG changes are characteristic of myotonia (see page 291). Calcification of subcutaneous tissue and renal parenchyma, an enlarged clitoris from excessive androgen levels, and osteoporosis may be seen.[59]

The laboratory findings, other than lymphopenia and eosinopenia, include elevated serum alkaline phosphatase, serum glutamic-pyruvic transaminase, plasma cholesterol, and a urine specific gravity of less than 1.012. The standard method of procuring a more definitive diagnosis is to measure the 17-ketogenic steroids in an accurate 24-hour collection of urine, which may be difficult to obtain in a veterinary hospital. Schechter recommends determinations of plasma cortisol and corticosterone utilizing the competitive protein-binding technique of Murphy and Pattee. Normal resting corticosteroid levels in dogs are 1 to 2.5 mg/100 ml, while in dogs with Cushing's syndrome normal levels usually range from 2.5 to 12.5 mg/100 ml. It is best to analyze two or three specimens for greatest accuracy. Another test is to measure the plasma corticosteroid levels after administration of ACTH. Affected dogs may produce values of 20 to 60 mg/100 ml in this test, while normal dogs have levels of 9.5 to 22 mg/100 ml. If an adrenal tumor is present high resting levels with a lack of response to ACTH stimulation have been observed.[55]

Secondary hyperadrenocorticism can be assessed by determining pituitary reserve. Twenty-three mg of metyrapone per kg body weight is given orally and urine is examined for two 24-hour periods. Normally there will be increased 17-ketogenic steroid elimination in the urine during the first 24 hours. Hypopituitarism and negative feedback mechanism will produce a decreased metyrapone or pituitary reserve response, but a normal ACTH response is seen. A poor response to both ACTH and metyrapone injections is seen in adrenocortical neoplasms.[59]

TREATMENT. Since 1969, o,p′ DDD (Lysodren), a specific adrenocorticolytic drug, has been used successfully to treat Cushing's syndrome in dogs. This drug causes necrosis of the zona reticularis and zona fasciculata of the adrenal cortex, thereby decreasing the production of corticosteroids. Eighteen dogs were treated over a 3-year period, and 13 showed excellent response. Nine of the 13 were still alive with complete remission of signs at the time of the report. The longest observation time was 3 years.[55]

Before deciding on therapy, bilateral adrenocortical hyperplasia should be differentiated from adrenal neoplasia and from such secondary disorders as hypothyroidism, diabetes mellitus, infection, CNS disorders, and degenerative tissue changes owing to excessive use of corticosteroids. During o,p′ DDD therapy, water consumption should be monitored, and after 5 days of therapy lymphocyte and eosinophil counts should be made. Treatment should be continued until these three values are normal. After successful therapy the plasma corticosteroid levels should be less than 2 mg/100 ml, and the ACTH stimulation test should be normal. If signs of hypoadrenocorticism or Addison's disease develop, potassium and sodium blood levels should be measured. A weekly maintenance schedule of drug treatment and laboratory evaluations is recommended.[55]

Unilateral adrenalectomy should be performed for localized adrenocortical tumors. Total adrenalectomy can be used for bilateral adrenocortical hyperplasia. Such surgery demands extremely careful surgical management before and after the operation, as well as lifelong steroid therapy. Siegel[58] in 1970 reported on 27 dogs with Cushing's syndrome seen over a period of 4 years. Three of these dogs had functional unilateral adrenocortical neoplasms, and 24 had bilateral adrenocortical hyperplasia. Of these 24, 14 were treated surgically with bilateral adrenalectomy. Ten of the 14 were alive and had complete amelioration of clinical signs at the time of the report.[58]

The prognosis is somewhat unpredictable since a pituitary tumor may grow during or after the treatment. However, most dogs respond well to o,p′ DDD treatment if there are no other health problems.[55]

Hypoadrenocorticism (Adrenocortical Insufficiency, Addison's Disease)[59]

Hypoadrenocorticism is an insidious and usually progressive disease that is characterized by weakness, loss of weight, hypotension, dehydration, gastrointestinal disturbances, and occasional hypoglycemia. This disorder is frequently misdiagnosed because of its similarity to acute renal and gastrointestinal disease. Thirteen cases were seen at the University of Pennsylvania clinic from 1962 to 1965. Most cases occurred at less than 5 years of age and seemed to be more frequent in females.[69]

The usual signs were pronounced muscle weakness, depression, lack of appetite, and vomiting.

The most common cause is atrophy of the adrenal cortices, possibly from an autoimmune reaction. Stress from infections, parturition, and surgery may precipitate an acute crisis resulting in shock and death.

The *pathogenesis* of the disease in its chronic form involves the inability of the adrenal cortex to produce sufficient quantities of aldosterone, which is responsible for maintaining an electrolyte balance between sodium and potassium. Aldosterone regulates the renal tubular reabsorption of sodium and the secretion of potassium, and lack of it leads to a tendency toward hyponatremia and hyperkalemia.[69] The *diagnosis* of the disorder before renal failure occurs is based on findings of hyponatremia, hypochloremia, hyperkalemia, a relative increase in lymphocytes and eosinophils, and a decrease in urinary excretion of 17-ketogenic steroids.[59] Bradycardia and EKG changes occur in advanced hyperkalemia. The chronic disorder may last for several months with persistent progressive vomiting, diarrhea (occasionally bloody), dehydration, and collapse.

TREATMENT. Acute attacks require intravenous corticosteroid administrations. Initially, 50 to 200 mg of hydrocortisone sodium succinate in 5 per cent glucose and normal saline can be given intravenously. As cortisol is a glucocorticoid and supports only vascular responses, it is important to administer simultaneously a mineralocorticoid such as fludrocortisone acetate (Florinef acetate). Large quantities of intravenous fluids (without potassium) are indicated until hypovolemia is controlled and urinary function is stabilized. Administration of 2 to 5 mg of desoxycorticosterone acetate (DOCA) in oil intramuscularly helps establish a normal electrolyte balance. Administration of DOCA and cortisone acetate intramuscularly, and a glucocorticoid intravenously must be maintained until the acute crisis is passed. Regulations of maintenance doses for long-term therapy must be done carefully. In chronic replacement therapy, dogs can be maintained on mineralocorticoid alone if salt intake is adequate. Success has been obtained by implanting DOCA subcutaneously for more prolonged effect. Use of desoxycorticosterone pivalate produces a response similar to DOCA; however, it is effectively released for a period of 3 to 4 weeks. Wolland feels that most patients can be maintained on oral tablets of fludrocortisone acetate (Florinef acetate) and a salt supplement. Frequent laboratory checks for potassium, sodium, and blood sugar are necessary. Hypoglycemic patients should be maintained on oral prednisolone and fludrocortisone.[59, 69] For details on adrenocortical disorders, see publications by Siegel[59] and Wolland.[69]

Hypothyroidism[53]

Hypothyroidism is defined as the state resulting from inadequate quantities of circulating thyroid hormone. Nongoiterous hypothyroidism may be divided into (1) primary hypothyroidism, caused by an absence or destruction of functioning thyroid tissue, and (2) hypothyroidism due to pituitary insufficiency.

The congenital form of primary hypothyroidism seen as dwarfism is rare. The acquired primary form is most frequently seen when thyroid atrophy has occurred, the cause of which may be an autoimmune mechanism. In pituitary hypothyroidism, thyrotropin deficiency is the result of destruction of the pituitary by a tumor, such as a chromophobe adenoma. Pituitary hypothyroidism can be differentiated from primary hypothyroidism by the thyroid stimulating hormone (TSH) stimulation test. Thyroid function indices do not increase after administration of TSH when there is a primary lesion in the thyroid, but they do increase in pituitary insufficiency.[53]

Hypothyroidism associated with goiter or enlargement of the gland may be due to (1) compensatory action of TSH secretion because of lack of circulating thyroid hormone which causes a hyperplasia, (2) iodine deficiency, (3) bilateral thyroid cancer that causes destruction of the gland and reduced function, and (4) lymphocytic thyroiditis. Iodine deficiency goiter may be seen in dogs fed only meat for a long period of time.[53]

The clinical features of hypothyroidism are well recognized by clinicians and include lethargy, subnormal temperature, coarse and scanty hair coat, thickened skin, pigmentation, puffy appearance, weak apex cardiac beat and slow pulse, and bilateral alopecia usually seen in larger breed dogs aged 2 to 5 years. Neurological signs in advanced cases are dementia, weakness, coma in hypothermia (as in exposure to cold), and (in man) cerebellar syndrome.[10] Highly trained dogs are mentally dull and show physical deficits not typical of normal behavior. Recent evidence suggests that dogs with hypothyroidism have low conduction velocities in peripheral nerve testing.[60]

The diagnosis of the disorder is based on the clinical signs, cardiac and EEG changes, and, in current practice, the evaluation of serum T3 (triiodothyronine) and T4 (thyroxine) as determined by radioimmunoassay tests. These tests are accurate and are not influenced by iodine medications.[41, 68]

TREATMENT. The successful treatment of primary hypothyroidism is based on the results of the T3 and T4 tests. If T3 alone is deficient the treatment of choice is L-triiodothyronine (Cytobin), 6 micrograms per pound, divided into three or four doses daily. If both T3 and T4 are deficient, generally L-thyroxine (Synthroid) is given orally in doses of 0.1 mg/7 lb. body weight twice daily. Doses of these drugs are much larger than those suggested for man because of the dog's rapid peripheral breakdown of thyroxine and possible incomplete absorption.[41, 68] The prognosis of therapy is generally favorable in dogs with thyroid atrophy. Of course, in cases of thyroid neoplasia, surgical removal of the thyroid is difficult without destroying the parathyroid glands. In such an event, parathyroid hormone and calcium replacement therapies must also be given.

Hyperthyroidism

Hyperthyroidism may be referred to as thyrotoxicosis or Graves' disease. Reports indicate that this disease may occur in the dog, particularly in the Pekingese and French bulldog, which frequently have hyperplastic thyroid glands and are characteristically exophthalmic, nervous, hyperactive, restless, and excitable. However, typical clinical Graves' disease causing neurological signs in dogs is rare,[37] and workers who run serum T3 and T4 radioimmunoassay tests in patients undergoing replacement therapy see increased values only when therapy has been excessive.[41]

Diabetes Mellitus

Diabetes mellitus is a rather common disease characterized by a loss of the insulin-secreting cells, the islets of Langerhans, in the pancreas. In dogs, acute or chronic pancreatitis and atrophy or fibrosis of the pancreas are most frequently responsible for islet destruction.

CLINICAL SIGNS. The characteristic signs are polydipsia, polyuria, nocturia, polyphagia, loss of weight, dryness of skin, the development of cataracts, hyperglycemia, and glycosuria. When cataracts are absent, characteristic fundic abnormalities may be seen by careful examination.

Diabetes mellitus can cause a diffuse peripheral neuropathy which on the EMG shows fibrillation potentials and positive sharp wave activity. Motor as well as sensory nerve conduction velocities are reduced. Diabetic coma is the terminal event.

The diagnosis is confirmed by the characteristic glycosuria and hyperglycemia.

TREATMENT. Insulin (neutral protamine Hagedorn) is administered daily with concomitant dietary and stress control. Choline, methionine, or lecithin added to the diet will help prevent secondary liver changes. Treatment of a diabetic ketoacidosis is a true medical emergency and requires vigorous intensive care. Similarly, the blood hyperviscosity syndrome due to severe hyperglycemia that causes an intracellular CNS dehydration must be treated appropriately. Consult medical textbooks for complete discussions.

Diabetes Insipidus

Usually diabetes insipidus does not cause any direct neurological symptoms, but it is an example of neurological dysfunction causing physical symptoms. The hypothalamus is the control center of the autonomic nervous system.

The hypothalamus contains neurosecretory cells in at least three nuclei that are intimately associated with the pituitary gland. The lateral tuberal nuclei (and perhaps others) appear to secrete substances that stimulate the release of the tropic hormones of the anterior pituitary (pars distalis). These substances are transported from the hypothalamus to the pituitary gland via the hypophysal portal system.

The supraoptic and paraventricular nuclei apparently produce the hormones associated with the posterior pituitary (pars nervosa). Neural secretions traverse axons from the hypothalamic nuclei into the pars nervosa via the hypothalamo-hypophysial tracts. Damage to the neurons or the tract interferes with the production of antidiuretic hormone (ADH), resulting in diabetes insipidus. Since these centers are vital to normal neurological function, destructive lesions may cause characteristic neurological deficits as well as the polyuria and polydipsia typical of diabetes insipidus.

Diagnosis and treatment of diabetes insipidus are discussed in several textbooks of medicine. The clinician should always regard hypothalamic pituitary abnormalities as localizing signs of CNS disease as well as endocrine disorders.[9]

Hypoparathyroidism

Spontaneous hypoparathyroidism is said to be a somewhat rare disorder that may be seen more frequently in puppies.[9] Occasionally tetanic signs and hypocalcemia can be seen in mature dogs. Clinical signs include tetanic manifestations, such as neuromuscular excitability, fibrillary muscular twitching, local or general muscular spasms, hyperactive reflexes, and occasional convulsions. Laboratory examinations reveal hypocalcemia and hyperphosphatemia.

Treatment. The treatment of spontaneous hypoparathyroidism is designed to adjust calcium and phosphorus to normal levels by providing calcium, parathormone, and vitamin D. In the acute attack, intravenous calcium gluconate is given in 5 to 15 ml doses of a 10 to 20 per cent solution, followed by oral calcium gluconate in doses of 5 to 10 gm daily. More prolonged elevation of blood calcium is attained by giving 25 to 200 units of parathormone subcutaneously or intramuscularly. The elevation lasts for 18 to 20 hours after injection. In most cases, good control of signs and apparent cures may be seen with administration of calcium and vitamin D for several weeks. Daily administrations of 50,000 to 200,000 units of synthetic oleovitamin D, vitamin D_2, or dihydrotachysterol have considerable therapeutic effect. Overdosage of medicants should be avoided or hypercalcemia will result.[9]

A form of hypocalcemia known as eclampsia or puerperal tetany, seen in lactating bitches, may be a form of hypoparathyroidism. Hypocalcemia and signs characteristic of tetany are seen. Barbiturates are generally used to control severe convulsions, and tranquilizers may control hyperexcitability. Calcium injections are needed for acute cases, whereas oral calcium and vitamin D are generally used for long-term control or prevention.[9]

FUNCTIONAL DISORDERS

Hepatic and Nephrotic Neuropathies

Hepatocerebral intoxication is a syndrome characterized by progressive mental changes, deterioration and fluctuation in the stage of consciousness, and finally coma. Wilson's disease, or hepatolenticular degeneration, is a familial condition in man and sheep that is thought to be due to a disorder of copper metabolism. Cirrhosis of the liver and degeneration of the lenticular nucleus of the brain are seen. Wilson's disease has not been diagnosed in dogs. Other neurological manifestations of hepatic disease such as polyneuropathy, pruritus, psychosis, and delirium tremens occur, but these are not as dangerous nor as difficult to manage as the coma.[43]

Experimental portacaval shunts (Eck fistula) in dogs produced hepatic coma known as meat intoxication. A dog with a shunt, if fed meat, showed signs nearly identical to those of hepatic coma in man. It was thought that these signs were primarily due to high levels of blood ammonia, the result of bacterial degradation of protein in the gastrointestinal tract. In portacaval shunts, the liver, which ordinarily transforms ammonia into urea, is bypassed. In animals (and man) with cirrhosis, a passive congestion develops that is usually compensated for by natural shunts. In man, the veins in the esophagus become enlarged and help in the shunting procedure. The liver dysfunction also allows for an increase in blood ammonia, because ammonia is not transformed to urea normally.[43]

Other biochemical changes include alteration in Kreb's cycle in the brain and liberation of alpha-ketoglutarate, pyruvate, and lactate in the brain. A decrease of oxygen consumption in the brain occurs, metabolism of indolic phenolic compounds is disturbed, and intracellular shift of inorganic phosphate, potassium depletion, alkalosis, and low cerebral blood flow can occur in hepatic coma.[43]

Strombeck and co-workers[61] reported on 13 cases of hyperammonemia and hepatic encephalopathy seen in a veterinary teaching hospital (University of California) in a 10-month period. Nine of the 13 dogs were medium to large breeds; they were evenly distributed between the sexes and ranged in age from 3 months to 9 years (mean 3.2 years). Clinical signs included listlessness, depression, polydipsia, ataxia, aimless pacing, anorexia, vomiting, diarrhea, seizures, head pressing, and apparent blindness.[61]

Six dogs had abnormal portal circulatory systems and four had hepatic disease; the cause of hyperammonemia was undetermined in three dogs. Cranial mesenteric arteriograms were used in diagnosing portal shunts in addition to necropsy findings. Liver biopsies were used to aid in determining the cause of hyperammonemia. The important features of these case reports are the significance of measuring blood ammonia content in dogs with clinical signs of hepatic encephalopathy and the relative frequency of such clinical cases.[61]

Brain lesions seen in hepatic dysfunction include widespread astrocytosis and degeneration of white matter, neuronal loss, phagocyte formation, and reactive astrocytosis in the cerebral cortex. Diagnosis is based on hepatic function tests, EEG findings, and characteristic clinical signs. Blood ammonia level tests are difficult to run and evaluate. Liver biopsy and histological examination are of value. Ammonia tolerance test is useful in mild cases.[43]

The treatment must be based on the etiology and an understanding of physiological changes occurring in the body. A marked reduction of protein intake, a reduction of intestinal bacterial flora by use of enteric antibiotics are of value in decreasing levels of blood ammonia. Oral cation exchange resins show therapeutic promise for removing ammonia. Peritoneal dialysis is effective for temporarily reducing pathologic blood constituents. Supportive therapy including administration of glucose, vitamin K, choline and methionine, B-complex vitamins, and prednisone is of value.[43]

The role of nephrotic neurological disorders has not been widely reported in the literature. Papilledema with chronic nephritis is a characteristic finding because of the resultant arterial disease. Asbury has reported that multiple symmetrical sensorimotor neuropathy was associated with long-standing chronic renal failure.[2] Uremic coma is well known to all clinicians. Hyperirritability, muscle twitching, and convulsions precede uremic coma and death.

Electrolyte Imbalance[21]

Functions of the nervous system are delicately susceptible to imbalances of electrolytes and water. A critical factor is maintenance of the resting potentials of the neuronal membrane by the distribution of sodium, mainly extraneuronally, and of potassium, mainly intraneuronally. Many serious medical, post-traumatic, and postoperative disorders in veterinary practice are due to electrolyte imbalances that are not recognized or seriously considered as the cause of general and neurological signs. Some of these possibilities pertaining to body sodium, potassium, and water are considered here. Even though fluids and electrolytes are regulated to some extent by the nervous system itself, shifts in cationic balance have been found in association with cerebral seizures, alterations of consciousness, and peripheral neuromuscular paralysis.[21]

Hyponatremia with intact sodium stores (water intoxication) can occur in oliguric anuric states in patients with organic renal disease, renal ischemia, hypotension, and peripheral circulatory failure in shock and trauma. There may be a lack of capacity to excrete water during postoperative periods of 12 to 36 hours. The late stages of congestive heart failure, cirrhosis of the liver, and excessive thirst from use of thiazide diuretics could cause so-called water intoxication. The neurological signs are mental confusion, dysphagia, incoordination, lethargy, muscle weakness and cramps, seizures, stupor, and coma.[21]

Hyponatremia with body sodium depletion may be related to a reduction in sodium intake, improper fluid therapy such as excessive glucose-water infusions, diarrhea, excessive sweating, adrenocortical insufficiency, and severe trauma or body burns. Clinical signs are similar to those of water intoxication except that seizures are less common.[21]

Hypernatremia in man is seldom seen clinically unless the thirst mechanism is impaired or the comatose patient is denied access to water. In dogs and cats, surgical procedures on the head, jaw, and neck might make drinking so difficult (because of pain) that water intake is impaired and hypernatremia results. Gastroenteritis with severe vomiting and diarrhea (especially in puppies), prolonged use of hypertonic solutions such as urea or mannitol, excessive renal excretion, and accidental salt poisoning could also cause severe dehydration and hypernatremia.[21]

Potassium depletion and hypokalemia may be due to renal tubular disease; use of diuretics (thiazides and carbonic anhydrase inhibitors) and increased adrenal steroids and aldosteronism; Cushing's syndrome; use of exogenous steroids; and vomiting and diarrhea, especially in patients where potassium intake is low and insulin therapy in the initial regulation of the diabetic patient. Muscular weakness, paralytic ileus muscle cramps, and cardiac effects, especially in patients taking digitalis, are prominent clinical signs [21]

Potassium intoxication and hyperkalemia usually result from defective renal excretion of potassium in kidney disease, acute or chronic renal failure, and adrenal insufficiency. Early EKG changes—high peaked T waves, decreased P waves, and decomposition of QRS complex—are followed by cardiac arrhythmia, heart block, and ventricular fibrillation. Weakness, myotonia, and periodic paralysis are evident.[21]

There has been no attempt to go into great detail in this discussion of electrolyte imbalances. The author is endeavoring to show that such imbalances are frequent and should be recognized early in the course of disease if treatment is to be effective. Laboratory support for diagnosis and therapy is essential.[21]

Horner's Syndrome

Horner's syndrome, a lesion of the sympathetic innervation of the head and eye, can be caused by lesions in the cranial thoracic spinal cord, the cervical spinal area, or the brain. Since the signs pertain primarily to the eye, this syndrome will be discussed in the neuro-ophthalmology chapter (p. 647).

Subtle Encephalomyelopathies—Systemic Disease or Neoplasia

There are many evidences of encephalomyelopathies in man that are the result of systemic diseases or distant effects of neoplasia. We recognize that dementias in animals resulting from these disorders may be difficult to detect except in the pet who is treated as part of the family. Frequently these subtle changes in behavior, mental acuity, memory, and sophisticated motor capabilities are due to mild CNS hypoxia and abnormal glucose metabolism resulting from a disease process not related primarily to the CNS. Many of the metabolic disorders and environmental states causing such CNS changes has been discussed previously. Chronic lung, heart, renal, and hepatic diseases are frequent causes of these subtle CNS signs.[29]

It has been estimated that 1 to 2 per cent of all patients with neoplasia have neurological disorders due to non-CNS related tumors. So called "encephalomyelitis with carcinoma" is characterized by multiple foci of neuronal loss, microglial proliferation, and perivascular round cell infiltration in the brain, brain stem, spinal cord, and dorsal root ganglia. Lung tumors are a frequent cause. Memory loss, hypotonia, ataxia, abnormal spinal fluid, hypergammaglobulinemia, and abnormal EEG patterns may be observed. Disorders of muscle may precede evidence of malignancy by months in patients over 50 years of age. Myopathy associated with carcinoma is indistinguishable clinically from other illnesses that cause painless, subacute, progressive, symmetrical, proximal muscle weakness but no alteration of sensation or reflexes. Pseudomyasthenia or Eaton-Lambert syndrome is a specific clinical myopathy resulting from neoplasia in man. Peripheral neuropathy resulting from cancer of the lung, myeloma, or Hodgkin's disease is indistinguishable from that associated with thiamine depletion.

These well-recognized disorders in man no doubt exist in pets as well, and clinical awareness of such possibilities will promote better veterinary practice and service.[26]

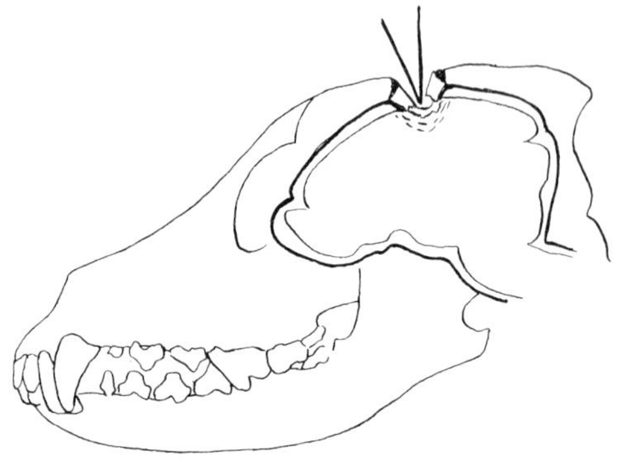

FIGURE 17–3 Penetrating wound into the cranial cavity. Such a wound causes bone fragments and foreign material to be driven into the brain substance, as well as hemorrhage.

COMPRESSIONS OF THE BRAIN[25]

Compressions of the brain are generally the result of fractures or neoplasia of the skull. Skull fractures frequently cause severe damage to the brain from fragmentation of bone and concomitant hemorrhage. If the dura mater has been penetrated by contaminated bone fragments, sepsis of the central nervous system frequently results. Since the blood-brain barrier may limit the levels of antibiotics in brain tissue, every effort should be made to minimize sepsis in brain fractures and injuries.

Skull fractures are easily diagnosed when there are exterior wounds, hematomas, or crepitation from palpation. Minute hairline fractures and those in nonpalpable areas may be difficult to diagnose even by radiography. Radiography is a necessary diagnostic aid in skull fractures and must be performed very carefully while the animal is being given critical intensive care for CNS or systemic shock injuries. Surgical removal of bone fragments, repositioning of compressive pieces of the skull, decompression of the brain, and control of intracranial hemorrhage may be necessary in patients with skull fractures (Figs. 17–2 to 17–4). These techniques are discussed in Chapters 12 and 20.

Cranial or skull neoplasia frequently develops gradually during a prolonged period of time. Abnormalities in conformation may be seen even before evidence of cerebral compression is noted. Brain compression frequently results from tumors originating in the nasal passages and sinus cavities. Radiography is essential for determining the diagnostic features as well as the prognosis of the lesion. Nonmalignant

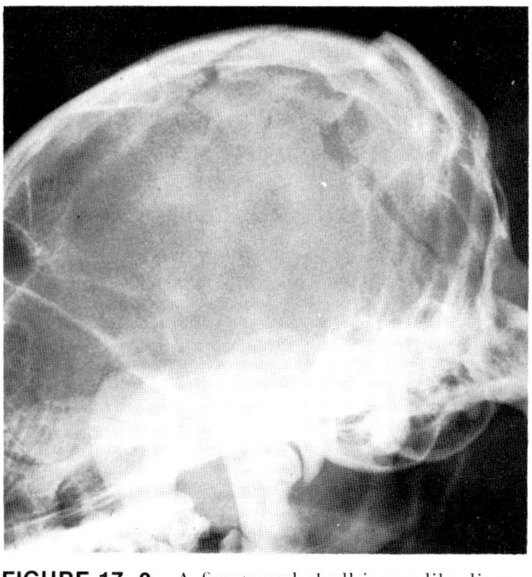

FIGURE 17–2 A fractured skull is readily diagnosable from this radiograph. The dog recovered with prompt craniotomy.

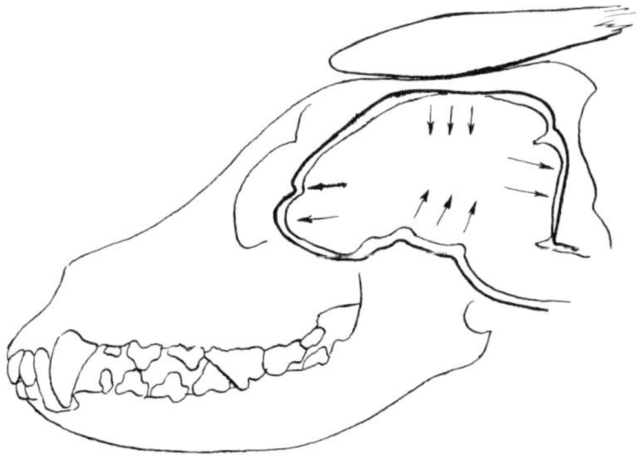

FIGURE 17–4 Trauma to the calvarium and brain from a flat object, causing a concussion with or without concomitant hemorrhage. Fissure fractures frequently occur in such traumas.

tumors can be removed surgically, but bone-related malignancies have an unfavorable prognosis. Accurate histopathological examination is essential to determine the efficacy of surgical or x-ray therapy.[25]

REFERENCES

1. Armistead, W. W.: Harmful effects of heat. *In* Catcott, E. J. (ed.): *Canine Medicine.* American Veterinary Publications, Inc., Santa Barbara, Cal., 1968, p. 261.
2. Asbury, A. K., Victor, M., and Adams, R. D.: Uremic polyneuropathy. Arch. Neurol. *8,* 413, 1963.
3. Averill, D. R.: Treatment of status epilepticus in dogs with diazepam sodium. J.A.V.M.A. *156,* 432, 1970.
4. Bardens, J. W.: Glycogen storage disease in puppies. Vet. Med. Small Anim. Clin. *61,* 1174, 1966.
5. Barker, J.: Epilepsy in the dog—a comparative approach. J. Small Anim. Pract. *14,* 281, 1973.
6. Bartels, K. P.: Treatment of epilepsy. Kleintier-Prax. *15,* 209, 1970 (Abstr. Int. Vet. Ref. Service, F-6-440, 1971).
7. Bielfelt, S. W., Redman, H. C., and McClellan, R. O.: Epileptiform seizures in beagles. Am. J. Vet. Res. *32,* 2039, 1971.
8. Blauch, B. S., and Case, W. C.: A brief review of narcolepsy with presentation of two cases in dogs. J. Am. Anim. Hosp. Assoc. *11,* 467–472, 1975.
9. Bloom, F.: Diseases of endocrine glands. *In* Catcott, E. J. (ed.): *Canine Medicine.* American Veterinary Publications, Inc., Santa Barbara, Cal., 1968, p. 430.
10. Bradley, W. G., and Walton, J. N.: Neurological manifestations of thyroid disease. Postgrad. Med. *50,* 118, 1971.
11. Courville, C. B.: Contribution to study of cerebral anoxia. Bull. Los Angeles Neurol. Soc. *15,* 99, 1950.
12. Croft, P. G.: Fits in dogs: A survey of 260 cases. Vet. Rec. *77,* 438, 1965.
13. Croft, P. G.: Conditions affecting the central nervous system in small animals. J. Small Anim. Pract. *6,* 261, 1965.
14. Croft, P. G.: The use of the electro-encephalograph in the detection of epilepsy as a hereditary condition in the dog. Vet. Rec. *82,* 712, 1968.
15. Cunningham, J. G.: Canine seizure disorders. J.A.V.M.A. *158,* 589, 1971.
16. Currie, T. T., Hayward, N. J., Campbell, P. C., Westlake, G., and Williams, J.: Epilepsy in dogs caused by large doses of penicillin and concurrent brain damage. Brit. J. Exp. Pathol. *51,* 492, 1970.
17. De Luca, K., Masotti, R. E., and Partington, M. W.: Altered calcium metabolism due to anticonvulsant drugs. Devel. Med. Child. Neurolog. *14,* 318, 1972.
18. Dennis, H. R.: Rickets following anti-convulsant therapy. Proc. R. Soc. Med. *65,* 12, 1972.
19. Egerton, N., Egerton, W. S., and Kay, J. H.: Neurologic changes following profound hypothermia. Ann. Surg. *157,* 366, 1963.
20. Falco, M. J., Barker, J., and Wallace, M. E.: The genetics of epilepsy in the British alsation. J. Small Anim. Pract. *15,* 685, 1974.
21. Glaser, G. H.: Neurologic symptoms with electrolyte and water imbalance. Postgrad. Med. *50,* 170, 1971.
22. Gottschalk, P. G., and Thomas, J. E.: Heat stroke. Mayo Clin. Proc. *41,* 470, 1966.
23. Guyton, A. C.: *Textbook of Medical Physiology,* 5th ed. W. B. Saunders Co., Philadelphia, 1976.
24. Hoerlein, B. F.: Heat stroke. *In* Kirk, R. W. (ed.): *Current Veterinary Therapy III.* W. B. Saunders Co., Philadelphia, 1968, p. 103.
25. Hoerlein, B. F.: *Canine Neurology, Diagnosis and Treatment,* 2d ed. W. B. Saunders Co., Philadelphia, 1971.
26. Horenstein, S.: Distant effects of neoplasms on the nervous system. Postgrad. Med. *50,* 85, 1971.
27. Jennings, P. B., Utter, W. F., and Fariss, B. L.: Effects of long-term primidone therapy in a dog. J.A.V.M.A. *164,* 1123, 1974.
28. Johnson, R. K.: Insulinoma in the dog. *In* Kirk, R. W. (ed.): *Current Veterinary Therapy V.* W. B. Saunders Co., Philadelphia, 1974, p. 818.
29. Karp, H. R.: Dementia in systemic diseases. Postgrad. Med. *50,* 202, 1971.
30. Kay, W.: Epilepsy. *In* Kirk, R. W. (ed.): *Current Veterinary Therapy V.* W. B. Saunders Co., Philadelphia, 1974, p. 686.
31. Kennedy, C., Grave, G. D., and Jekle, J. U.: Cerebral effects of hyperoxia in puppies. Pediatr. Res. *5,* 659, 1971 (Abst. Int. Vet. Ref. Service, F-6-476, 1972).
32. Kerem, D., and Elsner, R.: Cerebral tolerance to asphyxia. Am. J. Physiol. *225,* 593, 1973.
33. Kirk, R. W.: Hypoglycemia. *In* Kirk, R. W. (ed.): *Current Veterinary Therapy III.* W. B. Saunders Co., Philadelphia, 1968, p. 78.
34. Knecht, C. D., Oliver, J. E., Redding, R., Selcer, R., and Johnson, G.: Narcolepsy in a dog and a cat. J.A.V.M.A. *162,* 1052–1053, 1973.
35. Kutt, H., and McDowell, F.: Management of epilepsy with diphenylhydantoin sodium. J.A.M.A. *203,* 969, 1968.
36. Lovelace, R. E., and Horwitz, S. J.: Peripheral neuropathy in long-term diphenylhydantoin therapy. Arch. Neurol. *18,* 69, 1968.
37. Marine, D., and Lenhart, C. H.: Effects of the administration or the withholding of iodine-containing compounds in normal, colloid or actively hyperplastic (parenchymatous) thyroid of dogs. Arch. Int. Med. *4,* 253, 1909.
38. McGrath, J. T.: *Neurologic Examination of the Dog,* 2d ed. Lea and Febiger, Philadelphia, 1960.
39. Mitler, M. M.: Nacolepsy-cataplexy in a female dog. Exp. Neurol. *45,* 332–340, 1974.
40. Muir, W. W., Werner, L. L., and Hamlin, R. L.: Antiarrhythmic effects of diazepam during coronary artery occlusion in dogs. Am. J. Vet. Res. *36,* 1203, 1975.
41. Nachreiner, R. F.: Personal communication.
42. Neely, W. A., and Youmans, J. R.: Anoxia of canine brain without damage. J.A.M.A. *183,* 1085, 1963.
43. Oliver, J. E.: Hepatic neuropathies—a review with two case histories. Vet. Med. Small Anim. Clin. *60,* 499, 1965.

44. Oliver, J. E., and Hoerlein, B. F.: Convulsive disorders of dogs. J.A.V.M.A. *146,* 1126, 1965.
45. Palmer, A. C.: Pathological changes in the brain associated with fits in dogs. Vet. Rec. *90,* 167, 1972.
46. Palmer, A. C., and Walker, R. G.: Neuropathologic effects of cardiac arrest in animals; a study of 5 cases. J. Small Anim. Pract. *11,* 779, 1970.
47. Parker, A. J.: A preliminary report of a new antiepileptic medication for dogs. J. Am. Anim. Hosp. Assoc. *11,* 437, 1975.
48. Pochedly, C., and Ente, G.: Adverse hematologic effects of drugs. Pediatr. Clin. N. Am. *19,* 1095, 1972.
49. Redding, R. W., and Prynn, R. B.: Seizures. *In* Kirk, R. W. (ed.): *Current Veterinary Therapy III.* W. B. Saunders Co., Philadelphia, 1968, p. 463.
50. Redding, R. W.: Seizures, differential diagnosis, and therapy. Norden News *44,* 26, 1969.
51. Redding, R. W.: Diagnosis and therapy of seizures. J. Am. Anim. Hosp. Assoc. *5,* 79, 1969.
52. Reid, C. L.: Hypothyroidism. *In* Kirk, R. W. (ed.): *Current Veterinary Therapy III.* W. B. Saunders Co., Philadelphia, 1968, p. 555.
53. Rijnberk, A.: Hypothyroidism. *In* Kirk, R. W. (ed.): *Current Veterinary Therapy V.* W. B. Saunders Co., Philadelphia, 1974, p. 791.
54. Schechter, R. D.: Hyperadrenocorticism. *In* Kirk, R. W. (ed.): *Current Veterinary Therapy V.* W. B. Saunders Co., Philadelphia, 1974, p. 783.
55. Schechter, R. D., Stabenfeldt, G. H., Gribble, D. H., and Ling, G. V.: Treatment of Cushing's syndrome in the dog with an adrenocorticolytic agent (o, p′ DDD). J.A.V.M.A. *162,* 629, 1973.
56. Selhorst, J. B., Kaufman, B., and Horwitz, S. J.: Diphenylhydantoin-induced cerebellar degeneration. Arch. Neurol. *27,* 453, 1972.
57. Siegel, E. T.: Adrenal insufficiency. *In* Kirk, R. W. (ed.): *Current Veterinary Therapy IV.* W. B. Saunders Co., Philadelphia, 1971, p. 593.
58. Siegel, E. T., Kelly, D. F., and Berg, P.: Cushing's syndrome in the dog. J.A.V.M.A. *157,* 2081, 1970.
59. Siegel, E. T., and Belshaw, B. E.: Laboratory evaluation of adrenocortical and thyroid functions in the dog. *In* Kirk, R. W. (ed.): *Current Veterinary Therapy III.* W. B. Saunders Co., Philadelphia, 1968, p. 545.
60. Sims, M. H.: Personal communication.
61. Strombeck, D. R., Weiser, M. G., and Kaneko, J. J.: Hyperammonemia and hepatic encephalopathy in the dog. J.A.V.M.A. *166,* 1105, 1975.
62. Tufo, H. M., Ostfeld, A. M., and Shekelle, R.: Central nervous system dysfunction following open-heart surgery. J.A.M.A. *212,* 1333, 1970.
63. Wallace, M. E.: Keeshonds: a genetic study of epilepsy and EEG readings. J. Small Anim. Pract. *16,* 1, 1975.
64. Walton, J. N.: *Essentials of Neurology.* J. B. Lippincott Co., Philadelphia, 1961.
65. Ward, G. M.: Bovine cerebellar hypoplasia apparently caused by BVD-MD virus, a case report. Corn. Vet. *59,* 570, 1969.
66. Wechsler, I. S.: *Clinical Neurology,* 9th ed. W. B. Saunders Co., Philadelphia, 1963.
67. White, P. T., Plott, D., and Norton, J.: Relative anticonvulsant potency of primidone. Arch. Neurol. *14,* 31, 1966.
68. Wiggins, M. D.: Unpublished data.
69. Wolland, M.: Primary adrenocortical insufficiency. *In* Kirk, R. W. (ed.): *Current Veterinary Therapy V.* W. B. Saunders Co., Philadelphia, 1974, p. 789.
70. Zeft, H. J., Rembert, J. C., Curry, C. L., and Greenfield, J. C.: Effects of diphenylhydantoin on coronary and systemic haemodynamics in awake dogs. Cardiovasc. Res. *7,* 331, 1973.

CHAPTER 18

NEURO-OPHTHALMOLOGY

Stephen I. Bistner, B.S., D.V.M.

INTRODUCTION

Neuro-ophthalmology is the study of the sensory and motor innervation to the eye and adnexal structures. The visual pathways consists of the retina, optic nerve, and various structures of the brain that process visual information. A neuro-ophthalmologic examination in an animal is difficult because the animal cannot explain either visual or neurologic deficits. We must rely on a careful and systematic approach in examination of the ocular system and in interpreting the signs shown by the animal.

As in any medical examination, the detailed examination of the eyes should be preceded by a careful history. The following categories should be included in the history: chief complaint, present illness, review of systems, and past history.

In neuro-ophthalmology, the history of any visual impairment is extremely important. Questions regarding loss of vision include: Does the animal bump into objects or have difficulty going up and down stairs? Do visual difficulties seem worse in dim light or bright light? Do visual disturbances seem worse on one side or are they equal on both sides? Are there any personality changes accompanying the visual disturbances? The position of the head may indicate a possible visual field defect because the animal may be attempting to compensate for a visual problem. The use of a patch over one eye may help to distinguish which eye is affected.

A general inspection of the globe and external ocular structures should be conducted before any detailed examination of the eye is undertaken. Inspect the globe in normal daylight or roomlight and observe the relationship of the globe to the orbit and the eyelids. Note whether the eyes are in the same visual axis or whether a tropia is present. Note any undue prominence of one or both eyes. Note the presence of any other facial lesions (e.g., facial paralysis) which may affect the symmetry of the orbit.

INNERVATION OF THE EYE MUSCLES

EYELID

The size of the palpebral fissure is controlled by the following muscles of the eyelids. The *orbicularis oculi* is innervated by the auriculopalpebral branch of the facial nerve (cranial nerve VII). Contraction of this muscle closes the palpebral fissure. The *levator palpebrae superioris* is innervated by the oculomotor nerve (cranial nerve III). Contraction of the levator palpebrae elevates the upper lid, enlarging the palpebral fissure. Smooth muscle present in both eyelids is innervated by sympathetic postganglionic axons that enter the orbit with the ophthalmic nerve. Contracture of the smooth muscle enlarges the palpebral fissure.

In addition to controlling the orbicularis

oculi muscle and the muscles of facial expression, the seventh cranial nerve also carries parasympathetic fibers for the control of lacrimation. Inability to completely close the lid over the cornea (lagophthalmos) can result in exposure keratitis. Complete inability to close the lids is associated with seventh nerve damage and can result in neuroparalytic keratitis.

Lesions of the Facial Nerve

Lesions can affect the facial nerve at a number of sites: (1) at the level of the facial nerve nucleus; (2) as the nerve courses through the brain stem; (3) as the nerve leaves the brain stem to enter the inner ear through the internal acoustic meatus; or (4) as the nerve leaves the skull and separates into peripheral branches.

Lesions of the seventh nerve within the parenchyma of the brain stem usually result in damage to other nerves, and multiple signs can develop, including coma, paresis, nystagmus, ocular positional abnormalities, and pupillary changes. Brain stem lesions are likely to affect any combination of cranial nerves V, VI, VII, and VIII.

Peripheral facial nerve lesions may be present because of the intimate relationship of the seventh nerve to the inner ear. The facial nerve leaves the ventroloateral aspect of the brain stem and joins with both branches of the eighth cranial nerve to enter the internal acoustic meatus, coursing through the inner ear. The first branch to leave the facial nerve as it courses within the inner ear is the major petrosal branch, which contains parasympathetic fibers that help to control lacrimation. Inability to close the lids and abnormal tear production can be produced by facial nerve lesions caused by otitis interna.

Hemifacial Spasms

Roberts and Vainisi[176] have described hemifacial spasms in dogs in which there were unilateral spasms of the facial muscles that caused one side of the face to appear wrinkled. Additionally, Horner's syndrome was evident on the same side as the facial spasm. In each of the cases described in this report, there was severe otitis media that resulted in an extracranial lesion of the facial nerve.

Parker[159] has described hemifacial spasm associated with an intracranial lesion in a dog. In this case there was no associated Horner's syndrome, although intracranial damage to the third, fifth, seventh, and twelfth nerves was present. Parker also reported three cases of hemifacial spasms associated with severe otitis in dogs. True hemifacial spasms are supposed to be associated with irritative lesions of the seventh nerve and may be confused with a seventh nerve paralysis of the opposite side of the head.

Ptosis of the Eyelid

Inability to contract the *levator palpebrarum superioris* muscle is associated with damage to the third cranial nerve and results in ptosis of the lid. In internal ophthalmoplegia there is intranuclear (within the brain stem) damage to the third cranial nerve nuclei, resulting in paralysis of all fibers of the nerve; this produces ptosis of the lid, abnormalities of the extraocular muscles, widely dilated pupils, and paralysis of the ciliary muscle. In external ophthalmoplegia there is a more distal (peripheral) lesion of the third nerve, and only extraocular muscle or pupillary function may be affected.

A syndrome similar to myasthenia gravis in man has been reported in dogs and a cat.[68] The signs are those of generalized weakness, including weakness in the limbs, voice change, dribbling urine, drooping lids, and drooling from the mouth. One of the cardinal features of this syndrome is dilatation of the esophagus. The condition can be treated with neostigmine bromide, 15 mg orally three times a day.

The position of the membrana nictitans (third eyelid) in reference to the eyeball depends on the position of the eyeball in the orbit and the tone of the smooth muscle within the base of the membrana nictitans. Normal tone in the smooth muscle of the membrana nictitans is maintained by its sympathetic innervation. Normal tone keeps the membrana nictitans retracted in its normal position. Diseases of the sympathetic nervous system such as Horner's syndrome can cause the membrana nictitans to protrude and lie partly across the cornea.

CORNEA

The cornea has a large nerve supply derived from the ciliary plexus. The long ciliary nerves arise from the ophthalmic nerve, a branch of the trigeminal nerve. Nerves innervating the cornea are both myelinated and unmyelinated. Both sensory and trophic nerve fibers have been demonstrated in the cornea. Corneal sensation can be examined by touching the cornea with a cotton pledget or a corneal anesthesiometer, and can be evaluated by the blink response.

Alteration in the nerve supply to the cornea can cause pathologic findings in the cornea. Neurotrophic keratitis is associated with abnormalities in the ophthalmic branch of the fifth cranial nerve. Interruption of the normal trophic impulses to the corneal tissue results in corneal ulceration and loss of stromal tissue. Damage to the seventh cranial nerve, termed neuroparalytic keratitis, results in failure of the lids to close, leading to exposure keratitis. Both neurotrophic and neuroparalytic keratitis can be temporarily treated by a flap of membrana nictitans or a temporary tarsorrhaphy until nerve regeneration occurs.

EXTRAOCULAR MUSCLES

The dog and cat have seven extraocular muscles; (1) rectus medialis, (2) rectus lateralis, (3) rectus dorsalis, (4) rectus ventralis, (5) obliquus dorsalis, (6) obliquus ventralis, and (7) retractor bulbi. The oculomotor, trochlear, and abducens nerves innervate the extraocular muscles. It is important to check tonic neck and eye reflexes when evaluating the extraocular muscles. When the nose is elevated, the fore limbs extend and the hind limbs flex. As the nose is elevated, the eyes should remain focused within the center of the palpebral fissure.

Oculomotor Nerve Lesions

The oculomotor nerve (cranial nerve III) innervates the medial, dorsal, and ventral recti, the ventral oblique, and portions of the retractor oculi. Oculomotor nerve fibers also innervate the levator muscle of the upper lid and the constrictor pupillae muscle of the iris and ciliary musculature.

Complete oculomotor nerve paralysis produces a maximally dilated pupil that is unresponsive to direct and consensual light stimulation. The position of the eye in oculomotor paralysis depends on whether the eye is observed in its fixed position or in its field of movement. There is some difference of opinion regarding the static position of the eye . The classic description is a ventrolateral strabismus, although it has been stated that the eye is deviated medially due to partial action as an adductor of the superior oblique muscle.[177] In oculomotor palsy abnormalities in the tonic eye reflexes are characterized by a lack of downward motion of the eye when the head is raised and a lack of upward motion when the head is flexed. Lateral and medial movements of the globe are also limited.

Trochlear Nerve

The trochlear nerve (cranial nerve IV) innervates the dorsal oblique muscles, which normally causes intorsion of the eye. There may be no strabismus or functional deficit when damage occurs to this nerve.

Abducens Nerve

The abducens nerve (cranial nerve VI) innervates the retractor oculi and the lateral rectus muscles. Abnormalities of the abducens nerve result in a medial strabismus, incomplete ability to abduct the eyeball, and a decreased ability to retract the eyeball.

Strabismus

Strabismus refers to deviations of the eye. The various forms of strabismus are called tropias. Strabismus is observed in dogs which have disease in the vestibular system. When the head is in certain positions, the normal vestibular mechanism that adjusts the eyeball position to the position of the head is altered, causing the eye on the affected side to deviate ventrolaterally. This form of strabismus is transient, occurring only when the head is in certain positions. Movement of the head will alleviate the strabismus. Strabismus of this type is referred to as vestibular strabismus.

A bilateral, ventrolateral position of the eyes is commonly encountered in severely hydrocephalic dogs which have enlarged cranial cavities. This is assumed to result from the associated deformity of the orbit and not from bilateral oculomotor nerve compression. This conclusion is supported by the fact that the eyes can move in all directions with no associated mydriasis or ptosis. Brachycephalic breeds of dogs may show an exotropia which does not interfere with normal ocular movement or function (see Plate A).

Nystagmus

Nystagmus refers to the involuntary rhythmic oscillations or tremors of the eyes that occur independently of normal movements. Nystagmus may be either pendular (the movements occur at the same rate in each direction) or alternating (the movements are alternately rapid and slow). Alternating nystagmus, in which movement is chiefly in the horizontal plane, is classified accordingly to the direction of the rapid component (either right or left). Normal nystagmus can be induced through either the retina or the labyrinth of the inner ear. Abnormal vestibular nystagmus can be induced by flexing the head of the patient laterally from side to side in a dorsal plane. This produces nystagmus in the dorsal plane in the same direction as the movement. Flexion and extension of the head will induce a vertical nystagmus.

Abnormal nystagmus represents a disturbance in the symmetry of the tonic innervation of the extraocular muscles. Extraocular muscles receive tonic innervation from the labyrinth, the retina, the somatic musculature of the body, and the cerebrum.

Horizontal nystagmus is frequently seen in a variety of clinically significant conditions, including diseases of the inner ear, the eighth (vestibular) nerve, and the brain stem. Labyrinthitis secondary to otitis interna is commonly characterized by horizontal nystagmus, in which the rapid movement is directed away from the lesion. In disorders of the inner ear, the nystagmus is asymmetrical and disconjugate, meaning that nystagmus in one eye differs from that in the other eye. Nystagmus associated with peripheral or central nervous system lesions is usually transient and persists for only a few days unless exacerbation of the underlying cause occurs.

Vertical nystagmus is not commonly seen but may be associated with central disorders of the parenchyma of the brain stem and a variety of other causes, including trauma, neoplasms, hemorrhage, and infection.

A very fine, rotatory or oscillating type of nystagmus can be observed in animals with congenital defects in vision; it is associated with either retinal, optic nerve, or central nervous system lesions. Some Siamese cats have very fine rotatory nystagmus as a congenital defect.

INNERVATION OF THE PUPIL

The pupil of the eye is the classic example of antagonistic (reciprocal) autonomic innervation: parasympathetic innervation causes constriction of the pupil, while sympathetic innervation causes dilation of the pupil. Normal pupillary response involves cranial nerves II and III, and only brain stem connections are necessary. When light is directed toward the retina, the visual impulses created pass through the optic nerve to the optic chiasm, where they have an opportunity to cross to the opposite side. In the cat, about 66 per cent and in the dog about 75 per cent of the optic nerve fibers decussate at the optic chiasm. Optic nerve axons that conduct impulses initiated in the medial retina cross in the chiasm to the contralateral optic tract. Impulses originating in the lateral retina for

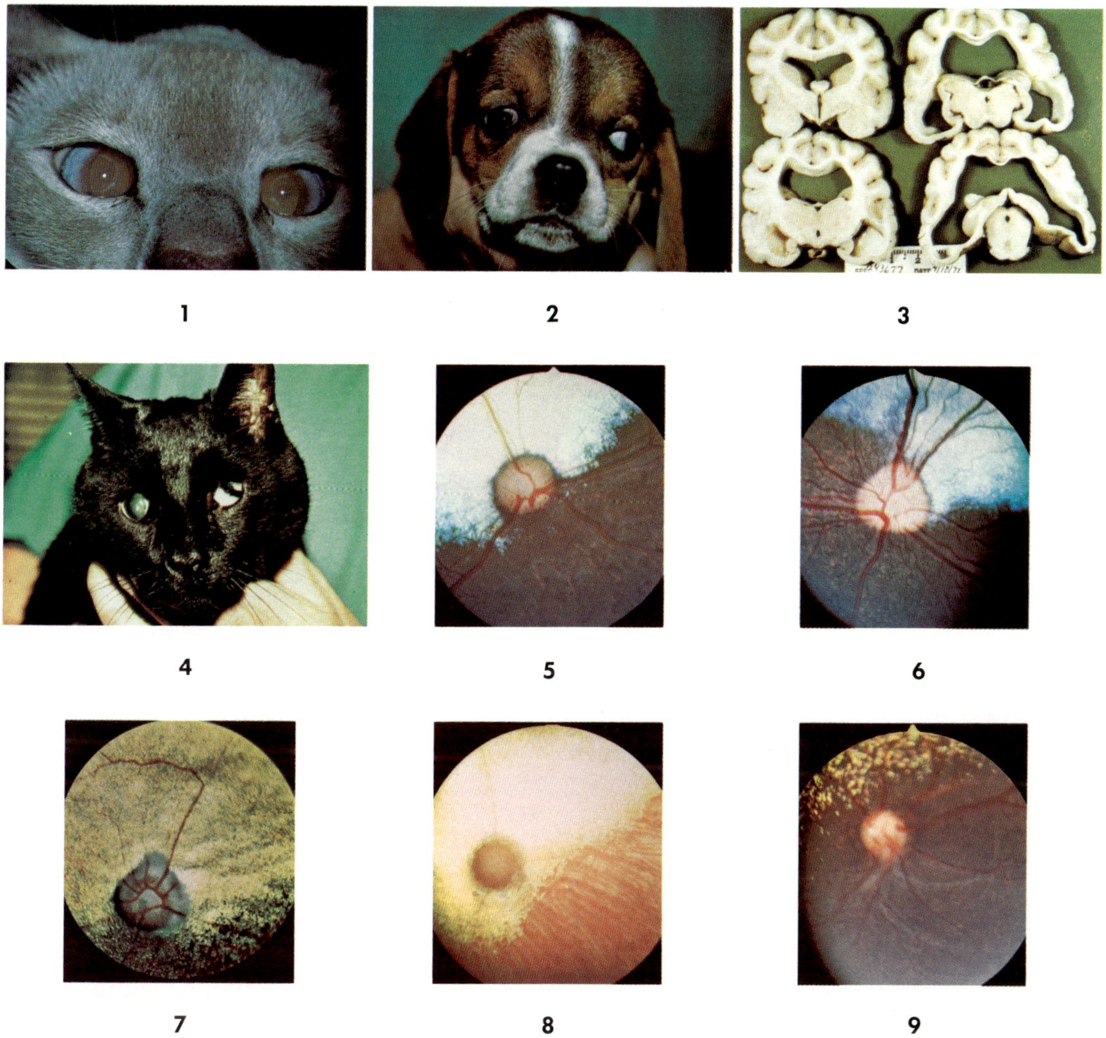

PLATE A (1) Siamese cat with congenital medial strabismus. This condition is not associated with a primary extraocular muscle abnormality but rather with abnormal neuroanatomical substrate for normal vision in the optic tracts and lateral geniculate body. (2) Lateral exodeviation of the eye associated with congenital hydrocephalus. (3) Brain sections from the beagle puppy in (2) showing lateral deviation of the globe and congenital hydrocephalus.

(4) Unilateral Horner's syndrome of the left eye characterized by miosis, protrusion of the nictitans membrane, ptosis, and apparent enophthalmos. (5) Normal fundus of the dog. The optic disk in this animal is located at the junction of the tapetum and nigral portions of the fundus. The optic nerve is surrounded by a peripapillary pigment ring. (6) Normal fundus of the dog. Note the venous anastomosis on the surface of the optic nerve head and the normal physiological cup in the center of the nerve. The optic nerve head is triangular in shape because of the amount of myelin in the optic nerve.

(7) Fundus of a 5-year-old miniature poodle with generalized progressive retinal atrophy. Note the loss of retinal vessel size, the abnormal "granularity" of the tapetum, and the paleness of the optic disk. (8) Advanced retinal degeneration in a cat. Note the loss of normal retinal vasculature, the hyperreflectivity of the tapetum, and the atrophy of the optic nerve. (9) Optic nerve hypoplasia in a dog. Normal retinal vasculature is present; however, the optic nerve is atrophic. A marked visual deficit was associated with this optic nerve hypoplasia.

the most part enter the ipsilateral optic tract from the chiasm (see Table 18–5).

PARASYMPATHETIC INNERVATION

The optic nerve has two components: one is composed of the fibers that pass to the pupillary centers within the brain stem, and the second is composed of those fibers that synapse in the thalamus and in turn project light impulses to the visual cortex of the brain. The pupillary fibers leave the optic tract and synapse in the midbrain, where crossing occurs. Impulses reach the rostral portion of the oculomotor nucleus, which contains cell bodies of preganglionic parasympathetic axons. Axons from the oculomotor nucleus project in the oculomotor nerve through the orbital fissure and periorbita, where synapse in the ciliary ganglion occurs between the preganglionic parasympathetic axons and the cell bodies of the postganglionic parasympathetic axons. The postganglionic nerves are continued as the short ciliary nerves to the eye and supply the constrictor pupillae muscle.

Because the light-stimulated axons have numerous opportunities to cross, stimulation of the retina of one eyeball affects the preganglionic parasympathetic neurons of each oculomotor nerve and thus induces pupillary constriction in both eyeballs. The response in the nonstimulated eyeball is called the consensual or indirect response.

Anisocoria is the condition of inequality of pupillary size. Pupils of unequal size can be associated with ocular disease, abnormalities of the sympathetic or parasympathetic peripheral innervation of the pupillary musculature, or central nervous system abnormalities.

Iris degeneration can result in atrophy of the constrictor pupillae musculature, which in turn leads to a dilated pupil that is unresponsive to light stimulation, although no visual abnormalities are present. The pupillary border is usually very irregular in appearance. Mydriasis of the pupil with poor response or no response to light may be associated with glaucoma, retinal detachment, retinal atrophy, or optic nerve atrophy. Miosis of the pupil is associated with uveitis.

Trauma to the skull is not infrequent in small animals. Pupillary and oculocephalic responses can be useful indicators of the extent of intracranial injury. The pupillary response is variable and depends on the severity of the injury and the degree of brain stem involvement. Constricted pupils may be associated with lesions in the diencephalon. Lesions of the oculomotor nucleus (midbrain) leave the pupils unresponsive to light. Brain stem lesions and increasing intraocular pressure are characterized by progressive loss of consciousness, decreasing voluntary motor activity, and dilated, nonresponsive pupils.

Tables 18–1 and 18–2 describe signs characteristic of severe damage to the brain stem and progressive unilateral tentorial herniation, and may be helpful in evaluating the traumatized animal.

SYMPATHETIC INNERVATION

The pathway for the sympathetic innervation of the dilator pupillae muscle in-

TABLE 18–1 SIGNS CHARACTERISTIC OF SEVERE DAMAGE TO THE BRAIN STEM AT VARIOUS LEVELS*

Level	Consciousness	Pupils	Eye Movements	Motor Function	Autonomic Responses
Early diencephalic	Apathy	Small but reactive	Normal	Hemiparesis	Normal to irregular respirations
Late diencephalic	Stupor	Small but reactive	Normal	Hemiparesis to tetraparesis	Cheyne-Stokes respiration
Midbrain	Coma	Bilateral dilation	Poor oculocephalic response	Decerebrate rigidity	Hyperventilation
Pons	Coma	Midposition, unresponsive	Oculocephalic response absent	Flaccid paralysis	Rapid shallow respirations
Medulla	Coma	Midposition, dilated terminally	Absent	Flaccid paralysis	Irregular to apnea, pulse slowing

*From Oliver, J. E., Jr.: Intracranial injury. *In* Kirk, R. W. (ed.): *Current Veterinary Therapy VI*. W. B. Saunders Co., Philadelphia, 1977.

TABLE 18–2 SIGNS CHARACTERISTIC OF PROGRESSIVE UNILATERAL TENTORIAL HERNIATION*

Level	Consciousness	Pupils	Eye Movements	Motor Function	Autonomic Responses
III N.	Normal to stupor	Ipsilateral dilation	Normal to slight lateral strabismus	Normal to hemiparesis	Normal
Early midbrain	Stupor	Ipsilateral to bilateral dilation	Ipsilateral ventro-lateral strabismus	Hemiparesis ipsi- or contralateral	Normal
Late midbrain to pons	Coma	Dilated bilateral to fixed mid-position	Ventrolateral strabismus to fixed midposition	Decerebrate rigidity	Hyperventilation
Pons	Coma	Midposition, unresponsive	Oculocephalic response absent	Flaccid paralysis	Rapid, shallow respirations
Medulla	Coma	Midposition, dilated terminally	Absent	Flaccid paralysis	Irregular to apnea, pulse slowing

*From Oliver, J. E., Jr.: Intracranial injury. *In* Kirk, R. W. (ed.): *Current Veterinary Therapy VI.* W. B. Saunders Co., Philadelphia, 1977.

volves both central and peripheral components. The central sympathetic component involves the hypothalamus and rostral midbrain, with projections through the pons, medulla, and descending lateral tectotegmentospinal system. The preganglionic neurons of the peripheral sympathetic pathway are located within the first three thoracic spinal cord segments. The axons from the thoracic and cervical sympathetic trunk course cranially to reach the cranial cervical ganglion ventromedial to the tympanic bulla. Synapse occurs, and the postganglionic nerves then travel via the long ciliary nerves to the dilator pupillae muscle. This same pathway also innervates the smooth muscle of the periorbita, eyelids and membrana nictitans.

Horner's Syndrome

A lesion anywhere along the pathway of this nerve can produce sympathetic denervation and the characteristic Horner's syndrome (miosis, ptosis, prolapse of the membrana nictitans, and apparent enophthalmos). In general, experience shows that central nervous system lesions cranial to the first thoracic segment rarely produce Horner's syndrome, with the exception of intracranial injury that involves contusion of the midbrain structures, including the origin of the lateral tectotegmentospinal system. Horner's syndrome is usually associated with a lesion of the lower motor neuron pathway, beginning possibly at the level of the first three thoracic segments (Table 18–3 and Plate A).

In the dog, supersensitivity to adrenergic amines may be helpful in localizing the lesion producing Horner's syndrome. When the lesion involves the postganglionic nerve pathway, the pupil will dilate after the topical instillation of 0.1 ml of 0.001 per cent epinephrine hydrochloride. When the lesion is preganglionic, a period of 30 to 40 minutes is required to obtain the same effect. Many postganglionic lesions are associated with trauma; in general, the prognosis for return of normal neural function with these injuries is better than with preganglionic lesions. The period of supersensitivity to adrenergic amines associated with postganglionic lesions is, however, short-lived, and the test described may be valuable only if performed one to two weeks following the initial injury.

The time period necessary for observation of spontaneous nerve regeneration in Horner's syndrome is variable and depends on the nature of the injury to the nerve. Symptomatic treatment of Horner's syndrome involves the topical instillation in the eye of an adrenergic amine such as 10 per cent phenylephrine. The dose of the medication may have to be adjusted because of its irritant effect on the eye when used over a prolonged period of time.

CENTRAL VISUAL PATHWAY

The central visual pathway begins with the photoreceptor cells of the retina. The many and varied diseases that can damage

TABLE 18–3 HORNER'S SYNDROME: SUMMARY OF LESIONS*

Location	Lesion	Associated Neurologic Deficit
T1–T3 spinal cord	External injury Neoplasm Focal poliomyelomalacia Diffuse myelomalacia (ascending and descending)	Pelvic and thoracic limb paresis or paralysis with lower motor neuron deficit in thoracic limbs and upper motor neuron deficit in pelvic limbs. Lower motor neuron deficit and analgesia of tail, anus, pelvic limbs, abdomen, and thorax with paretic thoracic limbs
T1–T3 ventral roots—proximal spinal nerves	Avulsion of roots of brachial plexus	Brachial plexus paresis or paralysis of the thoracic limb on the same side
Cranial thoracic sympathetic trunk	Lymphosarcoma Thyroid adenocarcinoma Neurofibroma	None if confined to the trunk
Cervical sympathetic trunk	Injury from surgical intervention in the area or from dog bites Neoplasm	None if unilateral. Bilateral lesions interfere with laryngeal and esophageal function because of vagal involvement
Middle ear cavity	Otitis media	Signs of peripheral vestibular disturbance—ipsilateral ataxia, head tilt, and nystagmus, and sometimes facial palsy
Retrobulbar	Contusion	Varies with degree of contusion to the optic and oculomotor nerves, which also influence pupillary size

*From de Lahunta, A.: Small animal neuro-ophthalmology. Vet. Clin. N. Am. *3* (3), 491–501, 1973.

the retina will not be discussed here. The reader is referred to Rubin's *Atlas of Veterinary Ophthalmoscopy** for a more complete discussion of retinal abnormalities.

OPTIC NERVE

Axons of ganglionic cells in the nerve fiber layer converge to form the optic nerve. The optic nerve (cranial nerve II) is a white nervous tract that connects the retina and the brain. It is not a peripheral nerve. The optic nerve can be divided into intraocular, intraorbital, intracanalicular, and intracranial segments. Like the brain, the optic nerve is surrounded by three layers: dura mater, arachnoidea, and pia mater. The subarachnoid space of the optic nerve is in communication with that of the brain.

*Rubin, L.: *Atlas of Veterinary Ophthalmoscopy.* Lea & Febiger, Philadelphia, 1974.

Abnormalities of the Optic Nerve

Lesions that affect the function of one optic nerve can cause severe visual abnormalities in the affected eye because of a dilated, unresponsive pupil. Light directed into the affected eye will produce no pupillary response in either eye. Light directed into the normal eye will elicit a response in both eyes. When an abnormality of the optic nerve affects only one eye, visual abnormalities may not be detected because visual acuity of the normal eye compensates for the defect (see Table 18–5).

There are numerous abnormalities of the optic nerve. Congenital optic nerve hypoplasia has been reported in numerous species of domestic animals, including cats, dogs, horses, cattle, and pigs. Optic nerve hypoplasia may be associated with multiple ocular abnormalities, or it may occur alone. Optic nerve hypoplasia is usually accompanied by normal numbers of retinal blood vessels, although the numbers of the retinal ganglion cells and the size

TABLE 18-4*

SUDDEN ACQUIRED BLINDNESS — **An Algorithm For Sudden Acquired Blindness**

Fundic Reflection → Present → Pupillary Response to Light → Hyporeflexic or Areflexic → Position of Iris → Mydriatic → Funduscopic Examination

1. ABSENT	2. NORMAL	3. MIOTIC	4. NORMAL	5. ABNORMAL
A. Abnormal opaque substance in aqueous or vitreous humor 1. Hemorrhage 2. Exudate B. Opacity of cornea 1. Edema C. Opacity of lens 1. Cataract D. Absence of pupil 1. Inflammation 2. Neoplasia	A. Lesions of lateral geniculate nucleus, optic radiations and occipital cortex 1. Trauma 2. Necrosis 3. Hydrocephalus 4. Toxicity 5. Infection 6. Mass 7. Degeneration 8. Biochemical	A. Iritis B. Cerebral edema	A. Lesions optic nerves, optic chiasm and optic tracts 1. Trauma 2. Mass 3. Infection 4. Degeneration 5. Inflammation B. Cortex and oculomotor nerve 1. Severe increased intracranial pressure	A. Papillitis 1. Optic nerve same as 4A B. Cupping of disc 1. Glaucoma C. Retinal detachment 1. Secondary to colobomas, ectasia 2. Trauma 3. Neovascularization 4. Inflammation 5. Infection 6. Toxicity 7. Idiopathic 8. Neoplasia

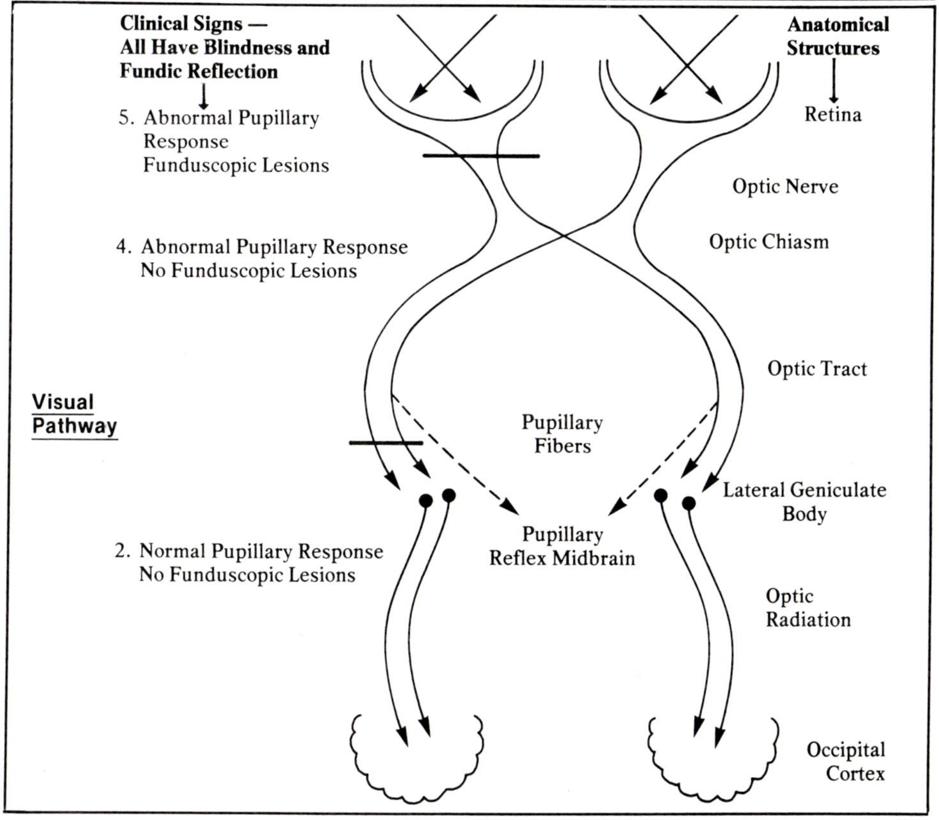

*From Schmidt, G.: An algorithm for sudden acquired blindness. Canine Pract., July-August, 1975, pp. 14–19.

of the nerve fiber layer may be reduced. True optic nerve hypoplasia must be distinguished from micropapilla (small optic nerve head). With only a small optic nerve head and a normal optic nerve, no visual abnormalities will be detected, and pupillary responses to direct light stimulation will be normal. Unilateral optic nerve hypoplasia is often not detectable on the basis of visual abnormalities unless the owner is very observant.

Optic Neuritis

Inflammation of the optic nerve (optic neuritis) may occur at any level of the nerve, at either an intraocular or a retrobulbar location. If the inflammation is intraocular, optic neuritis of the disk will be visible and is characterized by edema of the disk and surrounding retinal tissue, and hemorrhage on the surface of the disk. Retrobulbar optic neuritis may produce no ophthalmoscopically visible changes; however, sudden severe blindness may occur. Sudden blindness without any ophthalmoscopically visible abnormalities should make one suspect bilateral retrobulbar optic neuritis (Table 18–4).

Optic neuritis can be associated with a systemic disease, ingestion of toxic compounds, or ocular or central nervous system inflammation. Some of the systemic diseases that have been incriminated in optic neuritis are distemper, cryptococcosis, blastomycosis, feline infectious peritonitis, and generalized bacteremias.

Central nervous system inflammation such as meningitis or reactions of the reticulohistiocytic system (reticuloses) can also cause optic neuritis. Treatment of optic neuritis is directed at control of the inciting agent, if possible, and nonspecific reduction of the inflammation. Unfortunately, many cases of optic neuritis progress to optic nerve atrophy with the irreversible loss of vision.

Optic nerve atrophy may be secondary to optic neuritis, or it may be caused by compression of the optic nerve. Compression of the optic nerve may result from retrobulbar tumor, retro-orbital inflammation, or increased intraocular pressure in glaucoma (see Plates B and C).

Papilledema

Papilledema is not as commonly seen in dogs as it is in humans, where it is most often associated with increased intracranial pressure. Because the dog has ciliary vasculature around the optic nerve and no central retinal artery and vein, it is not subject to the same vascular abnormalities associated with increased intracranial pressure as in man. Unlike optic neuritis, papilledema does not result in severe visual loss. It is most often associated with inflammation in or around the optic nerve. Papilledema has also been associated with experimental production in dogs of malignant hypertension and venous congestion.

Optic Tract Lesions

The optic nerves cross at the optic chiasm, and the proportion of nerve fibers crossing varies depending on the species. In general, the axons that cross in the chiasm come from ganglionic cells on the medial (nasal) aspect of the retina. Axons from ganglionic cells on the lateral (temporal) aspect of the retina remain ipsilateral in their course through the central visual pathway. In the cat, 65 per cent of the optic nerve fibers decussate, and in the dog 75 per cent of them do. In the visual field of each eye, the neurons in the left optic tract are stimulated by light from the right half of the visual field. Because of the high percentage of optic nerve fibers that decussate in domestic animals, visual field deficits associated with optic tract lesions are mainly observed in the contralateral eye (Table 18–5).

Lesions of the optic chiasm and optic tracts may be associated with inflammation, degeneration, or tumor formation. The virus of canine distemper has a predilection for the optic tracts and visual pathways, causing inflammation and necrosis.

Pituitary neoplasms in animals, unlike those in man, rarely affect the visual pathways. The posterior position of the pituitary gland means that a pituitary tumor such as a chromophobe adenoma must be very large, invading the pituitary, hypothalamus, and thalamus before it encroaches on the optic tracts and produces bilateral hemianopsia.

(Text continued on page 660.)

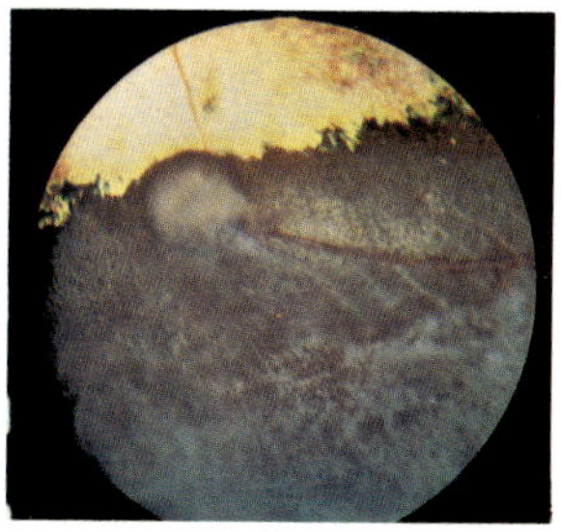

1

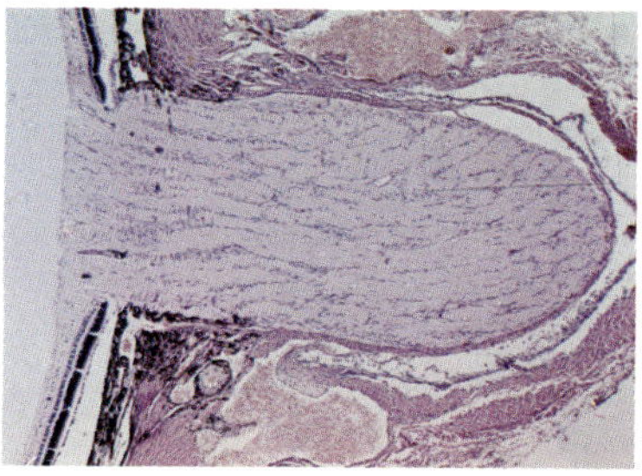

2

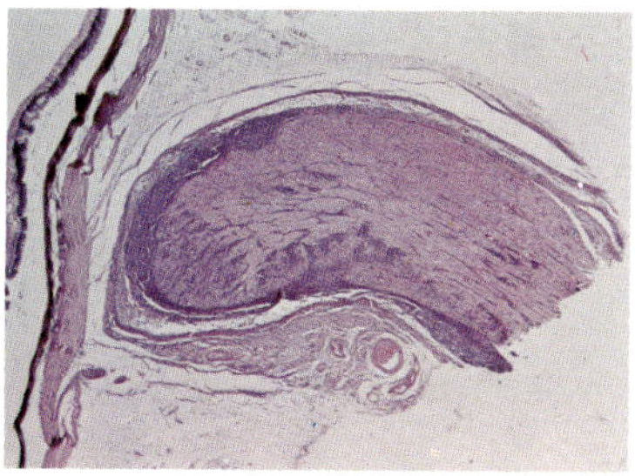

3

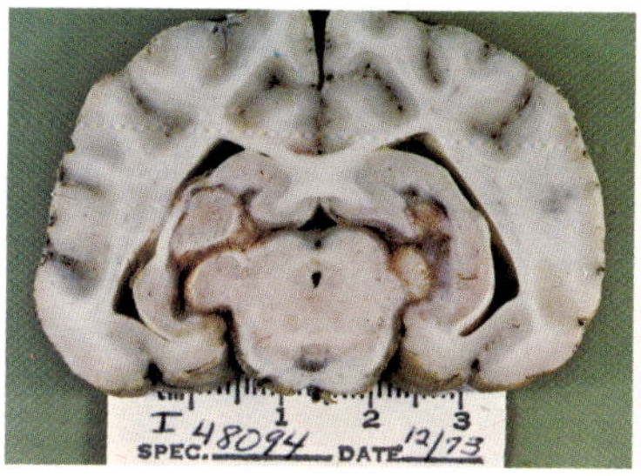

4

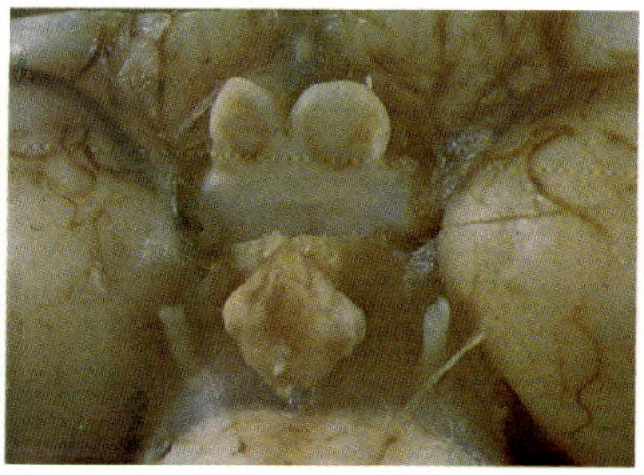

5

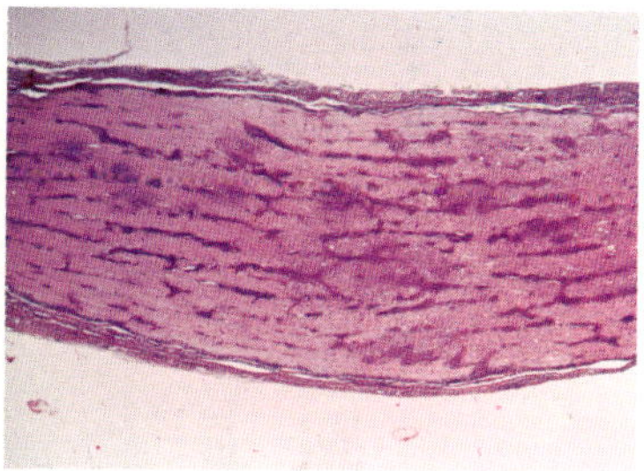

6

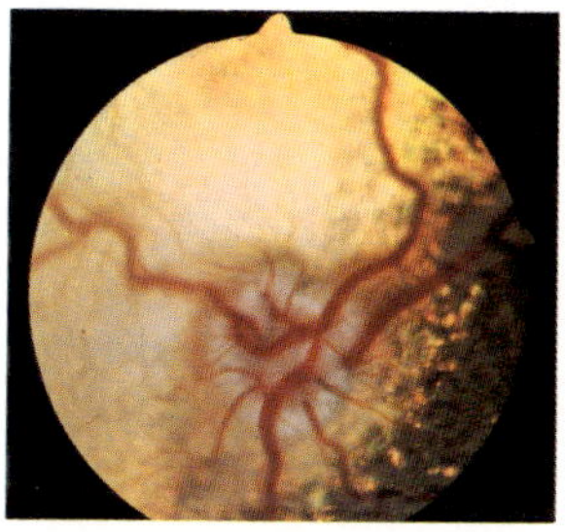

7

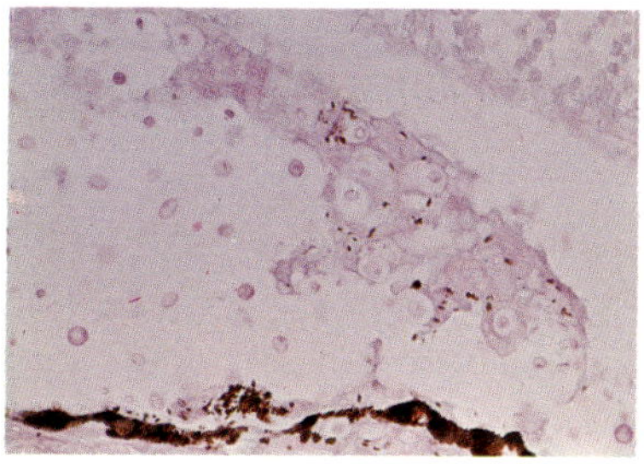

8

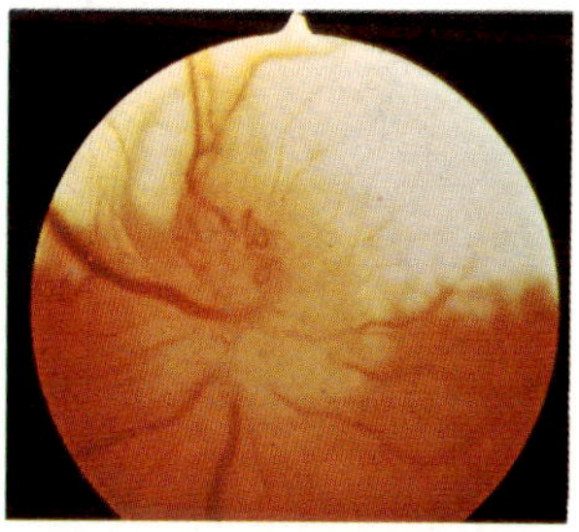

9

PLATE B (1) Severe retinal degeneration secondary to retinal inflammation with secondary optic nerve atrophy following an associated optic neuritis. (2) Longitudinal section of normal optic nerve. (3) Longitudinal section of optic nerve with transverse optic neuritis associated with feline infectious peritonitis. Visual loss is associated with this form of optic neuritis.

(4) Cross section of brain revealing severe meningitis associated with cryptococcal infection. (5) Severe edema and swelling of the optic nerves at the optic chiasm secondary to optic neuritis of unknown etiology. (6) Histological longitudinal section of the optic nerve depicted in B(5). The increase in amount of hematoxylin staining indicates severe inflammatory cell infiltrate and a transverse optic neuritis.

(7) Optic neuritis characterized by edema of the optic nerve head, increased vascularization of the optic nerve and peripapillary retinal edema. (8) Histological cross section of subretinal fluid from a cryptococcus infection in the dog. The organism is round or ovoid and measures up to 20 microns in diameter. It has a thin wall and is surrounded by a thick polysaccharide capsule. (9) Papilledema of the optic nerve in a dog. The retinal arterioles appear to bend where they pass over the edge of the elevated disk. Severe visual disturbances are not as frequently seen with papilledema as with papillitis.

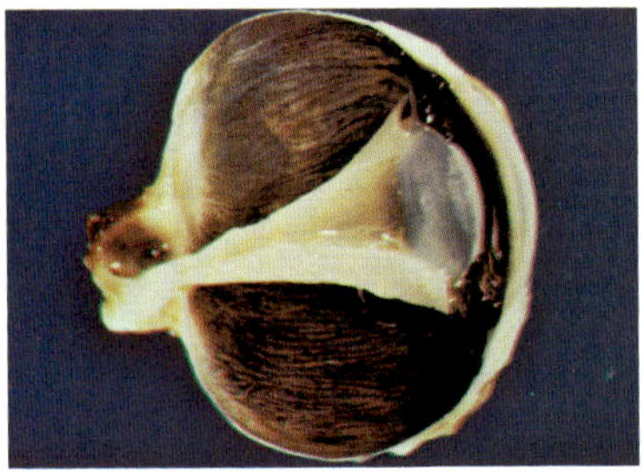

1

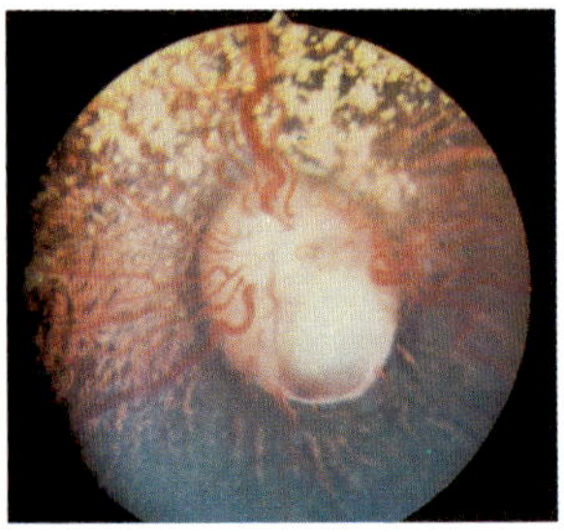

2

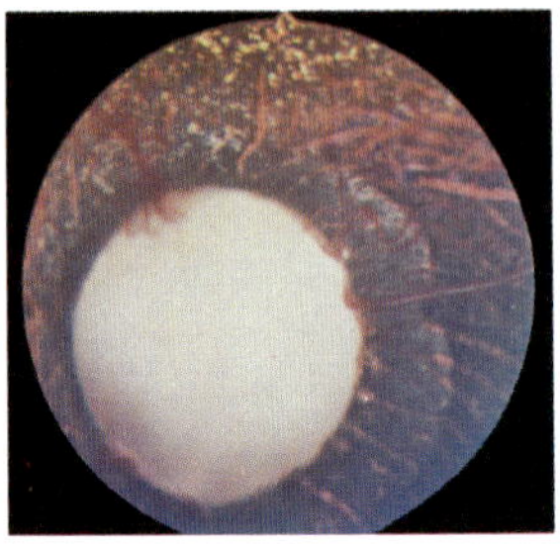

3

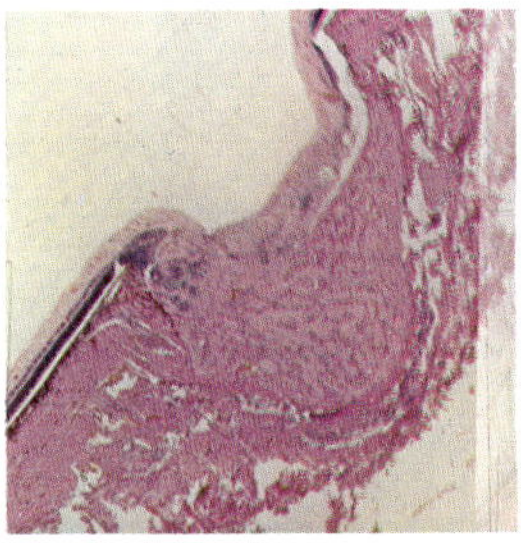

4

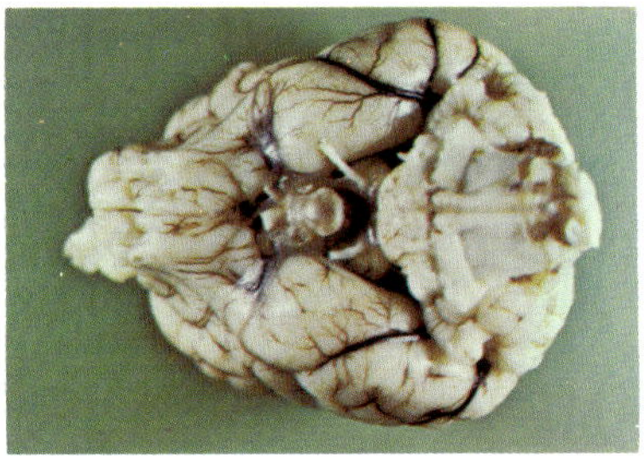

5

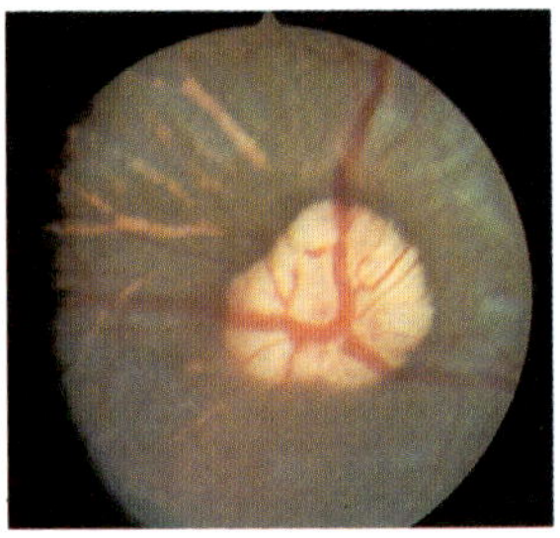

6

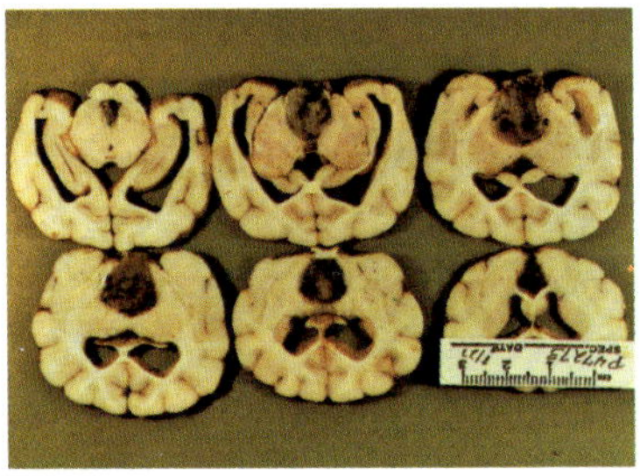

7

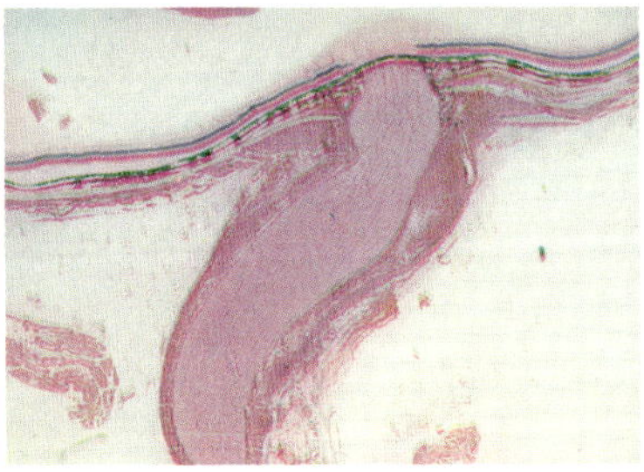

8

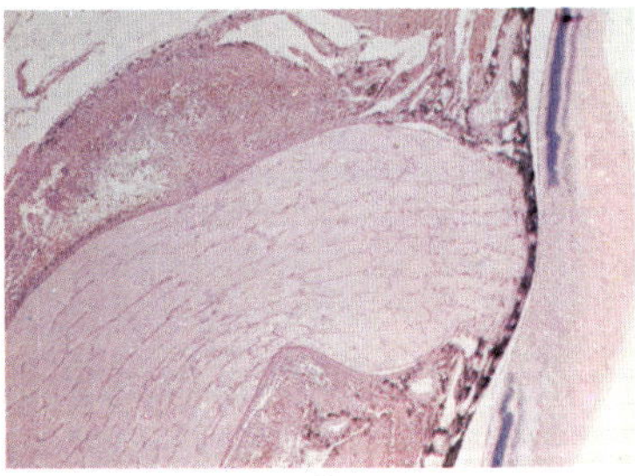

9

PLATE C (1) Congenital retinal detachment and large coloboma in a collie dog. A leukocoria (white pupillary reflex) was present, and no direct or consensual pupillary response could be elicited in this eye. (2) Optic nerve coloboma in a collie dog. This coloboma is in the typical position (6 o'clock). (3) Large colobomatous defect in a collie dog. Large colobomas can result in severe visual field defects or blindness.

(4) Histological section of the optic nerve of a collie with a colobomatous defect. Aberrant retinal tissue is present within the defect. (5) Ventral aspect of a brain from a collie dog with a severe coloboma of the left optic nerve. The left optic nerve as seen just anterior to the chiasm is atrophic. A severe visual deficit of the left eye was present. (6) Severe sudden onset of bilateral papilledema in a 12-year-old Chihuahua. The ophthalmoscopic appearance of the disk was characterized by edema formation with the major veins elevated over the disk surface. The point at which the veins pass over the disk is evident by a bend in the vein.

(7) Cross section of the brain from a 12-year-old Chihuahua that had a necrotic chromophobe adenoma of the pituitary gland. Ocular examination revealed bilateral papilledema. (8) Longitudinal section of the optic nerve from the case shown in (7). There is compression of the optic nerve by hemorrhage within the epidural space. (9) Longitudinal section of the optic nerve shows the compression of the nerve and resultant papilledema.

TABLE 18–5 SITES OF OPTIC LESIONS*

	① Right Optic Nerve	② Right Postorbital Area	③ Total Chiasm	④ Left Optic Tract	⑤ Left Visual Cortex	Left Cranial Nerve III
Left Eye						
Pupillary reaction (to light in left eye)	Both constrict	Only left pupil constricts	None—pupils dilated	Both constrict	Both constrict	Dilated—only right pupil constricts
Menace reaction	Normal	Normal	Absent	Mostly present	Mostly present	Present
Right Eye						
Pupillary reaction (to light in right eye)	Dilated—neither constricts	Dilated—neither constricts	None—pupils dilated	Both constrict	Both constrict	Only right pupil constricts
Menace reaction	Absent	Absent	Absent	Mostly absent	Mostly absent	Present

*Adapted from Allen, R., and Speakman, T. J.: Brain abscess and evaluation of current treatment. Canad. Med. Assoc. J. *86*, 852, 1962.

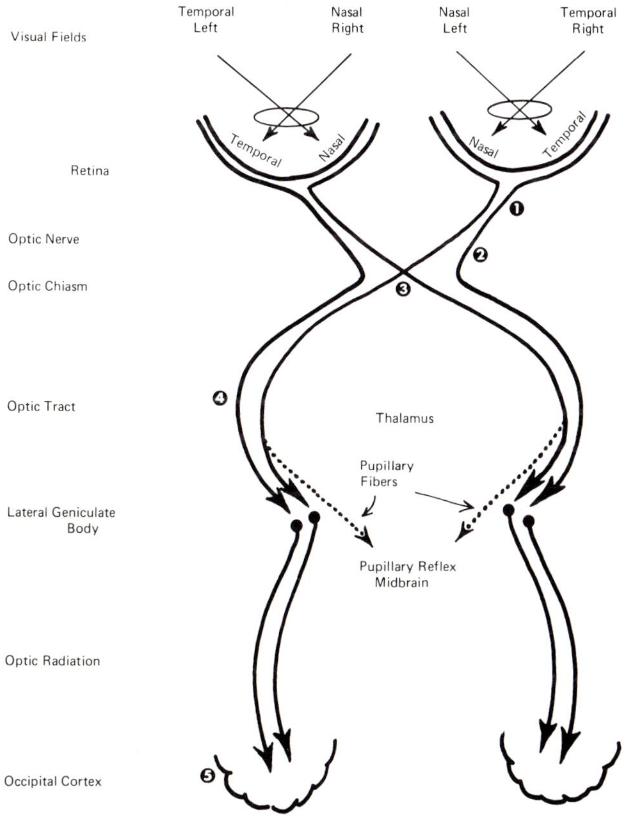

TABLE 18–6 PREDOMINANT CLINICAL SIGNS SHOWN BY 21 DOGS AFFECTED BY INTRACRANIAL NEOPLASMS*

Clinical Signs	No. of Cases
Change of temperament	17
Locomotor deficiency	17
Visual defect (including pupils)	15
Papilledema	10
Circling	10
Hemiplegia	8
Fits	8
Hemianopia	7
Head turn and/or tilt	7
Bulbar, including eye deviation and cranial nerve paralysis	7
Nystagmus	6
Sensory deficit	4
Pituitary	3

*From Palmer, A. C.; *Introduction to Animal Neurology*, 2d ed. Blackwell Scientific Publications, London, 1976.

INTRACRANIAL NEOPLASMS

Unilateral neoplasms in the hypothalamus and thalamus often encroach upon one optic tract, producing a contralateral visual deficit. Space-occupying lesions in the lateral hypothalamus or thalamus that affect the optic tract usually also affect the internal capsule or rostral crus cerebri. This results in a contralateral deficit in the limbs that will be evident on postural reaction testing.

The optic tracts run dorsally and caudally over the diencephalon to reach the lateral geniculate nucleus. A majority of optic tract axons synapse in this nucleus. Fibers pass from the lateral geniculate nucleus and terminate in the central (visual) cortex of the occipital lobe. The pathway from the optic tract to the visual cortex via the lateral geniculate nucleus and optic radiation must be intact for conscious visual perception to occur.

Unilateral lesions of the lateral geniculate nucleus, optic radiation, or visual cortex prodcue a contralateral visual field deficit. Pupillary response to direct light stimulation is normal. Abnormalities of the lateral geniculate nucleus, optic radiation, or visual cortex may be associated with trauma, neoplasms, hemorrhage, or optic degeneration.

TABLE 18–7 STORAGE DISEASES AFFECTING THE NERVOUS SYSTEM IN ANIMALS[a]*

Name of Disease	Material Stored	Deficient Enzyme	Species	Key References
Mannosidosis	Mannose, glucosamine	α-Mannosidase	Cattle	Jolly (1975)
GM_1 gangliosidosis type 1 (generalized gangliosidosis)	GM_1 gangliosides (brain and viscera) Mucopolysaccharides (viscera)	β-Galactosidase	Cat	Cheetham *et al.* (1974) Blakemore (1975)
GM_1 gangliosidosis type 2	GM_1 ganglioside (brain)	β-Galactosidase	Cattle Cat	Sheahan and Donnelly (1974) Farrell *et al* (1973)
GM_2 gangliosidosis (Tay-Sachs disease)	GM_2 ganglioside	Hexosaminidase A	Dog Pig (?)	Karbe (1973) Read and Bridges (1968)
Sphingomyelinosis (Niemann-Pick disease)	Sphingomyelin	Sphingomyelinase	Cat	Chrisp *et al.* (1970)
Glucocerebrosidosis (Gaucher's disease)	Glucocerebrosides	Glucocerebrosidase	Dog Sheep Pig	Hartley and Blakemore (1973a) Laws and Saal (1968) Sandison and Anderson (1970)
Ceroid lipofuscinosis (familial amaurotic idiocy)	Lipofuscins: ganglioside	Peroxidase (?)	Dog Cat	Patel *et al.* (1974) Green and Little (1974)
(Chediak-Higashi disease)	Lipofuscins (?)	Proteinase (?)	Cattle Mink	Padgett (1968)
"Neuronal lipodystrophy"	Lipids	?	Cattle	Read and Bridges (1969)
Globoid cell leukodystrophy (Krabbe's disease)	Cerebroside	β-Galactocerebrosidase	Dog Cat	Howell and Palmer (1971) Johnson (1970)
Metachromatic leukodystrophy	Sulfatide	Arylsulfatase A (?)	Mink	Andersen and Palludan (1968)
"Wobbler disease of mink"	Cerebroside, sulfatide ganglioside	?	Mink	Hirano *et al.* (1971)
Neurovisceral storage and dysmyelinogenesis in neonatal goats	Polysaccharides (?)	?	Goat	Hartley and Blakemore (1973b)

[a]Names in parentheses identify comparable disorders in man.
*From Done, J. T.: Developmental disorders of the nervous system in animals. *In Advances in Veterinary Science and Comparative Medicine*. Academic Press, New York, 1976.

The development of neoplasms and the associated signs they produce are closely related to the neuroanatomical position of the neoplasm. Visual deficits often accompany intracranial neoplasms. Other ocular abnormalities may also be present, depending on which ocular nerves are affected (Table 18–6).

METABOLIC DEFECTS WITH CNS MANIFESTATIONS

Numerous metabolic defects that may have central nervous system manifestations have been reported in animals.[118, 164] Lysosomal storage diseases result in a partial or complete failure to synthesize enzymes that are required for the catabolism and excretion of normal body constituents. The manifestations of these storage diseases depend on the enzymes involved and on the tissues that are most dependent on these enzymes. The central nervous system is prone to storage diseases that involve the catabolism of its glycoproteins. Deficiencies in the catabolism of myelin present as leukodystrophies and cerebrosidoses. Lipids assocated with general cell structure – i.e., sphingomyelin and gangliosides, are the substances stored in the lipidoses. Central nervous system storage diseases frequently involve some parts of the visual system. Abnormal accumulation of sphingomyelin, galactocerebrosides, lipofuscins, and GM_1 and GM_2 gangliosides have been found in ganglionic cells in the retina, brain, and peripheral nerves. Table 18–7 helps to classify some of the metabolic storage diseases of the central nervous system.

REFERENCES

1. Ades, H. W.: The acoustic projection system, a comparative study. J. Neurophysiol. *8*, 463, 1945.
2. Adrian, E. D.: Afferent discharges to the cerebral cortex from peripheral sense organs. J. Physiol. *100*, 159, 1941.
3. Allen, R., and Speakman, T. J.: Brain abscess and evaluation of current treatment. Canad. Med. Assoc. J. *86*, 852, 1962.
4. Alpers, B. J.: *Clinical Neurology*, 5th ed. F. A. Davis Co., Philadelphia, 1963.
5. Altman, H.: Histologic picture of inherited nerve deafness in man and animals. Arch. Otolaryng. *51*, 852, 1950.
6. Anderson, W. A., and Davis, C. C.: Congenital cerebellar hypoplasia in Holstein calf. J.A.V.M.A. *117*:470, 1950.
7. Antelyes, J.: Objectionable behavior in pet animals. Vet. Med. Small Anim. Clin. *62*, 774, 1967.
8. Armistead, W. W.: Harmful effects of heat. In Catcott, E. J., ed.: *Canine Medicine*. American Veterinary Publications, Inc., Santa Barbara, Cal., 1968, p. 261.
9. Asbury, A. K., Victor, M., and Adams, R. D.: Uremic polyneuropathy. Arch. Neurol. *8*, 413, 1963.
10. Averill, D. R.: Treatment of status epilepticus in dogs with diazepam sodium. J.A.V.M.A. *156*, 432, 1970.
11. Baker, A. B.: *An Outline of Neurology*. Wm. C. Brown, Dubuque, Iowa, 1958.
12. Baker, A. B. (ed.): *Clinical Neurology*, 2d ed. Hoeber, Medical Division of Harper and Row, New York, 1962.
13. Baker, J. A., and Gillespie, J. H.: Virus diseases. In *Canine Medicine*, 2d ed. American Veterinary Publications, Inc., Santa Barbara, Cal., 1959, Chap. 22.
14. Bardens, J. W.: Congenital malformation of the foramen magnum in dogs. Southwest. Vet. *18*, 1965.
15. Bardens, J. W.: Glycogen storage disease in puppies. Vet. Med. Small Anim. Clin. *61*, 1174, 1966.
16. Bistner, S., Rubin, L. F., Cox, T. A., and Condon, W. E.: Pharmacologic diagnosis of Horner's syndrome. J.A.V.M.A. *157*, 1220, 1970.
17. Blake, R., and Antoinetti, D. M.: Abnormal visual resolution in the Siamese cat. Science *194*, 109–110, 1976.
18. Bloom, F.: Diseases of endocrine glands. In Catcott, E. J. (ed.): *Canine Medicine*. American Veterinary Publications, Inc., Santa Barbara, Cal., 1968, p. 430.
19. Bradley, O. C., and Graham, T.: *Topographical Anatomy of the Dog*, 4th ed. Macmillan Co., New York, 1943.
20. Bradley, W. E., and Teague, C. T.: Cerebellar influence on the micturition reflex. Exp. Neurol. *23*, 399–411, 1969.
21. Breazile, J. E., Blaugh, B. D., and Nail, N.: Experimental study of canine distemper myoclonus. Am J. Vet. Res. *27*, 1375, 1966.
22. Breazile, J. E., and Thompson, W. D.: Motor cortex of the dog. Am J. Vet. Res. *28*, 1483–1486, 1967.
23. Brugghen, A. ver.: *Neurosurgery in General Practice*, Charles C Thomas, Springfield, Ill., 1952.
24. Brunner, F.: The application of behavior studies in small animal practice. In Fox, M. W. (ed.). *Abnormal Behavior in Animals*. W. B. Saunders Co. Philadelphia, 1968.
25. Brutkowski, S.: Functions of prefrontal cortex in animals. Physiol. Rev. *45*, 721–746, 1965.
26. Bucy, P. C.: The human neural mechanism controlling skeletal muscular activity. In Mosberg, W. H. (ed.): *Clinical Neurosurgery*. The Williams & Wilkins Co., Baltimore, 1962.
27. Buxton, D. F., and Goodman, D. C.: Motor function and the corticospinal tracts in the dog and raccoon. J. Comp. Neurol. *129*, 341–360, 1967.

28. Cassinari, V., and Pagni, V.: *Central Pain, a Neurosurgical Survey.* Harvard University Press, Cambridge, Mass., 1969.
29. Chang, H. T.: Choreiform movements in a dog suffering from cortico-striatal disease. J. Neurophys. *8*, 89, 1945.
30. Clark, E., and O'Malley, C. D.: *The Human Brain and Spinal Cord.* University of California Press, Los Angeles, 1968.
31. Cogan, D. G.: *Neurology of the Ocular Muscles.* Charles C Thomas, Springfield, Ill., 1948.
32. Coruville, C. B.: Contribution to study of cerebral anoxia. Bull. Los Angeles Neurol. Soc. *15*, 99, 1950.
33. Croft, P. G.: Fits in dogs: A survey of 260 cases. Vet. Rec. *77*, 438, 1965.
34. Croft, P. G.: Conditions affecting the central nervous system in small animals. J. Small Anim. Pract. *6*, 261, 1965.
35. Croft, P. C.: The use of the electro-encephalograph in the detection of epilepsy as a hereditary condition in the dog. Vet. Rec. *82*, 712, 1968.
36. Crosby, E. C., and Henderson, J. W.: The mammalian midbrain and isthmus region. II. Fiber connections of the superior colliculus. B. Pathways concerned in automatic eye movements. J. Comp. Neurol. *88*, 53–92, 1948.
37. Crosby, E. C., Yoss, R. E., and Henderson, J. W.: The mammalian midbrain and isthmus region. Part II. The fiber connections. D. The pattern for eye movements on the frontal eye field and the discharge of specific portions of this field to and through midbrain levels. J. Comp. Neurol. *97*, 357–383, 1952.
38. Crosby, E. C. Humphrey, T., and Laver, E. W.: *Anatomy of the Nervous System.* Macmillan Co., New York, 1962.
39. Crosby, E. C., Schneider, R., DeJonge, B., and Syonyi, P. The alterations of tonus and movements through the interplay betweeen the cerebral hemispheres and the cerebellum. J. Comp. Neurol. *127*, suppl. 1, 1–91, 1966.
40. Dahme, E., and Schiefer, B.: Intracranielle Geschwülste bei Tieren. Zbl. Vet. *7*, 341, 1960.
41. deLahunta, A.: Feline vestibular disease. In Kirk, R. W. (ed.): *Current Veterinary Therapy III, Small Animal Practice.* W. B. Saunders Co., Philadelphia, 1968, p. 466.
42. Denny-Brown, D.: *The Basal Ganglia.* University Press, Oxford, 1962.
43. Detweiler, K. K., Ratcliffe, H. L., and Luginbühl, H.: Significance of naturally occuring coronary and cerebral arterial disease in animals. Ann. N. Y. Acad. Sci. *149*, part 2, 868, 1968.
44. Dexler, H.: Über Pachymeningitis ossificans chronica und Compressions myelitis beim Hunde. Weim. Med. Presse *35*, 1998, 1893.
45. Dow, R. S., and Moruzzi, G.: *The Physiology and Pathology of the Cerebellum.* University of Minnesota Press, Minneapolis, 1958.
46. Drachman, D. A., Wetzel, N., Wasserman, M., and Naito, H.: Experimental denervation of ocular muscles. Arch. Neurol. *21*, 170–183, 1969.
47. Duke-Elder, S.: *System of Ophthalmology.* I. *The Eye in Evolution.* C. V. Mosby Co., St. Louis, 1950, pp. 688–689.
48. Dusser de Barenne, J. G.: Experimentelle Physiologie des Kleinhirns. Brmke W. Foerster's Handbook Neurol. *2*, 235–267, 1937.
49. Eccles, J. C., Ito, M., and Szentagothai, J.: *The Cerebellum as a Neuronal Machine.* Springer-Verlag, New York, 1967.
50. Egerton, N., Egerton, W. S., and Kay, J. H.: Neurologic changes following profound hypothermia. Ann. Surg. *157*, 366, 1963.
51. Elliott, H. C.: *Textbook of Neuroanatomy,* 2d ed. J. B. Lippincott Co., Philadelphia, 1969.
52. Emerson, J. D., Bruhn, J. M., Foley, J. O., and Emerson, G. M.: Autonomic responses to chronic electrode stimulation of cerebellum. Am. J. Physiol. *201*, 697–699, 1961.
53. Emmerson, J. L., and Deley, A. L.: Cerebellar hypoplasia, hypomyelinogenesis, and congenital tremors of fits associated with prenatal hog cholera vaccination of sows. J.A.V.M.A. *147*, 47, 1965.
54. Fankhauser, R., Luginbühl, H., and McGrath, J. T.: Cerebrovascular disease in various animal species. Ann. N. Y. Acad. Sci. *127*,817, 1965.
55. Fennegan, F. M., and Puiggari, M. J.: Influence on gastric motility in dogs. J. Neurosurg. *24*, 497–504, 1966.
56. Ferrier, D.: *The Functions of the Brain,* 2d ed. Smith, Elder, London, 1886.
57. Few, A. B.: The study of the clinical signs and necropsy findings resulting from experimentally produced intracranial lesions in the dog. Thesis, Auburn University, Auburn, Alabama, 1964.
58. Fisher, C. A., and Jones, G.; Optic neuritis in dogs. J.A.V.M.A. *160*, 68–79, 1972.
59. Fisher, C. A., and Liu, S.-K.: Neuro-opthalmologic manifestations of primary reticulosis of the central nervous system in a dog. J.A.V.M.A. *158*, 1240–1248, 1971.
60. Foldi, M., Csanda, E., Zoltan, O. T., and Dobranovics, I.: Oedema of the optic nerve and the retina as a consequence of experimental cervical lymphatic blockage. Angiologica *4*, 341–347, 1967.
61. Forman, D.: Responses to electrical stimulation of caudate nucleus in cats in chronic experiments. J. Neurophysiol. *20*, 230, 1957.
62. Fox, M. W.: Development abnormalities of canine skull. Canad. J. Comp. Med. Vet. Sci. *27*, 219, 1963.
63. Fox, M. W.: Otocephalic syndrome in the dog. Corn. Vet. *54*, 250, 1964.
64. Fox, M. W.: *Canine Behavior.* Charles C Thomas, Springfield, Ill., 1965.
65. Fox, M. W.: *Abnormal Behavior in Animals.* W. B. Saunders Co., Philadelphia, 1968.
66. Fox, C. A., and Snider, R. S.: *The Cerebellum.* Elsevier Publishing Co., New York, 1967.
67. Fox, J. G., and Gutnick, M. J.: Horner's syndrome and brachial paralysis due to lymphosarcoma in a cat. J.A.V.M.A. *160*, 977–980, 1972.
68. Fraser, D. C., Palmer, A. C., Senior, J. E. B., Parkes, J. D., and Yealland, M. F. T.: Myasthenia gravis in the dog. J. Neurol. Neurosurg. Psychiat. *33*, 431–437, 1970.

69. Frauchiger, E., and Fankhauser, R.: *Die Nervenkrankheiten Unserer Hunde.* Schmid and Cie, Bern, 1949.
70. Frauchiger, E., and Fankhauser, R.: *Vergleichende Neuropathologie.* Springer Publishing, Berlin, 1957.
71. Fritsch, G., and Hitzig, E.: Ueber die elektrische Erregbarkeit des Grosshirns. Arch. Anat. Physiol. Wissensch. Med. *37,* 300–322, 1870.
72. Gastaut, H., Bernard-Badier, M., Darraspen, M., and van Bozaert, L.: Anatomic and clinical study of 19 epileptic dogs. In Baldwin, M., and Bailey, P. (ed.); *Temporal Lobe Epilepsy.* Charles C Thomas, Springfield, Ill., 1958.
73. Gelatt, K. N., and Leopold, H. W.: Bilateral optic nerve hypoplasia in two dogs. Can. Vet. J. *12,* 91–96, 1971.
74. Geltzer, A. I.: Autonomic innervation of the cat iris. Arch. Ophth. *81,* 70–83, 1969.
75. Gol, A., and Faibish, G. M.: Effects of human hippocampal ablation. J. Neurosurg. *26,* 390–398, 1967.
76. Goltz, F.: Der Hunde ohne Grosshirn. Pflugers Arch. Ges. Physiol. *51,* 570–614, 1892.
77. Gottschalk, P. G., and Thomas, J. E.: Heat stroke. Mayo Clin. Proc. *41,* 470, 1966.
78. Gould, G. M. *Blakiston's New Gould Medical Dictionary.* Blakiston Co., Inc. New York, 1972.
79. Green, J. R., and Scheetz, D. G.: Surgery of epileptogenic lesions of the temporal lobe. Arch. Neurol. *10,* 135–148, 1964.
80. Green, J. R.: Temporal lobectomy, with special reference to selection of epileptic patients. J. Neurosurg. *26,* 584–593, 1967.
81. Grinker, R. R., and Sahs, A. L.: *Neurology.* Charles C Thomas, Springfield, Ill., 1966.
82. Guth, L., and Bernstein, J. J.: Selectivity in the reestablishment of synapses in the superior cervical sympathetic ganglion of the cat. Exp. Neurol. *4,* 59–69, 1961.
83. Guyton, A. C.: *Textbook of Medical Physiology,* 5th ed. W. B. Saunders Co., Philadelphia, 1976.
84. Hagen, L. O.: Lipid dystrophic changes in the central nervous system of dogs. Acta Path. Microbiol. Scand. *33,* 22, 1953.
85. Hamuy, T. Pinto, Bromiley, R. B., and Woolsey, C. N.: Somatic afferent areas I and II of dog's cerebral cortex. J. Neurophysiol. *19,* 485, 1956.
86. Harrinton, D. O.: *The Visual Fields.* C. V. Mosby Co., St. Louis, 1964, pp. 25–29, 83–87.
87. Henkind, P., Gould, H. B., and Bellhorn, R. W.: Optic nerve transection in cat's effector retinal vessels. Invest. Ophthalmol. *14,* 610–613, 1973.
88. Hjarre, A.: Über Tuberkulose bei Hunden und Katzen. Acta Tuberc. Scand. *13,* 125, 1939.
89. Hoerlein, B. F.: Cardiac resuscitation in a dog with cardiac arrest. J.A.V.M.A. *127,* 210, 1955.
90. Hoerlein, B. F.: Heat stroke. In Kirk, R. W. (ed.): *Current Veterinary Therapy III, Small Animal Practice.* W. B. Saunders Co., Philadelphia, 1968, p. 103.
91. Hoff, H. E., and Breckenridge, C. G.: Observations on the mammalian reflex prototype of the sign of Babinski. Brain *79,* 155, 1965.
92. Horsley, V., and Clarke, R. H.: The structure and function of the cerebellum examined by a new method. Brain *31,* 45–124, 1908.
93. Howard, D. R., and Breazile, J. E.: Optic fiber projections to the dorsal lateral geniculate nucleus in the dog. Am. J. Vet. Res. *34*:419–424, 1973.
94. Innes, J. R. M., and Saunders, L. Z.: *Comparative Neuropathology.* Academic Press, New York, 1962.
95. Innes, J. R. M.: Subacute diffuse sclerosing encephalitis in the dog. Neurology *18,* 161, 1968.
96. Jenkins, T. W.: *Functional Mammalian Neuroanatomy.* Lea & Febiger, Phialdelphia, 1972.
97. Jennet, W. B., and Stern, E. W.: Tentorial herniation, the midbrain and the pupil. J. Neurosurg. *17,* 598, 1960.
98. Jones, B. R., and Studdert, V.: Horner's syndrome in the dog and cat as an aid to diagnosis. Aust. Vet. J. *51,* 329–332, 1975.
99. Jubb, K. V., Saunders, L. Z., and Coates, H. V.: The intraocular lesions in canine distemper. J. Comp. Pathol. *67,* 21–29, 1957.
100. Kalil, R., Jhaveri, S., and Richards, W. R.: Anomalous retinal pathways in Siamese cats—An inadequate substrate for normal binocular vision. Science *174,* 302, 1971.
101. Kerr, F. W. L., and Hollowell, O. W.: Location of pupillomotor and accommodation fibers in the oculomotor nerve: Experimental observations on paralytic mydriasis. J. Neurol. Neurosurg. Psychiat. *27,* 473–481, 1964.
102. Kestenbaum, A.: *Clinical Methods of Neuro-ophthalmologic Examination,* 2d ed. Grune and Stratton, New York, 1961, pp. 189–191.
103. Kilham, L., and Margolis, G.: Cerebellar disease in cats induced by inoculation of rat virus. Science *148,* 244, 1965.
104. Kilham, L. G., Margolis, G., and Colby, E. D.: Congenital infections of cats and ferrets by feline panleukopenia virus manifested by cerebellar hypoplasia. Lab. Invest. *17,* 465, 1965.
105. Kirk, R. W.: Hypoglycemia. In Kirk, R. W. (ed.): *Current Veterinary Therapy III, Small Animal Practice.* W. B. Saunders Co., Philadelphia, 1968, p. 78.
106. Koestner, A., and Zeman, W.: Primary reticuloses of the central nervous system in dogs. Am. J. Vet. Res. *23,* 381, 1962.
107. Kluver, H., and Bucy, P. C.: Preliminary analysis of function of the temporal lobes in monkeys. Arch. Neurol. Psych. *42,* 979–1000, 1939.
108. Koppang, N.: Lipodystrophia cerebri in the English setter. J. Small Anim. Pract. *4, 37,* 1963.
109. Krakowka, S., McCullough, B., Koestner, A., and Olsen, R.: Myelin-specific autoantibodies associated with central nervous system demyelination in canine distemper virus infection. Infect. Immun. *8*(5), 819–827, 1973.
110. Kreiner, J.: The myeloarchitectonics of the frontal cortex of the dog. J. Comp. Neurol. *116,* 117, 1961.
111. Kreiner, J.: Myeloarchitectonics of the cingular cortex in dogs. J. Comp. Neurol. *119,* 255–267, 1962.

112. Kreiner, J., and Maksymowicz, K.: A three dimensional model of the striated nuclei in the dog's brain. Acta Biol. Exp. *22*, 69–79, 1962.
113. Kreiner, J.: Myeloarchitectonics of the parietal cortex in dog. Acta Biol. Exp. *24*, 195–212, 1964.
114. Kreiner, J.: Myeloarchitectonics of the sensorimotor cortex in dog. J. Comp. Neurol. *122*, 181–200, 1964.
115. Kreiner, J.: Myeloarchitectonics of the perisylvian cortex in dog. J. Comp. Neurol. *123*, 231–242, 1964.
116. Kreiner, J.: Myeloarchitectonics of the occipital cortex in dog and general remarks on the myeloarchitectonics of the dog. J. Comp. Neurol. *127*, 531–558, 1966.
117. Kreiner, J.: Homologies of the fissural and gyral pattern of the hemispheres of the dog and monkey. Acta Anta. *70*, 137–167, 1968.
118. Kurtz, H. J., and Fletcher, T. F.: The peripheral neuropathy of canine globoid-cell leukodystrophy (Krabbe-type). Acta Neuropathol. *16*, 226–232, 1970.
119. Kutt, H., and McDowell, F.: Management of epilepsy with diphenylhydantoin sodium. J.A.M.A. *203*, 969, 1968.
120. Langfitt, T. W., Weinstein, J. D., and Kassell, N. F.: Cerebral vasomotor paralysis produced by intracranial hypertension. Neurology *15*, 622, 1965.
121. Laties, A. M., and Sprague, J. M.: The projection of optic nerve fibers to the visual centers in the cat. J. Comp. Neurol. *127*, 35–70, 1966.
122. Leader, R. W.: The kinship of animal and human diseases. Sci. Am. *216*, 110, 1967.
123. Levinson, B. M.: Interpersonal relationships between pet and human being. In Fox, M. W. (ed.): *Abnormal Behavior in Animals*. W. B. Saunders Co., Philadelphia, 1968, Chap. 26.
124. Liles, S., and Davis, G. D.: Interrelation of caudate nucleus and lateral thalamus in regulation of somatic motor activity in anesthetized and awake cats. Fed. Proc. *27*, 387, 1968.
125. Liles, S. L., and Davis, G. D.: Athetoid and choreiform hyperkinesias produced by caudate lesions in the cat. Science *164*, 195–197, 1969.
126. Lorenz, M., de Lahunta, A., and Alstrom, D.: Neostigmine-responsive weakness in the dog, similar to myasthenia gravis. J.A.V.M.A. *161*, 795–800, 1972.
127. Luciani, L.: *Human Physiology* (5 vols.). Translated by Welby, F. A., Macmillan, London, 1915.
128. Luginbühl, H: Study of meningiomas in cats. Am. J. Vet. Res. *22*, 1031, 1961.
129. Luginbühl, H., Fankhauser, R., and McGrath, J. T.: Spontaneous neoplasms of the nervous system in animals. Progr. Neurol. Surg. *2*, 85, 1968.
130. Magnus, R.: *Korperstellung*. Springer-Verlag, Berlin, 1924.
131. Marine, D., and Lenhart, C. H.: Effects of the administration or the withholding of iodine-containing compounds in normal, colloid or actively hyperplastic (parenchymatous) thyroid of dogs. Arch. Int. Med. *4*, 253, 1909.
132. McGrath, J. T.: *Neurologic Examination of the Dog*, 2d ed. Lea and Febiger, Philadelphia, 1960.
133. McLaurin, R. L., and Helmer, F. A.: Errors in diagnosis of intracranial tumors. J.A.M.A. *180*, 1011, 1962.
134. Mettler, F. A., Finch, G., Girden, E., and Culler, E.: Acoustic value of the several components of the auditory pathway. Brain *57*, 475–483, 1934.
135. Mettler, F. A., and Goss, L. J.: Canine chorea due to strio-cerebellar degeneration of unknown etiology. J.A.V.M.A. *108*, 377–384, 1946.
136. Miller, M. E., Christensen, G. C., and Evans, H. E.: *Anatomy of the Dog*. W. B. Saunders Co., Philadelphia, 1964.
137. Monti, F.: Semiologia neuro-oftalmologica veterinaria. Annali della Facolta di Medicina Veterinaria di Torino *9*, 1–83, 1959.
138. Morgan, L. O.: Corpus striatum. A study of secondary degenerations following lesions in man and of symptoms and acute degenerations following experimental lesions in cats. Arch. Neurol. Psych. *18*, 495–549, 1927.
139. Moruzzi, G., and Magoun, H. W.: Brain stem reticular formation and activation of the E.E.G. EEG Clin. Neurophysiol. *1*, 445–473, 1949.
140. Mountcastle, V. B.: Somatic functions of the nervous system. Ann. Rev. Physiol. *20*, 487, 1958.
141. Neely, W. A., and Youmans, J. R.: Anoxia of canine brain without damage. J.A.M.A. *183*, 1085, 1963.
142. Newberne, J. W., Robinson, V. B., Estill, L., and Brinkman, D. C.: Granular structures in brains of apparently normal dogs. Am. J. Vet. Res. *21*, 782, 1960.
143. Newberne, P. M., and Hare, V.: Axon dystrophy in clinically normal dogs. Am. J. Vet. Res. *23*, 403, 1962.
144. Newman, P. P., and Paul, D. H.: The representation of some visceral afferents in the anterior lobe of the cerebellum. J. Physiol. *182*, 195–208, 1966.
145. Newman, P. P., and Paul, D. H.: The projection of splanchnic afferents on the cerebellum of the cat J. Physiol. *202*, 223–238, 1969.
146. Norrsell, U.: A conditioned reflex study of sensory defects caused by cortical somato-sensory ablations. Physiol. Behav. *2*, 73–81, 1967.
147. Oliver, J. E.: Hepatic neuropathies–a review with two case histories. Vet Med. Small Anim. Clin. *60*, 499, 1965.
148. Oliver, J. E., and Geary, J. C.: Cerebellar anomalies—two cases. Vet. Med. Small Anim. Clin. *60*, 697, 1965.
149. Oliver, J. E., and Hoerlein, B. F.: Convulsive disorders of dogs. J.A.V.M.A. *146*, 1126, 1965.
150. Oliver, J. E., Jr.: Canine cranial surgery. Thesis, Auburn University, Auburn, Alabama, 1966.
151. Oliver, J. E., Jr.: Principles of canine brain surgery. Animal Hosp. *2*, 73–88, 1966.
152. Oliver, J. E., Jr.: Brain tumor in a dog. Vet. Med. Small Anim. Clin. *61*, 29–34, 1966.
153. Oliver, J. E., Jr. Fletcher, T. F., and Purinton, P. T.: Unpublished data.
154. Palmer, A. C.: Clinical and pathological features of some tumors of the central nervous system in dogs. Res. Vet. Sci. *1*, 36, 1960.
155. Palmer, A. C.: The accident case. IV. C.N.S. J. Small Anim. Pract. *5*, 25, 1964.

156. Palmer, A. C.: *Introduction to Animal Neurology.* F. A. Davis Co., Philadelphia, 1965.
157. Palmer, A. C.: *Introduction to Animal Neurology,* 2d ed. Blackwell Scientific Publications, London, 1976.
158. Papez, J. W.: A proposed mechanism of emotion. Arch. Neurol. Psych. *38,* 725–744, 1937.
159. Parker, A. J., Cusick, P. K., Park, R. D., and Small, E.: Hemifacial spasms in a dog. Vet. Rec. *93,* 514–516, 1973.
160. Pavlov, I. P.: *Conditioned Reflexes, an Investigation of the Physiological Activity of the Cerebral Cortex.* Oxford University Press, London, 1927.
161. Penfield, W., and Rasmussen, T.: *The Cerebral Cortex of Man.* Macmillan Co., New York, 1950.
162. Percy, D. H., Olander, H. J., and Carmichael, L. E.: Encephalitis in the newborn pup due to a canine herpesvirus. Path. Vet. *5,* 135, 1968.
163. Percy, D. H., Munnel, J. F., Olander, H. J., and Carmichael, L. E.: Pathogenesis of canine herpesvirus encephalitis. Am. J. Vet. Res. *31,* 145, 1970.
164. Percy, D. H., and Jortner, B. S.: Feline lipidosis, Light and electron microscopic studies. Arch. Pathol. *92,* 136–144, 1971.
165. Plum, F., and Posner, J. B.: *The Diagnosis of Stupor and Coma.* F. A. Davis Co., Philadelphia, 1966.
166. Pribram, K. H., and Kruger, L.: Functions of the olfactory brain. Ann. N.Y. Acad. Sci. *58,* 109–138, 1954.
167. Prince, J. H.: *Comparative Anatomy of the Eye.* Charles C Thomas, Springfield, Ill., 1956, pp. 26–30.
168. Rademaker, G. G. J.: *Das Stehen.* Springer-Verlag, Berlin, 1931.
169. Redding, R. W., and Prynn, R. B.: Seizures. In Kirk, R. W. (ed.): *Current Veterinary Therapy III, Small Animal Practice,* W. B. Saunders Co., Philadelphia, 1968, p. 463.
170. Redding, R. W.: Seizures, differential diagnosis, and therapy. Norden News *44,* 26, Winter, 1969.
171. Redding, R. W.: Diagnosis and therapy of seizures. Animal Hosp. *5,* 79, 1969.
172. Reid, C. L.: Hypothyroidism. In Kirk, R. W. (ed.): *Current Veterinary Therapy III, Small Animal Practice.* W. B. Saunders Co., Philadelphia, 1968, p. 555.
173. Renfrew, S.: *An Introduction to Diagnostic Neurology.* Vol. 1, Livingstone, Edinburgh, 1967.
174. Ribelin, W. E., and Kinter, L. D.: Lipodystrophy of the central nervous system in a dog. A disease with similarity to Tay-Sachs disease of man. Corn. Vet. *46,* 532, 1956.
175. Roberts, T. D. M.: *Neurophysiology of Postural Mechanisms.* Plenum Press, New York, 1967.
176. Roberts, S. R., and Vainisi, S. J.: Hemifacial spasm in dogs. J.A.V.M.A. *150,* 381–385, 1967.
177. Rubin, L. F.: Neurophthalmology. In Hoerlein, B. F. (ed.): *Canine Neurology,* 2d ed. W. B. Saunders Co., Philadelphia, 1971.
178. Saunders, L. Z.: Congenital optic nerve hypoplasia in collie dogs. Corn. Vet. *42,* 67–90, 1952.
179. Sawyers, G. T., Webster, D. D., and Schut, L. J.: Treatment of uncontrolled seizure activity with diazepam. J.A.M.A. *203,* 913, 1968.
180. Schafer, E. A.: *Textbook of Physiology.* Vol. 2. Young J. Pentland, Edinburgh, 1900.
181. Schilder, P.: Loss of a brightness discrimination in the cat following removal of the striate area. J. Neurophysiol. *29,* 888, 1966.
182. Schlotthauer, C. F.: The nervous system, diseases of the brain. In *Canine Medicine,* 2d ed. American Veterinary Publications, Inc., Santa Barbara, Cal., 1959, Chap. 15.
183. Schmidt, G.: An algorithm for sudden acquired blindness. Canine Pract. July-August, 1975, pp. 14–19.
184. Schmidt, J. P.: Psychosomatics in veterinary medicine. In Fox, M. W. (ed.): *Abnormal Behavior in Animals.* W. B. Saunders Co., Philadelphia, 1968, Chap. 21.
185. Schneider, G. E.: Two visual systems. Science *163,* 895–902, 1969.
186. Schreiner, L., and Kling, A.: Behavioral changes following rhinencephalic injury in cat. J. Neurophysiol. *16,* 643–695, 1953.
187. Scott, F. W., and Gillespie, J. H.: Recent advances in feline leukopenia. Proc. 36th Ann. Animal Hosp. Assoc. *111,* 1969.
188. Scott, D. W., and Bistner, S. I.: Veterinary medicine. Small Anim. Clin. 1120–1122, Oct. 1973.
189. Sherman, S. M.: Visual judgment in cats. Invest. Ophthalmol. *11*(5), 394–401, 1972.
190. Sherrington, C. S.: In Denny-Brown, D. (ed.): *Selected Writings of Sir Charles Sherrington.* Hoeber, Medical Division of Harper and Row, New York, 1940.
191. Shultz, G., and Delay, P.: Losses in newborn lambs associated with bluetongue vaccinaton of pregnant ewes. J.A.V.M.A. *127,* 224, 1955.
192. Siegel, E. T., and Belshaw, B. E.: Laboratory evaluation of adrenocortical and thyroid functions in the dog. Kirk, R. W. (ed.) *Current Veterinary Therapy III, Small Animal Practice.* W. B. Saunders Co., Philadelphia, 1968, p. 545.
193. Singleton, M. C., and Peele, T. L.: Distribution of optic fibers in the cat. J. Comp. Neurol. *125,* 303–328, 1965.
194. Speck, R. V.: Mental health problems involving the family, the pet, and the veterinarian. J.A.V.M.A. *145,* 150, July, 1964.
195. Sprague, J. M.: Interaction of cortex and superior colliculus in mediation of visually guided behavior in the cat. Science *153,* 1544, 1966.
196. Sprague, J. M.: Visual, acoustic, and somesthetic deficits in the cat after cortical and midbrain lesions. In Purpura, D. P., and Yahr, M. (eds.): *The Thalamus,* Columbia University Press, New York, 1966.
197. Steinberg, S. A.: Idiopathic or primary demyelination of the brain stem and spinal cord. Cinicopathologic Conference. J.A.V.M.A. *143,*404, 1963.
198. Stockard, C. R.: The genetic and endocrinic basis for differences in form and behavior. Amer. Anat. Mem. No. 19., Wistar Inst. Anat. Biol., 1941.
199. Stone, A. B.: Variant lesions in the central nervous system of dogs and cats. J. Small Anim. Pract. *10,* 287, 1969.
200. Stone, A. B., and Fox, M. W.: Clinico-pathological studies of an encephalitic syndrome in dogs. J. Small Anim. Pract. *8,* 709, 1967.

201. Stone, J.: The naso-temporal division of the cat retina. J. Comp. Neurol. *126*, 585–600, 1966.
202. Tower, S. S., and Hines, M.: Dissociation of the pyramidal and extrapyramidal functions of the frontal lobe. Science *82*, 376, 1935.
203. Trevino, G. S.: Canine blastomycosis with ocular involvement. Path. Vet. *3*, 652–658, 1966.
204. Tunturi, A. R.: A study of the pathway from the medial geniculate body to the acoustic cortex in the dog. Am. J. Physiol. *147*, 311–319, 1948.
205. Tunturi, A. R.: Physiological determination of the arrangement of the afferent connections to the middle ectosylvian area in the dog. Am. J. Physiol. *162*, 489–502, 1950.
206. Turner, T.: Treatment of convulsions in dogs. Vet. Rec. *81*, 386, 1967.
207. Walsh, E. G.: *Physiology of the Nervous System.* 2d ed. Longmans, Green and Co., London, 1964.
208. Walton, J. N.: *Essentials of Neurology.* J. B. Lippincott Co., Philadelphia, 1961.
209. Waltz, T. A., and Ehni, G.: The thalamic syndrome and its mechanism. J. Neurosurg. *24*, 735, 1966.
210. Ward, G. M.: Bovine cerebellar hypoplasia apparently caused by BVD-MD virus, a case report. Corn. Vet. *59*, 570, 1969.
211. Wechsler, I. S.: *Clinical Neurology*, 9th ed. W. B. Saunders Co., Philadelphia, 1963.
212. Westphal, K., and Bär, R.: Ueber die Entstehung des Schlogenfalles. Deutsche Arch. Klin. Med. *151*, 31, 1926.
213. Weymouth, F. W.: The eye as an optical instrument. In Ruch, T. C., and Patton, H. D. (ed.): *Physiology and Biophysics*, 20th ed. 3 vol. W. B. Saunders Co., Philadelphia, 1973–1976.
214. Whisnant, J. P., Sayre, G. P., and Millikan, C. H.: Experimental intracerebral hematoma. Arch. Neurol. *9*, 586, 1963.
215. White, J. C.: Familial periodic nystagmus, vertigo, and ataxia. Arch. Neurol. *20*, 276, 1969.
216. White, P. T., Plott, D., and Norton, J.: Relative anticonvulsant potency of primidone. Arch. Neurol. *14*, 31, 1966.
217. Whittier, J. R.: Flexor spasm syndrome in the carnivore. I, II, III. Am. J. Vet. Res. *17*, 720, 1956.
218. Wilkins, R. H., Silver, D., and Odom, G. L.: The role of circulating substances in intracranial arterial spasm. I. Serotonin and histamine. Neurology *16*, 482, 1966.
219. Winans, S. S.: Visual form discrimination after removal of the visual cortex in cats. Science *158*, 944–946, 1967.
220. Wisniewski, H. K., Raine, C., and Kay, W.: Observations on viral demyelinating encephalomyelitis. Lab. Invest. *26*(5), 589–599, 1972.
221. Wright, N. G., and Cornell, H. J.: Symposium: Neonatal diseases of the dog. I. Viral induced neonatal disease in puppies. J. Small Anim. Pract. *9*, 449, 1968.
222. Woolsey, C. N.: Postural regulations of the frontal and motor cortex of the dog. Brain *56*, 353–370, 1933.
223. Woolsey, C. N.: Second somatic receiving area in the cerebral cortex cat, dog, and monkey. Fed. Proc. *2*, 55, 1943.
224. Woolsey, C. N.: Some observations on brain fissuration in relation to cortical localization of function. In Tower, D. B., and Schade, J. P. (eds.): *Structure and Function of the Cerebral Cortex.* Elsevier Publishing, Amsterdam, 1960.
225. Zimmerman, J. M., Nielson, H. C., King, T. C., and Colliver, J. C.: The effect of cerebral ischemia on learning and retention in dogs. J.A.M.A. *197*, 166, 1966.

CHAPTER 19

BEHAVIORAL DISORDERS

SECTION 1

PRINCIPLES OF BEHAVIOR

Victoria Lea Voith, D.V.M.
Benjamin L. Hart, D.V.M., Ph.D.

INTRODUCTION

When an animal exhibits behavior injurious to itself or unacceptable to its owner, the alternatives to existing with the unpleasant situation are either to change the behavior or to dispose of the pet. Unfortunately, until recently the most common way to eliminate a behavioral problem has been the latter. Frequently these pets are enjoyable companions but have acquired one trait which is intolerable. Perhaps it is because of this dual nature of the pet that the decision to dispose of it is so painful. It is frequently more emotionally disturbing for an owner to destroy a pet because of a behavioral problem than because of an infectious or traumatic physical disorder.

Animal behavior constitutes an integral part of veterinary practice, and veterinarians have many methods of treating behavioral problems. Veterinarians committed to promoting animal well-being will find that saving a life of an animal by correcting a behavioral disorder is as rewarding as treating it for an infectious or traumatic disease. Many behavioral problems, when properly diagnosed, can be treated effectively by using behavioral modification techniques, drugs, hormones, or even electroconvulsive shock therapy or neurosurgery.

Treating behavioral disorders creates a new dimension in practice and allows an expansion of the capacities of the practitioner. As with any new discipline, some clinicians may be hesitant to attempt it, but those who do will be surprised at the number of successes they experience. Again, because of the newness of this discipline, much is unknown. New and better approaches are constantly being developed. There are few guidelines for dosages of specific psychotropic drugs, yet ultimately precise utilization of such drugs may be commonplace. Incorporation of behavior modification techniques in a therapeutic regime may be awkward and tedious at first, but as expertise is developed the procedures can be done simply and quickly, and can be put into everyday use. Advising clients about the behavior of their pets has always been a part of veterinary practice, and veterinarians now can expand this role to a method of treatment.

CLASSIFICATION OF BEHAVIOR PROBLEMS

When there is a behavior problem, a primary diagnosis must be made before adequate treatment can be initiated. The major classifications of problems, which may be interrelated, are (1) objectionable species-typical behavior, (2) primary organic disorders, (3) genetically determined abnormal behavior, (4) adverse early experiences, (5) undesirable learned behavior, and (6) psychosomatic manifestations.

OBJECTIONABLE SPECIES-TYPICAL BEHAVIOR

One of the clinician's first tasks is to determine if the undesirable behavior is normal for that species. There are several natural and characteristic behavior patterns that owners may find undesirable in a pet. Such patterns include urine marking (leg lifting in dogs; spraying in cats), intermale fighting, and extreme forms of some types of aggression (competitive, maternal, or even pain-induced). Simply because a behavior is objectionable does not mean that it is abnormal, and, conversely, just because a behavior occurs naturally does not mean that it is unalterable. Manipulation of hormonal, neuronal, or environmental factors can alter the expression of normal behavior.

ORGANIC DISORDERS

Organic disorders of the nervous, somatic, or endocrine systems resulting from infectious, traumatic, neoplastic, or genetic diseases can cause abnormal behavior or create a predisposition to the acquisition of abnormal behavior. Polydipsia, polyphasia, aphasia, diarrhea, vomiting and hyperactivity are just a few examples of behavior that can be due to physiological abnormalities. Yet these same behavioral patterns may be the result of an emotional disturbance or a learning phenomenon.

GENETICALLY DETERMINED ABNORMAL BEHAVIOR

Physiological Disorders

Examples of behavior thought to be genetically acquired and due to physiological abnormalities are hyperkinesis and unprovoked aggressive attacks in certain breeds of dogs such as the Bernese Mountain dog and the St. Bernard.

Physiologically abnormal hyperkinetic dogs have been identified; like hyperkinetic children they respond to treatment with amphetamines.[8] The exact nervous system defect that results in the hyperkinetic syndrome has not been precisely identified or localized. The characteristic response to amphetamine is probably related to the drug's effect on the availability of norepinephrine or dopamine. Although hyperkinetic dogs do exist, it is unlikely that the number of genetically hyperkinetic animals in the present population is large, as dogs with such uncontrollable behavior are usually disposed of. The most prevalent reason for hyperactivity in dogs is that the animal has learned to get attention by such behavior.

Dogs which have a tendency toward unprovoked aggressive attacks are often described by their owners as having a glazed look in their eyes at the time of the attack and being unresponsive to auditory, visual, and tactile stimulation. These dogs usually act normally in all respects at other times. No lesions or EEG abnormalities have yet been found to be associated with this syndrome.[68] It is possible that this syndrome is a form of psychomotor epilepsy, and some practitioners have reported occasional success in treating such dogs with antiepileptic drugs such as diphenylhydantoin. However, because the drugs have sedative effects, the owners usually take other prophylactic measures, and since these attacks are manifested only sporadically, it is difficult to assess the value of antiepileptic treatment.

Functional Disorders

Inherited or genetically predisposed functional behavior abnormalities include such disorders as flank sucking in Doberman pinschers (Fig. 19–1) and wool chewing in Siamese cats. This kind of behavior may not be manifest except under certain environmental conditions, such as stress and high excitement, or unusual experiences in early life.

EARLY EXPERIENCE

Behavior is influenced at every stage of its development by genetic and environmental factors. It is important to keep in mind that although siblings and sometimes even sires and dams may exhibit similar undesirable behavior, it cannot be assumed that the behavior pattern is inherited. Exposure to the same environmental conditions, particularly early in life, can result in expression of similar behavior either in puppyhood or in adult life. The term experience refers to the exposure or lack of exposure to environmental events. The effects of early experience, which tend to be limited by critical age intervals and length of exposure time, are often manifest as general attitudinal or emotional alterations or the acquisition of maladaptive stereotypic behavior patterns.

LEARNING

Learning and experience are not the same. Learning can occur at any stage of life and is a more or less permanent modification of a specific response to a stimulus as a result of experience with that or similar stimuli. Although stimuli may elicit emotional responses via learning, such emotional responses, unlike those that result from early experience, are associated with relatively specific stimuli and are more amenable to change.

Many undesirable types of behavior of pets are a result of learning. The practitioner must become attuned to differentiating learned behavior from behavior that stems from a pathologic condition. He also needs to be aware of the contributing role that learning may play in manifestation of somatic disorders.

PSYCHOSOMATIC DISORDERS

Psychosomatic disorders are a manifestation of the reciprocal relationship between the emotions, learning, and somatic disease. Such disorders are commonly recognized in humans in the form of asthma, heart disease, peptic ulcers, gastrointestinal disorders, and neurodermatitis. That dogs, which are social creatures and live in the same environment as humans, can also develop psychosomatic disorders should not be surprising.

Psychosomatic medicine encompasses a knowledge of both the effects of physiolog-

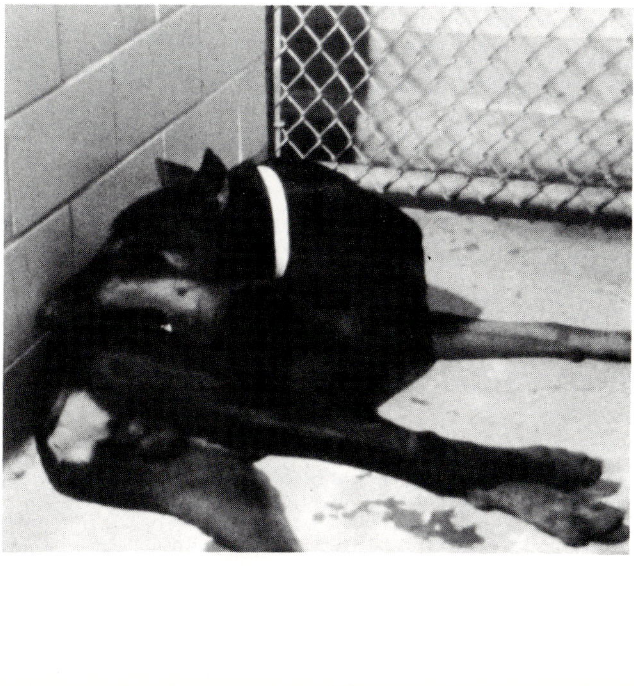

FIGURE 19–1 "Flank-sucking" in a Doberman pinscher.

ical variables on behavior and the effects of social and psychophysiological events on the predisposition, precipitation, time of onset, course, and outcome of the disease.

SUMMARY

These broad categories are not necessarily exclusive and are in fact frequently interrelated. Multiple etiologies and/or reinforcing causes must be considered. Each contributing factor must be noted in order to treat the animal effectively. A knowledge of normal animal behavior and the neuronal and endocrine control of behavior, and a careful and detailed anamnesis are prerequisites for making a reasonably accurate differential diagnosis. Observation of the animal, physical examination, and laboratory or therapeutic procedures are required to arrive at a more definite diagnosis.

THE BRAIN AND BEHAVIOR

Behavior is a function of the central nervous system, and there is great flexibility or plasticity in the neural mediation of behavior. Large areas of some parts of the brain can be destroyed and thousands of neurons may be lost with little perceptive change in behavior. Even the largest fiber tract in the brain, the corpus callosum, which contains axons that pass from one cerebral hemisphere to another, may be cut, yet the animal appears normal except when special tests are employed. But, there are other parts of the brain from which bilateral removal of an area only 2 mm in diameter will result in a major change in behavior such as the loss of sexual activity, a pronounced increase in eating, or an increase in aggressiveness.

Abnormalities in the brain that result from disease, trauma, drugs, or genetic defects may influence behavior. Tumors, for example, may suppress neural activity through pressure or destruction of neural tissue. Abnormal brain activity may be elicited by irritative processes resulting from the formation of scar tissue. Behavioral changes can be of diagnostic value in determining the location of pathological conditions in the brain. Conversely, if the site of the injury is known, it aids in understanding the behavioral changes in the animal.

There are several ways of affecting the brain indirectly and thereby altering normal behavior. Undesirable behavior such as aggressiveness or urine marking is commonly altered in domestic animals by castration. Castration of course, changes brain function, presumably by the withdrawal of testosterone. Another way of altering brain function is the systemic administration of drugs that influence behavior by acting upon certain parts of the brain through the blood supply. Blood-borne chemicals do not always reach the brain because of the blood-brain barrier, and this should be considered when deciding which hormonal or pharmacological preparations are necessary.

A more drastic way of changing brain function is by direct intervention. In experimental work the brain can be stimulated either electrically through implanted electrodes or chemically through the implantation of drugs or hormones. Brain function is also influenced by aspiration of tissue (especially cerebral cortex) or the creation of electrolytic or thermogenic lesions. Electroconvulsive shock or electroconvulsive therapy (ECT) also presumably directly alters cerebral neuronal activity but in a manner which is not understood.

The destruction of subcortical areas by electrodes lowered into the brain by the stereotaxic technique is being used more frequently as a method of changing some human behavioral patterns such as extremely violent or aggressive behavior. This approach has been utilized in clinical experiments in attempts to alter undesirable aggressive behavior in dogs[2] and urine spraying in cats.[28]

Although direct intervention in the brains of animals is not customary at the present time, there is no reason why such procedures could not be used at least in selected cases in specialized clinics. There is a great deal of information from basic research in animals that can serve as guidelines for this type of approach. Neurosurgery (psychosurgery), or ECT[48] at least offers an alternative to euthanasia.

INTERPRETING EXPERIMENTAL WORK ON BRAIN FUNCTION

Much of what is known about particular areas of the brain has been based on experiments involving the production of brain lesions or electrical and chemical stimulation of the brain. Some special considerations are pertinent in interpreting this information. Brain lesions are relatively permanent because the cells of the brain stop multiplying shortly after birth and neurons do not regenerate. Even axons in the brain that are severed do not regenerate enough to reestablish old conditions.

Brain lesions, whether caused experimentally or by disease or trauma, cause no pain except that arising from pain receptors in the skull periosteum, connective tissue, meninges, and skin. There are no pain receptors as such in the brain.

Many lesions alter a behavioral response when made bilaterally in homologous areas of the brain. These lesions can result in a behavioral deficit or an increase in a certain behavioral response. Removal of the hippocampus, for example, results in an increase in general activity.[34, 35] When a brain lesion reduces or eliminates some behavioral pattern there may be a tendency to think of the lesioned area as the "center" of that behavioral function. In the literature, for example, there are occasional references to a "sex center" or an "eating center." The word "center" is unfortunate because it implies a restricted localization of a behavioral function. Because many areas of the brain are involved in any particular behavioral pattern, the use of the term "system" is preferable. An appropriate analogy is the removal of a spark plug from an automobile engine.[19] With the spark plug out there may be vibration, spitting, coughing, and loss of power. Correspondingly, removal or sectioning of part of the brain can result in the impairment of motor control, memory loss, deficits in certain sensory functions, or elimination of a species-typical behavioral pattern. It is no more reasonable to ascribe the lost function to the destroyed brain area than to say that the function of the spark plug is to inhibit vibration, spitting, and coughing.

Care must also be taken in interpreting the results of experiments dealing with electrical brain stimulation.[53] Electrical current at the tip of an electrode acts indiscriminately on neurons and axons that project into many other brain areas. Some of the effects are excitatory and some are inhibitory. In the immediate zone of electrical stimulation neural function is undoubtedly highly distorted. In general, stimulation reveals the output effects on behavior from the stimulated area rather than the type of neural processing that occurs within the area. Another limiting characteristic of brain stimulation studies is that only a small proportion of a neural system is electrically activated. Behavioral patterns such as feeding, fighting, and sexual behavior involve the cerebral cortex, limbic system, hypothalamus, midbrain, and parts of the hindbrain. Usually in attempts to activate a certain behavior only one structural component on one side is electrically stimulated; thus only a fraction of the neurons involved in a certain behavioral pattern are directly excited.

Stimulus-Bound Behavior

Two general types of behavioral effects have been observed following electrical brain stimulation. One of the effects is referred to as "stimulus-bound" behavior, in which behavioral patterns such as eating, drinking, gnawing, hording, stalking, attacking, and copulation have been evoked by electrical stimulation, particularly in the basal forebrain. Because the behavior usually occurs when electrical stimulation is delivered, the behavior is referred to as stimulus-bound. Such stimulation seems to activate existing neural systems in the brain stem. Usually these behaviors occur only in appropriate situations—eating occurs if food is present, and copulation occurs if a female is present.

One interesting observation from such studies is that electrical stimulation of the same site does not always result in the same behavior. This may be explained by the fact that neural systems mediating behavior are not anatomically specific but intermeshed.[53] Chemical specificity may also exist.[55] In some hypothalamic sites an injection of norepinephrine through an implanted cannula evokes drinking behavior, but the injection of carbachol through the same cannula evokes eating response.

Experiments involving the activation of stimulus-bound behavior raise the question of what the animal feels. One school of thought is that stimulation is neither pleasurable nor unpleasurable to the animal; the neurological system is activated, and the behavior is superimposed upon the animal's concurrent activities with no particular mood or affect preceding it.

Electrical Self-Stimulation

Stimulation of many areas produces no behavioral response; such areas are sometimes referred to as "silent." When the appropriate experimental procedures are followed, it is apparent that the stimulation of some silent areas has a highly reinforcing or pleasurable effect on the animal. When allowed to control the electrical switch, rats with electrodes located in a number of structures will rapidly learn to deliver electrical shocks to their brains.[45] This phenomenon is referred to as self-stimulation behavior. Stimulation is reinforcing in the same manner that food or water is reinforcing for a hungry or thirsty animal. Animals will learn complex tasks in order to receive the stimulation. Every species studied so far, including cats, dogs, rats, monkeys, and even man, exhibits self-stimulation behavior. Even puppies during the first week of life have shown a type of electrical self-stimulation behavior.[3]

A number of subcortical brain areas contain self-stimulation sites. These include the hypothalamus, septum, hippocampus, and caudate nucleus.[45] Such areas are even found in some cortical sites, such as the cingulate gyrus and the piriform lobe (Fig. 19–2). The most powerful self-stimulation area is in the vicinity of the medial forebrain bundle in the lateral hypothalamus.

NEURAL BASIS OF SOME BEHAVIORAL PATTERNS

The purpose of this section is to review briefly the various brain areas that are involved in aggressive, sexual, feeding, and maternal behavior so that behavioral disturbances resulting from naturally occurring brain lesions may be related to the brain area involved.

Aggressive Behavior

Experiments dealing with brain stimulation have revealed the presence of several basic neural systems which, when stimulated, produce intense, stereotyped aggressive attacks. Electrical stimulation through implanted electrodes, of the lateral hypothalamus of cats, for example, evokes predatory aggression, in which a rat will be attacked and the experimenter ignored.[11] Stimulation of the medial hypothalamus, however, evokes aggressive behavior in which the cat attacks the experimenter and ignores the rat. It is assumed that the areas stimulated are part of the neural systems

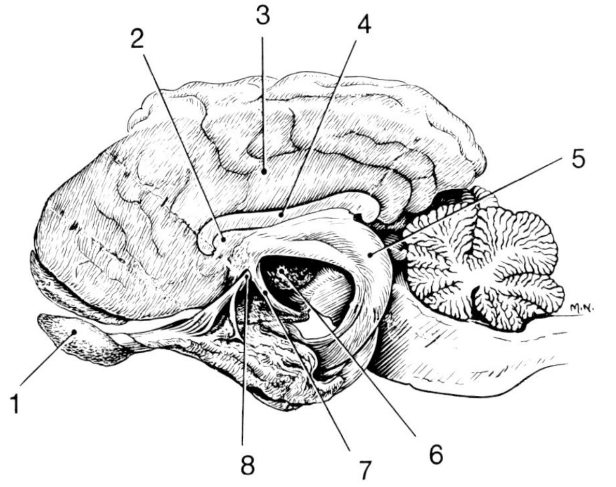

FIGURE 19–2 Lateral view of the brain showing the limbic system (rhinencephalic) structures. 1, Left olfactory bulb; 2, septal area; 3, cingulate gyrus; 4, corpus callosum; 5, hippocampus; 6, massa intermedia of thalamus; 7, column of fornix; 8, anterior commissure. (From Miller, M. E., Christensen, G. C., and Evans, H.: *Anatomy of the Dog*. W. B. Saunders Co., Philadelphia, 1964.)

that are activated when a cat is confronted with a natural stimulus such as prey or a predator. The amygdaloid nucleus is another brain area that can be stimulated either electrically or chemically; such stimulation elicits attack or fighting behavior.[15]

Stimulation can also suppress or arrest normal aggressive responses. Such effects have been seen with stimulation of the caudate nucleus and parts of the amygdaloid complex.[10]

Since stimulation of various areas of the brain may result in either excitation or suppression of aggressive or attack responses, it is not surprising that experimentally placed lesions may also result in increased or decreased aggressive behavior. One of the first neurological procedures to be discovered for making animals more aggressive was removal of the neocortex. If lest undisturbed, such animals may appear quite docile. However, the cats upon which these experiments were performed reacted with unmitigated violence to stimuli such as tail-pinching or a puff of air in the face which usually upset normal cats only moderately. Decortication is believed to produce these results because it removes the inhibitory influences that the neocortex normally exerts on subcortical neural systems which mediate aggressive reactions.[33]

Animals may also become overly aggressive following the removal of certain subcortical areas. Lesions in the septal and ventromedial hypothalamic nuclei of cats and rats make these animals aggressive to members of their own and other species. Immediately after the lesions occur the animals resist handling and bite indiscriminately. This behavior is probably more accurately referred to as hyperirritability.

The amygdaloid nuclei have played a prominent role in the lesion studies of aggressive behavior. The first most widely recognized study in which lesions of the forebrain proved effective in reducing aggression was that by Klüver and Bucy. They showed that bilateral removal of the temporal lobes, including the amygdala and part of the hippocampus, resulted in a surprising degree of tameness in previously vicious rhesus monkeys. In addition to this docility, Klüver and Bucy reported that their animals showed increased sexual activity, especially towards inappropriate objects, and a type of psychic blindness in regard to eating behavior.[36] Their monkeys attempted to eat objects such as meat, pieces of wood, and even feces.

Since this early work, it has been learned that many of the same behavioral effects can be produced by smaller lesions confined to the amygdala[56] and that the effects originally observed in monkeys can be produced in other species.[15] These effects are referred to as the Klüver-Bucy or temporal lobe syndrome. The most consistent changes in emotional behavior in several species studied are a loss of fear or timidity and a reduction in aggressive reactions.

The most extensive studies of amygdaloid lesions have been performed on cats.[17] Typically, during the first 2 postoperative weeks the cats are in a sort of stupor and eat very little voluntarily. Afterward, docility becomes very apparent. Predatory aggression as well as fear-induced and irritable aggression are reduced. These effects have also been observed in two Canadian lynxes which, of course, were more outwardly aggressive than domestic cats. The results of the same experiments in dogs have not been as striking as those in cats, although lesions of the amygdala and surrounding piriform and hippocampal areas in dogs have made the animals somewhat more docile to handlers.[2, 14]

The mechanism by which amygdaloidectomy changes aggressive, sexual, and feeding behavior is not understood. One fairly widely held hypothesis is that the amygdala normally exerts an inhibitory influence on brain stem areas mediating these behavioral patterns and that removal of this structure causes a release or disinhibition of this influence.

Sexual Behavior

The neocortex, amygdala, parts of the hypothalamus, preoptic region, and olfactory system all appear to play a role in the mediation of sexual behavior in males and females. Stimulation of several brain areas has been shown to evoke sexual responses, and lesions in a few limited areas may eliminate sexual responses. There does, however, appear to be a sexual dimorphism in that stimulation or ablation of the same areas produces different effects in males and females.

Sex hormones play a role in the neural mediation of sexual behavior. Testosterone, estrogen, and progesterone have an affinity for different neural sites. Thus, it is not surprising to find that the neural systems mediating male and female sexual behavior are different.

It should be emphasized that male and female sexual behavioral patterns are occasionally displayed by the opposite sex. For example, males may occasionally submit to being mounted by other males, and females may mount other females or males. Thus the neural "circuitry" for both kinds of behavior undoubtedly exists in both sexes.

Of the many subcortical areas in which experimental lesions have been produced in animals, only lesions of the medial preoptic–anterior hypothalamic continuum and related pathways have actually abolished copulatory responses of male mammals. In male cats,[27] dogs,[22] and rhesus monkeys[60] such lesions, when bilateral, can eliminate mating activity immediately and permanently. In male dogs the lesions markedly diminish urine marking responses as well.[22]

Lesions of the medial preoptic–anterior hypothalamic area do not impair receptivity in females. Lesions located more toward the ventromedial hypothalamus will apparently disrupt female sexual behavior that can normally be evoked by the administration of exogenous ovarian hormones.

Lesions in other areas of the brain have been reported to increase sexual activity. Sexual activity is increased in the Klüver-Bucy or temporal lobe syndrome, as are unusual or abnormal responses. This characteristic has been particularly noticeable in cats and monkeys. These animals mounted and attempted copulation with such inappropriate objects as dogs, teddy bears, and chickens.

Feeding and Drinking Behavior

Eating and drinking behavior can be evoked by electrical or chemical stimulation of specific hypothalamic sites. It is not surprising, therefore, that damage to certain hypothalamic areas also alters this behavior.[29]

It has been known for a long time that damage to the ventromedial hypothalamic nucleus results in obesity in many animals. The weight gain is not the result of inactivity but of overeating. This syndrome is referred to as hypothalamic hyperphagia. This syndrome has been observed in rats, cats,[32] and human patients (Fig. 19–3).

Lesions of the lateral hypothalamus have effects which are quite the opposite. Animals with such lesions refuse to eat and also refuse to drink. If the animals are kept alive by feeding through a stomach tube, most of them usually recover sufficiently to maintain normal weight.

Another brain area that has some role in feeding behavior is the amygdaloid nucleus. As mentioned previously, bilateral removal of this area in monkeys results in bizarre eating behavior such as ingestion of feces and pieces of wood.

Maternal Behavior

Work dealing with an analysis of neural mechanisms in maternal behavior has been almost completely limited to rodents. There is reason to believe that extrapolation from this work to dogs, cats, and other domestic animals may be inaccurate. This lack of information is unfortunate because female dogs and cats frequently show abnormal maternal behavior or are completely lacking in maternal responsiveness. A better understanding of the neural structures involved in the control of maternal behavior would help us decide whether neurological abnormalities were responsible for the behavioral disturbance.

Lesions of the cingulate cortex (septal, hippocampal, and accumbens) appear to affect maternal behavior by producing a hyperactivity or disorganization rather than a complete deficit in maternal responsiveness.[7, 35, 61–64] There are marked differences among rodents in the effect of these lesions.

The medial preoptic region does, however, appear to be essential to the mediation of maternal behavior in female rats. Bilateral lesions in this area result in immediate and complete cessation of nest building, retrieval, and nursing behavior.[44] In female cats, however, lesions of the medial preop-

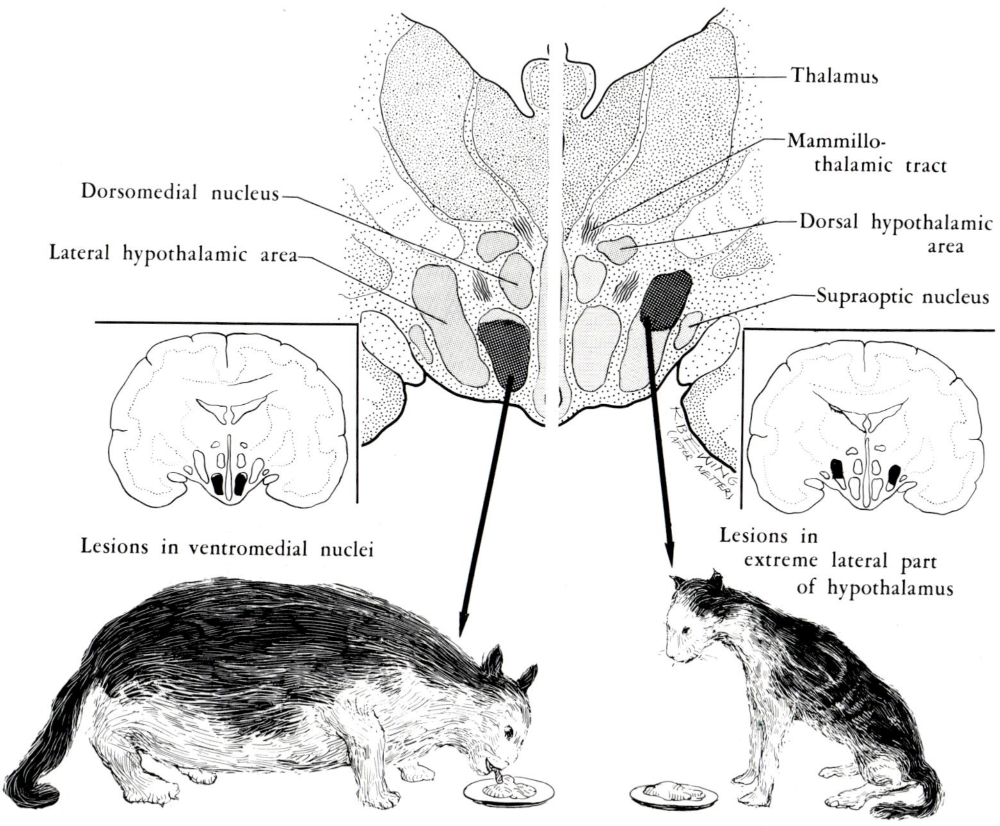

FIGURE 19–3 Effects of experimental lesions in the ventromedial and lateral areas of the hypothalamus on feeding behavior. (From Jenkins, T. W.: *Functional Mammalian Neuroanatomy.* Lea & Febiger, Philadelphia, 1972.)

tic region do not impair maternal behavior.[72]

The apparent species differences with regard to brain lesions in maternal behavior may be a reflection of the fact that maternal behavior is a complex system involving interaction between both mothers and the young and is influenced by multiple external stimuli and prior experience as well as by various hormonal factors.

EVALUATION OF NATURALLY OCCURRING BRAIN LESIONS

Suppressive Lesions

As evident from the preceding discussion, rather dramatic changes in behavior may follow the destruction of small areas of the brain. However, precautions are necessary in applying experimental studies to clinical problems. For example, almost all behavioral effects of experimentally induced lesions occur only if the lesions are bilateral. In areas bordering on the midline of the brain, a single naturally occurring lesion can cause bilateral damage. Hyperphagia has been observed in animals and human patients following damage (such as that produced by a tumor of the pituitary gland) to the ventromedial hypothalamic area. One would also expect impairment of male sexual behavior with a basal forebrain midline lesion which injured the preoptic area.

Increases in appropriate sexual responses and oral compulsive behavior associated with the Klüver-Bucy syndrome have been observed clinically in human patients in whom the temporal lobes and amygdala have been removed bilaterally to alleviate epilepsy. One would not expect these behavioral changes from naturally occurring lesions because the amygdala are so far from the midline that a single lesion could not cause bilateral damage. Even the aphasia and reduction in the need to drink that are caused by experimental lesions in the ventrolateral hypothalamus appear to be very unlikely in clinical situations for the same reason.

Irritative Lesions

Naturally occurring lesions of the brain such as tumors, cardiovascular damage, brain concussion, or other traumatic injury do not always act to suppress neural activity. With the appearance of scar tissue, neural excitation may occur and abnormal behavior can result from unilateral stimulation of certain areas.

One of the best examples of a behavioral disturbance from an excitatory lesion in the dog is temporal lobe or psychomotor epilepsy, in which the epileptogenic focus is in the temporal lobe. There is reason to believe that behavioral abnormalities may be associated with these lesions.[30] Typically, for a period of time prior to the seizure ranging from minutes to several hours, the dog may race about the house, howl excessively, or appear extremely frightened. Tumors of the piriform lobe, presumably also acting as an irritative focus, have been related to an unexplained increase in aggressiveness.

GONADAL HORMONES AND BEHAVIOR

The role of hormones is one of the most important considerations in dealing with behavioral problems of dogs and cats. Females of both species are routinely spayed to prevent the onset of estrous behavior as well as the physiological changes accompanying estrus. Male cats are generally castrated prepubertally to prevent the occurrence of objectionable masculine characteristics, especially urine spraying, roaming, and fighting. Castration of adult male dogs is being employed more frequently to change certain undesirable behavioral characteristics. In addition to gonadectomy to prevent or change undesirable behavior, castration is frequently requested by pet owners for pet population control. In these circumstances there is a concern, about the kinds of changes in behavior that may follow castration when no behavioral problem is involved.

An understanding of the kinds of changes induced by gonadectomy in the prepubertal and adult animal requires a discussion of the influences of hormones on the central nervous system in both the neonatal and the postpubertal stages.

SEXUAL DIFFERENTIATION

Evidence is now accumulating that there are anatomical and probably physiological and biochemical differences between males and females in some parts of the brain. This has been clearly shown in the medial preoptic region; both the termination of axons from other areas[47] and the cytoarchitecture[18] are different in the two sexes. These brain differences can probably be related to sexually dimorphic behavioral differences. With few exceptions males are more aggressive. This is especially true of interaction between adult males. Male cats have a much stronger predisposition to engage in urine spraying than female cats, and male dogs have a urination posture that is infrequently displayed by female dogs. The existence of sexually dimorphic differences such as these does not mean that males and females do not have the ability to display behavioral patterns typical of the opposite sex. Females certainly are capable of being fiercely aggressive and on occasion may display male-like urine marking. The difference between the sexes therefore is one of frequency or probability rather than one of quality.

The differences between the sexes in some behavioral patterns are reduced by removal of the testes or ovaries in adulthood. In males sexual behavior, urine marking, and fighting are often reduced by castration. However, castration does not bring either sex to some neural plane, and it is apparent that females are basically feminine in their behavior and males are basically masculine even following gonadectomy.

For the most part, the administration of the hormone of one sex to the opposite sex does not change behavioral characteristics accordingly. For example, administration of testosterone to a spayed female does not induce full masculine behavior, although it may enhance some aspects of masculine behavior such as mounting or urine marking. Administration of estrogen to castrated males may make them sexually attractive to normal males, but the estrogen-treated male does not behave like a female.

Recent research has shown that the sex-typical behavioral patterns are fundamentally a function of neonatal gonadal androgen secretion and the influence of androgen secretion upon certain brain areas. Before we consider this type of sexual differentiation, it is appropriate to give brief attention to the pattern of androgen secretion in the male.

Prior to and just after birth there is a surge in androgen production which then subsides within a couple of weeks. This surge in androgen production has been documented in the rat,[50] guinea pig,[49] and rhesus monkey[51] and presumably occurs also in cats and dogs. Androgen levels remain low until puberty, at which time there is a gradual increase in production; androgen reaches a rather steady level as the animal enters adulthood. This increase presumably stimulates complete masculine morphological development and activates certain behavioral patterns such as sexual behavior, aggressive behavior, and urine marking. If a male is castrated in adulthood, plasma testosterone declines rapidly within a few hours to very low and sometimes nondetectable levels.[49, 52]

It is believed that the surge in testosterone production that occurs just before and just after birth has an influence on the developing brain.[16] This influence apparently promotes or differentiates some type of neural development that predisposes the male to the display of masculine characteristics and sensitizes the brain to the effect of postpubertally secreted testosterone. The absence of testosterone production in females apparently leads to a different type of neural development which predisposes the animal to exhibit feminine behavior and sensitizes her to the secretion of estrogen at the time of puberty. Deprivation of androgen in the male neonatal dog by castration will cause a permanent reduction in masculine sexual behavior even if exogenous testosterone is given in adulthood.[6] The administration of testosterone to the fetal or neonatal female dog will result in various degrees of behavioral and genital masculinization and defeminization, depending upon the time of androgen treatment.[5]

SPECIFIC EFFECTS OF CASTRATION

Since androgens affect a number of morphological and physiological as well as behavioral characteristics in males, it is surprising that castration does not have more profound effects than it does. There is some evidence that castration makes males less active, but this is probably not a major effect. The most obvious behavioral changes relate to sexual, aggressive, and urine marking behavior.

Before discussing the changes in these behavioral patterns following castration in adulthood, some attention should be given to the behavioral differences between prepubertal and postpubertal castration. If males are castrated after the neonatal period but before the postpubertal increase in androgen production, sexual, aggressive, and urine marking behavior may never appear. This is the reason cats and occasionally dogs are castrated prepubertally. However, such animals still have the potential for masculine behavior; if, for example, they are given androgen at any time in later life they can display typical masculine behavior. Thus, sometimes anabolic steroids given to enhance weight gain and general condition may initiate undesirable urine marking or sexual behavior in prepubertally castrated animals.

There is very little experimental clinical information concerning the comparative effectiveness of castration prepubertally and postpubertally in preventing the undesirable aspects of masculine behavior. In fact, there is some evidence that prepubertal castration in dogs does not necessarily impair sexual mounting or aggressive behavior any more than is to be expected from postpubertal castration.[37] It could be that the main advantage of prepubertal castration is the time gained by castrating the animal early. That is, since the effects of castration seem to take place gradually, prepubertal castration simply allows more time for the effects of castration to occur. A possible disadvantage of prepubertal castration is that complete masculinization of such morphological characteristics as development of the hair coat, musculoskeletal system, body size, and penile structure may not occur. Thus, some dog and cat owners may wish to delay castration until after puberty.

Male Dogs

The effects of castration on the normal sexual behavior of adult male dogs has been studied fairly extensively. In general, castration usually results in some measurable decline in sexual activity almost immediately after castration, but certain individual dogs may continue to copulate, at least occasionally, for months or years after castration. This persistence is independent of any sexual experience prior to castration and is not due to compensatory secretion of androgen by the adrenal gland.[4, 20] Interestingly, among the several mammalian species studied, dogs have one of the greatest tendencies to persist in copulatory activity following castration.[21] In contrast to cats, male dogs usually do not develop undesirable masculine behavioral patterns sufficient to warrant routine prepubertal castration. However, there are problems in adult dogs that would be expected to be altered by castration, among them are mounting, urine marking in the house, aggressive behavior, and roaming. Puppies often go through a phase of mounting other dogs, people, or inanimate objects, but this usually ceases as they mature. If this behavior persists into adulthood or becomes pronounced at the time of puberty, it can be a serious problem. Urine marking may become a problem during or after puberty as male dogs develop the tendency to mark vertical objects in their environment, presumably as an expression of territorial identification. The motivation toward urine marking in the house may be so strong in some instances that even a well-housebroken dog may mark household furniture, draperies, or the walls.

Aggressive behavior is of particular concern because there are several types.[23] The one type of aggression that appears to be amenable to alteration by castration is fighting between males. This can be a problem for people who have two male dogs and for individuals who take their male dogs to public places where other males are encountered.

The effects of castration as determined by a clinical survey are represented in Figure 19–4.[31] Three categories of behavioral changes were used; rapid (occurring within approximately 2 weeks), gradual (occurring within a few months after castration), or no change. Intermale aggressive behavior, urine marking in the house, and mounting were reduced in 50 to 70 per cent of the dogs. In roughly half of the animals this change was rapid, and in the other half it was gradual. Using these figures as rough guidelines, it is probably safe to assume that changes in these types of behavior,

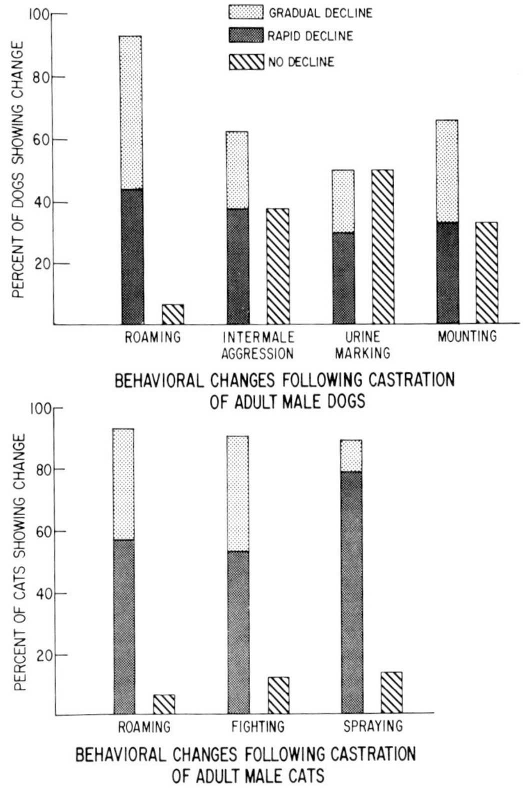

FIGURE 19–4 Percentage of dogs and cats in which castration was followed by a rapid decline, gradual decline, or no change in various objectionable behavior patterns. (Data on dogs from Hopkins, S. G., Schubert, T. A., and Hart, B. L.: Castration of adult male dogs: effects on roaming, aggression, urine marking, and mounting. J.A.V.M.A. *168*, 1108, 1976; data on cats from Hart, B. L.: Behavioral effects of castration. *Canine Pract. 3*, 17, 1976.)

though not 100 per cent effective, are sufficient to warrant castration as a therapeutic approach. With regard to roaming, the survey indicated that 90 per cent of the dogs showed either a rapid or a gradual decline in this behavior, probably as a reflection of diminished sexual drive or motivation.

Although urine marking in the house was altered gradually or rapidly in about 50 per cent of the dogs, some of the owners noticed that urine marking outside the house, when the dog was taken on walks or allowed to run loose, was not changed. This difference is probably related to the fact that olfactory stimuli from the urine of other dogs are the most important stimuli in evoking urine marking and are strongest outside the home.

The effect of castration on aggression deserves special attention, because in this survey it was found that territorial aggressiveness and fear-induced aggressiveness were not altered by castration. Aggressive behavior between male dogs was altered in about 60 per cent of the cases; these clinical results substantiate the feeling that it is basically only intermale aggressive behavior which is altered by castration in the adult.

Male Cats

Although cats are most frequently castrated prepubertally, there are a number of cat owners who do not request this operation until their animals are adults and have started to display some objectionable behavioral pattern. Cat owners may also ask about the behavioral consequences of prepubertal versus postpubertal castration, as they may wish to delay castration in order to get a more fully masculine development.

Behavioral patterns of male cats that are prevented or reduced by castration are fighting between males, roaming, and urine spraying. The results of a clinical survey conducted to determine the effectiveness of castration on these behavioral patterns in adult male cats are also presented in Figure 19–4.[26] It is evident that castration is generally more effective in altering undesirable masculine behavior in adult male cats than in male dogs. Basically, 80 to 90 per cent of the male cats castrated for roaming, fighting, or spraying showed either a gradual or a rapid decline in the behavior. Since the operation is so effective there may be little difference between prepubertal castration and postpubertal castration in preventing or eliminating these behavioral patterns.

GENERAL CHARACTERISTICS OF CASTRATION

There are substantial differences in the rate of decline of the various behavioral patterns following castration. It is also evident that a rapid decline in one behavioral pattern is not necessarily paralleled by a similar rate of decline in another. Since testosterone is metabolized almost completely within a few hours, the persistence of these behaviors is not due to retention of testicular androgens. Experimental work has revealed that adrenal androgens are probably not responsible for the persistence of the behavior either.

Some individual differences may relate to environmental circumstances. For example, male dogs living in homes or neighborhoods that are frequently visited by other males and are therefore likely to contain more pronounced stimuli to evoke urine marking or fighting, would not be expected to show the same probability of decline in the behavior as animals living under more isolated conditions.

Some individual differences in response to castration undoubtedly reflect genetic rather than experiential or age-related factors. Whether or not there are breed differences is an open question. The surveys revealed no correspondence between the age of the animals at the time of castration and a change in behavior following castration.

OTHER EFFECTS OF CASTRATION

Pet owners now are more frequently requesting that their animals be castrated for the purpose of pet population control. These people may wonder about the behavioral effects of castration other than the undesirable types of behavior previously discussed. There is no experimental evidence in either dogs or cats that castrated males become excessively fat, inactive, or lethargic following castration. This finding also corresponds with experimental work in laboratory animals that indicates that, if anything, castration results in a slight loss of body weight.[73] There is no indication that hunting ability or territorial defense in dogs is affected by castration.[26] If there is no apparent sexual dimorphism in the usual performance of a behavioral pattern, there is no reason to expect castration to alter that behavior. Since females, for example, are generally as good at hunting or acting as watchdogs as males, castration would not be expected to alter these qualities in males.

USE OF PROGESTINS IN MALES

If castration is not effective in altering one of the undesirable sexually dimorphic characteristics, the administration of a progestin such as medroxyprogesterone acetate (Depo-Provera) or megestrol acetate may have an effect. Progestins seem to have an effect similar to that of castration, and thus tend to extend the effects of castration.[24, 25] However, it is probably advisable to wait until the effects of castration on behavior are evident before administering progestin.

BEHAVIORAL EFFECTS OF OVARIAN HORMONES

In most animals estrogen has the effect of increasing general activity. Female dogs and cats during estrus usually move about more, vocalize more frequently, and may act nervous. The urine and vaginal secretions of females in proestrus and estrus are attractive to males. Sexual attractants in the vaginal secretions of urine are referred to as sex pheromones. They are undoubtedly noticed by males on their daily treks through the female's vicinity. It is not known whether the pheromones are metabolites of estrogen or a special secretion added to the urine and vaginal discharges.

The effects of progesterone in the sexual cycle are not clearly understood. In most females, probably including cats and dogs, progesterone has a suppressive effect on sexual behavior. Progesterone tends to make animals more calm and to some extent may reduce aggressiveness.

BEHAVIORAL EFFECTS OF OOPHORECTOMY

Although essentially oophorectomy makes a female anestrus, it does not necessarily make her less feminine. The basic patterns of masculine and feminine behavior are laid down in the early stages of the development of the nervous system.

Pet owners frequently wonder about the possible behavioral differences between spaying bitches before or after the first estrous cycle. At present there are no studies or other information that would indicate that the time of oophorectomy results in any behavioral differences.

There is a common feeling among dog owners that removal of the ovaries results in a tendency to become inactive and to gain weight. There is some experimental evidence from work on rats that indicates that oophorectomy does promote weight gain.[73] However, the main reason that some females become excessively fat and inactive is probably from lack of exercise and overfeeding rather than from some hormonally related cause.

EARLY EXPERIENCE

Just as androgens have an organizing influence on the nervous system of the prenatal and neonatal animal, various forms of early experiences can profoundly affect the development of the central nervous system and markedly alter behavioral patterns. Sometimes such behavior is not manifested until after the animal has reached adulthood.

RESTRICTED EARLY EXPERIENCE

Anatomical Changes

Rats exposed to an enriched, standard laboratory environment differ in brain chemistry and neuroanatomy from those in restricted environments.[54] There are differences in the activity of brain acetylcholinesterases, the ratio of cerebral cortical weight to the rest of the brain (most marked in the occipital region), the thickness of the cerebral cortex, and the length of cerebral hemispheres. There is a greater ramification of dendrites, particularly in the occipital cortex, of the rats reared in the enriched environment. The dendrites do not spread farther, but they show greater numbers of higher order branching. There are also a greater number of dendritic spines in the enriched experienced rat's cortex, especially on the basal dendrites. The net result of the enriched experience is that the number of functional synapses is greatly increased. These changes cannot be attributed to handling, locomotion, or stress. Social stimulation is not required, but can contribute to the effect. Passive watching by rats does not result in these effects—an active experience with a complex environment is necessary. The changes are not transitory but relatively long-lasting.

Behavioral Changes

In a series of studies at McGill University puppies were raised in restricted environments from 4 weeks of age to 9 months of age.[41-43, 65, 66] The puppies were housed either singly or with one or two peers. After 9 months the dogs were kept in normal laboratory conditions. When compared with the control dogs, the dogs reared in the restricted environment were just as physically healthy and vigorous, but they were also hyperactive, took longer to learn simple problems, were unable to learn avoidance tasks, tended to perseverate in their responses, and were less interested in social interactions with other dogs. These differences were still present as long as a year after removal from the restricted environment. Other investigators who have raised puppies in isolation have also noted that such dogs were inhibited in the development of escape responses and showed excessive fear when removed from their cages.[13]

Experiments conducted with kittens revealed similar results. Kittens raised in isolation from 2 weeks of age to 9 months (except for minimal contact for feeding) were hyperactive and more suspicious, fearful, and aggressive than were their littermates which had remained with the mother until 6 or 12 weeks of age.[59]

SOCIAL DEPRIVATION

Critical Period Hypothesis

J. P. Scott (1962) has suggested that there are major developmental critical periods in an animal's life that are optimal for learning, for infantile stimulation, and for the formation of basic social relationships.[58] The animal must be exposed to certain stimuli within a specific time interval in order to develop normally. If the animal does not experience the appropriate stimuli during these critical periods, it can develop abnormal behavior. The order in which these periods occur differs among mammals, and there is variation in behavior development within each species.

The imprinting phenomenon in precocial birds and the ewe lamb or goat kid affiliations after birth are dramatic examples of critical time periods. Exposure to the wrong stimulus not only affects the immediate relationships but can also influence later social relationships. Birds which have imprinted on a human being may later direct their courtship behavior toward humans. Bottle-reared lambs have difficulty establishing social and sexual relationships in adulthood.

Scott and his co-workers believe that the socialization period for dogs occurs between 3 and 10 weeks of age.[57] Within this somewhat flexible time period puppies develop social relationships with each other. This socialization process is not identical to imprinting in birds but does have long-term consequences. If a puppy is not exposed to other dogs or human beings during this time span, normal social behavior with peers or people may not develop. Puppies kept in large fields with limited exposure to people until 14 weeks of age show extreme fear of human beings and manifest escape reactions which are difficult if not impossible to overcome.[12]

The consequences of prolonged isolation from birth to adulthood on reproductive behavior of dogs and cats has not been studied extensively in laboratory situations. Reports from breeders indicate that there may be a wide range of variation among individuals and breeds in this respect, and that at least some animals exhibit reduced sexual receptivity toward members of their own species if reared without peer interaction.

PRACTICAL CONSIDERATIONS

Although deprivation and isolation experiments are not as intensely produced outside laboratory settings, similar situations can occur in natural settings. Occasionally dogs raised in kennels with little human interaction or exposure to the outside environment are extremely timid as adults. These dogs are afraid of people, strange places, and novel objects.

The veterinary practitioner is in a position to advise pet owners about the rearing of their animals and about precautions that should be taken. Puppies and kittens with a history of long neglect or adverse early experience are appealing but may not be the best animal to acquire as a pet. The probability that these animals will exhibit abnormal behavior is higher than that of animals known to have a normal relationship with littermates and positive interactions with people.

ORPHAN ANIMALS

Although it may be true that complete mother-infant-peer relationships are necessary for perfectly normal behavioral development, it has been shown that substitutions can be made for some functions of the mother, thus reducing the degree of manifestation of some abnormal forms of behavior. For example, rhesus monkeys reared with a stationary surrogate mother develop stereotypic rocking postures, bite themselves, and are extremely timid and either hypomotile or hypermotile. However, orphan rhesus monkeys reared with a mobile surrogate mother in the form of a cloth-covered swinging bottle or a dog do not develop these traits to the same degree.[39] Persons who desire to rear orphan puppies or kittens should be advised to handle them frequently, stroke them, pick them up, and move them about. Above all, they should not just feed the puppy or kitten and put it back down. If they do so, they could be carrying out their own deprivation experiments. An orphan raised with its littermates has a better chance of developing normally than if it were isolated. If the orphan has no littermates, it should be exposed to members of its own species, preferably peers, when the opportunity presents itself. Orphan puppies or kittens which are given a lot of attention, manipulation, and exposure to peers will probably become quite acceptable pets.

HANDLING

Early experiences are not always detrimental. Handling or early stimulation of neonatal laboratory animals has been intensely investigated and demonstrates the influence of early experiences on adult behavior. These experiments can take the form of picking up and stroking the neonate for a few minutes, exposing it to cold or shock, or simply removing it from the mother. The neonate is raised by its mother under standard conditions when it is not being handled. The manipulation time varies but is generally short, a matter of only a few minutes.

Although there are variations among species, most species handled in this way show accelerated development in growth. In an experiment with a litter of six Siamese kittens investigators reported that the handled kittens opened their eyes, emerged from the nest box, and developed EEG changes, coat pattern, and coloration sooner than littermates.[40]

In the majority of the investigations on handled neonates (rats) raised in conventional laboratory settings there has been an alteration in the adult animal's reactions, behaviorally and physiologically, to stress.[1] As adults, the rats handled as neonates are less emotional in novel situations than unhandled laboratory-reared rats. Handling also alters the adrenal responses of the adults, which have reduced adrenal cortical activity in response to environmental stresses.[38] Although both reduced emotionality and altered adrenal cortical function result from handling, it has not been proved that the pituitary-adrenal changes mediate the behavioral effects of early experience.[1]

It can be argued that the results of handling are not necessarily adaptive to wild animals.[9] However, a reduced level of excitement in dogs and cats in situations such as show rings, crowds, and changing living quarters would probably be looked upon as a benefit.

It should be pointed out that although behavior acquired as the result of early experience may be difficult to change, it is not impossible to modify the behavior somewhat. Fuller (1966) reported some success with behavior modification training and tranquilizers in reducing the fears of dogs reared in isolation.[13] Melzack (1954) also noted that after a year some of the behavioral effects of the restricted environmentally-reared dogs had diminished.[41] Rarely, however, are such animals completely normal.

The veterinarian should be aware of the effects of early experience to be able to make accurate prognoses, as well as to be able to advise owners in preventing behavioral problems from developing.

BEHAVIOR ACQUIRED THROUGH LEARNING

As mentioned earlier, experience and learning are not identical, although learning is dependent upon experience. If an unwanted behavior is tentatively diagnosed as the partial or total result of learning, several approaches are available to eliminate or reduce the frequency of occurrence. Since many of the concepts on which these techniques are based have been developed in experimental work with animals, the procedures used for human beings are easily adapted to treatment of animals. A few principles of learning can be applied to a great number of different cases. All cases will be slightly different, but individual variations in behavior can be accommodated within the general framework.

BEHAVIOR MODIFICATION TECHNIQUES

The frequency of occurrence of learned behavior can be reduced by extinction, reinforcement of alternative behavior, systematic desensitization, punishment, and flooding or response prevention. Application of these methods requires a clear understanding of the concepts of shaping (successive approximation), reinforcement (reward), punishment, schedules of reinforcement, and time contingencies. None of these principles is complex, but an understanding of them is essential. Familiarity with principles of learning is, of course, important in being able to change learned behavior, but it is equally important in determining whether the undesirable behavior is wholly or partially a learned reaction. One must be able to make a diagnosis.

DEFINITIONS

Positive Reinforcement

A reinforcer or reward is an event or state of affairs that tends to increase the probability that a certain response will recur. The reward is most effective when it is given 0.5 second after the response. In essence, the animal should be rewarded as soon as possible. This is most quickly accomplished by verbal praise. For added incentive the praise can be followed by a coveted food reward. The value of rewards and motivation influences acquisition and performance of a response. In treating behavioral problems the use of food rewards is almost always superior to verbal praise.

Extinction

Behavior that has been acquired or enhanced by association with positive reinforcement will be extinguished or reduced in frequency if positive reinforcement is withheld. More formally defined, extinction is the progressive weakening or diminishment in frequency of a response to a stimulus by repeatedly exposing the subject to the stimulus but never following the evoked response with positive reinforcement. Ignoring an animal that barks or scratches to get attention is an example of using extinction to eliminate a behavior.

Schedules of Reinforcement

The frequency and intervals at which the rewards are administered influence acquisition of a response and its rate of extinction—that is, how long the animal will later persist in the behavior without reinforcement.

For acquisition of a response immediate continuous reinforcement is best. This means that every response should be followed by a reinforcement. After a behavior is learned it can be sustained by reinforcements given at progressively longer intervals from the onset of the behavior. Initially, however, the reward should be immediate.

To maintain the response intermittent reinforcement is better than continuous reinforcement. This means that not every response is followed by a reinforcement. Two major types of intermittent reinforcement schedules are ratio and interval. In the fixed ratio schedule a set number of responses must be performed before the animal is rewarded. In a variable ratio schedule the reward is given to the animal after a varying number of responses have been performed. An animal on a fixed interval schedule is reinforced for the first response after a specific interval of time from the last reinforcement. On a variable interval schedule the animal is reinforced for the first response after a varying interval of time from the last reinforcement. All of the intermittent schedules result in increased resistance to extinction. Dogs with bad habits of barking or scratching on doors to get into the house are usually on a mixed variable ratio and interval schedule of reinforcement. Such a schedule produces very persistent behavior. Detailed questioning of owners about what they do when their animals engage in objectionable behavior frequently reveals that the animal is on an intermittent schedule of positive reinforcement of that behavior. The reinforcement may be in the form of access to the house or, most frequently, attention by the owner.

Delay of Reward

Although delay of reward retards acquisition of a response, varied delays of reward increase resistance to extinction of an acquired response. The optimum strategy in a training program is to employ immediate reinforcement when teaching the animal the desired response but then to use a schedule of varied delays of reinforcement after the animal has acquired the response.

Stimulus Generalization

Once an animal has acquired a response to one stimulus, it also acquires responses to similar stimuli. The more similar the other stimuli are to the original stimulus, the closer the responses resemble the response to the original stimulus. An animal afraid of men may also be apprehensive of boys. A dog terrified of firecrackers may be frightened by similar noises.

Generalization of Extinction

As an animal begins to extinguish its responses to a stimulus, it simultaneously extinguishes its responses to similar stimuli. If a fear response to boys is extinguished, the animal's response to men is also reduced.

Shaping

Shaping (successive approximation) is a technique used in training an animal to perform a desired behavior by initially reinforcing an approximation of the ultimately desired response. Once a certain approximation to the desired response has been reinforced and the animal is repeating it, progressively more exact approximations of the ultimately desired behavior are reinforced. Behavior that is progressively closer to the desired behavior is methodically reinforced. Finally, only the precise behavior is reinforced. Behavior which seems to be difficult to teach an animal can be easily acquired using this technique (Fig. 19–5). The key to success is immediate and frequent rewards at each step to change the behavior being rewarded in tiny increments.

Counter-Conditioning

Counter-conditioning is the training or conditioning of an animal to acquire a

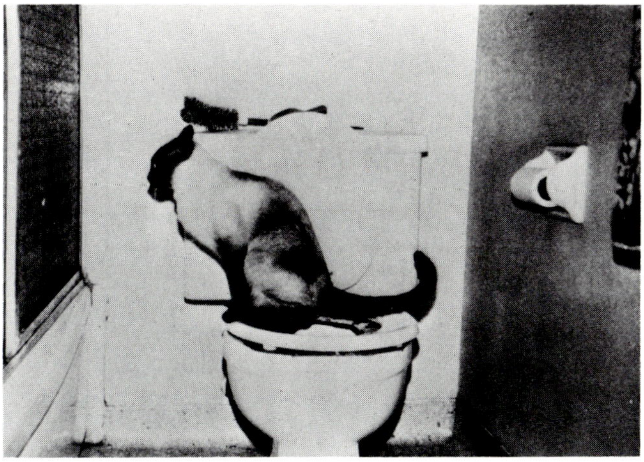

FIGURE 19-5 Animals can be taught useful behavior utilizing the technique of shaping. This cat was shaped to urinate and defecate into a toilet.

response to a stimulus which is incompatible with a response previously evoked by that stimulus. Classically, counter-conditioning is used to refer to reducing an animal's anxiety by teaching it to respond to the stimulus in a new way (physiologically incompatible with the undesired response) and pairing pleasant associations with the adverse stimulus. Frequently, the pleasant event can also be used as a reinforcer for the new behavior.

Systematic Desensitization

Gradually exposing an animal to increasing intensities of a stimulus without evoking the undesirable behavior is called desensitization. Systematic desensitization is used to break down anxiety and fear response habits in a piecemeal fashion by repeatedly exposing an animal to a weak fear-eliciting stimulus during a physiological state that is inhibitory of fear or anxiety.

Flooding

Flooding or response-prevention techniques are those in which the patient is forced to experience the intense anxiety of a phobic situation but is prevented from performing any avoidance behavior. The rationale behind such an approach is that once an individual has learned an avoidance or coping response to an adverse stimulus, it never again allows itself to be in the position of experiencing the stimulus without reacting to it. It therefore never has the opportunity to learn that the stimulus is not necessarily injurious. Flooding or response-prevention techniques have been fairly successful in eliminating learned avoidance responses in laboratory animals and reducing learned fear responses in people to phobic objects such as spiders which have previously been experienced for short intervals. These techniques might be tried with some forms of phobic reactions in animals.

Punishment

Punishment can be either the withdrawal of a pleasant stimulus or the application of an adverse one. The effect of punishment is to stop a behavior or prevent it from occurring.

EXAMPLES OF USING BEHAVIOR MODIFICATION

Perhaps the easiest way to explain these principles and techniques is to describe examples of using them in treating phobic reactions. Thunderstorms, firecrackers, trains, gunshots, and the appearance of uniformed men are examples of stimuli which frequently elicit fear reactions from animals. Some animals exhibit intense fear by shaking, salivating, pacing, seeking out

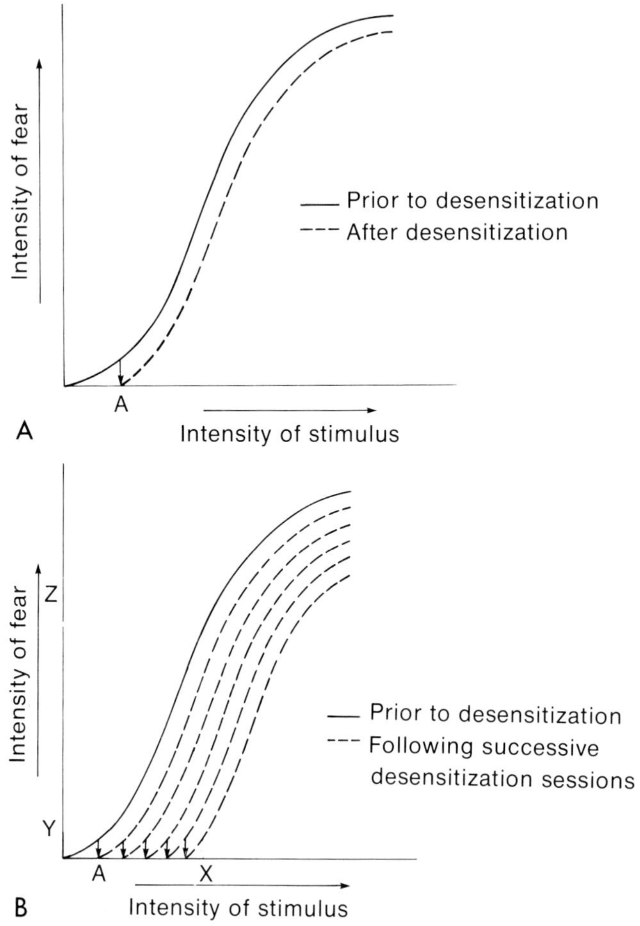

FIGURE 19–6 Theoretical representations of desensitization procedure. *A*. As the intensity of an aversive stimulus, such as the onset of a thunderstorm or approach of a person, increases, the intensity of the fear also increases as indicated in the response curve prior to desensitization. Following desensitization at a stimulus level A, the animal's fear may be reduced to zero. This desensitization may also result in reduction of fear at all higher levels of intensity of the aversive stimulus, as indicated by the new response curve. *B*. Several successive desensitization sessions given to an animal may result in successively lower response curves. Thus, a stimulus at point X will evoke a fear reaction of level Y after five desensitization sessions compared with a response at point Z prior to any desensitization.

their owners, or trying to hide. Frequently dogs react to fearful stimuli with aggression.

Fear of Noises

Dogs have been known to go through screen and glass doors, chew through wood, and sometimes even fracture their jaws in the process of trying to escape from the noise of firecrackers or thunderstorms. Heavy tranquilization (to the point where the animal cannot move) does prevent it from injuring itself but rarely results in alleviating the fear. Such an approach to controlling a phobic response also depends on a person being present when these stimuli occur.

However, the anxiety of the animal can be reduced by changing its behavioral response to the fear stimulus.[67] This can be done by gradually pairing pleasant associations with the noise and teaching the animal a new way of responding to it (sitting or lying down) that is incompatible with the undesired responses (panting, salivating, escape reactions).

If the intensity of the noise cannot be controlled, a facsimile must be substituted and the animal desensitized to it. This is done in the expectation that responses to the facsimile will be generalized to the real life situation. Thunderstorms are an example of this kind of stimulus. However, recordings can reproduce the sounds of an approaching storm, the height of the storm, and its departure. To maximize the probability of generalization, the recordings of the sounds should be real enough to elicit a fear reaction from the animal. Prior to beginning any desensitization series, the recording should be tested on the dog. As soon as the phobic reaction (nervousness, trembling, salivating) begins to appear, the test should be stopped. It is not necessary to produce a complete fear reaction, and in fact it could be detrimental. It is merely necessary to know if the artificial stimulus is real enough to elicit the phobic reaction.

Prior to beginning the desensitization procedure, the animal should be taught an alternative response to the detrimental behavior and learn to associate a pleasant event with this response. For example, a dog can be taught to sit or to lie down in anticipation of a reward. Appetizing food rewards are recommended because they are highly motivating. Eating also has a tendency to reduce anxiety.

At the first desensitization session the dog should be sitting or lying down and the sound recording turned on at a barely audible level, far below the volume that would elicit even a mild fear response from the dog. As long as the dog shows no fear reactions, it is frequently given food rewards. Gradually the intensity of the stimulus is increased, with pauses for several minutes at each progressively louder intensity. The dog is given tidbits every few seconds. (This procedure works well with one person manipulating the recording device and another attending to the animal.)

From the moment the desensitization program is initiated, only the new response (sitting or lying down) should be allowed to occur in conjunction with the recorded sounds. Both the sounds and the new response are thus paired with a pleasant, anxiety-reducing event (eating a delicious treat). Sitting during a thunderstorm recording in anticipation of a food reward is a new response to a previously fearful sound. Before the dog begins to manifest any fear reaction at all the sound intensity is slowly decreased while the dog continues to be rewarded.

If the dog should manifest a reaction to the sounds by getting up or shaking or trembling, the food reward is withheld until the dog stops the behavior and is again sitting attentively waiting for a food reward. The noise level may have to be decreased to achieve this. Ideally a fear reaction is never provoked.

If the dog gets up or begins to shake, no reassuring words or petting should be given. Such pleasant events, when paired with the undesired behavior, reinforce the fear reaction. Phobias or fear reactions, particularly those that get progressively worse, are frequently enhanced unwittingly by reinforcement from the owner trying to reduce the anxiety of the animal. Behavior that is acquired or facilitated by such association with positive reinforcement would be extinguished or reduced in frequency if the positive reinforcement were withheld. Verbal praise, petting, and food rewards should always be reserved for those times when the dog is not exhibiting the fear reaction. Never should a reinforcer be paired with any sign of the phobic reaction.

Once the dog has been desensitized to the recording and looks for a food reward in response to a thunderclap rather than shaking or shivering, the animal should be put on a variable intermittent schedule of reinforcement. Sometimes the dog must tolerate a sequence of two thunderclaps before being rewarded, sometimes four, and sometimes one. Occasionally the dog is rewarded immediately after hearing a noise, sometimes 5 or more seconds later. Such schedules encourage the new behavior to persist for a long time when reinforcement is not available, such as during a real storm, particularly when the owner is not present.

When desensitizing an animal to a phobic stimulus using an artificial stimulus it should not be expected that the dog will respond to a real storm or situation exactly as it did to the replicated sound. The degree to which the response will generalize is partly a function of the similarity of the two stimuli. This is why it is important to reproduce the phobic stimulus as closely as possible, particularly when approaching the end of the desensitization gradient. A storm has added properties such as atmospheric changes and light effects which cannot be duplicated.

Dogs which have previously reacted to storms or other noises with violent escape reactions will probably always be uneasy during storms or fireworks. They are still likely to be apprehensive in a real situation and will demonstrate this by moderate panting or salivation. However, they should be free of their previously injurious behavior.

Experiments have demonstrated that extinction takes place more rapidly if it is massed in a block of time rather than distributed among several very short intervals of time. Since a desensitization procedure includes extinction as part of the technique, a session should last ideally about 30 to 45 minutes. However, it should always be terminated before the animal becomes restless or tired of the game. If the animal has a short attention span, the length of the desensitization sessions must be accommodated to the individual's temperament.

Once an animal has been desensitized, it is advisable to reinforce the newly acquired way of responding to the stimulus by occasionally exposing the dog to either the stimulus or the replication thereof in practice sessions. If a long time elapses before exposure to some form of the stimulus, the animal may again manifest its original phobic reactions to the stimulus when it is presented.

Punishment is contraindicated as a primary or even an auxiliary method of eliminating fear and phobic reactions because it tends to increase anxiety. Pain can also elicit aggression.

Other Fears

The same techniques described for treatment of phobic reactions to noises can be employed in treating other fear reactions.[67, 70] The animal is first taught, using rewards, a response which is incompatible with the undesired response. It is conditioned to assume a different, nonfearful emotional attitude to the new response. A stimulus of reduced intensity is presented to the animal in graduated steps. The stimulus, the new response, and the reward are all paired. The animal soon learns that when the stimulus appears and it performs the new response it receives a reward. It is very important that the stimulus be introduced so slowly that the animal never has occasion to respond in an undesirable way. After the animal has learned the new response to the stimulus, it should be reinforced intermittently.

In many situations the actual stimulus that evokes the fear reaction can be used. The intensity of the stimulus can be decreased by keeping it at a distance to reduce its visual, auditory, or olfactory properties. The stimulus is slowly brought closer and closer to the animal or vice versa.

Animals that are apprehensive of children can be taught to sit quietly for a pleasant food reward and praise while a series of stimuli in the form of people of decreasing height and ages is presented. The intensity of the stimulus can be altered by distance as well as by size of the person. First an adult may be placed 20 feet away from the animal, then 18 feet, and so on until he or she is directly in front of the animal. The animal is rewarded for tolerating each step of the approach. The procedures are repeated, using progressively smaller people—first adults, then adolescents, then children. If an animal is more apprehensive of adults, the reverse sequence should of course be used. If an animal is afraid of men in uniform, women and then men wearing increasingly more formal-looking uniforms can gradually be introduced to the animal. If the dog is more afraid of the stimulus outside of the house, the techniques can be begun inside. Changing the environment can alter the intensity of the stimulus, and it is desirable to begin a desensitization program using the least intense stimulus.

In developing a desensitization program a variety of situations can be used to fit the specific problem. Basically, a continuum of stimuli is slowly introduced to the animal in an environmental setting that is made progressively more similar to the precise combination of events which elicit the fear response. At the beginning a situation is used which has never evoked a fear response; at the end the situation is the one which previously always evoked a severe fear response. The set of stimuli at the beginning are gradually transformed into the stimuli at the end without ever evoking a fear reaction.

Other Learned Behaviors

Gradual shaping of a new competing behavior, a method of introducing stimuli gradually, intermittent schedules of reinforcement, and extinction can effectively be applied to alter learned behaviors other than fears. Learned aggression related to fear or dominance,[70, 71] destructive behavior,[67, 69] and psychosomatic reactions are examples of types of behavior which can be approached using these techniques.

Destructive Behavior

Dogs that routinely destroy household items when the owner is absent can learn to refrain from such activities. Several times a day the owner presents the dog with a cue that signals a short departure; the owner then leaves but returns within a few minutes. The time of the absence varies but in general, steadily increases, and the dog is usually provided with an object that it is allowed to chew while the owner is away. Of course, once such a program is begun, temporary precautions must be taken to prevent the dog from engaging in destructive behavior if the owner is gone for long periods. Within a few weeks most animals can be safely left alone all day.

Hyperactive Dogs

Most dogs are hyperactive because they learn that such behavior gets attention. Such overactivity can be reduced by utilizing extinction (ignoring the dog's activity), and by reinforcing the animal for alternative behavior (for instance, being quiet, keeping all four feet on the floor, walking instead of running).

Punishment

Although punishment is not recommended for elimination of fears and phobias, it can be used to reduce the occurrence of other learned behavior, provided certain guidelines are followed. Punishment is most effective if (1) it is of maximum appropriate intensity from the onset, (2) it is capable of totally disrupting the behavior, (3) it is administered immediately after the onset of the behavior, and (4) it is administered after every occurrence of the behavior. Punishment is also more effective if the animal has learned that an alternative behavior exists.

Punishment always has the potential of inducing anxiety, and, if it is painful, of eliciting aggression. One of the greatest drawbacks of punishment is the potential misuse of it. The failure of punishment used either alone or in an inappropriate manner is quite evident to the veterinary practitioner. A client presenting an animal with a behavior problem generally has already tried punishment with no beneficial results.

SUMMARY

A large part of this section has concerned the application of learning principles to modify the behavior of animals because most types of undesirable behavior in dogs and many kinds of undesirable behavior in other companion animals are primarily or at least partially learned. Sometimes even after the primary cause of physiological behavior disorders or innate species-typical behavior patterns are treated, learned behavior may persist. This behavior can be changed using knowledge of learning principles.

If a clinician suspects that an undesirable type of behavior is primarily a learned phenomenon, he or she may try behavior modification techniques before exhaustive and expensive medical workups are undertaken. Expertise in behavior modification techniques requires experience. Many subtle skills are necessary in obtaining the anamnesis, observing the client and the animal, and explaining the technique and rationale behind them.

PSYCHOSOMATICS

Gastrointestinal disorders of animals are frequently correlated with emotional stress produced by specific environmental conditions. Chronic diarrhea at home may not be manifested when the animal is hospitalized or kenneled elsewhere. Sometimes the appearance of enteritis can be correlated with the presence of a certain individual or with a specific activity. For the animal's sake, a change in an aspect of the environment is preferable to a lifelong reliance on tranquilizing agents to control the disorder.

All practitioners have seen dogs exhibiting lameness long after the original injury is completely healed and there is no physical cause for the limping. When the owner is not in view, the animal walks normally. The owner's presence evokes the behavior, which is followed by sympathy and attention. A behavior followed by reinforcement tends to be repeated. Ignoring the lameness generally cures the malady within a few hours, and rewarding the pet for sound steps facilitates recovery. This is an example of utilizing extinction and reinforcement of an alternative response (sound steps). Actually, whether this type of lameness can be termed psychosomatic is questionable, because it may be that the animal has complete voluntary control over the behavior while it is manifested.

However, not all learned disorders are under voluntary control nor are they dependent on obvious positive reinforcement. A behavior may arise because it has been constantly paired with an event in the environment. Eventually this environmental factor can come to evoke the response. This is a classic example of conditioning—the behavior is a conditioned reflex. An interesting experiment illustrating the role this type of conditioning can play in the manifestation of a disease is learned asthma in guinea pigs.[46] Sensitized guinea pigs experienced asthmatic attacks when exposed to the antigen in a specific chamber. After several exposures, the animals continued to have asthmatic attacks when they were placed in the chamber without exposure to the antigen. The room itself came to elicit the asthmatic attacks. In another experiment in guinea pigs, asthma attacks which had been paired with an auditory stimulus could later be evoked by the sound.

Undoubtedly there are cases in veterinary medicine when a disability is frequently paired with specific environmental events, and after the original cause of the disease is gone a learned behavior persists.

CASE HISTORIES

Two examples of physiological abnormalities which could not be attributed to organic disorders but rapidly responded to behavior modification techniques are of interest. A small 3-year-old mixed breed dog had been vomiting every morning for several months shortly after the owners awakened. The dog had had two extensive clinical examinations, which included blood chemistry evaluations and gastroscopic and contrast gastrointestinal radiographic examinations. These procedures revealed no abnormalities which could explain the routine vomiting. The dog never vomited when hospitalized overnight. A detailed history revealed that the vomiting was always followed by attention from the owners. Generally this was in the form of sympathetic concern and lavish attention, but it also included disciplinary measures. Never had the owners ignored the vomiting. It was suggested to the owners that upon awakening they immediately pay attention to the dog before it had a chance to vomit. They were to play with the dog, teach it to do tricks, and reward it for acceptable behavior. The owners followed instructions, and the dog never vomited again. By giving the dog immediate attention in the morning they prevented him from demanding it by vomiting. It is probable that extinction of the emesis would also have occurred if the owners had consistently ignored the dog's behavior. Rewarding an alternate behavior, however, facilitated elimination of the undesired response.

A 10-week-old German shepherd was presented to a veterinary clinic with a history of sporadic posterior paresis. Several times a day the dog experienced episodes of dragging both hind legs. The dog appeared to have no control over the limbs. When the dog was hospitalized it was given a thorough examination, which revealed slightly luxating patellas. The dog was hospitalized for several days and for the first 3 days exhibited no posterior paresis. Toward the end of the hospitalization period, as the attendant left the dog after having fed and watered it, the puppy demonstrated the posterior paresis and vocalized loudly. Of course, the attendant usually turned around again and thus rewarded the dog with attention. When the owners returned for their dog, the puppy, which had walked into the discharge room on four normal limbs, became excited and immediately exhibited posterior paresis. The owners were instructed not to touch the dog when it manifested posterior paresis or any form of dragging its rear limbs. They were either to completely ignore the dog or, when possible, to walk away from it into another room. They were also instructed to spend some time teaching the dog behavioral responses which could be rewarded with attention, such as simple commands to sit, stay, and come. They were also encouraged to pet and praise the dog for walking toward them on four sound limbs. The owners agreed to do so and when contacted several months later reported that the dog had rapidly recovered from the posterior paretic syndrome. The dog only occasionally manifested posterior paresis for a few seconds when it was let into the house and was in a highly excited state. This particular case demonstrates again the utilization of both extinction of an undesirable behavior and reinforcement of an alternative behavior.

In both of these cases the behavior may have originally occurred for pathophysiological reasons. The manifested reactions were immediately paired with positive reinforcement by concerned owners. After the physiological cause was gone, the behavior persisted and continued to be reinforced.

Dramatic examples of body systems conditioned to react in an abnormal way are probably not the most common form of psychosomatic reactions that occur in animals. The most frequent forms are of a more insidious nature. Numerous reports in human medicine have correlated the onset of disease with stressful emotional events in the life history of an individual. Among patients experiencing emotional distress there is a slower recovery after illness, a higher incidence of death or a more rapid onset of death, and a higher incidence of complications following routine elective surgery or parturition. The same phenomenon undoubtedly applies to veterinary medicine.

PHARMACOLOGICAL APPROACHES TO BEHAVIORAL PROBLEMS

Psychoactive or psychotropic drugs are pharmacological agents which have behavioral effects and include stimulants, antidepressants, mood elevators, tranquilizers, and some of the hormonal steroids. At the present time tranquilizers and hormonal steroids are the main groups of drugs used in canine and feline practice. However, many of psychoactive drugs could be explored for use in dogs and cats even though the behavioral responses may be somewhat different from those in human patients. Limiting the choice of drugs to the few tranquilizers marketed for animal use eliminates the possibility of successful pharmacological treatments of several serious behavioral problems. More clinical reports of clinical successes and failures in administering different drugs for various problems are needed to assess the most valuable treatments.

TRANQUILIZERS

The calming action of tranquilizers has led to the rather widespread use of these drugs for restraint purposes. A tranquilized animal can be held for a physical examination, subjected to x-ray procedures, given medication, or transported in automobiles or planes. The anxiety and nervousness usually aroused on such occasions are suppressed.

One of the greatest values of tranquilizers has been control of an animal so that it does not engage in a particular behavioral pattern and therefore ceases to be reinforced for repetition of the behavior. It is highly beneficial to be able to simply stop an animal from repeating undesirable behavior while more lasting and therapeutic procedures are applied. For example, drugs might be used to suppress aggressive responses in an animal recovering from a painful surgical procedure or traumatic lesion, to reduce roaming tendencies while awaiting the behavioral effects of castration, or to prevent maternal aggression associated with pseudocyesis.

Tranquilizers may also be used in a desensitization program. The desensitizing process involves administering the drug to the point where the animal no longer shows the undesirable behavior. If the behavior is not affected or if pronounced side effects occur, a different type of drug should be tried.

When drugs are used simultaneously with a gradient extinction or desensitization program to control an animal it is best to start with the highest drug dose that can be tolerated by the animal. Gradually the dose is reduced over a period of weeks or months while the animal continues to be exposed to the stimuli which elicit the undesirable behavior. Positive reinforcement should be paired with an alternative behavior in the presence of the stimuli.

The use of tranquilizers is most appropriate in extreme situations when the intensity of the stimuli which elicit the undesirable behavior cannot be modified or controlled. It is possible that a behavioral pattern acquired under the influence of tranquilizer may not generalize to the nondrug state; therefore, if drugs are utilized in desensitization programs, the drug dosage should be reduced gradually while the presentation of the stimuli is continued.

Progestins

A group of drugs which has proved very useful in the treatment of behavioral problems is the progestins. Many of these compounds are still largely in the experimental stage, but one long-acting injectable form (medroxyprogesterone acetate, Depo-Provera) and one oral form (megestrol acetate) are frequently used in small animal practice.

Theoretically, the progestins act like the hormone progesterone in suppressing masculine behavioral patterns that occur in both intact and castrated males and females. They also seem to have a calming and tranquilizing effect. Long-acting progestins sustain effective systemic levels of the active steroid apparently for weeks or months, and therefore are more useful than progesterone itself. Spraying behavior in castrated and spayed cats will often be reduced or eliminated after a single injection of medroxyprogesterone in a dose of 10 mg/kg. The length of the therapeutic effectiveness is quite variable and probably depends on the animal's own genetic makeup and the environmental circumstances. The oral administration of megestrol acetate (5 mg per day for a week) will often have the same effect of reducing spraying in cats. It is recommended that the dose be gradually reduced to once a week or less, depending upon the reactions of the individual animal. Objectionable urine marking and fighting in male dogs have also been reduced by the injection of medroxyprogesterone at the rate of about 10 mg per kg.

REFERENCES

1. Ader, R.: Early experiences and hormones: emotional behavior and adrenocortical function. In Eleftheriou, B. E., and Spratt, R. (eds.): *Hormonal Correlates of Behavior.* Plenum Press, New York, 1975, p. 7.
2. Anderson, B., and Olson, K.: Effects of bilateral amygdaloid lesions in nervous dogs. J. Small Anim. Pract. *6,* 301, 1965.
3. Bacon, W. E., and Wong, I. G.: Reinforcement value of electrical brain stimulation in neonatal dogs. Devel. Psychobiol. *5,* 195, 1972.
4. Beach, F. A.: Coital behavior in dogs. VI. Long-term effects of castration upon mating in the male. J. Comp. Physiol. Psychol. *70,* 1, 1970.
5. Beach, F. A., and Kuehn, R. E.: Coital behavior in dogs. X. Effects of androgenic stimulation during development on feminine mating responses in females and males. Horm. Behav. *1,* 347, 1970.
6. Beach, F. A., Kuehn, R. E., Sprague, R. H., and Anisko, J. J.: Coital behavior in dogs. XI. Effects of androgenic stimulation during development on masculine mating responses in females. Horm. Behav. *3,* 143, 1972.
7. Carlson, N. R., and Thomas, G. J.: Maternal behavior of mice with limbic lesions. J. Comp. Physiol. Psychol. *66,* 731, 1968.
8. Corson, S. A., O'Leary, C. E., Kirilcut, V., Kirilcut, J., Knopp, W., and Arnold, L. E.: Differential effects of amphetamines on clinically relevant dog models of hyperkinesis and stereotypy: relevance to Huntington's chorea. In Barbeau, A., Chane, T. N., and Paulien, G. W. (eds.): *Advances in Neurology.* Vol. 1: *Huntington's Chorea, 1872–1972.* Raven Press, New York, 1973.
9. Daly, M.: Early stimulation of rodents: a critical review of present interpretations. Brit. J. Psychol. *64,* 435, 1973.
10. Delgado, J. M. R.: Free behavior and brain stimulation. Intern. Rev. Neurobiol. *6,* 349, 1964.
11. Flynn, J.: The neural basis of aggression in cats. In Glans, B. (ed.): *Neurophysiology and Evolution.* Rockefeller University Press, New York, 1967, p. 40.
12. Freeman, D. G., Elliot, E., and Kling, J. A.: Critical period in social development of dogs. Science *133,* 1016, 1961.
13. Fuller, J. L., and Clark, L. D.: Genetic and treatment factors modifying the postisolation syndrome in dogs. J. Comp. Physiol. Psychol. *61,* 251, 1966.
14. Fuller, J. L., Rosvold, H. E., and Pribiam, K. H.: The effect on affective and cognitive behavior in the dog of lesions of the pyriform-amygdala-hippocampal complex. J. Comp. Physiol. Psychol. *50,* 89, 1957.
15. Gloor, P.: Amygdala. In Field, J. (ed.): *Handbook of Physiology, Vol. 2: Neurophysiology.* Amer. Physiol. Soc., Washington, D.C., 1960.
16. Goy, R. W., and Goldfoot, D. H.: Hormonal influences on sexually dimorphic behavior. In Greep, R. O. (ed.): *Handbook of Physiology,* Section 7: *Endocrinology,* Vol. 2, Part I. Amer. Physiol. Soc., Washington, D.C., 1973.
17. Green, J. D., Clemente, C. D., and deGroot, J.:

Rhinencephalic lesions and behavior in cats. J. Comp. Neurol. *108*, 505, 1967.
18. Greenough, W. T., Carter, C. S., Steerman, C., and DeVougd, T. J.: Sex differences in dendritic pattern in hamster preoptic area. *Brain Res.* (in press, 1977.)
19. Gregory, R. L.: The logic of localization of function in the central nervous system. In *Biological Prototypes and Synthetic Systems.* Vol. I. Plenum Press, New York, 1962.
20. Hart, B. L.: Role of prior sexual experience in the effects of castration and sexual behavior of male dogs. *J. Comp. Physiol. Psychol. 66,* 719, 1968.
21. Hart, B. L.: Gonadal androgen and sociosexual behavior of male mammals: a comparative analysis. *Psychol. Bull. 81,* 383, 1974.
22. Hart, B. L.: Medial preoptic-anterior hypothalamic area and sociosexual behavior of male dogs. A comparative neuropsychological analysis. *J. Comp. Physiol. Psychol. 86,* 328, 1974.
23. Hart, B. L.: Types of aggressive behavior. *Canine Pract. 1,* 6, 1974.
24. Hart, B. L.: Behavioral effects of castration. *Canine Pract. 3,* 10, 1976.
25. Hart, B. L.: Urine spraying in cats. In Kirk, R. W. (ed.): *Current Veterinary Therapy VI.* W. B. Saunders Co. Philadelphia, 1977, p. 1259.
26. Hart, B. L., and Barrett, R. E.: Effects of castration on fighting, roaming, and urine spraying in adult male cats. *J.A.V.M.A. 163,* 290, 1973.
27. Hart, B. L., Haugen, C. M., and Peterson, D. M.: Effects of medial preopticanterior hypothalamic lesions on mating behavior of male cats. *Brain Res. 54,* 117, 1973.
28. Hart, B. L., and Voith, V. L.: Changes in urine spraying, feeding, and sleep behavior of cats following medial preoptic-anterior hypothalamic lesions in cats. Submitted to *Brain Res.*
29. Hoebel, B. G.: Feeding: neural control of intake. *Ann. Rev. Physiol. 33,* 533, 1971.
30. Holliday, T. A., Cunningham, J. G., and Gutnick, M. J.: Comparative clinical and electroencephalographic studies of canine epilepsy. *Epilepsia 11,* 281, 1970.
31. Hopkins, S. G., Schubert, T. A., and Hart, B. L.: Castration of adult male dogs: effects on roaming, aggression, urine marking and mounting. *J.A.V.M.A. 168,* 1105, 1976.
32. Ingram, W. R.: Brain stem mechanisms in behavior. *EEG Clin. Neurophysiol. 4,* 397, 1952.
33. Kaada, B.: Brain mechanisms related to aggressive behavior. In Clemente, C. E., and Lindsley, D. B. (eds.): *Aggression and Defences.* University of California Press, Berkeley, 1967.
34. Kim, C., Chai, H., Kim, J. K., Chang, H. K., Park, R. S., and Kang, I. Y.: General behavioral activity and its component patterns in hippocampectomized rats. *Brain Res. 9,* 379, 1970.
35. Kimble, D. P., Rogers, L., and Hendrickson, C. W.: Hippocampal lesions disrupt maternal not sexual behavior in the albino rat. *J. Comp. Physiol. Psychol. 63,* 401, 1967.
36. Klüver, H., and Bucy, P. C.: "Psychic blindness" and other symptoms following bilateral temporal lobectomy in rhesus monkeys. *Amer. J. Physiol. 119,* 352, 1937.
37. Le Boeuf, B. J.: Copulatory and aggressive behavior in the prepubertally castrated dog. *Horm. Behav. 127,* 1970.
38. Levine, S., Haltmeyer, G. C., Karas, G. G., and Denenberg, V. H.: Physiological and behavioral effects of infantile stimulation. *Physiol. Behav. 2,* 55, 1967.
39. Mason, W. A., and Berkson, G.: Effects of maternal mobility on the development of rocking and other behaviors in rhesus monkeys: a study with artificial mothers. *Devel. Psychobiol. 8,* 197, 1975.
40. Meier, G. W.: Infantile handling and development in Siamese kittens. *J. Comp. Physiol. Psych. 54,* 284, 1961.
41. Melzack, R.: The genesis of emotional behavior: an experimental study of the dog. J. Comp. Physiol. Psychol. *47,* 166, 1954.
42. Melzack, R., and Scott, T. H.: The effects of early experience on the response to pain. J. Comp. Physiol. Psychol. *50,* 155, 1957.
43. Melzack, R., and Thompson, W. R.: Effects of early experience on social behavior. *Canad. J. Psychol. 10,* 82, 1956.
44. Numan, M.: Medial preoptic areas and maternal behavior in the female rat. *J. Comp. Physiol. Psychol. 87,* 746, 1974.
45. Olds, J.: The central nervous system and the reinforcement of behavior. *Amer. Psychol. 24,* 114, 1969.
46. Ottenberg, P., Stein, M., Lewis, J., and Hamilton, C.: Learned asthma in the guinea pig. *Psychosom. Med. 20,* 395, 1958.
47. Raisman, G., and Field, P. M.: Sexual dimorphism in the neuropil of the preoptic area of the rat and its dependence on neonatal androgen. *Brain Res. 54,* 1, 1973.
48. Redding, R. W., and Walker, T. L.: Electroconvulsive therapy to control aggression in dogs. *Mod. Vet. Pract. 57,* 595, 1976.
49. Resko, J. A.: Androgens in systemic plasma of male guinea pigs during development and after castration in adulthood. *Endocrinology 86,* 1444, 1970.
50. Resko, J. A., Feder, H. H. and Goy, R. W.: Androgen concentrations in plasma and testis of developing rats. *J. Endocrinol. 40,* 485, 1968.
51. Resko, J. A., Malley, A., Begley, D., and Hess, D. L.: Radioimmunoassay of testosterone during fetal development of the rhesus monkey. *Endocrinology 93,* 156, 1973.
52. Resko, J. A., and Phoenix, C. H.: Sexual behavior and testosterone concentrations in the plasma of the rhesus monkey before and after castration. *Endocrinology 86,* 499, 1972.
53. Roberts, W. W.: Are hypothalamic motivational mechanisms functionally and anatomically specific? *Brain Behav. Ecol. 2,* 317, 1969.
54. Rosenzweig, M. R., Krech, D., Bennett, E. L., and Diamond, M. C.: Effects of environmental complexity and training on brain chemistry and anatomy: a replication and extension. *J. Comp. Physiol. Psychol. 55,* 429, 1962.
55. Routtenberg, A.: Intracranial chemical injection and behavior: A critical review. *Behav. Biol. 7,* 601, 1972.
56. Schreiner, L., and Kling, A.: Rhinencephalon and behavior. *Amer. J. Physiol.* 184, 1956.
57. Scott, J. P.: Critical periods in the development of social behavior in puppies. *Psychosom. Med. 20,* 42, 1958.
58. Scott, J. P.: Critical periods in behavioral development. *Science 138,* 949, 1962.

59. Seitz, P. F. D.: Infantile experience and adult behavior in animal subjects. II. Age of separation from the mother and adult behavior in the cat. *Psychosom. Med. 21*, 354, 1959.
60. Slimp, J. C., Hart, B. L., and Goy, R. W.: Heterosexual, autosexual, and social behavior of adult male rhesus monkeys with medial preoptic anterior hypothalamic lesions. *Brain Res.* (in press.)
61. Slotnick, M. B.: Disturbances of maternal behavior in rats following lesions of the dorsal limbic cortex. *Behaviour 29*, 204, 1967.
62. Slotnick, B. N., and Nigrosh, B. J.: Maternal behavior of mice with cingulate cortical, amygdala, or septal lesions. *J. Comp. Physiol. Psychol. 88*, 118, 1975.
63. Smith, M. O., and Holland, R. C. Effects of lesions of the nucleus accumbens on lactation and postpartum behavior. *Physiol. Psychol. 3*, 331, 1975.
64. Stamm, J.: The function of the median cerebral cortex in maternal behavior of rats. *J. Comp. Physiol. Psychol. 48*, 347, 1955.
65. Thompson, W. R., and Heron, W.: The effects of restricting early experience on the problem solving capacity of dogs. *Canad. J. Psychol. 8*, 17, 1954.
66. Thompson, W. R., and Heron, W.: The effects of early restriction on activity in dogs. *J. Comp. Physiol. Psychol. 47*, 77, 1954.
67. Tuber, P., Hothersal, D., and Voith, V. L.: Animal clinical psychology: a modest proposal. *Amer. Psychol. 29*, 762, 1974.
68. Van der Velden, N. A., De Weerth, C. J., Brooyman-Schallenberg, J. H. C., and Tielen, A. B.: An abnormal behavioral trait in Bernese mountain dogs (Bernes Sennenhund). *Tijdschr. Diergeneesk. 101*, 403, 1976.
69. Voith, V. L.: Destructive behavior in owner's absence. Parts I and II. *Canine Pract. 2(3)*, 11; *2(4)*, 8–12, 1975.
70. Voith, V. L.: Fear-induced aggressive behavior. Parts I and II. *Canine Pract. 3(5)*, 14–20; *3(6)*, 14–16, 1976.
71. Voith, V. L.: Aggressive behavior and dominance. *Canine Pract. 4(2)*, 8–15, 1977.
72. Voith, V. L., and Hart, B. L.: Medial preoptic-anterior hypothalamic ventral medial continuum and maternal behavior of female cats (unpublished observation, 1977).
73. Wade, G. N.: Sex hormones, regulatory behaviors, and body weight. In Rosenblatt, J. S., Hinde, R. A., Shaw, E., and Beer, C. G. (eds.): *Advances in the Study of Behavior.* Vol. 6. Academic Press, New York, 1976, p. 201.

SECTION 2
ELECTROCONVULSIVE THERAPY

R. W. Redding, D.V.M., Ph.D.

Chemotherapy, psychotherapy, and psychosurgery can be used as treatment for behavior disorders in the dog;[4] however, some animals fail to respond favorably to such treatment. An alternate method of behavior modification is electroconvulsive therapy (ECT) or multiple electroconvulsive therapy (MECT).[9] ECT is defined as one induced seizure in one day, whereas MECT consists of two or more successive induced seizures at one treatment period in one day.

EQUIPMENT FOR ECT AND MECT

Electroconvulsive therapy instruments such as Medcraft Mark 11 B24,* which is designed for human use, may also be used on dogs. By using standard 115 volt AC input, the treatment time can be varied from 0.1 to 1.0 second and the voltages from 70 to 170 volts. Two-inch stainless steel electrodes attached to a rubber head band are used to administer either ECT or MECT.

*Medcraft Incorporated, Skippack, Pa.

TREATMENT METHOD

Each patient should be given a complete physical and neurological examination, including electroencephalographic analysis, to eliminate the possibility of organic brain diseases that may be responsible for the behavior abnormality.

The patient is anesthetized with an ultrashort intravenous anesthetic prior to treatment. Methohexital (Brevane) is the agent of choice. Daily repeated use of thiobarbiturates will result in depression and prolonged anesthesia due to incomplete detoxification. Methohexital is used because it is more rapidly detoxified. Atropine (0.01 mg/kg) is administered prior to MECT to prevent cardiac arrhythmias and excessive salivation. An endotracheal tube is mandatory to insure an adequate airway, and a soft mouth gag is used to prevent injury to the tongue during the convulsive stage of the treatment.

Electrode jelly is applied bilaterally to the frontotemporal region of the head and rubbed into the skin to obtain low-resistance contact with the electrode disks. The patient leads are attached to the instrument output junction and to the terminals of the electrode disks.

In man, the voltage and current largely determine the success or failure of ECT or MECT. For optimum effectiveness, the stimulus must be of sufficient magnitude to surpass the patient's variable seizure threshold.[1, 3, 5, 7, 11] Voltages of from 90 to 140 will surpass the seizure threshold in dogs. Small animals require lower voltages and large ones need higher voltages. However, certain breeds such as the greyhound respond to lower voltages than would be expected. The treatment time for maximal effectiveness in dogs is 1 second. Three sequential seizures (MECT) are induced. The second and third successive seizures are induced immediately after the previous seizure has subsided. These treatments are administered for 5 or 6 successive days. After the third or fourth day of MECT a marked personality change usually becomes evident in dogs that have been belligerent. Patients that are selectively belligerent (to other dogs or to children, women, or men only) and whose behavior is not hostile toward the clinician show very little change during the treatment period.

INDICATIONS FOR MECT

In veterinary medicine MECT has been found to be effective in the treatment of aggression toward:[9] (1) the owner, (2) children, (3) other dogs, and (4) men or women. Other indications may be fear biting, neurodermatitis, destructive tendencies, flank sucking, tail biting, and excessive fear of loud noises. However, the effect of MECT on these behavior abnormalities has not been evaluated.

INDICATIONS FOR ECT

ECT has been used for various mental disorders in man since 1938.[3, 5, 7, 10] It has been primarily used in man for treatment of depression and hyperexcitable conditions such as mania.[3, 7, 8, 10] Occasionally, aggression has been treated.[1, 6] The following are the disorders in man for which ECT has been used and may be indicated:[7]

1. Affective disorders, including (a) depression with psychosomatic changes when suicide is a serious risk, and while awaiting responses to antidepressants; and (b) mania, when acute management is difficult.
2. Schizophrenia, including catatonic and schizo-affective patients and those reluctant to take medication.
3. Others: anxiety, panic, delirium tremens, neurodermatitis, ulceration colitis, tic douloureux, pain of phantom limbs, epilepsies, psychotic symptoms of general paresis, narcotic withdrawal, and aggression.

The effectiveness of ECT in the treatment of depression in man is superior to that of antidepressant drug therapy or psychotherapy.[1, 5, 7]

The contraindications for ECT or MECT in man are brain tumors; cardiovascular disease, including aneurysms, myocardial infarctions, congestive heart failure, and cerebrovascular accidents; and disorders of bone that may predispose to fractures at the time of a convulsion. The same contraindications are true for dogs.

COMMENTS

Retreatments may be necessary to maintain normal behavior. It is not uncommon in the treatment of humans for additional ECT to be instituted to maintain desired results.

After ECT treatment an "aura" of confusion and apparent loss of memory is observed in all patients. Owners report that their dogs are confused at times for 2 to 4 weeks after the treatment, after which there is a gradual return of memory. Following treatment and release from the hospital, the dog may show no more interest in the owner than in any other person. The ability to recognize the owner returns relatively rapidly, however. Such a memory loss has also been observed following ECT in man.[1, 3, 5, 8, 11]

There is considerable controversy concerning the relationship between memory loss and effectiveness of ECT in man.[3, 5, 8, 11] Administering unilateral ECT on the nondominant hemisphere has been recommended to reduce the amount of memory loss in special cases.[1, 5, 7] The author believes that the memory loss that occurs is associated with the improvement noted in the dog's behavior.

Although the mechanism of action of MECT is not completely understood,[1, 2, 6–8, 11] the following theories have been suggested (1) alteration of acetylcholine and catecholamines in the central synapses of the brain; (2) alteration of cellular permeability to electrolytes and amines; and (3) an increased permeability of the blood–brain barrier.

The reported human fatality rate following ECT is fewer than 1 in 10,000 treatments.[1] Deaths have not been directly related to the seizure but occur in the postseizure period.[1]

ECT and MECT are easily administered to dogs when proper equipment and general anesthesia are used.[9] A repeated series of treatments may be required in some cases.

REFERENCES

1. Abrams, R., and Fink, M.: Answers to questions frequently asked about ECT. Sem. Psychiat. *4*, 33–38, 1972.
2. Aird, R. B., Striat, L. A., Pace, J. W., Hrenoff, M. K., and Bowritch, S. C.: Current pathway and neurophysiologic effects of electrically induced convulsions. J. Nerv. Ment. Dis. *123*, 505–512, 1956.
3. Arnot, R. E.: Observations on the effects of electric convulsive treatment in man. Psycholog. Dis. Nerv. System *36*, 499–502, 1975.
4. Campbell, W. E.: *Behavior Problems in Dogs*. American Veterinary Publications, Santa Barbara, Calif., 1975.
5. Dornbush, R. L.: Memory and induced ECT convulsions. Sem. Psychiat. *4*, 47–54, 1972.
6. Fink, M.: The therapeutic process in ECT. Sem. Psychiat. *4*, 39–46, 1972.
7. Hurwitz, T. D.: Electroconvulsive therapy: A review. Comprehensive Psychiatry *15*, 303–314, 1974.
8. Ottosson, J.: Psychological or Physiological theories of ECT. Int. J. Psychiat. *5*, 170–174, 1968.
9. Redding, R. W., and Walker, T. L.: Electroconvulsive therapy to control aggression in dogs. Mod. Vet. Pract. *57*, 595–597, Aug. 1976.
10. Robitscher, J. B.: Psychosurgery and other somatic means of altering behavior. Bull Am. Acad. Psych. Law 7–33, March 1974.
11. Volavka, J.: Neurophysiology of ECT. Sem. Psychiat. *4*, 55–65, 1972.

CHAPTER 20

BRAIN SURGERY

B. F. Hoerlein, D.V.M., Ph.D.
J. E. Oliver, Jr., D.V.M., M.S., Ph.D.*

Once a lesion of the central nervous system has been diagnosed, treatment must then be considered. In some instances, surgery is the method of choice and may, in fact, offer the only hope for survival. This is so particularly with some of the brain injuries mentioned in Chapter 11.

Surgery for brain lesions has been performed for many years in man. The techniques and knowledge needed in brain surgery have developed considerably, and the resulting proficiency of surgeons is reflected in the decreasing mortality rate in brain surgery. Mullan[41] reported a 2.6 per cent mortality rate in 100 consecutive cases of surgery for brain tumors. Of 34 patients who had benign tumors, 76 per cent returned to their former jobs; of 28 patients who had slowly progressive infiltrative tumors, 68 per cent returned to their jobs; of 38 patients who had malignant tumors, 10 per cent returned.

Brain surgery is still a developing field in veterinary medicine, and most of the difficulties stem from inadequate diagnostic techniques. One must determine the type of lesion, the tentative diagnosis, and the precise location before surgery can be performed effectively. However, owing to current progress in physical diagnostics, radiography, angiography, ventriculography, and electroencephalography, brain surgery is becoming increasingly practical in small animals. The economic or sentimental value of the animal, which must be considered in veterinary surgery, will probably always hinder progress in brain surgery.

Chapter 8 dealt with basic considerations of neurosurgery and stressed the peculiarities of the CNS as compared with other systems. The principles of anesthesia, physiological monitoring, shock, positioning, equipment, control of hemorrhage, and means of combating edema and brain swelling were discussed. It was stressed that a knowledge of neuroanatomy, basic neurology, and surgery was fundamental to the specialized art and science of neurosurgery. Finally, an interest in and compassion for the postsurgical patient is necessary for his rehabilitation and recovery. This chapter will stress specific surgical procedures that have proved to be of value in alleviating the various brain disorders that cannot be handled satisfactorily by medical methods. These techniques have been developed by several workers at this clinic and all deserve a great deal of recognition. Besides the authors, these workers include Drs. Albert Few, E. D. Gage, S. F. Swaim, and R. W. Redding.

*Contributions from an experimental study; Canine Cranial Surgery, Master's Thesis, Auburn University, Auburn, Alabama, 1966, and subsequent publications.

ANATOMICAL CONSIDERATIONS

It has been mentioned that the brain is a unique organ that in man amounts to only 2.2 per cent of the total body weight and requires up to 15 per cent of the total circulating blood.[21] In man, the shape of the skull and brain are fairly consistent regardless of race or age. In the dog, the size, shape, contour, and thickness of calvarium vary tremendously in the different breeds. The breed with a cranium and calvarial musculature that are most similar to those in man is probably the Chihuahua. One must therefore continuously review the characteristic anatomy of the breed of each dog that is a candidate for brain surgery, or anatomical confusion can easily occur. In addition to consulting anatomy texts, one should palpate the patient's skull structures and study radiographs carefully for accurate location of surgical landmarks for that particular patient (Figs. 20–1 to 20–3).

The vascular supply to the pericalvarial tissues is not uniquely significant. The nerve supply to these structures is primarily from the trigeminal, facial, and second cervical nerves. The musculature is composed of superficial layers which control action of the eyelids and ears, whereas the heavy temporal muscle overlies the lateral craniotomy approach to the calvarium. The musculature involved in the approach to the cerebellum is massive, consisting of several dorsal cervical spinal muscles attached to the caudal surface of the occipital bone.[33, 39]

The blood vessels of the brain and skull

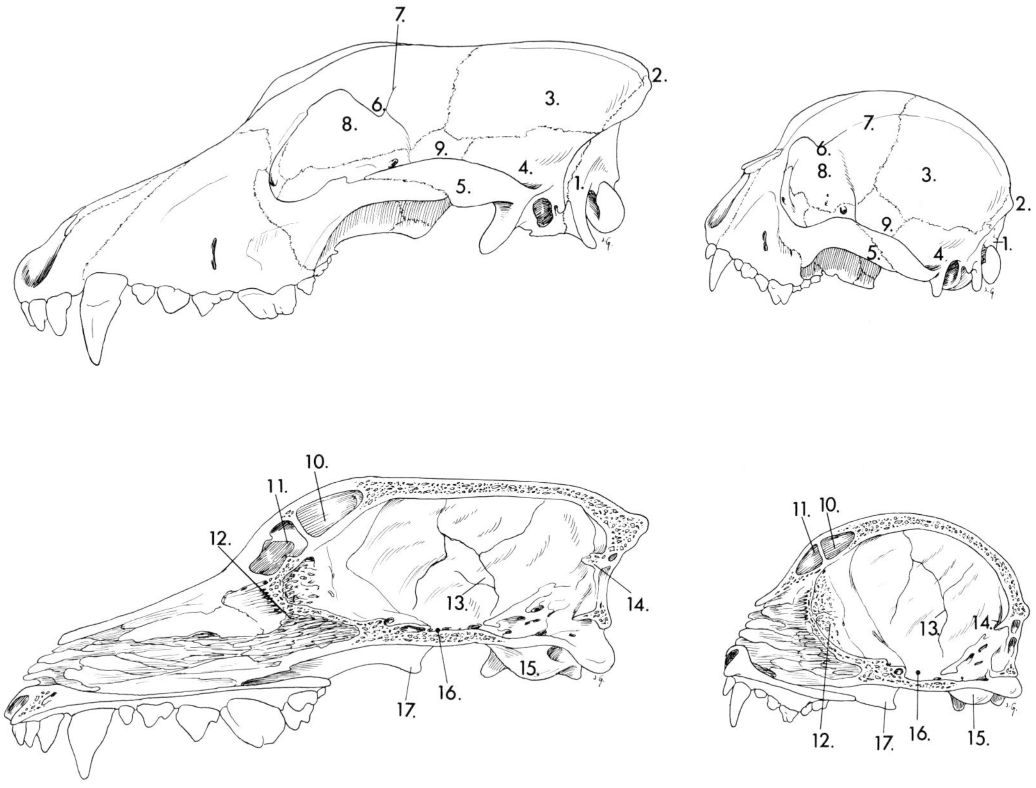

A B

FIGURE 20–1 Anatomical landmarks that are important in brain surgery. *A*. Dolichocephalic. *B*. Brachycephalic. (1) Occipital bone; (2) external occipital protuberance; (3) parietal bone; (4) temporal bone; (5) zygomatic arch; (6) zygomatic process of the frontal bone; (7) external frontal crest; (8) frontal bone; (9) sphenoid bone; (10) lateral part of frontal sinus; (11) medial part of frontal sinus; (12) cribriform plate; (13) groove for middle meningeal artery; (14) tentorium osseum; (15) bulla ossea; (16) hypophyseal fossa; (17) pterygoid bone. (After Seiferle, E.: Zur Topographie des Gehirns bei lang- und kurzköpfigen Hunderassen. Acta Anat., *63*:346, 1966; and Miller, M. E., Christensen, G. C., and Evans, H. E.: *Anatomy of the Dog*. Philadelphia, W. B. Saunders Co., 1964.)

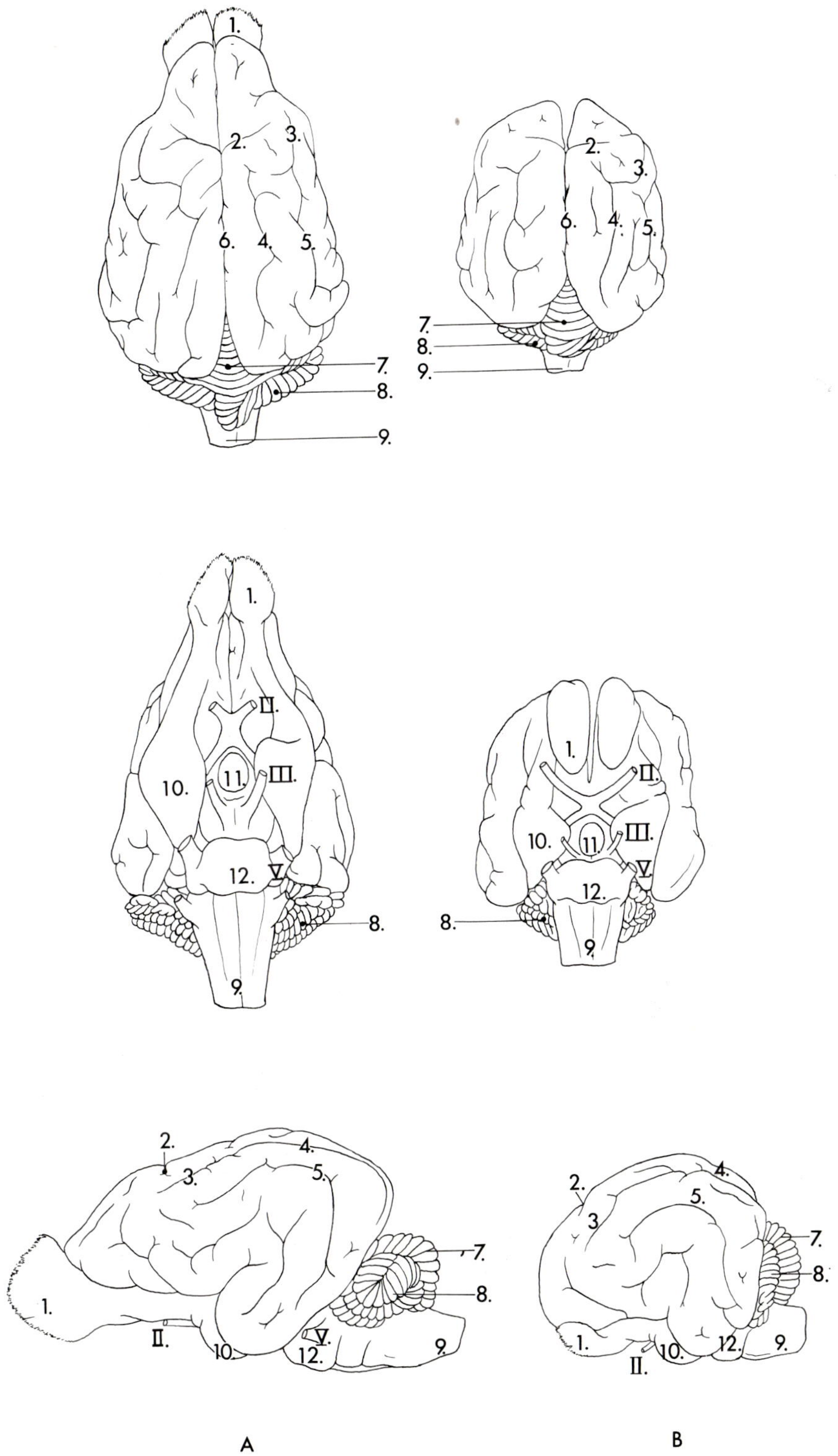

FIGURE 20–2 Brains from dolichocephalic skulls (*A*) compared to brains from brachycephalic skulls (*B*). (1) Olfactory bulb; (2) cruciate sulcus; (3) coronal sulcus; (4) lateral sulcus; (5) middle suprasylvian sulcus; (6) longitudinal fissure; (7) cerebellar vermis; (8) cerebellar hemisphere; (9) medulla oblongata; (10) pyriform lobe; (11) hypophysis; (12) pons; (II) optic nerve; (III) oculomotor nerve; (V) trigeminal nerve. (After Seiferle, E.: Zur Topographie des Gehirns bei lang- und kurzköpfigen Hunderassen. Acta Anat., *63*:346, 1966; and Miller, M. E., Christensen, G. C., and Evans, H. E.: *Anatomy of the Dog*. Philadelphia, W. B. Saunders Co., 1964.)

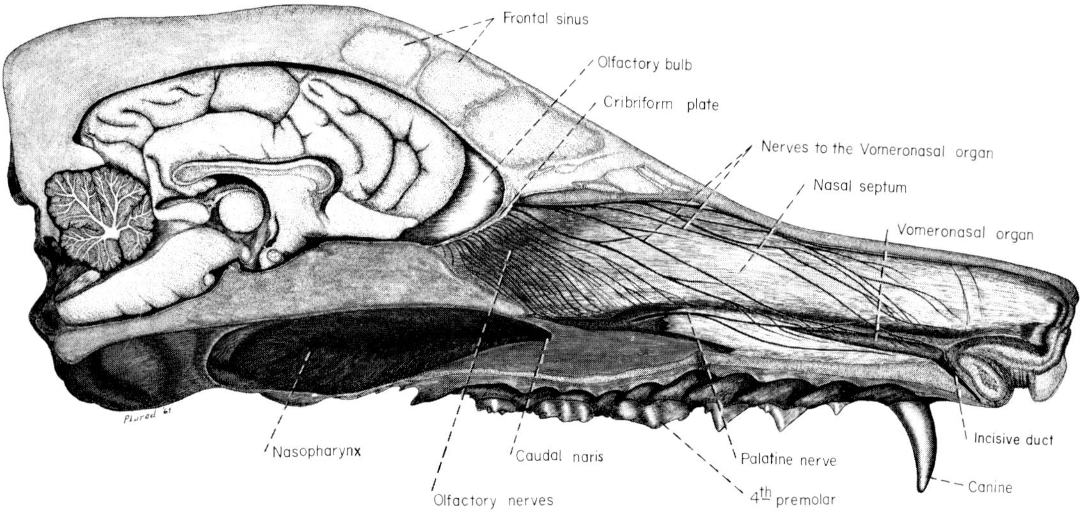

FIGURE 20–3 Sagittal section of the skull of the dog. Note position of the cerebrum, cerebellum, olfactory bulb, cribriform plate, and sinuses. (Courtesy of Getty, R.: *Sisson and Grossman's Anatomy of the Domestic Animal,* 5th ed, W. B. Saunders Co., Philadelphia, 1975.)

are of major importance to the neurosurgeon. Improper hemostasis and major bleeding from arterial or venous intervention can be disastrous. The venous sinuses lack a tunica adventitia and have no valves.[39] The sinus system is complex. It consists dorsally of the dorsal sagittal sinus, the transverse sinuses, and the straight sinus. Three sinuses—the temporal, the superior petrosal, and the sigmoid—join the transverse sinuses at their lateral extremity. The large paired cavernous sinuses lie on either side of the floor of the middle cranial fossa and communicate caudally with the ventral petrosal sinuses.

The venous drainage eventually involves the following routes: (1) the ophthalmic veins, which communicate with the cavernous sinus, and which are tributaries of the external maxillary vein; (2) the temporal, retroglenoid, and middle meningeal veins, which drain into the internal maxillary; (3) the sigmoid and ventral petrosal sinuses and some small veins, which drain into the internal jugular; and (4) the vertebral veins and sinuses. In the dog, the external jugular is the largest route of venous drainage; the internal jugular is smaller. In man, the internal jugular is the larger drainage route (Figs. 20–4 to 20–6).[39, 56, 65]

The arterial supply to the brain consists primarily of the internal carotid, the vertebral, and the ventral spinal arteries.[39] A significant anastomosis is present between the internal maxillary and the internal carotid arteries.[11, 27] In the dog, life is sustained if one of the aforementioned supply routes is maintained. There are no functional disturbances if only the carotid or vertebral arteries are destroyed.[6, 8, 9] The branches of these major vessels are pictured in Figures 20–7 to 20–11.

The paired rostral, middle, and caudal cerebral arteries supply the cerebral hemispheres and deep structures. The rostral and caudal cerebral arteries may be occluded without functional disturbance, but ligation of the middle cerebral results in contralateral hemiparesis and contralateral homonymous hemianopsia, due to necrosis of a large part of the cerebral hemisphere. Functional recovery from ligation will usually occur in 3 weeks.[49, 53] Collateral circulation, both arterial and venous, develops rapidly in most cases of vascular occlusion (Fig. 20–12).

The gross functional anatomy has been discussed in Chapters 2 and 4 and is effectively described in detail in various textbooks.[39] The specific details of surgical anatomy are discussed with the appropriate procedure.

(*Text continued on page 706.*)

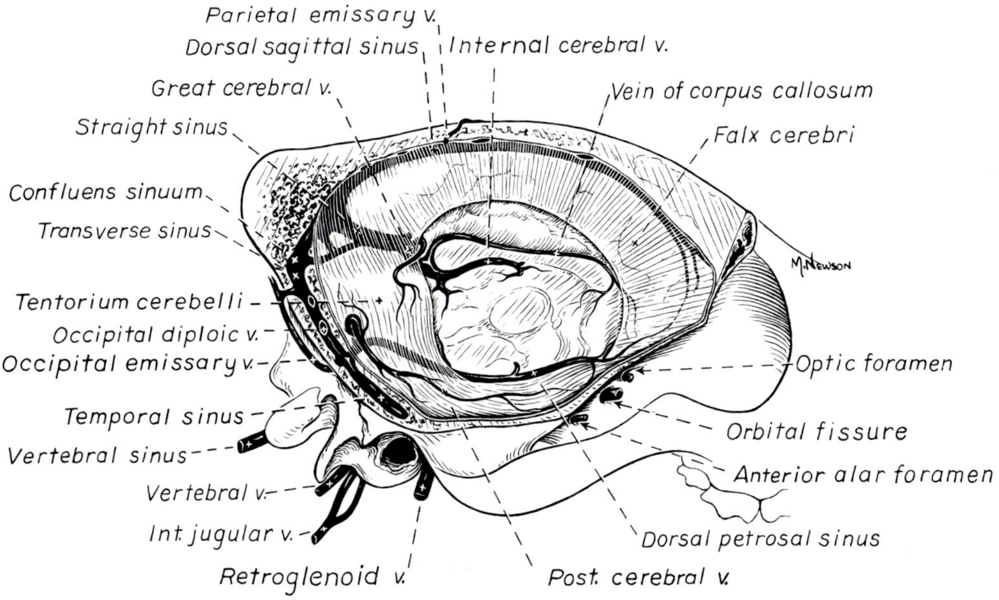

FIGURE 20–4 Cranial venous sinuses, lateral aspect (right cerebral hemisphere removed). (From Reinhard, K. R., Miller, M. E., and Evans, H. E.: The craniovertebral veins and sinuses of the dog. Am. J. Anat. *111*, 67, 1962.)

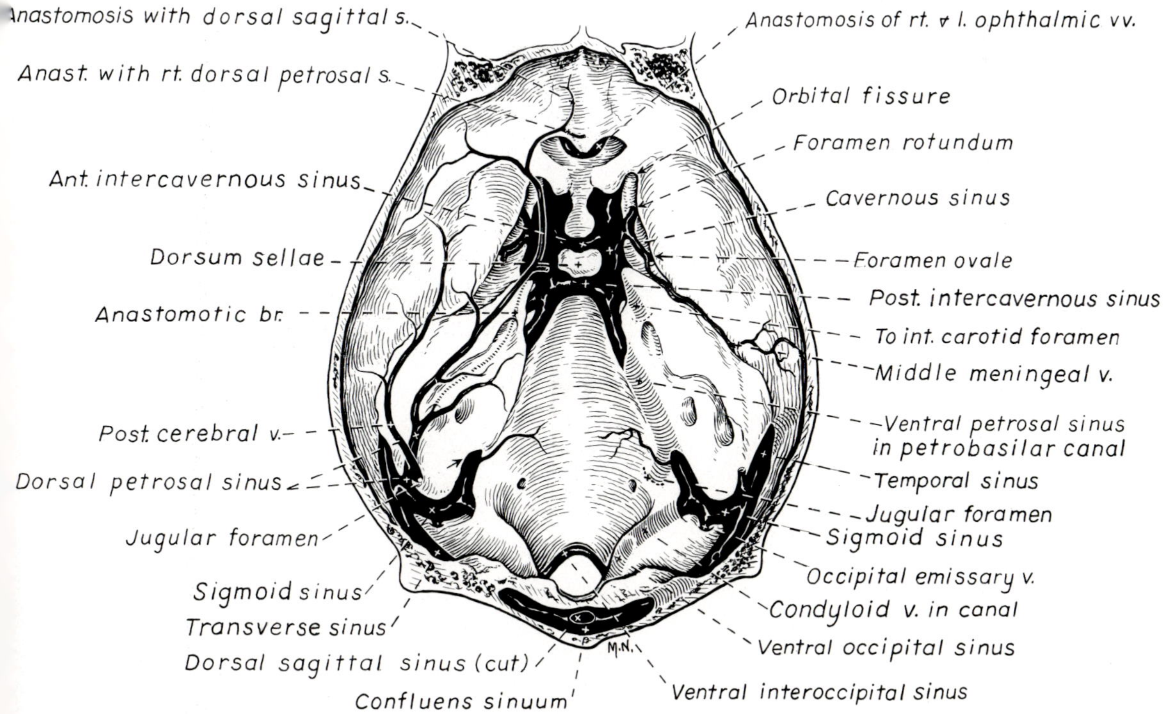

FIGURE 20–5 Cranial venous sinuses, dorsal aspect (calvarium removed). (From Reinhard, K. R., Miller, M. E., and Evans, H. E.: The craniovertebral veins and sinuses of the dog. Am. J. Anat. *111*, 67, 1962.)

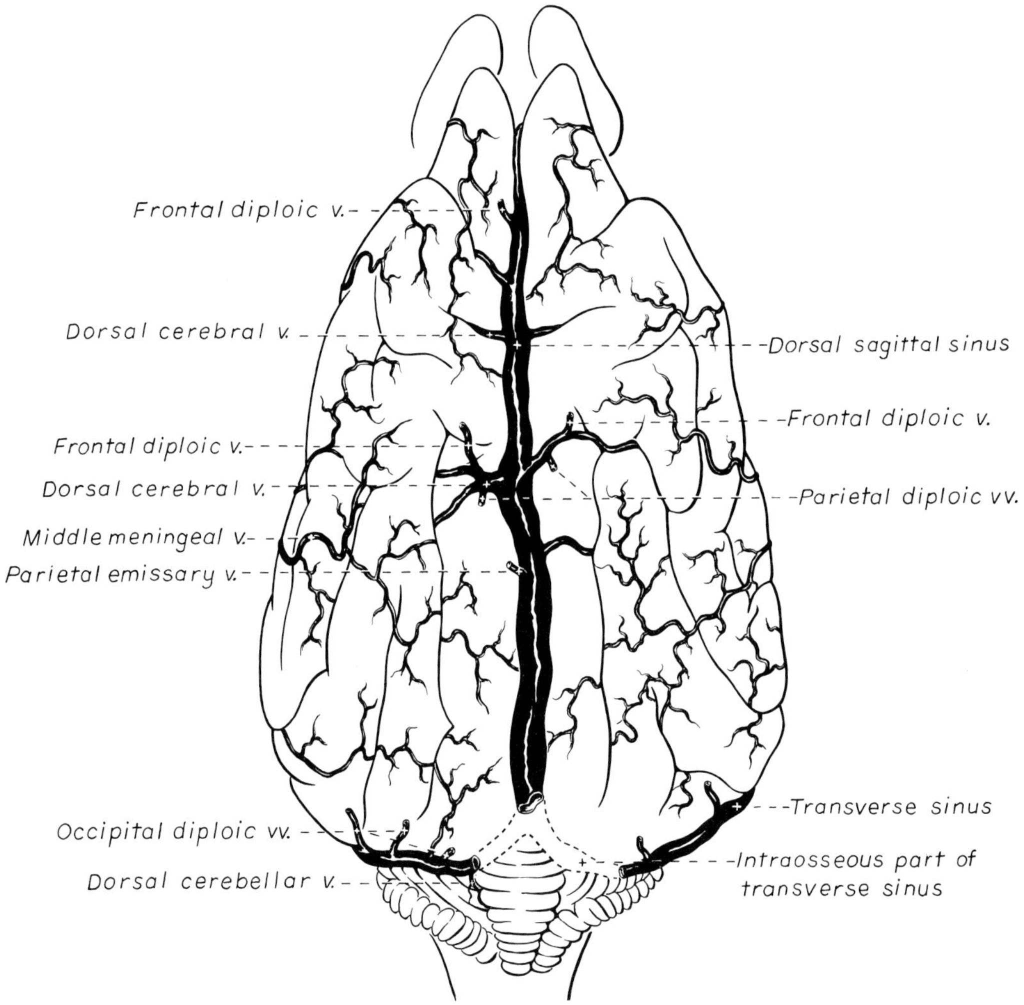

FIGURE 20–6 Veins of the brain, dorsal aspect. (From Miller, M. E., Christensen, G. C., and Evans, H. E.: *Anatomy of the Dog*. Philadelphia, W. B. Saunders Co., 1964.)

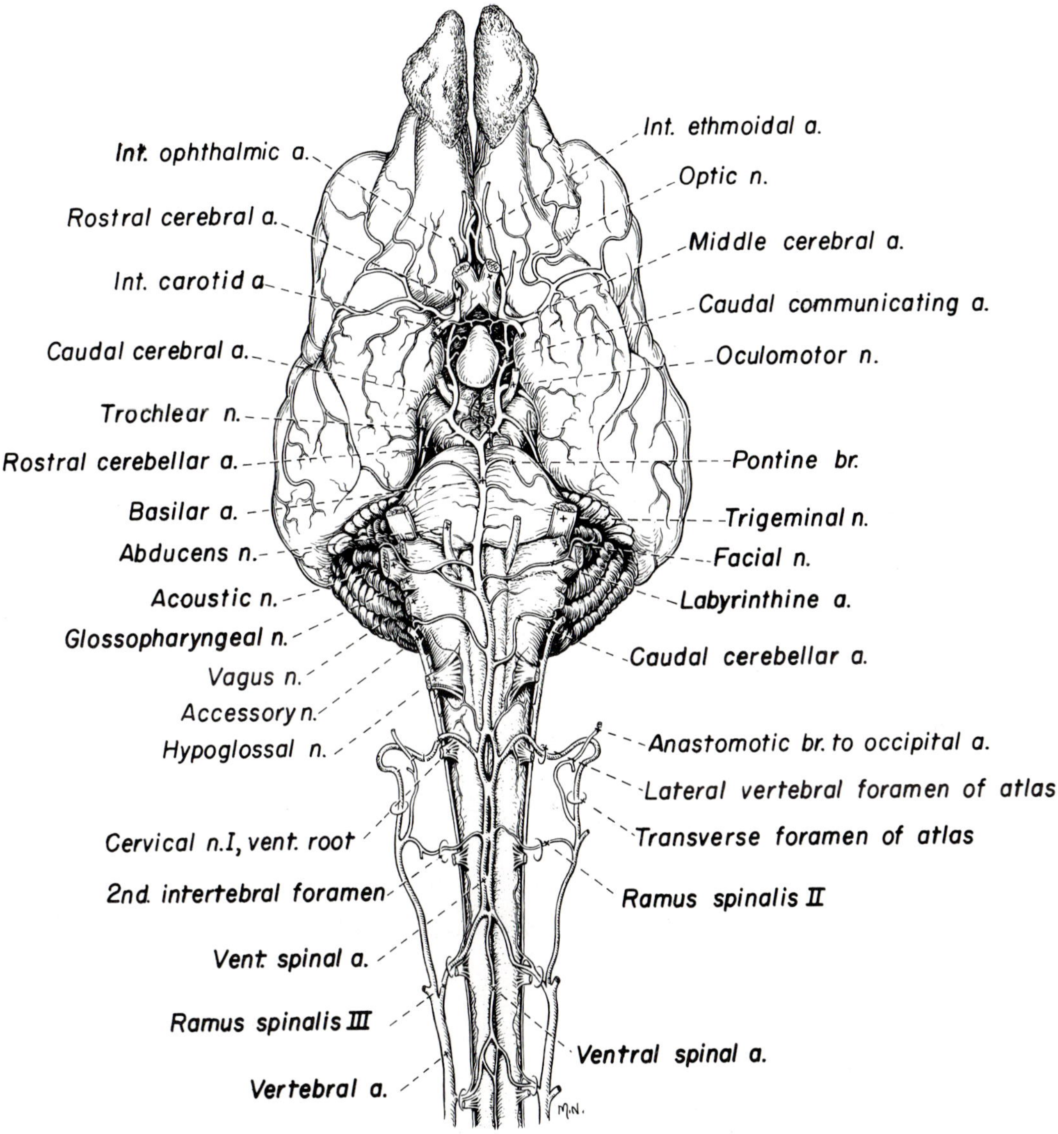

FIGURE 20–7 Arteries of the brain and cervical spinal cord, ventral aspect. (From Miller, M. E., Christensen, G. C., and Evans, H. E.: *Anatomy of the Dog*. Philadelphia, W. B. Saunders Co., 1964.)

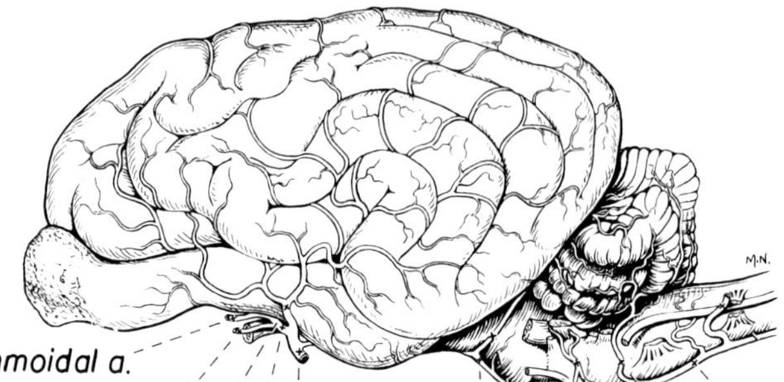

FIGURE 20–8 Distribution of the middle cerebral artery, lateral aspect. (From Miller, M. E., Christensen, G. C., and Evans, H. E.: *Anatomy of the Dog*. Philadelphia, W. B. Saunders Co., 1964.)

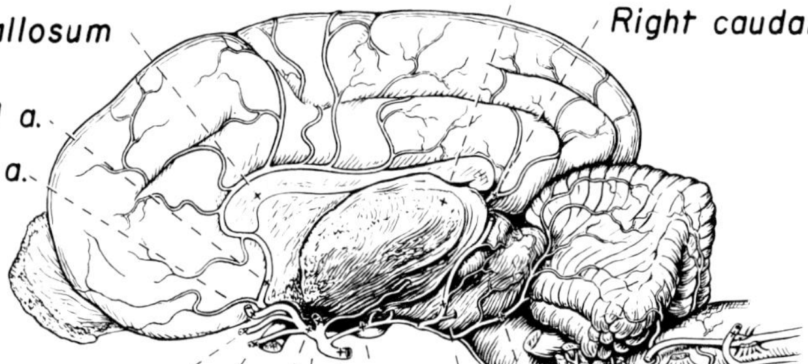

FIGURE 20–9 Arteries of the cerebellum and medial surface of cerebrum. (From Miller, M. E., Christensen, G. C., and Evans, H. E.: *Anatomy of the Dog*. Philadelphia, W. B. Saunders Co., 1964.)

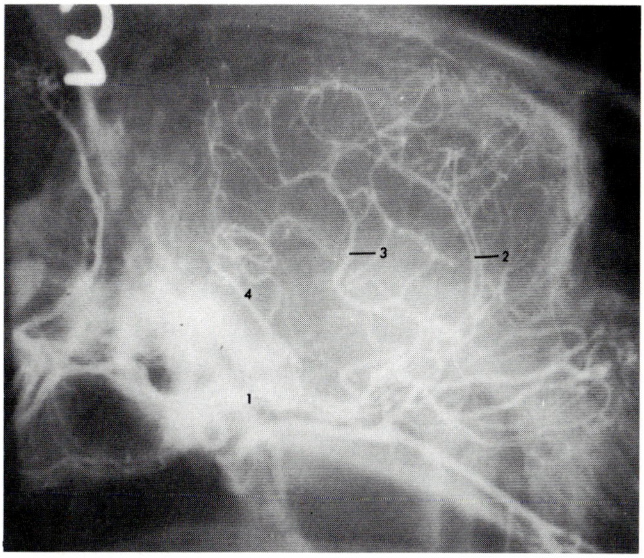

FIGURE 20–10 Cerebral arteriogram—lateral position. (1) Internal carotid artery; (2) rostral cerebral artery; (3) middle cerebral artery; (4) caudal cerebral artery. (See Chapter 2 for detailed anatomical circulation.)

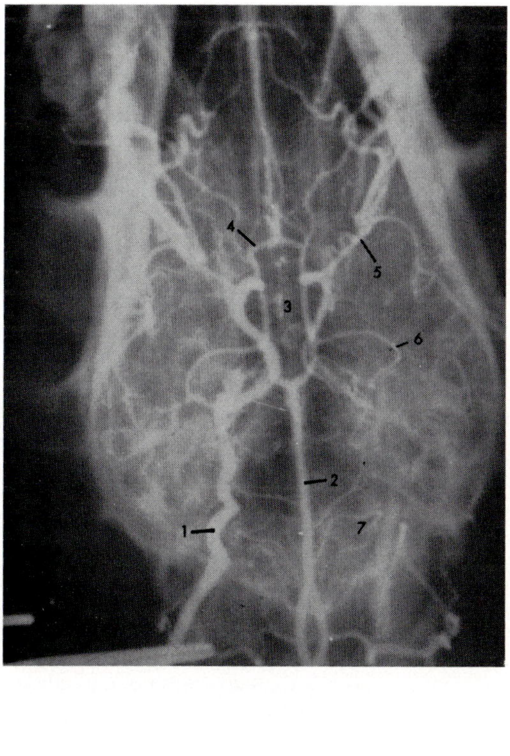

FIGURE 20–11 Cerebral arteriogram—ventrodorsal position. (1) Internal carotid artery; (2) basilar artery; (3) circle of Willis; (4) rostral cerebral artery; (5) middle cerebral artery; (6) caudal cerebral artery; (7) posterior cerebellar artery.

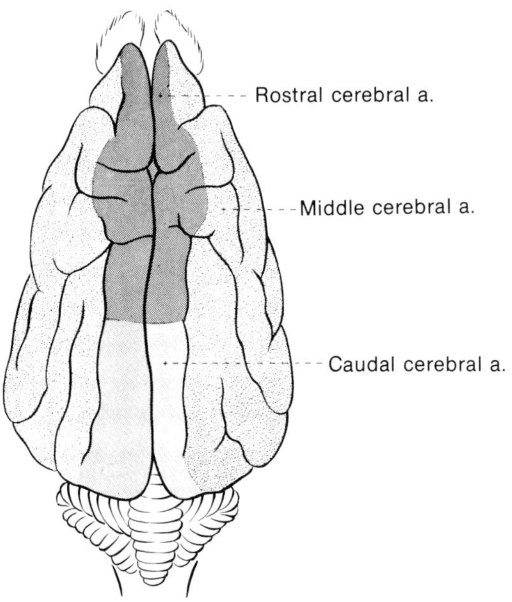

FIGURE 20–12 Areas supplied by the cerebral arteries, dorsal aspect. (From Miller, M. E., Christensen, G. C., and Evans, H. E.: *Anatomy of the Dog*. Philadelphia, W. B. Saunders Co., 1964.)

SURGICAL APPROACHES TO THE BRAIN

The cranial vault is divided anatomically into two compartments, the rostral and caudal fossae, which are separated by the tentorium cerebelli. These areas are often referred to as rostrotentorial (supratentorial in man) and caudotentorial (infratentorial in man). The caudal fossa or compartment contains the cerebellum, the medulla, and the fourth ventricle; the rostral compartment contains the cerebral hemispheres; and the midbrain is located at the junction of the two compartments. The surgical approaches developed to expose these areas are the lateral (lateral rostrotentorial), the bilateral (rostrotentorial), the suboccipital (caudotentorial), and the ventral (Figs. 20–13 to 20–17).[24, 25, 44, 46]

LATERAL (LATERAL ROSTROTENTORIAL) CRANIOTOMY

This approach involves an opening into the cranial cavity through portions of the frontal, parietal, temporal, or sphenoid bones, depending on the amount of exposure desired. This approach can expose the frontal, parietal, temporal, and occipital lobes. The pituitary gland, the anterior aspect of the cerebellum, and the lateral ventricles may also be approached via this route. The craniotomy can be extended caudally to expose the tentorium cerebelli and the midbrain. By surgically splitting the tentorium, the rostral aspect of the cerebellum can be explored. The craniotomy defect can be extended ventrally to expose the basilar artery, the pituitary gland, and other ventral structures. The lateral ventricle can be explored through a cortical incision in the suprasylvian gyrus (Fig. 20–18).

Technique

The skin incision can be made on the dorsal midline, but to afford a more spacious approach it is generally made in the shape of a horseshoe, extending from the lateral canthus of the eye to the dorsal midline and carried caudally to curve behind the ear. The skin should be carefully draped around the edges and folded back with some compression in order to in-

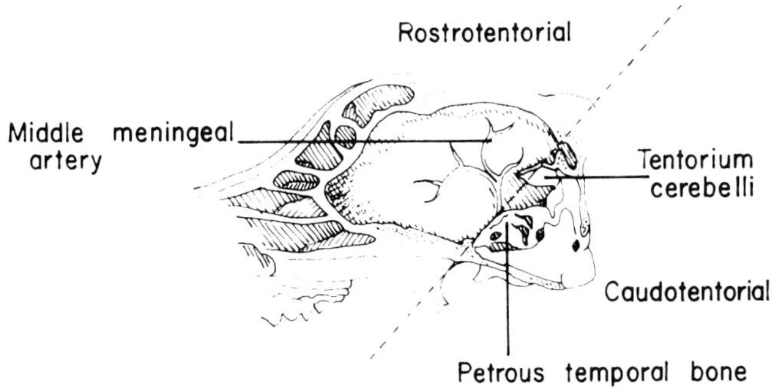

FIGURE 20–13 The cranial vault is divided into rostrotentorial and caudotentorial compartments by the tentorium cerebelli and petrous ridge. (From Oliver, J. E., Jr.: Surgical management of acute head injury. Proc. 19th Gaines Vet. Symposium, 1969.)

hibit bleeding. Ligation of major vessels and coagulation cautery of minor ones are always indicated (Fig. 20–19).

The superficial muscles are severed slightly lateral to the external sagittal crest. The dissection is continued along the nuchal crest and the muscles are reflected ventrolaterally. In preparing the isolated bone flap, the heavy temporal muscle is incised slightly lateral to its dorsal attachment and is bluntly dissected from the entire lateral aspect of the cranium. The muscle is removed by means of a periosteal elevator or the scalpel handle; care must be taken not to tear the periosteum. If maximum exposure is required, the superficial temporal artery and palpebral nerve can be ligated and severed at the rostral portion of the zygomatic arch near the lateral canthus of the eye. The caudal deep temporal artery and nerve are located at the dorsocaudal margin of the zygomatic arch. For greater exposure, it is then possible to transect the zygomatic arch at its rostral attachment and caudally just lateral to the mandibular articulation. Portions of the temporal muscle can be severed for a wider exposure; however, subsequent atrophy of this muscle will result in a cosmetic defect (Figs. 20–20 and 20–21).

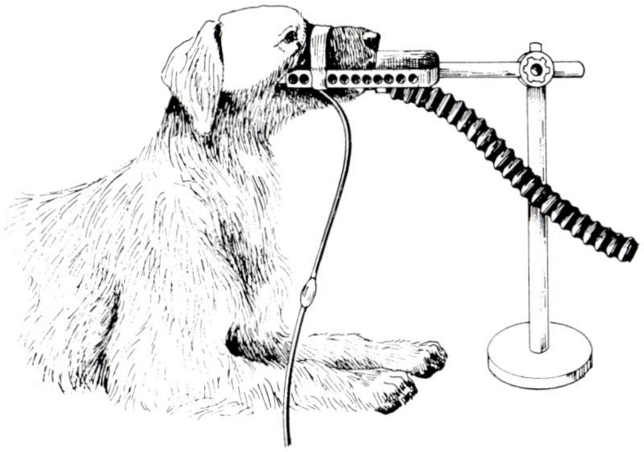

FIGURE 20–14 A device designed to stabilize the head in an elevated position for cranial surgery. The device allows for adjustments in height as well as any oblique position of the head. This position inhibits cerebral venous congestion, edema, and subsequent brain swelling that could occur if the head were in a lower position. It also inhibits pressure on the jugular, which might tend to raise intracranial pressure owing to impaired venous drainage.

Bone Flap

The bone over the lateral calvarium should generally be preserved by means of a flap or bone replacement. When the defect is covered with the bone flap, it is part of a craniotomy procedure. If the bone is not preserved and a permanent defect re-

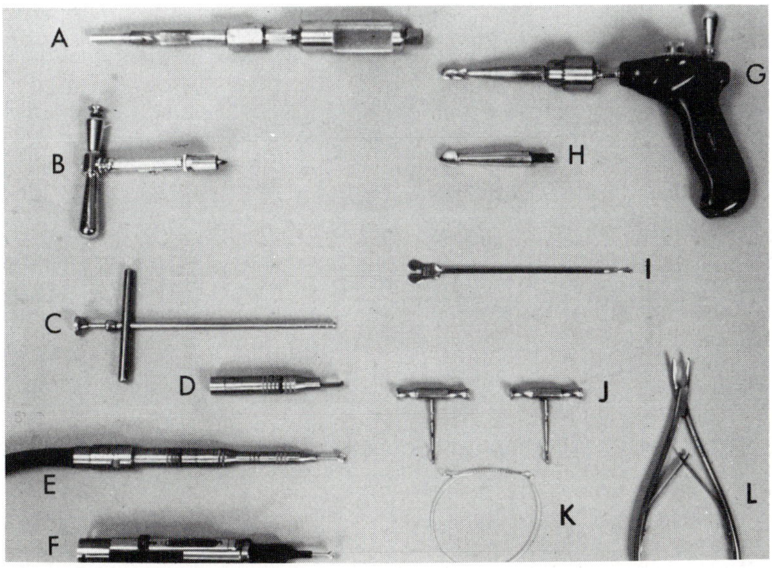

FIGURE 20–15 Various instruments used in entering the calvarium in brain surgery. A, Micrometer trephine; B, Galt trephine; C, Michelle laminectomy trephine; D, craniotome; E, Stryker air drill; F, Hall air drill; G, hand drill and bur; H, pointed bur; I, grooved director; J, handles for wire saw; K, wire saw; L, Lampert rongeur.

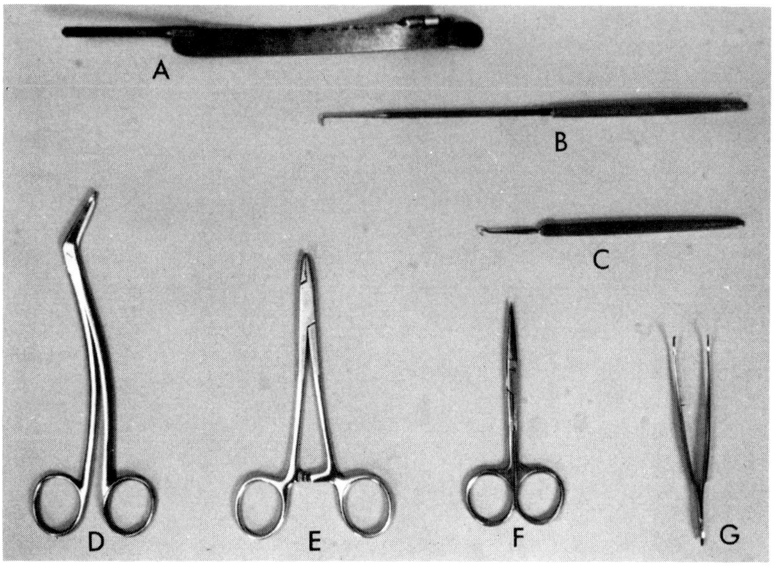

FIGURE 20–16 Various instruments useful in handling intracranial tissue. A, Brain retractor; B and C, dural hooks; D, dural scissors; E, ophthalmic needle holder; F, iris scissors; G, iris forceps.

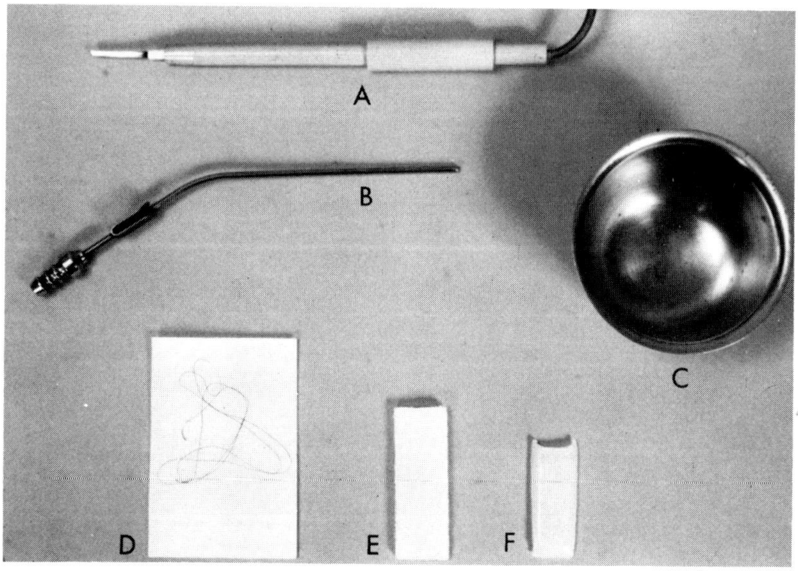

Figure 20–17 Agents and equipment useful in controlling intracranial hemorrhage. A, Low tension cautery; B, aspirator tip for removing warm saline; C, bowl for warm saline, which is used to continuously bathe brain tissue; D, cotton flannel patches (Cottonoid) with 6–0 ophthalmic silk suture for ligations; E, absorbable gelatin sponge (Gelfoam); F, bone wax. Silver clips (not shown) are also useful.

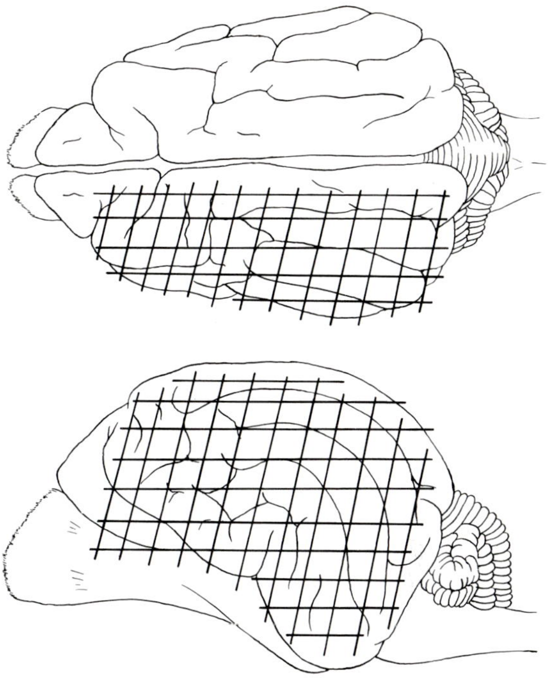

FIGURE 20–18 Dorsal and lateral views of the brain. Cross-hatching indicates approximate areas of exposure using a lateral supratentorial craniotomy.

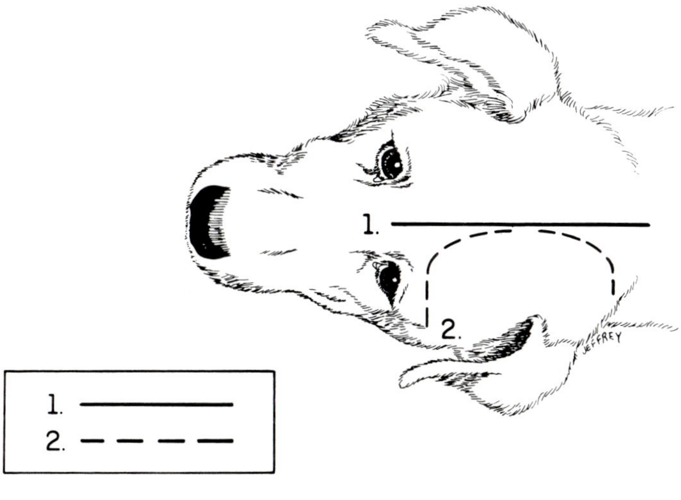

FIGURE 20–19 Skin incision patterns for a lateral supratentorial craniotomy. (1) Midline; (2) horseshoe. (After Oliver, J. E., Jr.: Surgical approaches to the canine brain. Am. J. Vet. Res. *29*, 366, 1968.)

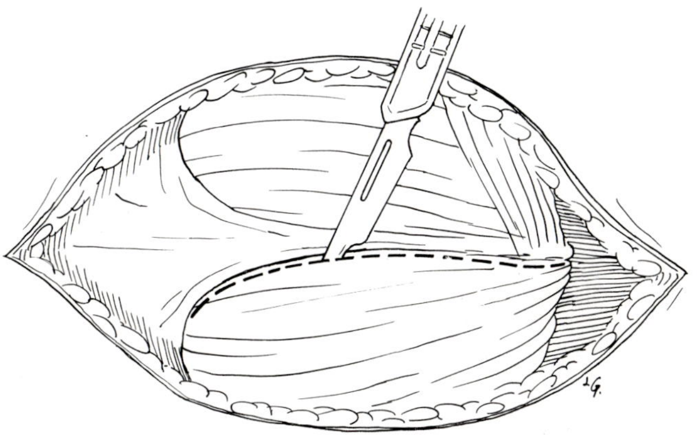

FIGURE 20–20 The incision in the temporal fascia is made approximately 3 to 4 mm from its calvarial attachment in order to facilitate later suturing.

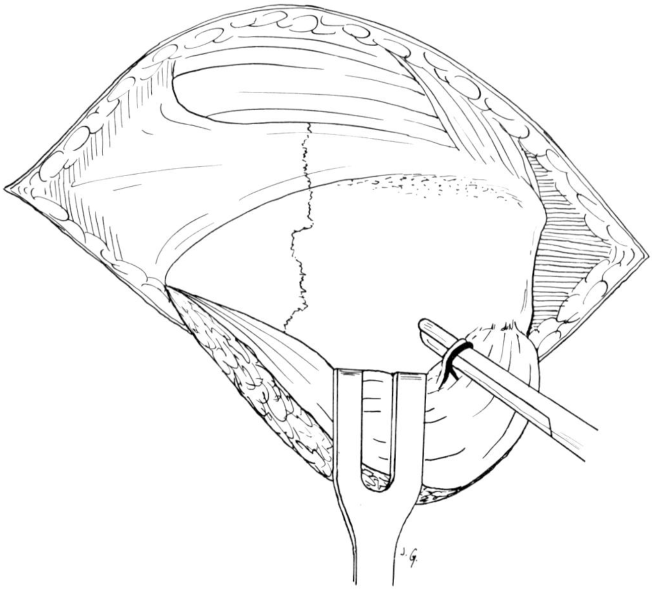

FIGURE 20–21 The temporal muscle is reflected ventrally. The hemostat demonstrates the caudal deep temporal artery and nerve.

sults, the procedure is termed a craniectomy.[3] The bone flap can be of two types, the isolated bone flap or the combined muscle-bone (hinged) flap.[10] The advantage of the latter procedure is that less muscle is transected and that the blood supply to the bone is perhaps better maintained by the attached muscle. In dolichocephalic breeds, exposure is more of a problem with this technique because the ventral aspects of the temporal muscle are so thick. In the brachicephalic breeds, such as the Chihuahua, the combined flap is a satisfactory technique. However, the isolated bone flap, if kept warm and moist during the isolation period, is a satisfactory method and usually gives more satisfactory exposure.

The technique of making the flap involves four bur, drill, or trephine holes placed in the extreme corners of the desired exposure area. If hand equipment is used, the bur technique is preferable, starting with a pointed bur and finishing with a round one until the endosteal layer of dura is exposed. Bur holes made with the ultra-high-speed drill (Hall or Stryker air drill) are faster, easier, and safer. The time involved is a fraction of that needed with hand equipment, which is also more traumatic. If a craniotome attachment is used with the air-driven drill, only one drill hole is needed and the flap is promptly cut from it. The outermost boundaries of the bone flap are located 0.5 cm rostral to the nuchal crest, to avoid the transverse sinus; 1.0 cm lateral to the dorsal midline, to avoid the dorsal sagittal sinus; at the orbit and frontal sinus rostrally; and at the temporal musculature, coronoid process of mandible, and zygomatic arch ventrally (Figs. 20–22 to 20–27).

If a craniotome attachment is not used, the dura mater must be separated from the calvarium by means of a curved, grooved director or a flat probe passed between the dorsal and lateral holes. The bur holes generally need additional shaping by means of a rongeur forceps to facilitate passing the director. Using high-speed equipment, the flap between the drill holes is cut with a fine pointed drill bit on the dorsal, caudal, and cranial sides of the proposed flap. Without the power equipment, a wire saw is then passed between the holes, and the grooved director is passed ventral to the wire in order to protect the dura during the sawing procedure. The bone is sawed or burred in as diagonal a direction as possible, producing a beveled edge, so that the flap will sit firmly when replaced. After the dorsal, rostral, and caudal sides are sawed, the ventral border is broken by means of prying the dorsal border. The act of sawing the ventral border increases the chance of lacerating the middle meningeal artery close to its origin. The ventral aspect of the craniotomy is enlarged by rongeurs as needed (Fig. 20–28).

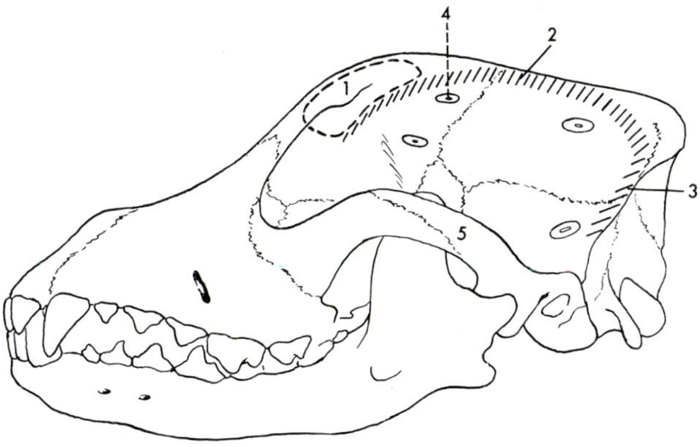

FIGURE 20–22 The usual positioning of bur holes preparatory to making an isolated bone flap in the lateral supratentorial craniotomy. (1) Frontal sinus; (2) midsagittal sinus; (3) transverse sinus; (4) bur holes; (5) zygomatic arch.

The air-driven equipment is the least traumatic and least time-consuming means of performing a craniotomy. In larger canine skulls the craniotome attachment may be used, assuring even greater reduction in operating time. The craniotome end is inserted in a suitably placed bur hole—the attachment works best when a curved rather than a straight rectangular cut is made. The blunt rounded guard pushes the dura away from the calvarium as the bur cuts the bone. Also, the procedure of making holes in the flap and adjacent skull needed for wiring the flap back in place is facilitated with the power equipment. This power equipment is now also used widely in veterinary hospitals doing orthopedic surgery.[59]

The diploic hemorrhage is controlled by rubbing bone wax over the cut bone edges. The isolated bone flap is kept warm and moist in saline-soaked sponges. Generally, greater exposure is needed ventrally, and this is obtained by careful use of the rongeur, which leaves a permanent defect in this area. The thick temporal muscle and zygomatic arch protect the brain underlying this defect from injury.

Handling the Dura Mater

The dura mater must be preserved from laceration during the burring, sawing, and rongeuring procedures. It is emphasized that the dura mater is one of the chief barriers to pyogenic sepsis, and that once it is invaded, asepsis must be strictly maintained. In a leading human neurosurgical clinic, postoperative infections were seen in 3.06 per cent of the so-called clean procedures (noncontaminated before surgery).[5] This report should demonstrate the need

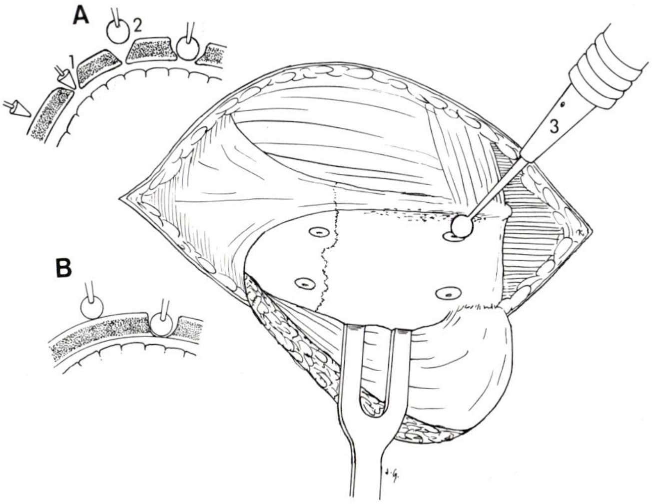

FIGURE 20–23 *A.* Using the hand-powered drill or bit, bur holes can be started more easily with a pointed bur and finished with the spherical bur. The burring should stop when the endosteum is exposed and should be finished with a rongeur. *B.* Using the air-powered drill, only the spherical bur is needed. Bur holes can be made with a hand drill, but an air drill facilitates the procedure. (1) Pointed bur; (2) spherical bur; (3) air drill.

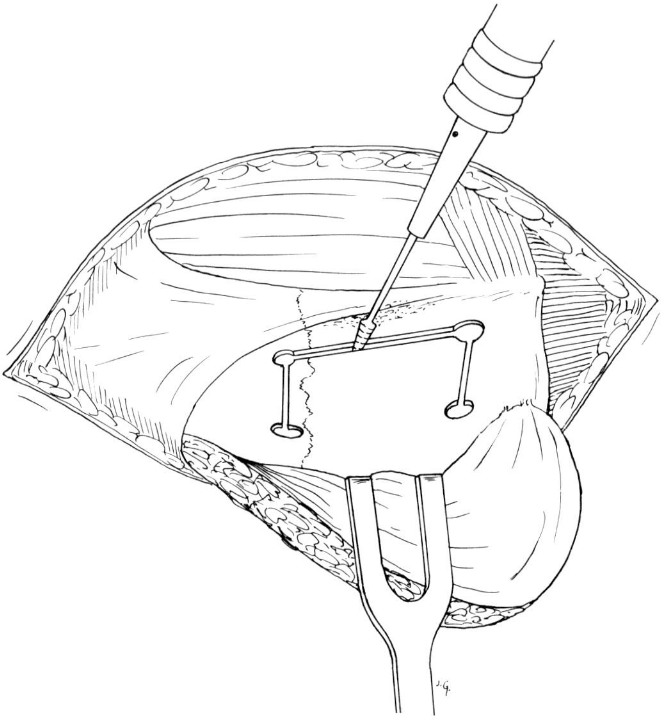

FIGURE 20–24 The bur holes are joined by grooving and carefully penetrating the bone with a small pointed bur. The ventral side of the flap is broken and generally not cut.

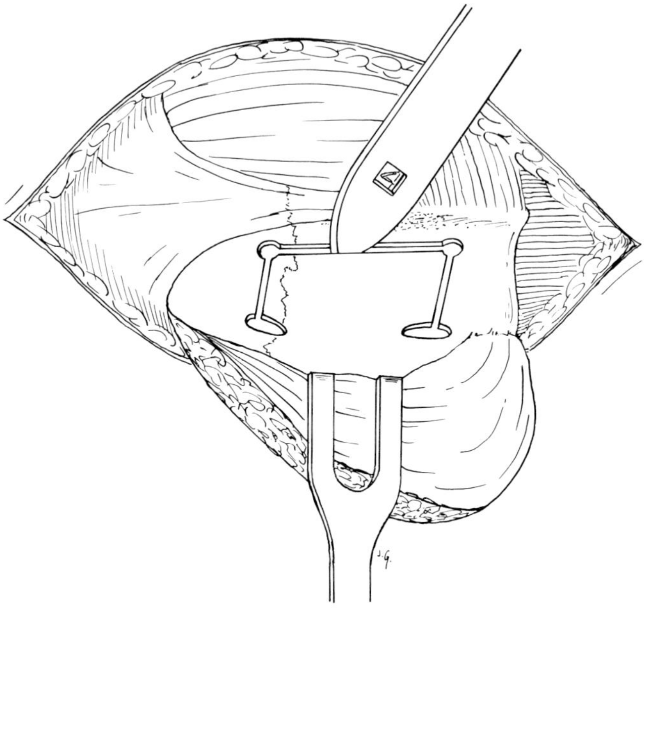

FIGURE 20–25 The bone flap is carefully pried open. The ventral border of the flap breaks straight because the lower bur holes are notched inward with the rongeur.

for strict asepsis. The dura can be retracted from the calvarium in young dogs, but occasionally it adheres so closely to the calvarial bone in old patients that separation is very difficult. One must be extremely careful not to lacerate or damage the cerebral cortex in such patients.[60]

In preparing the dural flap, the dura mater is incised 2 to 4 mm inward from the margin of the craniotomy defect. A dural hook, a small sharp suture needle placed in a needle holder, or a 23 to 25 gauge injection needle with the point bent into a hook, can be used to elevate the dura mater in order to facilitate making a small incision with a scalpel. The incision is enlarged in a rectangular fashion with small dural scissors, taking care not to incise the very soft fragile brain tissue. The middle meningeal artery is ligated by means of 6–0 silk or silver clips wherever it might be severed. The flap can be reflected dorsally or ventrally to suit the surgeon's need. The flap may be easier to suture when it is reflected ventrally. Usually, if a ventral exploration is necessary, the flap is made dorsally (Figs. 20–29 and 20–30).

The dura is a tough but still a very delicate membrane that will shrink if it is not kept moist and under stretching tension during the procedure. If such care isn't taken, the flap will not be large enough to close the dural defect at the time of closure. Therefore, 5–0 to 6–0 silk sutures are placed in the extreme corners of the flap, and the atraumatic needles are allowed to remain attached so that they can be used later to facilitate replacement of the flap.

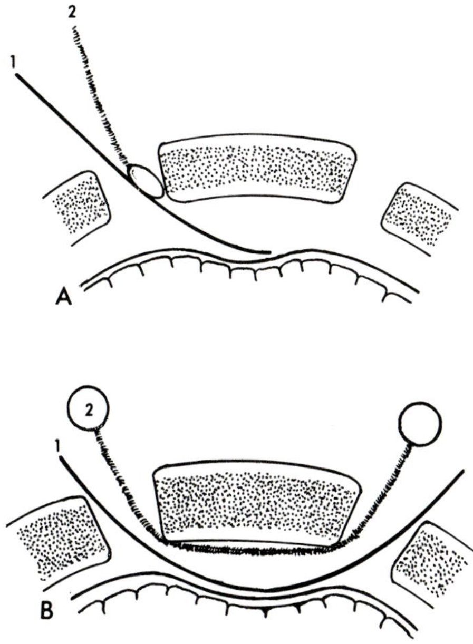

FIGURE 20–26 If an air drill is not available, the bur holes can be joined by using a grooved director to separate the dura from the bone, and to protect the dura from the wire saw that is used to cut the bone. (1) Grooved director; (2) wire saw.

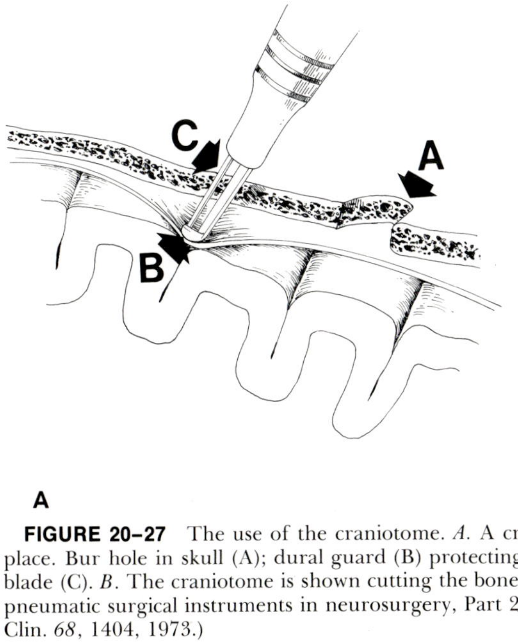

A

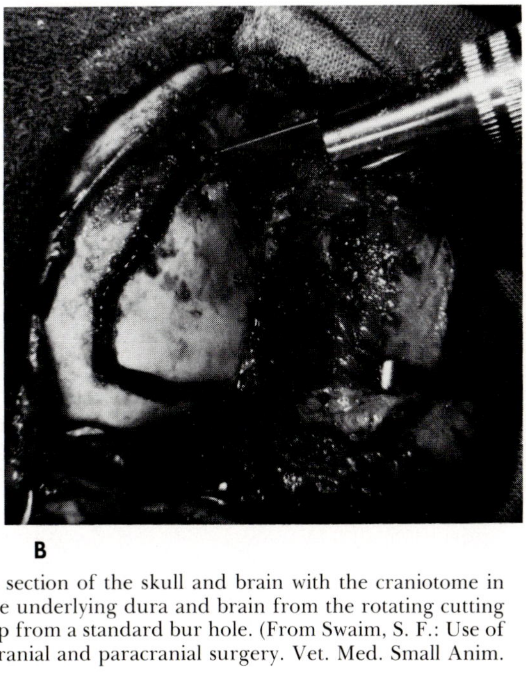

B

FIGURE 20–27 The use of the craniotome. *A*. A cross section of the skull and brain with the craniotome in place. Bur hole in skull (A); dural guard (B) protecting the underlying dura and brain from the rotating cutting blade (C). *B*. The craniotome is shown cutting the bone flap from a standard bur hole. (From Swaim, S. F.: Use of pneumatic surgical instruments in neurosurgery, Part 2. Cranial and paracranial surgery. Vet. Med. Small Anim. Clin. *68*, 1404, 1973.)

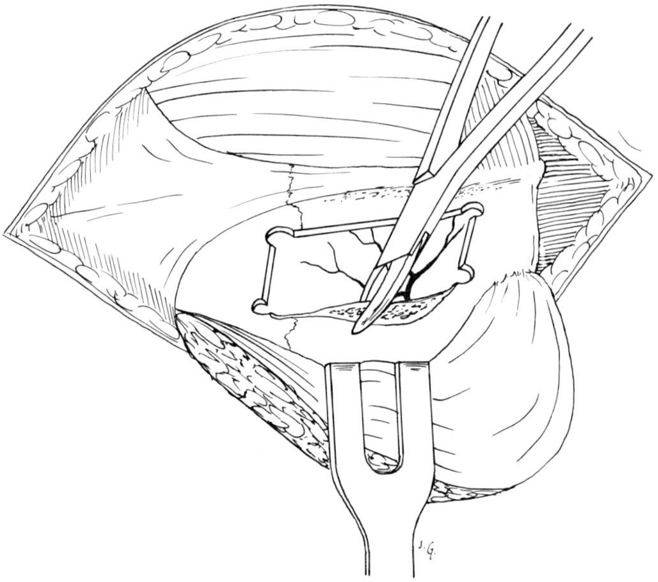

FIGURE 20–28 For a more complete exposure of the cranial cavity, the rongeur is used to enlarge the craniotomy opening. The resulting bone defect is of no consequence as long as the bone flap is replaced securely. (Courtesy of E. D. Gage.)

The reflected flap is sandwiched between cotton flannel strips that are kept moist with saline, and forceps are attached to the corner stay sutures. The forceps are allowed to hang over the edge of the surgical area and provide tension to the flap, and it is constantly bathed in saline. This care of the dural flap will facilitate later closure of the dural defect.

When operating time is prolonged, the dura and brain tissue must be kept moist and warm and must not be exposed excessively to air. Recently, a collagen sponge material (Biocol) has been used in over 300 patients in operations lasting from 1 to 13 hours. The material is soft, white, and pliable and has excellent wet strength; it absorbs 100 times its weight in water compared to an absorbing power of 30 times for most available gelatin sponges (Gelfoam). It reportedly protects the brain tissue from the trauma of contact retraction by instrumentation. It

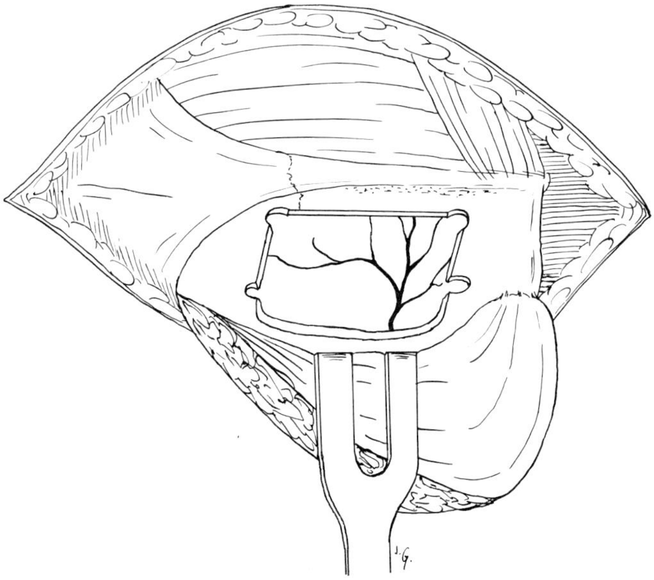

FIGURE 20–29 The ventral craniectomy is completed.

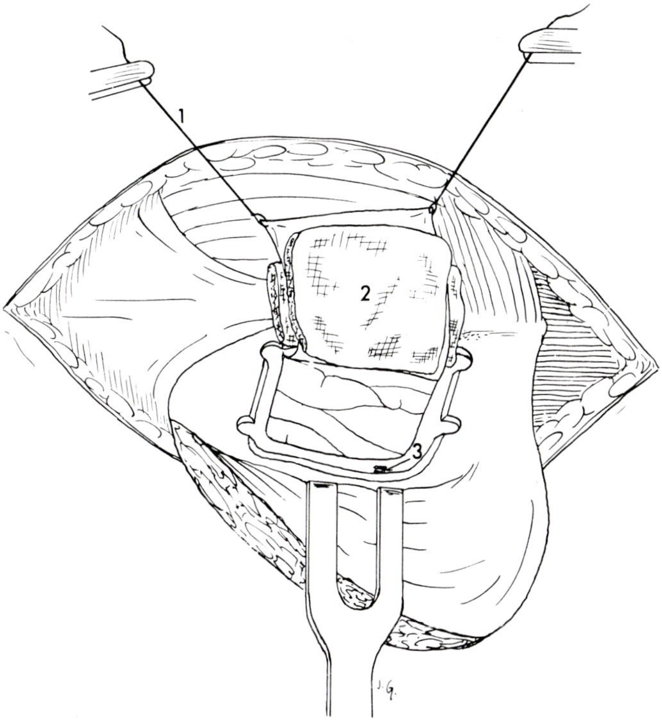

A

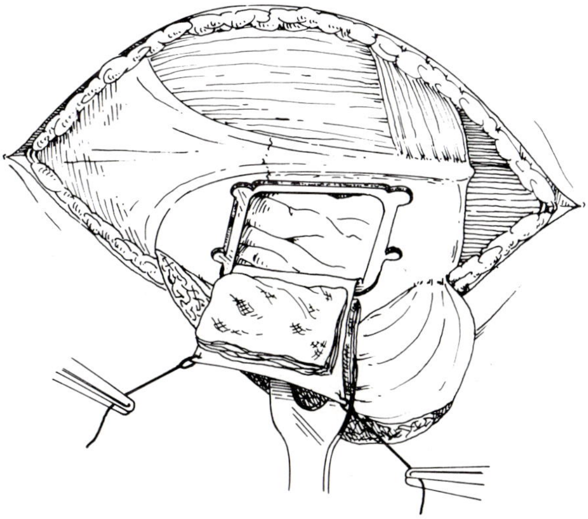

B

FIGURE 20–30 After the middle meningeal artery has been ligated, the dural flap is carefully protected from the calvarial edge by a surgical sponge or cotton flannel moistened with warm saline. In order to preserve the integrity of the dural flap for subsequent closure, continuous tension is applied to the stay sutures in each corner of the flap. Warm saline should be applied periodically to the dural flap to prevent shrinkage. (1) Tension sutures; (2) surgical sponge or cotton flannel applied to both sides of the dural flap; (3) middle meningeal artery ligation. *A*. Dural flap is hinged toward the midline to facilitate surgery in this area. *B*. Usually the dural flap is hinged downward in order to facilitate surgery in areas that are not near the midline. This facilitates the resuturing of the dura.

is nonabsorbable and should be removed after use.[32]

The usual surgical sponge materials may leave lint on CNS tissues that is said to promote connective tissue reactions. Therefore, use of lint-free sponges should probably be considered, especially when controlling hemorrhage in the brain and cord tissue itself. Lint-free sponges (Weck-Cel) are commonly used in peripheral nerve surgery.

The question that arises is whether the dural flap is that important. Most neurosurgeons feel that it is essential to maintain a water-tight dura mater even if a graft or substitute material has to be used. It is true that if there is no major damage to the pia-arachnoid, a neo-dura will form with no apparent adhesions in approximately 2 weeks.[28, 52, 57] This is particularly true in the absence of a bone flap.[29] However, in the neurosurgical procedure, at least minimal injury to the pia-arachnoid will occur, and a dural and bone flap should be preserved if at all possible.

The chief purpose of the dural closure is to prevent cerebral adhesions, CSF leaks, and infections.[1, 28] As stated previously, the dura must be closed under a bone flap or adhesions will occur.[29] The method of suturing will be discussed later in the chapter. A recent report states that fat tissue sutured on the inside of a small dural tear in the spinal dura will promote a watertight seal and is quickly invaded by connective tissue.[36] If the dura cannot be closed, the craniotomy should be left open. Autogenous transplants from temporal fascia or fascia lata have proved successful.[16, 44] Homologous dura mater is sterilized and stored in Hank's solution for 8 to 10 weeks or lyophilized and stored for 2 to 3 years.[35] Plastic adhesives have been proposed for nonsuture sealing of the dura but have proved to be irritating to neural tissues.[31] Plastic materials such as polythene film,[7] polyvinyl sponges,[12] Vinyon "N,"[61] Orlon,[26] Teflon,[1] and Silastic rubber dural replacement have been used. Charged gold leaf has been used clinically to help seal dural lacerations and defects.[15] In our practice, we have found temporal or subcutaneous fascia available and satisfactory when a graft is necessary to complete the closure (Fig. 20–31).

Examination of the Brain Cavity

It has already been mentioned that reduction of the brain volume is necessary when the cranial cavity needs examining or exploration, or if edema and brain swelling exist. If a gaseous anesthetic and oxygen mixture is employed, the simplest and most effective means of performing such a reduction is hyperventilation. Hyperventilation in conjunction with the elevated position of the head, administration of glucosteroids prior to surgery, and hypertonic mannitol prior to, during, and even after surgery will generally be highly effective in controlling brain swelling.[17, 19, 22] However, mannitol has been incriminated in promoting occasional intracranial hemorrhage during surgery. In the future, the addition of regional or systemic hypothermia to these procedures should make them even more efficacious.[14]

Controlled ventilation is generally started at the time of skin incision in an exploratory craniotomy. Since it requires 30 to 40 minutes of hyperventilation to produce maximal reduction in brain volume, the brain is already shrinking at the time of exposure. An increased rate of hyperventilation is started at this point (one and a half times the normal rate and in sufficient volume to visibly expand the chest). If the surgeon retracts the brain toward the midline and carefully aspirates the CSF from the ventral cisterns, the brain rapidly recedes from the cranial walls, and surgical examination with a lighted brain retractor is facilitated. Hyperventilation for long periods of time will result in a lowering of blood carbon dioxide levels, systemic alkalosis, and cerebral vascular constriction (producing cellular hypoxia). These effects have not generally been a problem in our experience.[45]

The brain should be bathed almost continuously in warm saline. Moist cotton flannel sponges overlying its surface will help prevent inflammation resulting from retraction and aspiration. One should never aspirate directly against nervous tissue, but only against cotton, absorbable or lint-free sponges overlying the tissue. The use of gelatin sponge pledgets pressed in place with cotton flannel, combined with saline irrigations and patience, will prove to be an ef-

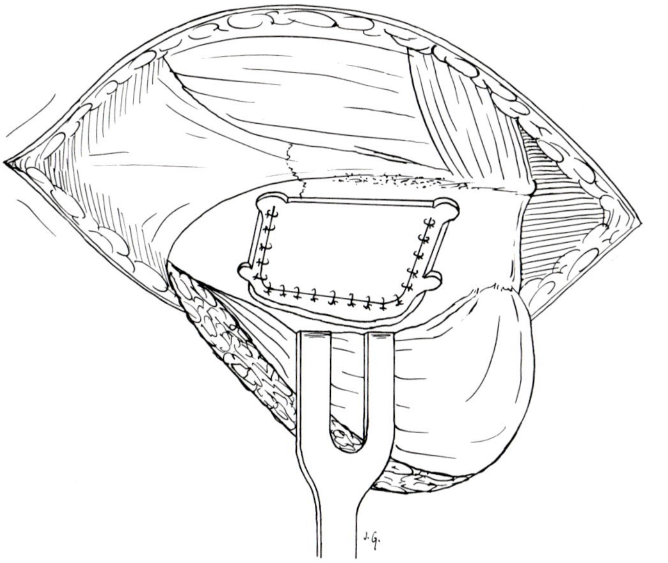

FIGURE 20–31 The dura should be securely closed with 6–0 surgical silk interrupted sutures. The dura should be closed when possible in order to inhibit sepsis and cortical adhesions.

fective means of controlling surface hemorrhage (Fig. 20–32).[45]

Incisions into the cortex should be made through a gyrus, because relatively large vessels are located in a sulcus. Hemorrhage from the pia mater can be controlled by use of low-intensity electrocautery, and the invasion of brain tissue should be as delicate as possible. Occasional cautery with separation of tissues rather than flagrant incising should be tried. Separated surfaces should be protected with gelatin sponge material. Many lesions will have undergone necrosis and liquefaction; this tissue can frequently be removed by aspiration. Hemorrhage in any cavity in the brain after removal of pathologic tissue must be controlled before closure. It is also best not to leave excessive gelatin sponge material in the area, since the clot formation in its substance makes an excellent cultural medium for any bacterial contamination and could be the focus for future seizure discharges. (Fig. 20–33).

Closure

After surgical correction in the brain, the dura is closed with interrupted sutures of 5–0 or 6–0 silk. The stay sutures in the flap corners are secured initially. The same material can be used for the rest of the closure. If the flap has been well cared for

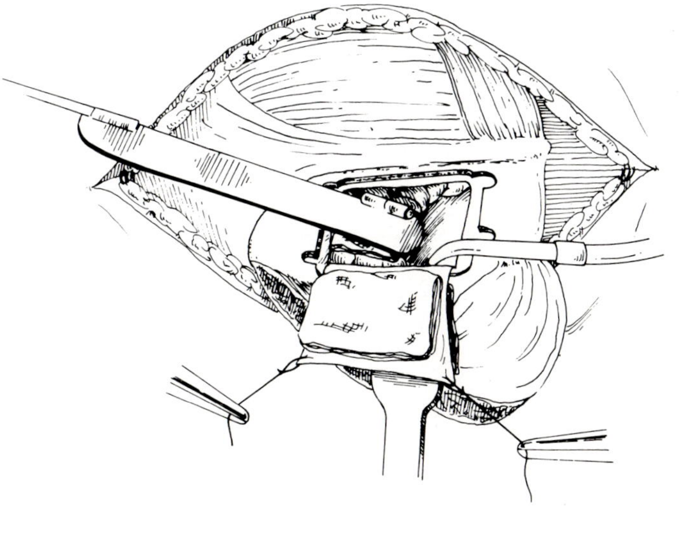

FIGURE 20–32 Exploration of the ventral cerebral areas is facilitated by moderate hyperventilation, gentle retraction of brain tissue with a padded retractor, and continuous aspiration of CSF from basal cisterns. Notice that the dural flap is hinged away from the midline.

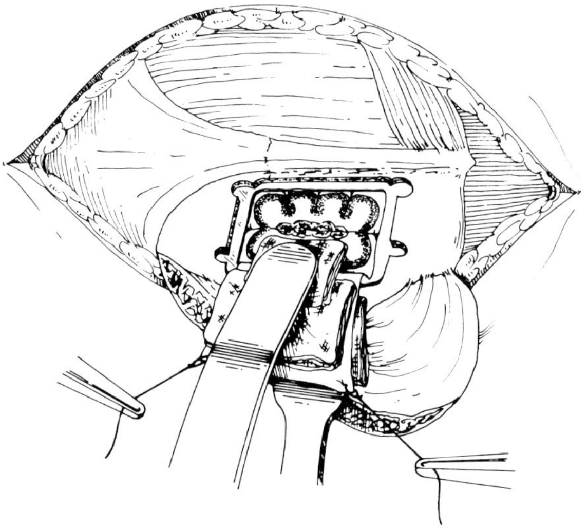

FIGURE 20–33 To expose deep lesions, the invasion of brain tissue should be done with blunt instruments or low tension cautery. Edges of incised tissue should always be protected from instruments by cotton flannel soaked in warm saline. Notice the pathological lesion just above the padded retractor.

during surgery, the closure is routine (Fig. 20–31). The bone flap is secured by means of orthopedic stainless steel wire through appropriate drill holes in the cranium and flap. Either a high-speed drill or a small Steinmann pin in a hand drill will suffice. One must be careful not to damage the dura or underlying brain when drilling these holes. The human drill guides and protectors are too large for most dogs; however, a scalpel handle or brain retractor placed beneath the cranial edges will afford the desired protection (Fig. 20–34).

In cases of cranial fractures, cranial bone pathology, or severe traumatic brain damage, a craniectomy defect may be indicated. A myoplastic flap can be cosmetically satisfactory and in some cases may even afford ample protection against future injury, especially if the defect is in a ventrolateral area and the dog is dolichocephalic. However, a prosthetic bone flap can be fashioned from acrylic, plastic, or metal.[15, 63] Gage has found stainless steel screen material satisfactory for maintaining a cosmetic appearance as well as affording more protection to the area.[13] Such a cranioplasty can be performed at the time of the initial surgery or at a later time to give protection to the brain. Caution is again advised in

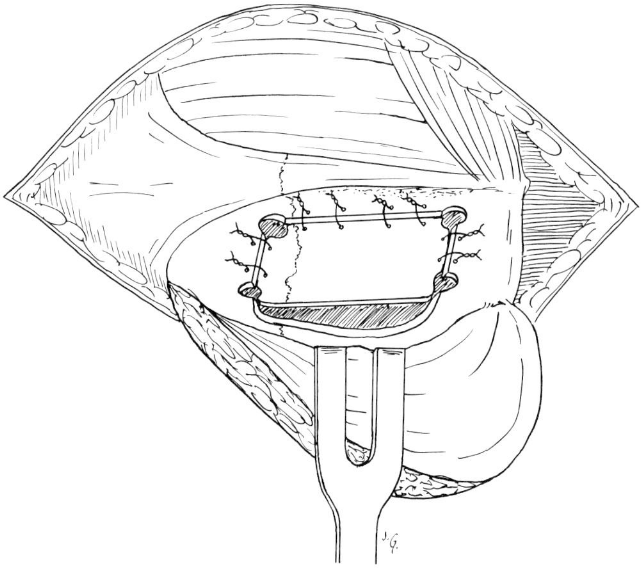

FIGURE 20–34 The bone flap is replaced and secured with stainless steel orthopedic wire. Notice the ventral craniectomy made to facilitate further examination.

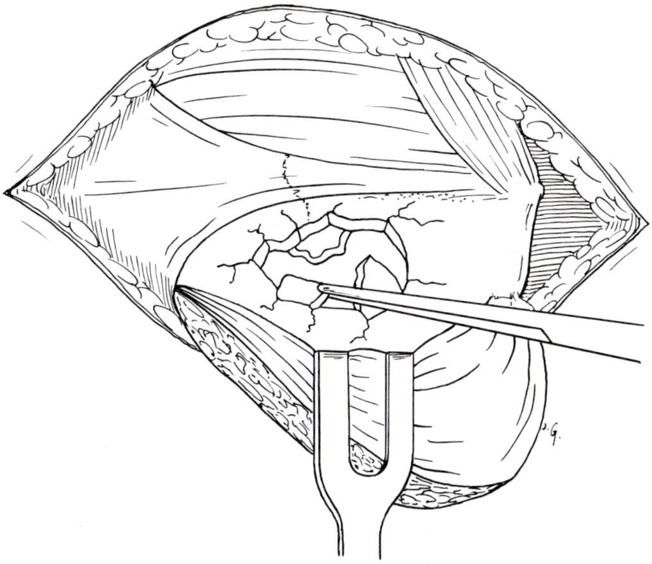

FIGURE 20–35 Comminuted cranial fractures require the removal of all fragments and a subsequent craniectomy.

making certain that the dura or dural substitute completely shields the cerebral cortex from the calvarium (or the calvarial prosthesis) in order to prevent cortical adhesions and future seizure episodes (Figs. 20–35 to 20–42).

The temporal muscle, superficial muscles, subcutis, and skin are closed routinely. Careful suturing of layers of tissue, maintaining proper hemostasis, and obliterating any dead space will reduce the possibility of formation of a subcutaneous hematoma or seroma. A snug but loose bandage using elastic adhesive will also aid in preventing a seroma. Maintaining a patent airway, preventing postsurgical delirium and self-mutilation, good nursing care, and other immediate postsurgical considerations have been discussed in detail in Chapters 8 and 12 (Fig. 20–43).

TRANSFRONTAL CRANIOTOMY[51]

In the lateral craniotomy, lesions of the prefrontal cerebrum, which is adjacent to the frontal sinus and olfactory areas, are difficult to expose. If there is a small focal

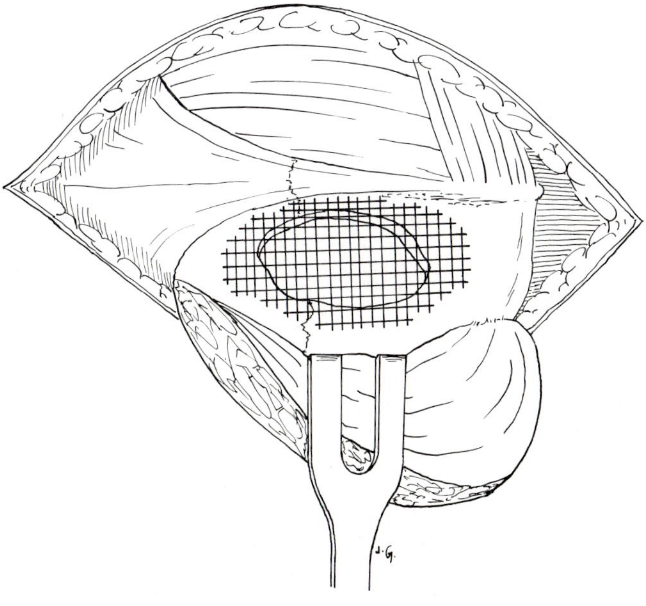

FIGURE 20–36 In a comminuted fracture of the skull, a bone flap usually cannot be preserved. Various types of surgical mesh can be used over the bone defect to help protect the brain from further trauma.

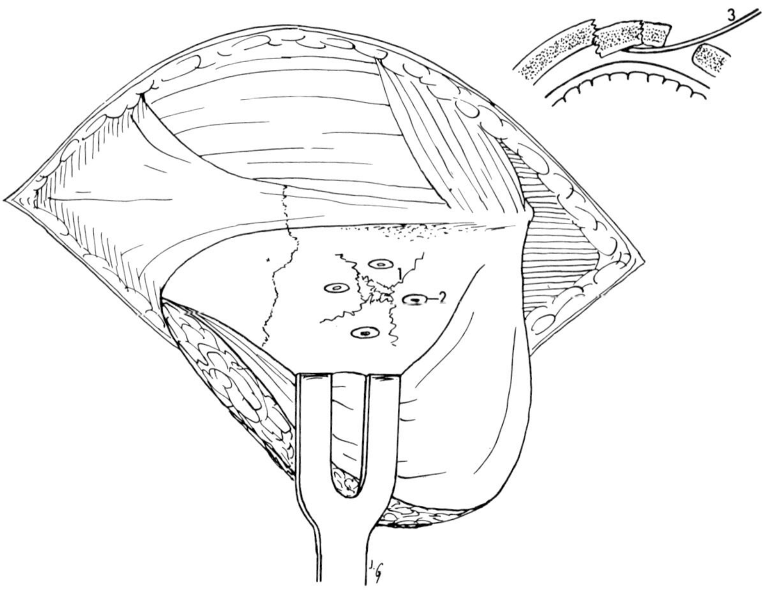

FIGURE 20–37 Depressed fragments must be carefully elevated in an effort to lessen meningeal and vascular injury. Appropriately placed bur holes can facilitate examination for subdural hemorrhage as well as providing access to these fragments. (1) Fracture; (2) bur holes; (3) elevating fragments through a bur hole.

lesion in this area, an isolated approach through the frontal sinus may be large enough to correct it. Probably a combination of the transfrontal and lateral craniotomies will be necessary for adequate exposure of most lesions in this area.

In the transfrontal approach, the midline skin incision commonly made for the lateral exposure is extended between the eyes sufficiently to expose the frontal sinus properly. The skin, subcutis, musculature (where present), and periosteum are removed from the area of the frontal sinus and the part of the calvarium involved in the exposure. The limits of the frontal sinus in the patient's particular type of skull are determined, and a triangular flap of outer frontal bone is removed by means of the smallest available drill bur for the air-powered drill (the small Stryker saw blade or hand saw may be used instead). The flap is wrapped in warm saline-soaked sponges

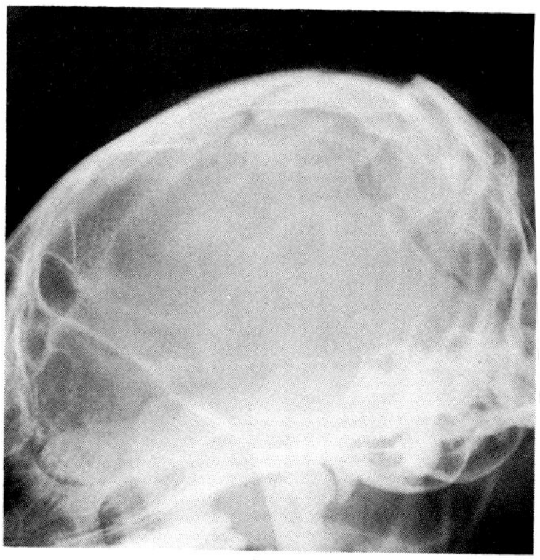

Fig. 20–38

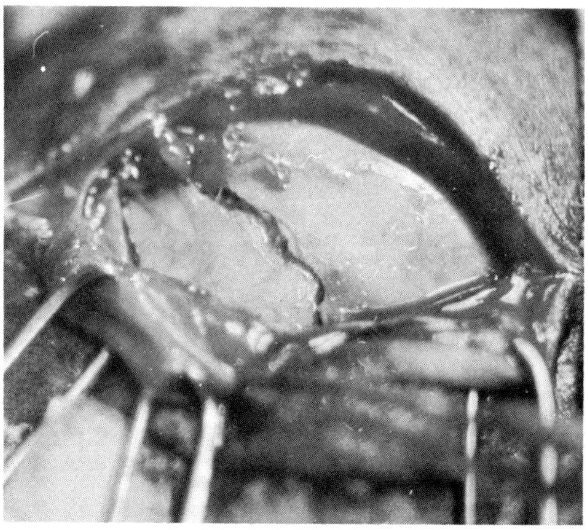

Fig. 20–39

FIGURE 20–38 A 3-year-old Manchester terrier had been struck by a car and lost consciousness within 2 hours. Note the badly fractured skull.

FIGURE 20–39 The fractured area of the calvarium.

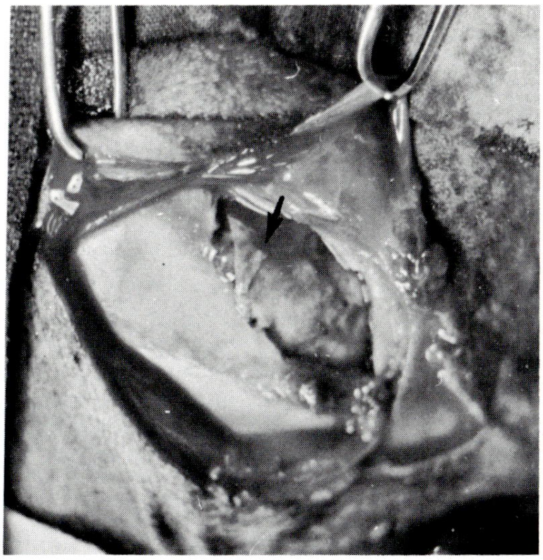

Fig. 20–40

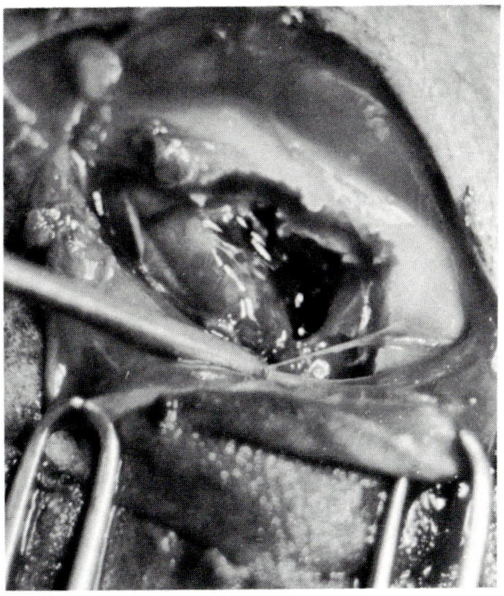

Fig. 20–41

FIGURE 20–40 The bone fragments are removed, and a dural laceration is noted.
FIGURE 20–41 Subdural hematoma can be seen, as well as lacerated cortical tissue.

or towel and preserved for final replacement. The exposed frontal sinus is thoroughly flushed with sterile saline and the mucosal lining is removed. At this point all previously used pieces of equipment are removed from the surgical area, surgical gloves are replaced with sterile ones, and new linen is draped in the area. Every effort is made to alleviate the chances of introducing infection from the sinus area into the cranial cavity (Fig. 20–44).

The cranial cavity is entered at least ½ cm from the midline and as far distal to the caudal limit of the frontal sinus as deemed necessary for proper exposure. If a complete unilateral cerebral and transfrontal approach is desired, there should be three bur holes (two caudal holes and the ventrocranial one) for the lateral flap previously described, and the dorsal bone incision should be extended to remove the inner or ventral (frontal bone) plate of the frontal sinus. The smallest air-driven bur drill should be used if at all possible. If the inner frontal bone plate in the sinus is diseased and cannot be removed for a flap, it should be carefully removed with a rongeur; the bone defect will then remain. If the small frontal sinus approach is sufficient, only the ventral flap of bone in the sinus is cut with the drill bit. Great care is needed to avoid lacerating the dura (Fig. 20–45).

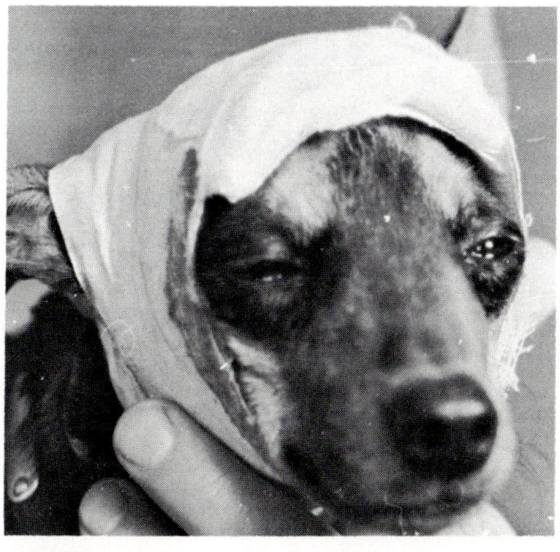

FIGURE 20–42 The hemorrhage was controlled, and dehydrating solutions were administered during and after surgery. The dog was conscious 12 hours later, and ambulatory 24 hours later.

The dural flap is cut at least 1 to 2 mm smaller than the bone flap so that it can be securely sutured after correction of the lesion. Since contamination is more likely in this approach, the suture material generally used is surgical gut. If the dura cannot be securely closed, temporal muscle fascia is removed and grafted over the dural defect to insure a watertight closure. All bone flaps are securely wired in place to prevent secondary compression of brain tissue from loose flaps. If necessary, a small tube into the frontal sinus can be left exposed for postoperative antibiotic infusions

The dangers of this surgery are (1) the

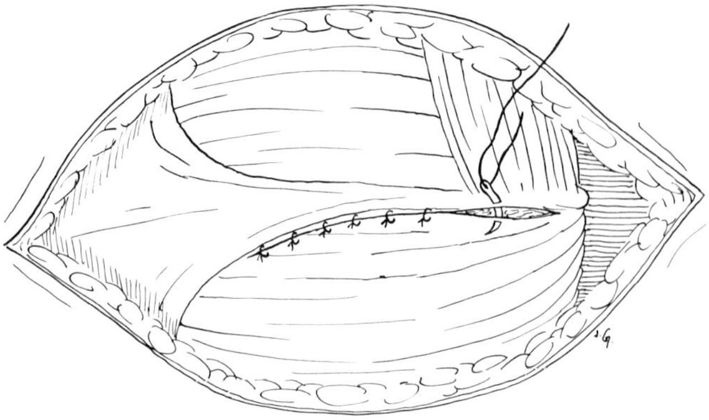

FIGURE 20–43 Suturing the temporal fascia. The superficial tissues and skin are closed in routine fashion.

chance of recurring infection because of the invasion of the frontal sinus, and (2) the possibility that dural defects will promote leakage of CSF into the sinus. However, this approach should be utilized when exposure of a cranial frontal lesion is expected to be difficult.[51]

THE BILATERAL (ROSTROTENTORIAL) CRANIOTOMY

This approach can be used for midline lesions or for massive cerebral decompressions in trauma. At the present time, the author prefers to use lateral craniotomies involving both sides separately rather than disturbing the dorsal sagittal sinus and possibly injuring it in a dorsal single bone flap.[48] Of course, midline pathologic lesions, such as lacerations of the sagittal sinus, tumors, and abscesses demand the midline approach.[3, 20, 38] The anatomical considerations already described are appropriate for this approach. The sagittal sinus is the primary problem (Fig. 20–46).

Technique

The incision can be a midline, a bilateral horseshoe, or an H incision. The H incision consists of a dorsal midline incision with transverse incisions at its extremities. The

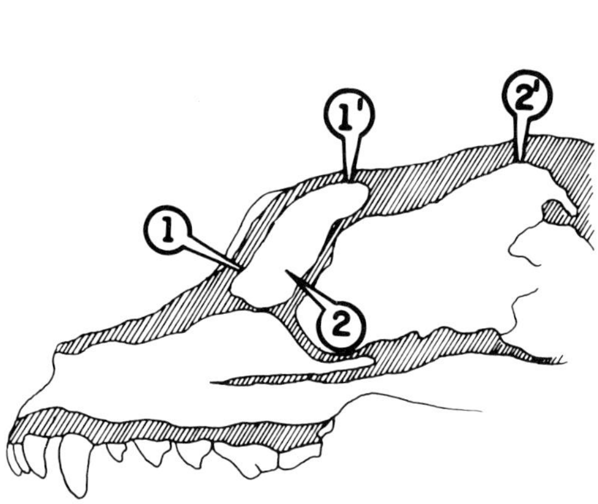

Fig. 20–44

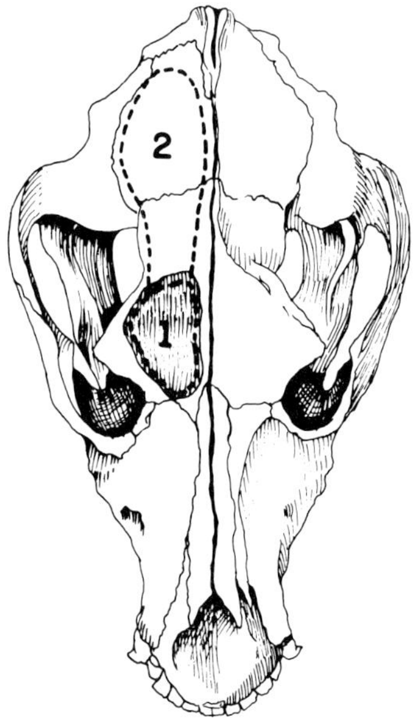

Fig. 20–45

FIGURE 20–44 In transfronal craniotomy (lateral view), access to the frontal sinus of the brain is made through the frontal sinus (2). An initial bone flap is made through the frontal sinus (1–1′). If necessary, the craniotomy flap is made in the areas indicated by 1′-2′.

FIGURE 20–45 In a transfrontal craniotomy (dorsal view) there is a frontal sinus bone flap (1) and a cranial bone flap through the inner plate of the frontal sinus, indicated by the dotted line in 1. If necessary, the calvarial bone flap of an appropriate size is made to effect an additional surgical correction (2).

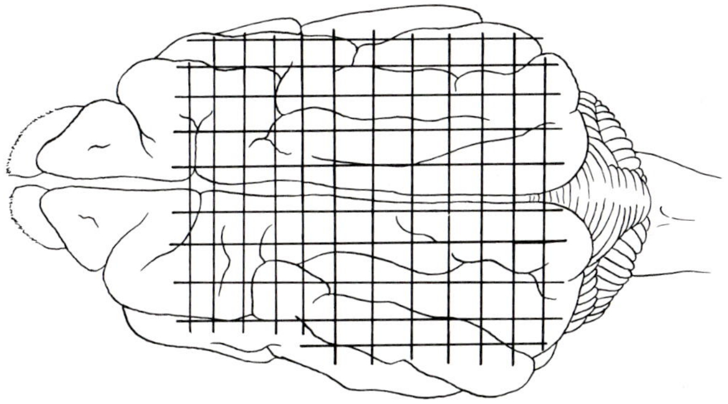

FIGURE 20–46 Dorsal view of brain. Cross-hatching indicates the area of the brain that can be exposed through the bilateral (rostrotentorial) craniotomy.

H incision unquestionably gives the best exposure (Fig. 20–47). The skin and musculature are retracted as in the lateral approach. The amount of temporal muscle reflected per side depends on the need for exposure. Perhaps one side will need complete reflection but the other will need to extend only 2 to 3 cm from the midline.

The bone flap differs somewhat from that in the unilateral approach. Bur holes are made at the extreme corners of the proposed area on the side of largest exposure, but the dorsal holes are closer to the midline (0.5 cm instead of 1.0 cm). Two more dorsal bur holes are made in like fashion on the opposite side, for a total of six bur holes. If a larger dorsal exposure is desired, a total of eight holes can be made, four on each side. On the side with the four holes, the rostral and caudal pairs are joined by sawing. The two dorsal holes on this side are enlarged with a rongeur forceps so that the endosteal layer of the dura can be separated from the bone over the sagittal sinus. This will provide for less damage to the sinus when the bone flap is lifted. The bur holes on the opposite side of the midline are united by a rostrocaudal cut. The sagittal sinus must be protected while the rostral pair of dorsal bur holes (one on each side of the midline) are joined across the midline by sawing or rongeuring. The caudal dorsal pair of holes are likewise joined across the midline. Finally, the bone flap is carefully lifted upward from the side with the two bur holes; any remaining dura is separated from bone, and the ventral border of the flap is broken on the side with four holes (Fig. 20–48).

Bleeding emissary veins that have been ruptured between the skull and the sagittal sinus are covered with pieces of crushed muscle or gelatin sponge and held in place by cotton flannel moistened with saline. Bone wax is used on cut bone edges to control diploic hemorrhage. The dural flap is prepared on the larger side of the opening. It is reflected dorsally to the midline. If a

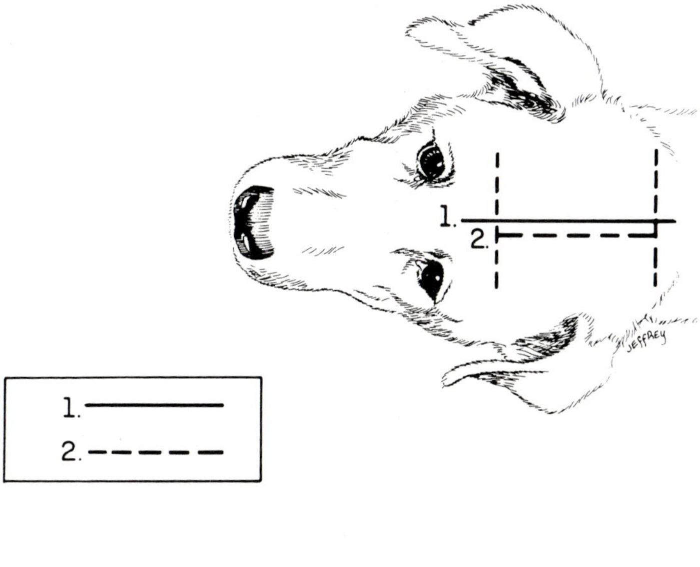

FIGURE 20–47 The skin incisions for the bilateral rostrotentorial craniotomy. (1) Midline incision; (2) H-shaped incisions. (After Oliver, J. E., Jr.: Surgical approaches to the canine brain. Am. J. Vet. Res. *29*, 371, 1968.)

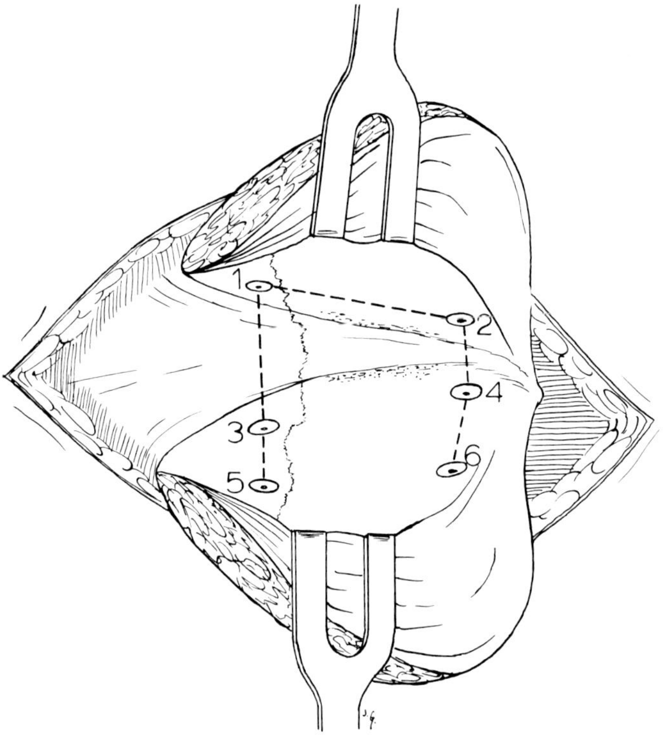

FIGURE 20–48 The bur holes for a bilateral craniotomy. Holes 3 and 4 are enlarged so that the dura and sagittal sinus can be carefully separated from the calvarial bone. Sawing between holes 1 and 3 and holes 2 and 4 is carefully performed in order not to lacerate the sagittal sinus. After sawing is completed, the flap is lifted from saw line 1–2 toward holes 5 and 6 until it breaks at this point, separating the dura from bone during the procedure. Dotted line indicates saw lines.

complete exposure of the midline and the longitudinal fissure is needed, it may be necessary to ligate and sever one or more of the dorsal cerebral veins that enter the sagittal sinus in the frontal area. Cauterization or gelatin sponge may be necessary to stop bleeding from some of these small vessels.

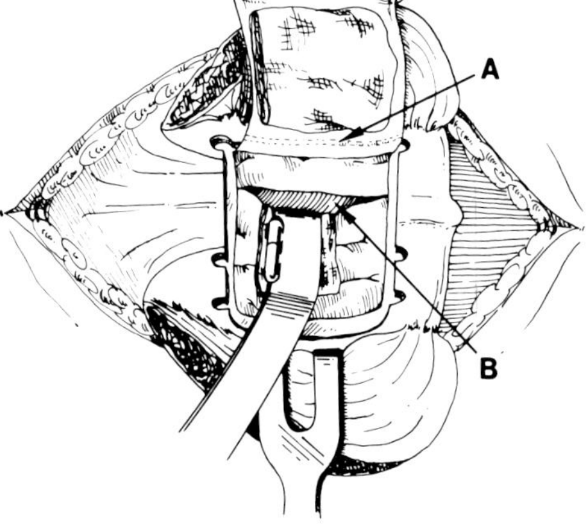

FIGURE 20–49 Retracting the cerebral hemisphere in order to examine the area for a midline lesion. *A*. The dural flap containing the midsagittal sinus (dotted line). *B*. The longitudinal fissure between the hemispheres.

In this manner, even such deep midline structures as the cingulate gyrus, the corpus callosum, the third ventricle, and posteriorly the tentorium cerebelli can be exposed. The dura, bone muscle, and skin can be closed as described earlier (Fig. 20–49).

CAUDAL SUBOCCIPITAL OR CAUDOTENTORIAL CRANIECTOMY

The suboccipital approach to the brain is used to expose the caudal aspect of the cerebellum, the dorsal aspect of the medulla, the fourth ventricle, and the rostral portions of the spinal cord if necessary. Since the bone is irregularly thin and the musculature is extremely heavy, one does not generally attempt to preserve a bone flap (Fig. 20–50).

Technique

The head should be flexed nearly at a right angle to the cervical vertebrae. The skin incision may be either a midline incision or a crossbow incision (midline and curved incision over the nuchal crest) (Fig. 20–51). The superficial fascia is severed on the midline to expose the dorsal cervical muscles, which are removed from the caudal aspect of the occiput about 0.5 cm from their tendinous attachments. These stumps of insertion will facilitate suturing at the time of closure. The caudal aspect of the occipital bone is cleaned of all muscle by using blunt dissection or cautery, or both. Greater exposure can be obtained by splitting the dorsal musculature on the midline at least to the level of the atlas. Electrocautery coagulation will control bleeding from the smaller vessels in the muscle (Fig. 20–52).

One or more bur holes can be made in the base of the skull lateral to the midline. The rongeur is used to expand the craniectomy defect carefully up to the transverse sinuses laterally, the occipital protuberance dorsally, and the foramen magnum ventrally. Since the bone is irregular and the dura adheres tightly to it, the dura is frequently torn and a flap is not possible. The cerebellum is exposed and examined, and the correction is accomplished as necessary. The dorsal aspect of the medulla and the area of the fourth ventricle can be exposed by lifting the vermis of the cerebellum (Figs. 20–53 to 20–55).

The dura is sutured, if possible, or a graft can be furnished, if necessary. Since a bone flap is not preserved, the dural closure is not a critical problem to prevent adhesions. Occasionally, gelatin sponge is used over the dural remnants. The musculature is securely sutured, and the remainder of the closure is routine. An appropriate brace placed either ventrally or dorsally will promote healing of the supporting muscles.

When the cerebellar exposure was inadequate, Oliver tried three different procedures to solve the problem.[44] He found that removal of the nuchal crest resulted in invasion of the transverse sinus, which had to be ligated. Even though good exposure of the lateral aspects of the cerebellum was achieved, the patient rarely survived. Exposure of the tentorium through a lateral craniotomy, splitting it to expose the anterior portions of the cerebellum, is possible, but very time-consuming.[40] An approach made by separate suboccipital and lateral rostrotentorial openings affords good exposure of the cerebellum and tentorium. A cerebellar lesion could be exposed initially with a suboccipital approach, and then if necessary the lateral flap could be made, leaving the nuchal crest and its transverse sinus intact.

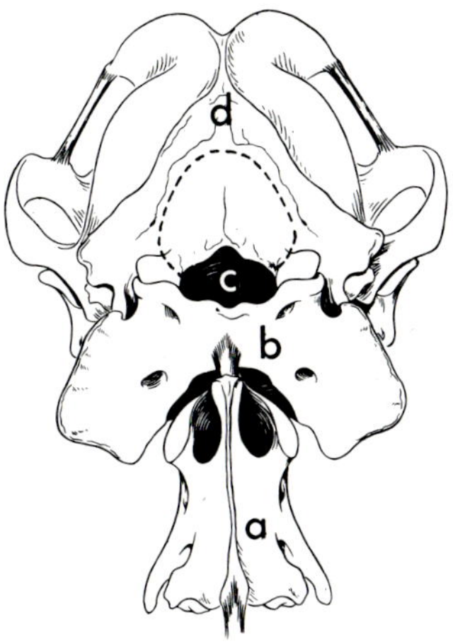

FIGURE 20–50 Base of the skull. The dotted line indicates the maximum extent of the usual craniotomy defect for an approach to the cerebellum: (a) axis, (b) atlas, (c) foramen magnum, (d) occipital protuberance. (After Miller, M. E.: *Guide to the Dissection of the Dog,* 3rd ed. Edwards Bros., Ann Arbor, Mich., 1952, © Dr. Malcolm E. Miller.)

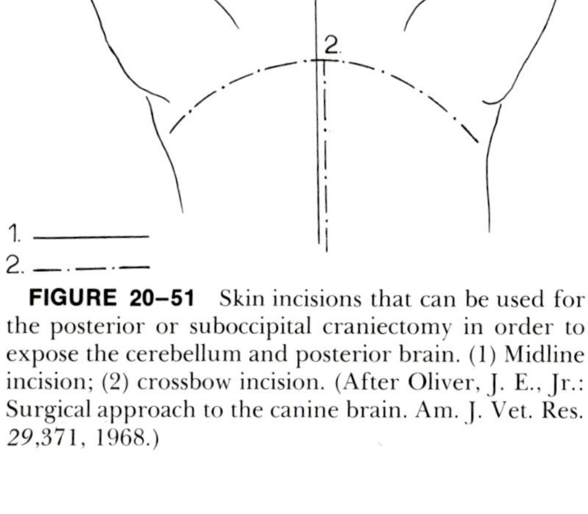

FIGURE 20–51 Skin incisions that can be used for the posterior or suboccipital craniectomy in order to expose the cerebellum and posterior brain. (1) Midline incision; (2) crossbow incision. (After Oliver, J. E., Jr.: Surgical approach to the canine brain. Am. J. Vet. Res. *29*,371, 1968.)

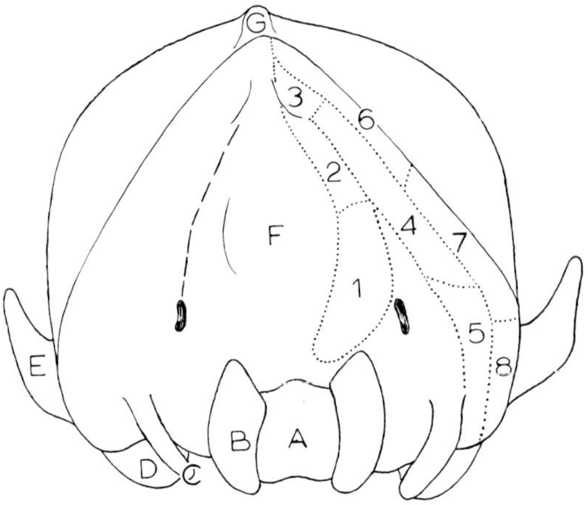

FIGURE 20–52 The muscular attachments to the caudal surface of the occipital bone encountered in a posterior craniectomy. (A) foramen magnum; (B) occipital condyle; (C) jugular process; (D) tympanic bulla; (E) zygomatic process; (F) occipital bone; (G) external occipital protuberance; (1) M. rectus capitis dorsalis major; (2) M. rectus capitis dorsalis minor; (3) M. semispinalis capitis and M. biverter cervicus; (4) M. complexus; (5) M. obliquus capitis cranalis; (6) M. rhomboideus capitis; (7) M. splenius capitis; (8) M. sternomastoideus and M. cleidomastoideus.

THE VENTRAL CRANIECTOMY

The ventral approach seems to have limited clinical value, since only the pituitary gland, the ventral surfaces of the medulla, and the pons can be exposed (Fig. 20–56).

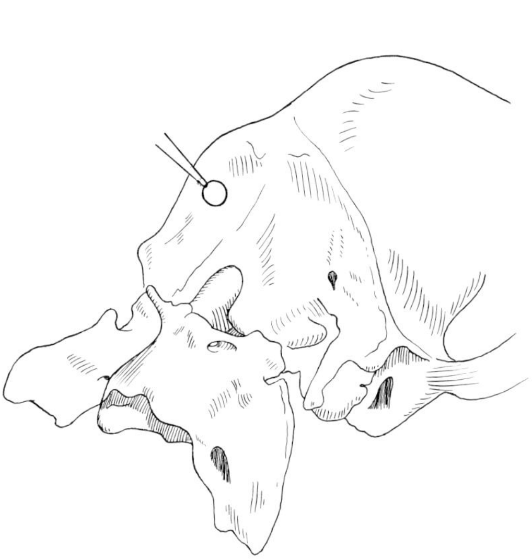

FIGURE 20–53 A bur hole is made to observe the area for subdural hemorrhage and as a possible beginning point for a posterior craniectomy. A bone flap is seldom indicated in the posterior approach.

Technique

The usual approach to this area of the brain is through either the mouth[23, 34, 37] or the ventral midline.[62, 64] For the oral approach, the dog is placed in a dorsal recumbent position with his mouth wide open. An endotracheal or tracheotomy tube is essential. The pharynx is packed with gauze sponges to prevent aspiration of fluid, and the oral cavity is swabbed with antiseptic solution. The incision is made with an electrocautery knife, through the mucosa and soft palate and down to the base of the skull. A palpable landmark is the pterygoid process, which is located directly even with the intersphenoid suture. The periosteum and mucosa are removed caudally over the basisphenoid bone until the occipitosphenoid suture is exposed. The pituitary gland lies directly dorsal to the middle of the basisphenoid bone. The available craniectomy area is limited, in most cases, to a section about 0.5 cm wide and 0.7 cm long because of the ventral petrosal sinuses caudally and the cavernous sinuses laterally and rostrally.

The bur is used directly over the pituitary, and the hole is enlarged appropriately with the rongeurs. Lesions of the pituitary can frequently be removed by aspiration, as can the pituitary gland itself. A large tumor of the gland would be difficult to remove via this approach.

In closure, the dura might be sutured, if that is possible, but it can be left open. Gelatin sponge may be left as a dural and bone substitute. The mucosa is securely sutured with 3–0 medium chromic gut. This approach is difficult and has the disadvantage that asepsis is nearly impossible.

In the neck approach, the dog is placed in the dorsal recumbent position with the head extended and firmly immobilized. An endotracheal catheter is essential. A midline incision is made from the body of the mandible to the level of the third and fourth cervical vertebrae. The trachea, the sternohyoideus, and the sternothyroideus muscles are retracted from the carotid sheath to allow for dissection in fascial planes. The larynx can be palpated at the level of the occipital condyles. Blunt dissection is extended to the base of the skull, where the bodies of the atlas and axis can be palpated. A self-retaining retractor is applied and the rectus capitis ventralis and longus capitis are elevated from their insertions on the basioccipital bone.

The bur hole is made just rostral to the rim of the foramen magnum and is enlarged rostrally up to the pituitary gland. The total lateral craniectomy dimension can be only about 1 cm because of large venous sinuses. To expose the pituitary gland adequately, the pharyngeal mucosa must be elevated, but one must be careful not to enter the oral cavity and permit contamination. The dura is opened, and the area is examined as necessary. The dura is closed where possible, and gelatin sponge may be left as a dural and bone substitute. The closure is made routinely. The large basilar artery would make surgical corrections in this area difficult.

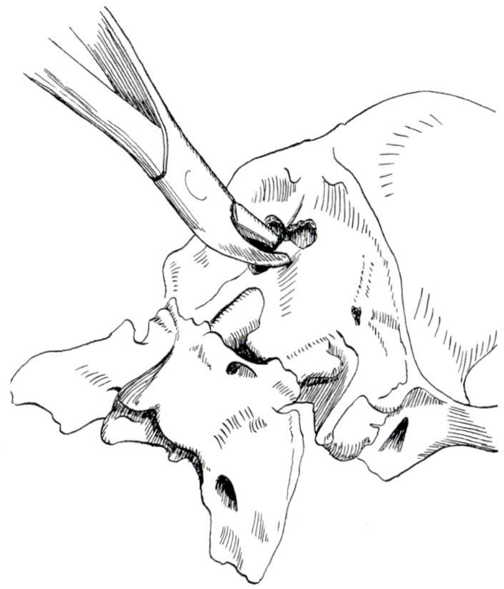

FIGURE 20–54 For more extensive exploration, the rongeur can be used either from the trephine hole or from the foramen magnum. Care should be used not to lacerate the dura mater.

PREFRONTAL LOBOTOMY[54, 55]

The prefrontal lobotomy has been developed by Redding as a possible means of altering overaggressiveness, destructive behavior, fear-biting, and self-mutilation in dogs. As discussed in Chapter 19, Redding is currently treating more behavioral disorders with electroconvulsive shock therapy than with surgery. Prefrontal lobotomy is then used as a "last resort."

The animal is prepared as for any brain surgery, positioned in a head holder, and given gaseous anesthetics as previously described. The skin incision and resection of the temporal muscle are performed in the same way as in the lateral craniotomy. To provide good exposure of the craniotomy site, the temporal muscle should be freed as far cranially and ventrally to the zygomatic arch as possible. An air-driven spherical bur is used to remove a vertical section of bone medial to the widest part of the zygomatic arch on the cranial portion of the calvarium. The slotlike opening is generally one cm wide and 1.5 to 3.0 cm long vertically. A trephine and rongeur can be used

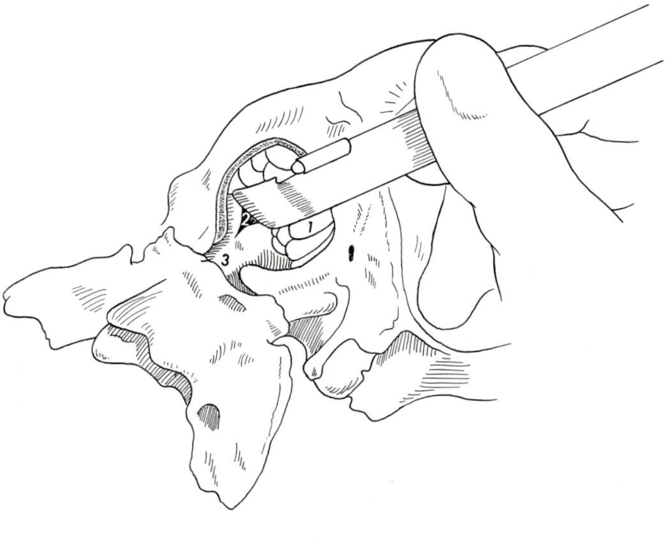

FIGURE 20–55 The posterior cranial compartment can be examined by using gentle retraction, hyperventilation, and aspiration of subarachnoid fluids, as explained under the lateral cerebral approach. The cerebellum is being elevated to demonstrate the fourth ventricle. (1) Cerebellum; (2) fourth ventricle; (3) medulla oblongata.

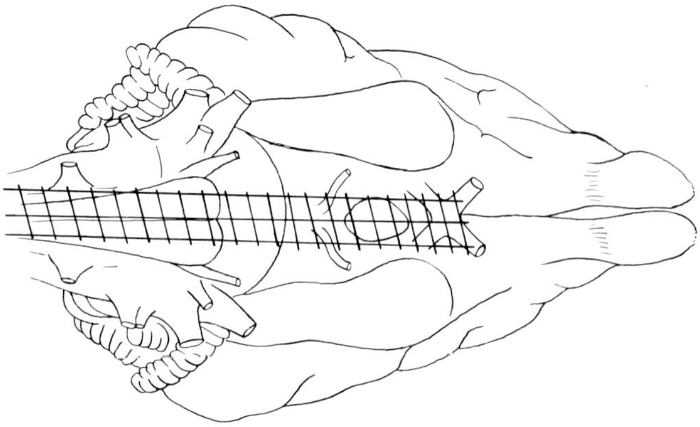

FIGURE 20–56 The cross-hatching represents the approximate area of the ventral brain that can be exposed in a ventral craniectomy.

cautiously, since this area of the calvarium is extremely thin, and accidental laceration of the dura can easily occur. The dura is elevated by a dural hook, and a 3 to 4 mm incision is made with a small scalpel blade (Figs. 20–57 and 20–58).

A lobotomy "knife" is fashioned from a blunt probe and is bent at a 35 degree angle. The length of the cutting portion of the probe is equal to the mediolateral depth of the frontal lobe in this area, usually 4 to 6 cm. The knife should be long enough to reach the midline but not cross it. An imaginary line is drawn transversely across the brain at the caudalmost aspect of the zygomatic process through the slotlike opening in the skull. The knife is inserted through the slot and dural incision, and the cutting edge is angled at 15 degrees cranially to the imaginary line. The lobotomy knife blade is inserted just to the midline and is rotated upward and downward to sever the neuronal fibers to the frontal lobe. The cutting action is repeated until no resistance from brain tissue is felt. Substantial resistance indicates a blood vessel has been encountered; in this case the knife can be withdrawn and reinserted after another bearing on the imaginary line and 15-degree angle has been determined (Figs. 20–59 to 20–61).

After cutting, a small amount of blood may flow from the incision, but this rapidly ceases. No attempt is made to close the tiny dural incision, and the bone defect remains open. The temporal muscle is replaced and sutured, and the subcutis and skin are closed. In a bilateral prefrontal lobotomy the same procedure is repeated on the opposite side.

If restlessness occurs immediately after surgery, an analgesic such as meperidine hydrochloride (Demerol) can be used to prevent self-mutilation. The dog may need hand feeding for a few days because of postsurgical confusion or memory loss. Ti-

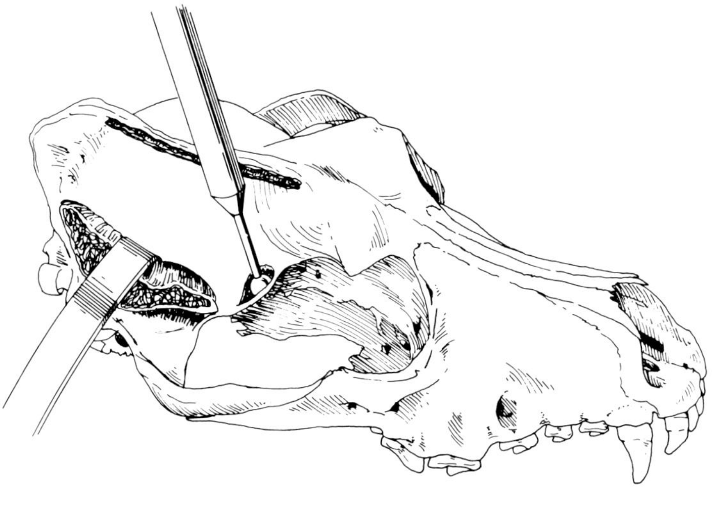

FIGURE 20–57 In the prefrontal lobotomy, the craniotomy is performed after the temporal muscle in this area of the skull has been reflected. (From Redding, R. W.: Prefrontal lobotomy. *In* Bojrab, M. J. (ed.): *Current Techniques in Small Animal Practice I.* Lea & Febiger, Philadelphia, 1975.)

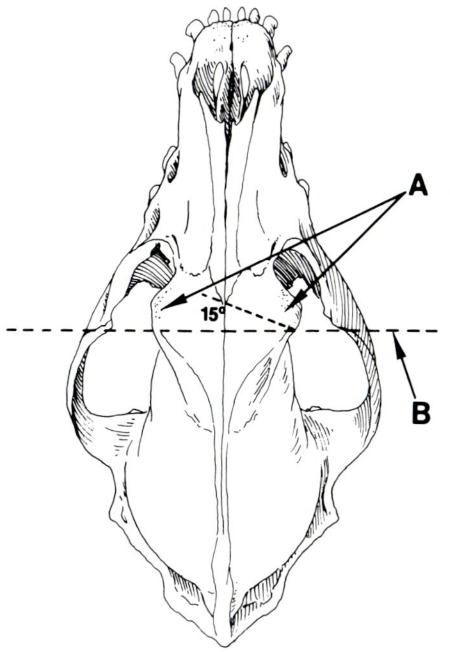

FIGURE 20–58 Dorsal view of the skull. A, Zygomatic processes of the frontal bones. B, Imaginary reference line. The incision in brain tissue is placed at a 15-degree angle from the reference line. (From Redding, R. W.: Prefrontal lobotomy. *In* Bojrab, M. J. (ed.): *Current Techniques in Small Animal Practice I.* Lea & Febiger, Philadelphia, 1975.)

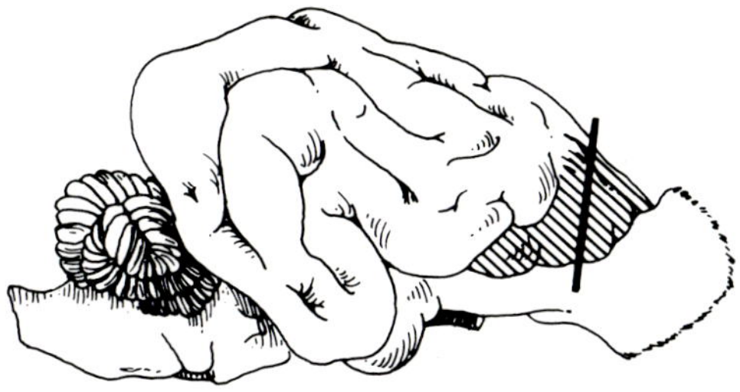

FIGURE 20–60 Lateral view of the leukotomy incision and isolated portion of brain. (From Redding, R. W.: Prefrontal lobotomy. *In* Bojrab, M. J. (ed.): *Current Techniques in Small Animal Practice I.* Lea & Febiger, Philadelphia, 1975.)

midity and disorientation gradually subside after a few days, and the dog is usually normal in a few weeks.

The postsurgical sequelae include injury to the basal nuclei when the incision has been too far caudal, and motor deficits may occur. Accidental invasion of the frontal sinus can be prevented by study of radiographs and anatomical landmarks for the type of skull involved.

Redding has performed this operation in eight patients and has had good results in four cases, fair results in two cases, and poor results in two cases.

Allen and co-workers report moderate to good success in four out of six Alaskan malamutes who could work together in harness after lobotomies. Four of five house pets showed considerable improvement in behavior, but the operation was unsuccessful in one cat. The behavior traits after surgery in some instances were so abnormal that the authors share Redding's

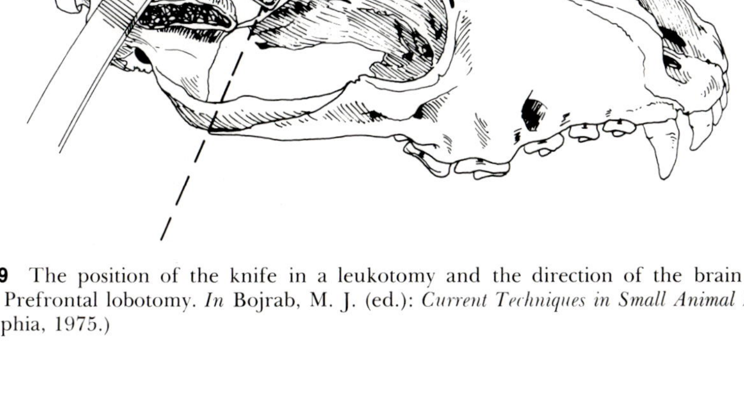

FIGURE 20–59 The position of the knife in a leukotomy and the direction of the brain incision. (From Redding, R. W.: Prefrontal lobotomy. *In* Bojrab, M. J. (ed.): *Current Techniques in Small Animal Practice I.* Lea & Febiger, Philadelphia, 1975.)

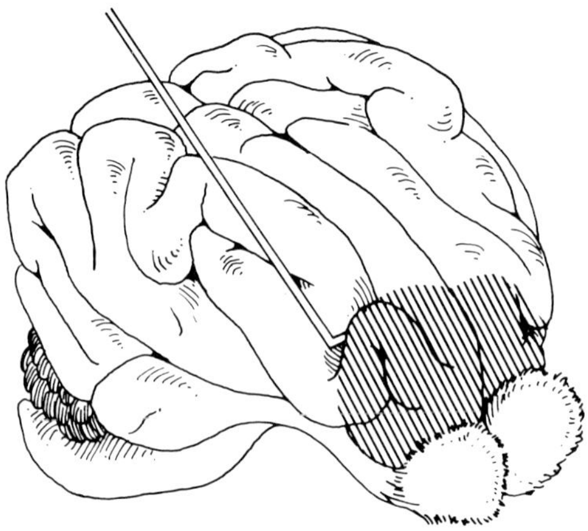

FIGURE 20–61 Anterior oblique view showing the prefrontal areas of the brain isolated by the leukotomy. (From Redding, R. W.: Prefrontal lobotomy. *In* Bojrab, M. J. (ed.): *Current Techniques in Small Animal Surgery I.* Lea & Febiger, Philadelphia, 1975.)

opinion that the surgery should be reserved for a last resort.[2]

APPLICATION OF BRAIN SURGERY

After numerous cranial surgical procedures performed by various of the workers originally or presently associated with this clinic (Drs. Few, Oliver, Gage, Swaim, Redding, and Hoerlein), we have concluded that there are many indications for craniotomies and craniectomies in veterinary practice.

In cranial trauma, the patient can progressively lose consciousness and neurological function.[50] In such cases, it is apparent that intracranial hemorrhage or edema and swelling is progressive and that corrective measures must be taken promptly to preserve life. The most efficient way to differentiate edema from hemorrhage is the appropriate use of bur holes in the calvarium.[47] Removal of depressed bone fragments and hemorrhage, ligation of bleeding vessels, and decompression are performed as needed.[42] The response has been dramatic and most rewarding. Very frequently, such emergency surgery can be performed with the training, personnel, equipment, and facilities available in many current veterinary practices.[58]

The importance of radical decompression in severe cerebral edema in human neurology has been emphasized by Kerr. He stated that the chronic or "malignant" variety of cerebral edema characteristically responds only transiently to nonsurgical methods (steroids, hypertonic solutions, etc.) and that radical or extensive decompression of the brain is indicated in such a case. He proposed an excision of both calvaria, incision of the dura, and the insertion of large homologous dural grafts. Bone defect replacements can be performed at a later date.[30]

The need for diagnosis may be another indication for brain surgery, after the standard physical, radiographic, laboratory, and EEG procedures. In such cases, the surgical *correction* is made if possible. If the problem cannot be solved surgically, the dog is destroyed on the surgical table according to prior agreement with the owner. This proves to be a satisfactory way of terminating a case and gives the owner the best available service. It also enhances progress in neurology because the body is available for a complete necropsy. In our experience, cortical adhesions or necrosis may be present as a result of past injuries. Frequently such cases can be helped. Obviously, tumors, abscesses, and vascular abnormalities can frequently be corrected by brain surgery.[43] In this "nonemergency" category of brain surgery, practice personnel should have equipment and general competence beyond that needed for the previously described emergency cases. This type of surgery must be based on a good understanding of neurological and diagnostic phenomena.

We conclude that brain surgery may be within the realm of competent general practitioners, particularly in cases of acute traumatic cranial fractures and hemorrhage. Probably the diagnosis of chronic lesions, such as tumors, may demand more specialized competence, but this can be secured through interest, additional training, and experience. The field of brain surgery in veterinary practice is a most rewarding, challenging, and rapidly developing one.

REFERENCES

1. Albin, M. S., D'Agostino, A. N., White, R. J., and Grindlay, J. H.: Nonsuture sealing of a dural substitute utilizing a plastic adhesive, Methyl-2-cyanoacrylate. J. Neurosurg. *19,* 545, 1962.

2. Allen, D. B., Cummings, J. F., and de Lahunta, A.: Effects of lobotomy on aggressive behavior. Cornell Vet. *64,* 201, 1974.
3. Asenjo, A.: *Neurosurgical Techniques.* Charles C Thomas, Springfield, Ill., 1963.
4. Averill, D. R.: Intracranial injuries. *In* Kirk, R. W. (ed.) *Current Veterinary Therapy V.* W. B. Saunders Co., Philadelphia, 1974.
5. Balch, R. E.: Wound infections complicating neurosurgical procedures. J. Neurosurg. *26,* 41, 1967.
6. Boyd, R. J., and Connolly, J. E.: Total cerebral ischemia in the dog. Arch. Surg. *84,* 434–438, April, 1962.
7. Brown, M. H.: Use of polythene film as a dural substitute. Surg. Gynec. Obstet. *86,* 663–668, 1948.
8. Bunce, D. F. M.: Survival of dogs following section of carotid and vertebral arteries. Proc. Soc. Exp. Biol. *103,* 581–585, 1960.
9. Bunce, D. F. M.: Arterial supply to the brain of the dog. Anat. Record *136,* 172–173, 1960.
10. Cone, W. V., and Penfield, W. C.: Myoplastic craniotomy. Arch. Neurol. Psychiat. *35,* 1–11, 1936.
11. de la Torre, E., Netsky, M. G., and Meschan, I.: Intracranial and extracranial circulations in the dog. Anatomic and angiographic studies. Amer. J. Anat. *105,* 343–382, 1959.
12. Dodge, H. W., Jr., Grindlay, J. H., Craid, W. McK., and Ross, P. J.: Use of polyvinyl sponge in neurosurgery. J. Neurosurg. *11,* 258, 1954.
13. Gage, E. D.: Unpublished data.
14. Galbraith, J. G.: Hypothermia in the management of brain injuries. J. Med. Assoc. *30,* 197, 1960.
15. Gallagher, J. P., and Geschickter, C. F.: The use of charged gold leaf in surgery. J.A.M.A. *189,* 928–933, 1964.
16. Glaser, M. A., and Thienes, C. H.: Dural defects: How important is their surgical repair? An experimental and clinical study upon heteroplastic autoplastic dural grafts. Calif. West. Med. *48,* 163–166, 1938.
17. Goluboff, B., Shenkin, H. A., and Haft, H.: The effects of mannitol and urea on cerebral hemodynamics and cerebrospinal fluid pressure. Neurology *14,* 891, 1964.
18. Gotoh, F., Meyer, J. S., and Takagi, Y.: Cerebral effects of hyperventilation in man. Arch. Neurol. *12,* 410, 1965.
19. Gunn, C. G., Williams, G. R., and Parker, I. T.: Edema of the brain following circulatory arrest. J. Surg. Res. *2,* 141, 1962.
20. Gurdjian, E. S.: *Operative Neurosurgery,* 2nd ed. Williams and Wilkins, Baltimore, 1964.
21. Guyton, A. C.: *Textbook of Medical Physiology,* 4th ed. W. B. Saunders Co., Philadelphia, 1971.
22. Hayes, G. J., and Slocum, H. C.: The achievement of optimal brain relaxation by hyperventilation technics of anesthesia. J. Neurosurg. *19,* 65–70, 1962.
23. Himwich, W. A., Costa, E., Canham, R. G., and Goldstein, S. L.: Isolation and injection of selected arterial areas in the brain. J. Appl. Physiol. *15,* 303, 1960.
24. Hoerlein, B. F., Few, A. B., and Petty, M. F.: Brain surgery in the dog—preliminary studies. J.A.V.M.A. *143,* 21–29, 1963.
25. Hoerlein, B. F.: *Canine Neurology, Diagnosis and Treatment,* 2nd ed. W. B. Saunders Co., Philadelphia, 1971.
26. Huertas, J.: The use of Orlon for dural replacement. J. Neurosurg. *12,* 550, 1955.
27. James, C. W.: The radiographic anatomy of the arterial system of the dog. Thesis, Auburn University, Auburn, Alabama, 1963.
28. Keener, E. B.: Regeneration of dural defects, a review. J. Neurosurg. *16,* 415, 1959.
29. Keener, E. B.: An experimental study of reactions of the dura mater to wounding and loss of substance. J. Neurosurg. *16,* 424, 1959.
30. Kerr, F. W. L.: Radical decompression and dural grafting in severe cerebral edema. Mayo Clin. Proc. *43,* 852–864, 1968.
31. Kline, D. G., and Hayes, G. J.: Experimental evaluation of the effect of a plastic adhesive, methyl-2-cyanoacrylate, on neural tissue. J. Neurosurg. *20,* 647, 1963.
32. Kurze, T., Apuzzo, M. L. J., Weiss, M. H., and Heiden, J. S.: Collagen sponge for surface brain protection. J. Neurosurg. *43,* 637, 1975.
33. Leahy, J. R.: Muscles of the head, neck, shoulder and forelimb of the dog. Thesis, Cornell University, Ithaca, N.Y., 1949.
34. Markowitz, J., Archibald, J., and Downie, H. G.: Central nervous system. In *Experimental Surgery,* 5th ed. Willaims and Wilkins, Baltimore, 1960.
35. Mason, M. S., and Reaf, J.: Homologous dura mater grafts. Ann. Surg. *153,*423, 1961.
36. Mayfield, F. H., and Kurokawa, K.: Watertight closure of spinal dura mater. J. Neurosurg. *43,* 639, 1975.
37. McLean, A. J.: Transbuccal approach to encephalon in experimental operations upon carnivoral pituitary, pons and ventral medulla. Ann. Surg. *88,* 985–993, 1928.
38. Meirowsky, A. M.: Wounds of dural sinuses. J. Neurosurg. *5,* 496, 1953.
39. Miller, M. E., Christensen, G. C., and Evans, H. E.: *Anatomy of the Dog.* W. B. Saunders Co., Philadelphia, 1964.
40. Morrell, R. M.: Effect of cutting the tentorium cerebelli on the response to craniocerebral trauma. J. Neurosurg. *17,* 374, 1960.
41. Mullan, S.: Current mortality of the surgical treatment of brain tumors. J.A.M.A. *182,* 601, 1962.
42. Oliver, J. E., Jr.: Surgical decompression in a cranial fracture. Auburn Vet. *20,* 78–79, 1964.
43. Oliver, J. E., Jr.: Surgical relief of epileptiform seizures in a dog. Vet. Med. Small Anim. Clin. *60,* 367, 1965.
44. Oliver, J. E., Jr.: Canine cranial surgery. Thesis, Auburn University, Auburn, Alabama, 1966.
45. Oliver, J. E., Jr.: Principles of canine brain surgery. Animal Hosp. *2,* 73–88, 1966.
46. Oliver, J. E., Jr.: Surgical approaches to the canine brain. Am. J. Vet. Res. *29,* 353–378, 1968.
47. Oliver, J. E., Jr.: Management of the patient with acute head injury. The newer knowledge about dogs. Gaines Dog Research Center, October, 1969.
48. Owens, G.: Experimental occlusion of dural sinuses. Surg. Forum *8,* 521, 1957.
49. Owens, G.: Evaluation of cerebral venous hypertension as therapy for cerebral infarction. Surg. Forum *10,* 764, 1959.

50. Palmer, A. C.: The accident case. IV. The significance and estimation of damage to the central nervous system. J. Small Anim. Pract. *5*, 25, 1964.
51. Parker, A. J., and Cunningham, J. G.: Transfrontal craniotomy in the dog. Vet. Rec. *90*, 622, 1972.
52. Penfield, W. G.: Meningocerebral adhesions. Surg. Gynec. Obstet. *39*, 803–810, 1924.
53. Rasmussen, T. B.: Experimental ligation of the cerebral arteries of the dog. Thesis. University of Minnesota, St. Paul, Minn., 1938.
54. Redding, R. W.: Prefrontal lobotomy. *In* Bojrab, M. J. (ed.): *Current Techniques in Small Animal Surgery I*, Lea and Febiger, Philadelphia, 1975.
55. Redding, R. W.: Prefrontal lobotomy of the dog. Scientific Presentations. Am. Anim. Hosp. Assoc. *374*, 1972.
56. Reinhard, K. R., Miller, M. E., and Evans, H. E.: The craniovertebral veins and sinuses of the dog. Am. J. Anat. *111*, 67, 1962.
57. Sayad, W. Y., and Harvey, S. C.: The regeneration of the meninges. The dura mater. Ann. Surg. *77*, 129–141, 1923.
58. Smith, H. A.: Subdural hematoma and cerebral contusion: A case report. The Veterinarian *6*, 9, 1961.
59. Swaim, S. F.: Use of pneumatic surgical instruments in neurosurgery, part 2: Cranial and paracranial surgery. Vet. Med. Small Anim. Clin. *68*, 1404, 1973.
60. Swaim, S. F.: Personal communication.
61. Teng, P., and Feigin, I.: Vinyon "N" as a dural substitute. J. Neurosurg. *12*, 591, 1955.
62. Verdura, J., White, R. J., and Albin, M.: New technique for aseptic hypophysectomy in the dog. J. Surg. Res. *3*, 174–175, 1963.
63. Walker, A. E.: The late results of cranioplasty. Arch. Neurol. *9*, 105, 1963.
64. White, R. J., and Donald, D. E.: Basilar artery ligation and cerebral ischemia in dogs. Arch. Surg. *84*, 108–113, 1962.
65. Worthman, R. P.: The longitudinal vertebral venous sinuses of the dog. I. Anatomy. II. Functional aspects. Am. J. Vet. Res. *17*, 341, 1956.

CHAPTER 21

HYDROCEPHALUS*

B. F. HOERLEIN, D.V.M., PH.D.
E. D. GAGE, D.V.M., M.S.

CEREBROSPINAL FLUID

In Chapter 6, the pressure, normal composition, and alterations of cerebrospinal fluid (CSF) in disease were discussed. The physiological characteristics of CSF are described in this chapter on hydrocephalus.

FORMATION OF CSF

The clear, watery CSF envelops and bathes the brain and spinal cord internally in the cerebral ventricles and the central canal of the spinal cord and externally in the subarachnoid spaces and cisterns. The CSF is produced primarily by the choroid plexuses and ependymal linings of the ventricles, but extraventricular sources, such as the leptomeninges and subarachnoid spaces, constitute at least 30 per cent of the total CSF production. Sato determined that only 42 per cent of the CSF was formed in the ventricles.[43, 61, 65] Bering reported that in the normal 15-kg dog, CSF was produced at the rates of 0.016 ml/min in the lateral and third ventricles, 0.011 ml/min in the fourth ventricle, and 0.020 ml/min in the subarachnoid space (total—0.047 ml/min). Also, the intraventricular formation of CSF was calculated to take place at the rate of 0.24 ml/min/gm from the choroid plexus and 0.3×10^{-3} ml/min/cm^2 from the ependymal surface.[5]

The two mechanisms of formation are diffusion and secretion. Substances pass by diffusion into the fluid from the plasma and across the membranes (including the ependyma) that line the CSF-containing spaces. Recent work suggests that a major fraction of the CSF is formed within the cerebral parenchyma because the extracellular fluids in the brain and CSF are identical or very similar. Therefore, it is felt that CSF is formed in part by the drainage of brain interspaces into the CSF spaces.[41] The rate of entry is largely determined by particle size, but it also depends to some extent on lipoid solubility. The latter is a consideration because of the identity of cerebrospinal and extracellular fluid of the neuraxis. Certain substances, in addition to entering by diffusion, are actively *secreted* into the CSF by the choroid plexus. When compared to plasma, CSF contains higher concentrations of magnesium and chloride ions and lower levels of glucose, proteins, amino acids, uric acid, calcium, potassium, and PO_4 ions. Therefore, CSF is also said to be a secretion in that its formation depends upon the expenditure of energy.[41] Water can enter and leave the system freely at all points in sufficient quantity to render the secreted sodium isotonic with the plasma.[7]

*Much credit is due to Drs. A. B. Few, J. E. Oliver, and S. F. Swaim for their unselfish contributions.

Bering studied formation, flow, and absorption of CSF by "steady-state" ventricular perfusion. He concluded that the formation of CSF was constant, independent of hydrostatic pressure, and unaffected by the development of hydrocephalus.[4] Rubin and co-workers studied CSF production and absorption in persons with CNS malignancies. They concluded that CSF production was unaffected by intracranial pressure or by the age of the subject, and that acetazolamide (Diamox) caused a reduction in CSF production.[60] Garcia-Benogochea found that both the gonads and cortisone influence the formation and absorption of CSF in adult cats and that these influences were interrelated. Intramuscular injections of cortisone in noncastrated adult cats produced a significant reduction in the amount of CSF collected by spinal catheterization; the same injections in castrated cats caused an increase of CSF.[22] Sato and co-workers found that in dogs the CSF production rate began to decline immediately after the injection of 0.15 mg/kg of dexamethasone; it attained a maximal reduction of 50 per cent in 50 minutes. There were no significant differences between the treated and control dogs in CSF and serum chemical constituents that would influence the flow of CSF. The role of steroids will be discussed later in this chapter under treatment.[62]

CIRCULATION

CSF flows from the relatively large paired lateral ventricles through the interventricular foramina (foramina of Monro), and into the midline third ventricle. It continues from the third ventricle into the fourth ventricle by way of the cerebral aqueduct (aqueduct of Sylvius). From here, most of the fluid leaves the ventricular system and passes by means of the lateral apertures (lateral foramina of Luschka) into the subarachnoid cavity. The median aperture of the fourth ventricle in man (foramen of Magendie) is absent in the dog and other animals lower than the anthropoid apes.[6, 43, 65] A small amount of fluid passes into the central canal of the spinal cord from the fourth ventricle. The greater part of the fluid surges forward into the cerebral subarachnoid spaces and basal cisterns; the balance circulates in a restricted fashion in the spinal subarachnoid space. In dog experiments, after iodine-131 or iodine-125 radioiodinated human serum albumin cisternal or intravenous injections cisternograms and ventriculograms as well as fluids collected from the nasal cavities demonstrated considerable leakage of CSF into the submucous space, local lymphatics, and the nasal cavity itself.[12] In man, the bulk of fluid in the spinal subarachnoid space appears to follow a downward route behind the cord, posterior to the dentata ligaments, to the lumbar theca, and upward in front of the cord to the basilar cisterns [41]

Bering determined that in the dog, the amount of CSF in the cerebral subarachnoid and cisternal areas was 5.8 to 7.9 ml when perfusions were determined using creatinine and inulin. The mean volumes of CSF in the ventricular system, determined by similar perfusion methods, were 3.9 ml for creatinine, 3.0 ml for inulin, 5.2 ml for RISA, and 7.6 ml for urea[5].

Bowsher and Oldendorf have accumulated interesting data on the circulation of CSF. The total rate of production is about 0.5 per cent of the total CSF volume per minute. In man, ½ to 1 liter of CSF is formed daily. In addition to the propulsive force generated by CSF production in the ventricle, mixing is probably aided by cilia and by changes in cranial blood volume that result from cardiac systole and respiratory movements. Distinct lateral displacement of the walls of the third ventricle synchronous with heart action has been demonstrated by ultrasonic studies, suggesting a to-and-fro surge of fluid in the third ventricle with systole. Since the foramen magnum represents the major vent for displacement of intracranial fluid when the systolic surge of blood enters the cranial cavity, there is a substantial surge (probably more than 1 ml in man) of CSF past the medulla with each systole. The large exchange of fluid past the fourth ventricular foramina must serve to accelerate mixing and disposal throughout the subarachnoid space with fresh ventricular fluid. The bulk flow of fluid in the low-concentration CSF compartment supports a "sink action" as a function of CSF; this will be discussed later under CSF functions.[7, 48, 49]

It is well to emphasize at this point that the subarachnoid space has some important extensions that are also supplied with CSF. These include the cranial and spinal nerves, especially the optic and acoustic nerves. For instance, the eye has a direct pathway to the cranial vault, since the optic nerves are sheathed by an extension of the cerebral meninges and are therefore bathed in CSF. Each lateral ventricle has an anterior projection known as the olfactory tract, and the cavity of the olfactory bulb. Therefore, the CSF can be in intimate contact with or even mixed with the lymph fluid of the eye, ear, and olfactory areas of the nose. In addition, other minute extensions, known as Virchow-Robin spaces,[43] occur around the blood vessels entering the brain.

In man, the main route by which CSF is returned to the blood is across the arachnoid villi, although subsidiary sites of absorption probably include the ventricular ependyma, the leptomeninges, and the lymphatics of the spinal and cranial nerves.[41] The routes or areas of absorption of CSF in the dog probably are much the same, since dogs do have arachnoid villi,[52] which Fankhauser[15] describes as similar to those in the horse but smaller. Pollay and Welch[52] compare the function of the villus mechanism in dogs to that of a ball valve. In perfusion experiments these authors saw open flow of fluid in only one direction from the meninges to the dorsal sagittal sinus.[52]

ABSORPTION

Water leaves and enters the CSF cavities freely and with great rapidity across all lining membranes. In the ventricles, absorption occurs mainly across the ependyma, but under some circumstances the choroid plexuses can undoubtedly take up injected materials.[39]

Since output of fluid in the ventricles exceeds absorption, the CSF flows from the ventricles into the subarachnoid spaces, where absorption normally takes place at the nearest point. Cerebrospinal fluid is contained in a rigid system (the cranial vault), to which elasticity is given largely by the subarachnoid venous bed. This elasticity is responsible for the resting pressure of the CSF. Fluctuations in resting pressure are in fact volumetric changes due to filling of the valveless subarachnoid veins in inspiration, straining, and coughing.[7] No doubt another factor is the local force generated through the pressure wave transmitted to the CSF by choroid plexus arterial pulsation.[4, 71] These changes in volume are in phase throughout the system. In the closed system, an increase in volume of the semipermeable subarachnoid veins results in displacement of substances in the CSF into the interior of the veins, resulting in their removal from the subarachnoid space. This is the force responsible for normal CSF absorption by the leptomeningovascular route. The slow component of absorption is due to a perineurolymphatic pathway.[7]

Even though it has been shown that CSF *production* is unaffected by intracranial pressure, the rate of *absorption* from the subarachnoid space is directly proportional to intracranial pressure within the range of zero to 100 mm water. Absorption capacity exceeds CSF production by at least fourfold.[60]

FUNCTIONS

The functions of CSF are important to the integrity of the central nervous system and therefore to that of the animal. In its function as a "stress" or "cushion" mechanism, it is particularly essential to the brain. The ventricles and the subarachnoid space serve as the internal and external fluid cushions of the brain. CSF serves an important function by providing a chemical environment for the central nervous system. There is strong evidence that the intraventricular administration of biogenic amines stimulates the letdown of pituitary-releasing factors from cellular elements in contact with CSF. The tanycyte, a special cell which projects from the ventricular surface into the infundibular recess, may form an essential link in the control of pituitary function by responding as a sensor to substances circulating in CSF.

The so-called sink action of CSF was mentioned previously. CSF performs this sink or lymphatic role because it is the only system sufficiently nonspecific to transport all the substances that must be removed from the brain, such as lipid-insoluble substances, foreign bodies, red cells, protein, and bacteria.[41] If this sink action of the low concentration CSF compartment is to be effective, the CSF must have close contact with all portions of the CNS tissues. In the adult human, there is no point in the brain at which the CSF is more than 2 cm from the ependyma or the pia mater. The gray cortical matter, which has an exceptionally high metabolic rate, is located within a few millimeters of the CSF. This proximity is probably even more pronounced in smaller mammals such as the dog. The need for CSF to have access to tissues may be a factor in the odd shape of the brain, with its sulci, gyri, ventricles, and other odd formations. The brain is highly irregular instead of having a gross morphological simplicity, as does the liver or kidney. The sink action may therefore be a prime function of CSF.[48, 49]

HYDROCEPHALUS

INCIDENCE

Hydrocephalus is one of the most frequently encountered neurological disorders seen in clinical small animal practice. In the veterinary medical data program,* 708 cases of congenital hydrocephalus among 1186 cases of various congenital diseases (59.7 per cent) were recorded in institutional teaching hospitals. If these 708 cases of congenital hydrocephalus are related to the total of 1014 cases of congenital neurological diseases, a 69.8 per cent incidence is noted. Of the 708 cases, 384 (54.2 per cent) occurred in the 0 to 1-year age group. About 51 per cent of patients were males.

In the Auburn clinic from 1969 to 1975, hydrocephalus was diagnosed in 165 dogs and 11 cats, based on clinical signs, EEG findings, radiographic signs, and necropsy observations. The majority of these cases were observed in Chihuahuas, toy poodles, Yorkshire terriers, and other miniature breeds. Ages of affected animals ranged from 5 weeks to 6 years, with some 30 per cent being over 1 year of age. Many mature animals probably had subclinical hydrocephalus; and trauma, infections, or other stress precipiated the clinical syndrome.

*Courtesy of Dr. William Priester, National Cancer Institute, Bethesda, Maryland.

TYPES OF HYDROCEPHALUS

The accumulation of fluid in the brain is called hydrocephalus. Such accumulation of fluid occurs in all conditions in which there is a diffuse cerebral atrophy, but in these conditions the disorder is compensatory and of little clinical significance in itself. Hydrocephalus usually produces clinical signs only when the fluid is under increased pressure. In the classic definition, *obstructive hydrocephalus* occurs when the raised pressure ensues from an obstruction at some point in the course of circulation of CSF between the choroid plexuses and its exit from the fourth ventricle. This is the most common type of hydrocephalus in the dog. In the other main type, *communicating hydrocephalus,* there is increased pressure of CSF but no observable source of obstruction; the fluid circulates freely between the ventricular and subarachnoid areas. Obstructive hydrocephalus typically causes accumulation of fluid in the ventricles and may be called ventricular dropsy or internal hydrocephalus. When the accumulation of fluid is greatest in the subarachnoid areas, the condition may be called external hydrocephalus.[3]

Congenital Hydrocephalus

Congenital hydrocephalus is present at the time of or shortly after birth and is usually due to a congenital malformation which interferes with CSF circulation at one or several points. It is characterized by an enlarged cranium. The cerebral aqueduct may be narrowed, or a cerebellar herniation through an enlarged foramen magnum may constrict CSF outflow from the fourth ventricle (occipital dysplasia, Arnold-Chiari syndrome) (Fig. 21–1). The condition may occur concurrently with atlantoaxial subluxation in both humans and dogs. In other cases, there is impaired upward flow of CSF above the tentorium from the ventricles, leaving free circulation around the spinal cord. Birth trauma re-

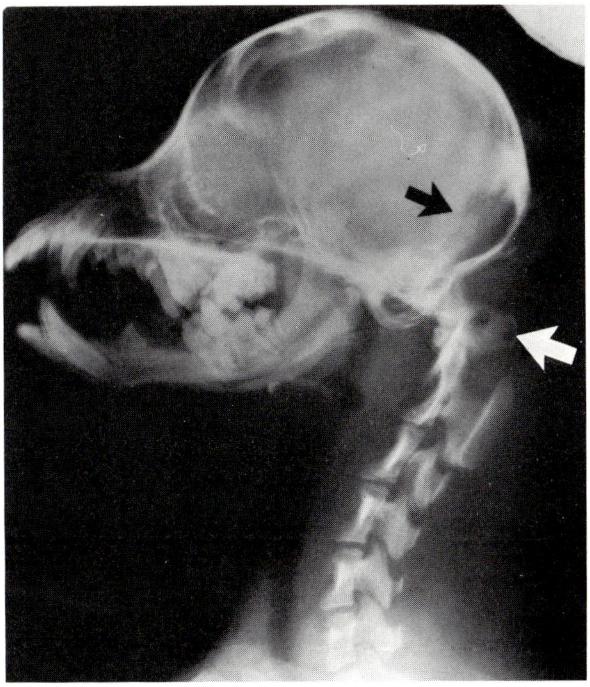

FIGURE 21–1 A case of occipital dysplasia (enlarged foramen magnum), shortened Cl vertebra, partial spina bifida of the cervical vertebrae, and clinical hydrocephalus. The arrow points to the very large foramen magnum.

sulting in hemorrhages and adhesions may be the cause of infantile hydrocephalus.[3].

Acquired Hydrocephalus

Acquired hydrocephalus may be seen at any age. When it occurs after skeletal maturity, there is typically no enlargement of the skull. It can occur with inflammatory or neoplastic lesions that occlude CSF circulation. Adhesions following meningitis or arachnoiditis may occlude the outlet of the fourth ventricle or obliterate the cerebrospinal channels in the cisterns above the tentorium. Parasitic cysts can be a cause. Thrombosis of the dorsal sagittal sinus and other venous sinuses can impair absorption of fluid.[3]

The definitions given here are classically academic, and many clinicians and pathologists have broader concepts of obstructive and communicating hydrocephalus. If one does not see any obstruction in the free flow of CSF and yet the accumulation of fluid is primarily ventricular, is it a case of obstructive or communicating hydrocephalus? If acute hydrocephalus occurs in a 12-week-old puppy, should it be classified as congenital in spite of the lack of evidence of a narrow aqueduct or other deformity? Could it not be acquired? In another case, a 2-year-old Chihuahua with an acute decompensation of CSF pressure and an acute ventricular distention but no evidence of obstruction to CSF flow might have a subclinical congenital form of the disease, even though clinical signs recurred after maturity, and it might be communicative rather than obstructive hydrocephalus. Perhaps the classification of disease types should be abolished or de-emphasized unless the obstruction of CSF flow has been proved. The following discussion, however, will make use of the classic definitions, and obstructive hydrocephalus is discussed according to its two types, congenital and acquired (Figs. 21–2 to 21–6).

CAUSES OF HYDROCEPHALUS

The causes of hydrocephalus have already been cited briefly. In the *congenital* forms, nutrition may play a role. It has been shown that a vitamin A deficiency in rabbits can cause an increase in the amount of CSF and thus produce hydrocephalus.[42] It has also been shown that hypervitaminosis A causes, among other things, a decrease in CSF pressure, probably by an

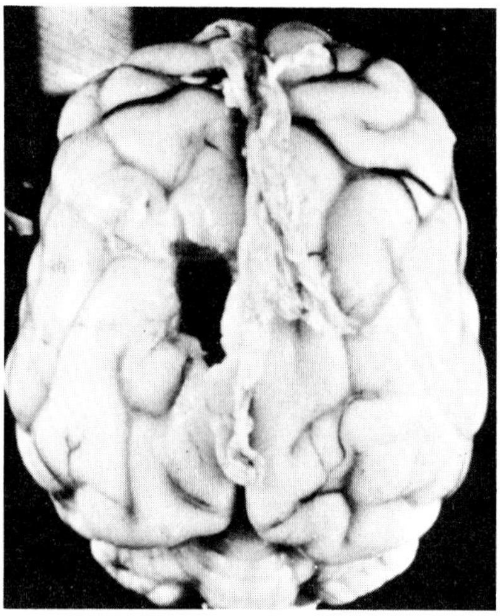

FIGURE 21–2 Communicating hydrocephalus, in which the lateral ventricle communicates with the subarachnoid space.

increased permeability to CSF outflow.[23] Rickets has been incriminated in other cases.[7] Newberne and co-workers have reported hydrocephalus in rats that ate a diet deficient in vitamin B_{12}; an even higher incidence resulted from deficiency of vitamin B_{12} and cobalt.[46] Based on experiments in which hydrocephalus was produced in immature laboratory animals by various viruses, there is evidence that neonatal infectious agents may cause clinical congenital hydrocephalus.[44] Cerebral atrophy and resultant dilatation of the ventricles are common in older animals. However, this is not true hydrocephalus, since there is no increased pressure of CSF in the ventricles.

Malformations of the brain have been reported as causes of congenital hydrocephalus.[16] Finally, there may be a familial or hereditary aspect in the etiology of congenital hydrocephalus.[31, 68]

It is a well-known fact that most of the clinical cases of both congenital and acquired forms of hydrocephalus occur in certain types of dogs, such as the miniature breeds with dome-shaped heads. The Chihuahua and Manchester terrier are commonly affected, as are the Pekingese and brachycephalic breeds.[31] In the Chihuahua particularly, hydrocephalus should be considered in any animal showing neurological signs attributable to the brain.

Redding[58] studied a large kennel of Chihuahuas in which hydrocephalus, predominantly acquired, was a common occurrence. All dogs had periodic electroencephalograms to determine subclinical as well as clinical cases. The dogs with mild clinical disease usually showed signs of an ill-natured disposition, probably due to chronic pain, manifested by difficulty in training, nervousness, and degrees of aggressiveness. Animals which were affected, judging by abnormal signs and electroencephalograms, seemed to produce a high percentage of affected offspring. The selective breeding program has been helped tremendously by using the EEG as a screening device and the evidence of hydrocephalus as a hereditary disorder has been substantiated.[58] Redding has concluded that many of the miniature breeds in which open fontanelles are almost constant are suffering from a subclinical (com-

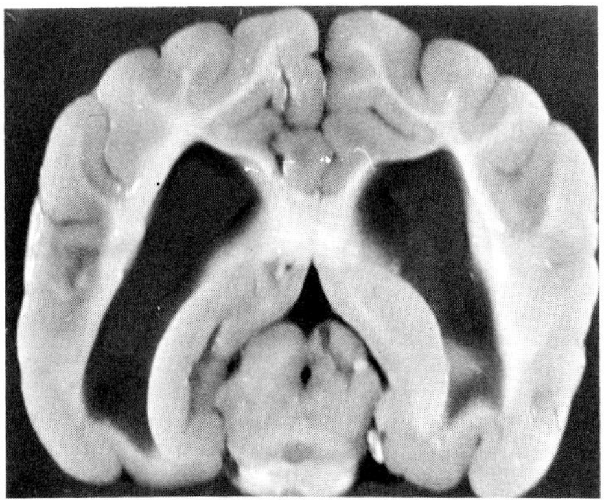

FIGURE 21–3 A case of obstructive ventricular dropsy (internal hydrocephalus) in which the two lateral ventricles are grossly enlarged. They are bilaterally symmetrical.

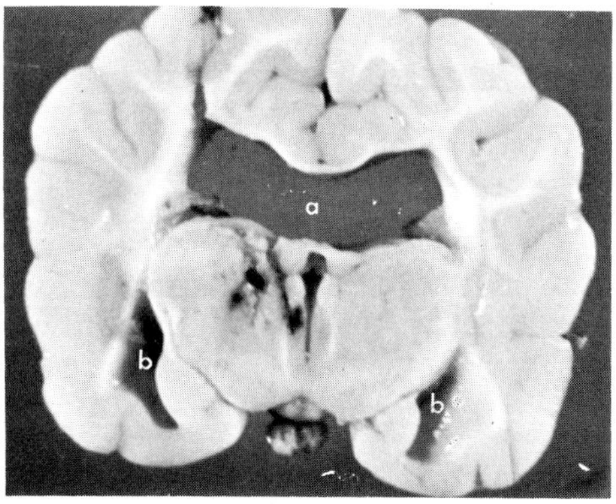

FIGURE 21–4 The two lateral ventricles are communicating freely (a), as though only one ventricle existed. Extremities of the lateral ventricles (b).

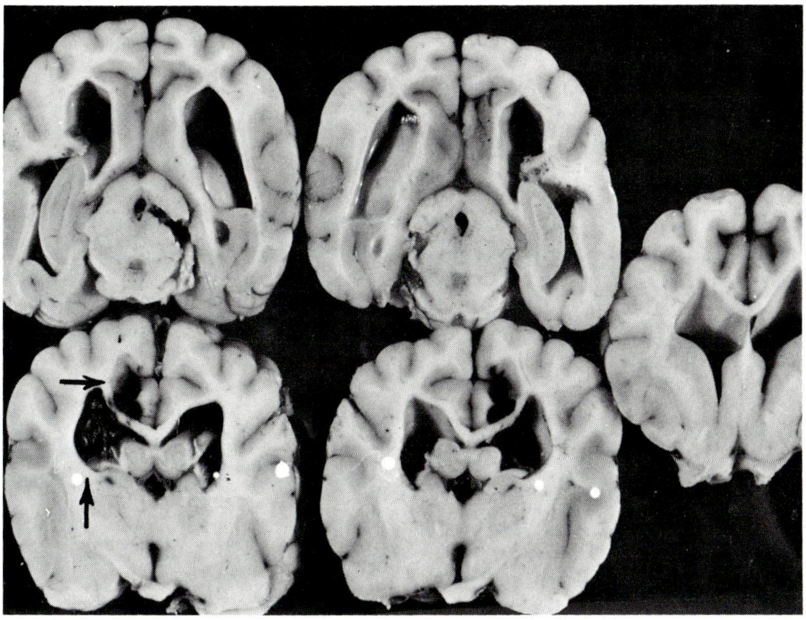

FIGURE 21–5 Ventricular dropsy associated with a brain tumor.

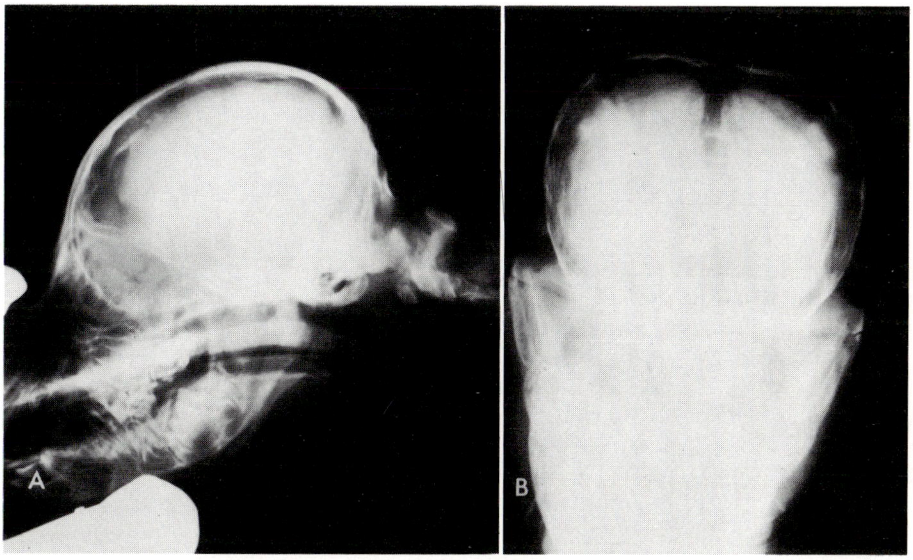

FIGURE 21–6 Ventriculograms using meglumine iothalamate as the contrast medium. Notice the severe dilatation of both lateral ventricles.

pensated) form of hydrocephalus. Trauma, infection, or some generally nonpathogenic stress "triggers" the disorder and results in an acute attack of hydrocephalus. There is a high incidence of an enlarged foramen magnum in these breeds, occasionally combined with longitudinal shortening of the first cervical vertebra (also called occipital dysplasia); this may be a contributing factor in the cause of hydrocephalus. If occipital dysplasia is accompanied by cervical spina bifida and syringomyelia, the disorder is called the Arnold-Chiari syndrome (Fig. 21–1).

In attempts to study experimentally produced hydrocephalus in healthy mongrels and beagles, Cammermeyer observed a high percentage of cases in which hydrocephalus occurred naturally. Pathologic changes involved diffuse meningoencephalitis.[8] The cause of these changes was undetermined, but possibly a previous high incidence of distemper in the experimental group was a factor.

The causes of acquired or secondary hydrocephalus are varied. Any condition that contributes to overproduction of fluid by the choroid plexuses, obstruction in the flow of fluid, or deficiency of fluid absorption will produce hydrocephalus.[39] Cranial trauma, infectious agents such as toxoplasma, bacteria, and viruses causing encephalitis and meningitis, and neoplasia are frequent causes of clinically acquired hydrocephalus.

Vandevelde and Higgins[69] have observed five puppies from 7 to 12 weeks of age representing large and small breeds of dogs who were affected with acute neurological clinical disease. Electroencephalograms and other clinical signs were abnormal. Grossly, the brains showed marked ventricular enlargement and compressed cortical and subcortical tissue. Microscopically, severe periventricular lesions were noted, especially around the olfactory canal and lateral ventricles. Irregularly shaped false diverticula projected into the surrounding nervous tissues from the lateral ventricles. The changes were characteristic of suppurative bacterial infection, possibly by the olfactory route. There was no evidence of viral involvement. Bacterial infections in the brain and meninges are not considered common in the dog; however, pigs, cows, and lambs frequently incur streptococcal infections which cause varied neurological lesions including hydrocephalus. It is probable that infectious agents cause so-called congenital hydrocephalus, but this disorder should be called acquired hydrocephalus instead.[69]

So-called "normal pressure" hydrocephalus in man has received considerable attention in past years. This disorder, usually seen in older patients, is characterized by dementia, awkward movement, normal CSF pressure, and enlarged ventricles without cortical atrophy. Marked improvement in this disorder has been obtained with ventriculoatrial shunting.[32, 33, 74]

In an effort to explain the pathophysiological mechanisms of clinical hydrocephalus, including the "normal pressure" type, hydrocephalus has been experimentally produced by injecting kaolin, lampblack, hot paraffin, iodized oil, silicone in oil, or Silastic somewhere in the spaces occupied by CSF (usually the intraventricular[25, 32, 33] spaces). James and co-workers[32] produced chronic communicating hydrocephalus in dogs by injecting Silastic into the lumbar subarachnoid space. The progressive changes were seen by cisternography, isotope transfer determinations, CSF pressure measurements, radioautography, and light and electron microscopy. This study was stimulated by the dramatic relief afforded by surgical shunting of chronic communicating or normal pressure hydrocephalus in man.

Silastic-produced hydrocephalus develops very slowly, and there is no generalized meningeal and ependymal inflammatory response as long as ventricular circulation is maintained. When radiopharmaceuticals are injected into the lumbar subarachnoid space in normal subjects, the CSF flows over the brain convexities to the arachnoid villi and not into the ventricles. In patients with hydrocephalus, the material enters the ventricle (reversed flow) and remains there for 24 to 72 hours or longer. Before the occurrence of reversal flow and stasis, CSF pressure increases but then decreases when the flow of CSF changes and ventricular enlargement occurs. These facts remain unexplained.[32, 33]

Pathologically, loss of cilia and flattening of the normal cuboidal cells of the ependymal linings at the angles of the ventricles are among the first changes. Changes in the subependymal cells—so-called "rests"—soon follow. As the ventricles enlarge, changes in the periventricular cells occur. The normally loosely packed cells become compact, and an increase in nuclear density follows. Compression of the granule cells in the neuronal layers is present. In chronic hydrocephalus there is no effective ependymal barrier to movement of large labeled molecules. Loss of ependymal cells with frank tears and loss of cell junctions occurs. Myelinated fibers are sparsely distributed in the white matter, and acellular lakes representing edematous fluid appear. Perivascular edema is prevalent. The more severe the hydrocephalus, the more extensive the edema and the greater the "facilitated" diffusion. The pathological changes suggest that the transependymal movement is due to the loss of the ependymal barrier and separation between cells in the subependymal region. As edema increases, it may well create resistance to further ventricular enlargement, which leads to "compensation" by counter pressure from periventricular tissue.[33]

There were some clinical signs in these experimentally produced hydrocephalics. There was a progression from pelvic to pectoral limb motor involvement. The fibers that supply the lower limb course parallel to the ventricular surface, whereas those of the pectoral limbs enter the periventricular area at right angles. This arrangement may make the hind limb fibers more susceptible to ventricular pressures. Diversionary shunting in such cases in humans (and in canine communicating hydrocephalics) probably offers relief for many of the neurological signs by providing an efficient pathway for removal of CSF and thus lessening edema and ventricular enlargement.[33]

CLINICAL SIGNS

It has been stated previously that clinical hydrocephalus does not always fit the classic definitions. There is good evidence that hydrocephalus in the very young animal can be acquired and that congenital hydrocephalus may be present clinically without causing an enlarged calvarium, appearing later as a clinical entity.

In classic congenital hydrocephalus, clinical signs are apparent shortly after birth. The head is enlarged, the calvarium is prominent and rounded, and open fontanelles can be detected on palpation. Since the skull sutures are not ossified, the skull enlarges in proportion to the increased volume of fluid in the brain, so that the brain is less compressed than it would be otherwise. However, affected puppies may soon show depressed neurological activity, dullness, inactivity, stupidity, and locomotor weakness or incoordination. Occasionally, the puppy may become vicious, have convulsions, and whine continuously. Brain reflexes as well as spinal reflexes become abnormal. Percussion of the skull produces a tympanic sound like that of a ripe watermelon. Visual deficits, an outward-downward strabismus, resting nystagmus, abnormal muscle rigidity, spasms, pupillary dilatation, and intermittent clonus have also been observed in congenital cases.[11, 40]

Hydrocephalus occurring in mature animals does not present such characteristic clinical signs. If the ventricular dilation is unilateral, abnormal motor disturbances such as unilateral circling and falling and abnormal reflexes can be seen. The cause of such signs must be differentiated from other unilateral cerebral lesions. If the ventricular enlargement is generalized, weakness and more subtle motor deficits occur first in the rear limbs and progress to the front limbs, as mentioned earlier. Dullness, sleepiness, depressed mentality, and convulsive seizures are frequently encountered. A choked optic disk is seen occasionally in an ophthalmoscopic examination. In mild clinical cases there may be signs of head pain, irritability, and restlessness. A dog may hold his head low and rigid as if he were suffering from a cranial cervical compression such as disk protrusion or an atlantoaxial subluxation. One must conclude that acquired ventricular dropsy produces a great variety of clinical signs (Figs. 21–7 to 21–13).

DIAGNOSIS

Acquired hydrocephalus is characterized by the most varied and multiple clinical manifestations of all neurological disorders. In any neurological disturbance in small or miniature breeds, such as Boston terriers,

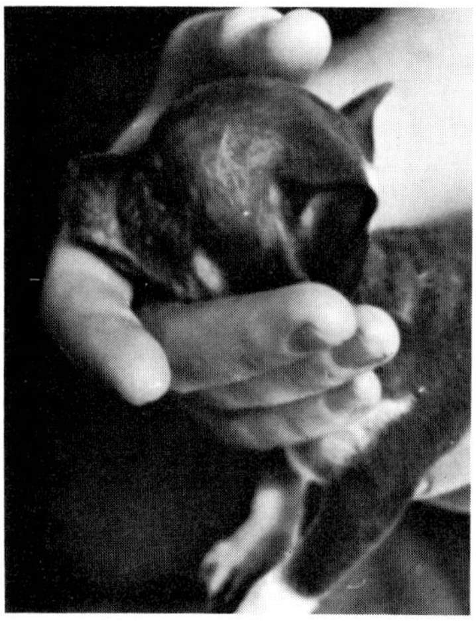

Fig. 21–7

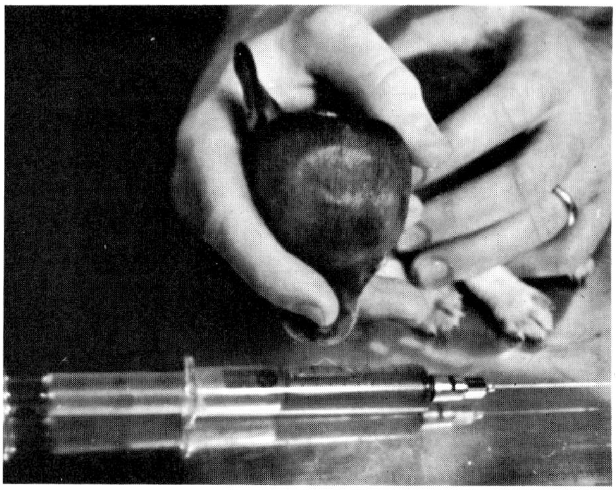

Fig. 21–8

FIGURE 21–7 A 3-month-old Chihuahua puppy has congenital ventricular dropsy. At this stage, the puppy showed signs of depression, dullness, and incoordination. Notice the enlarged head.

FIGURE 21–8 Ten milliliters of ventricular fluid was easily withdrawn through a fontanelle puncture. Notice the depression in the skin overlying the calvarial defect.

Chihuahuas, Pekingese, Yorkshire terriers, miniature schnauzers, toy poodles, and Manchester terriers, one should always consider the possibility of hydrocephalus. A detailed history frequently shows a slowly developing pattern of neurological signs, starting with head pain, mild changes in behavior, listlessness, and weakness in the hind limbs. Frequently a slight stress or trauma causes an acute neurological motor deficit, a state of depressed consciousness, or even seizures. In susceptible breeds, a fall from bed or a disease may precipitate a neurological syndrome with several of these clinical signs.

The neurological examination should be detailed and complete, especially in regard to traumatic skull or spinal injuries that cause compressive disease, infectious diseases, and neoplasia. Occasionally the ocular fundic examination reveals a choked or edematous optic disk, which could point

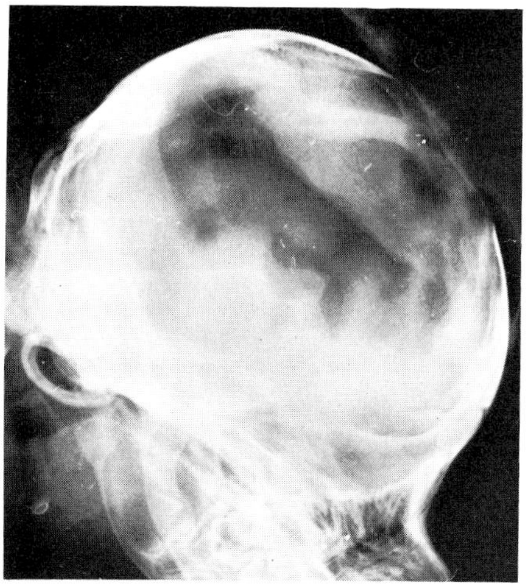

Fig. 21–9

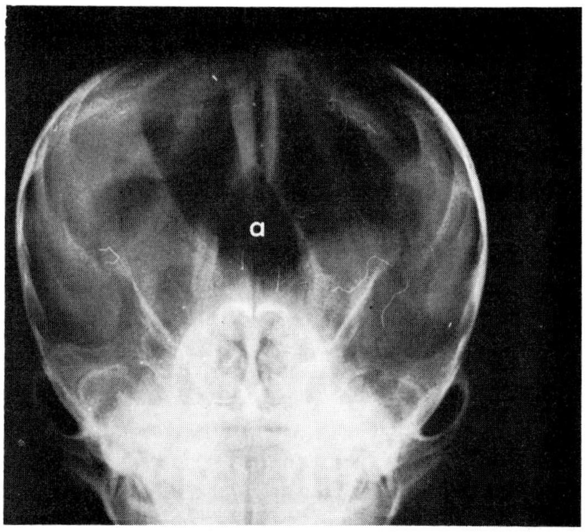

Fig. 21–10

FIGURE 21–9 Same case as shown in Figure 21–7. Air was injected into the lateral ventricle after withdrawal of fluid. Air can be seen in the ventricles as well as in the subarachnoid space.

FIGURE 21–10 Same case as shown in Figure 21–7, frontal view. This view demonstrates a communicating hydrocephalus between the lateral ventricles (a).

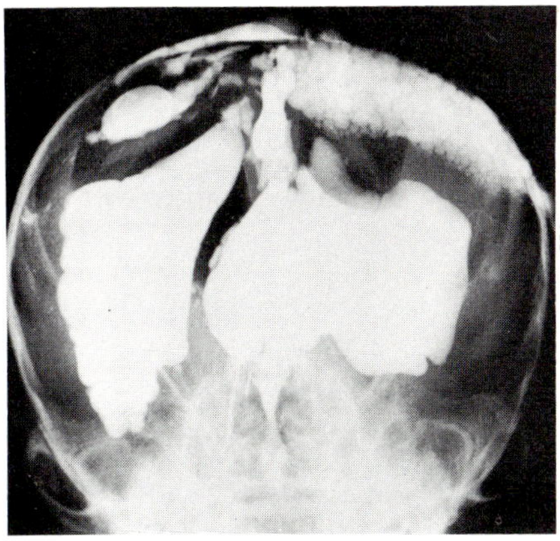

Fig. 21-11

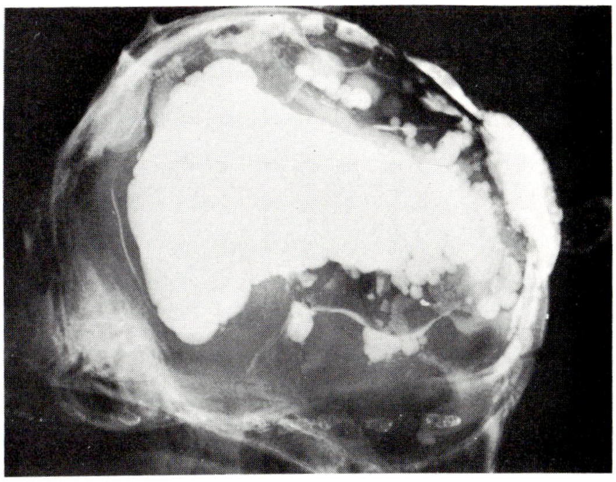

Fig. 21-12

FIGURE 21-11 Same case as shown in Figure 21-7. Pantopaque was injected into the lateral ventricles a few days later.

FIGURE 21-12 Same case as shown in Figure 21-7, lateral view.

toward a diagnosis of hydrocephalus. At the Auburn clinic, the sequence of special tests includes an EEG examination followed by a radiographic examination. If EEG is not available, flat film radiography is the recommended procedure.

Accurate interpretation of the electroencephalogram is a superb aid in the diagnosis of acquired hydrocephalus, since the neurological signs are so diversified. Large group practices find this equipment a necessity, not only for this disorder but also for other cerebral diseases. These recordings reveal high amplitude (25–200 mV) slow waves (1–5 Hz) on which often a fast frequency of 10 to 12 Hz is superimposed. Many EEG tracings in patients with hydrocephalus are so characteristic that if there is no indication of infectious, compressive, or neoplastic diseases, no further laboratory or radiographic procedures are necessary at this time. Medication is prescribed on an outpatient basis or, in severe cases, hospitalization is recommended (Fig. 21-14).[54, 57]

When EEG recordings are questionable or when other disorders are suspected from a physical examination, flat film radiography is performed, using an appropriate chemical restraint unless the animal is unusually docile or comatose. Lateral, ventrodorsal, right angle anteroposterior (AP), open mouth, and oblique AP views are usually taken according to the methods most suitable for showing brain densities, the ventricles, and the size of the foramen magnum. The radiographs should include at least the cranial cervical vertebrae. Open fontanelles and cranial sutures may persist after the normal age for closure, and a homogeneous "ground glass" appearance of the cerebrum is evidence of cerebral convolutional atrophy and an abnormally large area of fluid density. Occasional cortical thinning can be seen in advanced cases.

In most cases, the significant changes noted in the EEG and radiographic examinations constitute a confirmative diagnosis. If these examinations are not conclusive, the CSF pressure and volume may be measured, and the spinal fluid may be examined by ventricular tap. If the fontanelles are open, surgical preparation of the site

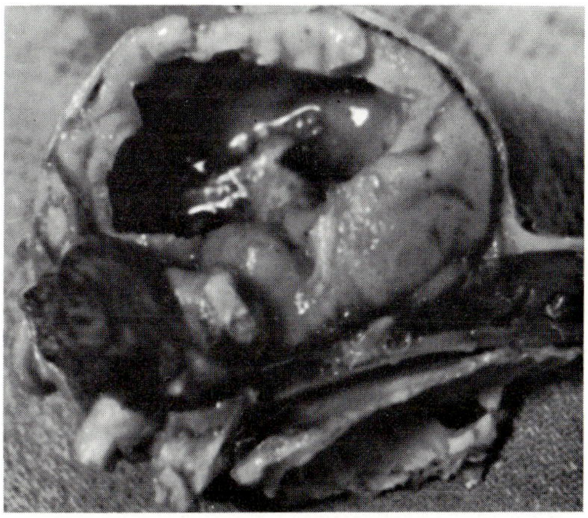

FIGURE 21-13 Same case as shown in Figures 21-7 to 21-12, necropsy specimen. Notice the large communication between the lateral ventricles and the absence of cerebral brain tissue.

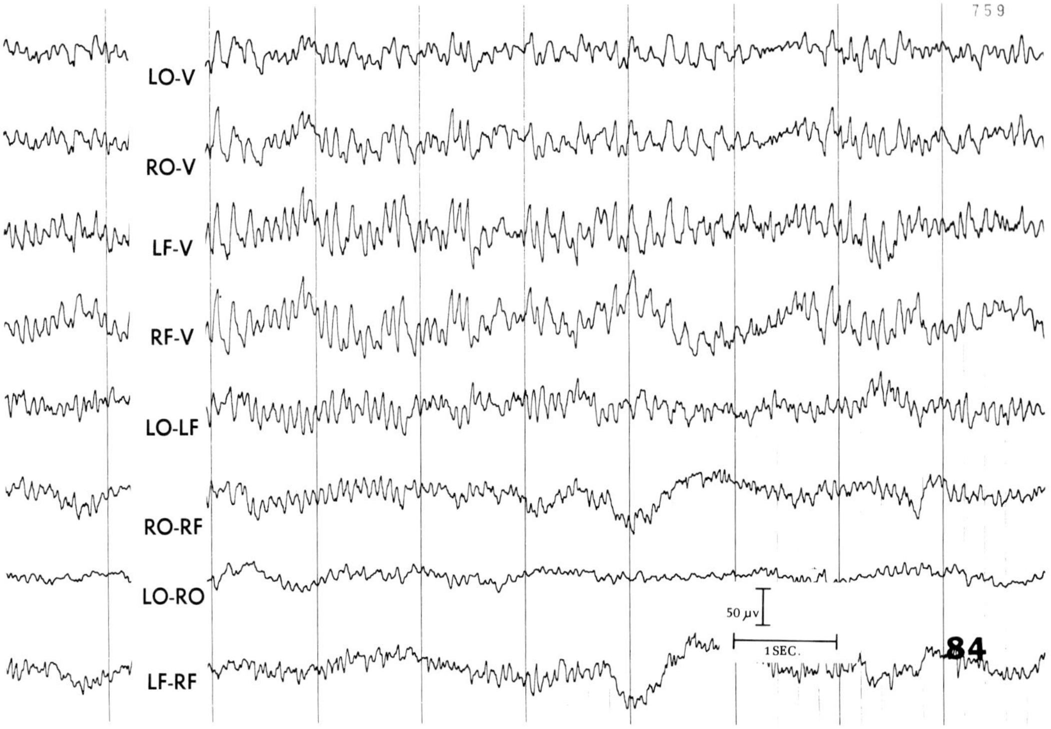

A

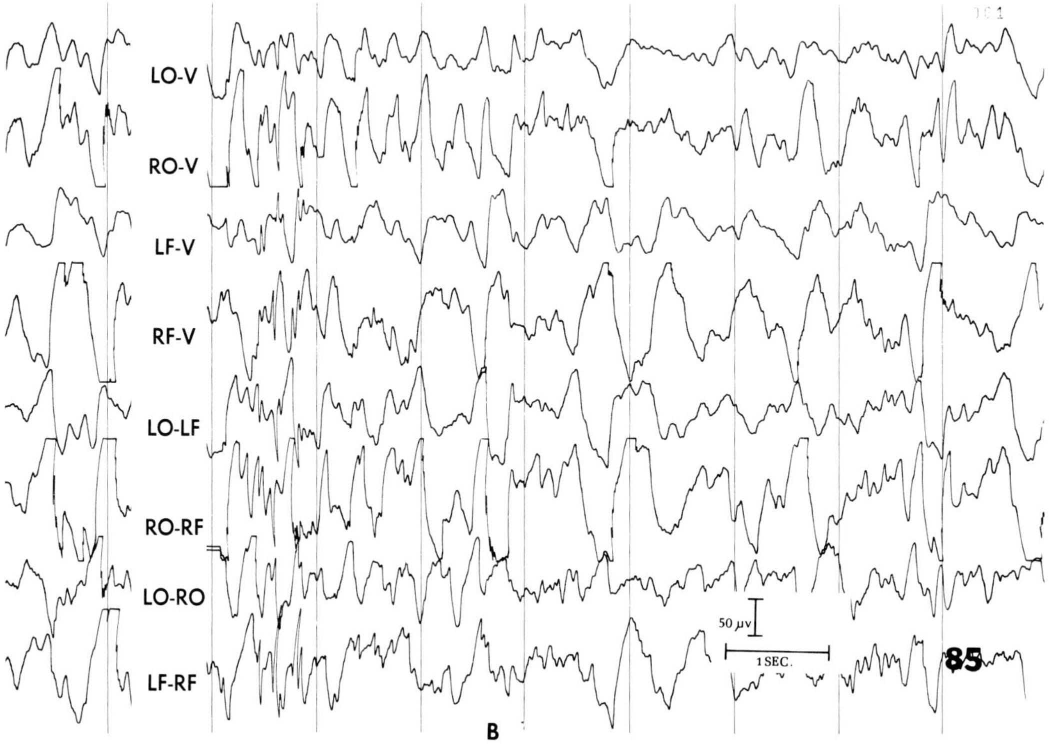

B

FIGURE 21–14 *A*. EEG pattern characteristically seen in hydrocephalus. This tracing displays activity of 6 to 15 Hz, 25 to 70 microvolts, which is hypersynchronous in leads common to the vertex lead. *B*. This pattern is also characteristic of hydrocephalus with 2 to 4 Hz and some overriding higher frequencies; 50 to 150 microvolts is hypersynchronous but is not as evident as the pattern in *A*.

and ventricular introduction of a small gauge injection needle can be accomplished easily and safely. In normal small dogs (less than 10 pounds), very little CSF is present on the tap—perhaps 0.1 ml to not more than 1 ml. The fluid should be allowed to drip into a vial under its own pressure. Marked negative pressure on a syringe plunger would collapse the ventricle and result in hemorrhage and injury to the brain (or it might cause quick death). If abnormal amounts (0.5 to 2 ml, depending on the size of the dog) of CSF are collected from patients with neurological signs, there is a good chance that hydrocephalus is present. If there are no open fontanelles ventricular taps can be easily made, as described in Chapters 5 and 6. In such a case a ventriculogram may also be made, since anesthesia and more extensive surgical invasion are necessary (Fig. 21–15)[28, 29, 51] (see Chapter 5). Pressure readings can be obtained from ventricular taps if desired but they are usually obtained from spinal taps. Observations of greater availability of fluid and increased flow rate are at least clinical evidence of hydrocephalus. Cerebrospinal fluid should be examined for evidence of neoplastic or inflammatory disease (Chapter 6). Culture of fluid should be performed when indicated.[63]

In man, cisternography is a relatively safe, effective, and convenient method of diagnosing acquired hydrocephalus when physical signs are not as apparent as in the congenitally enlarged skull. The scan sequence of CSF flow and the comparative ventricular size are diagnostic. This equipment is costly and is currently available only to institutional or institutionally affiliated practices. Uptake by blood of radioactive isotopes injected into spaces occupied by CSF can be used as an aid in diagnosing hydrocephalus, but this method is not widely used in clinical practice.

In our practice, cisternal or lumbar spinal taps are performed infrequently as a diagnostic procedure in patients with acquired hydrocephalus. When they are performed, the CSF pressure is recorded. In the obstructive type of hydrocephalus, the availability and pressure of CSF are depressed; after removal of 1 to 2 ml of fluid, a very slow or incomplete recovery to the original pressure is seen. In communicating hydrocephalus, on the other hand, a high

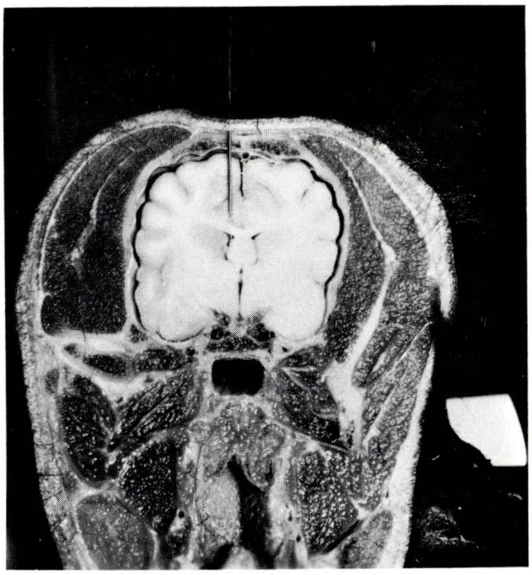

FIGURE 21–15 The site of ventricular puncture is approximately 1 cm from the midline, 2 to 3 cm deep, and midway between the lateral canthus of the eye and the occipital protuberance.

pressure reading and rapid recovery is characteristic after removal of an aliquot of CSF. A sudden release of high CSF pressure and large quantities of CSF in patients with large space-occupying masses in the cranial cavity will cause herniation of the tentorium or foramen magnum and may result in sudden death. Great care should be exercised in performing cisternal taps in patients with severe depression of CSF, since anesthesia is dangerous, careless manipulation of the needle can cause damage to the cord, and sudden release of CSF can cause respiratory and circulatory collapse.

General hematologic and pathologic tests may be helpful in diagnosing disorders causing neurological signs (Figs. 21–16 to 21–19).

TREATMENT

Medical Treatment

The treatment of hydrocephalus has been primarily surgical. It has been reported that cisternal or ventricular tap, or both, and use of dehydrating agents or diuretics may promote relief in clinical hydrocephalus. It is possible that temporary removal of fluid will allow a rearrangement of the system of drainage so that a deformity may be corrected. It has been shown

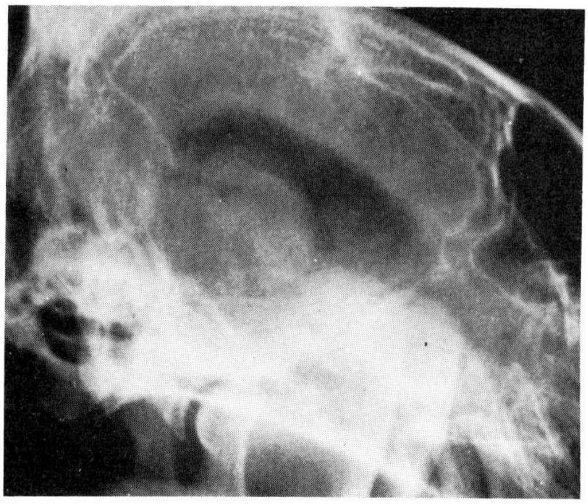

Fig. 21–16

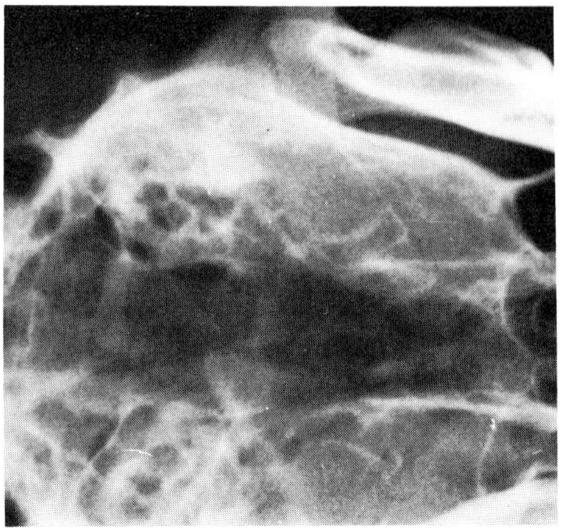

Fig. 21–17

FIGURE 21–16 Pneumoventriculogram showing the lateral view of a normal ventricle.
FIGURE 21–17 Same case as shown in Figure 21–16, VD view. Notice that the lateral ventricles are poorly defined.

that in the dog, a considerable amount of CSF may leak into the nasal submucosal space, local lymphatics, and the nasal cavity itself.[12] Therefore, some cases of hydrocephalus may be stabilized by enhancing this type of flow mechanism. Also, removal of cellular debris that may have been drained off by tapping may promote normal absorption. Usually, cisternal or ventricular tap and drainage plus the use of hypertonic or dehydrating solutions will promote temporary relief but will not provide a permanent cure. The therapeutic use of vitamins should always be employed, and excellent general nutrition should be maintained.

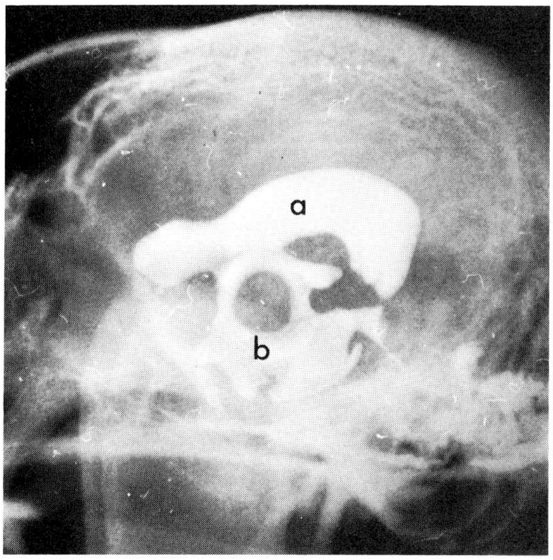

FIGURE 21–18 Same case as shown in Figure 21–16. Pantopaque ventriculogram taken 3 weeks later. Notice the definition in the lateral (a) and third (b) ventricles.

One agent that has been shown to decrease CSF pressure is acetazolamide (Diamox), which decreases the total amount of CSF by inhibiting the activity of carbonic anhydrase and secondarily alters ion ratios and fluid production. Mannitol and urea solutions administered intravenously have been used extensively to relieve cerebral edema and to reduce intracranial pressure and brain volume. Leonard[37] demonstrated that both solutions at 25 to 30 per cent concentrations produced immediate and profound reduction in CSF pressures when given at a rate of 1.5 gm/kg body weight. The reduced pressure lasted an average of 1.5 hours.[37] Hypertonic solutions afford temporary relief in an acute attack of clinical hydrocephalus. Other agents such as isosorbide (Hydronal) (2.5–3 mg/kg every 6 to 12 hours) have been used for short-term administration in man.

It has been shown that calves with chronic hypervitaminosis A have a marked decrease in CSF pressure. Light and electron microscopic examination revealed that the arachnoid granulations were reduced to two-thirds their normal size, and the height of the epithelial cells of the lateral and third ventricular plexuses decreased significantly.[23] Possibly avitaminosis A might also influence the formation of hydrocephalus.

Glucocorticosteroids have been used extensively in the control of traumatic inflam-

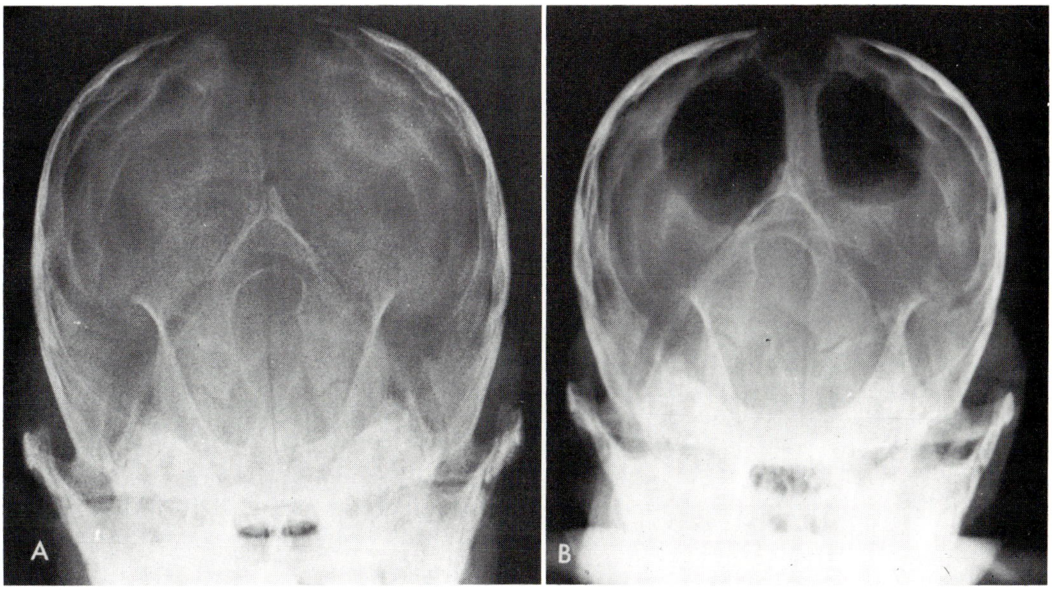

Figure 21–19 *A.* Anteroposterior view of a hydrocephalic. *B.* Anteroposterior pneumoventriculogram. Notice the enlarged ventricles.

mation in the CNS, to "shrink" brain tissue, and lower CSF pressure. Sato studied the effect of intravenous administration of dexamethasone on CSF production in dogs using a method of caudocephalad perfusion of the spinal subarachnoid space with an insulin-containing buffer. The CSF production rate began to decline immediately after the injection of 0.15 mg/kg dexamethasone and attained a maximal reduction of 50 per cent in 50 minutes. The data presented by Sato showed that a profound reduction in the production of CSF was maintained 130 minutes after administration. However, his observations on the duration of therapeutic action were not conclusive because of the methods used. The precise method of action of steroids on CSF production also remains a mystery.[62]

It has been observed that some patients with initially normal intracranial pressure have developed intracranial hypertension after prolonged steroid therapy. In an effort to explain this, Johnston and coworkers studied the effects on dogs of CSF absorption when steroids were chronically administered and then suddenly withdrawn. It was found that steroid withdrawal was associated with marked reduction in CSF absorption and an increase in resistance to CSF flow. Dogs on steroids also showed reduced CSF absorption, although the reduction was not significant statistically.[34]

Many questions about the effect of steroids on the production and absorption of CSF remain unanswered. Johnston[34] concluded that their work substantiated the premise that steroids affect primarily brain bulk and CSF production and not CSF absorption. Since the future control of hydrocephalus probably lies in the use of medications and other control methods rather than surgical treatments, the long-range effect of a below normal or "scanty" amount of CSF on the neurological and mental activity of the CNS might be considered. Scientific research will eventually answer many of these medical mysteries.

The effect of glucocorticosteroids on CSF pressure has led to more emphasis on the nonsurgical control of hydrocephalus in dogs. Harrison[26] has promoted the clinical use of steroids as a mode of therapy in hydrocephalus, and many clinicians have found that surgical shunts are needed much less frequently. The initial nonsurgical treatment consists of slowly removing excess CSF by means of a ventricular tap, through an open fontanelle if possible. This fluid should be allowed to drip slowly from the needle hub, since suction by syringe will promote ventricular collapse, cerebral hemorrhage, and demise of the patient. A ventricular tap frequently stabilizes the clinical status of a hydrocephalic for several weeks to months.

Harrison[26] subsequently administers dexamethasone 0.25 mg per 5 kg (11 lb) body weight twice daily. If signs stabilize, the dose is reduced by one-half after 7 days. If the clinical signs have largely disappeared—that is, those which developed at the last acute episode—the medication is discontinued after 3 weeks of the reduced dosage schedule. Generally, clinical signs are relieved early (1 to 3 days) in the treatment schedule.

If several exacerbations have occurred upon cessation of treatment, continuous therapy may be necessary. In such cases, Harrison suggests that medication be given only in the morning and that the patient be monitored for signs of Cushing's disease every 2 to 4 months. Usually ACTH should be given by the end of 6 months of steroid therapy. In some patients, steroids can be discontinued during ACTH therapy, while in others, clinical signs of hydrocephalus will appear in a few days if oral steroids are not administered. The recommended dose of ACTH gel is 20 units per 5 kg once or twice a week for 1 month, given in the late evening hours.[26]

Harrison has treated 118 cases of hydrocephalus and has estimated that the results in 60 per cent of these cases are very favorable. In puppies less than 8 weeks of age, the results are poor, but in patients aged 3 months or older the success ratio climbs. In general, the older the dog, the better the results. Animals respond equally when motor or seizure signs predominate; however, minor motor deficits frequently persist. Oral dexamethasone is used, since depression occurs frequently after initial intramuscular injections of the drug.[26]

Swaim's modified dosage regimen for a 2½ kg dog (5 lb) is a 0.25-mg dexamethasone tablet orally twice daily for 4 days, three-fourths tablet twice a day for 4 days, one-half tablet twice a day for 4 days, and one-fourth tablet for 1 to 3 weeks. Medication then ceases until the dog has a recurrence. If given, iurosemide could be started at 2 to 4 mg/kg two or three times daily as needed; the dose is decreased over a 1 to 2 week period. Anticonvulsants are occasionally given for more complete control of seizures.[67]

Surgical Treatment

Various surgical procedures have been used to relieve hydrocephalus. In communicating hydrocephalus, many procedures to direct CSF into suitable channels or locations for absorption have been evaluated. Tubes and cannulae have been used from the ventricles into the subarachnoid space, under the pericranium, and to the longitudinal sinus, the jugular vein, the pleural cavity, the middle ear, and the epidural space. The CSF from the spinal subarachnoid space has been shunted to the peritoneum, the retroperitoneum, the intestine, the kidney, the pelvis, and the ureter. Interventriculostomy and choroid plexectomy have been performed.[2, 9, 14, 17, 20, 25, 27, 45, 50, 53, 55, 56, 59, 64]

Ventriculoatrial Shunt

Since the brain of the dog is relatively small when compared to that of man, surgical shunts are the simplest and most effective means of surgical correction. The usual shunts currently used in humans consist of a catheter placed in a CSF space above the block, extending to a CSF area immediately below the blockage or to the cervical CSF space; to a body cavity from which the fluid is readily absorbed, as in pleural and peritoneal shunts; to the blood stream itself with an appropriate intervening valve system, as in atrial shunts; or to the urinary bladder for complete elimination from the body. Each method has advantages in certain cases and each has frequent complications.[74] According to the voluminous literature concerning complications of surgical shunting in man, there is a 30 to 75 per cent rate of revision of the apparatus and a fairly high incidence (30 to 50 per cent) of eventual failure.[30] In spite of these statistics, surgical shunting is the procedure of choice in man for long-term control of hydrocephalus.

In veterinary medicine, ventriculoatrial shunts using the Holter and, more recently, the Denver valve have been selectively performed since the first surgery by Few[17] in 1961 (Fig. 21–20). More recently, a few surgeons have been using the ventriculoperitoneal shunt procedure on selected cases. Each method has its advantages. The atrial shunt procedure will be described in

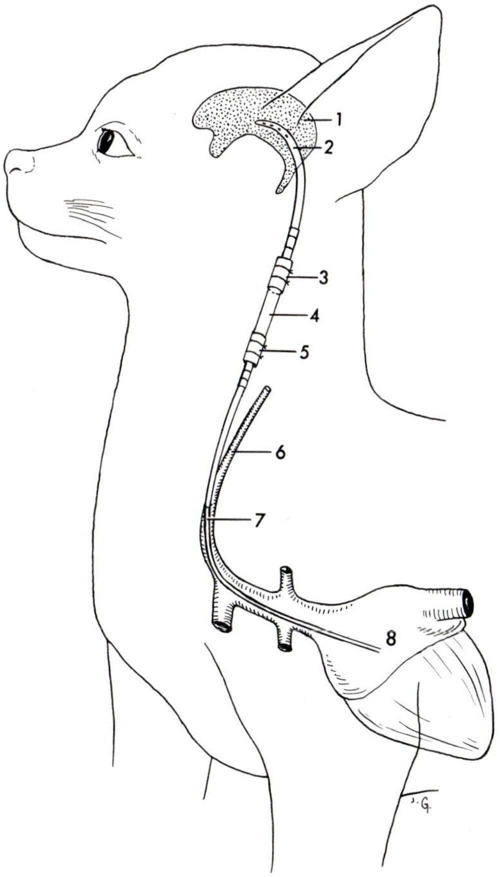

FIGURE 21–20 A sketch showing a ventriculoatrial shunt. (1) Lateral ventricle; (2) ventricular catheter made of siliconized rubber; (3) proximal Holter one-way valve; (4) intermediate silicone rubber tube that can be manipulated by hand to stimulate CSF flow in case of temporary occlusion of system; (5) distal Holter one-way valve; (6) jugular vein; (7) venous catheter ligated in place in the jugular vein over a connector apparatus so as not to diminish lumen of tube; (8) right atrium.

detail, and then the differences in the peritoneal shunt will be discussed. Although the ventriculoatrial shunt is perhaps the simplest of neurosurgical techniques, success will depend on several primary considerations.[17, 20, 27, 50] Many of these have been emphasized in previous chapters.

Adherence to strict asepsis in all details is again a necessity for this procedure. Perhaps the most pressing problem is proper anesthesia. Since many hydrocephalics are neurologically depressed or even comatose, little anesthesia is necessary. Methoxyflurone (Metofane) or halothane (Fluothane) in an oxygen mixture administered in a closed or semiclosed system should be standard. An ultrashort barbiturate (Pentothal) can be very carefully administered for induction in order to properly pass an endotracheal tube. However, induction with gaseous anesthesia (mask) and a local anesthetic applied to the epiglottis and laryngeal aperture are generally safer in critically ill patients. The level of anesthesia and the assessment of vital functions should be monitored very carefully throughout the entire procedure, as suggested in Chapter 8. Presurgical medication with atropine and broad spectrum antibiotics is routine, and preoperative administration of adrenal corticosteroids may be desirable in critical patients.

The positioning of the patient is also an important consideration. As was emphasized previously, cranial surgery should generally be performed with the head elevated in order to limit cerebral congestion, edema, and swelling. In this procedure, the head is placed on a moderately large cushion and occasionally the table is tilted slightly also to promote elevation of the head. The dog should be placed in the lateral recumbent position with the head rotated slightly toward an oblique lateroventral position. Site preparation should include all of the calvarium and the entire

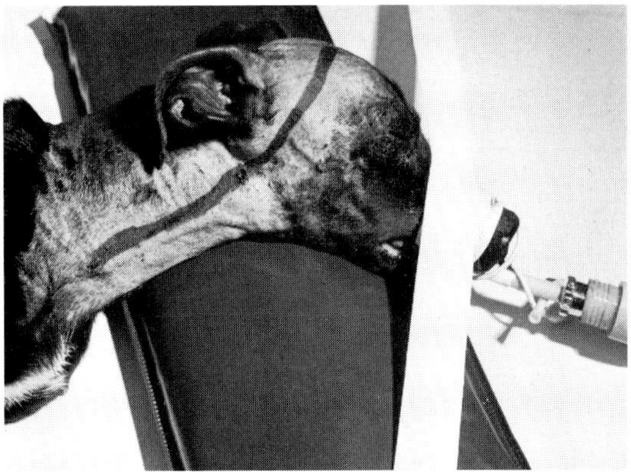

FIGURE 21–21 Dog in proper position for surgery, with proposed incision line marked by the solid line. (From Gage, E. D., and Hoerlein, B. F.: Surgical treatment of canine hydrocephalus by ventriculoatrial shunting. J.A.V.M.A. *153*:1423, 1968.)

lateroventral cervical area, terminating on the chest at least 6 cm caudal to the thoracic inlet (Fig. 21–21).

The skin incision starts on the calvarial midline and courses posteroventrally in front of the ear and along the jugular furrow to a site somewhat beyond the thoracic inlet. The subcutaneous tissues are routinely severed and retracted. The temporal muscle is incised 2 to 4 mm from its dorsal attachment and bluntly dissected from the dorsolateral skull. A hole is made in the skull about 2 to 4 cm from the midline at a point halfway between the widest part of the zygomatic arch and the occipital protuberance. This hole can be made with a highspeed bur, a hand bur, a trephine, or an intramedullary pin. Much care should be employed in young animals, as the bone may be extremely thin. The hole may be enlarged and shaped with a small rongeur in order to facilitate a nonrestrictive opening for the ventricular catheter. This catheter (radiopaque silicone) has an outside diameter of 2.5 mm.

The lateral ventricle is carefully located with a 22-gauge spinal needle. The depth of the ventricle will depend on the degree of ventricular distention. The needle is removed, the depth needed for free flow of fluid is observed, and the dura is carefully incised so as to facilitate the passage of the proximal catheter. When a clear, free flow of fluid is obtained from the proximal catheter, it is ligated or clamped in order to prevent a marked or rapid loss of CSF. Excessive removal of fluid is dangerous to the patient and might promote a subdural hematoma. Blood, debris, and other material might obstruct the valve; therefore, occasional irrigation of the ventricle with warm saline may be necessary in order to remove such material (Figs. 21–22 to 21–24).

The distal end of the ventricular catheter is placed through a stab incision in the thickened ventral portion of the reflected temporal muscle. This incision is considerably more ventral than the cranial opening for the ventricular end of the catheter, so that the catheter will lie for some distance

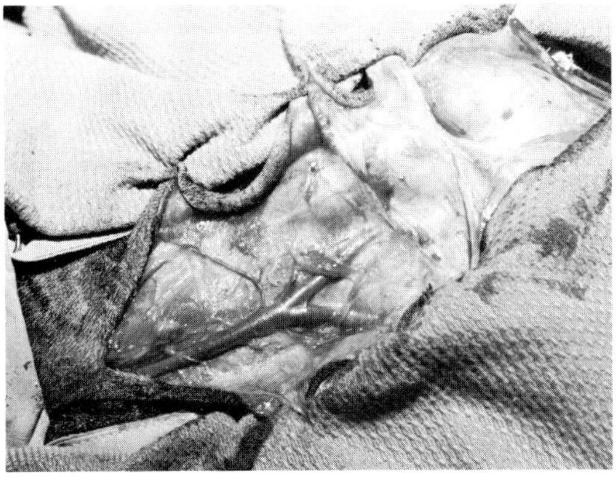

FIGURE 21–22 Exposure of cranial musculature and jugular vein prior to surgical implantation of the shunt system. (From Gage, E. D., and Hoerlein, B. F.: Surgical treatment of canine hydrocephalus by ventriculoatrial shunting. J.A.V.M.A. *153*:1423, 1968.)

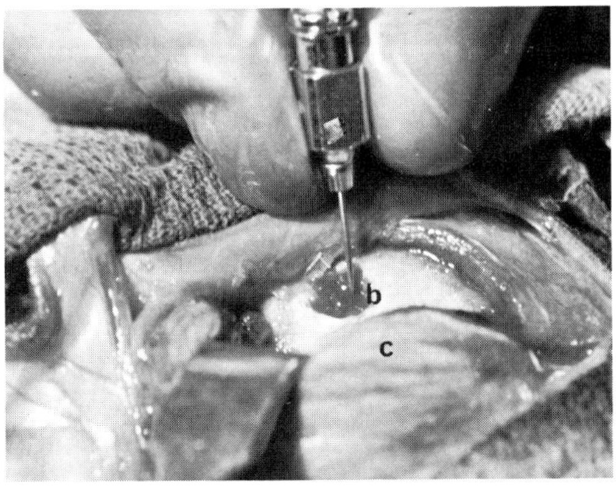

FIGURE 21–23 Tapping of the lateral ventricles with a 22-gauge spinal needle. (b) Opening in the skull: (c) retracted temporal muscle. (From Gage, E. D., and Hoerlein, B. F.: Surgical treatment of canine hydrocephalus by ventriculoatrial shunting. J.A.V.M.A. *153*: 1423, 1968.)

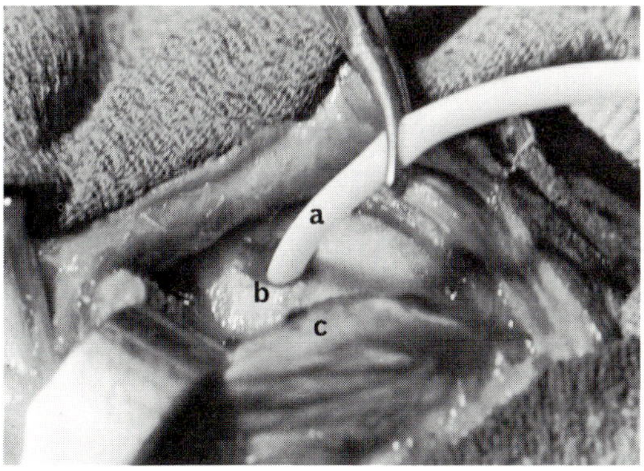

FIGURE 21–24 Insertion of ventricular catheter into the lateral ventricles. (a) ventricular catheter; (b) opening in the skull; (c) retracted temporal muscle. (From Gage, E. D., and Hoerlein, B. F.: Surgical treatment of canine hydrocephalus by ventriculoatrial shunting. J.A.V.M.A. *153*:1423, 1968.)

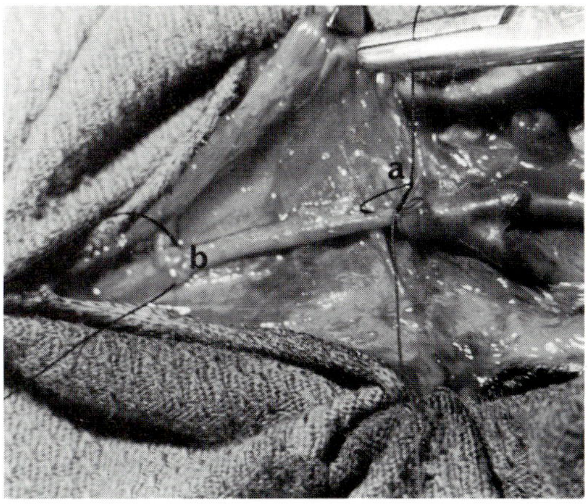

FIGURE 21–26 Isolation and ligation of the jugular vein. Ligature is tied just below bifurcation (a) and is held taut to prevent back flow of blood (b). (From Gage, E. D., and Hoerlein, B. F.: Surgical treatment of canine hydrocephalus by ventriculoatrial shunting. J.A.V.M.A. *153*:1423, 1968.)

along the skull in a stationary but unrestricted fashion. The temporal muscle is resutured to its dorsal attachment with 2-0 medium chromic catgut. It is felt that this procedure will allow for stable placement of the catheter and will discourage subsequent malpositioning (Fig. 21–25).

The jugular vein is isolated and permanently ligated below its bifurcation from the internal and external maxillary branches. An incision in the jugular vein is made and three 6–0 silk stay sutures are placed in the opening to facilitate passage of the distal siliconized catheter (outside diameter is 1.3 mm). If back flow of blood is occurring, a bulldog clamp or taut suture can be placed temporarily on the jugular vein posterior to the opening. The proper length for the distal catheter is estimated by measuring from a previously taken lateral thoracic and cervical radiograph. The catheter should extend into the mid-atrium for optimal performance (Figs. 21–26 to 21–28).

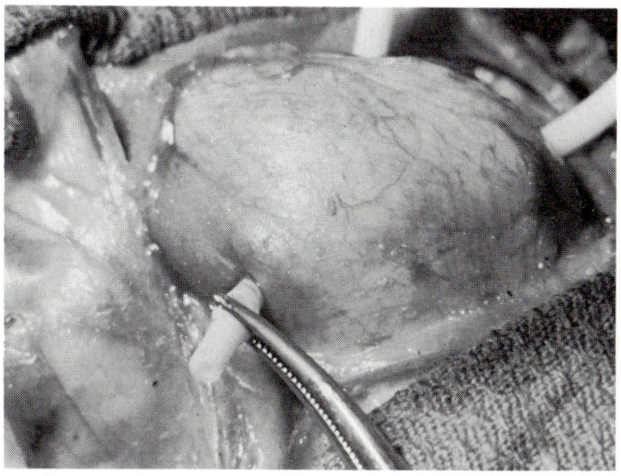

FIGURE 21–25 Placing the ventricular catheter under the temporal muscle for added stability. (From Gage, E. D., and Hoerlein, B. F.: Surgical treatment of canine hydrocephalus by ventriculoatrial shunting. J.A.V.M.A. *153*:1423, 1968.)

The end of the distal catheter is beveled at a 45-degree angle and lubricated with a sterile saline-heparin solution to promote venous catheterization. Care should be taken not to leave a sharp point on the bevel, for the vessel may be lacerated or the passage may be difficult. An area of apparent constriction is frequently encountered at the thoracic inlet and can be overcome by direct manipulation of the vein within the operative area. A special stylet placed inside the catheter will also aid in its passage. After the calculated length has been passed, another radiograph should be taken to determine proper atrial position. If the catheter tip is still in the terminal jugular vein, it may cause fibrinous occlusion. If it has been inserted into the cardiac ventricle, ventricular fibrillation or cardiac insufficiency due to mechanical interference with the AV valves may occur.

After proper placement has been established, the catheter is prepared for permanent fixation in the vein. Since the catheter

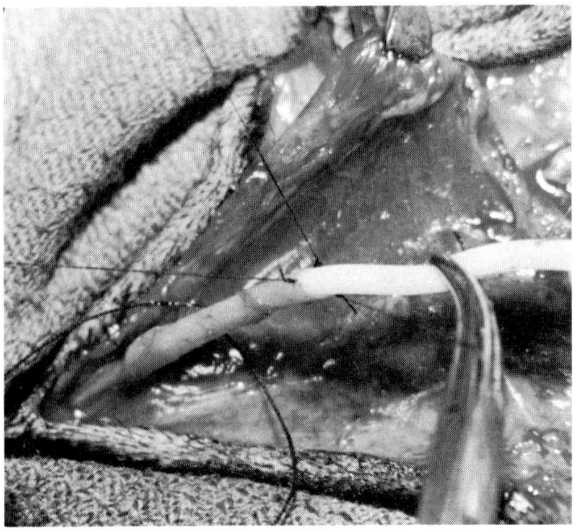

FIGURE 21–27 Catheterization of the atrium through the jugular vein. Notice the use of stay sutures. (From Gage, E. D., and Hoerlein, B. F.: Surgical treatment of canine hydrocephalus by ventriculoatrial shunting. J.A.V. M.A. *153*:1423, 1968.)

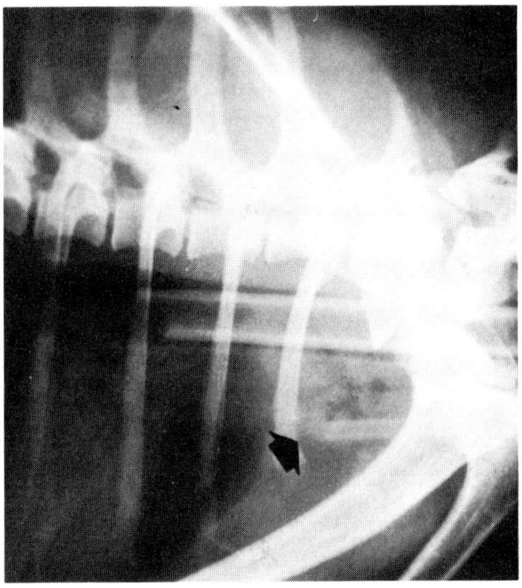

FIGURE 21–28 Radiograph taken during surgery indicating that the atrial catheter (arrow) needs to be inserted farther to reach the right atrium. (From Gage, E. D., and Hoerlein, B. F.: Surgical treatment of canine hydrocephalus by ventriculoatrial shunting. J.A.V. M.A. *153*:1423, 1968.)

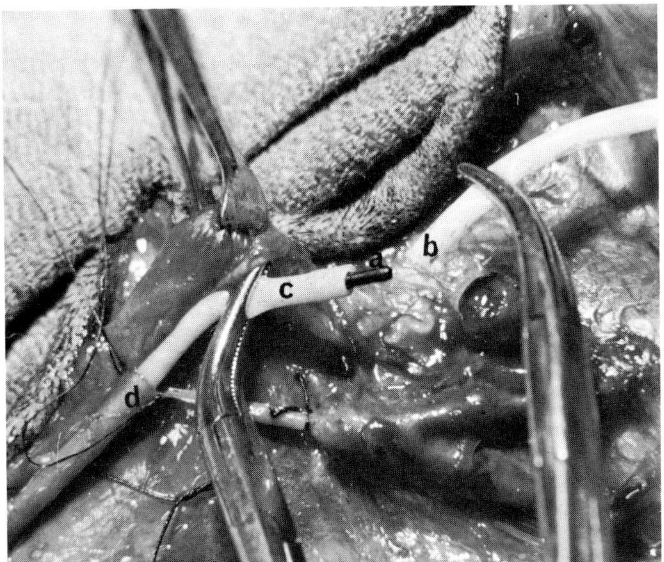

FIGURE 21–29 Placement of connector to allow ligation of jugular vein upon catheter. (a) Connector; (b) proximal segment of atrial catheter; (c) segment of atrial catheter already inside jugular vein; (d) catheterized jugular vein. (From Gage, E. D., and Hoerlein, B. F.: Surgical treatment of canine hydrocephalus by ventriculoatrial shunting. J.A.V.M.A. *153*:1423, 1968.)

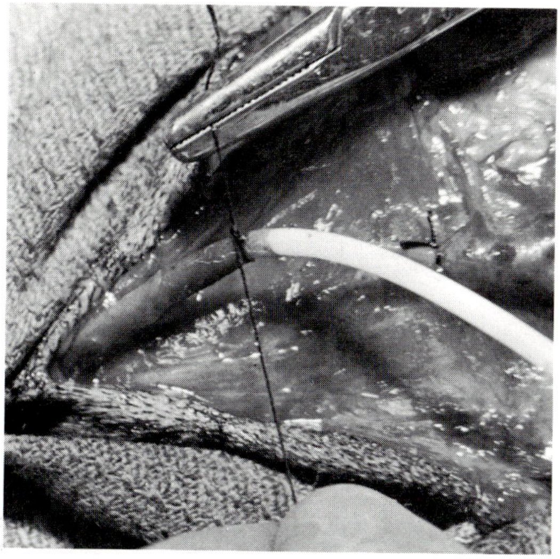

FIGURE 21–30 Ligation of the jugular vein over the connector and catheter. (From Gage, E. D., and Hoerlein, B. F.: Surgical treatment of canine hydrocephalus by ventriculoatrial shunting. J.A.V.M.A. *153*: 1423, 1968.)

is soft and flexible, direct ligation of it in the vein would promote constriction. Therefore, a metal adapter is inserted into cut segments of the catheter, and the segments are secured by ligating the adapter with 3–0 monofilament, nonabsorbable material such as nylon. The adapter is reinserted into the jugular vein and securely positioned by means of another 3–0 perivas-

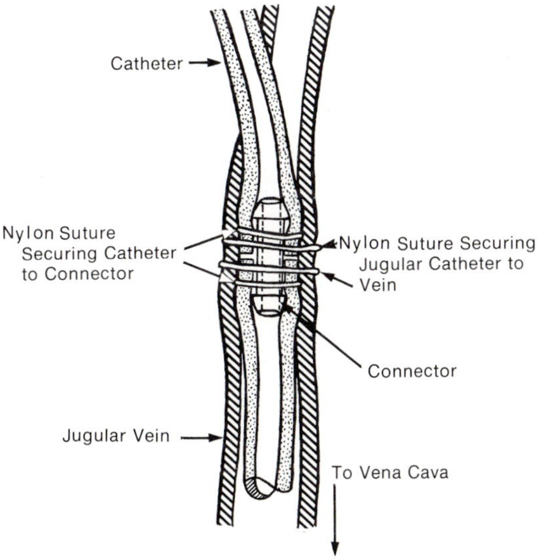

FIGURE 21–31 Drawing showing technique and position of the connector and catheter inside the jugular vein. (From Gage, E. D., and Hoerlein, B. F.: Surgical treatment of canine hydrocephalus by ventriculoatrial shunting. J.A.V.M.A. *153*:1423, 1968.)

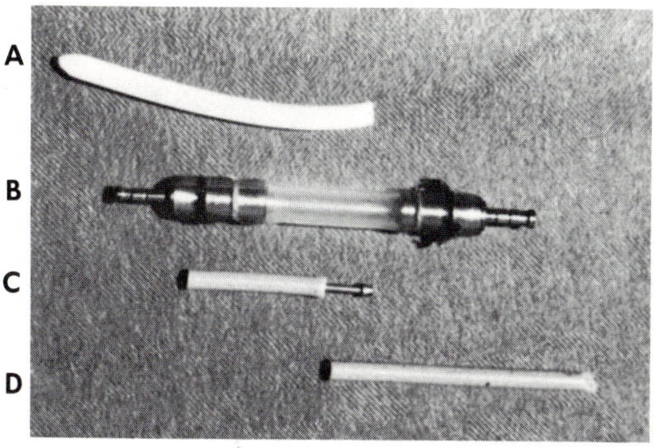

FIGURE 21–32 The two-valve Holter assembly: (A) Ventricular catheter that fits on an adapter; (B) the proximal and distal one-way valves with an intermediate silicone tube, which is designed for subcutaneous manipulation if necessary to maintain flow; (C) connector of catheter segments inside the jugular vein to provide secure positioning and ligation to the vein; (D) atrial catheter.

cular ligation. A sterile saline-heparin solution has been used to flush the distal catheter periodically during these manipulations. After a final flush, the distal catheter is clamped to prevent back flow (Figs. 21–29 to 21–31). A telescopic ventriculoatrial shunt that elongates longitudinally with growth of the child has recently been reported. This has proved successful in 15 of 18 cases during the observation period of 1 to 4 years.[72]

The unidirectional valves we have used are the Holter and Denver valves. The Holter valve is currently made in two parts with an intermediate flexible tube that can be massaged to promote flow if a temporary minor occlusion has occurred or if the system is not draining at an adequate rate. The valve is connected to the open ventricular catheter, and when clear CSF is flowing freely, it is secured to the unclamped venous catheter. The entire apparatus is anchored by appropriately suturing adjacent subcutaneous tissues around it. The skin incision is closed in a contour fashion. The operative area is generally bandaged (Figs. 21–32 to 21–38). Postoperative care should include the administration of antibiotics (chloromycetin), corticosteroids, and vitamins and intensive nursing care. Some cases will necessitate hand-feeding and fluid administrations for a few days. Restricted exercise for 3 to 6 days postsurgically is recommended if the dog is active. Epiphora is an occasional postoperative sequela, but it usually subsides in

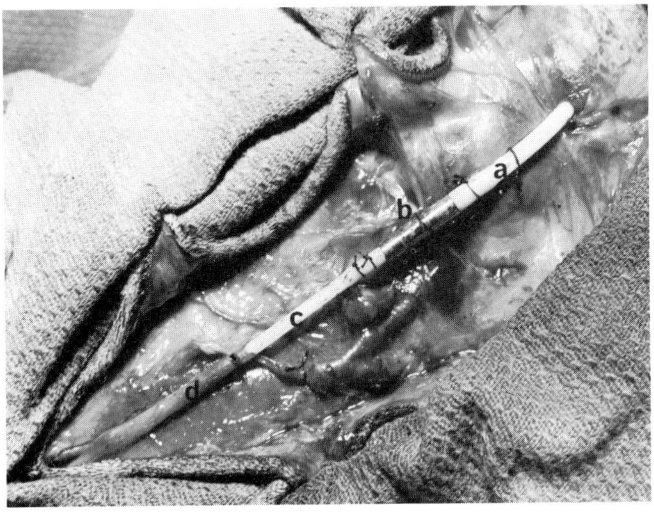

FIGURE 21–33 The Holter ventriculoatrial shunt completed and ready for closure of the wound. (a) Ventricular catheter; (b) Holter valve; (c) atrial catheter; (d) jugular vein. (From Gage, E. D., and Hoerlein, B. F.: Surgical treatment of canine hydrocephalus by ventriculoatrial shunting. J.A.V.M.A. *153*:1423, 1968.)

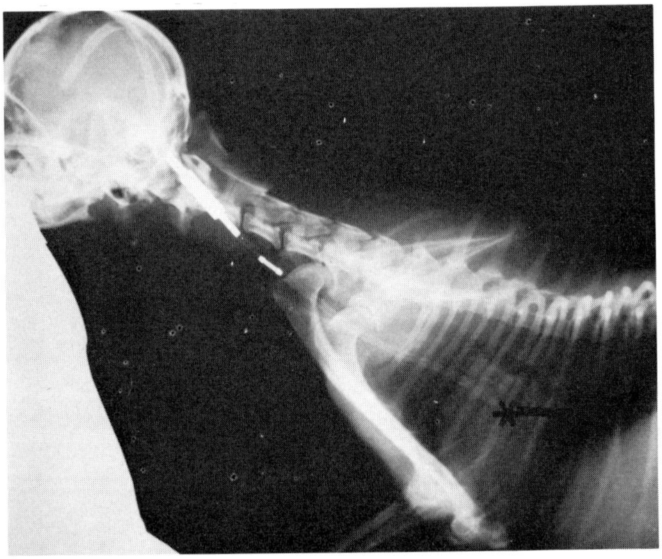

FIGURE 21–34 Postoperative radiograph showing the shunt unit in place in the dog. (From Gage, E. D., and Hoerlein, B. F.: Surgical treatment of canine hydrocephalus by ventriculoatrial shunting. J.A.V.M.A. *153*:1423, 1968.)

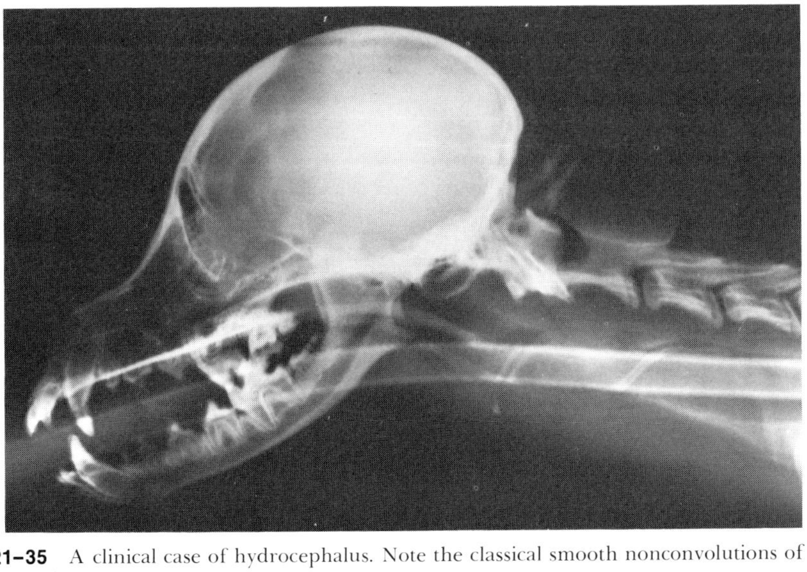

FIGURE 21–35 A clinical case of hydrocephalus. Note the classical smooth nonconvolutions of the cerebrum; this is the "ground glass" appearance.

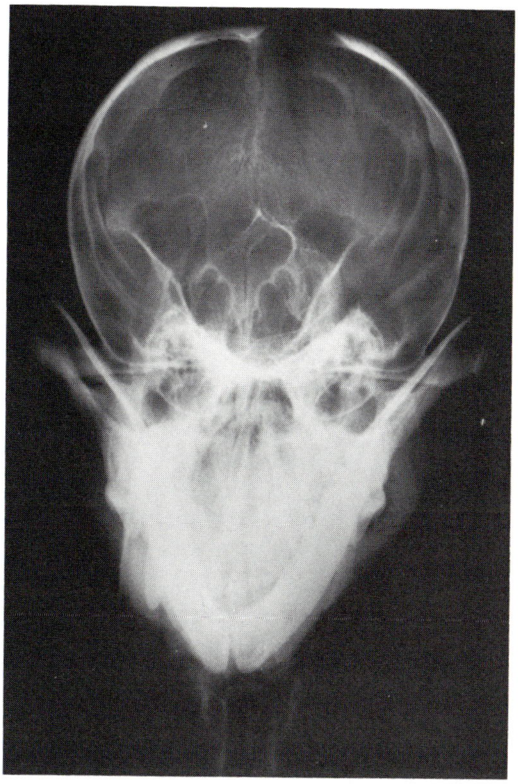

FIGURE 21–36 AP view of the case shown in Figure 21–35. Notice the extremely enlarged foramen magnum and the open cranial sutures.

a few days. Clinical observations should determine if the valve is functioning, and an occasional massage of the flexible portion may be necessary. We have found that frequent massage by overzealous clients is contraindicated, as the patient may become hyperirritable from such efforts. Massage should be performed by the surgeon, possibly under sedation or tranquilization. If the patient tends to relapse at any time after the operation, the placement of valve and catheter should be checked radiographically or surgically. Adjustment of the catheter has occasionally been necessary (Figs. 21–31 to 21–33).[17, 20, 27, 50]

Ventriculoperitoneal Shunt[35]

In the ventriculoperitoneal (VP) shunt the ventricular catheter may be placed either laterally or paramedially in the calvarium. The catheter is inserted through the brain tissue in the same way as in the ventriculoatrial shunt, and the shunt tubing is fixed in place with nonabsorbable suture material.

An incision is made in the paralumbar skin, and the subcutaneous tissue is bluntly dissected from the craniocervical area back to the incision in the paralumbar skin. The peritoneal catheter is now introduced through the subcutaneous channel from the cranial cervical incision to the paralumbar incision, allowing an additional 8 to 12 cm of tube length. The peritoneal catheter is attached to the shunt tubing with nonabsorbable suture material, and the subcutis and skin are then closed in a routine fashion. A small incision is made in the paralumbar region through the abdominal mus-

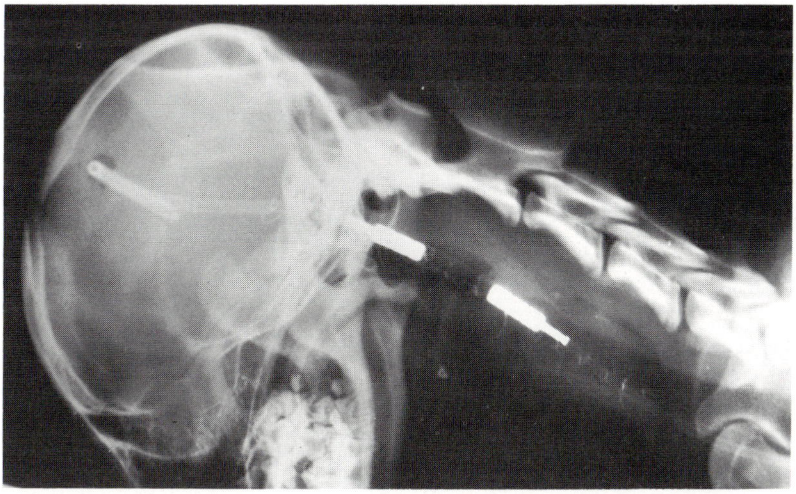

FIGURE 21–37 The Holter valve in place. This is the two-valve Holter assembly pictured in Figure 21–32. Same case as shown in Figure 21–35.

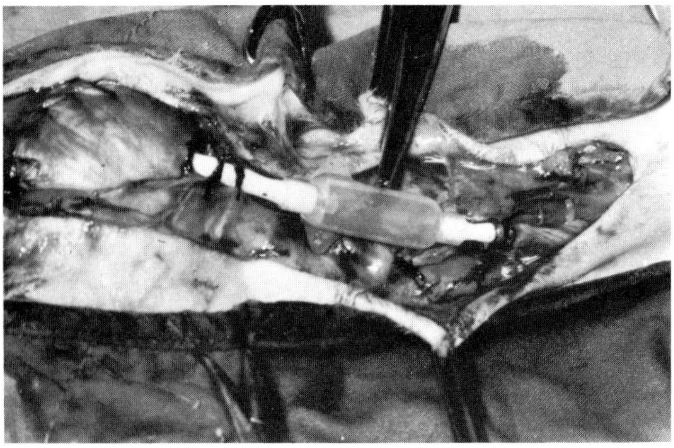

FIGURE 21–38 The Denver valve sutured in place. This valve is sutured in place in the same way as the Holter valve described in other figures and in the text.

cles into the peritoneal cavity. To prevent injury to the peritoneal catheter by traction, the proximal end (which is trimmed before attachment to the ventricular tubing) should be used for traction subcutaneously. A special springed catheter (Raimondi spring catheter) which tends to prevent kinking is now available; it facilitates penetration of musculature prior to introduction into the peritoneal cavity.

Before the catheter is inserted into the peritoneal cavity, the function of the slit valve should be checked. The tube is filled with sterile saline and allowed to drain. If the valve is functioning properly, the column of saline falls to 6 to 10 cm above the valve in 30 to 60 seconds. The valve should drain freely when pressure in the tube exceeds 6 to 10 cm of water. Adhesions in the valve resulting from heat sterilization may be broken by rolling the valved end between the thumb and index finger. After testing the valve, approximately 8 to 12 cm of the valved end of the catheter is inserted into the peritoneal cavity. The abdominal incision is closed with simple interrupted 2-0 or 3-0 catgut sutures, and the subcutis and skin are closed routinely (Fig. 21–39).

One advantage of ventriculoperitoneal shunting compared to ventriculoatrial shunting is that it can accommodate growth in the animal if the proximal end is firmly

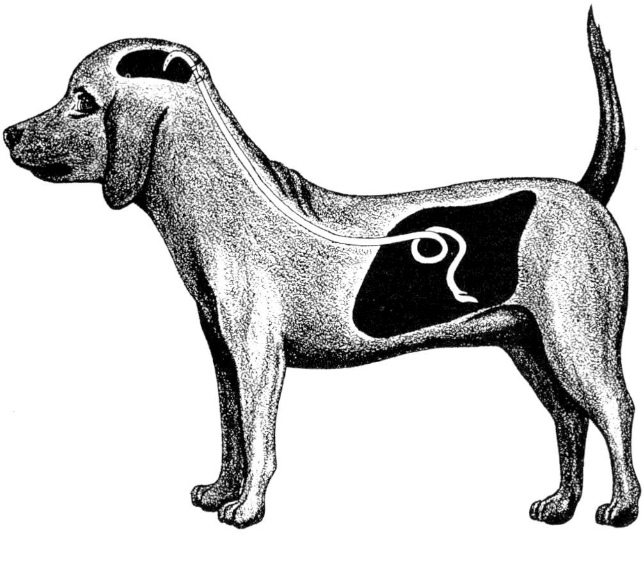

FIGURE 21–39 Ventriculoperitoneal shunt. Notice that the distal catheter is extended subcutaneously from the head area into the peritoneal cavity. (From Knecht, C. D.: Ventriculoperitoneal shunt for hydrocephalus. *In* Bojrab, M. J. (ed.): *Current Techniques in Small Animal Surgery I.* Lea & Febiger, Philadelphia, 1975.)

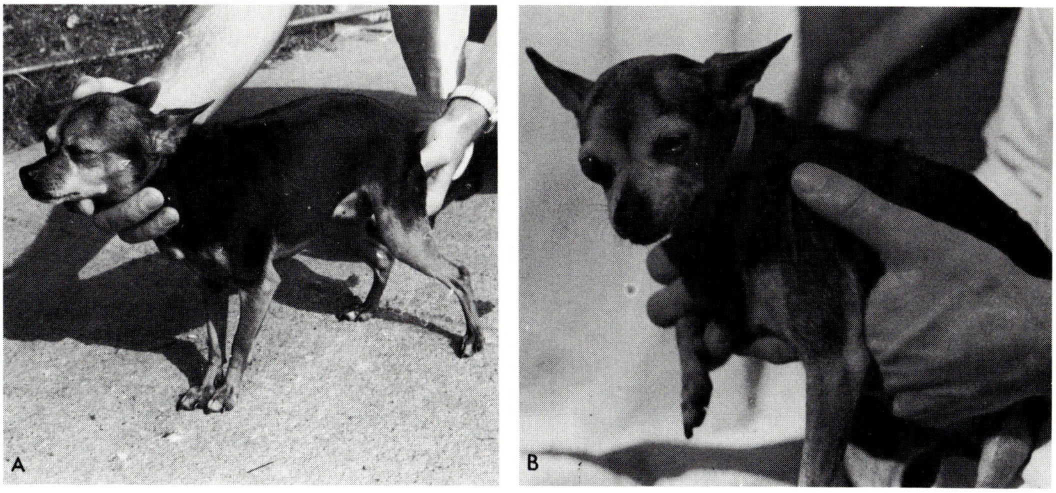

FIGURE 21–40 A 4-year-old Chihuahua had acquired obstructive ventricular dropsy. A Holter valve and ventriculoatrial shunt were installed in August, 1962. This picture was taken in April, 1965. *B*. Picture taken in November, 1969. The dog was still normal at this time. It eventually died of other causes in 1971 at 13 years of age (9 years after shunting). A second operation, consisting of a shunt on the other side, was performed in 1970.

anchored to the cranial tissue. This allows the excess peritoneal catheter to slip with growth. In ventriculoatrial shunts a jugular vein is sacrificed, whereas in the ventriculoperitoneal method it is preserved. Cost is about the same for both methods.

The disadvantage of the ventriculoperitoneal method is that the extensive subcutaneous dissection and additional incisions necessary for the placement of tubing increase the chances of infection.[25] A comparative study of the results of 300 cases of ventriculoperitoneal and ventriculoatrial shunts in humans was made. The differences in primary and total revision rates between the two methods were not statistically significant, although 58 per cent of the ventriculoperitoneal shunts and 48 per cent of the ventriculoatrial shunts needed at least one revision.[30]

Results of Surgery

In the previous reports by Few[17], Oliver[50], Hoerlein[27, 29], and Gage[20], a total of 21 dogs were given surgical ventricular shunts, 13 of which were successful. In the 1969–1975 period, Gage treated surgically 25 dogs with hydrocephalus; their ages varied from 6 weeks to 3 years. Eighteen of the 25 dogs (72 per cent) were toy poodles or Chihuahuas. The Holter valve was used in 21 dogs, the Denver valve in four. Twenty-four of the shunts were ventriculoatrial, and one was a ventriculoperitoneal shunt. The results were classified as follows: good – 1 year survival or more – 12 dogs (48 per cent); fair, 4; died within 1 week after surgery, 4; died after 1 week due to complications, 5.

In six cases of ventriculoatrial shunting with the Holter valve in Auburn (1969–1975),[67] good to satisfactory results were achieved in four, while in the other two cases multiple adjustments of catheters and valves were necessary.

Failures in surgical shunting are frequently related to irreversible neurological disease which existed before surgery was attempted. Some animals succumb during or shortly after surgery due to other organ dysfunctions. Deaths due to anesthesia are less frequent when proper assessment of organ functions has been made previously and when skilled monitoring of vital signs during surgery has been performed. Postsurgical infections may occur, and abnormal cerebrospinal fluid may promote plugging of the valve. The ventricular catheter may change position in time; for instance, it may invade the opposite hemisphere or migrate through the cerebrum to the calvarium. Surgical readjustments of catheters may be necessary due to excessive activity or growth of the animal (Fig. 21–40).

In man, ventricular valves and shunts

have given significant results. Yashon compared surgical and nonsurgical treatment in infantile hydrocephalus. Of 147 patients, 58 were treated nonsurgically and had a survival rate of 40 to 50 per cent, whereas in 69 patients treated surgically, the survival rate was 70 per cent. A 20 to 30 per cent decrease in mortality indicates that the ventriculovenous shunt is of value.[73]

In Foltz's 5-year study of 65 surgical cases, 64.4 per cent were successful; of these, 33.8 per cent had competent I.Q.'s and 27.6 per cent had deficient I.Q.'s. In nonsurgical cases, the survival rate was 22.2 per cent; of these, 5.5 per cent had competent scores and 16.7 per cent had incompetent scores.[18]

In man, the main complications have been secondary infection; catheter displacements; catheter thrombosis or occlusion; subdural hematoma from rapid collapse of the ventricles causing rupture of bridging meningeal veins; breaks in tubing; and perforation of the atrial wall by the distal catheter, which caused pericardial effusion and cardiac tamponade.[13, 19, 36, 47, 73] In one study in children, blockage of the valve system occurred occasionally after closure of the fontanelles. Ten per cent of the children died from causes directly related to valve failures, and 78 per cent needed one or more revisions of the valve system.[19]

The advent of more satisfactory means of clinical stabilization of hydrocephalus with steroid therapy has decreased the necessity for surgical shunting. However, in our experience, surgical shunting is still a satisfactory procedure if the dog is mature and the owner can afford the rather expensive equipment needed. Several of our patients have lived normal lives from 2 to 8 years after surgery. Selective breeding of individuals of susceptible breeds that display good temperament and have normal EEGs and radiographs should be investigated further. Sincere breeders will make special efforts to help control this disorder by proper breeding practices.

REFERENCES

1. Albert, R. A.: Canine ventriculography and encephalography. Thesis, Auburn University, Auburn, Alabama, 1967.
2. Anderson, F. M.: Ventriculo-auriculostomy in treatment of hydrocephalus. J. Neurosurg. *16*, 551, 1959.
3. Bannister, R.: *Brain's Clinical Neurology*, 4th ed. Oxford University Press, New York, 1973.
4. Bering, E. A., Jr.: Circulation of the cerebrospinal fluid. J. Neurosurg. *19*, 405, 1962.
5. Bering, E. A., and Sato, O.: Hydrocephalus: Changes in formation and absorption of cerebrospinal fluid within the cerebral ventricles. J. Neurosurg. *20*, 1050, 1963.
6. Blake, J. A.: The roof and lateral recesses of the fourth ventricle, considered morphologically and embryologically. J. Comp. Neurol. *10*, 79, 1906.
7. Bowsher, D.: *Cerebrospinal Fluid Dynamics in Health and Disease.* Charles C Thomas, Springfield, Ill., 1960.
8. Cammermeyer, J.: Frequency of meningoencephalitis and hydrocephalus in dogs. J. Neuropath. Exp. Neurol. *20*, 386, 1961.
9. Dandy, W. E.: Ventriculography following injection of air into the cerebral ventricles. Ann. Surg. *68*, 5, 1918.
10. de Lahunta, A., and Cummings, J. F.: The clinical and electroencephalographic features of hydrocephalus in three dogs. J.A.V.M.A. *146*, 954, 1965.
11. DiChiro, G., and Grove, A. S., Jr.: Evaluation of surgical and spontaneous cerebropsinal fluid shunts by isotope scanning. J. Neurosurg. *24*, 743, 1966.
12. De Chirco, G., and Harrington, T.: Spontaneous cerebrospinal fluid rhinorrhea in normal dogs. Radioisotope studies of an alternate pathway of CSF drainage. J. Neuropath. Exp. Neurol. *31*, 447, 1972.
13. Dzenitis, A. J., Mealey, J., Jr., and Waddell, J. R.: Myocardial perforation by ventriculoatrial shunt tubing. J.A.M.A. *194*, 1251, 1965.
14. Elvidge, A. R.: Treatment of obstructive lesions of the aqueduct of Sylvius and the fourth ventricle by interventriculostomy. J. Neurosurg. *24*, 11, 1966.
15. Fankhauser, R.: Untersuchungen über die arachnoidalen Zotten und Granulationen bei Tieren. Schweiz. Arch. Tierheilkd. *104*, 13, 1962.
16. Fankhauser, R.: Drei Verbildungen des Gehirns. Schweiz. Arch. Tierheilkd. *107*, 1, 1965.
17. Few, A. B.: The diagnosis and surgical treatment of canine hydrocephalus. J.A.V.M.A. *149*, 286, 1966.
18. Foltz, E. L., and Shurtleff, D. B.: Five year comparative study of hydrocephalus in children with and without operation (113 cases). J. Neurosurg. *20*, 1064, 1963.
19. Forrest, D. M., and Cooper, D. G. W.: Complications of ventriculoatrial shunts: Review of 455 cases. J. Neurosurg. *29*, 506, 1968.
20. Gage, E. D., and Hoerlein, B. F.: Surgical treatment of canine hydrocephalus by ventriculoatrial shunting. J.A.V.M.A. *153*, 1418, 1968.
21. Gage, E. D.: Surgical treatment of canine hydrocephalus. J.A.V.M.A.. *157*, 1729, 1970.
22. Garcia-Bengochea, F.: The effect of cortisone on cerebrospinal fluid production in castrated adult cats. Neurology *16*, 512, 1966.
23. Gorgacz, E. J., Nielsen, S. W., Frier, H. I., Eaton, H. D., and Rousseau, J. E.: Morphological alterations associated with decreased cerebrospinal fluid pressure in chronic bovine hypervitaminosis A. Am. J. Vet. Res. *36*, 171, 1975.

24. Greene, H. J., Leipold, H. W., and Vestweber, J. E.: Experimentally induced hydrocephalus in calves. Am. J. Vet. Res. *35*, 945, 1974.
25. Gurdjian, E. S.: *Operative Neurosurgery,* 2nd ed. The Williams and Wilkins Co., Baltimore, 1964.
26. Harrison, E. O.: Unpublished data.
27. Hoerlein, B. F., and Few, A. B.: Brain surgery in the dog—preliminary studies. J.A.V.M.A. *143*, 21, 1963.
28. Hoerlein, B. F., and Petty, M. F.: Constant encephalography and ventriculography in the dog—preliminary studies. J.A.V.M.A. *22*, 1041, 1961.
29. Hoerlein, B. F.: *Canine Neurology, Diagnosis and Treatment,* 2nd ed. W. B. Saunders Co., Philadelphia, 1971.
30. Ignelzi, R. J., and Kirsch, W. M.: Follow-up analysis of ventriculoperitoneal and ventriculoatrial shunts for hydrocephalus. J. Neurosurg. *42*, 679, 1975.
31. Innes, J. R. M., and Saunders, L. Z.: *Comparative Neuropathology.* Academic Press, New York, 1962.
32. James, A. E., Jr., Burns, B., Flor, W. F., Strecker, E. P., Merz, T., Bush, M., and Price, D. L.: Pathophysiology of chronic communicating hydrocephalus in dogs (*Canis familiaris*). J. Neurol. Sci. *24*, 151, 1975.
33. James, A. E., Jr., De Land, F. H., Hodges, F. J., and Wagner, H. N.: Normal-pressure hydrocephalus: Role of cisternography in diagnosis. J.A.M.A. *213*, 1615, 1970.
34. Johnston, I., Gilday, D. L., and Hendrick, E. B.: Experimental effects of steroids and steroid withdrawal on cerebrospinal fluid absorption. J. Neurosurg. *42*, 690, 1975.
35. Knecht, C. D.: Ventriculoperitoneal shunt for hydrocephalus *In* Bojrab, M. J. (ed.): *Current Techniques in Small Animal Surgery I.* Lea and Febiger, Philadelphia, 1975, p. 7.
36. Kurlander, G. J., and Chua, G. T., Roentgenology of ventriculo-atrial shunts for the treatment of hydrocephalus. Am. J. Roentgenol. *101*, 157, 1967.
37. Leonard, J. L., and Redding, R. W.: Effects of hypertonic solutions on cerebrospinal fluid pressure in the lateral ventricle of the dog. Am. J. Vet. Res. *34*, 212, 1973.
38. McCarthy, L. E., and Borison, H. L.: Volumetric compartmentalization of the cranial cerebrospinal fluid system determined radiographically in the cat. Anat. Rec. *155*, 305, 1966.
39. McGrath, J. T.: *Neurologic Examination of the Dog.* 2nd. ed. Lea and Febiger, Philadelphia, 1960.
40. Messert, B., and Baker, N. H.: Syndrome of progressive spastic ataxia and apraxia associated with occult hydrocephalus. Neurology *16*, 440, 1966.
41. Milhorat, T. H.: The third circulation revisited. J. Neurosurg. *42*, 628, 1975.
42. Millen, J. W., and Woolan, D. H.: The effect of vitamin A deficiency in female rabbits on the incidence of hydrocephalus in the young. J. Neurol. Psychiat. *19*, 17, 1956.
43. Miller, M. E., Christensen, G. C., and Evans, H. E.: *Anatomy of the Dog.* W. B. Saunders Co., Philadelphia, 1964, p. 542.
44. Mims, C. A.: An analysis of the toxicity for mice of influenza virus I. Intracerebral toxicity. Brit. J. Exp. Pathol. *41*, 586, 1960.
45. Murtagh, F., and Lehman, R.: Peritoneal shunts in the management of hydrocephalus. J.A.M.A. *202*, 1010, 1967.
46. Newberne, P. M., and O'Dell, GB. L.: Histopathology of hydrocephalus resulting from a deficiency of vitamin B_{12}, Proc. Soc. Exp. Biol. Med. *97*, 62, 1958.
47. Noonan, J. A., and Ekmke, D. A.: Complications of ventriculovenous shunts for control of hydrocephalus. New Eng. J. Med. *269*, 70, 1963.
48. Oldendorf, W. H., and Davson, H.: Brain extracellular space and the sink action of cerebrospinal fluid. Arch. Neurol. *17*, 196, 1967.
49. Oldendorf, W. H.: Why is cerebrospinal fluid? Bull, Los Angeles Neurol. Soc. *32*,, part I, 169, 1967.
50. Oliver, J. E., Jr.: Surgical approaches to the canine brain. Am. J. Vet. Res. *29*, 353, 1968.
51. Oliver, J. E., Jr., and Conrad, C. R.: Cerebral ventriculography. In Ticer, J. W. (ed.): *Radiographic Technique in Small Animal Practice.* W. B. Saunders Co., Philadelphia, 1975.
52. Pollay, M., and Welch, K.: The function and structure of the canine arachnoid villi. J. Surg. Res. *2*, 307, 1962. Cited by Jenkins, T. W.: *Functional Mammalian Neuroanatomy.* Lea and Febiger, Philadelphia, 1972.
53. Poppen, J. L.: *An Atlas of Neurosurgical Techniques.* W. B. Saunders Co., Philadelphia, 1960.
54. Prynn, R. B., and Redding, R. W.: Electroencephalogram in occult canine hydrocephalus. J.A.V.M.A. *152*, 1651, 1968.
55. Pudenz, P. H., Russell, F. E., Hurd, A. H., and Shelden, C. H.: Ventriculo-auriculostomy. A technique for shunting cerebrospinal fluid into the right auricle; preliminary report. J. Neurosurg. *14*, 771, 1957.
56. Pudenz, R. H.: Experimental and clinical observations on the shunting of cerebrospinal fluid into the circulatory system. Proc. Congr. Neurol. Surg. *5*, 98, 1958.
57. Redding, R. W.: Canine electroencephalography. In Hoerlein, B. F. (ed.): *Canine Neurology, Diagnosis and Treatment,* 2d ed. W. B. Saunders Co., Philadelphia, 1971.
58. Redding, R. W.: Unpublished data.
59. Robertson, J. T., Schick, R. W., Morgan, F. and Matson, D. D.: Accurate placement of ventriculoatrial shunt for hydrocephalus under electrocardiographic control. J. Neurosurg. *18*, 255, 1961.
60. Rubin, R. C., Henderson, E. S., Ommaya, A. K., Walker, M. D., and Rall, D. P.: The production of cerebrospinal fluid in man and its modification by acetazolamide. J. Neurosurg. *25*, 430, 1966.
61. Sato, O., Asai, T., Amano, Y., Hara, M., Tsugane, R., and Yogi, M.: Formation of cerebrospinal fluid in spinal subarachnoid space. Nature *233*, 129, 1971.
62. Sato, O., Hara, M., Asai, T., Tsugane, R., and Kageyama, N.: The effect of dexamethasone phosphate on the production rate of cerebrospinal fluid in the spinal subarachnoid space of dogs. J. Neurosurg. *39*, 480, 1973.
63. Savell, C. M.: Cerebral ventricular tap: An aid to diagnosis and treatment of hydrocephalus in

the dog. J. Am. Anim. Hosp. Assoc. *10*, 500, 1974.
64. Scarff, J. E.: Third ventriculostomy by puncture of the lamina terminalis and floor of third ventricle. J. Neurosurg. *24*, 933, 1966.
65. Schaltenbrand, G., and Putman, T.: Untersuchungen zum Kreislauf der Liquor cerebrospinalis mit Hilfe intravenose Fluorescineinspritzungen. Dtsch. Z. Nervenheilk. *96*, 123, 1927.
66. Strecker, E. P., Bush, M., and James, A. E.: Cerebrospinal fluid imaging as a method to evaluate communicating hydrocephalus in dogs. Am. J. Vet. Res. *34*, 101, 1973.
67. Swaim, S. F.: Unpublished data.
68. Urman, H. K., and Grace, O. D.: Hereditary encephalomyopathy. A hydrocephalus syndrome in newborn calves. Cornell Vet. *54*, 229, 1964.
69. Vandelelde, M., and Higgins, R. J.: Unpublished data.
70. Wechsler, I. S.: *Clinical Neurology*, 9th ed. W. B. Saunders Co., Philadelphia, 1963.
71. Wilson, C. B., and Bertan, V.: Interruption of the anterior choroidal artery in experimental hydrocephalus. Arch. Neurol. *17*, 614, 1967.
72. Wise, B. L.: A telescopic ventriculoatrial shunt that elongates with growth. J. Neurosurg. *40*, 665, 1974.
73. Yashon, D.: Prognosis in infantile hydrocephalus. J. Neurosurg. *20*, 105, 1963.
74. Youmans, J. R.: *Neurological Surgery*, Vol. 1. W. B. Saunders Co., Philadelphia, 1973, p. 573.

GLOSSARY OF TERMS*

Compiled by
Tommy L. Walker, D.V.M., M.S.
and
Steven F. Swaim, D.V.M., M.S.

Abiotrophy – The premature and endogenous loss of vitality or tissue substance.

Achondroplasia – A hereditary, congenital, familial disturbance of epiphyseal chondroblastic growth and maturation causing inadequate enchondral bone formation and resulting in a peculiar type of dwarfism with short limbs, normal trunk, small face, normal vault, lordosis, and trident hands or paws.

Adnexa – Appendages or adjunct parts; e.g., the adnexa oculi are the lacrimal apparatus and other appendages of the eye.

Afferent – Conveying toward a center; e.g., afferent nerves convey impulses from the periphery toward the central nervous system.

Agenesis – Absence of an organ; frequently used to designate such absence resulting from failure of appearance of the primordium of an organ in embryonic development.

Algorithm – A rule of procedure for solving a mathematical problem (such as finding the greatest common divisor) that frequently involves repetition of an operation.

Amaurosis – Blindness, especially blindness occurring with no apparent lesion of the eye. Blindness may be due to disease of the optic nerve, retina, or brain.

Amblyopia – A dimness of vision with no detectable organic lesion of the eye.

Amphiarthrosis – A form of articulation permitting little motion, the apposed surfaces of bone being connected by fibrocartilage.

Anamnesis – The collected data concerning a patient, including data about his family, previous environment, and experiences; any abnormal sensations, moods, or acts observed by the patient himself or by others, with the dates of their appearance and duration; and any results of treatment.

Anesthesia – The loss of feeling or sensation. Although the term can be used to mean loss of tactile sensibility or of any of the other senses, it is applied especially to loss of the sensation of pain, as induced to permit performance of surgery or other painful procedures.

Angiography – The roentgenological visualization of blood vessels.

Anisocoria – Inequality of the diameters of the pupils.

Anlage – Primordium.

Annulus fibrosus – A fibrous ring consisting of bands of parallel fibers that run obliquely from one vertebral body to the next. They provide a means for the transmission of stresses and upward movements.

Anodyne – A medicine that relieves pain.

Anopia – An absence or rudimentary condition of the eye.

Anosmia – Absence of the sense of smell.

---

*Dorland's Illustrated Medical Dictionary, 25th edition, and various physiology, neurology, and neurosurgery texts were used as a basis for defining terms in this glossary. Modification of some terms was necessary for veterinary application.

Aplasia—The lack of development of an organ; frequently used to designate complete suppression or failure of development of a structure from the embryonic primordium.

Apoplexy—A condition caused by acute vascular lesions of the brain, such as hemorrhage, thrombosis, or embolism; it is marked by coma and followed by paralysis.

Arachnoidea—A delicate membrane interposed between the dura mater and the pia mater, being separated from the pia mater by the subarachnoid space.

Areflexia—Absence of the reflexes.

Arnold-Chiari syndrome—A congenital anomaly in which the cerebellum and medulla oblongata, which is elongated and flattened, protrude down into the spinal canal through the foramen magnum; it may be associated with many other defects, including spina bifida occulta and meningomyelocele.

Arteriography—Roentgenography of arteries after injection of radiopaque material into the blood stream.

Arthrodesis—The surgical fixation of a joint by fusion of the joint surfaces; artificial ankylosis.

Ascending—Having an upward course, i.e., toward the brain.

Astasia—Motor incoordination with inability to stand.

Asthenia—A lack or loss of strength and energy; weakness.

Astrocyte—A neuroglial cell of ectodermal origin, characterized by fibrous or protoplasmic processes. Collectively, such cells are called astroglia.

Asynergy—Lack of coordination among parts or organs normally acting in harmony. A disturbance of that proper association in the contraction of muscles that assures that the different components of an act follow in proper sequence, at the proper moment, and are of the proper degree, so that the act is executed accurately.

Ataxia—Failure of muscular coordination; irregularity of muscular action.

Athetoid—Affected with athetosis.

Athetosis—A derangement marked by ceaseless occurrence of involuntary, slow, sinuous, writhing movements.

Atonic—Lacking normal tone or strength; pertaining to or characterized by atony.

Atrophy—A wasting away or diminution in the size of cell, tissue, organ, or part. Denervated muscle atrophy results from severance of the motor nerve supplying the muscle.

Axon—The central core that forms the essential conducting part of a nerve fiber.

Axonotmesis—Damage to nerve fibers of such severity that complete peripheral degeneration follows; the internal architecture, however, is fairly well preserved, so that recovery is spontaneous and of good quality.

Azoturia—Excess of urea or other nitrogen compounds in the urine.

Babinski's response—Dorsiflexion of the big toe on stimulating the sole of the foot. It occurs with lesions of the pyramidal tract of the central nervous system or with damage to the foot region of the motor cortex. It is more marked if the foot region of the premotor cortex is damaged as well as the motor cortex.

Basal nuclei (ganglia)—Masses of gray matter centrally embedded with the thalamus in the cerebral hemisphere. The basal nuclei are the caudate nucleus, putamen, globus pallidus, amygdaloid nucleus, and claustrum. The subthalamus, substantia nigra, and red nucleus are considered by some to be part of the basal nuclei. These nuclei are mainly concerned with the motor functions.

Bell's palsy—A flaccid paralysis due to a lesion of the facial nerve and resulting in a characteristic distortion of the face.

Blood-brain barrier—The barrier separating the blood from the parenchyma of the central nervous system. It consists of the walls of the blood vessels of the central nervous system and the surrounding glial membranes.

Blood-cerebrospinal fluid barrier—The barrier separating the blood from the cerebrospinal fluid. The anatomical location of this barrier is considered to be in the choroid plexus.

Brachycephalic—Having a short wide head.

Bradycardia—An abnormal slowness of the heart beat. Central bradycardia is due to disease of the central nervous system; vagal bradycardia is due to disturbed vagal tone.

Bulbar paralysis—Paralysis due to changes in the motor centers of the medulla oblongata.

Bundle—A collection of fibers or strands, such as a fasciculus or band of nerve fibers.

Caloric test—When a normal ear is irrigated with hot water (110° to 120° F), a rotatory nystagmus is developed toward the side of the irrigated ear; if the ear is irrigated with cold water, a rotary nystagmus is developed away from the irrigated side. There is no nystagmus if the labyrinth is diseased.

Calvarium—The domelike superior portion of the cranium, composed of portions of the frontal, parietal, and occipital bones. It is also called the skullcap.

Catalepsy—A condition characterized by a waxy rigidity of the muscles so that the patient tends to remain in any position in which he is placed.

Catatonia—A form of schizophrenia characterized by negativistic reactions, phases of stupor or excitement, and impulsive or stereotypic behavior.

Cataplexy—A state of immobility and rigidity seen in some animals as a result of certain forms of stimulation.

Cauda equina—The sheaf of roots of the lower spinal nerves that descend in the spinal canal from their point of attachment to the spinal cord to the site of their emergence between the vertebrae.

Caudal (caudad)—Denoting a position more toward the cauda, or tail, than some specified point of reference.

Caudotentorial—Referring to that portion of the cranial vault that is caudal to the extension of the dura mater that forms a partition between the cerebrum and the cerebellum.

Cerebellar nystagmus—A pathological tremor of the eyeballs due to damage to the deep nuclei of the cerebellum. If the flocculonodular lobe is involved, the nystagmus will be associated with loss of equilibrium.

Cerebrospinal fluid (CSF)—The fluid contained within the four ventricles of the brain, the subarachnoid space, and the central canal of the spinal cord; it is formed by the choroid plexus and brain parenchyma, circulated through the ventricles into the subarachnoid space, and absorbed into the venous system.

Cerebrospinal fluid-brain barrier—The barrier that separates the cerebrospinal fluid from the parenchyma of the central nervous system. The anatomical location of this barrier is considered to be the pia mater and ependyma.

Chondrodystrophy—A morbid condition characterized by abnormal development of cartilage.

Chorea—The occurrence of frequent, jerky, but well-coordinated movements, performed involuntarily.

Choreiform—Resembling chorea.

Chromatolysis—The disintegration of the Nissl (chromophil) bodies of a nerve cell as the result of injury, fatigue, or exhaustion; it is a part of the so-called axon reaction.

Chronaxy—The time required for the excitation of a nervous element by a definite stimulus; the minimum time at which a current just doubles the rheobase will excite contraction.

Clonus—A spasm in which rigidity and relaxation alternate in rapid succession.

Coloboma—An apparent absence or defect of some ocular tissues, especially a congenital fissure of any part of the eye.

Coma—A state of unconsciousness from which the patient cannot be aroused, even by powerful stimulation.

Comitant strabismus—Deviation of an eye due to a faulty insertion of the eye muscles, resulting in a constant amount of deviation in whatever direction the eyes are looking (see also *Incomitant strabismus*).

Concussion—A violent jar or shock, or the condition that results from such injury.

Consensual—Excited by reflex stimulation; used especially to designate the similar reaction of both pupils to a stimulus applied to only one.

Contralateral—Situated on or pertaining to the opposite side.

Contre coup lesion—Injury resulting from a blow on another side, such as a fracture of the skull caused by a blow on the opposite side.

Contusion – A bruise.
Coordination – The harmonious functioning of interrelated organs and parts; applied especially to the process of the motor apparatus of the brain that provides for the cooperation of particular groups of muscles for the performance of definite adaptive useful responses.
Craniectomy – Excision of a part of the skull.
Cranioplasty – Any plastic operation on the skull; surgical correction of defects of the skull.
Craniotomy – Any operation on the cranium.
Curettage – The removal of growths or other material from the wall of a cavity or other surface, as with a curet.

Decerebration – Transection of the brain stem between the superior and inferior colliculi, resulting in extensor rigidity of the limbs due to lack of inhibitory impulses from higher centers.
Decompression – The removal of pressure. (1) Cerebral decompression is done by removing a flap of skull and incising the dural mater for the purpose of relieving intracranial pressure. (2) Decompression of the spinal cord is done by removing the dorsal or lateral elements, or both, of the vertebral arch to relieve pressure on the spinal cord.
Decorticate – Signifies that portions of the cortical substance of a structure or organ (e.g., the brain) have been removed.
Decussation – Referring to the crossing of nerve fibers or tracts from one side of the central nervous system to the opposite side. The optic chiasm is the crossing of some fibers of the optic nerve to the opposite side of the brain.
Deficiency – A transient or permanent loss of function due to a lesion of a part of the nervous system.
Delirium – A mental disturbance with a comparatively short course and marked by illusions, hallucinations, short unsystematized delusions, cerebral excitement, physical restlessness, and incoherence. Delirium may occur in the course of a more prolonged mental disorder or as a result of fever, disease, or injury.
Dementia – A general designation for mental deterioration.
Demyelination – The destruction or removal of the myelin sheath of a nerve or nerves.
Dendrite – A branched (tree-shaped) protoplasmic process from a nerve cell that conducts impulses toward the cell body.
Dentate ligament (denticulate ligament) – A fold of pia mater of the spinal cord, beginning in a longitudinal line along the spinal cord between the lines of attachment of the ventral and dorsal roots. The lateral edge is scalloped and has about 21 pointed processes that extend laterally and fuse with the arachnoid and dura mater.
Depolarization – The process of neutralizing polarity. In nerve fiber depolarization, a stimulus to the nerve fiber alters the permeability of the cell membrane and results in an influx of positively charged sodium ions from the extracellular fluid into the nerve fiber, thus initiating an action potential in the nerve fiber.
Dermatome – A sensory root field on the skin. The area of skin supplied with afferent nerve fibers by a single dorsal spinal root.
Descending – Extending downward, e.g., away from the brain.
Diarthrodial joint – A synovial joint.
Diencephalon – The posterior part of the prosencephalon, consisting of the hypothalamus, thalamus, metathalamus, and epithalamus.
Diplegia – Paralysis affecting like parts on both sides of the body; bilateral paralysis.
Diploë – The trabecular osseous tissue between two tables of the cranial bones.
Discrimination – The quality or power of finely distinguishing; e.g., the ability of the central nervous system to distinguish between various sensory impulses.
Discospondylitis – An inflammation of the intervertebral disk and the adjacent vertebrae.
Disinhibition – The abolition of inhibition; in an experimental animal, the revival of an extinguished conditioned reflex or response by giving a stimulus to which the animal is unaccustomed.
Diskectomy – Excision of an intervertebral disk.

Diskography—Roentgenography of the spine, for visualization of an intervertebral disk, after injection into the disk itself of an absorbable contrast medium.
Dolichocephalic (mesocephalic)—Having a long narrow head.
Dura mater—The outermost, toughest, and most fibrous of the three membranes (meninges) covering the brain and spinal cord.
Durotomy—The operation of cutting the dura mater; usually a longitudinal division.
Dyscrasia—Formerly used to indicate a depraved state of the humor, the term is now used generally to indicate a morbid condition, especially one which involves an imbalance of component elements. Blood dyscrasia is an abnormal or pathological condition of the blood.
Dyskinesthesia (dyskinesia)—Impairment of the power of voluntary movement, resulting in a fragmentary or incomplete movement.
Dysmetria—A condition in which there is improper measuring of distance in muscular acts. It is a disturbance of the power to control the range in muscular movements and is commonly associated with cerebellar disease—e.g., hypermetria is overstepping.
Dysmyelination—Abnormal myelin synthesis in the developing central nervous system.
Dysphagia—Difficulty in swallowing.
Dysphonia—An impairment of voice; a difficulty in vocalization.
Dysrhaphia—An incomplete closure of the primary neural tube.
Dyssynergia—A disturbance of muscular coordination.
Dystrophy—Any disorder arising from defective or faulty nutrition.

Effector—A muscle or gland that contracts or secretes, respectively, in direct response to nerve impulses.
Efferent—Conveying away from a center; e.g., efferent nerves convey impulses away from the central nervous system toward the periphery.
Electroencephalography—The recording of electric currents developed in the brain by means of electrodes applied to the scalp or to the surface of the brain, or placed within the substance of the brain.
Electromyography—The recording of the changes in electric potential of muscle by means of (1) surface or needle electrodes to determine merely whether the muscle is contracting or not (useful in kinesiology); (2) insertion of a needle electrode into the muscle and observation by cathode-ray oscilloscope and loud-speaker of the action potentials that are spontaneously present in a muscle (abnormal) or induced by involuntary contractions, to detect the nature and location of motor unit lesions; or (3) recording the electrical activity evoked in a muscle by stimulation of its nerve (this is useful for the study of several aspects of neuromuscular function, neuromuscular conduction, extent of nerve lesions, and reflex responses, among other purposes).
Embolus—A clot or other plug brought by the blood from another vessel and forced into a smaller one, thus obstructing the circulation.
Encephalitis—Inflammation of the brain.
Encephalization—The developmental process by which the cerebral cortex has taken over the functions of the lower (spinal) centers.
Encephalomalacia—Morbid softness, or softening, of the brain.
Encephalomeningitis—Inflammation of the brain and its membranes.
Encephalomyelitis—Inflammation involving both the brain and the spinal cord.
Encephalopathy—Any degenerative disease of the brain.
Enchondrosis—An outgrowth from cartilage; an enchondroma.
Endoneurium—The interstitial connective tissue in a peripheral nerve, separating the individual nerve fibers.
Enophthalmos—Abnormal retraction of the eye into the orbit.
Ependyma—The lining membrane of the ventricles of the brain and of the central canal of the spinal cord.
Epicritic—Relating to or serving the purpose of accurate determination; applied to cutaneous nerve fibers that serve the purpose of perceiving fine variations of touch or temperature.
Epidural—Situated upon or outside the dura.

Epidurography—Radiography of the spine after a radiopaque medium has been injected into the epidural space.
Epilepsy—The uncontrolled excessive activity of a part or all of the central nervous system. (1) Generalized epilepsy involves essentially all parts of the brain at once. (2) Partial epilepsy involves either a minute focal point or a moderate portion of the brain.
Epileptic focus (epileptogenic focus)—The area of cortex responsible for causing epileptic seizures as revealed in the encephalogram.
Epineurium—The connective tissue covering of a peripheral nerve.
Epiphora—An abnormal overflow of tears down the cheek, mainly due to stricture of the lacrimal passages.
Equilibrium—A state of balance of the body. The maintenance of equilibrium is mainly controlled by the vestibular apparatus (utricle and semicircular canals), the reticular nuclei of the brain stem, and the flocculonodular lobes of the cerebellum.
Erben's reflex—The slowing of the pulse upon bending the head and trunk strongly downward; said to indicate vagal excitability.
Esotropia—Deviation of a visual axis toward that of the other eye when fusion is a possibility.
Evoked response—To call forth or bring about an action or movement by the application of a stimulus.
Exotropia—Deviation of a visual axis away from that of the other eye when fusion is a possibility.
Extensor rigidity—Rigid extension of an animal's limbs, as in decerebrate rigidity.
Extrapyramidal system (extracorticospinal tracts)—Collectively, all the tracts in addition to the corticospinal tract that transmit motor signals from the brain to the spinal cord.

Facilitation—The passage of an impulse through nerve tissue that diminishes the resistance of the nerve so that following impulses will evoke a reaction more easily.
Faradic stimulation—Stimulation induced by a rapidly alternating current; repetitive pulses of short duration, usually at a rate ranging between 3 per second and 200 per second.
Fasciculation—A small local contraction of muscles, visible through the skin, representing a spontaneous discharge of a number of fibers innervated by a single motor nerve filament.
Fasciculus—A small bundle or cluster; used as a general term in anatomical nomenclature to designate a small bundle of nerve or muscle fibers, e.g., the fasciculus of cuneatus and gracilis of the spinal cord are a part of the spinal dorsal column system.
Feedback—The method by which a central nervous system structure such as the cerebellum aids in coordinating voluntary muscle movements. In this case the afferent impulses return for feedback to the cerebellum from the peripheral proprioceptors and allow the cerebellum to compare intended actions (the impulses for which were initiated in the cerebral cortex) with performed actions. The cerebellum can initiate corrective impulses as needed.
Fenestration—The act of perforation. Disk fenestration is the removal of intervertebral disk material by perforation and curettage of the intervertebral disk space.
Fibrillation—A small, local involuntary contraction of muscle, invisible under the skin, resulting from spontaneous activation of single muscle cells or muscle fibers.
Filum terminale—A slender, threadlike prolongation of the spinal cord from the conus medullaris to the apex of the dural sac, where it fuses with the filum of the dura mater and extends to the back of the coccyx, where it blends with the periosteum.
Flaccid—Weak, lax, or soft.
Flaccid paralysis—Paralysis with loss of tone in the muscles of the paralyzed part and absence of reflexes.
Fontanelle—A soft spot, such as one of the membrane-covered spaces remaining in an incompletely ossified skull.
Foraminotomy—The operation of removing the roof of the intervertebral foramina, done for the relief of nerve root compression.
Funiculus—A general term for a cordlike structure or part.

Galvanic stimulation – Single pulses of long duration, ranging from 100 milliseconds to several seconds.

Gangliosidosis – A lipid storage disorder marked by accumulation of gangliosides in tissues due to an enzyme defect.

Glioma – A tumor composed of tissue which represents neuroglia in any one of its stages of development. The term is sometimes extended to include all of the primary intrinsic neoplasms of the brain and spinal cord, including astrocytomas, ependymomas, neurocytomas, and others.

Gliosis – An excess of astroglia in damaged areas of the central nervous system.

Grand mal – A type of generalized epileptic seizure characterized by extreme neuronal discharges in the mesencephalic portion of the reticular activating system. These discharges spread throughout the entire central nervous system. They cause generalized tonic convulsions followed by clonic convulsions and terminate in a postseizure state of depression of the entire nervous system.

Guillain-Barré syndrome (Landry's paralysis) – A syndrome characterized by pain or tenderness in the muscles, motor weakness, and abolition of tendon reflexes. In dogs, a similar disorder has been called polyradiculoneuritis (coon dog paralysis).

Gyrus – One of the tortuous elevations (convolutions) of the surface of the brain caused by infolding of the cortex.

Hematomyelia – An effusion of blood within the spinal cord.

Hematorrhachis – Hemorrhage into the vertebral canal.

Hemeralopia – Day blindness; defective vision in bright light.

Hemianopia – Defective vision or blindness in half of the visual field.

Hemiballismus – A violent form of motor restlessness involving only one side of the body and being most marked in the upper extremity, resulting from a destructive lesion of the hypothalamic nucleus.

Hemilaminectomy – Removal of the vertebral laminae on one side only.

Hemiplegia – Paralysis of one side of the body.

Hemiparesis – Muscular weakness affecting one side of the body.

Hemivertebra – A developmental anomaly characterized by incomplete development of one side of a vertebra.

Hemorrhagic myelomalacia – Morbid softening of the spinal cord associated with hemorrhage.

Hepatoencephalopathy (hepatic encephalopathy) – A condition usually occurring secondarily to advanced disease of the liver but also seen in the course of any severe disease or in patients with portal canal shunts. It is marked by disturbances of consciousness that may progress to deep coma (hepatic coma), psychiatric changes of varying degrees, flapping tremor, and fetor hepaticus.

Heterograft (xenograft) – A graft of tissue transplanted from one animal to another of a different species.

Hippus – An abnormal exaggeration of the rhythmic contraction and dilation of the pupil. This occurs independent of changes in illumination or fixation of the eyes.

Homograft (allograft) – A graft of tissue from an individual to another of the same species but of disparate genotype.

Hopping reaction – A reflex used to evaluate the cerebellar and cortical areas of a dog's brain. The subject is advanced in a horizontal position with one foot on a flat, nonslippery surface. The normal response is accurate placement of the foot to support weight.

Horner's syndrome – Damage to the sympathetic pathway that supplies sympathetic nerves to the eye. It is characterized by unilateral enophthalmos, persistent miosis, ptosis of the upper palpebra, and a transitory dilation of the conjunctival, choroidal, and retinal blood vessels.

Hydrocephalus – A condition characterized by an abnormal accumulation of fluid in the cranial vault.

Hydromyelia – A pathologic condition characterized by the accumulation of fluid in the enlarged central canal of the spinal cord.

Hypalgesia – Diminished sensitivity to pain.

Hyperalgesia – A condition of excessive sensitivity or sensibility to pain. Auditory hyperalgesia means that slight noises cause pain. In muscular hyperalgesia, slight exertion causes great weariness or pain.

Hyperesthesia—An abnormally increased sensitivity of the skin or an organ of special sense.

Hyperkinesia—Abnormally increased motor function or activity.

Hypermetria—A form of dysmetria in which voluntary muscular movement overreaches the intended goal. It is commonly associated with diseases of the cerebellum.

Hyperopia—That error of refraction in which rays of light entering the eye parallel to the optic axis are brought to a focus behind the retina, as a result of the eyeball being too short from front to back. Also called farsightedness.

Hyperoxia—An excess of oxygen in the system resulting from exposure to high oxygen concentrations, especially to hyperbaric pressures of oxygen.

Hyperphagia—The ingestion of a greater than optimal quantity of food.

Hypersomnia—Uncontrollable drowsiness or pathologically excessive sleep.

Hypersthenia—Great strength or tonicity.

Hyperthermia—An abnormally high body temperature or fever.

Hypertonus—A condition of excessive tone, tension, or activity—e.g., excessive muscle tone.

Hyperventilation—Abnormally prolonged, rapid, and deep breathing in which an increased amount of air enters the pulmonary alveoli, resulting in reduction of carbon dioxide tension.

Hypesthesia (hypoesthesia)—Abnormally decreased sensitivity of the skin or an organ of special sense.

Hypometria—A form of dysmetria in which voluntary muscular movement falls short of reaching the intended goal. It is commonly associated with diseases of the cerebellum.

Hypomyelinogenesis—A form of dysmyelinogenesis characterized by a decreased quantity of myelin.

Hypophagia—The ingestion of a less than optimal quantity of food.

Hypoplasia—Incomplete development of an organ so that it fails to reach adult size; hypoplasia is less severe in degree than aplasia.

Hyporeflexia—Weakening of the reflexes.

Hyposmia—An abnormally decreased sensitivity to odors.

Hypothermia—An abnormally low body temperature.

Hypotonus—A condition of abnormally diminished tone, tension, or activity—e.g., a reduction in muscle tone.

Hypoxia—A low oxygen content or tension; deficiency of oxygen in the inspired air.

Hysteria—A psychoneurosis, the symptoms of which are based on conversion. It is characterized by a lack of control over acts and emotions, morbid self-consciousness, anxiety, exaggeration of the effect of sensory impressions, and simulation of various disorders.

Idiopathic—Of the nature of an idiopathy; self-originated; of unknown cause.

Incomitant strabismus—Deviation of an eye such that the amount of deviation of the affected eye is not the same in all directions in which the eyes are looking (see also *Comitant strabismus*).

Incontinence—The inability to control excretory functions, as defecation (fecal incontinence) or urination (urinary incontinence). Fecal incontinence is the failure of voluntary control of the anal sphincters, with involuntary passage of feces or flatus. Urinary incontinence is the failure of voluntary control of the vesical and urethral sphincters, with constant or frequent involuntary passage of urine.

Incoordination—A lack of the normal adjustment of muscular motions; failure of organs to work harmoniously.

Inhibition—Arrest or restraint of a process. Reflex inhibition is a condition in which a negative response is evoked by a stimulus.

Integration—A combination of different acts so that they contribute toward a common end.

Intention tremor—A tremor that arises or is intensified when a voluntary coordinated movement is attempted. It is associated with lack of cerebellar control of coordination.

Interarcuate ligament (yellow ligament)—Thin, elastic sheaths between arches of adjacent vertebrae.
Internuncial cells—Neurons within the central nervous system that serve as a medium of communication among neurons or nerve centers.
Ipsilateral—Situated on or pertaining to the same side.
Ischemia—Deficiency of blood in a part due to functional constriction of a blood vessel.
Intraneural—Within or into a nerve.

Jacksonian seizure—A type of partial epilepsy characterized by an extremely rapid discharge from a focal organic lesion of the brain. When the discharge rate is high enough, synchronous waves spread over adjacent cortical areas, resulting in a progressive "march" of involuntary muscle contractions throughout the opposite side of the body that may progress to a grand mal seizure.

Kinesiology—The sum of what is known regarding human motion; the study of motion of the human body.
Kinesthesia—The sense by which movement, weight, position, etc., are perceived; commonly used to refer specifically to the perception of changes in the angles of joints.
Kyphosis—A condition characterized by an abnormally increased convexity in the curvature of the thoracic spine as viewed from the side.

Labyrinthitis—Inflammation of the intercommunicating cavities or canals constituting the internal ear. Also called otitis interna.
Laminectomy—Excision of the dorsal arch of a vertebra.
Latency—A state of seeming inactivity, such as that occurring between the instant of stimulation and the beginning of response.
Lemniscus—A general term for a band or bundle of fibers in the central nervous system.
Leptomeninx—The pia and arachnoid of the brain and spinal cord.
Lethargy—A condition of drowsiness or indifference.
Leukodystrophy—Disturbance of the white substance of the brain.
Leukoencephalitis—Inflammation of the white substance of the brain.
Leukomyelitis—Inflammation of the white substance of the spinal cord.
Limbus (limbic system)—A ring of cerebral cortex that lies on the medioventral surface of each cerebral hemisphere (limbic lobe of the cortex) and surrounds a group of deeper structures. It is concerned with overall behavior and emotions of the animal.
Lobotomy—An incision into a lobe; in psychosurgery, surgical incision of all the fibers of a lobe of the brain.
Lordosis—An abnormally increased concavity in the curvature of the lumbar spine as viewed from the side.
Lower motor neuron—Neurons whose cell bodies are located in the brain stem and spinal cord, while the axons from the motor fibers form outside the central nervous system to innervate muscular structures.
Lumbarization—A condition in which the first segment of the sacrum fails to fuse with the second, so that there is one additional articulated vertebra, and the sacrum consists of only two segments.
Luxation—A dislocation with major displacement but without concurrent fractures.

Malacia—The morbid softening or softness of a part or tissue.
Mania—A phase of mental disorder characterized by an expansive emotional state, elation, hyperirritability, and increased motor activity.
Menace reaction—A threatening gesture toward the eye will result in a blink response of the eye and simultaneous head recoil. The menace reaction is mediated by cranial nerves II and VII.

Meninges—The three membranes that envelop the brain and spinal cord: the dura mater, pia mater, and arachnoid.

Meningitis—Inflammation of the meninges. When it affects the dura mater, the disease is termed pachymeningitis; when the arachnoid and pia mater are involved, it is called leptomeningitis or meningitis proper.

Meningocele—A hernial protrusion of the meninges through a defect in the skull or vertebral column.

Meningomyelocele—A hernial protrusion of a part of the meninges and substance of the spinal cord through a defect in the vertebral column.

Microglia—The small, non-neural, interstitial cells of mesodermal origin that form part of the supporting structure of the central nervous system. They are of various forms and may have slender branched processes. They are migratory and act as phagocytes to waste products of nerve tissue. Called also Hortega cells, gitter cells, mesoglia, and microgliocytes.

Micturition—The passage of urine; urination.

Miosis—Excessive contraction of the pupil.

Mirror focus—A secondary epileptogenic focus in the contralateral hemisphere resulting from a primary epileptogenic focus. When present, seizures may persist after the primary focus has been removed.

Modality—A specific sensory entity—e.g., taste, touch, pain, and sight.

Motor—Pertaining to a muscle, nerve, or center that produces movement.

Motor point—That region of a muscle into which its motor nerve enters or in which there is a high density of nerve terminals.

Multisegmental—Involving the neurons of more than one segment of the spinal cord (see *Segment*).

Myasthenia—A muscular debility; any constitutional anomaly of muscle.

Mydriasis—Extreme dilation of the pupil.

Myelin—The fatlike substance forming a sheath around certain nerve fibers.

Myelination (myelinization)—The act of taking on myelin.

Myelitis—Inflammation of the spinal cord.

Myelodysplasia—Defective development of any part (especially the lower segments) of the spinal cord.

Myelography—Roentgenography of the spinal cord after injection of a contrast medium into the subarachnoid space.

Myelomalacia—A morbid softening of the spinal cord.

Myelopathy—A general term denoting a functional disturbance and/or pathological changes in the spinal cord. The term is often used to designate nonspecific lesions in contrast to inflammatory lesions (myelitis).

Myelotomy—The operation of severing tracts in the spinal cord.

Myoclonus—Shocklike contractions of a portion of a muscle, an entire muscle, or a group of muscles. They may be restricted to one area of the body or appear synchronously or asynchronously in several areas.

Myopathy—A term used to describe a disease of the muscles.

Myopia—An error of refraction in which rays of light entering the eye parallel to the optic axis come to focus in front of the retina because the anterior-posterior measurement of the eyeball is too long. Also called nearsightedness.

Myositis—An inflammation of a voluntary muscle.

Myotome—A group of muscles innervated from a single spinal segment.

Myotonia—Increased muscular irritability and contraction with decreased power of relaxation; tonic spasm of muscle.

Myringotomy—A surgical incision of the tympanic membrane.

Narcolepsy—A condition marked by an uncontrollable desire to sleep or by sudden attacks of sleep occurring at intervals; often associated with cataplexy.

Neuralgia—Paroxysmal pain that extends along the course of one or more nerves.

Neurapraxia—A nerve injury in which paralysis occurs in the absence of structural changes.

Neuraxis—An axon.

Neurilemma (neurolemma)—The thin membrane spirally enwrapping the myelin layers of a myelinated nerve fiber or the axon of an unmyelinated nerve fiber.

Neuritis—Inflammation of a nerve. The condition is attended by pain and tenderness over the nerves, anesthesia and paresthesia, paralysis, wasting, and disappearance of the reflexes.

Neuroglia—The supporting structure of nervous tissue (Virchow, 1854). It consists of a fine web of tissue made up of modified ectodermic elements, in which are enclosed peculiar branched cells known as neuroglial cells or glial cells. The neuroglial cells are of three types: macroglia or astroglia, oligodendrocyte or oligodendroglia, and microglia. Astrocytes and oligodendrocytes appear to play a role in myelin formation, transport of material to neurons, and maintenance of the ionic environment of neurons.

Neurology—That branch of medical science that deals with the nervous system, both normal and diseased.

Neuroma—A tumor or new growth largely made up of nerve cells and nerve fibers; a tumor growing from a nerve.

Neuromatosis—A disease condition characterized by the presence of many neuromas.

Neuron—Any of the conducting cells of the nervous system. A typical neuron consists of a cell body, which contains the nucleus and the surrounding cytoplasm (perikaryon); several short radiating processes (dendrites); and one long process (the axon), which terminates in twiglike branches (telodendrons) and may have branches (collaterals) projecting along its course. The axon together with its covering or sheath forms the nerve fiber.

Neuronophagia—The destruction of nerve cells by phagocytic action.

Neuropathy—A general term denoting functional disturbances and/or pathological changes in the peripheral nervous system.

Neuropil—A dense feltlike network of interwoven cytoplasmic processes of nerve cells (dendrites and neurites) and of glial cells in the central nervous system and in some parts of the peripheral nervous system.

Neurorrhaphy—The suturing of a cut nerve.

Neurotmesis—Nerve injury in which all essential structures have been sundered, despite apparent maintenance of anatomic continuity.

Nissl substance—Large granular bodies that stain with basic dyes, forming the substance of the reticulum of the cytoplasm of a nerve cell. Ribonucleoprotein has been found to be one of the main constituents.

Node of Ranvier—Constrictions occurring on myelinated nerve fibers at regular intervals of about 1 mm; at these sites the myelin sheath is absent, and the axon is enclosed only by Schwann cell processes.

Nociceptive—Receiving injury; said of a receptive neuron for painful sensations. A nociceptor is a receptor for pain.

Normotonia—Normal tone or tension.

Nucleus—A general term used to designate a group of nerve cells ordinarily located in the central nervous system. These have a direct relationship to the fiber of a particular nerve.

Nucleus pulposus—A semifluid mass of white and elastic fibers that forms the central portion of an intervertebral disk; it has been regarded as the persistent remains of the embryonic notocord.

Nyctalopia—Night blindness; failure or imperfection of vision at night or in a dim light, with good vision only on bright days.

Nystagmus—An involuntary rapid movement of the eyeball that may be horizontal, vertical, rotatory, or mixed. (1) Optokinetic nystagmus is normal. In it, the eyes fixate on successive points in a continuously moving scene. (2) Nystagmus with activated semicircular canals is also normal. The head turns, activates the semicircular canals, and produces a slow movement of the eyes in a direction opposite to that of the head rotation, followed by a fast eye movement in the direction of rotation. (3) Vestibular nystagmus is pathological. Damage to the vestibular apparatus causes continuous tremor of the eyes. (4) In cerebellar nystagmus (also pathological), damage to deep nuclei of the cerebellum causes continuous nystagmus. There is loss of equilibrium if the flocculonodular lobe is affected. (5) Nystagmus with ocular lesions is also pathological. In it, damage to the fovea regions of both eyes results in the eyes moving back and forth, trying to fix an object at a central visual point.

Occipital dysplasia—A malformation of the occipital bone characterized by an enlarged foramen magnum, which exposes the brain stem and cerebellum.
Oligemia—A deficiency in the volume of blood.
Oligodendroglia—The non-neural cells of ectodermal origin forming part of the adventitial structure (the neuroglia) of the central nervous system. The vinelike prolongations of these cells form an incomplete investment for the myelin sheaths in the white matter, and with the microglia they form the perineuronal satellites in the gray matter.
Opisthotonos—A form of tetanic spasm in which the head is bent backward and the spine is in a position of lordosis.
Osteophyte—A bony excrescence or osseous outgrowth.
Otorrhea—A discharge from the ear, especially a purulent one. Cerebrospinal fluid otorrhea is escape of cerebrospinal fluid through the external auditory meatus due to fracture of the temporal bone.

Pachymeninx—The dura mater.
Palmar—Pertaining to the ventral surface of the front paw.
Palsy—Paralysis.
Panniculus reflex—Characterized by a localized reflex contraction of the cutaneous muscles over the thoracic and lumbar spine in response to a painful stimulus. The pathway of cutaneous sensation begins at the spinal cord at each segment (dermatome) and ascends to the brachial plexus (C8–T1) and to the lateral thoracic nerve, which innervates the cutaneous trunci (panniculus carnosus) muscles. A segmental lesion will block the ascending afferent stimulus, thus abolishing the reflex.
Panophthalmitis—An inflammation of all the structures or tissues of the eye.
Papilledema—Edema of the optic papilla.
Papillitis—Inflammation of the optic papilla.
Paralysis—The loss or impairment of motor function of a part due to a lesion of the
Paraplegia—Paralysis of the hind limbs and the lower (caudal) part of the body; both motion and sensation are affected.
Paresis—Slight or incomplete paralysis.
Paresthesia—A morbid or perverted sensation; an abnormal sensation—e.g., burning or prickling.
Paroxysm—A sudden recurrence or intensification of symptoms; a spasm or seizure.
Pathways—(1) Afferent pathways are the nerve structures through which a sensory impulse is conducted to the central nervous system. (2) Efferent pathways are the nerve structures through which an impulse passes from the central nervous system to the periphery.
Perineurium—The connective tissue sheath surrounding each bundle of fibers (fasciculus) in a peripheral nerve.
Perithelium—The layer of connective tissue that surrounds the capillaries and smaller vessels.
Perocormus (perosomus)—A fetus with a greatly deformed body or trunk.
Petit mal—A form of generalized epilepsy. (1) The myoclonic form is characterized by a burst of neuronal discharges lasting a fraction of a second throughout the central nervous system. It results in a single muscle jerk. (2) In the absence form, the victim loses consciousness for a few seconds, during which there may be twitchlike contractions of the muscles.
Phlebography—Roentgenography of a vein or veins by the use of contrast medium.
Phobic—The nature of or pertaining to phobia or morbid fears.
Pia mater—The innermost of the three membranes (meninges) covering the brain and spinal cord, investing them closely and extending into the depths of the fissures and sulci. It consists of reticular, elastic, and collagenous fibers.
Placing reaction—There are two types. (1) Tactile or touch placing is used to evaluate the sensory peripheral nerves, spinal cord, brain stem, motor cortex, and efferent peripheral nerves. The dog's eyes are covered and the dorsal surface of the paw is allowed to touch the edge of a table. Normally the foot is lifted and placed correctly on the table top. (2) Optical or sight placing is used to evaluate optic nerves and visual

pathways to the cerebral cortex as well as regions in the brain stem, spinal cord, and efferent peripheral nerves. The dog's eyes are not covered, and the dorsal surface of the paw is advanced to the table's edge. Normally the foot is raised to the table top before it touches the table edge.

Pneumoencephalography—The radiographic visualization of the fluid-containing structures of the brain after cerebrospinal fluid is intermittently withdrawn and replaced by air, oxygen, or helium.

Polarization—A nerve cell in its resting electrical state (polarized state). The inside of the cell membrane is negatively charged with respect to the outside of the cell membrane, where there is a concentration of positively charged ions.

Polio—Denotes relationship to the gray matter of the nervous system.

Poliomyelopathy—Any disease primarily affecting the gray matter of the spinal cord.

Polydipsia—Excessive thirst persisting for long periods of time.

Polyradiculoneuritis—An acute inflammation involving multiple peripheral nerves, the spinal nerve roots, and possibly the spinal cord (coon dog paralysis). (see *Guillain-Barré syndrome.*)

Polyuria—The passage of a large volume of urine in a given period.

Proprioception—Information concerning the movements and position of the body and its parts as conducted by sensory nerve impulses to the central nervous system. Sensory nerve terminals that transmit this information are located principally in the muscles, tendons, and labyrinth of the ear.

Proptosis—A forward displacement. Ocular proptosis is bulging of the eyeball, or exophthalmos.

Protopathic—Primary; idiopathic.

Pseudomeningocele—A diverticulum-like structure extending through tissues of the neck. It may arise from complete or incomplete avulsion of the nerve roots with a concomitant tear of the arachnoid or dura.

Pseudopapilledema—An anomalous elevation of the optic disk.

Psychosis—A general term for any major mental disorder of organic and/or emotional origin characterized by derangement of the personality and loss of contact with reality, often with delusions, hallucinations, or illusions.

Psychosomatic—Pertaining to the mind-body relationship; having bodily symptoms of psychic, emotional, or mental origin; commonly used to refer to a group of disorders thought to be caused in part or in whole by emotional disturbances but presenting a physiologic derangement.

Psychotropic—Exerting an effect upon the mind; capable of modifying mental activity; usually applied to drugs that affect the mental state.

Ptosis—Drooping of the upper eyelid from paralysis of the third cranial nerve (oculomotor nerve) or from sympathetic innervation.

Pyramidal system (corticospinal tracts)—A major pathway for transmission of motor impulses from the motor areas of the cerebral cortex to the ventral motor neurons of the spinal cord. It is of less importance in animals than in man.

Pyrexia—A fever or a febrile condition; abnormal elevation in body temperature.

Quadrantanopsia (quadrantanopia)—Defective vision or blindness in one fourth of the visual field, bounded by a vertical and a horizontal radius.

Quadriplegia (tetraplegia)—Paralysis of all four limbs.

Rachischisis—A congenital fissure of the spinal column.

Radiculoneuritis—Acute febrile polyneuritis.

Radiculopathy—Disease of the nerve roots.

Reflex—A response that is simple, practically invariable, inherited, and usually useful to the organism. Reflexes depend on a neuronal connection from a sense organ to an effector organ called the reflex arc.

Reflex arc—A neural arc utilized in a reflex action; an impulse travels centrally over afferent fibers to a nerve center, and the response travels outward to an effector organ or part over efferent fibers.

Release—When a lower level of the central nervous system is separated from a higher level, excessive activity or other signs that are normally held in check by the higher centers may be seen. (1) In the classic decerebrate animal, a facilitory area of the brain is separated (released) from the influence of higher inhibitory centers, resulting in excessive muscle tone. (2) Transection of the medulla below the vestibular nuclei separates (releases) an inhibitory area from the influence of a higher facilitory area, resulting in flaccid muscles and inhibited cord reflexes.

Reticulosis—An abnormal increase in cells derived from or related to the reticuloendothelial system.

Reticulum—A network—e.g., the reticular formation of the brain—is composed of areas of diffuse neurons located in the medulla, pons, mesencephalon, and portions of the diencephalon. The formation contains small nuclei, which are associated with motor and sensory function.

Rheobase—The minimum potential of electric current necessary to produce stimulation.

Rhinencephalon—A term generally applied to certain parts of the human brain previously thought to be concerned entirely with olfactory mechanisms, including the olfactory nerves, bulbs, tracts, and subsequent connections (all olfactory in function) and the limbic system (not primarily olfactory in function); it is homologous with the olfactory portions of the brain in lower animals. Called also olfactory brain or smell brain. One of the portions of the telencephalon in the embryo.

Rhinitis—An inflammation of the mucous membrane of the nose.

Rhizotomy—Interruption of the roots of spinal nerves within the spinal canal, usually by surgical division.

Rigidity—An abnormal stiffness or inflexibility of body parts due to hypertonus of extensor or flexor muscles or both. Decerebrate rigidity is a rigid extension of an animal's limbs that results from sectioning the brain stem between the rostral and caudal colliculi.

Risus sardonicus—A grinning expression produced by spasm of the facial muscles.

Rostral (rostrad)—Denoting a position situated nearer the nose in relation to a specific point of reference.

Rostrotentorial—Referring to that portion of the cranial vault that is anterior or cranial to the extension of dura mater that forms a partition between the cerebrum and cerebellum.

Sacralization—Anomalous fusion of the seventh lumbar vertebrae to the first segment of the sacrum so that the sacrum consists of four segments.

Sarcolemma—The delicate plasma membrane that invests every striated muscle fiber.

Schiff-Sherrington reaction—The phenomenon characterized by hyperextension of the fore limbs pain the axillary region, and flaccid paralysis in the hind limbs. The condition is due to a spinal lesion in the thoracic or lumbar area (between T2 and L4).

Schmorl nodes—Nodules seen in radiographs of the spine. They are caused by prolapse of a nucleus pulposus into an adjoining vertebra.

Schwann cell—One of the large nucleated masses of protoplasm lining the inner surface of the sheath of Schwann or neurilemma.

Schwannoma—A neoplasm of the white substance of a nerve sheath.

Sclerosis—An induration, or hardening, especially hardening of a part from inflammation and in diseases of the interstitial substance. The term is used chiefly for such a hardening of the nervous system due to hyperplasia of the connective tissue or to designate hardening of the blood vessels.

Scoliosis—An appreciable lateral deviation in the normally straight vertical line of the spine.

Segment—A portion of the spinal cord contained between two imaginary sections, one cranial and one caudal to a pair of spinal nerves.

Segmental—Referring to a reflex whose nerve components are present within a segment of spinal cord.

Seizure—An attack of epilepsy; the sudden attack or recurrence of disease.

Semicoma—A stupor from which the patient may be aroused.

Sensory—Pertaining to a nerve, pathway, or center that subserves sensation.

Sinusitis—Inflammation of a sinus. The condition may be purulent or nonpurulent, acute or chronic. Depending on the site of involvement, it is known as ethmoid, frontal, maxillary, or sphenoid sinusitis.

Sitz bath—A tub in which one bathes in a sitting posture, usually for therapeutic reasons.

Somnolence—Sleepiness; unnatural drowsiness.

Spasm—A sudden, violent, involuntary contraction of a muscle or group of muscles, attended by pain and interference with function, producing involuntary movement and distortion.

Spastic—Of the nature of or characterized by spasms. Hypertonic, so that the muscles are stiff and the movements awkward.

Spastic paralysis—Paralysis characterized by extension of the limbs and heightened deep muscle reflexes.

Spasticity—A state of increased muscle tension, resulting in continuous increase of resistance to stretching. In quadrupeds it is manifested by extension of the limbs. It is usually due to a hyperactive stretch reflex.

Spina bifida—A developmental anomaly characterized by defective closure of the bony encasement of the spinal cord, through which the cord and meninges may (s. bifida cystica) or may not (s. bifida occulta) protrude.

Spinal animal—An animal in which all connections of the spinal cord to the brain have been severed, leaving only the reflexes inherent to the spinal cord (flexor reflex, crossed extensor reflex, stretch reflex, and reflexes that control the basic rhythm and pattern of locomotion).

Spinal shock—The loss of spinal reflexes after injury to the spinal cord. The loss of reflexes appears in the muscles innervated by the cord segments located below the site of the lesion. Immediate and complete flaccid paralysis, loss of sensibility, and retention of urine and feces are also signs of spinal shock. It lasts only a short time in domestic animals.

Spondylectomy—The surgical removal of a vertebra.

Spondylitis—Inflammation of the vertebrae.

Spondyloarthrosis—Degenerative spinal arthritis.

Spondylolisthesis—Displacement of one vertebra with respect to its adjacent vertebra due to an unstable joint. It usually occurs at the lumbosacral articulation and may result in prolific exostosis and ankylosis of the joint.

Spondylosis—Ankylosis of a vertebral joint.

Stereotaxic—Referring to the technique used to create lesions in a precise area of the brain by means of fixing the head in a rigid apparatus and inserting probes into the brain at a predetermined distance from fixed reference points.

Stoic—One apparently or professedly indifferent to pleasure or pain.

Strabismus—Deviation of the eye that the patient cannot overcome. The visual axes assume a position relative to each other different from that required by the physiological conditions. It is also called manifest deviation, squint, cast, and heterotropia.

Stroke—A condition that has a sudden onset caused by acute vascular lesions of the brain, such as hemorrhage, embolism, thrombosis, or rupturing aneurysm, which may be marked by hemiplegia or hemiparesis, vertigo, numbness, aphasia, and dysarthria; it is often followed by permanent neurological damage. Called also cerebrovascular accident or stroke.

Stupor—A state of partial or nearly complete unconsciousness.

Subarachnoid—Situated in or occurring between the arachnoid and the pia mater.

Subluxation—A dislocation with minor displacement but without concurrent fractures.

Suboccipital—A position located below the occiput.

Sulcus—A groove, trench, or furrow; a general term for such a depression, especially one on the surface of the brain separating the gyri.

Synapse (synaptic junction)—The anatomical relation of one nerve cell to another. The junction between the processes of two adjacent neurons, where a nervous impulse is transmitted from one neuron to another. Impulses pass from the terminal arborization of one axon to the dendrites of an adjacent neuron at the synapse.

Syncope—A temporary suspension of consciousness due to cerebral anemia; a faint or swoon.

Syndrome—A set of symptoms that occur together; the sum of signs of any morbid state; a symptom complex.

Syringomyelia—A condition marked by abnormal cavities filled with liquid in the substance of the spinal cord.

Tactile—Pertaining to the sensation of touch.
Tanycyte—A special cell that projects from the ventricular surface into the infundibular recess. Its function has been postulated as that of a sensor to substances circulating in the CSF.
Tectum—The roof of the mesencephalon: that part of the mesencephalon dorsal to the cerebral (mesencephalic) aqueduct, comprising the quadrigeminal plate and the rostral and caudal colliculi.
Tegmentum—The part of the cerebral peduncle dorsal to the substantia nigra, consisting of an upward extension of the pontine tegmentum; it is made up of various nuclei, fiber tracts, and the reticular formation and is separated dorsally from the tectum by the cerebral (mesencephalic) aqueduct.
Telencephalon—The paired cerebral vesicles, which are the anterolateral evaginations of the prosencephalon, together with the median, unpaired portions, the lamina terminalis; from it the cerebral hemispheres are derived.
Temporal lobe seizure—A type of partial epilepsy that originates from a focal lesion in the ventrolateral lobe of a cerebral hemisphere.
Tenesmus—Ineffectual and painful straining at stool or in urination.
Tentorium—An anatomical part resembling a tent or covering.
Tentorium cerebelli—The process of dura mater that supports the occipital lobes and covers the rostral surface of the cerebellum. Its internal border is free and bounds the tentorial notch; its external border is attached to the skull and encloses the transverse sinus behind.
Tetany—A syndrome manifested by sharp flexion of the carpal and tarsal joints, muscle twitching, cramps, and convulsions, sometimes with attacks of stridor.
Tetraparesis—Muscular weakness in all four extremities.
Tetraplegia (quadriplegia)—Paralysis of all four extremities.
Tic—Any spasmodic movement or twitching.
Tic douloureux—Chronic paroxysmal trigeminal neuralgia.
Tonotopic—Organization of an area according to sensitivity to a certain range of tones (frequency), as in the auditory cortex.
Tone—The normal degree of vigor and tension; in muscle, the resistance to passive elongation, or stretch.
Tonic—Characterized by continuous tension.
Tonic–clonic (tonoclonic)—Both tonic and clonic; said of a spasm consisting of a convulsive twitching of the muscles.
Tonus—The slight continuous contraction of muscle, which in skeletal muscles aids in the maintenance of posture and in the return of blood to the heart.
Torticollis—Wryneck; a contracted state of the cervical muscles, producing a twisting of the neck and an unnatural position of the head.
Tracheostomy—Surgical creation of an opening into the trachea through the neck and insertion of a tube to facilitate the passage of air to the lungs or the evacuation of secretions.
Tracheotomy—Incision of the trachea through the skin and muscles of the neck for purposes of exploration, removal of a foreign body or local lesion, or obtaining a biopsy specimen.
Tract—A collection or bundle of nerve fibers having the same origin, function, and termination.
Transverse myelopathy—A myelopathy involving one or a few segments of the spinal cord. The clinical signs are similar to those produced when the cord is transected.
Tremor—An involuntary trembling or quivering.
Trismus—Motor disturbance of the trigeminal nerve, especially spasm of the masticatory muscles that results in difficulty in opening the mouth (lockjaw); a characteristic early symptom of tetanus.

Upper motor neuron (UMN)—Motor neurons whose cell bodies and axons lie totally within the CNS, the axons forming the descending fasciculi.
Uncus—The medially curved anterior end of the parahippocampal gyrus.

Vasomotor—Any element or agent that affects the caliber of a blood vessel.
Venography (phlebography)—Roentgenography of the veins after injection of a contrast medium into bone marrow at an appropriate site, such as the iliac crest, ischium, pubic bones, greater trochanter, spinous processes of the vertebrae, or sternum; this is intra-osseous venography.
Vermicular—Wormlike in shape or appearance.
Vertigo—An illusion of movement; a sensation as if the external world were revolving around the patient (objective vertigo) or as if he himself were revolving in space (subjective vertigo). The term is sometimes erroneously used as a synonym for dizziness. Vertigo may result from diseases of the inner ear or may be due to disturbances of the vestibular centers or pathways in the central nervous system.
Vestibular apparatus—That portion of the inner ear composed of the semicircular canals and utricle that functions to maintain equilibrium.
Veterinary ethology—A scientific study of animal behavior.

Xanthochromia—Any yellowish discoloration, as of the skin or cerebrospinal fluid.

INDEX

Note: Page numbers in italics refer to illustrations; those followed by t indicate tables.